MDE | 15

MODERN DRUG ENCYCLOPEDIA

AND THERAPEUTIC INDEX

A COMPENDIUM

YORKE MEDICAL BOOKS
666 FIFTH AVENUE, NEW YORK, NEW YORK

MDE | 15

MODERN DRUG ENCYCLOPEDIA

AND THERAPEUTIC INDEX

EDITOR

Arthur J. Lewis, M.D.

Associate Dean and Professor of Medicine, University of Tennessee College of Medicine, Memphis, Tennessee.

EXECUTIVE EDITOR

Gertrude Dittus Gonzales, B.S.Phar., R.Ph.

CONTRIBUTING EDITOR

Charles L. Winek, Ph.D.

Professor of Pharmacology and Toxicology, Duquesne University School of Pharmacy, Pittsburgh, Pennsylvania

Chief Toxicologist, Allegheny County Coroner's Office, Pittsburgh, Pennsylvania

A COMPENDIUM

The composition of most of the preparations described in this work is protected by U. S. Letters Patent; many of the proprietary names of the products are trade-marked and registered at the U. S. Patent Office by the firms whose names are mentioned with these products.

Published 1979

Fifteenth Edition

Library of Congress Catalog Card Number: 34-12823

International Standard Book Number: 0-914316-17-6

FOREWORD

Therapeutics is a dynamic aspect of medicine, restricted only by the ingenuity of the physician and the responsibility of governmental agencies. Both must document efficacy and safety. At present both efficacy and safety are under review by Federal agencies in collaboration with scientific advisory committees.

As a result of our commitment to accuracy and timeliness, the Fifteenth Edition of THE MODERN DRUG ENCYCLOPEDIA AND THERAPEUTIC INDEX is still intended to be primarily a ready reference to the many therapeutic preparations presently available to physicians rather than a textbook of pharmacology or a manual of therapeutics.

All preparations are listed alphabetically; descriptive monographs appear only under the generic name of individual drugs or of the primary ingredient of combination products. The trade names of generic drugs are given at the end of each monograph in the section on availability. Multiple combination products, however, are described under their trade names. In addition, a number of pharmacologically similar preparations, such as the penicillins and the phenothiazines, are discussed in one comprehensive monograph rather than in separate sections. The therapeutic indications listed are those provided by the manufacturer and approved by the U.S. Food and Drug Administration.

There has been increasing concern about the problem of drug interactions in the treatment of patients, and numerous books and articles have been published recently providing comprehensive lists of such interactions. This has produced in many physicians what has been called the "drug interaction anxiety syndrome." Many of these lists include interactions based on observations which may not be clinically significant and are the result of isolated reports or mere impressions. Admittedly, there are many real and potentially serious interactions such as the effect of some pharmaceuticals on anticoagulant metabolism, which may result in serious hemorrhage. However, we have resisted the temptation to provide another comprehensive list which might only exacerbate the "interaction syndrome" and have incorporated potentially adverse interactions in the individual monographs.

Except for certain diagnostic agents, only the prescription products of manufacturing pharmaceutical firms having more than local distribution are included. We have been as accurate as is humanly possible; however, should you find any discrepancy, we would appreciate your notifying us so that the correction can be included in the supplement, MODERN DRUGS.

In addition to the listing of pharmaceuticals and biologicals, a Therapeutic Index, a Manufacturers' Index and a General Index are included. The appropriate Drug Enforcement Administration (DEA) schedule is given for preparations under DEA control. Although we have made every effort to keep the listings up-to-date, the schedule is frequently revised. The manufacturer or the DEA should be consulted if there is uncertainty. A review of the Controlled Substances Act of 1970 (PUBLIC LAW 91-513) is included.

An important feature of the ENCYCLOPEDIA is the Glossary of Pharmaceutical Dose Forms prepared, as for prior editions, by Dr. Charles L. Winek. In addition to updating the Glossary, Dr. Winek has provided a section on Drug Blood Levels for use in both therapeutic and toxicologic situations.

The introduction of new, potent medications imposes an enormous responsibility on the physician. Not only must he be aware of the availability, method of use and the indications and contraindications of these agents, but through continuing education he must also be familiar with unusual problems that may be encountered.

THE MODERN DRUG ENCYCLOPEDIA attempts to compile this necessary information into a concise, up-to-date, quick reference form and to that end we have added an addendum to the text to make it as timely as possible. To keep the ENCYCLOPEDIA current a supplementary publication, MODERN DRUGS, is provided. This supplement contains descriptions of new preparations released after publication of the ENCYCLOPEDIA, and also provides new information about older preparations if it becomes available.

THE MODERN DRUG ENCYCLOPEDIA and MODERN DRUGS provide the physician with complete and authoritative information on all pharmaceutical agents whether established or newly released.

Arthur J. Lewis, M.D.

Memphis, Tennessee, 1979

CONTENTS

THE MODERN DRUG ENCYCLOPEDIA—FEATURES AND USE

For your convenience, THE MODERN DRUG ENCYCLOPEDIA AND THERAPEUTIC INDEX is divided into four basic reference sections, cross referenced to lead you directly to the information you need. They are:

PHARMACEUTICALS AND BIOLOGICALS

Listed in alphabetical order by generic or trade name are the descriptions of the products of manufacturers whose nationally distributed prescription drugs are included. When the preparation is a single substance, the trade name will indicate the generic name under which the full product description can be found. When a combination product has a principal ingredient, there is a cross reference to the listing of that generic ingredient under which the complete product description is given. Use this section if you know the generic or trade name of the drug and wish to verify its composition, action, usage, administration, contraindications, warnings, adverse reactions and availability.

THERAPEUTIC INDEX

This section provides an alphabetical listing of products by therapeutic indication. All pharmaceuticals and biologicals described in this edition are classified under their therapeutic functions and the page number of the complete description is given. Use this section to locate the drugs available for the specific treatment required.

MANUFACTURERS' INDEX

This is an alphabetical listing of the manufacturers and their products. It is a complete list of all the drugs described in the first section of the Encyclopedia, followed by the page number on which the product description appears. Use this section if you know the name of the manufacturer, but not the name of the drug or its therapeutic use.

GENERAL INDEX

This section is a combined index, containing alphabetized reference to all the preparations described in the first section, listing both generic and trade names with page locations. Use this section as your master index to any description or reference in THE MODERN DRUG ENCYCLOPEDIA.

TO LOCATE A DRUG NOT IN THE ENCYCLOPEDIA

Refer to MODERN DRUGS, supplement to THE MODERN DRUG ENCYCLOPEDIA. New drugs made available since publication of this volume are described in this supplement.

GLOSSARY

A directory of pharmaceutical trade-name dosage forms and their definitions.
Compiled by Charles L. Winek, Ph.D., Duquesne University, School of Pharmacy.

General Terms: LA = long-acting
LP = long-acting principle
RA = repeat-action
SA = sustained-action
TC = time coat
TD = time-disintegration
UF = ultrafine particles for greater absorption, in capsule form

Abboject *(Abbott):* Disposable syringe for injection.
Abbo-Liter *(Abbott):* A type container for sterile solutions.
Abbo-Vac *(Abbott):* A type vacuum container with solution for collecting blood.
Aerohaler *(Abbott):* A device for administering powders in aerosols to the upper respiratory tract and lungs, consisting of a discharge chamber with interchangeable mouth and nose pieces.
Aerotrol *(Abbott):* Controlled-dose nebulizer for oral inhalation.
Aspirol *(Lilly):* Breakable, cloth-covered, thin, glassed, inhalant container.
Bitab *(Merrell-National):* Double-strength tablet.
Buccalet *(Ciba):* Kidney-shaped tablet for buccal or sublingual absorption.
Calendar Pak *(Searle):* Dosage-reminder container for patient convenience.
Caplet *(Winthrop):* Elongated, uncoated tablet.
Capsulette *(Armour):* Capsule-shaped tablet.
Cartrid *(Lilly):* Single-dose cartridge (injectable).
Centri-Vac *(Baxter):* Sterile, nonpyrogenic, vacuum container for collecting blood and for preparing plasma or serum by centrifugation.
Cherro-Chew Tab *(Philips Roxane):* Flavored, chewable tablet.
Chewable *(Squibb):* Soft, soluble tablet.
Chronosule *(Schering):* Sustained-release capsule.
Chronotab *(Schering):* Sustained-action tablet.
Clipsule *(Lederle):* Squeezable gelatin capsule, convenient for administration to children.
Color-Break Ampul *(Astra):* Ampul with colored line at point of breakage.
Compack *(Searle):* Purse-container dispenser for oral contraceptives with patient schedule reminder.
Dialpak *(Ortho):* Plastic tablet-dispenser with visible dosage schedule for patient reminder.
Disket *(Lilly):* Inscribed tablet.
Dispensajar *(Dome):* Special-design plastic jar with disc allowing delivery of a small amount of ointment or cream.
Dospak *(Upjohn):* Unit package of scheduled medication.
Dospan *(Merrell-National):* Continuous-release tablet.
Dosule *(Organon):* Measured dose of hormone-containing ointment in a tube
Dri-Cap *(Lederle):* Dry-filled, sealed capsule.
Dropperette *(Cooper):* Sterile, disposable plastic tube containing sterile solution specifically designed for aseptic technic in ophthalmic surgery.
Drop-Tainer *(Alcon):* Plastic container of ophthalmic solution with built-in tip.
Duchette *(Purdue Frederick):* Individual package of douche powder.
Dulcet *(Abbott):* Soluble, candy-flavored, cube-shaped sugar tablet.

Durabond *(Mallinckrodt):* Long-acting medication—usually tannate salts.
Duracap *(Meyer):* Long-acting capsules.
Dura-Tab *(Cooper):* Sustained-action tablet.
Emplet *(Parke-Davis):* Enteric-coated tablet with a distinctive flame-colored coating.
Encoat *(Merrell-National):* Enteric-coated tablet.
Enduret *(Geigy):* Prolonged-action tablet.
Enkeric *(Rorer):* Special brand of enteric coating.
Enseal *(Lilly):* Time-disintegrating enteric-coated tablet.
Enterab *(Abbott):* Enteric-coated tablet.
Envule *(Glenwood):* Pure, drug "envelope" sealed against contamination, moisture and light.
Extentab *(Robins):* Extended-action tablet.
Filmtab *(Abbott):* A tablet coated with a thin film for rapid disintegration in the stomach.
Flexidose *(Squibb):* Controlled-dose calibrated dropper.
Flo-Pak *(Burroughs Wellcome):* Dry, sterile powder in flexible plastic bottle with piercing device to introduce drug into intravenous solutions.
Fluor-I-Strip *(Ayerst):* Sterile individual ophthalmic applicators.
Gelseal *(Lilly):* Sealed gelatin capsule.
Glosset *(Winthrop):* Sublingual tablet.
Gradumet *(Abbott):* Long-release tablet.
Granucap *(Tutag):* Sustained-release capsule.
Hafgram *(Warner-Chilcott):* 0.5 gram coated tablet.
Hafs *(Breon):* Half-strength compressed tablet.
Hypoglossal *(Carnrick):* Capsule for sublingual or buccal administration.
Hypoloid *(Burroughs Wellcome):* Identifying trademark for injectable solutions.
Immunogen *(Parke-Davis):* Identifying trademark for specific antigenic substances obtained from the surface of bacterial cells (ecto-antigens) substantially free of bacterial autolysates and extraneous protein.
Infatab *(Parke-Davis):* Triangular-shaped, grooved tablet, flavored and intended for pediatric use.
Inlay-Tab *(Dorsey):* Oblong, capsule-shaped, flat tablet with two medications, one inlayed in the other, involving two different colors.
Ion-O-Trate *(Abbott):* Special vial of concentrated solution to be added to solutions in Abbo-Liters.
Isoject *(Pfizer):* A prefilled, sterile, disposable injection system.
Jetomizer *(Wyeth):* A convenient and effective device for application of medication high in the nasal passages.
Juvelet *(Dorsey):* Time-release tablet for children, with a special tasteless coating.
Kapseal *(Parke-Davis):* A hard capsule that is sealed by a band of gelatin at the points of closure.
Koff-Ball *(Philips Roxane):* A chewable, gelatin capsule containing liquid medication.
Lacrivial *(Cooper):* Sterilized, plastic container of ophthalmic solution with dropper top.
Linguet *(Ciba):* Tablet for mucosal absorption.
Lingusorb *(Ayerst):* Buccal and sublingual tablet.
Liquifilm *(Allergan):* Ophthalmic drops with a plastic polymer vehicle that forms a clear, elastic film on the lid and lid margins releasing the active ingredients over a prolonged period.
Lontab *(Ciba):* Long-acting tablet.
Lozi-Tab *(Davies Rose Hoyt):* Lozenge type.
Loz-Tablet *(Warren-Teed):* Tablet designed to be dissolved in mouth for 5 minutes before swallowing.
Lyovac *(Merck Sharp & Dohme):* Vacuum-desiccated, lyophilized preparation restored to original volume by addition of accompanying diluent.
Mandet *(Lederle):* Flavored, chewable tablet.
Medihaler *(Riker):* Aerosol device.
Medilet *(Schering):* Color-flecked tablet for children.
Medule *(Upjohn):* Medication coated for prolonged action.
Melet *(Dow):* Troche-type chewable tablet.

Membrette *(Wyeth):* Soluble tablet for administration of hormone substances by mouth.
Memorette *(Syntex):* Plastic tablet dispenser with visible dose schedule.
Merseal *(Merck Sharp & Dohme):* Film-coated tablet.
Micropellet *(Schering):* Microscopic crystalline form.
Mistometer *(Winthrop):* Oral inhalation apparatus.
Mix-O-Vial *(Upjohn):* A two-compartment vial
Mono-Drop *(Winthrop):* A plastic, squeezable, dropper-container.
Mucorette *(Schering):* Tablet for oromucosal absorption.
Oret *(Smith, Miller & Patch):* Compressed tablet.
Ovoid *(Winthrop):* Sugar-coated, oval-shaped tablet.
Pakette *(Mead Johnson):* Purse dispenser with dosage schedule.
Pediatab *(Philips Roxane):* Flavored, compressed tablet.
Pharynget *(Lederle):* Troche.
Pilpak *(Wyeth):* Purse-compack dispenser with visible day/dosage schedule.
Plasma-Vac *(Baxter):* Sterile, nonpyrogenic, vacuum-container for pooling, storing and administering plasma or serum aspirated from other containers.
Plastule *(Ives):* Compressed tablet.
Plateau Cap *(Marion):* Sustained-release capsule.
Pliapak *(Abbott):* Disposable, plastic bag for blood.
Pressule *(Squibb):* Individual dose of medication in a squeezable plastic container.
Pressure Pak *(Abbott):* An aerosol-type container.
Prestab *(McNeil):* Prolonged-duration tablet.
Pulvo-Cap *(Dow):* Dry-filled capsule.
Pulvule *(Lilly):* Filled, bullet-shaped, hard-gelatin capsule.
Purogenated *(Lederle):* A highly refined biological product which has been purified by chemical and physical means.
Radiocap *(Abbott):* Capsule containing a radioactive isotope.
Rectisert *(Ayerst):* Single-dose rectal applicator.
Repetab *(Schering):* Repeat-action tablet.
Respihaler *(Merck Sharp & Dohme):* Aerosol for oral inhalation.
Saftiflask *(Cutter):* Flask for storage and administration of intravenous solution.
Saftifuge *(Cutter):* Completely-closed, vacuum flask for withdrawal of blood for preparation of plasma by centrifugation.
Saftivac *(Cutter):* Completely-closed, vacuum flask for withdrawal of whole blood.
Savoret *(Lilly):* Medicated, flavored tablet.
Secule *(Ayerst):* Sealed vial containing an injectable in dry form.
Sequel *(Lederle):* Sustained-release capsule.
Serobacterin *(Merck Sharp & Dohme):* Identifying trademark for sensitized bacterial vaccine (bacterial vaccine treated with its corresponding immune serum).
Sheroid *(Cooper):* Special, gelatin-coated vitamin tablet.
Sifter Cartridge *(Abbott):* Small, plastic, disposable cartridge containing dry, powdered medicament to be used with the Aerohaler.
Singlet *(Dow):* Continuous-release dosage form.
Sofcream *(Merrell-National):* Foamed cream medication dispensed from an aerosol can.
Softab *(Stuart):* Soft tablet that melts in the mouth (no water needed).
Solodose *(Cooper):* Individual packette of powdered drug.
Soloid *(Burroughs Wellcome):* Identifying trademark for quickly-soluble product.
Solvet *(Lilly):* Soluble tablet.
Spansule *(Smith Kline & French):* Sustained-release capsule containing tiny colored pellets.
Spersoid *(Lederle):* Soluble, dispersible powder.
Sprayomizer *(Ayerst):* Special, squeeze container of throat spray.
Spraypak *(Smith Kline & French):* Soft, plastic container with spray top.
Steraject *(Pfizer):* Single-dose, disposable cartridge with sterile needle affixed, ready for injection.
Sterap *(Lilly):* Sterile envelope of powder medication for topical application.
Sterilope *(Abbott):* Sterilized, double envelope of powdered medication.
Steri-Tainer *(Ophthalmos):* Autoclaved container of ophthalmic solution with dropper top.

Steri-Vial *(Parke-Davis):* Sterilized, injectable vial of medication.
Sub-U-Tab *(Abbott):* Sublingual tablet.
Supposicone *(Searle):* Special-base suppository that needs no refrigeration.
Suppositab *(Dorsey):* Special-shaped tablet for insertion into the vagina.
Supprette *(Webcon):* Water soluble base suppository.
Tabloid *(Burroughs Wellcome):* Trademarked name for tablet.
Tabule *(Mallinckrodt):* Elongated, capsule-shaped tablet.
Tastitab *(Roerig):* Soluble, flavored tablet.
Tembid *(Ives):* Special-base matrix tablet which allows controlled, gradual release of drug.
Tempule *(Armour):* Proportionate-release medication form.
Ten-Tab *(Merrell-National):* Continuous-release tablet.
Testpac *(Upjohn):* A trial package of tablets to start medication.
Timecap *(Kremers-Urban):* Sustained-release capsule.
Timespan *(Roche):* Sustained-release tablet.
Timetab *(Kremers-Urban):* Tablet constructed for timed release of active ingredient. The therapeutic effect extends over a 10-12 hour period.
Titradose *(Ives):* Easily broken scored tablets.
Trablet *(Ames):* Trapezoid-shaped, enteric-coated tablet.
Transfuso Vac *(Baxter):* Sterile, nonpyrogenic, vacuum-container with anticoagulant; for drawing, storing, transporting and administering blood and for preparing plasma.
Trinidex *(Baxter):* Parenteral solution in Vacoliter Container which contains the vitamins: niacinamide, riboflavin and thiamine hydrochloride.
Tubex *(Wyeth):* Closed injection system with cartridge and needle unit.
Tubule *(Warren-Teed):* A single-dose, gelatin container of ointment for rectal application.
Turbinaire *(Merck Sharp & Dohme):* Intra-nasal applicator.
Tymcap *(Amfre-Grant):* Timed-disintegration capsule.
Tymtab *(Amfre-Grant):* Timed-disintegration tablet.
Unimatic *(Squibb):* Disposable syringe for intramuscular injection.
Univial *(Abbott):* A double-chambered, sterile vial usually containing in each chamber an active ingredient and diluent or agents which are not compatible on long standing. The chambers are separated by a diaphragm. When the material is to be used, one chamber is depressed, breaking the diaphragm. After solution or mixing, the material is withdrawn as in a rubber-stoppered vial.
Vaccine-Vial *(Cooper):* Rubber-capped, rubber-diaphragm vial containing injectable solution.
Vacoliter *(Baxter):* Dispensing container with ready-to-use, sterile, nonpyrogenic, parenteral solution under vacuum.
Vacule *(Merck Sharp & Dohme):* Rubber-diaphragm-capped vial containing injectable solution.
Vaporole *(Burroughs Wellcome):* Cloth-covered, breakable, thin-glassed inhalant container.
Wyseal *(Wyeth):* Special-coated tablet.
Zestab *(Roche):* Chewable flavored tablet for pediatric use.

DRUG & CHEMICAL BLOOD LEVEL DATA*

This table has been prepared by Dr. Charles L. Winek, Chief Toxicologist of Allegheny County Coroner's Office and Professor of Toxicology, Duquesne University School of Pharmacy, Pittsburgh, Pennsylvania.

The data contained in the table has been gathered from the literature and from personal experience. The values are not considered absolute, but are to be used as a guide in evaluating a given case. The values can be affected by dose, route of administration, absorption differences, age and sex, tolerance, method of analysis, pathological or disease state, etc. Users of the table are referred to Wecht's Legal Medicine Annual 1973 and Winek's Toxicology Annual 1974 for chapters discussing the data, references to the data, and factors affecting blood level values.

DEFINITION OF BLOOD LEVELS

Therapeutic Blood Level: Fochtman and Winek defined a therapeutic blood level as that concentration of drug present in the blood (its serum or plasma) following therapeutically effective dosage in humans.

Toxic Blood Level: The concentration of drug or chemical present in the blood (its serum or plasma) that is associated with serious toxic symptoms in humans.

Lethal Blood Level: The concentration of drug or chemical present in the blood (its serum or plasma) that has been reported to cause death, or is so far above reported therapeutic or toxic concentrations that one can judge that it might cause death in humans.

COMPOUND	Therapeutic or Normal	Toxic	Lethal
Acetaminophen (Tylenol)	1 - 2 mg%	40 mg%	150 mg%
Acetazolamide (Diamox)	1 - 1.5 mg%	. . .	. . .
Acetohexamide (Dymelor)	2.1 - 5.6 mg%	. . .	. . .
Acetone	. . .	20 - 30 mg%	55 mg%
Aluminum	0.013 mg%	. . .	. . .
Aminophylline (Theophylline)	1 - 2 mg%	. . .	. . .
Amitriptyline (Elavil)	5 - 20 mcg%	40 mcg%	1.0 - 2.0 mg%
Ammonia	50 - 170 mcg%	. . .	. . .
Amobarbital (Amytal)	0.1 mg%	0.7 mg%	2 mg%
Amphetamine	2 - 3 mcg%	. . .	0.2 mg%
Arsenic	0.0 - 0.002 mg%	0.1 mg%	1.5 mg%
Barbiturates			
short acting	0.1 mg%	0.7 mg%	1 mg%
intermediate acting	0.1 - 0.5 mg%	1 - 3 mg%	3 mg% & >
phenobarbital	ca. 1.0 mg%	4 - 6 mg%	8 - 15 mg% & >
barbital	ca. 1.0 mg%	6 - 8 mg%	10 mg% & >

Cont'd

DRUG & CHEMICAL BLOOD LEVEL DATA (Cont'd)

COMPOUND	Therapeutic or Normal	Toxic	Lethal
Benzene	. . .	any measurable	0.094 mg%
Beryllium	tissue levels generally used (lung & lymph)	. . .	. . .
Boron (Boric acid)	0.08 mg%	4 mg%	5 mg%
Bromide	5.0 mg%	50 - 150 mg% (17 mEq./L)	200 mg%
Brompheniramine (Dimetane)	0.8 - 1.5 mcg%	. . .	. . .
Butabarbital (Butisol)	0.1 - 0.5 mg%	1 - 3 mg%	> 3 mg%
Cadmium	0.01 - 0.02 mcg%	0.005 mg%	. . .
Caffeine	0.5 - 1 mg%	. . .	. . .
Carbamazepine (Tegretol)	0.2 mg%	0.8 - 1.0 mg%	. . .
Carbon monoxide	1 %	15 - 35%	50%
Carbon tetrachloride	. . .	2 - 5 mg%	. . .
Carisoprodol (Rela, Soma)	1.0 - 4.0 mg%	. . .	. . .
Chloral hydrate (Noctec)	1.0 mg%	10 mg%	25 mg%
Chlordiazepoxide (Librium)	0.1 - 0.3 mg%	0.55 mg%	2 mg%
Chloroform	. . .	7 - 25 mg%	39 mg%
Chlorpheniramine	. . .	2 - 3 mg%	. . .
Chlorpromazine (Thorazine)	0.05 mg%	0.1 - 0.2 mg%	0.3 - 1.2 mg%
Chlorpropamide (Diabinese)	3.0 - 14.0 mg%	. . .	. . .
Chlorprothixine (Taractan)	0.004 - 0.03 mg%	. . .	. . .
Codeine	2.5 mcg%	. . .	20 - 60 mcg%
Copper	100 - 150 mcg%	540 mcg%	. . .
Cyanide	0.015 mg%	. . .	0.5 mg% & >
DDT	1.3 mcg%	. . .	. . .
Desipramine (Norpramin)	.059 - 0.14 mg%	. . .	1 - 2 mg%
Dextropropoxyphene (Darvon)†	5 - 20 mcg%	0.5 - 1 mg%	5.7 mg%
Diazepam (Valium)	0.05 - 0.25 mg%	0.5 - 2.0 mg%	2.0 mg% & >
Dieldrin	0.15 mcg%	. . .	. . .
Digitoxin	2 - 3.5 mcg%	. . .	32 mcg%
Digoxin	0.06 - 0.13 mcg%	0.20 - 0.90 mcg%	. . .
Dinitro-o-Cresol	. . .	3 - 4 mg%	7.5 mg%
Diphenhydramine (Benadryl)	0.5 mg%	1 mg%	. . .
Diphenylhydantoin (Dilantin)	0.5 - 2.2 mg%	5 mg%	10 mg% & >
Diphenoxylate (Lomotil)	1.0 mcg%	. . .	. . .
Disopyramide (Norpace)	0.3 - 0.8 mg%	. . .	. . .
Disulfiram (Antabuse)	0.25 mg%	. . .	. . .
Divinyl Oxide	. . .	. . .	70 mg%
Doxepin	15 mcg%	. . .	1.5 mg%
Ephedrine	10.0 mcg%	. . .	. . .
Ethanol	. . .	150 mg%	350 mg% & >
Ethchlorvynol (Placidyl)	ca. 0.5 mg%	2 mg%	15 mg%
Ethinamate (Valmid)	0.5 - 1.0 mg%	. . .	. . .
Ethosuximide (Zarontin)	2.5 - 7.5 mg%	. . .	. . .
Ethyl chloride	. . .	. . .	40 mg%
Ethyl ether	90 - 100 mg%	. . .	140 - 189 mg%
Ethylene glycol	. . .	150 mg%	200 - 400 mg%
Fluoride	0 - 0.05 mg%	. . .	0.2 mg%
Flurazepam (Dalmane)	0.05 - 0.15 mg%	0.25 mg%	. . .
Glutethimide (Doriden)	0.02 mg%	1 - 8 mg%	3 - 10 mg%
Gold (Sodium aurothiomalate)	300 - 600 mcg%	. . .	. . .

Cont'd

DRUG & CHEMICAL BLOOD LEVEL DATA (Cont'd)

COMPOUND	Therapeutic or Normal	Toxic	Lethal
Haloperidol (Haldol)	0.05 - 0.9 mcg%	1 - 4 mg%	
Halothane (Fluothane)	0.18 mg%	...	20 mg%
Hydrogen sulfide	...	...	0.092 mg%
Hydromorphone (Dilaudid)	...	...	0.01 - 0.03 mg%
Imipramine (Tofranil)	0.005 - 0.016 mg%	> 0.07 mg%	0.2 mg%
Iron	50 mg% (RBC)	0.6 mg% (serum)	...
Isopropanol	...	340 mg%	...
Lead	0.005 - 0.07 mg%	0.13 mg%	...
Lidocaine	0.2 - 0.6 mg%	0.90 mg%	2.5 mg%
Lithium	0.42 - 0.83 mg% (0.6 - 1.2 mEq./L)	1.39 mg% (2.0 mEq./L)	1.39 - 3.47 mg% (2.0 - 5.0 mEq./L)
Lorazepam (Antivan)	2.0 mcg%	...	...
L.S.D.	...	0.1 - 0.4 mcg%	...
Magnesium	1.5 - 2.5 mg%	...	5 mg%
Manganese	0.015 mg%	0.46 mg%	...
Meperidine (Demerol)	60 - 65 mcg%	0.5 mg%	ca. 3 mg%
Meprobamate	1 mg%	10 mg%	20 mg%
Mercury	0.006 - 0.012 mg%	...	...
Methadone	48 - 86 mcg%	0.2 mg%	0.4 mg% & >
Methamphetamine	...	0.5 mg%	4 mg%
Methanol	...	20 mg%	89 mg% & >
Methapyrilene	0.2 - 0.4 mg%	3 - 5 mg%	5 mg% & >
Methaqualone (Quaalude)	0.5 mg%	1 - 3 mg%	3 mg% & >
Methsuximide (Celontin)	0.25 - 0.75 mg%	...	...
Methylene chloride	...	...	28 mg%
Methylenedioxyamphetamine (MDA)	...	...	0.4 - 1.0 mg%
Methyprylon (Noludar)	1.0 mg%	3 - 6 mg%	10 mg%
Morphine	0.01 mg%	...	0.005 - 0.4 mg% (free morphine from heroin)
Nickel	0.041 mg%	...	...
Nicotine	...	1 mg%	0.5 - 5.2 mg%
Nitrofurantoin (Furadantin)	0.18 mg%	...	...
Nortriptyline (Aventyl)	12 - 16 mcg%	0.5 mg%	1.3 mg%
Orphenadrine	0.2 mg%	...	0.4 - 0.8 mg%
Oxalate	0.2 mg%	...	1.0 mg%
Oxazepam (Serax)	0.1 mg%	...	...
Papaverine	0.1 mg%	...	...
Para-methoxyamphetamine (PMA)	...	...	0.2 - 0.4 mg%
Paraldehyde	ca. 5.0 mg%	20 - 40 mg%	50 mg%
Pentazocine (Talwin)	0.014 - 0.016 mg%	0.2 - 0.5 mg%	1 - 2 mg%
Perphenazine (Trilafon)	...	0.1 mg%	...
Phencyclidine	...	...	0.1 mg%
Phensuximide (Milontin)	1 - 1.9 mg%	...	...
Phenylbutazone (Butazolidin)	ca. 10 mg%	...	...
Phosphorus	tissue levels usually used		
Primidone (Mysoline)	1.0 mg%	5 - 8 mg%	ca. 10 mg%
Probenecid (Benemid)	10 - 20 mg%	...	...
Procainamide	0.6 mg%	1 mg%	...
Prochlorperazine (Compazine)	...	0.1 mg%	...
Promazine (Sparine)	...	0.1 mg%	...

Cont'd

DRUG & CHEMICAL BLOOD LEVEL DATA (Cont'd)

COMPOUND	Therapeutic or Normal	Toxic	Lethal
Propoxyphene	5 - 20 mcg%	0.5 - 2 mg%	5.7 mg%
Propranolol (Inderal)	0.0025 - 0.02 mg%	...	0.8 - 1.2 mg%
Propylhexedrine (Benzedrex)	...	...	0.2 - 0.3 mg%
Quinidine	0.3 - 0.6 mg%	ca. 1.0 mg%	3 - 5 mg%
Quinine	...	...	1.2 mg%
Salicylate (acetylsalicylic acid)	2 - 10 mg%	15 - 30 mg%	50 mg%
Sulfadiazine	8 - 15 mg%	...	...
Sulfadimethoxine (Madribon)	8 - 10 mg%	...	...
Sulfaguanidine	3 - 5 mg%	...	...
Sulfanilamide	10 - 15 mg%	...	...
Sulfisoxazole (Gantrisin)	9 - 10 mg%	...	...
Strychnine	...	0.2 mg%	0.9 - 1.2 mg%
Theophylline	1 - 2 mg%	...	...
Thiocyanate	8 - 14 mg%	...	...
Thiothixene (Navane)	1.0 mcg%	...	...
Thioridazine (Mellaril)	0.10 - 0.15 mg%	1.0 mg%	2 - 8 mg%
Tin	0.012 mg%	...	...
Tolbutamide (Orinase)	5.3 - 9.6 mg%	...	...
Toluene	...	...	1.0 mg%
Tribromoethanol	...	...	9 mg%
Trichloroethane	...	...	10 - 100 mg%
Trimethadione (Tridione)	1.2 mg%	...	...
Trimethobenzamide (Tigan)	0.1 - 0.2 mg%	...	...
Uric Acid	3 - 7 mg%	...	...
Valproic Acid/Sodium Valproate (Depakene)	1 - 10 mg%	20 mg%	...
Warfarin	0.1 - 1.0 mg%	...	...
Zinc	68 - 136 mcg%	...	...
Zoxazolamine (Flexin)	0.3 - 1.3 mg%	...	...

* Modified from Clinical Toxicology, 3(4), pp. 541-549, Dec., 1970 by C. L. Winek

† Liver levels are about 20 × higher than blood levels.

DEFINITIONS:

Therapeutic blood level—The concentration of drug present in the blood (serum or plasma) following therapeutically effective dosage.

Toxic blood level—The concentration of drug present in the blood (serum or plasma) that has been reported to cause serious toxic symptoms.

Lethal blood level—The concentration of drug present in the blood (serum or plasma) that has been reported to cause death or is so far above reported therapeutic and toxic levels that one can judge that it might cause death.

THE DRUG ENFORCEMENT ADMINISTRATION

A REVIEW OF THE CONTROLLED SUBSTANCES ACT OF 1970, AND THE REORGANIZATION PLAN OF 1973, REVISED AS OF APRIL 1, 1977

In April 1968 the Federal Bureau of Narcotics in the Treasury Department was merged with the Bureau of Drug Abuse Control of the Food and Drug Administration to form the Bureau of Narcotics and Dangerous Drugs (BNDD). This new Bureau, based in the Justice Department, functioned under the regulations of the two older agencies until May 1971 when the Controlled Substances Act of 1970 became law. The 1970 Act replaced the earlier amendments and acts under which the previous Bureaus operated. As a result the Internal Revenue Service was no longer responsible for the annual registration of those distributing narcotics or for issuing narcotics order forms. These functions became the sole responsibility of the Bureau of Narcotics and Dangerous Drugs (BNDD) of the U.S. Department of Justice.

On July 1, 1973 the Presidential Reorganization Plan No. 2 of 1973 established the Drug Enforcement Administration to combat drug abuse. This agency, which merged the Bureau of Narcotics and Dangerous Drugs, the Office of National Narcotic Intelligence, the components of the Bureau of Customs having investigative drug responsibilities, the Office of Drug Abuse Law Enforcement and the components of the Office of Science and Technology which were related to drug enforcement, was set up to oversee the enforcement of proper control of narcotic and dangerous drug abuse.

Under the former provisions, medications were classified primarily on the basis of prescribing characteristics. The class depended on somewhat arbitrary distinctions as to whether narcotics order forms and written prescriptions were required (Class A), whether oral prescription by a physician or dentist was permissible (Class B), whether the preparation was an "exempt narcotic" for which a narcotics registry number was required but for which over-the-counter sale for bona fide medical use was permitted (Class X), or whether the preparation was considered to have little addicting properties and no record-keeping below the manufacturer's level was required (Class M).

The Controlled Substances Act of 1970 reclassified appropriate substances into five schedules based upon accepted medical use and the potential for abuse. In brief, the findings for each of these schedules as outlined in PUBLIC LAW 91-513, with examples, are as follows:

Schedule I—

A—The drug or other substance has a high potential for abuse.

B—The drug or other substance has no currently accepted medical use in treatment in the United States.

C—There is a lack of accepted safety for use of the drug or other substance under medical supervision.

Examples in this schedule are marihuana, peyote, mescaline and lysergic acid diethylamide (LSD).

Schedule II—

A—The drug or other substance has a high potential for abuse.

B—The drug or other substance has a currently accepted medical use in treatment in the United States or a currently accepted medical use with severe restrictions.

C—Abuse of the drug or other substance may lead to severe psychological or physical dependence.

Examples in this schedule include opium, morphine, codeine, dihydromorphinone (Dilaudid), the amphetamine group, phenmetrazine (Preludin) and methylphenidate (Ritalin).

Schedule III—

A—The drug or other substance has a potential for abuse less than the drugs or other substances in Schedules I and II.

B—The drug or other substance has a currently accepted medical use in treatment in the United States.

C—Abuse of the drug or other substance may lead to moderate or low physical dependence or high psychological dependence.

Drugs in this schedule include preparations formerly known as "Class B narcotics" (such as various combinations which included codeine), paregoric (formerly an "exempt narcotic"), and non-narcotic drugs such as methyprylon (Noludar), glutethimide (Doriden), amobarbital (Amytal), secobarbital (Seconal), amobarbital and secobarbital (Tuinal) and pentobarbital (Nembutal).

Schedule IV—

A—The drug or other substance has a low potential for abuse relative to the drugs or other substances in Schedule III.

B—The drug or other substance has a currently accepted medical use in treatment in the United States.

C—Abuse of the drug or other substance may lead to limited physical dependence or psychological dependence relative to the drugs or other substances in Schedule III.

Examples of drugs in this schedule include phenobarbital, chloral hydrate, chlordiazepoxide (Librium), diazepam (Valium), ethchlorvynol (Placidyl) and meprobamate.

Schedule V—

A—The drug or other substance has a low potential for abuse relative to the drugs or other substances in Schedule IV.

B—The drug or other substance has a currently accepted medical use in treatment in the United States.

C—Abuse of the drug or other substance may lead to limited physical dependence or psychological dependence relative to the drugs or other substances in Schedule IV.

Drugs in this schedule include preparations formerly considered "exempt narcotics," such as codeine-containing cough preparations.

The refilling of a prescription by a pharmacist for a controlled substance listed in Schedule II is prohibited. No prescription for a controlled substance listed in Schedule III or IV can be filled or refilled more than six months after the date on which the prescription was written and no such prescription may be refilled more than five times.

It is necessary to register with the Drug Enforcement Administration for each of these five schedules on an annual basis. The subsequent prescribing of listed drugs is restricted to that schedule for which the physician or dentist has previously registered.

We have indicated the appropriate schedule for preparations listed in THE ENCYCLOPEDIA when it has been so indicated by the manufacturer or when it is obvious from the Drug Enforcement Administration (DEA) regulations.

PHARMACEUTICALS

AND

BIOLOGICALS

ACCELERASE-PB

Description: Each grey and white capsule contains:

Pancrelipase*	(approx.) 165 mg
Conjugated bile salts, mixed	65 mg
Cellulase	2 mg
Calcium carbonate	20 mg
Phenobarbital	16 mg
Belladonna alkaloids** (total)	0.2 mg

* Includes 1000 Organon units lipase, amylase equivalent to 750 mg pancreatin, N.F.; trypsin equivalent to 600 mg pancreatin, N.F., and other pancreatic enzymes derived from hog pancreas.

** 87.5% hyoscyamine and 12.5% atropine (as sulfates).

Indications: Symptomatic relief of functional digestive disorders characterized by bloating, belching, flatulence and other symptoms resulting from inadequate secretion of enzymes and diminished motor activity of the upper digestive tract. Recommended especially for geriatric patients with declining production of digestive enzymes or reduced secretory response due to temporary stresses.

Contraindications: Known hypersensitivity to any of the components. Other contraindications are bile salts in the presence of complete biliary obstruction, and belladonna alkaloids in the presence of acute glaucoma, urinary bladder neck obstruction, pyloric obstruction, pyloric stenosis with significant gastric retention, prostatic hypertrophy, duodenal obstruction, cardiospasm (megaesophagus), achalasia of the esophagus, and severe cardiac disease.

Warnings: Phenobarbital may be habit-forming.

Precautions: Use with caution in patients with suspected ocular pressure, partial intestinal obstruction and/or diverticulitis, renal or hepatic disease, and known sensitivity to pork protein.

Adverse Reactions: Blurred vision, dry mouth, difficult urination, and allergic reactions manifested by skin rash, urticaria or other symptoms of hypersensitivity may occur.

Dosage and Administration: *Orally.* Adults: One capsule 3 times daily with meals. Three capsules provide sufficient lipase activity to digest 25 gm of dietary fat; trypsin activity to digest 50 gm of dietary protein; amylase activity to digest 125 gm of starch and cellulase activity to digest 0.24 gm of cellulose.

Availability:
ACCELERASE®-PB Capsules in bottles of 60 and 500. **(Organon)**

ACENOCOUMAROL

Chemical Name: 3-(α-acetonyl-4-nitrobenzyl)-4-hydroxycoumarin.

Description: Acenocoumarol, one of the intermediate-type anticoagulants, is a potent, synthetic coumarin-type compound. It occurs as a white crystalline powder, is tasteless, odorless, almost insoluble in water or in organic solvents, and forms water-soluble salts with alkalis.

The drug acts by inhibiting the synthesis of prothrombin in the liver, thereby reducing the concentration of prothrombin in the blood and increasing prothrombin time. The inhibition of prothrombin involves interference with the action of vitamin K, and it has been suggested that acenocoumarol, like bishydroxycoumarin, competes with vitamin K for an enzyme essential for prothrombin synthesis. The drug also interferes with the production of factors VII, IX, X, so that their concentration in the blood is lowered during therapy.

It is readily absorbed from the gastrointestinal tract and reaches a peak effect within 30 to 48 hours. The decline of activity is rapid, and normal prothrombin levels are restored within 48 hours after the drug's withdrawal. Its onset of action is faster than that of bishydroxycoumarin, but not quite so fast as that of ethyl biscoumacetate.

Indications: Prophylaxis and treatment of venous thrombosis and its extension, treatment of atrial fibrillation with embolization, the prophylaxis and treatment of pulmonary embolism, and as an adjunct in the treatment of coronary occlusion.

Contraindications: As with any drug that induces hypoprothrombinemia, acenocoumarol is contraindicated in patients with hemorrhagic diathesis or subacute endocarditis

Warnings: Use with extreme caution, if at all, in patients with hepatic or renal disease, which might impair the detoxication and excretion of the drug. Extremely careful usage is also necessary in patients with subacute bacterial endocarditis, ulcerating or granulomatous lesions, toxic-infectious syndromes and generally in the presence of severe debilitation and severe illness. Anticoagulant therapy may be used in these patients only if urgently indicated and then only with utmost care to avoid overdosage. Acenocoumarol is a potent drug and utmost care should be exercised when it is administered in any condition where added risk of hemorrhage is present; therefore, it is advised that the drug be withdrawn at the earliest sign of bleeding. Treatment of each patient is highly individualized. Dosage should be controlled only by periodic determination of prothrombin time since determinations of clotting and bleeding times are not effective measures for control of therapy. When heparin sodium, which prolongs the one-stage prothrombin time, is given with acenocoumarol, a period of at least 5 hours after the last intravenous dose and 24 hours after the last subcutaneous dose of heparin sodium should elapse in order to obtain a valid prothrombin time. Fetal or neonatal hemorrhage, which can lead to death *in utero,* is a possibility, since oral anticoagulants pass through the placental barrier; acenocoumarol may pass into the milk of the mother and cause hypoprothrombinemia in the nursing infant. Therefore, when indicated for pregnant patients or lactating mothers, the risk of withholding the drug should be carefully weighed against the potential hazards entailed in administering it. Surgical procedures should be avoided in patients with lowered prothrombin activity; in an emergency, the prothrombin level may be restored rapidly by transfusion of fresh whole blood, and the administration of vitamin K in full doses.

Precautions: The action of anticoagulants may be affected by the concurrent use of other drugs. Fatalities have been reported from interactions affecting the metabolism of coumarin anticoagulants or their binding to plasma proteins. Thus, salicylates or phenylbutazone may accentuate the effect of acenocoumarol while barbiturates may antagonize it. Antibiotics which alter the intestinal bacterial flora may decrease the normal supply of vitamin K and consequently may increase the effect of acenocoumarol. Therefore, if a drug is to be added to or withdrawn from a patient's therapeutic regimen, it is essential that the prothrombin time be carefully checked. Alterations in diet, too, may modify the response to anticoagulant therapy. Other factors which may alter the activity of this drug are fever, alcoholism, ascorbic acid deficiency, x-ray therapy, and diarrhea. Care in patient selection is desirable to ensure cooperation, particularly from alcoholic, emotionally unstable or psychotic, or senile patients. The physician should be aware that bleeding during oral anticoagulant therapy may not always correlate with the prothrombin time.

For complete information on potential drug interactions, see monograph on Bishydroxycoumarin.

Adverse Reactions: The principal adverse reaction is hemorrhage due to overdosage. Hemorrhage usually is evident, but the possibility of intestinal hemorrhage must be considered when a patient has abdominal symptoms. In the absence of hemorrhage, the drug should be withheld until the prothrombin time returns to safe levels. Mild to severe bleeding can be controlled by either oral or parenteral administration of vitamin K. Intravenous injection should be slow and should not exceed a rate of 10 mg/min. Local skin necrosis has occurred on very rare occasions, even when the prothrombin time was within apparently safe limits. Other possible adverse reactions include alopecia, urticaria, dermatitis, hypersensitivity reactions primarily related to individual patient reactivity, fever, nausea, vomiting, cramps, diarrhea, leukopenia, agranulocytosis, mouth ulcers, and nephropathy. Patients should be told that urine may turn red-orange.

Dosage and Administration: *Orally.* **It is essential that therapy be controlled by periodic prothrombin time determinations.** A dosage of 16 to 28 mg the first day and 8 to 16 mg the second day may be followed by a maintenance dosage of 2 to 10 mg daily, depending upon prothrombin time determinations. These should be done daily the first 7 to 10 days. Once stability has been achieved, determinations may be required only once a week thereafter. Heparin may be given at the start of treatment if considered necessary.

Availability:
SINTROM® Tablets, 4 mg (white, double-scored) in bottles of 50. **(Geigy)**

ACETAMINOPHEN with BUTABARBITAL SODIUM

Chemical Name: *N*-acetyl-*p*-aminophenol.

Description: Acetaminophen is a nonsalicylate analgesic-antipyretic agent. It occurs as a white, odorless, crystalline powder with a slightly bitter taste; it is slightly soluble in water. Acetaminophen is the principal metabolite of both acetanilid and phenacetin.

Indications: For the treatment of headache and mild to moderate pain in muscles and joints. Also for the treatment of fever associated with childhood. Formulations with butabarbital are indicated for relief of tension headaches, head pain associated with upper respiratory tract infections and discomfort and pain associated with tension.

Contraindications: Hypersensitivity to acetaminophen or to any other component of the drug.

Warnings: Butabarbital may be habit-forming.

Precautions: Should be used with caution in patients with severe hepatic disease. It has been reported that acetaminophen may augment the activity of anticoagulants. This should be considered when the drug is administered to patients taking anticoagulant medication.

Adverse Reactions: In rare instances, drowsiness, nausea, constipation, dizziness, and skin rash have been noted. Prolonged use of acetaminophen may cause little or no methemoglobinemia. Although large doses have been noted to potentiate the action of oral anticoagulants, small doses have little or no effect on prothrombin time. Whether or not prolonged use of acetaminophen can cause a phenacetin-induced type of renal damage is not known. Hepatic necrosis has been observed following overdosage. For adverse effects associated with the use of butabarbital, see monograph on Butabarbital Sodium.

Dosage and Administration: *Orally.* The usual dosage for adults is 1 or 2 tablets every 4 hours; not to exceed 8 tablets in a 24-hour period. Children 8 to 12 years of age, 1/2 tablet every 4 to 6 hours; not to exceed 2 tablets in a 24-hour period.

Availability:
MINOTAL Tablets, 325 mg with butabarbital sodium, 15 mg in bottles of 100. **(Carnrick)**
PHRENILIN Tablets, 325 mg with butabarbital sodium, 15 mg and caffeine, 40 mg in bottles of 100. **(Carnrick)**

ACETAMINOPHEN with CODEINE (C-III)

Description: Acetaminophen alone is used as an analgesic to relieve pain in a variety of arthritic and rheumatic conditions involving musculoskeletal pain, as well as in headache, dysmenorrhea, myalgia and neuralgia. Acetominophen has no antiinflammatory properties in usual dosage. Codeine is selective in its action by inhibiting perception of pain centrally and altering the physiologic reaction associated with pain perception. Codeine also acts as an antitussive by centrally depressing the cough reflex. Each white tablet, imprinted with the number 1, 2, 3 or 4, contains:

	No. 1	*No. 2*	*No. 3*	*No. 4*
Codeine phosphate	7.5 mg	15 mg	30 mg	60 mg
Acetaminophen	300 mg	300 mg	300 mg	300 mg

Indications: The combination of the two drugs provides analgesia in a variety of conditions requiring the control of moderate or chronic pain. It is also indicated as an analgesic-antipyretic-antitussive agent in the acute stages of the common cold and in other acute respiratory diseases.

Contraindications: Hypersensitivity to either of the components.

Warnings: Codeine may be habit-forming. Although rare, psychic dependence, physical dependence and tolerance may develop upon repeated administration of preparations containing codeine. Mental and/or physical abilities of the patient may also be impaired; therefore, they should be advised to use special care when undertaking activities requiring alertness and physical coordination. The concomitant use of codeine with other CNS-depressant agents such as analgesics, general anesthetics, phenothiazines, other tranquilizers, sedative-hypnotics (including alcohol) may produce an additive CNS-depressant effect. When such combined therapy is contemplated, the dose of one or both agents should be reduced. When prescribed for pregnant patients, the physician should carefully consider the benefits versus the risks to the fetus.

Precautions: The respiratory depressant effects of narcotics and their capacity to elevate cerebrospinal fluid pressure may be markedly exaggerated in the presence of head injury, other intracranial lesions, or a preexisting increase in intracranial pressure. Furthermore, narcotics can produce side effects which may obscure the diagnosis and clinical course of patients with head injuries, or those with acute abdominal conditions. Utmost care is advised in elderly or debilitated patients, and in those with severe impairment of hepatic or renal function, hypothyroidism, Addison's disease, and prostatic hypertrophy or urethral stricture.

Adverse Reactions: The most frequently observed complications include lightheadedness, dizziness, sedation; nausea and vomiting. These effects appear to be more prominent in ambulatory than in nonambulatory patients, and some of these reactions may be alleviated if the patient lies down. Other reported reactions include euphoria, dysphoria, constipation, and pruritus. Serious overdosage is characterized by hepatoxicity due to the acetaminophen component and narcosis and cardiorespiratory depression due to the codeine component.

Dosage and Administration: *Orally.* For adults, 1 or 2 tablets or capsules or 1 or 2 teaspoonsful of elixir every 4 hours as required. Children 7 to 12 years of age, 2 teaspoonsful 3 or 4 times daily; 3 to 6 years of age, 1 teaspoonful 3 or 4 times daily.

Availability:

Ⓒ III **Acetaminophen w/Codeine**

Tablets, 300 mg with codeine phosphate, 30 mg in bottles of 100 and 1000. **(ICN)**

Tablets, 325 mg with codeine phosphate, 15 and 30 mg in bottles of 1000. **(Lederle)**

Tablets, 300 mg with codeine phosphate, 15 (No. 2), 30 (No. 3) and 60 mg (No. 4) in bottles of 1000 and in unit-dose cartons of 100. **(Philips Roxane)**

Ⓒ III CAPITAL® with CODEINE: **(Carnrick)**

Suspension, 120 mg with codeine phosphate, 12 mg/5 ml in bottles of 1 pint and 1 gallon.

Tablets, 325 mg with codeine phosphate, 30 mg in bottles of 100 and 1000.

Ⓒ III EMPRACET® Tablets, 300 mg with codeine phosphate, 30 and 60 mg in bottles of 60, 500 and in Dispenserpak® (unit-dose) packages of 25. **(Burroughs Wellcome)**

Ⓒ III HASACODE Strong Tablets, 300 mg with codeine phosphate, 32 mg in bottles of 100. **(Arnar-Stone)**

Ⓒ III LIQUIX-C Capsules, 320 mg with codeine phosphate, 32 mg in bottles of 100 and 1000. **(Elder)**

Ⓒ III PHENAPHEN® with CODEINE: **(Robins)**

Capsules, 325 mg with codeine phosphate, 15 mg (No. 2); 30 mg (No. 3); and 60 mg (No. 4) in bottles of 100 and 500 and in Dis-Co (unit-dose) packages of 96 (4 x 24).

Tablets, 650 mg with codeine phosphate, 30 mg in bottles of 50.

Ⓒ III SK-APAP™ with CODEINE Tablets, 325 mg with codeine phosphate, 15, 30 and 60 mg in bottles of 100. **(Smith Kline & French)**

Ⓒ III TYLENOL® with CODEINE: **(McNeil)**

Elixir, 120 mg with codeine phosphate, 12 mg/5 ml in bottles of 1 pint.

Tablets, No. 1, 2 and 4 in bottles of 100 and 500; No. 2 and 4 in Dispensit® (unit-dose) cartons of 500; No. 3 in bottles of 100, 500 and 1000 and in Dispensit® (unit-dose) cartons of 500.

ACETAZOLAMIDE

Chemical Name: 5-Acetamido-1,3,4-thiadiazole.

Description: Acetazolamide is a nonbacteriostatic sulfonamide possessing a chemical structure and pharmacologic activity distinctly different from those of the antibacterial sulfonamides. It functions by suppressing the enzyme carbonic anhydrase in the renal tubules. Its diuretic effect is due to the retardation of the reversible hydration of carbon dioxide and dehydration of the carbonic acid reaction in the kidney. The result is renal loss of bicarbonate ion along with sodium, potassium and water. Diuresis and alkalinization of the urine thus occur.

Although its diuretic activity may play a small part, acetazolamide is effective in various forms of glaucoma by virtue of its inhibitory action upon carbonic anhydrase in the eye which results in a decrease in the amount of secretion of aqueous humor. This decrease in ocular inflow produces a decrease in intraocular tension. This is in contrast to standard miotics which act to lower intraocular tension by influencing outflow. A complementary effect frequently is obtained by using acetazolamide adjunctively with miotics. Its usefulness in epilepsy has been attributed to inhibition of carbonic anhydrase in the central neurons thus retarding any abnormal, paroxysmal, or excessive discharge.

Indications: In chronic simple (open-angle) glaucoma, secondary glaucoma and, preoperatively, in acute congestive (closed-angle) glaucoma. The drug is of little use in severe glaucoma due to peripheral anterior synechiae or in hemorrhagic glaucoma. The drug is useful in the treatment of edema due to congestive heart failure. Patients with chiefly left-sided decompensation usually obtain relief after several days. Acetazolamide has been used successfully in cardiac patients with renal disease, and with decompensation of varying degrees. However, patients with pronounced renal failure usually do not respond although therapy in these patients has not been proved to be hazardous. Acetazolamide has also found application either alone or as an adjuvant in the treatment of epilepsy and, for its diuretic action, in drug-induced edema.

Contraindications: In situations involving depressed sodium and/or potassium blood serum levels, marked renal and hepatic disease or dysfunction, adrenal gland failure and hyperchloremic acidosis. Long-term use is contraindicated in patients with chronic noncongestive angle-closure glaucoma, since it may permit organic closure of the angle to occur while the deteriorating glaucoma is masked by lowered intraocular pressure.

Warnings: Studies with acetazolamide in rats and mice have demonstrated teratogenic and embryocidal effects at exceedingly large doses. Although evidence of these effects in clinical use is lacking, the drug should not be used during pregnancy, especially during the first trimester, unless the anticipated benefits are greater than the potential adverse effects.

Precautions: Increasing the dose does not increase the diuresis and may increase the incidence of drowsiness and/or paresthesia. However, in the presence of complete refractory renal failure, very large doses have been employed in conjunction with other diuretics in order to promote diuresis. In common with all sulfonamides, the following adverse reactions may occur: fever, rash, crystalluria, renal calculus, bone marrow depression, thrombocytopenic purpura, hemolytic anemia, leukopenia, pancytopenia, and agranulocytosis. The drug should be discontinued and appropriate therapy instituted at the first sign of such reactions.

Adverse Reactions: During short-term therapy, side effects are minimal and may include paresthesias, particularly in the extremities; some loss of appetite; polyuria and occasional instances of drowsiness and confusion. During long-term therapy, an acidotic state may supervene. This usually can be corrected by administering bicarbonate. Transient myopia has been reported, which invariably subsides upon reduction of dosage or withdrawal of therapy. Other occasional reactions include urticaria, melena, hematuria, glycosuria, hepatic insufficiency, flaccid paralysis and convulsions.

Dosage and Administration: *Glaucoma*—Acetazolamide should be used as an adjunct to the usual therapy. In the treatment of chronic simple (open-angle) glaucoma, the dosage ranges from 250 mg to 1 gm in 24 hours, usually in divided doses for amounts in excess of 250 mg/dose. In the treatment of secondary glaucoma and in the preoperative treatment of some cases of acute congestive (closed-angle) glaucoma, the preferred dosage is 250 mg every 4 hours; some patients have responded to 250 mg twice a day on short-term therapy. When the Sequels are employed, the recommended dose is 1 capsule (500 mg) 2 times daily (morning and evening). *Epilepsy*—the suggested total daily dose is 8 to 30 mg/kg in divided doses. Although some patients respond to a low dose, the optimum range is reported to be from 375 mg to 1 gm daily. When used in combination with other anticonvulsants, the suggested initial dose is 250 mg once daily. *Congestive heart failure, to induce diuresis*—the initial dose appears to be 250 to 375 mg (approximately 5 mg/kg) once daily in the morning. This dosage is most effective when given on alternate days. For those who cannot take acetazolamide by mouth, the sodium salt may be given parenterally. The direct intravenous route of administration is preferred. The intramuscular route may be used but is painful because of the alkaline pH of the solution. *Drug-induced edema*—the recommended dosage is 250 to 375 mg once daily for 1 or 2 days, alternating with a day of rest.

Availability:
DIAMOX®: **(Lederle)**
Tablets, 125 mg in bottles of 100; 250 mg in bottles of 100, 1000 and in unit-dose packages of 30, 60 and 100 (10 × 10) in cartons of 50.
Sustained Release Capsules (Sequels®), 500 mg in bottles of 30 and 100.
Parenteral (sodium salt) in vials of 500 mg.
HYDRAZOL Tablets, 250 mg in bottles of 100. *For oral ophthalmic use only.* **(Parke-Davis)**

ACETOHEXAMIDE

Chemical Name: N-(*p*-acetylphenylsulfonyl)-N′-cyclohexylurea.

Description: Acetohexamide is a sulfonylurea compound that is characterized by the presence of an acetyl group in the para position of the phenyl ring and the incorporation of a cyclohexyl group on the urea moiety. It occurs as a crystalline substance that is insoluble in water and soluble in alcohol.

Acetohexamide has essentially the same pharmacologic action and clinical uses as chlorpropamide and tolbutamide. It is an oral antidiabetic agent that appears to be effective in lowering the blood sugar level in carefully selected patients with maturity-onset diabetes. It acts by stimulating the beta cells of the pancreas to release insulin. In addition, acetohexamide appears to exert some action on the liver in that the output of glucose is inhibited and the deposition of glycogen is increased. In large doses, the sulfonylureas appear to potentiate the hypoglycemic effect of insulin.

Acetohexamide is partially acetylated by the liver and the metabolites, which retain some hypoglycemic action, are excreted by the kidneys. Following a single oral dose, the maximal drop in blood sugar occurs usually in 3 hours; however, optimal levels may not be attained for 5 to 6 days when the drug is administered daily or twice daily. The half-life of this agent and its metabolites is 6 to 8 hours, and the duration of effects is 12 to 24 hours.

Indications: For the treatment of mild, stable, maturity-onset or adult-type diabetes that is uncomplicated by ketosis or acidosis. The use of this drug in insulin-dependent patients may necessitate a reduction of their insulin requirements.

Contraindications: In patients with hyperglycemia and glycosuria due to primary renal disease, and in those who are hypersensitive to the sulfonylurea compounds.

Warnings: Since safe use in pregnant women has not been established, the use of acetohexamide is not recommended for the management of diabetes during pregnancy. Also, serious consideration should be given to the potential hazards of its use in women of childbearing age who may become pregnant. The drug is of no value in diabetes complicated by acidosis and coma, and if complicated by fever of any cause, trauma, infection or surgical procedures, it may be necessary to return the patient to insulin therapy or to use insulin in addition to acetohexamide.

Precautions: In patients with impaired liver and/or kidney function, and in debilitated or malnourished individuals, careful observation of the patient and adjustment of dosage are essential to prevent the occurrence of hypoglycemia. Thiazide-type diuretics may aggravate diabetes, thereby altering the dosage of acetohexamide required. Phenylbutazone, probenecid, and the antimicrobial sulfas may enhance the action of acetohexamide, resulting in prolonged hypoglycemia. Sulfonylurea compounds have been observed to aggravate hepatic porphyria, and also to decrease tolerance to alcohol manifested as a disulfiram reaction. The possible occurrence of secondary failures and the spontaneous tendency of diabetes to fluctuate in severity should be considered. Therefore, patients should be carefully supervised and their diabetes regularly evaluated in order to avoid hyperglycemic and hypoglycemic episodes.

Adverse Reactions: All the standard measures indicated during diabetes therapy should be followed so that extreme and prolonged hypoglycemia may be avoided. Other reactions noted were gastrointestinal disturbances (nausea, epigastric fullness, heartburn), and headache; they appear to be dose-related and may disappear when the dosage is reduced. Allergic skin manifestations (pruritus, erythema, urticaria, morbilliform or maculopapular eruptions) occur but are usually transient and may disappear with continued dosage. If the skin reactions persist, therapy with this drug should be terminated. Photosensitivity reactions have been observed; also jaundice of both the cholestatic and mixed hepatic types. Rarely noted were leukopenia, thrombocytopenia, pancytopenia, agranulocytosis, aplastic anemia, and hemolytic anemia.

Dosage and Administration: *Orally.* Daily dosage may range from 250 mg to 1.5 gm. No loading dose is required. Doses in excess of 1.5 gm daily are not recommended. Most patients receiving 1 gm or less daily can be controlled on a convenient once-daily dosage schedule. Patients who need 1.5 gm daily usually benefit from twice-daily dosage given before the morning and evening meals. Acetohexamide may be used in combination with insulin. For full prescribing information, see package literature.

Availability:
DYMELOR® Tablets, 250 and 500 mg in bottles of 50, 200, and 500, and in individual blister-strips of 10 in packages of 10 strips. **(Lilly)**

ACETOPHENAZINE MALEATE: see The Phenothiazines

ACETRIZOATE SODIUM

Chemical Name: Sodium 3-acetamido-2,4,6-triiodobenzoate.

Description: Sodium acetrizoate is a contrast medium which contains 65% iodine. It is a viscous water-soluble medium that is nonirritating, leaves no radiopaque residue and permits adequate visualization of the uterus and fallopian tubes when employed in a 50% concentration. Each ml of the solution contains sodium acetrizoate, 0.53 gm and polyvinylpyrrolidone, 0.23 gm compounded with calcium ethylenediaminetetraacetate and potassium phosphate.

Indications: Hysterosalpingography.

Contraindications: Should not be used for hysterosalpingography in the presence of severe vaginal or cervical infections, existing or recent pelvic infection, marked cervical erosion or endocervicitis, or during pregnancy. The procedure should not be attempted during the immediate pre- or postmenstrual phase.

Warnings: Not intended for intravenous administration.

Dosage and Administration: Standard procedures for hysterosalpingography, as described in gynecological literature, should be observed. If indicated in the patient's history, an intracutaneous skin test or sublingual absorption observation may be performed with 0.1 ml of the solution.

Availability:
SALPIX Solution in vials of 10 ml in packages of 6. **(Ortho)**

ACETYLCARBROMAL

Chemical Name: *N*-Acetyl-*N*-bromodiethylacetylurea.

Description: Acetylcarbromal is a nonbarbiturate, fast-acting nonsoporific sedative suitable for daytime use. It occurs as crystals, has a slightly bitter taste and is slightly soluble in water, but is freely soluble in alcohol and in ethyl acetate.

It acts on the higher centers, producing a calming, nonhypnotic effect. Perception and alertness are said to remain unimpaired. It is converted to urea and is readily eliminated.

Indications: For the relief of tension and anxiety. The effects are achieved without impairing muscular coordination or causing drowsiness, sluggish reflexes or dulling of sensorium. Rapid onset of action and relatively rapid elimination are cited as lessening the tendency to cumulative effects and toxicity thus permitting long-term administration.

Contraindications: When used at recommended doses, there are no known contraindications except in those patients who are sensitive to bromides.

Warnings: Acetylcarbromal may be habit-forming.

Precautions: Excessive doses may produce narcosis and respiratory depression. Prolonged use at usual dosage levels or gross overdosage may result in bromism, which may aggravate alcoholism, arteriosclerotic states and low-salt syndromes.

Adverse Reactions: As with all sedative drugs, large doses may cause drowsiness. However, no significant untoward side effects have been reported with recommended doses.

Dosage and Administration: *Orally.* For adults, 1 to 2 tablets up to 4 times daily. For children, proportionately less, according to age and weight.

Availability:
SEDAMYL® Tablets, 250 mg in bottles of 100. **(Riker)**

ACETYLCHOLINE CHLORIDE

Description: Acetylcholine chloride is a parasympathomimetic agent that acts directly on the postjunctional effector cells of the eye. This action produces intense miosis by stimulating contraction of the sphincter muscle of the iris. This effect is transient since the compound is rapidly hydrolyzed by acetylcholine esterase to choline and acetic acid. It occurs as an odorless, hygroscopic, white, crystalline powder that is freely soluble in water and in alcohol.

Indications: To obtain complete miosis in seconds by irrigation of the iris after delivery of the lens in cataract surgery, as well as in penetrating keratoplasty, iridectomy and other anterior segment surgery where rapid, complete miosis may be required.

Contraindications: None known at the present time.

Precautions: To obtain the desired effect quickly and completely, any anatomical obstruction to miosis, such as anterior or posterior synechiae, may require surgical removal prior to the administration of acetylcholine chloride. In cataract surgery, the drug should be applied only after delivery of the lens. Since the solution is unstable, it should be prepared immediately prior to instillation. Any solution that has not been used should be discarded.

Adverse Reactions: Probably due to its rapid inactivation, acetylcholine appears to have no systemic or local reactions.

Dosage and Administration: *Intraocular.* Instill ½ to 2 ml into the anterior chamber before or after securing 1 or more sutures. Instillation should be parallel to the iris face and tangential to the pupil border. Pilocarpine may be applied *topically* before dressing to maintain miosis.

Availability:
MIOCHOL® Solution, 20 mg with mannitol, 100 mg in 2-chamber vials (the lower chamber contains the 2 components and the upper chamber contains 2 ml of sterile water for injection). **(Smith, Miller & Patch)**

ACETYLCYSTEINE

Chemical Name: *N*-Acetyl-*L*-cysteine.

Description: Acetylcysteine is the generic name for the N-acetyl derivative of the naturally occurring amino acid, L-cysteine. The compound is a white crystalline powder which melts at 104-110° C and has a very slight odor. It has a molecular weight of 163.2.

The viscosity of pulmonary mucous secretions depends on the concentrations of mucoprotein and to a lesser extent deoxyribonucleic acid (DNA). The latter increases with enhanced purulence owing to cellular debris. The mucolytic action of acetylcysteine is related to the sulfhydryl group in the molecule. This group probably "opens" disulfide linkages in mucus thereby lowering the viscosity. The mucolytic activity of acetylcysteine is unaltered by the presence of DNA, and increases with increasing pH. Significant mucolysis occurs between pH 7 and 9.

Indications: As adjuvant therapy for patients with abnormal, viscid, or inspissated mucous secretions, in such conditions as: chronic bronchopulmonary disease, characterized by chronic emphysema, emphysema with bronchitis, chronic asthmatic bronchitis, tuberculosis, bronchiectasis and primary amyloidosis of the lung; acute bronchopulmonary disease such as pneumonia, bronchitis, tracheobronchitis; pulmonary complications of cystic fibrosis; tracheostomy care; pulmonary complications associated with surgery; during anesthesia; post-traumatic chest conditions; atelectasis due to mucous obstruction; diagnostic bronchial studies such as bronchograms, bronchospirometry, and bronchial wedge catheterization.

Contraindications: Acetylcysteine is contraindicated for those patients who are sensitive to it.

Warnings: After proper administration of acetylcysteine, an increased volume of liquefied bronchial secretions may occur. When cough is inadequate, the open airway must be maintained by mechanical suction if necessary. When there is a large mechanical block due to foreign body or local accumulation, the airway should be cleared by endotracheal aspiration, with or without bronchoscopy. Asthmatics under treatment with acetylcysteine should be watched carefully. If bronchospasm progresses, this medication should be discontinued immediately.

Precautions: With a face mask there may be stickiness on the face after nebulization. This is easily removed by washing with water. Under certain conditions, a light purple color may develop in the solution of acetylcysteine. This does not significantly affect safety or mucolytic effectiveness. To prevent the concentration of acetylcysteine in the solution remaining after prolonged nebulization, dilute with an equal volume of Sterile Water for Injection, when 3/4 of the initial volume has been nebulized.

Adverse Reactions: Occasionally, stomatitis, nausea or rhinorrhea may develop. Rarely, sensitivity and sensitization reactions occur. A few susceptible patients, particularly asthmatic patients, may experience varying degrees of bronchospasm associated with the administration of nebulized acetylcysteine. Most patients with bronchospasm are quickly relieved by the use of a bronchodilator given by nebulization.

Dosage and Administration: May be administered by nebulization, direct application, or by intratracheal instillation. Inhalation *(nebulization)*, 2 to 20 ml of a 10% solution or 1 to 10 ml of a 20% solution nebulized into a face mask or mouth piece may be given every 2 to 6 hours, and for instillation into the trachea by tracheostomy or bronchoscope, 1 to 2 ml of a 10 to 20% solution every 1 to 4 hours. The recommended dose for most patients is 6 to 10 ml of the 10% solution or 3 to 5 ml of the 20% solution 3 or 4 times daily. **Acetylcysteine should not be placed directly into the chamber of a heated (hot pot) nebulizer.**

Availability:
MUCOMYST® Solution, 10 and 20% in vials of 4, 10 and 30 ml. **(Mead Johnson)**

ACI-JEL

Description: A bland, nonirritating, water-dispersible, buffered acid jelly, containing acetic acid, 0.92%; oxyquinoline sulfate, 0.025%; boric acid, 3%; ricinoleic acid, 0.7% and glycerin, 5%. Compounded with tragacanth, acacia, propylparaben, potassium hydroxide, stannous chloride, egg albumen, potassium bitartrate, perfume and water.

Indications: In any case where the restoration and maintenance of vaginal acidity is desirable as in the treatment of nonspecific vaginal infection and in the milder forms of simple cervicitis. It is also useful prophylactically after courses of more specific therapy. In these cases, maintenance of vaginal acidity will largely prevent recurrences of the infection. In those patients demonstrating a tendency to constantly recurring vaginitis, the jelly in minimal doses affords a method of prophylaxis.

Contraindications: None known.

Dosage and Administration: *Intravaginally.* In the average case, 1 applicatorful inserted into the vaginal vault in the morning and upon retiring. In those cases where there is a tendency to vaginal discharge or leakage, a vulvar pad is recommended. The frequency of application and duration of treatment depend upon the type of case and the degree of progress.

Availability:
ACI-JEL® Therapeutic Vaginal Jelly in tubes of 85 gm with the measured-dose applicator.
(Ortho)

ACRISORCIN

Chemical Name: 9-Aminoacridine compound with 4-hexylresorcinol.

Description: Acrisorcin is a synthetic compound prepared from 9-aminoacridine and hexylresorcinol. It occurs as a yellow, crystalline powder and is slightly soluble in water and soluble in alcohol.

In vitro tests suggest that acrisorcin is bacteriostatic or bactericidal to a variety of bacteria. These tests also show that in a concentration of 31.25 mcg/ml, acrisorcin is fungistatic to a variety of fungi.

Indications: Topical treatment of tinea versicolor. Since a reliable technique for the culture of the causative organism, *Malassezia furfur,* has not been established, diagnosis must be made and therapeutic response evaluated from clinical appearance and scrapings of the lesions. Clinical use of acrisorcin for various topical bacterial infections and fungal infections other than those caused by *M. furfur* has produced variable results, and the drug is recommended only for use in the treatment of tinea versicolor.

Contraindications: Known hypersensitivity to any of the components.

Precautions: Do not use around the eyes. If irritation or sensitization develops, use of the drug should be discontinued and appropriate therapy instituted. *Store away from heat.*

Adverse Reactions: Blisters, erythematous vesicular eruptions, hives, pruritus following exposure to ultraviolet light, and a burning sensation in a case of eczema have been reported. Also, in a case of eczema, the tinea versicolor became slightly worse after treatment with this drug.

Dosage and Administration: *Topically.* Apply a small amount of cream on affected area twice daily: once in the morning and again at night. The evening application should follow a warm soapy bath and use of a stiff bath brush on the lesions. All soap must be removed by thorough rinsing and followed by thorough drying with a towel before the cream is applied. Towels and all clothing worn next to the skin must be laundered after each use. Traditionally, tinea versicolor has shown a strong tendency to relapse when treated by conventional therapy, and there is no evidence that the infection produces immunity in the host. In most cases, all evidence of the disease will disappear in a matter of days following initiation of therapy with acrisorcin. However, treatment should be continued twice daily for at least 6 weeks.

Availability:
AKRINOL® Cream, 2 mg/gm in tubes of 50 gm. **(Schering)**

ACUTUSS with CODEINE Ⓒ

Description: Contains in each 5 ml (teaspoonful):

Codeine phosphate	10 mg
Phenylpropanolamine hydrochloride	5 mg
Phenylephrine hydrochloride	5 mg
Chlorpheniramine maleate	2 mg
Guaifenesin	100 mg
Alcohol	5%

Indications: Symptomatic treatment of acute coughs and related aches and discomforts associated with colds, allergy, and common upper respiratory tract infections.

Contraindications: Sympathomimetic amines are contraindicated in patients with severe hypertension or with coronary artery disease, in those taking MAO inhibitors, in nursing mothers, and in patients with known hypersensitivity or idiosyncrasy to any of the components.

Warnings: Codeine phosphate may be habit-forming, and should be administered with the same degree of caution as with all oral medications containing narcotic analgesics. Sympathomimetic amines (phenylpropanolamine and phenylephrine) should be administered with extreme caution in the presence of hypertension, cardiac or peripheral vascular disease, diabetes mellitus, hyperthyroidism, or glaucoma. These agents may cause mild stimulation in sensitive patients.

Precautions: Patients taking antihistamines should be cautioned not to drive a car or operate dangerous machinery. Antitussives should be used judiciously in sedated or debilitated patients. Patients with a productive cough should not have their cough reflex severely inhibited so that retention of secretions may be avoided.

Adverse Reactions: Reactions occur occasionally and are mild. Nausea, dizziness and dry mouth occur infrequently; vomiting and drowsiness, rarely. Also, hypersensitivity, urticaria, visual disturbances, urinary retention, vertigo, rare blood dyscrasias (agranulocytosis, thrombocytopenia, pancytopenia), hyperexcitability, nightmares, hallucinations, nervousness, palpitation and tremors.

Dosage and Administration: *Orally.* Adults, 1 or 2 teaspoonsful 3 or 4 times daily.

Availability:
Ⓒ ACUTUSS® with CODEINE Elixir in bottles of 90 ml. **(Philips Roxane)**

AD-CEBRIN w/FLUORIDE: see The Fluoride-Vitamins

ADEFLORS (THE): see The Fluoride-Vitamins

ADENOSINE PHOSPHATE

Synonym: Adenosine-5-monophosphate (AMP).

Chemical Name: 5′-Adenylic acid.

Description: Adenosine phosphate, a monophosphorylated adenine riboside, is a natural component of muscle tissue. Directly or as a part of adenosine triphosphate (ATP), AMP has been identified in many stages of metabolism. It is also associated with many normal biochemical processes. Studies have indicated that it is essential in phosphorylation reactions and in certain enzyme reactions. Also, it appears to be a necessary agent for carbohydrate and fat metabolism. It occurs as white crystals that are readily soluble in boiling water and practically insoluble in alcohol.

Although the exact mechanism by which adenosine phosphate provides certain therapeutic benefits is not known, it has been proposed that its usefulness may result from the correction of either biochemical imbalances or cellular deficiencies or both. The clinical benefits from therapy may be due in part to the drug's vasodilating action and reduction of tissue edema and inflammation.

When administered, adenosine phosphate produces increased blood levels of adenosine triphosphate. Following a 20 mg injection (intramuscularly), 90% of the total blood adenine compounds are converted into ATP with peak levels attained in 24 hours, and above normal levels maintained for 48 hours.

Indications: As adjunctive therapy to alleviate the edema, pruritus, pain, erythema, and scaling associated with varicose vein complications (ulceration, chronic thrombophlebitis and stasis dermatitis). It has been employed preoperatively, postoperatively, and in the therapeutic management of these conditions. Although it is not considered as initial or primary therapy for acute and chronic bursitis, tenosynovitis, and intractable pruritus, a favorable response has been observed in some patients.

Contraindications: Patients with a history of myocardial infarction, and in the presence of cerebral hemorrhage.

Warnings: Since occasional cases of an anaphylactoid reaction have been reported following administration of the sustained-action solution, the drug should be discontinued if the patient experiences dyspnea or tightness in the chest. A history of allergy implies greater than usual risk to the patient. The drug should be used in women of childbearing potential and particularly during early pregnancy only if the expected benefits clearly justify the possible risk to the unborn child. The drug is presently not recommended for use in children because documented clinical experience has not been sufficient to establish safe use and a suitable dosage regimen in this age group.

Adverse Reactions: Because of the vasodilating effects of the drug when absorbed rapidly, patients may experience slight flushing, dizziness and palpitation. Other reported complaints include hypotension, dyspnea, epigastric discomfort, nausea, occasional local rash and diuresis; augmentation of bursitis and tendinitis.

Dosage and Administration: *Intramuscularly or Sublingually. For varicose vein complications*—the dosage of the sustained-action solution is 100 mg (1 ml) daily for 3 days followed by 100 mg (1 ml) 3 times a week. When reduction of edema, inflammation and pruritus is achieved, a dosage of 20 mg (1 ml) of the sustained-action solution may be administered 1, 2 or 3 times a week depending upon the response of the patient. For maintenance therapy, 1 tablet, sublingually or placed in the buccal pouch, 5 to 7 times daily for 4 to 7 days, then 2 to 5 tablets daily as required. Patient should be instructed to refrain from admixing the tablet with saliva, food or liquid while the tablet is being absorbed. *For bursitis, tenosynovitis, and intractable pruritus*—the dosage of the aqueous solution is 20 mg (1 ml) to 100 mg (5 ml) daily. The dosage should not exceed 100 mg/day. Alternately, the sustained-action solution may be given in dosages of 20 to 100 mg daily or 3 times a week. For maintenance, 1 tablet every hour up to 5 to 7 tablets daily as required.

Availability:
MY-B-DEN®: **(Dome)**
Aqueous Solution, 20 mg/ml in vials of 1 ml.
Sublingual Tablets, 20 mg in bottles of 50.
Sustained-Action Solution (in gelatin), 20 and 100 mg/ml in vials of 10 ml.

THE ADRENAL CORTICOSTEROIDS

Description: The basic structure of the adrenal steroids is the cyclopentanophenanthrene nucleus, which consists of three 6-carbon rings and a single 5-carbon ring. All the corticosteroids are 21-carbon compounds with a 2-carbon side chain at C-17. A ketone group at C-3 and a double bond between carbons 4 and 5 of the steroid molecule are required for glucocorticoid activity. Essential also is the maintenance of such features as the 11-hydroxyl and the 20-keto groups. Spatial orientation of the groups attached to the steroid molecule is importantly related to their pharmacologic functions. In the body the corticosteroidal hormones are synthesized from dietary cholesterol which is enzymatically converted to 21-carbon corticosteroids and 19-carbon weak androgens.

The adrenal cortex secretes a number of steroidal hormones, the most important of which are hydrocortisone (cortisol) and aldosterone. All other secreted cortical hormones are probably inactive precursors, metabolites, or end products of those two. Hydrocortisone and its companion synthetic preparations are glucocorticoids which have as their primary action resistance to many types of stress and maintaining the integrity of various body enzyme systems. The mineralocorticoid aldosterone has a primary effect on the stability of the body's electrolytes, especially sodium and potassium. Both hydrocortisone and aldosterone are able to suppress the stimuli which initiate their secretion by specific feed-back mechanisms.

Hydrocortisone is the secretory product of the zona fasciculata of the adrenal following stimulation by the adrenocorticotrophic hormone (ACTH). ACTH release is controlled by the plasma level of hydrocortisone, a diurnal rhythm and stress. Following secretion, hydrocortisone enters the circulation where it is reversibly bound to transcortin, an α_2-globulin. Metabolic inactivation occurs primarily in the liver where the hydrocortisone is converted into glucuronides which are excreted by the renal route.

The adrenocortical zona glomerulosa secretes aldosterone, primarily in response to changes in blood volume, the primary stimulating agents being angiotensin, sodium and potassium. ACTH plays a secondary role and is probably operative only in acute situations. Aldosterone is metabolized in the liver to an inactive derivative with an additional 10% being converted to an active glucuronide by the liver and kidneys.

The effects of hydrocortisone on the functions of the body are widespread and significant. It suppresses secretion of ACTH and the melanocyte-stimulating hormone of the pituitary; it has a stimulating effect on protein catabolism, and impairs glucose utilization of muscle cells while stimulating hepatic gluconeogenesis. Hydrocortisone has an antiinflammatory action partly explained by its stabilization of lysosomes, and it also has an effect on electrolyte systems which, like aldosterone, result in sodium retention and potassium excretion.

Aldosterone produces its effects on the body physiology by acting on the electrolyte transport of the epithelial cells of the kidney as well as those of the sweat glands and the gastrointestinal tract. Under the influence of this hormone, sodium is retained and potassium is secreted.

Indications: In most cases, adrenal corticosteroids are used in supraphysiologic amounts with the intention of influencing favorably a variety of clinical conditions by the suppression of inflammatory or immunologic processes. However, their antiinflammatory action is inseparable from their metabolic effects which, upon prolonged administration, result in signs and symptoms similar to those of Cushing's syndrome. Corticosteroids have been used systemically in the treatment of connective tissue diseases (e.g., psoriatic arthritis, rheumatoid arthritis, postraumatic osteoarthritis, epicondylitis, rheumatic fever, acute nonspecific tenosynovitis, acute and subacute bursitis, ankylosing spondylitis, disseminated lupus erythematosus, periarteritis nodosa, dermatomyositis and scleroderma); by local injection in the treatment of inflamed joints, tendons, bursae and soft tissues; in the symptomatic treatment of systemic lupus erythematosus, for the relief of symptoms due to systemic allergic states (e.g., allergic rhinitis, bronchial asthma; reactions to drugs, serum, and transfusions) and dermatoses with an allergic component; topically, for the relief of symptoms of allergic, inflammatory and pruritic dermatoses; cutaneous manifestations of systemic collagen diseases (e.g., systemic lupus erythematosus, acute rheumatic carditis, dermatomyositis and pemphigus); by intralesional injection in psoriasis, alopecia areata, keloids, atopic dermatitis and stasis dermatitis; by local application or instillation in inflammatory ocular diseases (e.g., allergic blepharitis and certain types of anterior and posterior uveitis, choroiditis, iritis, iridocyclitis, chorioretinitis, optic neuritis, sympathetic ophthalmia, conjunctivitis, keratitis and acute glaucoma) or inflammatory otic conditions (e.g., allergic otitis externa); to produce symptomatic relief or temporary remission in numerous miscellaneous conditions, including ulcerative colitis, nephrotic syndrome, nonsuppurating thyroiditis; sarcoidosis; Loeffler's syndrome; berylliosis; fulminating or disseminated pulmonary tuberculosis (with concurrent antituberculous chemotherapy); acute Bell's palsy; severe acute trichinosis; idiopathic and thrombocytopenic purpura; autoimmune hemolytic anemia, erythroblastopenia (RBC anemia), congenital (erythroid) hypoplastic anemia; tuberculous meningitis with subarachnoid block; diagnostic testing of adrenocortical hyperfunction; the hypercalcemia of malignancy, and such neoplastic diseases as acute leukemia (especially in children), chronic lymphocytic leukemia, lymphosarcoma, reticulum cell sarcoma and metastatic breast cancer. Corticosteroids have also been used in meningococcemia, which often is associated with adrenal insufficiency and collapse. Large doses of soluble corticosteroids have been given parenterally for the treatment of severe hypotension unresponsive to standard treatment for shock. Large doses, parenterally, have also been used in various other emergency situations, including acute hypersensitivity reactions (e.g., anaphylactic shock, status asthmaticus, organ transplantation, and drug or transfusion reactions).

Contraindications: In the absence of a life-threatening situation, the glucocorticoids should be avoided in patients with active peptic ulcer disease; virus diseases, such as varicella or herpes simplex of the eye; infectious diseases without antibiotic coverage, such as active tuberculosis; myasthenia gravis, and emotional disorders especially those of a psychotic character.

Topical steroids are contraindicated in vaccinia and varicella, in the presence of skin infections of bacterial and fungal character, acute purulent infections of the eye(s), fungal infection of the ear(s) and perforation of the tympanic membrane.

Hypersensitivity to the adrenal corticosteroids or to any of the components formulated with it is an obvious contraindication.

Warnings: Mineralocorticoids should be accompanied by adequate glucocorticoid therapy in adrenal insufficiency or the salt-losing form of the adrenogenital syndrome. Corticosteroids may mask some signs of infection, and new infections may appear during their use due to decreased resistance and an inability to localize infection. Prolonged use may produce posterior subcapsular cataracts, glaucoma with possible damage to the optic nerves, and may enhance the establishment of secondary ocular infections due to fungi or viruses. Normal or large doses of these hormones, particularly hydrocortisone or cortisone, can cause elevation of blood pressure, salt and water retention, and increased excretion of potassium; these effects are less likely to occur with the synthetic derivatives except when used in large doses. Therefore, dietary salt restrictions and potassium supplementation may be necessary. All corticosteroids increase calcium excretion. *While on therapy with these drugs patients should not be given a smallpox vaccination. Other immunization procedures should not be undertaken because of possible neurological complications and a lack of antibody response.* The use of these agents in patients with active tuberculosis should be restricted to those cases of fulminating or disseminated tuberculosis in which these drugs are used in conjunction with an appropriate antituberculous regimen. If corticosteroids are indicated in patients with latent tuberculosis or in those reacting to tuberculin, close observation is necessary as the disease may become active; during prolonged corticosteroids therapy, these patients should receive chemoprophylaxis. Concomitant use of an anticonvulsant drug may cause an acceleration of hepatic conjugation and biliary excretion of the corticosteroid which may lead to lower levels of the free drug or its metabolites and thus less inhibition of ACTH secretion. Since anaphylactoid reactions have occurred in a few patients receiving parenteral corticosteroid therapy, it is advised that appropriate precautionary measures be taken prior to administration, especially when the patient has a history of allergy to any drug. These preparations should be administered with caution, if at all, to pregnant and lactating women and to women of childbearing potential unless its use is an absolute one. If it is necessary to administer steroids during pregnancy, the newborn infant should be observed closely for signs of hypoadrenalism and appropriate therapy instituted if such signs are present.

Precautions: The adrenal corticosteroids are capable of producing serious side effects. Prolonged administration of these preparations will produce the clinical picture of Cushing's syndrome with all its side effects. Associated with this is suppression of ACTH secretion with resultant adrenal atrophy. This atrophy of the adrenal glands makes gradual withdrawal of therapy mandatory when treatment with the glucocorticoids is to be discontinued. Abrupt cessation may not only result in a rebound of the condition being treated, but also results in acute adrenal insufficiency with vascular collapse. The status of alternate day therapy in minimizing this is currently being evaluated. Glucocorticoid therapy should be used with extreme caution in the presence of diabetes mellitus; osteoporosis; active or latent peptic ulcer, diverticulitis, and nonspecific ulcerative colitis; probability of impending perforation, abscess or other pyogenic infection; recent intestinal anastomoses; myasthenia gravis; vascular disease such as severe hypertension, left ventricular failure, and thrombophlebitis; glaucoma; convulsive disorders, and chronic renal disease, especially in the presence of uremia. Evidence of serious infection may be masked by the administration of the glucocorticoids and the clinician must follow patients on such therapy closely. Prolonged administration of the glucocorticoids in high dosage may result in osteoporosis with resultant vertebral collapse. The effects of corticosteroids may be enhanced in patients with hypothyroidism and in those with cirrhosis of the liver. They should be used cautiously in the presence of ocular herpes simplex because of possible corneal perforation. The lowest possible dose should be used to control the condition under treatment, and when reduction in dosage is possible, the reduction should be gradual. Psychic disorders ranging from euphoria, insomnia, mood swings, personality changes, and severe depression, to frank psychotic manifestations may appear; also, existing emotional instability or psychotic tendencies may be aggravated by corticosteroids. In the presence of hypoprothrombinemia, aspirin should be used with caution in conjunction with these preparations. Also, growth and development of infants and children on prolonged corticosteroid therapy should be carefully followed. Suitable precautions should be taken during topical application, particularly if extensive areas are treated or if the occlusive technique is applied since the possibility exists that increased absorption of the corticosteroid may occur.

Adverse Reactions: The adrenal glucocorticoids are important preparations which are both potent and potentially dangerous. Two general types of adverse reactions are seen: Those of an acute nature related to true hypersensitivity, or more commonly on an irritant basis such as that following topical, intralesional or intraarticular administration. In addition, the adrenal insufficiency following sudden cessation of therapy in patients on a prolonged course of medication can also be considered acute. A second type of adverse reaction resulting from chronic administration of the adrenal steroids is related either to the production of Cushing's syndrome or one of the complications of that disease such as collapse of vertebrae secondary to osteoporosis, hypertension, etc. Posterior subcapsular cataracts have been described in patients on prolonged glucocorticoid therapy. Other ophthalmic manifestations noted were increased intraocular pressure, glaucoma, and exophthalmos. Complications that may also occur with these preparations include *fluid and electrolyte disturbances* such as sodium retention, fluid retention, congestive heart failure in susceptible patients, potassium loss, and hypokalemic alkalosis. *Musculoskeletal disorders* are manifested by muscle weakness, steroid myopathy, loss of muscle mass, osteoporosis, vertebral compression fractures, aseptic necrosis of femoral and humeral heads, and pathologic fracture of long bones. *Gastrointestinal disorders* include peptic ulcer with possible perforation and hemorrhage, pancreatitis, abdominal distention, and ulcerative esophagitis. *Dermatologic disorders* are manifested by impaired wound healing, thin fragile skin, petechiae and ecchymosis, facial erythema, increased sweating, and reactions to skin tests may be suppressed. Topical application may cause burning, itching, irritation, dryness, folliculitis, secondary infections, skin atrophy, striae, miliaria, masceration of the skin, hypertrichosis, acneiform eruptions, and hypopigmentation. *Endocrine disorders* include menstrual irregularities; development of Cushingoid state; suppression of growth in children; secondary adrenocortical and pituitary unresponsiveness, particularly in times of stress as in trauma, surgery or illness; decreased carbohydrate tolerance; manifestations of latent diabetes mellitus; and increased requirements of insulin or oral hypoglycemic agents in diabetes. *Metabolic disorders* are manifested by a negative nitrogen balance due to protein catabolism. *Neurologic disorders* are usually manifested by convulsions, vertigo and headache. A reversible pseudo-brain tumor syndrome, related to steroid therapy, has been reported in children; the entity is characterized by oculomotor nerve signs, headache, and papilledema.

The adverse reactions related to the mineralocorticoids are essentially involved with salt and water retention. These will be discussed under the individual preparation.

Dosage and Administration: The dosage of each of the adrenal corticosteroids generally is wide. This is necessarily so, because dosage of these drugs is dependent upon the acuteness, prognosis, and the probable duration of the disease, as well as upon the diagnosis.

The preceding pages discussed, in brief, the physiologic, clinical and therapeutic similarities of the adrenal corticosteroids as a group. In the pages that follow, the individual monographs will discuss specifically each of the following adrenal corticosteroids:

Beclomethasone Dipropionate
Betamethasone
Cortisone Acetate
Desonide
Desoximetasone
Desoxycorticosterone
Dexamethasone
Diflorasone Diacetate
Fludrocortisone Acetate
Flumethasone Pivalate
Fluocinolone Acetonide
Fluocinonide
Fluorometholone
Fluprednisolone
Flurandrenolide
Halcinonide
Hydrocortisone
Medrysone
Meprednisone
Methylprednisolone
Paramethasone Acetate
Prednisolone
Prednisone
Triamcinolone

BECLOMETHASONE DIPROPIONATE

Chemical Name: 9-Chloro-11β, 17, 21-trihydroxy-16β-methylpregna-1, 4-diene-3, 20-dione 17,21-dipropionate.

Description: Beclomethasone dipropionate is a synthetic adrenal glucocorticoid that is chemically related to prednisolone, differing only in that it has a halogen [chlorine] at the 9-alpha position and a methyl group in place of the hydrogen at the 16-beta position on the prednisolone nucleus. These modifications in the molecule tend to enhance its antiinflammatory action while attenuating its sodium-retaining activity. Although the mode of antiinflammatory action is uncertain, it has been found to exert a selective topical action on the bronchial mucous membrane thereby providing relief of the distressing signs and symptoms of bronchial asthma in patients who have not been adequately controlled by bronchodilators or other nonsteroidal preparations. Response to the drug is usually evident in 1 week with beneficial effects occurring in 2 to 4 weeks. When administered in the recommended dosage, it has been reported to produce little or none of the undesirable hormonal effects usually associated with oral or parenteral corticosteroids. After the medication is inhaled, the drug is deposited in the respiratory and gastrointestinal tissues where it is readily absorbed and metabolized and is excreted primarily in the feces (over 90%) as free drug and metabolites. Less than 10% is recoverable from the urine. There is, at present, no evidence of tissue storage of beclomethasone dipropionate or its metabolites.

Indications: Symptomatic control of bronchial asthma. Its use should be limited to patients who are steroid-dependent in order to reduce or eliminate the systemic dose administration, to those not on corticosteroid therapy who have not responded adequately to other treatment, and in patients in whom the relative contraindications to systemic steroid therapy have prevented their use, or in whom undesirable hormonal effects have occurred. The drug is not indicated for patients with non-asthmatic bronchitis, those who are not completely steroid-dependent, and those whose condition can be adequately controlled by bronchodilators or other nonsteroidal medications.

Contraindications: Primary treatment of status asthmaticus or other acute episodes of asthma where intensive measures are required, or an unusual sensitivity to the drug or to any ingredient in the preparation are contraindications to its use.

Warnings: Particular care is needed when patients who previously received systemic corticosteroids are transferred to beclomethasone since deaths due to chronic adrenocortical insufficiency have occurred during and after the transfer. Additionally, these patients may also be at high risk when exposed to trauma, surgery or infections, particularly gastroenteritis, since the drug does not provide the systemic steroidal requirement necessary for coping with these emergencies. Therefore, it is important for the physician to warn patients who have discontinued or reduced their oral steroid requirement while on beclomethasone to resume taking or increasing the oral dosage during periods of stress or acute exacerbations of their asthma. Patients should also be instructed to carry a warning card indicating that they may need supplementary systemic steroids should a crisis arise. To assess the risk of adrenal insufficiency in emergency situations, routine tests of adrenal cortical function, including measurement of early morning resting cortisol levels, should be performed periodically in all patients. An early morning resting cortisol level may be accepted as normal only if it falls at or near the normal mean level. Localized infections with *Candida albicans* or *Aspergillus niger* have occurred frequently in the mouth and pharynx and occasionally in the larynx. Positive cultures for oral Candida may be present in up to 75% of patients. Should this develop, it may be necessary to discontinue therapy and/or to institute appropriate antifungal therapy. Since doses greater than those recommended appear to provide no further benefits, higher dosage regimens are unwarranted. Transfer of patients previously receiving oral steroids to beclomethasone inhaler may unmask allergic conditions such as rhinitis, conjunctivitis, and eczema, and may precipitate withdrawal symptoms such as joint and/or muscular pain, lassitude and depression. See general statement

Precautions: The replacement of a systemic steroid with beclomethasone inhaler has to be gradual and should be carefully supervised by the physician. During long-term administration it is advised that hypothalamic-pituitary-adrenal status be periodically assessed. Studies with pregnant animals strongly suggest that the drug causes congenital abnormalities in the fetus; therefore, use in pregnant and lactating women and in those of childbearing potential requires that the possible benefits of the drug be weighed against the potential hazards to the mother and fetus. Infants born to mothers who have received substantial doses of corticosteroids during pregnancy should be carefully observed for hypoadrenalism. Until further clinical trials establish safe use and proper dosage, it is not recommended for use in children under 6 years of age. See general statement.

Adverse Reactions: No major side effects attributable to the use of recommended doses have been reported, and no observable systemic effect has been noted when the daily dosage was below 1 mg (20 puffs). Above this amount, reduction of plasma cortisol, indicating adrenocortical suppression, may occur. (See Warnings.) A few patients have complained of hoarseness or dry mouth. See general statement.

Dosage and Administration: *Oral inhalation.* Adults: The usual dosage is 2 inhalations (0.1 mg) 3 or 4 times daily. In patients with severe asthma, it is advisable to start with 12 to 16 inhalations daily, and then adjust the dosage downward according to the response of the patient. The maximal daily intake should not exceed 20 inhalations (1 mg). Children 6 to 12 years of age: The usual dosage is 1 or 2 inhalations 3 or 4 times daily. The maximal intake should not exceed 10 inhalations. Patients receiving systemic corticosteroids: Initially, the aerosol should be used concurrently with the patient's usual maintenance dose of systemic steroid. In these cases, no reduction in oral steroid should be attempted until after 1 or 2 weeks of aerosol use. Following this interval, gradual withdrawal of the systemic steroid is started by reducing the daily or alternate daily dose. The next reduction is made after an interval of 1 or 2 weeks, depending on the patient's response. Generally, these decrements should not exceed 2.5 mg of prednisone or its equivalent.

Availability:
VANCERIL® Suspension (microcrystalline) in aerosol containers of 10 mg, designed so that each actuation releases approximately 50 mcg of beclomethasone dipropionate. One inhaler usually delivers 200 oral inhalations. **(Schering)**

BETAMETHASONE

Chemical Name: 9-Fluoro-11β, 17, 21-trihydroxy-16β-methylpregna-1, 4-diene-3, 20-dione.

Description: Betamethasone is a synthetic corticosteroid which is structurally related to dexamethasone. This is said to enhance the antiinflammatory action of the molecule and reduce the sodium- and water-retaining properties of the fluorine atom bond at carbon 9.

Orally, 600 mcg of betamethasone is approximately equivalent to 750 mcg of dexamethasone, to 5 mg of prednisone or prednisolone, or to 20 mg of hydrocortisone.

Betamethasone *disodium phosphate,* a soluble and rapidly acting ester, is combined with betamethasone acetate, a slightly soluble and repository type ester, to facilitate rapid control as well as steady maintenance of corticosteroid effects.

Betamethasone *diproprionate,* a 17,21-dipropionate ester, 0.64 mg of which is equivalent to 0.5 mg of betamethasone has been incorporated into a hydrophylic, emollient cream base to provide antiinflammatory, antipruritic and vasoconstrictive activity in the topical management of corticosteroid-responsive dermatosis.

Betamethasone *valerate,* a 17-valerate ester, 1.2 mg of which is equivalent to 1 mg of betamethasone, has been incorporated into a moisturizing cream base and into a moisturizing ointment base to provide antiinflammatory, antiallergic and antipruritic activity in the topical management of corticosteroid-responsive dermatoses.

Indications: Betamethasone shares the actions and uses of other adrenal corticosteroids (see general statement). As with all corticosteroids, some patients show a better response to betamethasone than to other agents and vice versa. After intramuscular injection, the effects of a combination of betamethasone acetate and betamethasone disodium phosphate appear within 2 to 3 hours and persist for 3 to 7 days. Following intraarticular, intrasynovial or soft tissue injection, the effects of the combination appear within a few hours and may persist for 1 to 4 weeks. Betamethasone is inadequate therapy for Addison's disease or the salt-losing form of the adrenogenital syndrome; if used for these diseases, supplementation with a mineralocorticoid is necessary. Topical application is indicated for the relief of the inflammatory manifestations of corticosteroid-responsive dermatoses.

Contraindications: In general, the same as those for other adrenal corticosteroids. Local injections of betamethasone disodium phosphate with betamethasone acetate are generally contraindicated in the presence of acute infection.

Warnings: See general statement.

Precautions: See general statement. Patients should be observed closely for the development of less obvious reactions indicating hypercorticalism. As with dexamethasone, diuresis may develop in patients transferred to betamethasone from steroids other than dexamethasone.

Adverse Reactions: Reactions to betamethasone are similar in nature and in frequency and severity to those of other corticosteroids, and the same precautions apply. With short-term therapy in therapeutic dosage, sodium and water retention or potassium depletion rarely occurs. Betamethasone appears to produce weight gain. For further information on adverse reactions, see general statement.

Dosage and Administration: Betamethasone is administered *orally* in divided doses. A suspension containing the acetate and disodium phosphate may be utilized by *intraarticular, intradermal, intramuscular, intrasynovial* or *soft tissue* injection. The package literature should be consulted for specific dosage.

In the treatment of rheumatoid arthritis and other rheumatic conditions, the recommended initial *oral* dosage averages 1.2 to 2.4 mg daily, but the daily dosage should be reduced to 0.6 to 1.2 mg as rapidly as possible. Similar dosage is used in treating bursitis on a short term basis. Acute rheumatic fever may be treated with an initial *oral* dosage of 6 to 8.4 mg of betamethasone daily, if indicated. An initial *oral* daily dose of 3.6 to 4.8 mg of betamethasone is recommended in managing acute lupus erythematosus, but a higher dose may be necessary to control the clinical and laboratory manifestations. Maintenance therapy usually requires between 1.2 to 3.6 mg daily. In the management of chronic pulmonary disease characterized by obstruction and fibrosis an initial daily dosage in the range of 2.4 to 3.6 mg is recommended. A dose of 1.2 to 2.4 mg of betamethasone is used for maintenance therapy. A similar dosage range is utilized for the management of inflammatory eye disease, dermatologic conditions and allergic conditions such as hay fever and asthma; the manufacturer's package literature should be consulted for specific recommendations.

The parenteral preparation containing the disodium phosphate and the acetate may be used in an *intramuscular* dose of 6 to 12 mg. This may be repeated every 3 to 7 days depending on the response. A maintenance dose of 6 mg weekly is usually sufficient.

The size and location will determine the amount of betamethasone to be utilized for *intrasynovial* or *intraarticular* administration. Ordinarily, 1 to 2 ml (6 to 12 mg) is injected into the large joints with 0.25 to 1 ml (1.5 to 6 mg) utilized for the smaller ones. An average dose of 0.5 ml (3 mg) is used for ganglia and 1 ml (6 mg) for bursal injection. A dose of 0.6 to 1.2 mg of betamethasone daily is utilized to diagnose the adrenogenital syndrome by its effect on the urinary 17-ketosteroid excretion.

Intralesional administration should be based on the expected response of the dermatological condition, but a single dose should not exceed 6 mg. The package literature should be consulted for specific details.

Topically, the cream or ointment is gently rubbed into the cleansed affected area 1 to 3 times daily; more frequent applications may be necessary in the treatment of stubborn cases. Occlusive dressing may be used for the management of refractory lesions of psoriasis and other deep-seated dermatoses, such as neurodermatitis.

Availability:

Betamethasone

CELESTONE®: **(Schering)**

Cream, 0.2% in tubes of 15 gm.

Syrup, 0.6 mg/5 ml in bottles of 120 ml. Protect from light.

Tablets, 0.6 mg in bottles of 100 and 500 and in tablet-packs of 21.

Betamethasone Acetate and Betamethasone Disodium Phosphate

CELESTONE® SOLUSPAN® Injection, 6 mg/ml in multiple-dose vials of 5 ml. Shake well before using and store away from heat. **(Schering)**

Betamethasone Benzoate

BENISONE® Cream & Gel, 0.025% in tubes of 15 and 60 gm. **(Warner-Chilcott)**

UTICORT® Gel, 0.025% in tubes of 15 and 60 gm. *Contains 13.8% alcohol.* **(Parke-Davis)**

Betamethasone Dipropionate

DIPROSONE®: **(Schering)**

Cream, 0.05% in tubes of 15 and 45 gm.

Lotion, 0.05% in plastic squeeze bottles of 20 and 60 ml. *Contains 46.8% isopropyl alcohol.*

Ointment, 0.05% in tubes of 15 and 45 gm. *Not for ophthalmic use.*

Topical Aerosol, 0.1% in containers of 85 gm.

Betamethasone Phosphate

CELESTONE® PHOSPHATE Injection, 3 and 4 mg/ml in vials of 1 and 5 ml. **(Schering)**

Betamethasone Valerate

VALISONE®: **(Schering)**

Cream, 0.01% (reduced strength) in tubes of 15 and 60 gm; 0.1% in tubes of 5, 15 and 45 gm.

Lotion, 0.1% in plastic squeeze bottles of 20 and 60 ml.

Ointment, 0.1% in tubes of 5, 15 and 45 gm.

Topical Aerosol, 0.15% in containers of 85 gm.

CORTISONE ACETATE

Synonym: Kendall's Compound E.

Chemical Name: 17,21-Dihydroxypregn-4-ene-3,11,20-trione-21 acetate.

Description: In vivo, cortisone is an oxidation product of hydrocortisone (cortisol), a natural hormone of the adrenal cortex. Cortisone acetate is produced synthetically, occurring as a white or practically white, crystalline powder that is insoluble in water and only slightly soluble in alcohol.

Indications: Cortisone acetate shares the actions and uses of other adrenal corticosteroids. See general statement.

Contraindications: In general, the same as those for other adrenal corticosteroids.

Warnings: See general statement.

Precautions: See general statement.

Adverse Reactions: Reactions to cortisone acetate are similar to those of other corticosteroids. See general statement.

Dosage and Administration: Cortisone acetate may be administered *orally* or *intramuscularly*. The dosage by either route is similar and is related to the condition being treated. The onset of action when the drug is administered *orally* is more rapid, but that administered *intramuscularly* lasts longer. Orally, the total daily dose is divided into 3 or 4 doses while the same total amount need only be given once daily intramuscularly. *It should not be used intravenously.*

When used in the management of rheumatoid arthritis and associated conditions, the usual initial daily dose is 100 mg orally. That dose is rapidly reduced to arrive at a maintenance dose which will control evidence of disease activity. This reduction is accomplished by periodic reductions of not more than 10 to 12.5 mg/day. A similar approach is utilized in allergic problems involving skin and eyes, as well as nonallergic inflammatory eye disease.

Cortisone acetate has also been used in the management of acute rheumatic fever (up to 400 mg daily initially with subsequent reduction based on evidence of clinical and laboratory activity), acute lupus erythematosus (where 200 to 300 mg are used initially) as well as in scleroderma and the leukemias and lymphomas. The medical literature as well as the manufacturers' information should be consulted for the details of managing these diseases with this potent preparation.

When utilized in the management of chronic adrenal insufficiency (Addison's disease) 10 to 25 mg of cortisone are administered daily with supplemental desoxycorticosterone or synthetic mineralocorticoid and sodium chloride. In acute adrenal insufficiency, either precipitated by stress plus Addison's disease or on the basis of adrenal atrophy produced by prior steroid administration, 100 to 300 mg of cortisone should be administered daily until the precipitating cause has been removed.

Topically, in severe inflammatory conditions of the eye, treatment may be initiated with the 2.5% ophthalmic suspension and the 0.5% suspension used for maintenance. In less severe conditions, the 0.5% suspension may be used initially. One or 2 drops of suspension are instilled into the conjunctival sac every hour during the day and every 2 hours during the night. After a favorable response is obtained, the frequency of instillation may be reduced to every 4 hours and then to 3 or 4 times daily. Alternatively, the 1.5% ophthalmic ointment may be applied 3 or 4 times daily. The ointment may be particularly useful in cases which require the use of an eye pad, or for application at night in conjunction with daytime therapy with the suspension.

Availability:

Cortisone Acetate

Suspension, 25 mg/ml in vials of 20 ml. **(Upjohn)**

Tablets, 5 mg in bottles of 50; 10 mg in bottles of 100; 25 mg in bottles of 100 and 500. **(Upjohn)**

CORTONE®: **(Merck Sharp & Dohme)**

Suspension, 25 mg/ml in vials of 20 ml; 50 mg/ml in vials of 10 ml.

Tablets, 5 mg in bottles of 50; 25 mg in bottles of 100.

w/Neomycin

NEOSONE® Ophthalmic Ointment 1.5% w/neomycin sulfate, 0.5% (equiv. to 3.5 mg of base) in tubes of 3.5 gm with applicator tip. **(Upjohn)**

DESONIDE

Chemical Name: 16α-Hydroxyprednisolone-16,17-acetonide.

Description: Desonide is a non-fluorinated corticosteroid that provides the antiinflammatory, antipruritic and vasoconstrictive activity associated with other adrenal corticosteroids. Each gm of cream or ointment and each ml of otic solution provides 0.5 mg of desonide. The cream is microdispersed in an acid mantle vehicle buffered to the pH range of normal skin and the ointment is microdispersed in white petrolatum; the otic solution contains 2% acetic acid.

Indications: As adjunctive therapy for the relief of inflammatory manifestations in acute and chronic steroid responsive dermatosis.

Contraindications: Hypersensitivity to any of the components, and in the presence of vaccinia and varicella.

Precautions: If reactions indicating sensitivity are encountered, the cream should be discontinued. In the presence of an infection, appropriate antifungal or antibacterial therapy should be instituted. If a favorable response does not occur promptly, the use of the corticosteroid cream should be discontinued until the infection has been adequately controlled. Application to extensive areas or under occlusive dressings may result in systemic absorption; therefore, adequate precautions are essential. Since the safe use of topical steroids in pregnant patients has not been established, they should not be used extensively, in large amounts, or for prolonged periods during pregnancy. **Note:** *Should not be used in the eyes.*

Adverse Reactions: Burning sensations, itching, irritation, dryness, folliculitis, hypertrichosis, acneform eruptions, and hypopigmentation have been observed. Reactions occurring more frequently with occlusive dressings are maceration of the skin, secondary infection, skin atrophy, striae, and miliaria.

Dosage and Administration: *Topically.* Apply a thin film of cream or ointment to the affected area and massage lightly. The usual dosage schedule is 2 or 3 times daily.

Availability:
TRIDESILON®: **(Dome)**
Creme, 0.05% in tubes of 15 and 60 gm and in jars of 5 lbs.
Ointment, 0.05% in tubes of 15 and 60 gm.
Otic Solution, 0.05% in bottles of 10 ml with dropper.

DESOXIMETASONE

Chemical Name: 9α-Fluoro-11β, 21-dihydroxy-16α-methylpregna-1,4-diene-3,20-dione.

Description: A synthetic corticosteroid primarily effective for its antiinflammatory, antipruritic and vasoconstrictive actions.

Indications: Topically for the relief of inflammatory manifestations of corticosteroid-responsive dermatosis.

Contraindications: Hypersensitivity to any of the components and in the presence of vaccinia and varicella. **Note:** Not for ophthalmic use.

The warnings, precautions and adverse reactions are generally the same as those for other topical steroids. See general statement.

Dosage and Administration: *Topically.* Apply a small amount and massage gently into the cleansed affected area twice daily.

Availability:
TOPICORT® Cream, 0.25% in tubes of 15 and 60 gm. **(Hoechst)**

DESOXYCORTICOSTERONE

Chemical Name: 21-Hydroxypregn-4-ene-3,20-dione.

Description: Desoxycorticosterone, an active mineralocorticoid secreted by the zona glomerulosa of the adrenal cortex, is a metabolic precursor of aldosterone. It has about one-thirtieth the mineralocorticoid potency of aldosterone. It is usually prepared synthetically as either the acetate or pivalate ester. It is administered intramuscularly or implanted as a pellet subcutaneously.

The pharmacology of desoxycorticosterone is similar to that of aldosterone since it is concerned with the metabolism of sodium and potassium, conserving the body stores of the former with the excretion of the latter. It is also involved with the regulation of body water. As indicated in the general statement, it acts on the epithelial cells of the kidney, sweat glands, and the gastrointestinal tract to accomplish this effect. It has no glucocorticoid activity and, therefore, has no actions of an antiinflammatory nature; neither does it have any direct effect on protein or carbohydrate metabolism. Desoxycorticosterone does not suppress ACTH or MSH secretion by the pituitary gland. It can produce hypertension.

Indications: Desoxycorticosterone may be used in treating chronic adrenal insufficiency (Addison's disease) where it restores electrolyte and water balance to normal. Sodium is retained, the blood volume is restored to normal and potassium excretion is increased. As a corollary to the normalization of the blood volume, cardiac output is improved. In the presence of acute adrenal insufficiency, glucocorticoid therapy should accompany the administration of desoxycorticosterone.

Contraindications: Hypersensitivity to the compounds; in patients with cardiac disease or hypertension.

Warnings: No more than 10 mg of the *acetate* should be given at one time. Because of its high potency and prolonged duration of activity, the *pivalate* should not be given more frequently than once a month. Mineralocorticoids should be accompanied by adequate glucocorticoid therapy in treating adrenal insufficiency or the salt-losing form of the adrenogenital system. When prescribed for pregnant patients, the physician should carefully consider the benefits versus the risk to the fetus, and the newborn infant should be carefully observed for hypoadrenalism.

Precautions: As with other adrenocortical hormones, desoxycorticosterone *acetate* may cause severe reactions if dosage is too high or prolonged. It causes the retention of sodium and, therefore, associated retention of water. Thus, it may cause increased blood volume, edema, elevated blood pressure and enlargement of the heart. Decreased excretion of sodium is accompanied by increased excretion of potassium. Retention of sodium and the loss of potassium are accelerated by a high intake of sodium. Hence, it may be necessary to restrict intake of sodium and increase that of potassium. In patients with essential hypertension or a tendency toward its development, a marked rise in blood pressure may follow administration of this drug. Addisonian patients are more sensitive to the action of the hormone and may exhibit, in exaggerated degree, the adverse reactions mentioned. On rare occasions, irritation at the site of injection or pellet implantation has been reported. As with any medication, hypersensitivity may occur. The possible reactions to the *pivalate ester* are those which may be encountered with any preparation of desoxycorticosterone. Generally, they are the direct result of excessive retention of salt and water and excretion of potassium: excessive weight gain, edema, hypertension and, eventually, cardiac failure. Successful compromise between dosage and undesirable effects usually can be reached. Only if absolutely necessary should a glucose tolerance test (particularly intravenously) be performed, as addisonian patients—whether or not taking desoxycorticosterone—have the tendency to develop severe hypoglycemia within 3 hours, whereas such a reaction in normal individuals has not been observed. In all instances, it is advisable to support the effect of desoxycorticosterone acetate therapy by the oral administration of extra amounts of sodium chloride.

Adverse Reactions: Headache, arthralgia, weakness, ascending paralysis, low potassium syndrome, and hypersensitivity may occur; rarely irritation at the site of injection.

Dosage and Administration: In treating Addison's disease, the initial dosage usually is 5 to 6 mg of the acetate by *deep intramuscular injection* for 3 or 4 days. In treating or preventing an addisonian crisis, it should be remembered that the acetate injectable solution is slowly absorbed and does not manifest a maximal effect until 6 to 12 hours after injection. As a rule, a crisis can be avoided when the patient is under control with desoxycorticosterone acetate and sodium chloride, in association with proper adjustment of diet and muscular activity. Maintenance dosage is adjusted on the basis of clinical and serum electrolyte response, but is usually 1 to 5 mg daily. After the daily maintenance dose is determined with acetate in oil, 1 ml (25 mg) of the pivalate suspension is given for each mg of the solution in oil required for daily maintenance; the calculated dose (average 25 to 100 mg) is administered every 4 weeks. For the pellet implantation and use of the pivalate form (intramuscular repository), the physician is urged to study the package literature carefully. Glucocorticoid therapy may be necessary for crisis situations or to control hypoglycemia.

Availability:

Desoxycorticosterone Acetate

DOCA® Acetate Solution in Oil, 5 mg/ml in multiple-dose vials of 10 ml. **(Organon)**

PERCORTEN® Acetate: **(Ciba)**

Pellets (for implantation), 125 mg in cartons of 1. The exact weight of each sterile pellet is stated on the individual container. Available to hospitals and clinics only.

Solution in Oil, 5 mg/ml in multiple-dose vials of 10 ml.

Desoxycorticosterone Pivalate

PERCORTEN® Pivalate Aqueous Suspension (IM only), microcrystalline, 25 mg/ml in multiple-dose vials of 4 ml. **(Ciba)**

DEXAMETHASONE

Chemical Name: 9-Fluoro-11β, 17, 21-trihydroxy-16α-methylpregna-1, 4-diene-3, 20-dione.

Description: Dexamethasone is a synthetic adrenal glucocorticoid. While the parent compound is practically insoluble in water, its disodium phosphate ester is freely soluble. On a dose basis, 0.75 mg of dexamethasone is equivalent to 5 mg of prednisone or 20 mg of hydrocortisone.

Indications: Dexamethasone shares the actions and uses of other corticosteroids. It may be used for the treatment of cerebral edema associated with primary or metastatic brain tumors; in the preoperative preparation of patients with increased intracranial pressure secondary to brain tumors; as a palliative for inoperable or recurrent brain neoplasm, and for the management of cerebral edema associated with neurosurgery. Also for the management of endocrine, rheumatic, collagen and dermatologic disorders, allergic states, ophthalmic, respiratory, gastrointestinal, and neoplastic diseases, hematologic disorders, and edematous states. Dexamethasone phosphate injection may be beneficial in patients with cerebral edema due to head injury or pseudotumor cerebri. Dexamethasone is not indicated as substitute therapy for careful neurological evaluation and for definitive management such as neurosurgery or other specific therapy.

For more detailed information on the actions, indications, contraindications and warnings for therapy with dexamethasone, see general statement.

Contraindications: In general, the same as those for other adrenal corticosteroids. Topical steroids are contraindicated in the presence of vaccinia and varicella.

Warnings: Decadron-LA should not be administered *intravenously.*

Precautions: Dexamethasone has minimal sodium or water retaining properties. The development of overadministration may therefore be quite subtle. See general statement for other precautions.

Adverse Reactions: In general, they are the same as those with other adrenal corticosteroids. Those noted with topical application include burning sensations, itching, irritation, dryness, follicultis, hypertrichosis, acneform eruptions, and hypopigmentation. Reactions occurring more frequently with occlusive dressings are maceration of the skin, secondary infection, skin atrophy, striae, and miliaria.

Dosage and Administration: Severity, prognosis and expected duration of the disease and the reaction of the patient are the basis for individualized therapy. As with other adrenal corticosteroids, dosage should be increased or decreased gradually. *Orally.* One 0.75-mg tablet of dexamethasone will replace 4 mg of triamcinolone or methylprednisolone, 5 mg of prednisone or prednisolone, 20 mg of hydrocortisone or 25 mg of cortisone. In other words, dosage usually can be determined on a tablet for tablet replacement basis. When individual variations from the suggested dosage occur, the 0.5-mg tablet may be included in the dosage regimen. *Topically,* 0.1% dexamethasone is as effective as 1% hydrocortisone in the treatment of susceptible skin conditions. For use in the *eye,* 1 or 2 drops of an 0.1% solution or suspension may be instilled into the conjunctival sac every hour during the day and every 2 hours during the night for initial therapy. Alternatively, an 0.05% ointment may be instilled 3 or 4 times daily initially and once or twice daily for maintenance. For application to the *ear,* 3 or 4 drops of solution may be instilled into the clean, dry aural canal 2 or 3 times daily, or a thin film of an ointment may be applied in the ear 2 or 3 times daily. For application to the *nasal mucosa,* a nasal solution may be sprayed once or twice into each nostril 2 or 3 times a day. For application to the *skin,* gently massage a small amount on the affected area 3 or 4 times daily. *Parenterally* or into soft tissue, 4 to 20 mg, *intravenously* or *intramuscularly,* repeated as necessary, but not exceeding 80 mg a day. The size and interval of dosage should be based on the patient's response. For *cerebral edema,* initially 2.5 ml (10 mg) *intravenously* followed by 1 ml (4 mg) *intramuscularly* every 6 hours until symptoms subside. Response is usually noted within 12 to 24 hours. Dosage may be reduced after 2 to 4 days of therapy and gradually discontinued over a period of from 5 to 7 days. *For the palliative management of recurrent or inoperable brain tumors,* 2 mg *orally* or *by injection* 2 or 3 times daily. The usual precautions in regard to corticosteroid therapy should be employed, and antacids, anticholinergic drugs and diet measures to prevent gastrointestinal ulcer or hemorrhage should be considered. *For intralesional injection,* 0.8 to 1.6 mg/injection site. *For intraarticular and soft tissue injection,* the dose varies, depending on the location and the severity of the inflammation. The usual dose is 4 to 16 mg. If further treatment is needed, dosage may be repeated at intervals of 1 to 3 weeks. See package literature for details.

Availability:

Dexamethasone

AEROSEB-DEX® Topical Aerosol, 1.66 mg/15 gm in aerosol cans of 90 gm. **(Herbert)**

DECADERM® Ointment, 0.1% in Estergel® (specially formulated vehicle consisting of gelled isopropyl myristate, wool alcohols B.P., refined lanolin alcohol, microcrystalline wax, anhydrous citric acid and anhydrous sodium phosphate dibasic) in tubes of 15 and 30 gm. **(Merck Sharp & Dohme)**

DECADRON®: **(Merck Sharp & Dohme)**

Elixir, 0.5 mg/5 ml in bottles of 100 ml with calibrated dropper assembly and in bottles of 237 ml.

Tablets: 0.25 mg in bottles of 100; 0.5 mg in bottles of 100 and 1000 and in single-unit packages of 100; 0.75 mg in bottles of 100 and 1000 and in single-unit packages of 100, and in individual Paks® of 12; 1.5 and 4 mg in bottles of 50 and in single-unit packages of 100.

DECADRON-LA® Suspension (as acetate), 8 mg/ml in vials of 1 and 5 ml. *Not for IV use.* **(Merck Sharp & Dohme)**

DECASPRAY® Topical Aerosol, 10 mg/90 gm in aerosol cans of 90 gm. **(Merck Sharp & Dohme)**

DERONIL® Tablets, 0.75 mg in bottles of 50. **(Schering)**

DEXAMETH® Tablets, 0.75 mg in bottles of 100. **(USV)**

DEXONE™ Tablets, 0.5, 0.75, 1.5 and 4 mg in bottles of 100 and 1000 and in unit-dose packages of 100. **(Rowell)**

HEXADROL®: **(Organon)**

Cream, 0.04% in tubes of 10 and 30 gm.

Elixir, 0.5 mg/5 ml in bottles of 120 ml.

Tablets, 0.5 mg (yellow, scored) in bottles of 30 and 500; 0.75 mg (white, scored) in bottles of 100 and 500; 1.5 mg (peach, scored) in bottles of 50; 4 mg (green, scored) in bottles of 100. All potencies in strip-packages of 100.

MAXIDEX® Ophthalmic Suspension, 0.1% in DropTainer® dispensers of 5 and 15 ml. **(Alcon)**

SK-DEXAMETHASONE™ Tablets, 0.5 and 1.5 mg in bottles of 100; 0.75 mg in bottles of 100 and 1000. **(Smith Kline & French)**

w/Neomycin

MAXITROL®: **(Alcon)**

Ophthalmic Ointment (sterile), 0.1% w/neomycin sulfate, 0.5% (equiv. to 0.35% of base) and polymyxin B sulfate, 6000 units/gm in tubes of 3.5 gm.

Ophthalmic Suspension (Sterile), 0.1% w/neomycin sulfate, 0.5% (equiv. to 0.35% of base) and polymyxin B sulfate, 6000 units/ml in dropper bottles of 5 ml.

NeoDECASPRAY® Topical Aerosol, 10 mg w/neomycin sulfate, 50 mg/90 gm (equivalent to 35 mg of base) in aerosol cans of 90 gm. **(Merck Sharp & Dohme)**

Dexamethasone Sodium Phosphate

DECADRON® Phosphate: **(Merck Sharp & Dohme)**

Injection, 4 mg/ml in disposable syringes of 1 ml and rubber-capped vials of 1, 5 and 25 ml; 24 mg/ml in vials of 5 and 10 ml.
Injection, 4 mg w/lidocaine hydrochloride, 10 mg/ml in vials of 5 ml (Decadron with Xylocaine®)
Ophthalmic Ointment, 0.05% in tubes of 3.5 gm.
Ophthalmic Solution, 0.1% in dropper bottles of 2.5 and 5 ml.
Ophthalmic Solution (Ocumeter®), 0.1% in plastic dispenser bottles of 5 ml.
Respihaler®, 18 mg/12.6 gm in aerosol containers of 12.6 gm with or without oral attachment.
Topical cream, 0.1% in tubes of 15 and 30 gm.
Turbinaire®, 18 mg/12.6 gm in aerosol containers of 12.6 gm with or without nasal attachment.
DEXAMETHASONE SODIUM PHOSPHATE Injection, 4 mg/ml in Tubex® (sterile cartridge-needle unit) of 1 ml in packages of 10. **(Wyeth)**
HEXADROL® Phosphate Injection, 4 mg/ml in vials of 1 and 5 ml and in prefilled disposable syringes of 1 ml; 10 mg/ml (IV only) in vials of 10 ml. **(Organon)**
MAXIDEX® Ophthalmic Ointment, 0.05% in tubes of 3.5 gm. **(Alcon)**
w/Neomycin
NeoDECADRON®: **(Merck Sharp & Dohme)**
Ophthalmic Ointment, 0.05% w/neomycin sulfate, 0.5% in tubes of 3.5 gm.
Ophthalmic Solution, 0.1% w/neomycin sulfate, 0.5% in dropper bottles of 2.5 and 5 ml.
Ophthalmic Solution (Ocumeter®), 0.1% w/neomycin sulfate, 0.5% plastic dispenser bottles of 5 ml.
Topical Cream, 0.1% w/neomycin sulfate, 0.5% in tubes of 15 and 30 gm.

DIFLORASONE DIACETATE

Chemical Name: 6α,9α-Difluoro-11β,17,21-trihydroxy-16β-methylpregna-1,4-diene-3,20-dione 17,21 diacetate.

Description: A synthetic, fluorinated, topical corticosteroid that has been found useful in the treatment of such distressing skin disorders as psoriasis and most eczematous dermatoses including atopic, neuro-, contact, and nummular dermatitis and seborrhea. The cream is recommended for application to moist lesions or moist body areas and the ointment to dry and scaly lesions. Both formulations are paraben-free.

Indications: Provides antiinflammatory action in steroid-responsive dermatoses as an adjunctive measure.

Contraindications: In vaccinia, varicella, and in those patients who manifest undue hypersensitivity to any of the components. **Note:** Not for ophthalmic use.

The warnings and precautions are generally the same as those for other topical corticosteroids. See general statement.

Adverse Reactions: Those that may occur include burning, itching, irritation, striae, skin atrophy, secondary infection, dryness, folliculitis, hypertrichosis, acneform eruptions, and hypopigmentation; and with the use of occlusive dressings, masceration of the skin, secondary infection, skin atrophy, striae, and miliaria.

Dosage and Administration: *Topically.* The cream may be applied 2 to 4 times daily and the ointment 1 to 3 times daily, as directed by the physician.

Availability:
FLORONE®: **(Upjohn)**
Cream, 0.05% in tubes of 15 and 30 gm.
Ointment, 0.05% in tubes of 15 and 30 gm.

FLUDROCORTISONE ACETATE

Chemical Name: 9α-Fluoro-11β,17α,21-trihydroxy-4-pregnene-3,20-dione 21-acetate.

Description: The 9-*alpha*-fluoro derivative of hydrocortisone acetate, fludrocortisone acetate occurs as a white, crystalline powder very slightly soluble in water and sparingly soluble in alcohol.

Although the physiologic activity of fludrocortisone is similar in nature to that of hydrocortisone, its effects—particularly on electrolyte balance, but also on carbohydrate metabolism—are considerably heightened and prolonged.

Small oral doses produce marked sodium retention and increased urinary potassium excretion. Fludrocortisone acetate also causes a rise in blood pressure, apparently because of these effects on electrolyte levels. In larger doses, the steroid inhibits endogenous adrenal cortical secretion, thymic activity and pituitary corticotropin excretion; promotes the deposition of liver glycogen; and, unless protein intake is adequate, induces negative nitrogen balance. When used topically or locally, fludrocortisone acetate reduces inflammation due to such factors as bacterial infection, allergy or chemical and physical irritants. It relieves itching, smarting and burning and inhibits otic discharge and secretion.

Indications: Replacement therapy for frank adrenal insufficiency, such as Addison's disease and for the treatment of salt-losing adrenogenital syndrome. **Note:** Because of the marked effect on sodium retention, use in treatment of conditions other than those indicated is not recommended.

Contraindications: Those conditions which are usually considered absolute contraindications to the use of adrenal corticosteroids. Because of its marked effect on sodium retention, fludrocortisone should not be used to treat conditions other than Addison's disease and adrenal hyperplasia.

For adverse reactions and further cautions in therapy with fludrocortisone acetate, see general statement.

Dosage and Administration: *Orally,* in the treatment of Addison's disease, the usual dosage is 0.1 mg daily, although dosages ranging from 0.1 mg 3 times a week to 0.2 mg daily have been employed. If hypertension develops as a consequence of therapy, the dose should be reduced to 0.05 mg daily. Concomitant oral administration of cortisone or hydrocortisone may be advisable. In the treatment of salt-losing adrenogenital syndrome, the usual dosage is 0.1 to 0.2 mg daily. Administration of supplemental potassium chloride and restriction of salt intake may be necessary.

Availability:
FLORINEF® Acetate Tablets, 0.1 mg (light-pink, scored) in bottles of 100. **(Squibb)**

FLUMETHASONE PIVALATE

Chemical Name: 6α, 9α-Difluoro-11β, 17α-dihydroxy-16α-methyl-21-trimethylacetoxy-1, 4-pregnadiene-3, 20-dione.

Description: Flumethasone pivalate is a topical corticosteroid, which is said to be effective in the treatment of dermatoses because of its antiinflammatory, antipruritic and vasoconstrictive activity.

Animal studies have shown that the local antiinflammatory effects of flumethasone were more than 800 times than that of cortisol acetate, about 70 times than that of prednisolone pivalate, and about 10 times than that of dexamethasone pivalate. Further studies indicated that systemic effects were virtually absent.

Indications: For relief of the inflammatory manifestations of corticosteroid-responsive dermatosis. May be useful in the treatment of a variety of dermatoses, such as sunburn, anogenital pruritus, atopic dermatitis, contact dermatitis (dermatitis venenata), eczema of hands and feet including dyshidrosis and pompholyx, nummular eczema, neurodermatitis, lichen simplex chronicus, eczematous dermatitis, infantile eczema, intertrigo, psoriasis, seborrheic dermatitis, lichen planus, otitis externa, miliaria (ointments are not recommended), stasis dermatitis, insect bites, exfoliative dermatitis and diaper rash.

Contraindications: Vaccinia, varicella and hypersensitivity to any ingredient.

Precautions: If irritation develops, treatment should be discontinued and appropriate countermeasures instituted. An infection, if present, should be treated with a suitable antifungal or antibacterial agent. In the absence of a favorable response, the steroid should be discontinued until the infection has been brought under control. Suitable precautions should be taken to circumvent the possibility of increased systemic absorption when extensive areas are treated or if an occlusive dressing is used. Since the safety of their use during the gestation period has not been established, topical corticosteroids should not be used extensively during pregnancy, either in large amounts or for prolonged periods. **Note:** This product is not intended for ophthalmic use.

Adverse Reactions: The following local reactions have been reported with topical corticosteroids: burning sensation, pruritus, irritation, dryness, folliculitis, hypertrichosis, acneiform eruptions, hypopigmentation. The following may occur more often with occlusive dressings than without: macerated skin, atrophy of skin, secondary infection, striae and miliaria.

Dosage and Administration: *Topically.* Gently rub in the cream on affected areas until it disappears. This should be done 3 or 4 times daily for at least a few days until the lesions have been cleared. Occlusive dressings may be used to manage psoriasis or stubborn conditions such as chronic neurodermatitis, lichen planus or lichen simplex conditions. Usually, the longer the patient is treated by the occlusive technique, the more rapid is the rate of response. Consult package literature for details relating to the occlusive-dressing method of treatment.

Availability:
LOCORTEN® Cream (in water-washable base), 0.03% in tubes of 15 and 60 gm. **(Ciba)**

FLUOCINOLONE ACETONIDE

Chemical Name: 6α,9α-Difluoro-16α-hydroxyprednisolone-16, 17-acetonide.

Description: Fluocinolone acetonide is a synthetic corticosteroid related to triamcinolone acetonide except that an additional fluorine atom is present in the 6-*alpha* position on the nucleus.

It is claimed that topical application of 0.025% fluocinolone acetonide is more effective than 1% hydrocortisone and about as effective as 0.1% triamcinolone acetonide in the management of appropriate skin diseases.

Indications: Topically, for the relief of the inflammatory manifestations of dermatoses. The combination product may be of help in treating those skin disorders that are or have become infected by organisms susceptible to neomycin. These include atopic dermatitis, neurodermatitis, contact dermatitis, seborrheic dermatitis, eczematous dermatitis, pruritus ani, lichen simplex chronicus, postanal surgical infections, nummular eczema, stasis dermatitis, intertrigo, exfoliative dermatitis and intertriginous psoriasis. Products containing fluocinolone are not intended for ophthalmic use.

Contraindications: Hypersensitivity to any of the components and in the presence of vaccinia and varicella. In general, they are the same as those for other adrenal corticosteroids.

Precautions: The cream containing 0.2% of fluocinolone acetonide should be used for restricted periods, and the quantity used/day should not exceed 2 gm.

Adverse Reactions: Burning sensations, itching, irritation, dryness, folliculitis, hypertrichosis, acneform eruptions, and hypopigmentation have been noted. Reactions occurring more frequently with occlusive dressings are maceration of the skin, secondary infection, skin atrophy, striae, and miliaria.

For further precautions and adverse reactions in therapy, see general statement.

Dosage and Administration: *Topically.* Fluocinolone acetonide should be applied in small amounts and rubbed into the cleansed affected area 2 to 4 times daily. The 0.2% concentration should be used with care and only for restricted periods. The physician is urged to consult the package literature for specific prescribing recommendations.

Availability:

Fluocinolone Acetonide

FLUONID®: **(Allergan)**
Cream, 0.01 and 0.025% in tubes of 15 and 60 gm and in jars of 425 gm.

Ointment, 0.025% in tubes of 15 and 60 gm.
Topical Solution, 0.01% in plastic squeeze bottles of 20 and 60 ml.
SYNALAR®: **(Syntex)**
Cream, 0.01% 115% in tubes of 15, 45 and 60 gm and in jars of 120 and 425 gm; 0.025% in tubes of 15 and 60 gm and in jars of 120 and 425 gm.
Cream, 0.2% (SYNALAR-HP®) in tubes of 5 and 12 gm.
Ointment, 0.025% in tubes of 15 and 60 gm and in jars of 425 gm.
Topical Solution, 0.01% in plastic squeeze bottles of 20 and 60 ml.
SYNEMOL® Cream, 0.025% in tubes of 15 and 60 gm. **(Syntex)**
w/Neomycin
NEO-SYNALAR® Cream, 0.025% w/neomycin sulfate, 0.5% (equiv. to 0.35% neomycin base) in tubes of 15 and 60 gm. **(Syntex)**

FLUOCINONIDE

Chemical Name: 6α, 9-Difluoro-11β, 16α, 17,21-tetrahydroxypregna-1,4-diene-3, 20-dione, cyclic 16,17-acetal with acetone 21-acetate.

Description: Fluocinonide is the 21-acetate ester of fluocinolone acetonide. Fluocinonide appears to be completely soluble in a hydrophylic, water-miscible cream base, as offered for clinical use, consisting of stearyl alcohol, polyethylene glycol 6000, propylene glycol, 1,2,-6-hexanetriol and citric acid.

Indications: Topically, as adjunctive therapy for the relief of inflammatory manifestations of acute and chronic dermatoses and psoriasis.

Contraindications: Topical steroids are contraindicated in vaccinia and varicella, and in those patients with a history of sensitivity to any of the components.

Precautions: Systemic absorption may occur when extensive areas are treated. Since safe use in pregnant women has not been established, fluocinonide should not be used extensively, in large amounts, or for prolonged periods of time.

Adverse Reactions: Burning sensations, itching, irritation, dryness, secondary infection, folliculitis, acneform eruptions, hypopigmentation, striae, and skin atrophy have been reported.

For further precautions and adverse reactions, see general statement.

Dosage and Administration: *Topically.* Apply a small amount and massage gently into the cleansed affected area 3 or 4 times daily, as needed.

Availability:
LIDEX®: **(Syntex)**
Cream, 0.05% in tubes of 15, 30 and 60 gm.
Ointment, 0.05% in tubes of 15, 30 and 60 gm.
LIDEX-E Cream, 0.05% in tubes of 15 and 60 gm. **(Syntex)**
TOPSYN® Gel, 0.05% in tubes of 15 and 60 gm. **(Syntex)**

FLUOROMETHOLONE

Chemical Name: 9-α-Fluoro-11β,17α-dihydroxy-6α-methylpregna-1,4-diene-3,20-dione.

Description: A synthetic corticosteroid related to the natural hormones of the adrenal cortex, fluorometholone occurs as a white or yellowish crystalline powder sparingly soluble in alcohol and insoluble in water.

In general, topical application of fluorometholone appears to be 40 times as effective as hydrocortisone. With such a potency ratio, a response can be expected and the possibility of systemic activity minimized. In clinical studies on patient's eye(s) treated with both dexamethasone and fluoromethasone, the latter drug showed a lower propensity to increased intraocular pressure than did dexamethasone.

Indications: Various dermatoses such as contact dermatitis, atopic dermatitis, seborrheic dermatitis and neurodermatitis, anogenital pruritus. The combinations product affords therapeutic control of secondary infections caused by neomycin-sensitive organisms. Also for antiinflammatory action in the palpebral and bulbar conjunctiva, cornea and anterior segment of the globe. Ocular conditions which benefit from therapy include allergic conjunctivitis, acne rosacea keratitis, superficial punctate keratitis, herpes zoster keratitis, iritis, cyclitis, and selected infective conjunctivitis. Additionally, it is of value for the treatment of corneal injury due to chemical or thermal burns, or penetration of foreign bodies.

Contraindications: Acute superficial herpes simplex keratitis; fungal diseases of the ocular structures; vaccinia, varicella and most other viral diseases of the cornea and conjunctiva; tuberculosis of the eye, and hypersensitivity to any of the constituents of the preparations.

Warnings: Steroid medication in the treatment of herpes simplex keratitis (involving the stroma) requires great caution; frequent slit-lamp microscopy is mandatory. Prolonged use may result in glaucoma, damage to the optic nerve, defects in visual acuity and fields of vision, posterior subcapsular cataract formation, or may aid in the establishment of secondary ocular infections from fungi or viruses liberated from ocular tissue. Also, in those diseases causing thinning of the cornea or sclera, perforation has been known to occur with the use of topical steroids. Acute purulent untreated infection of the eye may be masked or activity enhanced by the presence of steroid medication. Safe use in children under 2 years of age and in pregnant women has not been established.

Precautions: As fungal infections of the cornea are particularly prone to develop coincidentally with long-term use, fungal invasion must be suspected in any persistent corneal ulceration when a steroid has been administered or is being administered. Intraocular pressure should be checked frequently.

Adverse Reactions: Glaucoma with optic nerve damage, visual acuity or field defects, posterior subcapsular cataract formation, secondary ocular infection from pathogens liberated from ocular tissue, and perforation of the globe.

For other contraindications, precautions and adverse reactions, see general statement.

Dosage and Administration: *Topically,* 1 to 3 applications daily after thorough cleansing of the affected skin area. The cream should be rubbed gently into the skin; the ointment should be applied in a thin film. Ophthalmic suspension, 1 to 2 drops instilled into the conjunctival sac 2 to 4 times daily. During the initial 24 to 48 hours, the dosage may be increased to 2 drops every hour. Care should be taken not to discontinue therapy prematurely.

Availability:

FML® Ophthalmic Suspension, 0.1% with polyvinyl alcohol, 1.4% (Liquifilm®) in dropper bottles of 5 and 10 ml. **(Allergan)**

OXYLONE® Cream, 0.025% in tubes of 15 and 60 gm and in jars of 120 gm. **(Upjohn)**

NEO-OXYLONE® Ointment, 0.025% w/neomycin sulfate, 0.5% (equiv. to 0.35% neomycin base) in tubes of 7.5 gm. **(Upjohn)**

FLUPREDNISOLONE

Chemical Name: 6α-Fluoro-11β,17α,21-trihydroxypregna-1,4-diene-3,20-dione.

Description: Fluprednisolone is a synthetic adrenal glucocorticoid related structurally to both paramethasone and prednisolone.

On a dosage basis, 2 mg of fluprednisolone is the equivalent of 5 mg of prednisolone or 20 mg of hydrocortisone.

For the actions, indications, contraindications, warnings, precautions and the usual adverse reactions associated with fluprednisolone, see general statement.

Adverse Reactions: Response to fluprednisolone generally is identical to other corticosteroids. However, short-term courses of treatment minimize sodium and water retention and potassium depletion. Negative nitrogen balance occurs. Weight gain is common and hyperactivity of the central nervous system has been reported.

Dosage and Administration: *Orally.* The initial dosage may vary from 1.5 to 30 mg daily. For maintenance, the initial dosage should be reduced by small amounts at appropriate intervals until the lowest dose that maintains an adequate clinical response is achieved. In the absence of a satisfactory response, reevaluation should be made to review the diagnosis.

Availability:
ALPHADROL® Tablets, 1.5 mg in bottles of 100 and 500. **(Upjohn)**

FLURANDRENOLIDE

Chemical Name: 6α-Fluoro-16α-hydroxyhydrocortisone 16, 17-acetonide.

Description: A synthetic adrenal glucocorticoid which is related structurally to triamcinolone; it is very slightly soluble in water and soluble in alcohol.

In general, topical application of flurandrenolide appears to be approximately 20 times as potent as hydrocortisone and about twice as potent as triamcinolone acetonide.

Indications: Adjunctive topical management of those dermatologic disorders which may be expected to respond to corticosteroids. The skin disorders include various dermatoses, folliculitis and infectious eczematous dermatitis. It is used under occlusive dressings for the management of resistant nummular dermatitis, psoriasis, and chronic neurodermatitis. The addition of neomycin sulfate broadens the usefulness of flurandrenolide so that dermatoses complicated by infection may be treated more effectively. Topical preparations are recommended only as a supplement to and not as a substitute for other treatments (lotions, wet dressings, etc.) used in the conventional management of skin lesions.

Contraindications: Topical steriods are contraindicated in vaccinia and varicella and in those hypersensitive to any of the components.

Precautions: Any superimposed bacterial infection should first be treated with a suitable antibiotic until infection has been brought under control. The same precaution, of course, applies equally to a preparation containing neomycin. Flurandrenolide should not be used in the eyes, and care should be exercised when it is applied near the eyes.

For contraindications, warnings, adverse reactions and further precautions, see general statement.

Dosage and Administration: *Topically.* Dry, scaly lesions: a small amount of ointment is applied in a thin film to affected areas 2 or 3 times daily. Moist, weeping lesions: a small amount of cream should be rubbed gently into affected area 2 or 3 times daily. The lotion is usually applied to intertriginous areas, such as the axilla and groin. Some persistent dermatoses may be treated more effectively by applying the medication under an occlusive, non-permeable dressing. The tape is applied after the skin is cleansed and dried, and it is usually replaced every 12 hours or may be left in place for 24 hours if it is well tolerated. When necessary, the tape may be used at nighttime and removed during the day. If irritation or infection develops, the tape should be removed and the physician consulted.

Availability:

Flurandrenolide

CORDRAN®: **(Dista)**

Cream (CORDRAN® SP), 0.025% (half-strength) in tubes of 30 and 60 gm and in jars of 225 gm; 0.05% in tubes of 7.5, 15 and 60 gm and in jars of 225 gm.

Lotion, 0.05% in plastic squeeze bottles of 15 and 60 ml.

Ointment 0.025% (half-strength) in tubes of 30 and 60 gm and in jars of 225 gm; 0.05% in tubes of 7.5, 15 and 60 gm and in jars of 225 gm.

Tape, 4 mcg/sq cm in rolls of 7.5 cm (3 inches) wide and 200 cm (80 inches) long.

w/Neomycin Sulfate

CORDRAN®-N: **(Dista)**

Cream, 0.05% w/neomycin sulfate, 0.5% (equiv. to 0.35% (3.5 mg) neomycin base) in tubes of 7.5, 15 and 60 gm.

Ointment, 0.05% w/neomycin sulfate, 0.5% (equiv. to 0.35% (3.5 mg) neomycin base) in tubes of 7.5, 15 and 60 gm.

HALCINONIDE

Chemical Name: 21-Chloro-9-fluoro-11β, 16α, 17-trihydroxypregn-4-ene-3, 20-dione, cyclic 16, 17-acetal with acetone.

Description: A synthetic corticosteroid primarily effective for its antiinflammatory, antipruritic and vasoconstrictive actions.

Indications: Adjunctive therapy and symptomatic relief of inflammatory manifestations of acute and chronic dermatosis that respond to corticosteroid treatment.

Contraindications: Hypersensitivity to any of the components and in the presence of vaccinia and varicella. **Note:** Not for ophthalmic use.

The warnings, precautions and adverse reactions are generally the same as those for other topical corticosteroids. See general statement.

Dosage and Administration: *Topically.* Apply a small amount and massage gently into the cleansed affected area 2 to 3 times daily. Some resistant cases of psoriasis and neurodermatitis may be treated more effectively by applying the cream under an occlusive, nonpermeable dressing.

Availability:
HALOG®: **(Squibb)**
Cream, 0.025 and 0.1% in tubes of 15 and 60 gm and in jars of 240 gm.
Ointment, 0.1% in tubes of 15 and 60 gm and in jars of 240 gm.
Solution, 0.1% in plastic squeeze bottles of 20 and 60 ml.

HYDROCORTISONE

Synonym: Kendall's Compound F.

Chemical Name: 11β, 17, 21-Trihydroxypregn-4-ene-3, 20-dione.

Description: Hydrocortisone (cortisol) is the most important glucocorticoid secreted by the adrenal cortex since it corrects most of the pathophysiology following adrenalectomy when administered in amounts comparable to that normally secreted. It is closely related chemically and pharmacologically to cortisone. Cortisone, however, lacks specific pharmacological activity; its effects on body function result only because of its conversion to hydrocortisone in vivo. Pharmacologically, 20 mg of hydrocortisone is the equivalent of 25 mg of cortisone.

Hydrocortisone *acetate,* a derivative of hydrocortisone (free alcohol), differs structurally from cortisone acetate by a hydroxyl rather than a ketone radical at carbon-11 in the steroid nucleus. Because it is less soluble than the free alcohol [hydrocortisone], the acetate, in the form of an aqueous suspension, is used intraarticularly, producing a prolonged local effect. In special circumstances, however, where a rapid and profound hormonal effect is required, the free alcohol may be administered intravenously; the insoluble acetate never should be administered intravenously.

The water-insoluble *cypionate ester* of hydrocortisone is tasteless and odorless and has the same metabolic and antiinflammatory activity as hydrocortisone with equal activity on an equimolar basis. Given orally, it is more slowly absorbed from the gastrointestinal tract than hydrocortisone.

The *sodium succinate ester* of hydrocortisone has the same metabolic and antiinflammatory actions as hydrocortisone and, because of its extreme solubility in water, permits the immediate intravenous administration of high doses in a small volume of diluent and is particularly useful where high blood levels are required rapidly. When given parenterally and in equimolar amounts, the two compounds are equivalent in biologic activity. Following the intravenous injection of the sodium succinate, demonstrable effects are evident within 1 hour and persist for a variable period. Excretion of the administered dose is nearly complete within 12 hours. Thus, if constantly high blood levels are required, injections should be given every 4 to 6 hours. The sodium succinate is also rapidly absorbed when given intramuscularly and is excreted in a pattern similar to that observed after intravenous injection.

For indications, contraindications, warnings, precautions and adverse reactions, see general statement.

Dosage and Administration: *Orally,* the administered dosage of hydrocortisone will depend on both the individual and the condition being treated. In general, the initial dosage should be large enough to suppress all signs of the condition being treated. This is usually followed by a period during which the dosage is reduced to a level high enough to suppress evidence of disease activity, but low enough to minimize complications of therapy. The total daily dosage administered will depend on the condition being treated and the duration of therapy. In life-threatening situations, such as acute lupus erythematosus, the initial dosage may be high whereas in chronic conditions, such as rheumatoid arthritis, the initial daily oral dose may range between 40 and 80 mg. The daily dosage is usually given 4 times daily.

Intraarticularly, the acetate or butylacetate derivative of hydrocortisone is usually utilized; the amount used depends primarily on the size of the joint to be injected. A dose of 5 to 10 mg is usually injected into small joints such as those of the fingers, while 15 to 35 mg are used for large joints such as the hip and knee.

Properly diluted solutions of *hydrocortisone* (free alcohol) should be given *intravenously only,* never intramuscularly or subcutaneously. The *sodium succinate* ester may be given *intravenously* or *intramuscularly.* The dosage is 100 mg, infused slowly intravenously over a period of 2 to 10 hours, depending upon the severity of the condition. In certain emergency situations, hydrocortisone may be combined with intramuscular cortisone acetate.

Rectally, as a retention enema or as a foam for the treatment of ulcerative colitis and proctitis and as an adjunct to other measures. Before instituting therapy, a complete rectal examination to rule out serious pathology should be performed.

Topically, a thin film of the steroid is applied in a suitable ointment, cream, lotion or spray, 1 to 4 times daily in concentrations of 0.125% in mild or recent skin lesions up to 2.5% in severe or chronic lesions, or 3 to 4 drops of otic suspension in the ear 3 or 4 times daily.

For more detailed information on dosage and administration, the manufacturers' package literature should be consulted.

Availability:

Hydrocortisone

Tablets, 10 and 20 mg in bottles of 1000. **(Lederle)**

Tablets, 10 and 20 mg in bottles of 100. **(McKesson)**

Tablets (HYDROCORTONE®), 10 and 20 mg in bottles of 100. **(Merck Sharp & Dohme)**

AEROSEB-HC® Topical Aerosol, 225 mg in aerosol containers of 90 gm. After evaporation of the propellant, the solution contains 0.5% of hydrocortisone. **(Herbert)**

ALPHADERM® Cream, 1% in tubes of 30 and 100 gm. **(Norwich-Eaton)**

BARSEB® HC Scalp Lotion, 1% w/salicylic acid, 0.5% in plastic-squeeze bottles of 60 ml. **(Barnes-Hind)**

BARSEB® THERA-SPRAY® Topical Spray, 360 mg w/salicylic acid, 288 mg in aerosol bottles of 120 gm with applicator tube. **(Barnes-Hind)**

CORT-DOME®: **(Dome)**

Creme, 0.125 and 0.25% in tubes of 30 gm and Dispensajar®s of 120 gm and 1 lb; 0.5% in tubes of 15 and 30 gm and Dispensajar®s of 120 gm and 1 lb; 1% in tubes of 15 and 30 gm.

Lotion, 0.125% in bottles of 180 ml; 0.25% in bottles of 120 ml; 0.5% in bottles of 15, 30 and 120 ml; 1% in bottles of 15 and 30 ml.

CORTEF®: **(Upjohn)**

Sterile Suspension (IM), 50 mg/ml in vials of 5 ml.

Tablets, 5 mg in bottles of 50; 10 and 20 mg in bottles of 100.

CORTENEMA® Aqueous Suspension (retention enema), 100 mg in disposable units of 60 ml with lubricated rectal tip in cartons of 7 single-dose units. **(Rowell)**

CORTRIL® Topical Ointment, 1% in tubes of 15 gm. **(Pfipharmecs)**

DERMACORT®: **(Rowell)**

Cream, 1% in jars of 1 lb.

Lotion, 0.5% in plastic-squeeze bottles of 120 ml with dispensing top; *p*H is 5.5.

ELDECORT Cream, 0.5, 1 and 2% in tubes of 15 and 30 gm and in jars of 1 lb. **(Elder)**

HEB®-CORT: **(Barnes-Hind)**

Cream, 0.25% in tubes of 30 gm and in jars of 120 gm; 0.5% in tubes of 30 gm; 1% in tubes of 30 gm and jars of 1 lb.

Lotion, 0.25% in plastic-squeeze bottles of 120 ml.

HEB-CORT MC Lotion, 0.25% w/menthol and camphor in plastic-squeeze bottles of 60 ml. **(Barnes-Hind)**

OPTEF® Eye Drops, 0.2% in dropper bottles of 2.5 ml. **(Upjohn)**
PANTHO-F® Cream, 1% w/panthenol, 2% in tubes of 20 gm. **(USV)**
PROCTOCORT™ Cream, 1% in tubes of 30 gm with 12 finger cots. **(Rowell)**
RECTOID® Aqueous Suspension (for retention enema), 100 mg in disposable units of 60 ml with applicator tip in cartons of 7 single-dose units. **(Pharmacia)**

w/Pramoxine Hydrochloride

DROTIC Otic Suspension, 1% w/pramoxine hydrochloride, 1% and acetic acid, 2% in plastic dropper bottles of 10 ml. **(Ascher)**

w/Neomycin Sulfate and/or Iodochlorhydroxyquin

CORT-QUIN® Creme, 0.25% w/diiodohydroxyquin, 1% in tubes of 30 gm; 0.5% (microdispersed) w/diiodohydroxyquin, 1% in tubes of 15 gm. **(Dome)**
DOMEFORM-HC® Creme, 0.5% w/iodochlorhydroxyquin, 3% in tubes of 15 gm. **(Dome)**
NEO-CORT-DOME®: **(Dome)**
Creme, 0.25, 0.5 and 1% w/neomycin sulfate, 0.5% (equiv. to 0.35% neomycin base); 0.25% in tubes of 30 gm and Dispensajar®s of 120 gm; 0.5 and 1% in tubes of 15 gm.
Lotion, 0.25 and 0.5% w/neomycin sulfate, 0.5% (equiv to 0.35% neomycin base); 0.25% in bottles of 120 ml; 0.5% in bottles of 30 ml.
Otic Suspension, 1% w/neomycin sulfate, 0.5% (equiv. to 0.35% neomycin base) and acetic acid, 2% in bottles of 10 ml with dropper.

w/Neomycin Sulfate and Nystatin

NEO-NYSTA-CORT® Ointment, 1% w/neomycin sulfate, 0.5% and nystatin, 100,000 units/gm in tubes of 15 gm. **(Dome)**

Hydrocortisone Acetate

CORTRIL® Acetate Aqueous Suspension, 25 mg/ml in vials of 5 ml. **(Pfizer)**
CORTEF®: **(Upjohn)**
Sterile Injectable Suspension, 50 mg/ml in vials of 5 ml.
Topical Ointment, 1 and 2.5% in tubes of 5 and 20 gm.
CORTIFOAM® Rectal Foam, 10% in aerosol containers of 20 gm with rectal applicator. **(Reed & Carnrick)**
ORABASE® HCA Oral Paste, 0.5% in an oral paste vehicle containing pectin, gelatin, sodium carboxymethylcellulose dispersed in a plasticized hydrocarbon gel composed of 5% polyethylene in mineral oil in tubes of 5 gm. **(Hoyt)**
HYDROCORTONE®: **(Merck Sharp & Dohme)**
Ophthalmic Ointment, 1.5% in tubes of 3.5 gm.
Ophthalmic Suspension, 2.5% in dropper bottles of 5 ml.
Saline Suspension, 25 and 50 mg/ml in vials of 5 ml. *For intrasynovial use.*
Topical Ointment, 1% in tubes of 15 and 30 gm.
CORT-DOME® Suppositories, 15 mg (regular) and 25 mg (high potency) in cartons of 12. **(Dome)**

w/Lidocaine and/or iodochlorhydroxyquin

LIDAFORM-HC®: **(Dome)**
Creme and Lotion, 0.5% w/lidocaine, 3% and iodochlorhydroxyquin, 3% in tubes of 15 gm and bottles of 30 ml.

w/Neomycin Sulfate

NEO-CORTEF: **(Upjohn)**
Lotion, 1% w/neomycin sulfate, 5 mg (equiv. to 3.5 mg neomycin base) in plastic squeeze bottles of 15 ml.
Ophthalmic Ointment, 0.5 and 1.5% w/neomycin sulfate, 5 mg (equiv. to 3.5 mg neomycin base) in tubes of 3.5 gm with applicator tip.
Ophthalmic Suspension, 0.5 and 1.5% w/neomycin sulfate, 5 mg (equiv to 3.5 mg neomycin base); 0.5% in dropper bottles of 5 ml; 1.5% in dropper bottles of 2.5 and 5 ml.
Topical Cream, 1 and 2.5% w/neomycin sulfate, 5 mg (equiv. to 3.5 mg neomycin base) in tubes of 20 gm.
Topical Ointment, 0.5, 1 and 2.5% w/neomycin sulfate, 5 mg (equiv. to 3.5 mg neomycin base); 0.5 and 2.5% in tubes of 5 and 20 gm; 1% in tubes of 5, 20 and 120 gm.
LIDA-MANTLE-HC® Creme, 0.5% w/lidocaine, 3% in tubes of 15 and 30 gm. **(Dome)**

w/Pramoxine Hydrochloride

PROCTOFOAM®-HC Rectal Foam, 1% w/pramoxine hydrochloride, 1% in aerosol containers of 15 gm with rectal applicator. **(Reed & Carnrick)**

Hydrocortisone Cypionate

CORTEF® Oral Suspension, 10 mg/5 ml in bottles of 120 ml. **(Upjohn)**

Hydrocortisone Sodium Phosphate

HYDROCORTONE® Phosphate Injection, 50 mg/ml in disposable syringes of 2 ml and in multiple-dose vials of 2 and 10 ml. **(Merck Sharp & Dohme)**

Hydrocortisone Sodium Succinate

A-HYDROCORT™ Sterile Powder for Injection in Univial®s of 100, 250 and 500 mg and 1 gm. **(Abbott)**

SOLU-CORTEF® For Injection: **(Upjohn)**

Sterile Powder in vials of 100 mg with or without diluent.

Sterile Powder, 100 and 250 mg in Mix-O-Vials® of 2 ml; 500 mg in Mix-O-Vials of 4 ml; 1 gm in Mix-O-Vials of 8 ml.

Hydrocortisone Valerate

WESTCORT™ Cream, 0.2% in tubes of 15 and 60 gm. **(Westwood)**

MEDRYSONE

Chemical Name: 11β-Hydroxy-6α-methylpregn-4-ene-3,20-dione.

Description: Medrysone is a steroid related structurally to progesterone, differing from the latter in that a 6-methyl and an 11-hydroxyl group have been added to provide antiinflammatory and antiallergic activity with little or no effect on intraocular pressure. Medrysone occurs as a white, crystalline powder sparingly soluble in water.

Although the antiinflammatory potency of medrysone is less than that of 0.1% dexamethasone, its potential to increase intraocular pressure is less than that of either dexamethasone or betamethasone.

Indications: Treatment of allergic conjunctivitis, vernal conjunctivitis, episcleritis and epinephrine sensitivity. Since the drug's effectiveness in iritis or uveitis has not been demonstrated, it should not be used in these conditions.

Contraindications: Acute, untreated, purulent ocular infections; acute herpes simplex (dendritic) keratitis; viral diseases of the conjunctiva and cornea; ocular tuberculosis; fungal diseases of the eye; hypersensitivity to any component of the preparation.

Warnings: (1) Steroids may mask, enhance or activate infectious diseases of the eye; (2) perforation of the cornea or sclera has been reported occasionally following prolonged use of topical steroids. With high dosage, they have been associated with thinning of the cornea; (3) prolonged use of topical steroids may increase intraocular pressure with possible resultant glaucoma, damage to the optic nerve, and defects in visual acuity and fields of vision, although this effect is not as great with medrysone as it is with other steroids; (4) prolonged use of topical steroids may, on rare occasions, be associated with the development of posterior subcapsular cataracts; (5) systemic absorption and systemic side effects are possible with the use of topical steroids; (6) it is not recommended for use in iritis and uveitis; (7) steroid medication in the presence of stromal herpes simplex requires considerable caution; frequent slit-lamp microscopy is suggested; (8) prolonged use may aid in the establishment of secondary ocular infections from fungi and viruses liberated from ocular tissue.

Precautions: When this drug is used for extended periods, the intraocular pressure and the lens should be examined periodically. If ulceration of the cornea persists, particularly when a steroid has been used or is presently being used, fungal infection should be suspected. The use of topical steroids during pregnancy should be limited to conditions sufficiently serious to warrant their use, so that the potential risk to the fetus could be justified by the anticipated benefit to the mother.

Adverse Reactions: Occasional, transient stinging and burning may occur on instillation of the preparation.

Dosage and Administration: *Topically.* Instill 1 drop into the conjunctival sac up to every 4 hours.

Availability:

HMS® LIQUIFILM® Ophthalmic Suspension, 1% with polyvinyl alcohol (Liquifilm), 1.4%, in plastic dropper bottles of 5 and 10 ml. **Note:** The 5 ml bottles are filled to 1/2 capacity and the 10 ml bottles are filled to 2/3 capacity for proper drop control. *Do not freeze.* **(Allergan)**

MEPREDNISONE

Chemical Name: 17,21-Dihydroxy-16β-methylpregna-1,4-diene-3,11,20-trione.

Description: Meprednisone is a synthetic compound with antiinflammatory, antiallergic, antirheumatic, diuretic and natriuretic activity. Laboratory and clinical experience indicate that the antiinflammatory effect of 4 mg of meprednisone is approximately equivalent to that of 0.6 mg of betamethasone, 0.75 mg of dexamethasone, 2 mg of paramethasone, 4 mg of methylprednisolone or triamcinolone, 5 mg of prednisone or prednisolone, 20 mg of hydrocortisone, and 25 mg of cortisone. Salt and water retention appears to be less than that of prednisone.

Indications: Meprednisone shares the action and uses of other adrenal corticosteroids. See general statement.

Contraindications: Active, healed or incompletely healed tuberculosis; pregnancy, particularly during the first trimester. For other contraindications; also warnings, precautions and adverse reactions, see general statement.

Dosage and Administration: *Orally.* Dosage must be individualized according to the severity of the disease and the response of the patient. Suggested *daily* dosages in diseases requiring prolonged treatment: *Rheumatoid arthritis:* Severe—initially 20 to 24 mg; maintenance 4 to 10 mg; moderate—initially 8 to 12 mg; maintenance 2 to 6 mg. *Chronic refractory asthma:* Severe—initially 32 to 48 mg; maintenance 4 to 12 mg; moderate—initially 12 to 16 mg; maintenance 4 to 12 mg. *Pulmonary emphysema:* Initially 16 to 24 mg; maintenance 8 to 16 mg. *Allergic* and *inflammatory dermatoses:* Initially 16 to 24 mg; maintenance 4 to 12 mg. *Disseminated lupus erythematosus:* Initially 48 to 64 mg; maintenance 8 to 20 mg. *Adrenogenital syndrome:* Maintenance 4 to 12 mg (to maintain urinary 17-ketosteroid level within the normal range). *Nephrosis:* Initially 20 to 60 mg (for 10 to 14 days or until diuresis occurs); maintenance 12 to 40 mg (3 consecutive days of each week for 6 to 12 months). **Note:** In severe, acute disease, when rapid corticosteroid effects are desired, the patient may be treated with an injectable steroid; for maintenance, the patient can then be given meprednisone orally.

Availability:
BETAPAR® Tablets, 4 mg in bottles of 100. **(Parke-Davis)**

METHYLPREDNISOLONE

Chemical Name: 11β, 17, 21-Trihydroxy-6α-methylpregna-1,4-diene-3,20-dione.

Description: Methylprednisolone is a synthetic corticosteroid related structurally to prednisolone. On a weight basis, 4 mg of methylprednisolone is equivalent to 5 mg of prednisolone or prednisone and to 20 mg of hydrocortisone.

Compared with more soluble steroid salts, the **acetate ester** of methylprednisolone is claimed to have a longer duration and more rapid onset of activity. Used as intraarticular therapy, the therapeutic effect is usually evident by 12 to 24 hours, and lasts for more than 7 days.

The **sodium succinate ester** is characterized by a prompt onset of action, and is intended for emergency therapy of short duration. This ester should be administered within 48 hours of its preparation as a solution.

The general statement should be consulted for basic information including indications, contraindications and warnings for this substance.

Precautions: Acute and chronic infection should cause the physician to critically evaluate the need for the administration of steroids generally. However, it has been used in association with appropriate antibiotics in cases of shock associated with gram-negative septicemia. Intraarticular administration should not be used if infection is suspected or demonstrated.

Since sodium and water retention is minimized with administration of methylprednisolone, patients must be carefully evaluated for more subtle signs of overdosage.

Adverse Reactions: The myopathy seen with all steroid preparations also occurs with methylprednisolone.

Dosage and Administration:

Orally. The proper dose will depend on the condition under therapy and the response of the patient. Usually, the daily dose is divided into 4 parts.

Intraarticularly. The joint involved and the extent of activity will determine the intraarticular dosage. Large joints may require 20 to 80 mg while 4 to 10 mg will suffice for smaller ones. Depending on the location, 4 to 30 mg can be administered in the management of bursitis and soft-tissue problems.

Intracutaneously or intralesionally. The clinical condition and the response to therapy will determine the frequency of injection, 20 to 60 mg of the acetate ester being used.

Intramuscularly. The **acetate** salt may be used intramuscularly as either a single weekly dose or as a daily dose, the dosage being dependent on the clinical status. The weekly dose will usually vary from 40 to 120 mg.

Intravenously or intramuscularly. The **sodium succinate** salt should only be used for intravenous administration but may be used intramuscularly. When used intramuscularly, the usual dose is 10 to 40 mg and may be repeated every 6 to 24 hours. The intravenous preparation usually is utilized for emergency therapy, and is used in a dose of 10 to 500 mg depending on the condition and the response and it can be repeated every 6 hours if necessary. The larger dose has been recommended in treating the shock of septicemia where appropriate antibiotic therapy and other adjunctive measures are also utilized.

Topically. The **succinate ester** is utilized as a retention enema in the management of ulcerative colitis. An 0.25 or 1% ointment prepared from the **acetate ester** is used in the management of appropriate dermatologic conditions.

For specific information on indications and dosage, the literature including the manufacturers' package circular should be consulted.

Availability:

Methylprednisolone

MEDROL®: **(Upjohn)**

Medules® (sustained release capsules), 2 mg in bottles of 100.

Tablets, 2 mg in bottles of 30 and 100; 4 mg in bottles of 30, 100 and 500 and in unit-dose packages of 100; 8 mg in bottles of 25 and 100; 16 mg in bottles of 50; 24 and 32 mg in bottles of 25.

Dosepaks®, 4 mg in packages of 21 tablets.

ADTpaks, 16 mg in packages of 14 tablets.

Methylprednisolone Acetate

DEPO-MEDROL® Sterile Aqueous Suspension, 20 mg/ml in vials of 5 ml; 40 mg/ml in vials of 1, 5 and 10 ml; 80 mg/ml in vials of 1 and 5 ml and in U-Ject® (disposable syringes) of 1 ml. **(Upjohn)**

MEDROL®: **(Upjohn)**

Acetate Topical Ointment, 0.25 and 1% in tubes of 7.5, 30 and 45 gm with applicator tip.

Enpaks® (for rectal instillation), 40 mg/bottle, with or without administration unit.

w/Neomycin Sulfate

NEO-MEDROL®: **(Upjohn)**

Ophthalmic Ointment (sterile), 0.1% w/neomycin sulfate, 5 mg (equiv. to 3.5 mg neomycin base) in tubes of 3.5 gm with applicator tip.

Topical Ointment, 0.25 and 1% w/neomycin sulfate, 5 mg (equiv. to 3.5 mg neomycin base) in tubes of 7.5, 30 and 45 gm with applicator tip.

Methylprednisolone Sodium Succinate

A-METHAPRED™ Sterile Powder for Injection in Univial®s of 40 and 125 mg w/o diluent and 500 mg and 1 gm w/diluent. **(Abbott)**

SOLU-MEDROL® Sterile, 40 mg in Mix-O-Vials® of 1 ml; 125 mg in Mix-O-Vials of 2 ml; 0.5 gm with 8 ml vial of diluent; 1 gm with 16 ml vial of diluent. **(Upjohn)**

PARAMETHASONE ACETATE

Chemical Name: 6α-Fluoro-11β, 17α, 21-trihydroxy-16α-methyl-1,4-pregnadiene-3,20-dione 21-acetate; 6α-Fluoro-16α-methylprednisolone.

Description: Paramethasone is a synthetic adrenal steroid structurally related to dexamethasone which is readily absorbed from the gastrointestinal tract following oral administration.

On a weight basis, 2 mg of paramethasone is equivalent to 0.75 mg of dexamethasone, 5 mg of prednisone and 20 mg of hydrocortisone.

Since paramethasone is similar in action and usage to other similar adrenal steroids, the general statement should be consulted for basic information. The combination product provides relief of pain, stiffness and inflammation associated with mild to moderately severe rheumatoid arthritis.

Contraindications: Therapy with paramethasone is contraindicated in the presence of systemic fungal infections and in the presence of ocular herpes simplex because of possible corneal perforation.

Precautions: These are similar to all the adrenal corticosteroids. Psychic derangement may appear. Also a significant increase in appetite has been seen.

Dosage and Administration: *Orally.* The initial dosage may vary from 2 to 24 mg daily depending on the condition being treated. The dosage requirement is quite variable and must be individualized. If the drug is to be discontinued following therapy of long duration, it is mandatory that it be withdrawn gradually.

Availability:
HALDRONE® Tablets, 1 mg (yellow, capsule-shaped) in bottles of 100; 2 mg (orange, capsule-shaped, scored) in bottles of 30 and 100. **(Lilly)**
STERO-DARVON® with A.S.A. Tablets, 0.25 mg with propoxyphene hydrochloride, 32 mg and aspirin, 500 mg in RxPaks of 50. **(Lilly)**

PREDNISOLONE

Chemical Name: 11β,17,21-Trihydroxypregna-1,4-diene-3,20-dione.

Description: Prednisolone is a synthetic chemical derivative of hydrocortisone which has increased antiinflammatory properties without an accompanying increase in salt and water retention. On a weight basis, 5 mg of prednisolone is equivalent to 20 mg of hydrocortisone.

The slightly soluble **acetate** and **butylacetate** esters of prednisolone are utilized for intraarticular and soft-tissue injection in treating diseases of the joints and nonarticular structures.

Aqueous solutions of the **sodium phosphate** and **hemisuccinate** preparations are used intramuscularly or intravenously for the management of emergency situations where urgent systemic therapy is necessary.

The prednisolone base as well as the **sodium phosphate** compound are used for topical therapy in dermatological, nasal and ophthalmological disorders.

The general statement should be consulted for an overview of actions, indications, contraindications and uses of prednisolone.

Warnings: In diseases due to microorganisms, infection may be masked, enhanced or activated by the steroid; extended use may cause increased intraocular pressure in susceptible individuals. Therefore, it is advised that the intraocular pressure be checked frequently. In diseases that cause thinning of the cornea, perforation has occurred with the use of topical steroids.

Precautions: The precautions to be observed are those of the steroids in general.

Adverse Reactions: Adverse effects are those noted with other steroids. It has been suggested that gastric disturbances are more common with prednisolone in comparison with hydrocortisone. Other complications noted were sensitivity to heat; fat embolism; adverse effects on growth and development of the individual and on spermatozoa; hypotensive and shock-like reactions, also anaphylactoid or hypersensitivity reactions.

Dosage and Administration: The dosage and the method of administration will depend on the condition being treated and the response of the patient. Prednisolone can be administered *orally, topically* and *parenterally.* In the latter instance, it can be given intramuscularly, intravenously, intraarticularly or directly into a bursa or periarticular tissue.

Orally, the usual initial dose is 30 to 50 mg daily in serious cases and 5 to 25 mg in less serious situations in 4 doses with subsequent reduction to a level sufficient to control the disease being treated.

The same daily dosage is indicated when the acetate or butylacetate preparation is used *intramuscularly.* The usual dose for *intraarticular* administration is 20 to 30 mg for large joints such as the knee and 5 to 10 mg for smaller joints; 10 to 30 mg are used in bursitis with smaller amounts injected for tendonitis and treatment of ganglion cysts.

The sodium succinate ester may be given *intravenously,* 25 to 50 mg being injected initially with the same dose being repeated in 3 to 4 hours if necessary. It may also be given by continuous intravenous drip, 100 mg being given every 12 hours.

Topically, as a 0.5% cream, lotion or solution used up to 4 times daily. Solutions of prednisolone may be applied topically to the *eye, ear* or *nose.* Application to the eye is administered by solutions of 0.1 to 0.5%, rarely 1% or by ointments of 0.2 to 0.5% 3 to 4 times daily. Application to the ear, the 0.25 to 0.5% solution or the ointment may be applied into the aural canal 2 or 3 times daily. An 0.1 to 0.2% suspension or solution should be sprayed into each nostril every 4 hours where *nasal* therapy is indicated.

The medical literature and the manufacturers' recommendations should be consulted for specifics.

Availability:

Prednisolone

Tablets, 5 mg in bottles of 1000. **(Lemmon)**

Tablets, 5 mg in bottles of 100 and 1000. **(McKesson)**

DELTA-CORTEF® Tablets, 5 mg in bottles of 100 and 500. **(Upjohn)**

METI-DERM®: **(Schering)**

Aerosol, 0.33 mg/gm in spray dispensers of 150 gm.

Cream, 0.5% in tubes of 10 and 25 gm.

PREDNIS® Tablets, 5 mg in bottles of 100. **(USV)**

STERANE® Tablets, 5 mg in bottles of 100 and 1000. **(Pfipharmecs)**

Combinations

ATARAXOID® Tablets, 2.5 and 5 mg w/hydroxyzine hydrochloride, 10 mg in bottles of 100. **(Pfizer)**

NEO-DELTEF® Eye Drops, 0.2% w/neomycin sulfate, 0.5% (equiv. to 0.35% neomycin base) in dropper bottles of 2.5 ml. **(Upjohn)**

METI-DERM® with NEOMYCIN: **(Schering)**

Aerosol, 0.33 mg/gm with neomycin sulfate, 0.33 mg/gm in aerosol containers of 150 gm.

Ointment, 5 mg/gm with neomycin sulfate, 5 mg/gm (equiv. to 3.5 mg neomycin base) in tubes of 10 gm.

Prednisolone Acetate

ECONOPRED® Ophthalmic Suspension, 0.125 and 1% in Drop-Tainer® dispensers of 5 ml. **(Alcon)**

ECONOPRED® FORTE Ophthalmic Suspension, 1% in Drop-Tainer® dispensers of 5 and 10 ml. **(Alcon)**

METICORTELONE® Injection, 25 mg/ml in multiple-dose vials of 5 ml. **(Schering)**

PRED MILD® Ophthalmic Suspension, 0.12% in dropper bottles of 5 and 10 ml. **(Allergan)**

PRED PLUS® Ophthalmic Suspension, 1% in dropper bottles of 5 and 10 ml. **(Allergan)**

STERANE® Injection, 25 mg/ml in vials of 5 ml. *For IM and intraarticular use.* **(Pfizer)**

w/Atropine Sulfate

MYDRAPRED Ophthalmic Solution, 0.25% w/atropine sulfate, 1% in Drop-Tainer® bottles of 5 ml. **(Alcon)**

w/Neomycin Sulfate

NEO-DELTA-CORTEF®: **(Upjohn)**

Ophthalmic Ointment, 0.25 and 0.5% w/neomycin sulfate, 0.5% (equiv. to 0.35% neomycin base) in tubes of 3.5 gm with applicator tip.

Ophthalmic Suspension, 0.25% w/neomycin sulfate, 0.5% in dropper bottles of 5 ml.

Topical Ointment, 0.5% w/neomycin sulfate, 0.5% (equiv. to 0.35% neomycin base) in tubes of 5 and 20 gm.

w/Sodium Sulfacetamide

BLEPHAMIDE® Liquifilm® Ophthalmic Suspension, 0.2% w/sodium sulfacetamide, 10% and phenylephrine hydrochloride, 0.12% in dropper bottles of 5 and 10 ml. **(Allergan)**

BLEPHAMIDE S.O.P. Ophthalmic Ointment, 0.2% w/sodium sulfacetamide, 10% in tubes of 3.5 gm. **(Allergan)**
CETAPRED® Ophthalmic Ointment (sterile) 0.25% w/sodium sulfacetamide, 10% in tubes of 3.5 gm. **(Alcon)**
Isopto CETAPRED Ophthalmic Solution, 0.25% w/sodium sulfacetamide, 10% in Drop-Tainer® bottles of 5 and 15 ml. **(Alcon)**
METIMYD®: **(Schering)**
Ophthalmic Ointment, 0.5% w/sodium sulfacetamide, 10% in tubes of 3.5 gm.
Ophthalmic Suspension, 0.5% w/sodium sulfacetamide, 10% in dropper bottles of 5 ml.

Prednisolone *tertiary*-**Butylacetate**
HYDELTRA®-T.B.A. Injectable Suspension, 2% in rubber-capped vials of 1 and 5 ml. **(Merck Sharp & Dohme)**

Prednisolone Sodium Phosphate
HYDELTRASOL®: **(Merck Sharp & Dohme)**
Injection, 20 mg/ml in vials of 2 and 5 ml.
Ophthalmic Ointment, 0.25% in tubes of 3.5 gm.
Ophthalmic Solution, 0.5% in dropper bottles of 5 ml.
INFLAMASE® Solution, 0.125 and 1% (FORTE) in plastic squeeze bottles of 5 ml with dropper tip. **(Smith, Miller & Patch)**
METRETON® Ophthalmic Solution, 0.5% in dropper bottles of 5 ml. **(Schering)**

w/Neomycin Sulfate
NEO-HYDELTRASOL®: **(Merck Sharp & Dohme)**
Ophthalmic Ointment, 0.25% w/neomycin sulfate, 0.5% in tubes of 3.5 gm.
Ophthalmic Solution, 0.5% w/neomycin sulfate, 0.5% in dropper bottles of 2.5 and 5 ml.

w/Sodium Sulfacetamide
OPTIMYD® Ophthalmic Solution, 0.5% w/sodium sulfacetamide, 10% in plastic dropper bottles of 5 ml. **(Schering)**

PREDNISONE

Chemical Name: 17,21-Dihydroxypregna-1,4-diene-3,11,20-trione.

Description: Prednisone is a synthetic chemical derivative of cortisone which is equivalent to prednisolone both in dosage and response.

The indications, contraindications, warnings, precautions, uses and dosage of prednisone are essentially identical to those for prednisolone and the general statement should be consulted for an overview.

On a weight basis, 5 mg of prednisone is equivalent to 5 mg of prednisolone, 20 mg of hydrocortisone and 25 mg of cortisone.

Prednisone is only available as an oral preparation.

Availability:

Prednisone
Tablets, 5 mg in bottles of 500. **(Lederle)**
Tablets, 5 mg in bottles of 1000. **(Lemmon)**
Tablets, 2.5 mg in bottles of 100; 5 mg in bottles of 100, 1000 and 5000. **(McKesson)**
Tablets, 5, 10, 20 and 50 mg in bottles of 100 and 1000 and in unit-dose packages of 100 (10 x 10). **(Philips Roxane)**
Tablets, 5 mg in bottles of 100. **(USV)**
DELTASONE® Tablets, 2.5 mg in bottles of 100; 5 mg in bottles of 100 and 500 and in Dosepak® (unit-dose) packages of 100; 10 and 20 mg in bottles of 100 and 500 and in unit-dose packages of 100; 50 mg in bottles of 100 and in unit-dose packages of 100. **(Upjohn)**
METICORTEN® Tablets, 1 mg in bottles of 100, 5 mg in bottles of 100, 500 and 1000. **(Schering)**
ORASONE Tablets, 1, 5, 10 and 20 mg in bottles of 100, 1000 and 5000 and in unit-dose packages of 100 (10 x 10); 50 mg (film-coated) in bottles of 100 and in unit-dose packages of 100. **(Rowell)**
PARACORT® Tablets, 5 mg in bottles of 1000 and in unit-dose packages of 100 (10 x 10). **(Parke-Davis)**
SK-PREDNISONE™ Tablets, 5 mg in bottles of 100 and 1000. **(Smith Kline & French)**

TRIAMCINOLONE

Chemical Name: 9-Fluoro-11β, 16α, 17, 21-tetrahydroxypregna-1, 4-diene-3, 20-dione; 9α fluoro-11β, 16α, 17,21-tetrahydroxypregna-1,4-diene-3,20-dione cyclic 16, 17-acetal with acetone.

Description: Triamcinolone is a synthetic fluorinated adrenal corticosteroid structurally related to dexamethasone. It is primarily a glucocorticoid in properties, possessing minimal sodium and water retention when used in therapeutic dosage.

When administered orally, 4 mg of triamcinolone is equivalent to 0.75 mg of dexamethasone, 4 mg of methylprednisolone, 5 mg of prednisone or prednisolone and 20 mg of hydrocortisone on a weight basis; also 4 mg of triamcinolone is equivalent to 5 mg of the diacetate preparation.

The **acetonide** salt of triamcinolone has a longer duration of action and is used in preparations for topical, intramuscular, intraarticular and intralesional use. It is not used for intravenous administration.

The **diacetate** preparation is utilized orally as well as for intramuscular, intraarticular, and intralesional use. It is not for intravenous use.

When the acetonide or diacetate preparations are administered by introduction into a joint or bursa, pharmacological activity begins within a few hours and may persist for a number of weeks.

Combined with nystatin for specific anticandidal activity and with neomycin and gramicidin for antibacterial activity. Since triamcinolone produces effects similar to the other adrenal corticosteroids, the general statement should be consulted for an overview.

Precautions: These are similar to those seen with the other glucocorticoids. Tissue atrophy at the site of injection may follow administration of both the acetonide and diacetate preparations. Skin infection should be excluded before administering triamcinolone by the intralesional route.

Adverse Reactions: In general, these are similar to those seen with other adrenal corticosteroids, especially the glucocorticoids. It is claimed, however, that triamcinolone neither stimulates the appetite nor does it cause weight gain. It does not usually cause sodium and water retention. There are also suggestions that the incidence of muscle weakness and loss of muscle mass may be higher in patients treated with triamcinolone on a long-term basis than those treated with other steroids. Syncope and episodes of an anaphylactoid character have been reported to follow intramuscular, intraarticular and intralesional administration. Masceration of the skin, secondary infection, skin atrophy, striae, and miliaria may occur with the application of an occlusive dressing following topical administration. For adverse reactions to the component drugs, see their specific monographs.

Dosage and Administration: Both triamcinolone and its diacetate salt are given *orally.* The hexacetonide and the diacetate preparations may be administered by the *intraarticular* or *intrabursal* route. The latter preparations can also be given *intradermally* and *intramuscularly.* There is no intravenous preparation available. The acetonide salt is used *topically.*

The range of dosage is wide and will depend on the condition being treated and the response of the individual patient. The usual initial dose for adults will vary from 8 to 32 mg daily. The dose may be divided or given as a single dose. Subsequent reduction of the dose is in order consistent with the patient's response and the physician's evaluation based on the status of the patient.

The intramuscular dose will also reflect the problem of the patient being treated.

The dosage of triamcinolone diacetate for local injection will depend on the activity of the disease and the extent of the area to be injected. A dose of 25 mg is suggested for knee joint management.

Dermatological problems susceptible to steroid therapy can be managed either by *topical* application or, where indicated, by *intralesional* administration. Neurodermatitis, keloids, and psoriasis have been treated by the latter method wherein 2 to 3 mg of triamcinolone acetonide or diacetonide per injection site have been administered. Triamcinolone acetonide cream, lotion or foam is applied *topically* usually 2 to 4 times daily. A 0.1% ointment can also be instilled in the ear, eye or mouth 2 to 4 times daily.

Subcutaneous injection of 25 to 50 mg of triamcinolone diacetate 1 to 2 times a week has been used to treat alopecia areata.

For specific information, the physician is directed to the literature and to the manufacturers' instructions.

Availability:

Triamcinolone

ARISTOCORT® Tablets, 1 mg (yellow, scored) in bottles of 50; 2 mg (pink, scored) and 4 mg (white, scored) in bottles of 30, 100 and 500; 8 mg (yellow, scored) in bottles of 50; 16 mg (white, scored) in bottles of 30. **(Lederle)**

KENACORT® Tablets, 1 and 2 mg (white, scored) in bottles of 50; 4 mg (white) in bottles of 30, 100 and 1000; 8 mg (buff-colored) in bottles of 50. **(Squibb)**

SK-TRIAMCINOLONE™ Tablets, 2 and 8 mg in bottles of 100; 4 mg in bottles of 100 and 500. **(Smith Kline & French)**

Triamcinolone Acetonide

ARISTOCORT®: **(Lederle)**

Topical Cream, 0.025 and 1% in tubes of 15 and 75 gm and in jars of 240 gm and cans of 5.25 lbs; 0.5% in tubes of 15 gm and in jars of 240 gm.

Topical Ointment, 0.1% in tubes of 15 and 75 gm and in jars of 240 gm and in cans of 5 lbs; 0.5% in tubes of 15 gm and in jars of 240 gm.

ARISTOCORT® A: **(Lederle)**

Lotion, 0.1% (releases 0.15 mg/spray) in pressurized containers of 15 gm.

Topical Cream, 0.025 and 0.1% with Aquatain® (hydrophilic base) in tubes of 15 and 75 gm and in jars of 240 gm; 0.5% with Aquatain in tubes of 15 gm and in jars of 240 gm.

Topical Ointment 0.1% in tubes of 15 and 75 gm and in jars of 5 lbs; 0.5% in tubes of 15 gm.

ARISTODERM® Foam, 0.1% in pressurized bottles of 15 gm. **(Lederle)**

ARISTOGEL® Gel, 0.1% in tubes of 15 and 75 gm. **(Lederle)**

KENALOG®: **(Squibb)**

Cream, 0.025% in tubes of 15 and 80 gm and in jars of 240 gm and 5.25 lbs; 0.1% in tubes of 15, 60 and 80 gm and in jars of 240 gm and 5.25 lbs; 0.5% in tubes of 20 gm and in jars of 240 gm.

Dental Paste (in Orabase®), 0.1% in tubes of 5 gm.

Lotion, 0.025% in bottles of 60 ml; 0.1% in bottles of 15 and 60 ml.

Ointment, 0.025% in tubes of 15 and 80 gm and in jars of 240 gm; 0.1% in tubes of 15, 60 and 80 gm and in jars of 240 gm; 0.5% in tubes of 20 gm and in jars of 240 gm.

Suspension (IM), 40 mg/ml in vials of 1, 5, and 10 ml.

Suspension (parenteral; not for IV use), 10 mg/ml in multi-dose vials of 5 ml.

KENALOG-H Cream, 1% (hydrophilic base) in tubes of 15 and 60 gm and in jars of 240 gm. **(Squibb)**

TRAMACIN Cream, 0.025 and 0.1% in tubes of 15 and 80 gm and in jars of 280 gm and 5.25 lbs; 0.5% in tubes of 20 gm. **(Johnson & Johnson)**

w/Gramicidin and/or Neomycin Sulfate

MYCOLOG® Cream and Ointment, 0.1% w/neomycin sulfate, 0.25%; gramicidin, 0.025% and nystatin, 100,000 units in tubes of 15, 30 and 60 gm and in jars of 120 gm. **(Squibb)**

Triamcinolone Diacetate

ARISTOCORT®: **(Lederle)**

Suspension Forte, Parenteral (not for IV use), 40 mg/ml in vials of 1 and 5 ml.

Suspension, Intralesional (not for IV use), 25 mg/ml in vials of 5 ml.

Syrup (cherry-flavored), 2 mg/5 ml in bottles of 120 ml.

KENACORT® Syrup (fruit-flavored), 4 mg/5 ml in bottles of 120 ml. **(Squibb)**

Triamcinolone Hexacetonide

ARISTOSPAN® PARENTERAL Suspension, 5 mg/ml in vials of 5 ml contained in a 12.5 ml vial *for intralesional use;* 20 mg/ml in vials of 1 and 5 ml and in Lederject® disposable syringes of 1 ml *for intraarticular use.* **(Lederle)**

AEROLONE COMPOUND

Description: A combination of bronchodilators, each 100 ml of which contain cyclopentamine hydrochloride, 500 mg and isoproterenol hydrochloride, 250 mg, with propylene glycol, ascorbic acid, coloring and purified water. Sodium hydroxide is added to adjust the pH.

Indications: Treatment of bronchospasm associated with acute and chronic bronchial asthma, pulmonary emphysema, bronchitis, and bronchiectasis.

Contraindications: Known hypersensitivity to any of the components or cardiac arrhythmias associated with tachycardia.

Warnings: Occasional patients have been reported to develop severe paradoxical airway resistance with repeated excessive use of isoproterenol inhalation preparations. The cause of this refractory state is unknown. It is advisable that in such instances, the use of this preparation be discontinued immediately and alternative therapy instituted. Deaths have been reported following excessive use of isoproterenol inhalation preparations, and the exact cause is unknown. Cardiac arrest was noted in several instances. Safe use during pregnancy has not been established relative to possible adverse effects on fetal development; therefore, it should not be used in pregnant women unless, in the judgment of the physician, the potential benefits outweigh the possible hazards.

Precautions: This preparation should be used with caution in patients with serious cardiac disease, hypertension or hyperthyroidism.

Adverse Reactions: Insomnia, nervousness, vertigo, tachycardia and palpitation may occur on rare occasions as an indication of overdosage. There is no specific treatment; general management consists of controlling the symptoms of CNS stimulation by using sedatives, such as barbiturates.

Dosage and Administration: *Inhalation.* A nebulizer which produces a fine mist is necessary. The mist is inhaled through the mouth, after which the breath is held for a moment. Usually, 6 to 12 inhalations will bring adequate relief. The technique is the same as that for administering epinephrine, 1:100. Mild cases may require only 1 treatment/day, whereas very severe cases may need the medication every 15 minutes. Ordinarily, the number of treatments for repeated attacks should not exceed 8/24 hours.

Availability:
AEROLONE® COMPOUND Solution in bottles of 30 ml. **(Lilly)**

ALBUMIN, NORMAL HUMAN SERUM

Description: Normal human serum albumin is a sterile preparation of serum albumin obtained by cold alcohol fractionation from pooled whole human plasma that is nonreactive for hepatitis B surface antigen. Not less than 96% of its total protein is albumin. Each 100 ml of the solution contains 25 gm of serum albumin osmotically equivalent to 500 ml, or 5 gm equivalent to 100 ml, of normal human plasma. It contains no added preservative, but may contain stabilizing agents. The product is low in salt content; 20 ml contain only 60 mg of sodium ion rather than the 420 mg normally present in plasma.

Normal human serum albumin reduces edema by its osmotic diuretic effect, raises the serum protein level in hypoproteinemic states, and reduces hemoconcentration and blood viscosity by its osmotic effect. Each 20 ml of the 25% solution injected intravenously into a well hydrated patient draws approximately 70 ml of additional fluid into the circulation within 15 minutes. If hemorrhage is present, the hemodilution results in anemia which, if severe, should be corrected by blood transfusion.

Indications: Primarily as replacement therapy in hypoproteinemic states; for emergency treatment of hypovolemic shock due to burns, trauma, hemorrhage and infection and to promote diuresis in cases of edema due to chronic renal disease and hepatic cirrhosis. The preparation has been reported useful in treating hyperbilirubinemia associated with erythroblastosis fetalis by transferring bilirubin from the extravascular to the intravascular space, binding it to albumin, and eliminating it in the subsequent exchange transfusion. It has also been reported useful in the prevention or treatment of cerebral edema due to neurosurgical procedures or following anoxia. Normal human serum albumin may be used as a vehicle for diluting and transfusing packed red blood cells. Serum hepatitis reportedly has not occurred following this method of transfusion. In general, serum albumin may be given in conjunction with whole blood, plasma, isotonic saline solution, glucose or sodium lactate solutions.

Contraindications: Severe anemia or cardiac failure.

Warnings: If shock is due to hemorrhage, concomitant administration of whole blood or red blood cells should be considered to maintain adequate oxygen-carrying capacity of the blood. Large amounts of fluid lacking in clotting factors may dilute the patient's clotting factors. Patients receiving large amounts of albumin for plasma replacement following blood loss may need in addition, fresh platelet-rich plasma or whole blood if prothrombin levels are low because of dilution.

Precautions: Since no preservatives are used, this product should be used promptly after opening the bottle. It should not be used if the solution is turbid when viewed with transmitted light. Caution should be used when administering the 25% concentration to patients with low cardiac reserve, in order to prevent hypervolemia with subsequent cardiac failure and/or pulmonary edema. If dehydration accompanies shock, additional intravenous fluids must be administered in conjunction with normal serum albumin. The loss of blood due to hemorrhage necessitates evaluation of the need for transfusion of red blood cells. In the management of shock due to hemorrhage, it is imperative that all severed blood vessels be ligated, since the correction of hypotension may cause recurrence of hemorrhage.

In the presence of edema and in those situations where the administration of sodium is contraindicated, normal serum albumin may be administered slowly undiluted, or may be diluted in glucose solution rather than in saline. In patients who have approximately normal blood volumes, the rate of administration should not exceed 1 ml/minute of the 25% concentration, as more rapid infusion or injection could result in circulatory embarrassment and pulmonary edema.

Adverse Reactions: Chills, dyspnea, fever, urticaria, and changes in blood pressure, pulse rate, and respiration have been associated with the administration of this product. If such reaction occurs and the patient requires additional serum albumin, material from a different lot should be used. Pulmonary edema and/or respiratory distress may be due to protein overload caused by too rapid or repeated administration.

Dosage and Administration: *Intravenously.* The dosage for hypoproteinemia, with or without edema, is 1 ml/lb (2.2 ml/kg) daily, given slowly at a rate not exceeding 2 ml/minute. In hypertension or cardiac failure, 20 ml of serum may be added to 30 ml of 10% dextrose solution and injected at a slow rate. Administration of serum albumin in hypoproteinemia is considered supportive and the underlying pathology of the condition must be corrected.

In the treatment of shock, the initial dose is 1 ml/lb of body weight followed in 15 to 30 minutes if necessary with about 1/2 of this dose. In the presence of dehydration, other fluid must be given with serum albumin since its action is based upon an osmotic effect.

In the treatment of burns, the initial dose is 1 ml/lb of body weight, followed by a 5% solution of albumin (40 ml of albumin plus 160 ml of normal saline or 5% dextrose) in sufficient quantities to control hemoconcentration and to maintain electrolyte balance.

In the treatment and prevention of cerebral edema, 60 to 80 ml of serum albumin are administered within a period of 8 to 10 minutes and fluids are withheld completely during the succeeding 8 hours.

For more detailed information regarding dosage, the physician is urged to consult the manufacturers' package literature.

Availability:

ALBUMIN (PLASBUMIN™-5) Solution, 5% in vials of 50 ml w/o administration set and vials of 250 and 500 ml w/administration set; 25% (salt-poor) in vials of 20 ml w/o administration set and vials of 50 and 100 ml w/administration set. **(Cutter)**

ALBUMINAR-5 Solution, 5% in bottles of 250 and 500 ml w/administration set. **(Armour)**

ALBUMINAR-25 Solution (salt-poor), 25% in vials of 20, 50 and 100 ml w/administration set. **(Armour)**

ALBUMISOL® Solution, 5% in vials of 250 and 500 ml w/administration set; 25% (salt-poor) in vials of 50 ml w/administration set. **(Merck Sharp & Dohme)**

ALBUSPAN® Solution, 5% in vials of 250 and 500 ml w/administration set; 25% (salt-poor) in vials of 50 ml w/administration set. **(Parke-Davis)**

ALBUTEIN Solution, 5% in vials of 250 and 500 ml; 25% (salt-poor) in vials of 20, 50 and 100 ml w/administration set. **(Abbott)**

BUMINATE Solution, 5% in vials of 250 and 500 ml w/administration set; 25% (salt-poor) in vials of 20, 50 and 100 ml w/administration set. **(Hyland)**

ALKAVERVIR

Description: Alkavervir is a partially purified mixture of biologically standardized alkaloids extracted from the root of veratrum viride. It occurs as a light yellow powder that is practically insoluble in water and freely soluble in alcohol. The drug produces a hypotensive effect and concomitant bradycardia by affecting chemoreceptors of the circulatory system. The increase in afferent impulses leads to a negative feedback from the CNS which thereby decreases sympathetic tone, increases vagal tone and reduces blood pressure. Both systolic and diastolic pressures are lowered and the heart is slowed. Following oral administration, the onset of action usually occurs within 2 hours and the effects may continue for 4 to 6 hours.

Indications: Relief of mild to moderate essential hypertension.

Contraindications: Adams-Stokes disease; vasovagal syncope, pheochromocytoma, coarctation of the aorta, increased intracranial pressure, and idiosyncrasy or hypersensitivity to the drug.

Warnings: Caution must be employed when alkavervir is used in conjunction with surgery because of the additive effects of the anesthetic and preanesthetic agents on the blood pressure.

Veratrum alkaloids may accentuate the cardiac irritability produced by digitalis, and when used concurrently may induce ectopic cardiac rhythms. The bradycrotic effect of these alkaloids are additive to, but not synergistic with, that produced by morphine and related drugs. If a saluretic agent is to be added to the regimen of patients previously or currently receiving a veratrum alkaloid, a reduced dosage of both drugs is indicated since the combination results in a greater reduction in blood pressure than can be achieved by either one alone. Simultaneous use of ganglionic blocking agents, hydralazine, guanethidine, methyldopa, chlorthalidone, or thiazides with alkavervir necessitates an immediate dosage reduction of each drug by about 50%. Careful observation for changes in blood pressure must be made when combined therapy is used.

Safe use during pregnancy or lactation has not been established. Therefore, the drug should be used in pregnant or lactating patients or in women of childbearing age only when in the judgment of the physician, its use is deemed essential to the welfare of the patient.

Precautions: As with other hypotensive agents, special caution should be employed when treating patients with angina pectoris, coronary thrombosis, decreased renal function, or cerebrovascular disease. Hypertensive patients with chronic renal disease may adjust poorly to lowered blood pressure levels. Very large doses may be associated with reflex respiratory depression and direct bronchiolar constriction. Caution is warranted when treating patients with a history of bronchial asthma who may react adversely to the cholinergic effects of veratrum preparations. Discontinue therapy if signs of nausea and excessive slowing of the pulse rate are observed. Temporary lessening of dosage may be necessary during periods of excessively hot weather.

Adverse Reactions: Most adverse reactions seen during therapy with this drug have been of a minor and self-limiting nature. These include: bradycardia, anorexia, nausea and vomiting, excessive hypotension and prostration, epigastric and substernal burning, which may be mistaken for anginal pectoris, unpleasant taste, sialorrhea, salivation, sweating, blurring of vision, hiccups, mental confusion and cardiac arrhythmias, usually controlled with atropine. Very large doses have caused bronchiolar constriction and respiratory depression.

Dosage and Administration: *Orally.* Dosage must be adjusted according to the patient's response in order to achieve maximal therapeutic benefits with minimal toxicity. The recommended initial dose is 8 or 9 mg daily administered in 3 or 4 equally divided doses. The usual dosage ranges from 8 to 15 mg daily given in 3 or 4 divided doses at intervals of not less than 4 hours, preferably after meals and at bedtime.

Availability:
VERILOID® Tablets, 2 and 3 mg in bottles of 100. **(Riker)**

ALLOPURINOL

Chemical Name: 4-Hydroxypyrazolo(3,4-d) pyrimidine (HPP).

Description: Allopurinol is a structural analogue of the natural purine base hypoxanthine in which the carbon and nitrogen at the number 7 and number 8 positions in the purine nucleus are transposed. It occurs as a colorless, odorless, tasteless solid, insoluble in cold water and soluble in about 250 parts of hot water.

It is a potent inhibitor of xanthine oxidase, the enzyme responsible for the conversion of hypoxanthine to xanthine and of xanthine to uric acid, the end product of purine metabolism. It acts on purine catabolism, without disrupting the biosynthesis of vital purines, by inhibiting the production of uric acid by blocking the biochemical reactions immediately preceding its formation. Its action differs from that of uricosuric agents which lower the serum uric acid level by increasing urinary excretion of uric acid. It thereby avoids the hazard of hyperuricosuria in patients with gouty nephropathy or with a predisposition to the formation of uric acid stones. The drug possesses no uricosuric, antiinflammatory or analgesic activity.

The half-life of allopurinol in the body is determined both by renal excretion and by oxidation to 4,6-dihydroxypyrazolo (3,4-d) pyrimidine (oxypurinol). The renal clearance of oxypurinol is slower than that of allopurinol and since it is also an inhibitor of xanthine oxidase it contributes significantly to the enzyme inhibition. Both allopurinol and oxypurinol also tend to inactivate xanthine oxidase, which further controls the level of its activity.

The combined increase in hypoxanthine and xanthine excreted in the urine usually, but not always, is considerably less than the accompanying decline in urinary uric acid. This phenomenon may be due to a pseudo-feedback inhibition of purine biosynthesis by allopurinol ribotide. However, it has been demonstrated that reutilization of both hypoxanthine and xanthine for nucleotide and nucleic acid synthesis is markedly enhanced when their oxidations are inhibited by allopurinol. This reutilization and the normal feedback inhibition which would result from an increase in available purine nucleotides serve to regulate purine biosynthesis, and, in essence, the defect of the over-producer of uric acid is thereby compensated. Innate deficiency of xanthine oxidase, which occurs in xanthinuria as an inborn error of metabolism, has been shown to be compatible with normal well-being. While urinary levels of oxypurines attained with full doses of allopurinol may in exceptional cases equal those (250 to 600 mg/day) which in xanthinuric patients have caused formation of urinary calculi, they usually fall in the range of 50 to 200 mg. No evidence of renal damage or the formation of xanthine crystalluria has been observed clinically.

The serum concentration of oxypurines in patients receiving allopurinol is usually in the range of 0.3 to 0.4 mg% compared to a normal level of approximately 0.15 mg%. A maximum of 0.9 mg% was observed when the serum urate was lowered to less than 2 mg% by high doses of the drug. In one exceptional case a value of 2.7 mg% was reached. These amounts are far below the saturation level at which precipitation of xanthine or hypoxanthine would be expected to occur so that tissue deposition is unlikely. The solubilities of uric acid and xanthine in the serum are similar (about 7 mg%) while hypoxanthine is much more soluble. The finding that the renal clearance of oxypurines is at least 10 times greater than that of uric acid explains the relatively low serum oxypurine concentration at a time when the serum uric acid level has decreased markedly. At serum oxypurine levels of 0.3 to 0.9 mg%, the oxypurine:inulin clearance ratios were between 0.7 and 1.9. The glomerular filtration rate and urate clearance in patients receiving allopurinol do not differ significantly from those obtained prior to therapy. The rapid renal clearance of oxypurines suggests that allopurinol therapy should be of value in allowing patients with gout to increase their purine excretion.

Administration of allopurinol generally results in a fall in both serum and urinary uric acid usually within 2 to 3 days. The magnitude of this decrease can be manipulated since it is dose-dependent to a limited extent. A week or more of treatment with allopurinol may be required for the full effects of the drug to be manifest since the serum uric acid level falls gradually, similarly serum uric acid levels may return to pretreatment levels slowly, usually after a period of 7 to 10 days following cessation of therapy. This reflects primarily the slow accumulation and clearance of oxypurinol. In some patients, particularly those with tophaceous gout, a significant fall in urinary uric acid excretion may not occur. It has been postulated that this may be due to the mobilization of urate from the tissue deposits as the serum uric acid level begins to fall.

Allopurinol also inhibits the enzymatic oxidation of mercaptopurine, the sulfur-containing analogue of hypoxanthine, to 6-thiouric acid. This oxidation, which is catalyzed by xanthine oxidase, inactivates mercaptopurine. Hence, the inhibition of such oxidation by allopurinol may result in as much as 75% reduction in the therapeutic dose requirement of mercaptopurine when the two compounds are given simultaneously. However, salicylates may be administered together with allopurinol for their antirheumatic effect without compromising the action of allopurinol—unlike the status with other drugs which, unlike allopurinol, have a uricosuric effect. Results of reproductive studies in animals have shown that the drug does not produce teratologic effects in the offspring.

Indications: Allopurinol is a potentially harmful drug and strict attention should be given to the indications for its use. It is intended for the treatment of gout, either primary or secondary to the hyperuricemia associated with blood dyscrasias. It is also indicated in primary and secondary nephropathy, with or without accompanying symptoms of gout. It may be given prophylactically to prevent tissue urate deposition or renal calculi in patients with leukemias, lymphomas or other malignancies who are receiving cancer chemotherapy with its resultant elevating effect of serum uric acid levels. It is especially useful in patients with gouty nephropathy, in those who form renal urate stones, and in those with severe gouty arthritis. It is effective in preventing the occurrence and recurrence of uric acid stones and gravel, and in the treatment and prevention of acute urate nephropathy in patients with neoplastic disease. *Its use in other hyperuricemic conditions is not recommended at this time.*

Contraindications: Allopurinol is not recommended for nursing mothers or for children with the exception of those with hyperuricemia secondary to malignancy. **Patients who have developed a severe reaction to allopurinol should not be restarted on the drug.**

Warnings: A few cases of reversible clinical hepatoxicity have been noted in patients taking allopurinol and in some patients asymptomatic rises in serum alkaline phosphatase or serum transaminase have been observed. Accordingly, periodic liver function tests should be performed during the early stages of therapy, particularly in patients with preexisting liver disease. Due to the occasional occurrence of drowsiness, patients should be alerted to the need for due precautions when engaging in activities where alertness is mandatory. It is advised that iron salts should not be given simultaneously with allopurinol since animal studies have suggested an increase in hepatic iron accumulation. This drug should not be administered to immediate relatives of patients with idiopathic hemochromatosis. When employed to inhibit the oxidation of mercaptopurine or azathioprine, the dose of both these drugs should be reduced to $^1/_4$ to $^1/_3$ of the therapeutic requirement when used alone, and then adjusted to the observed effects. Since the effect of xanthine oxidase inhibition on the human fetus is still unknown, allopurinol should be used in pregnant women or women of childbearing age only if the potential benefits to the patient are weighed against the possible risks to the fetus.

Precautions: Allopurinol has been reported to prolong the half-life of the anticoagulant dicumarol; therefore, this interaction should be kept in mind when this drug is given to patients who are receiving anticoagulant therapy; also their coagulation time should be reassessed. Prophylactic administration of colchicine is advisable during the early stages of therapy to prevent precipitation of acute attacks of gout. A fluid intake sufficient to yield a daily urinary output of at least 2 liters and the maintenance of a neutral or, preferably, slightly alkaline urine are desirable to avoid the theoretic possibility of formation of xanthine calculi under the influence of allopurinol therapy, and to help prevent renal precipitation of urates in patients receiving concomitant uricosuric agents. Patients with impaired renal function should be carefully observed during the early stages of allopurinol administration and the drug withdrawn if increased abnormalities in renal function appear, since a few patients with preexisting renal disease have shown a rise in BUN levels. It is recommended that periodic determinations of liver and kidney function and complete blood counts be performed.

Adverse Reactions: The most common adverse reaction is skin rash which is most frequently maculopapular in type; exfoliative, urticarial and purpuric lesions as well as erythema multiforme and toxic epidermal necrolysis have also been reported. Occasionally, fever has accompanied the dermatitis. Therapy must be discontinued promptly at the first sign of a rash, since this reaction may become quite serious if treatment is continued after symptoms appear. After a drug-free period, it is generally possible to resume use of the drug at a lower dosage without untoward incident. Alopecia (few cases), drowsiness, nausea, vomiting, diarrhea and intermittent abdominal pain have been reported occasionally. Symptoms suggestive of drug idiosyncrasy characterized by fever, chills, leukopenia or leukocytosis, eosinophilia, arthralgias, skin rash, and pruritus have been reported in a few patients. There have been additional reports of agranulocytosis, anemia, aplastic anemia, bone marrow depression, leukopenia, pancytopenia, thrombocytopenia, single reports of peripheral neuritis, and a few reports of cataracts. The relationship of allopurinol to these events has not been confirmed. Although a generalized hypersensitivity vasculitis or necrotizing angiitis which can result in irreversible hepatotoxicity and death has been reported, these reactions are rare.

Dosage and Administration: *Orally.* To achieve full control of gout and to lower serum uric acid to normal or near-normal levels, the dosage will vary with the severity of the disease. The average is 200 to 300 mg/day for those with mild gout and 400 to 600 mg/day for those with moderately severe tophaceous gout, preferably taken after meals. The appropriate dosage may be administered in divided doses or as a single dose of 300 mg. Similar considerations govern the regulation of dosage for maintenance purposes in secondary hyperuricemia. To prevent uric acid nephropathy during vigorous therapy of neoplastic disease, 600 to 800 mg daily for 2 or 3 days is advisable together with a high fluid intake. The minimal effective dose is 100 to 200 mg daily and the maximal recommended dose is 800 mg daily. By selecting the appropriate dose, together with the use of uricosuric agents in certain patients, it is possible to reduce the serum uric acid level to normal and, if desired, to hold it as low as 2 to 3 mg% indefinitely. Children, 6 to 10 years of age, with secondary hyperuricemia associated with malignancies may be given 300 mg of allopurinol daily, while those under 6 years of age generally are given 150 mg. The response is evaluated after about 48 hours of therapy and dosage is adjusted if necessary. Patients taking uricosuric agents, colchicine and/or antiinflammatory agents should continue this therapy, while dosage of allopurinol is adjusted until a normal serum uric acid level and freedom from acute attacks have been maintained for several months. The physician is urged to study the package literature carefully for the complete prescribing information on this drug.

Availability:
ZYLOPRIM®: Tablets, 100 mg (scored) in bottles of 100 and 1000; 300 mg in bottles of 30, 100 and 500. Both potencies are also available in unit-dose packages of 1000.

(Burroughs Wellcome)

ALPHAPRODINE HYDROCHLORIDE Ⓒ II

Chemical Name: *dl*-1,3-Dimethyl-4-phenyl-4-piperidinol propionate hydrochloride.

Description: Alphaprodine hydrochloride is a rapid-acting, synthetic narcotic analgesic with a short duration of action. It is related to meperidine in chemical structure and pharmacologic action, and like meperidine it produces a generalized depression of the central nervous system with euphoric and sedative effect. It occurs as a white, crystalline powder that is freely soluble in water, soluble in alcohol, and is stable to heat, light, and air.

Alphaprodine is a potent narcotic agent that produces drug dependence of the morphine type; however, its analgesic and depressant actions are less intense but more prompt and of shorter duration than those of morphine.

Following subcutaneous administration, analgesia usually occurs within 5 minutes and persists for about 2 hours. When injected intravenously, the onset of action occurs within a few minutes and lasts for approximately 1½ to 2 hours.

Indications: Obstetrical analgesia, urological examinations and procedures, particularly cystoscopy, preoperatively in both major and minor surgery, and for renal or biliary colic, or cardiovascular pain.

Contraindications: In patients with known hypersensitivity to the drug.

Warnings: Alphaprodine is an addicting drug. The depressant effects are potentiated in the presence of drugs such as barbiturates, general anesthetic agents and some phenothiazines; accordingly, the dosage of alphaprodine should be reduced when used concomitantly with such agents. As with other opiates, this drug should be used with extreme caution in conditions such as increased intracranial pressure, hepatic insufficiency, severe CNS depression, myxedema, acute alcoholism, delirium tremens, convulsive disorders and Addison's disease; and in patients receiving MAO inhibitors because of the possibility of hypotension. It is not intended for relief of chronic pain because its short duration of action would require more frequent administration and might increase the possibility of addiction. While the safety and efficacy of the drug have been established as an analgesic agent in obstetrics, there is limited experience regarding its use earlier in pregnancy. As is true in all narcotic agents, particularly during the first trimester, use of this agent requires that its potential benefits be weighed against its possible hazards.

Precautions: Intramuscular administration is not recommended because of limited clinical experience with this route of administration. When the drug is given intravenously, special attention should be given to the possibility of respiratory depression. This condition develops most readily in patients with severe pulmonary disease and in the elderly or debilitated patients.

Adverse Reactions: Respiratory depression has been noted occasionally following the administration of alphaprodine preoperatively and during labor. This may be severe enough to warrant active measures, particularly in neonatal situations. It is recommended that levallorphan tartrate be administered in such cases to combat the respiratory changes. Dizziness, drowsiness, sweating, and urticaria have been reported. Nausea, vomiting, restlessness and confusion are rarely encountered. Coma, shallow respiration, cyanosis, hypotension, pinpoint pupils, and early unconsciousness are symptoms of severe toxic effects from overdosage. If these occur, either levallorphan tartrate or nalorphine hydrochloride should be administered intravenously. **Note:** The use of a narcotic antagonist in a patient addicted to narcotics may precipitate an acute withdrawal syndrome. In the presence of apnea, artificial respiration and oxygen therapy should be employed and a patent airway assured. The patient should be carefully observed during the first 24 hours.

Dosage and Administration: *Subcutaneously or intravenously. Obstetrics,* initially 40 to 60 mg subcutaneously after cervical dilation has begun; dose may be repeated as required at 2-hour intervals. May be combined with scopolamine or atropine, and may be used in conjunction with nerve block or inhalation analgesia as required. If barbiturates are used concomitantly, there is a greater risk of respiratory depression. *Minor surgery,* initially 40 mg subcutaneously or 20 mg intravenously. *Preoperative medication in major surgery,* initially 20 to 40 mg subcutaneously or 10 to 20 mg intravenously. *Renal or biliary colic, cardiovascular pain,* initially 20 to 60 mg subcutaneously or 20 to 30 mg intravenously. *Urologic procedures,* initially 20 to 30 mg intravenously. Levallorphan tartrate is an effective narcotic antagonist in the event of overdosage; it may be used to prevent narcotic-induced respiratory depression. Administered parenterally in the ratio of 1 part levallorphan to 50 parts alphaprodine. *Dosage for children under 12 years of age has not been established.*

Availability:
Ⓒ NISENTIL® Solution, 40 mg/ml in ampuls of 1 ml in cartons of 10 ampuls; 60 mg/ml in ampuls of 1 ml in cartons of 10 ampuls, and in vials of 10 ml. **(Roche)**

ALPHOSYL HC

Description: The cream and lotion contain allantoin, 2% and coal tar extract, 5%; in addition the cream contains 0.5% hydrocortisone, whereas the lotion contains 0.25% hydrocortisone. The formulation is said to enhance the ability of the skin to absorb and retain moisture, dissolve the cement substances in psoriatic scales and promote the retention of the amphoteric proteins of the stratum corneum.

Indications: Topical treatment of psoriasis, especially in acute inflammatory conditions in intertriginous areas where dry, scaly lesions may cause constant friction and irritation. May also be used to relieve the itching, scaling and erythema associated with other chronic dermatoses.

Contraindications: Preparations containing hydrocortisone should not be used on infected areas unless accompanied by appropriate antibacterial therapy; or in the presence of viral infections such as herpes simplex, vaccinia and varicella, or tuberculosis of the skin. Coal tar extracts are contraindicated in infected or impetiginized lesions.

Precautions: The use of coal tar for prolonged periods and continuously in contact with skin may cause irritation. If irritation or sensitization occurs, treatment should be discontinued. Contact with the eyes should be avoided.

For adverse reactions and further precautions associated with hydrocortisone, the general statement on the Adrenal Corticosteroids should be consulted.

Dosage and Administration: *Topically.* The cream or lotion is applied by rubbing into the lesion 2 to 4 times daily as indicated. Where heavy scaling or crusting occurs, the usual bath to soften and facilitate removal of scale is recommended before applying the lotion.

Availability:
ALPHOSYL® HC: **(Reed & Carnrick)**
Cream in tubes of 30 gm.
Lotion in bottles of 120 ml.

ALSEROXYLON

Description: Alseroxylon is the fat-soluble, extracted root fraction of *Rauwolfia serpentina.* It is referred to as the alseroxylon fraction and contains reserpine and other nonadrenolytic amorphous alkaloids.

It has been suggested that the drug probably produces its antihypertensive effect through depletion of tissue stores of catecholamines (epinephrine and norepinephrine) from peripheral sites. By contrast, its sedative and tranquilizing properties are thought to be related to depletion of 5-hydroxytryptamine from the brain.

Alseroxylon is characterized by a slow onset of action and by a sustained effect. Both its cardiovascular and central nervous system effects may persist following withdrawal of the drug. Orally, 1 mg of alseroxylon is approximately equivalent to 0.2 mg of reserpine.

Indications: Treatment of mild essential hypertension alone or as adjunctive therapy with other antihypertensive agents in the more severe forms of hypertension.

Since the pharmacologic actions of alseroxylon are essentially those of its major component, reserpine, see monograph on Reserpine for detailed information on contraindications, warnings, precautions and adverse reactions.

Dosage and Administration: *Orally.* For adults, the average initial dose is 2 to 4 mg daily. The usual maintenance dose is 2 mg daily. Higher doses should be used cautiously because severe mental depression and other side effects may be considerably increased. Concomitant use of alseroxylon and ganglionic blocking agents, guanethidine, veratrum, hydralazine, methyldopa, chlorthalidone, or thiazides necessitates careful titration of dosage with each one of these agents.

Availability:
RAUTENSIN® Tablets, 2 mg in bottles of 100 and 500. **(Dorsey)**
RAUWILOID® Tablets, 2 mg in bottles of 100 and 1000. **(Riker)**

ALUMINUM NICOTINATE

Description: Aluminum nicotinate is a chemical complex, 625 mg of which consists of aluminum hydroxydinicotinate, 450 mg and nicotinic acid (niacin), 155 mg equivalent in activity to 500 mg of niacin.

Aluminum nicotinate hydrolyzes uniformly in the gastrointestinal tract into free nicotinic acid with aluminum hydroxide splitting off to provide an effective buffering action. Nicotinic acid, in large doses, appears to cause a reduction in serum lipids. This effect is manifested on cholesterol, triglycerides, phospholipids and free fatty acids. The action appears to be both prompt and sustained. The mechanism of action of nicotinic acid is unknown, although a number of theories have been advanced. The hypocholesteremic action has been explained on the basis of increased oxidation of cholesterol or of inhibition of cholesterol synthesis. Nicotinic acid has also been shown to inhibit catecholamine-induced release of fatty acids from adipose tissue, and this action may account for its apparent hypolipemic effect.

The exact relationship of hyperlipidemia to atherosclerosis or coronary heart disease is not known. Although nicotinic acid appears to be effective in correcting serum lipid abnormalities, its influence on morbidity and mortality cannot be assessed at the present time.

Indications: As an adjunctive aid to diet and other measures in conditions where a reduction of serum cholesterol and total lipid levels in hypercholesteremia and hyperlipemia is desirable. It may also be useful in reducing xanthomatous tissue cholesterol deposits.

Contraindications: In patients with hepatic dysfunction, active peptic ulcer, or with arterial bleeding. Also, in those with known idiosyncrasy to nicotinic acid.

Warnings: Use of aluminum nicotinate during pregnancy or lactation or in women of childbearing age requires that the potential benefits of the drug be weighed against its possible hazards to the mother and child. Until further clinical experience is gained, its use in children is not recommended at the present time.

Precautions: Patients with peptic ulcer, liver or gallbladder disease should be under close medical supervision during therapy, and frequent monitoring of liver function tests and blood glucose levels should be performed at regular intervals. Diabetic patients may require an adjustment of diet and insulin dosage in the event of decreased tolerance. Patients taking hypotensive drugs of the adrenal-blocking type should be observed for signs of postural hypotension. Since elevated uric acid levels have been known to occur, patients predisposed to gout require special care.

Adverse Reactions: Occasional reactions to large doses of niacin are decreased glucose tolerance (resembling diabetic type curve) sometimes with glycosuria, temporary activation of peptic ulcer, transient jaundice, and metabolic disturbance of liver function without definitive hepatic pathology. These reactions, although not reported with this product, were found to be reversible when therapy with niacin had been discontinued. Certain transitory skin changes have been observed with niacin; these included dryness and keratosis nigricans, particularly in the axillae. Niacin may also produce temporary flushing, headache, hyperuricemia, toxic amblyopia, hypotension, pruritus, and mild gastrointestinal distress.

Dosage and Administration: *Orally.* The usual dosage schedule is 2 to 4 tablets 3 times daily with or after meals. The dosage should be individualized according to the effect on serum lipid levels.

Availability:
NICALEX® Tablets, 625 mg (white) in bottles of 100 and 1000. **(Merrell-National)**

AMANTADINE HYDROCHLORIDE

Chemical Name: 1-Adamantanamine hydrochloride.

Description: Amantadine hydrochloride is a stable, white, crystalline substance, readily soluble in water and in alcohol. Its synthetic chemical structure is unrelated to those of other chemotherapeutic antiinfective compounds, thus providing a different approach to the prevention (prophylaxis) of respiratory infections caused by influenza A_2 (Asian) virus strains.

Amantadine appears to exert its antiviral effect by preventing the release of infectious viral nucleic acid into the host cells rather than by viricidal activity. In tissue culture the drug inhibits several strains of influenza A_2 (Asian) virus. Its mechanism of action in the treatment of Parkinson's disease has not been determined. Animal studies show that the drug increases the release of dopamine from neuronal storage sites and, at comparable clinical doses, it did not produce anticholinergic activity. Clinical improvement is usually noted in 2 to 5 days; however, its therapeutic efficacy appears to be less than that of levodopa. Data are insufficient for recommending its safe and effective use in drug-induced parkinsonism.

Approximately 90% of an orally administered dose is recovered in the urine indicating complete absorption; about 50% is excreted in unchanged form within 20 hours. No evidence of metabolites has been found.

Laboratory and clinical studies with amantadine indicated no disturbances in the kidney, liver, bone marrow, or blood that were definitively related to the drug. Also, no significant pharmacological interactions of amantadine with other drugs, in particular penicillin, tetracycline, acetylsalicylic acid, antihistamines, oral antidiabetic drugs and cardiovascular agents have been demonstrated.

Indications: Prophylactic agent for influenzal respiratory infections caused by susceptible influenza A_2 virus strains. It is indicated in those individuals considered to be high-risk patients. These include individuals of all ages who suffer from chronic debilitating diseases such as cardiovascular, pulmonary, renal or metabolic disorders, and in older age groups. When respiratory illness is thought to be due to susceptible influenza A_2 virus strains, the drug should be used prophylactically in all those who have come in contact with the patient. There is no clinical evidence that this drug is effective in the prophylaxis of any influenzal or respiratory illness other than A_2 (Asian) influenza. Therefore, this drug should be restricted to the prophylaxis of influenza A_2 (Asian), and should not be used in the treatment of patients with established A_2 (Asian) influenza or viral infections. Also indicated in the treatment of idiopathic Parkinson's disease, postencephalitic parkinsonism, and symptomatic parkinsonism which may follow injury to the CNS caused by carbon monoxide poisoning, and in elderly patients who have developed parkinsonism in association with cerebral arteriosclerosis. In responsive patients, relief of the parkinsonian symptoms is usually evident within 48 hours. The drug has also been found useful in the treatment of drug-induced extrapyramidal reactions.

Contraindications: In patients hypersensitive to the drug.

Warnings: When amantadine hydrochloride is administered to patients with central nervous system disease, particularly geriatric patients with cerebral arteriosclerosis, and patients with a history of epilepsy or other "seizures," strict observation of the patients for possible untoward central nervous system effects of the drug is required (see adverse reactions). Because long-term experience with this medication has been limited in patients on psychopharmacologic therapeutic agents or central nervous system stimulants, careful observation is required if these patients are given amantadine. Intolerance has not been noted when medication followed alcohol ingestion; however, full consideration should be given to any symptoms that may occur. Patients who experience CNS effects or blurring of vision should be cautioned against operating a motor vehicle or working in situations in which complete alertness is important. Congestive heart failure may develop in patients with a history of cardiac failure or peripheral edema. Since laboratory studies with animals given excessive doses produced some embryotoxic and teratogenic effects in animal fetuses, the use of this drug in women of childbearing age should be undertaken only after weighing the possible risks to the fetus against the benefits to the patient. This drug should not be administered to nursing mothers.

Precautions: When amantadine is used concurrently with anticholinergic agents, the dose of either drug should be reduced if atropine-like symptoms develop. Therapy should not be abruptly terminated since a parkinsonian crisis may result. Careful adjustment of dosage is necessary in patients with renal impairment, congestive heart failure, peripheral edema, or orthostatic hypotension. Accumulation of the drug with toxic effects can occur when renal function is inadequate. Care should also be exercised when administering the drug to patients with liver disease, or to those with a history of recurrent eczematoid rash, or with psychosis or severe psychoneurosis uncontrolled by chemotherapeutic agents, and when used concurrently with CNS stimulants.

Adverse Reactions: The most frequently occurring serious complications include depression, congestive heart failure, orthostatic hypotensive episodes, psychosis, and urinary retention. Rarely observed were convulsions, leukopenia, and neutropenia. Those of a less serious nature include hallucinations, confusion, anxiety and irritability; anorexia, nausea, and constipation; ataxia and dizziness (lightheadedness); livedo reticularis, and peripheral edema. Less frequently occurring side effects include vomiting; dry mouth; headache; dyspnea; fatigue, insomnia, and a sense of weakness. Skin rash, slurred speech, and visual disturbance were infrequently observed and, rarely, eczematoid dermatitis and oculogyric episodes. There is no specific antidote for overdosage. General supportive measures should be employed along with immediate gastric lavage or induction of emesis. Fluids should be forced and, if necessary, given intravenously. Since the excretion rate of amantadine increases rapidly when the urine is acidic, the administration of urine acidifying fluids may help to increase its elimination from the body. The patient's vital signs should be monitored, and if hyperactivity and convulsions develop, sedatives and anticonvulsant agents should be administered. The patient should be observed for the possible development of arrhythmias and hypotension; and blood electrolytes, urine pH, and urinary output should be checked. If anuria develops, catheterization should be instituted.

Dosage and Administration: *Orally. For parkinsonism:* The daily dosage is 100 mg (1 capsule) 2 times daily. When combined with other antiparkinson drugs, the initial dose is 100 mg daily; may be increased to 200 to 400 mg (2 to 4 capsules) daily in divided doses if necessary. *For prophylaxis of influenza A_2:* **Adults**—The daily dosage is 200 mg (2 capsules or 4 teaspoonsful of syrup taken once a day or 1 capsule or 2 teaspoonsful of syrup taken twice a day). If untoward reactions of the central nervous system develop on a once-a-day dosage schedule, then a split dosage schedule is advisable. **Children, 1 to 9 years of age**—The total daily dose should be calculated on the basis of 2 to 4 mg/lb of body weight, but should not exceed 150 mg/day. The daily dose, *given as the syrup,* should be administered in 2 to 3 equal portions. **Children, 9 to 12 years of age**—The total daily dose is 200 mg given as 1 capsule (100 mg) or 2 teaspoonsful (100 mg) twice daily. Treatment should be started as soon as possible after contact with individuals suffering from Asian (A_2) influenzal respiratory illness and should be continued on a daily basis for at least 10 days following a known exposure, or up to 30 days in case of possible repeated and unknown exposures. Under circumstances where repeated, uncontrolled and unknown exposures to the infection are possible, amantadine can be given on a continuous daily regimen for up to 90 days. *For drug-induced extrapyramidal reactions:* The usual dosage is 100 mg twice daily; however, some patients may require up to 300 mg daily.

Availability:
SYMMETREL®: **(Endo)**
Capsules, 100 mg in bottles of 100 and 500.
Syrup, 50 mg/5 ml in bottles of 1 pint.

AMBENONIUM CHLORIDE

Chemical Name: [Oxalylbis(iminoethylene)]bis[(*o*-chlorobenzyl)diethylammonium] dichloride.

Description: Ambenonium chloride is a synthetic quaternary ammonium compound which occurs as a white, crystalline powder freely soluble in water.

The drug reversibly inactivates cholinesterase, thus potentiating the effects of endogenous acetylcholine. Evidence suggests that it may also stimulate the motor-end-plate. It appears to have a more prolonged effect than neostigmine, with less severe gastrointestinal reaction. Also, bronchial secretion of mucus appears to be less with this drug than with either neostigmine or pyridostigmine. Ambenonium chloride has been found useful in patients who cannot tolerate neostigmine bromide or pyridostigmine bromide because of hypersensitivity to the bromide ion.

Indications: Treatment of myasthenia gravis.

Contraindications: Ambenonium should not be administered concurrently with belladonna derivatives (atropine) since they may suppress the muscarinic symptoms of overdosage. It is also contraindicated in patients receiving mecamylamine.

Warnings: Other cholinergic agents should not be administered concomitantly with this drug except under strict medical supervision.

Precautions: Utmost care and supervision of the patient are required, since the warning of overdosage is slight and the requirements of patients vary tremendously. Constant consideration should be given to the fact that a narrow margin exists between the first appearance of side effects and serious toxic symptoms. Therefore, caution in increasing the dosage is essential. Ambenonium should be used with extreme caution in patients with bronchial asthma and in the presence of intestinal or urinary tract obstruction. If the drug is intended for use in pregnant women or in women of childbearing potential, the physician must evaluate the risk to the fetus versus the potential benefits to the patient.

Adverse Reactions: Those associated with systemic cholinergic activity such as sweating, miosis, muscular weakness, urinary symptoms, and an increase in the production of saliva. Gastrointestinal manifestations of a cholinergic nature, such as vomiting, diarrhea, and cramping are also seen. These are similar to those noted with neostigmine. In addition, CNS reactions such as nervousness, confusion, and headache may occur. Overdosage is usually manifested by excessive gastrointestinal stimulation, excessive salivation, miosis, and serious fasciculations of voluntary muscles. If these occur, the drug should be temporarily discontinued and 0.5 to 1 mg of atropine should be given intravenously; artificial respiration, endotracheal intubation, oxygen and other supportive measures may also be necessary.

Dosage and Administration: *Orally.* The patient's response will determine the precise dosage of the drug. The starting dose is usually 5 mg with a range of 5 to 25 mg 3 or 4 times daily being necessary in moderately severe disease. Other cholinergic medication should be discontinued when ambenonium therapy is instituted.

Availability:
MYTELASE® Caplets®, 10 mg in bottles of 100. **(Winthrop)**

AMBENYL EXPECTORANT Ⓒ

Description: Reduces the frequency of paroxysms of coughing. Each 5 ml contains:

Codeine sulfate	10 mg
Bromodiphenhydramine hydrochloride	3.75 mg
Diphenhydramine hydrochloride	8.75 mg
Ammonium chloride	80 mg
Potassium guaiacolsulfonate	80 mg
Menthol	0.5 mg
Alcohol	5 %

Indications: Antitussive and expectorant for the control of cough due to colds or allergy.

Contraindications: Ambenyl should not be given to premature or newborn infants. It is also contraindicated in patients who are hypersensitive to any of the components, in those who have asthmatic attacks, narrow-angle glaucoma, prostatic hypertrophy, stenosing peptic ulcer, pyloroduodenal obstruction, bladder neck obstruction, and in patients who are taking MAO inhibitors.

Warnings: Codeine sulfate may be habit-forming. Overdosage or accidental ingestion of large quantities of antihistamines may produce convulsions or death, especially in infants and children. As in the case of other preparations containing central nervous system depressant drugs, patients receiving Ambenyl should be cautioned about probable additive effects with alcohol and other central nervous system depressants (hypnotics, sedatives and tranquilizers). Patients who become drowsy should be cautioned against engaging in activities requiring alertness such as driving a car or operating heavy machinery or appliances when taking this drug. Although there is no evidence that the use of Ambenyl is detrimental to the mother or fetus, the use of any drug during pregnancy or lactation should be carefully assessed. Because of the anticholinergic effect of diphenhydramine hydrochloride, an inhibitory effect on lactation may occur.

Precautions: Bromodiphenhydramine and diphenhydramine have an atropine-like action which should be considered when prescribing Ambenyl. Use with caution in patients with a history of asthma.

Adverse Reactions: Patients sensitive to any of the components may experience drowsiness, confusion, nervousness, restlessness, nausea, vomiting, diarrhea, blurring of vision, diplopia, difficulty in urination, constipation, nasal stuffiness, vertigo, palpitation, headache, insomnia, urticaria, drug rash, photosensitivity, hemolytic anemia, hypotension, epigastric distress, tightness of the chest and wheezing, thickening of bronchial secretions, dryness of mouth, nose, and throat and tingling, heaviness, and weakness of hands.

Dosage and Administration: *Orally.* Adults, 1 to 2 teaspoonsful 4 times a day. Children, ½ to 1 teaspoonful 3 or 4 times a day.

Availability:
Ⓒ AMBENYL® Expectorant in bottles of 120 ml, pints and gallons, and in 5-ml unit-dose containers. **(Marion)**

AMESEC

Description: Each Pulvule or Enseal contains:

Aminophylline	130 mg
Ephedrine hydrochloride	25 mg
Amobarbital	25 mg

Indications: Antispasmodic and sedative for the prevention and treatment of asthma.

Contraindications: Hypersensitivity to any of the components.

Warnings: Amobarbital may be habit-forming.

Precautions: Administer with caution to patients who are overstimulated by ephedrine or other sympathomimetic drugs, and in the presence of severe cardiac disease, hypertension, or hyperthyroidism. The CNS-depressant effects of amobarbital may be additive with those of other similar acting drugs including alcohol.

Adverse Reactions: Patients hypersensitive to CNS stimulants may become hyperactive and emotionally upset and may complain of insomnia, nervousness, nausea, or vomiting. Tachycardia and extrasystoles may be produced.

Dosage and Administration: *Orally,* 1 to 5 Pulvules every 24 hours, or 1 Enseal once, twice, or 3 times in each 24-hour period. To prevent nocturnal asthmatic attacks, 1 Pulvule plus 1 Enseal at bedtime.

Availability:
AMESEC®: **(Lilly)**
Enseals® in bottles of 100.
Pulvules® (capsules) in bottles of 100 and 500.

AMIKACIN SULFATE

Description: Amikacin is a semisynthetic aminoglycoside antibiotic derived from kanamycin. In vitro studies indicate that the drug possesses a broad range of activity against gram-negative and gram-positive organisms. Some gram-negative strains that have shown resistance to other aminoglycosides including gentamicin, tobramycin, and kanamycin have been found to be susceptible to amikacin. Gram-negative organisms sensitive to the drug include Pseudomonas, *Escherichia coli,* Proteus (both indole positive and negative), Providencia, Klebsiella-Enterobacter-Serratia, Acinetobacter (formerly Mima-Herellea), and *Citrobacter freundii.* Sensitive gram-positive organisms include Staphylococcus (both penicillinase- and nonpenicillinase-producing strains) including those that have been found resistant to methicillin. Those less sensitive include *Streptococcus pyogenes,* enterococci and *Streptococcus pneumoniae* (formerly *Diplococcus pneumoniae).* An important characteristic of amikacin is that it resists degradation by most aminoglycoside-inactivating enzymes known to affect gentamicin, tobramycin and kanamycin. It has been reported to be clinically effective against such resistant organisms as *Proteus rettgeri, Providencia stuartii, Serratia marcescens,* and *Pseudomonas aeruginosa.*

Intramuscular injection of 250 mg of the drug yields a peak serum level of 12 mcg/ml at about 1 hour; this falls to 0.3 mcg/ml at approximately 10 hours. Intravenous infusion in doses of 500 mg yields a peak serum level of 38 mcg/ml in 30 minutes (end of infusion); this falls to 24 mcg/ml, 18 mcg/ml and 0.75 mcg/ml at 30 minutes, 1 hour and 10 hours respectively. Repeated injections do not lead to accumulation of the drug in the blood if renal function is normal. Pharmacokinetic studies in normal adult individuals reveal the mean serum half-life to be slightly over 2 hours with a mean total apparent volume of distribution of 24 liters (28% of body weight). By the ultrafiltration technique, reports on serum protein binding range from 0 to 11%. The mean serum clearance rate was found to be about 100 ml/min and the renal clearance rate to be 94 ml/min. The drug is excreted by the kidney primarily by glomerular filtration. When renal function is normal, about 92% of an intramuscular dose is excreted unchanged within 8 hours, and 98% within 24 hours. In the first 6 hours mean urine concentrations were reported to be 563 mcg/ml following a 250-mg dose, 697 mcg/ml following a 375-mg dose and 832 mcg/ml following a 500 mg dose. Amikacin diffuses into cerebrospinal, pleural and amniotic fluids and into the peritoneal cavity.

The drug is potentially nephrotoxic, ototoxic, and neurotoxic; therefore, simultaneous use of other drugs causing similar disturbances, particularly kanamycin, gentamicin, tobramycin, neomycin, streptomycin, cephaloridine, paromomycin, viomycin, polymycin B, colistin, and vancomycin should be avoided. Additionally, it should not be given concurrently with potent diuretics such as ethacrynic acid, furosemide, meralluride sodium, mercaptomerin sodium, or mannitol. Some diuretics themselves cause otoxicity, and intravenously administered diuretics enhance aminoglycoside toxicity by altering antibiotic concentrations in serum and tissue.

Indications: Clinical trials have demonstrated the drug's usefulness in treating such serious diseases as bacteremia, septicemia, including neonatal sepsis; serious infections of the respiratory tract, bones, joints, CNS, including meningitis, and of the skin and soft tissues; intraabdominal infections, including peritonitis, and in burns and postoperative infections, including postvascular surgery; and serious, complicated and recurrent urinary tract infections. Bacteriologic studies should be performed to identify the causative organisms and their susceptibility to the drug. Amikacin may be considered as initial therapy in suspected gram-negative infections, and therapy may be instituted before obtaining the results of susceptibility testing.

The contraindications, warnings, precautions and adverse reactions are generally those associated with other aminoglycoside antibiotics. See monographs on Gentamicin Sulfate, Tobramycin Sulfate, and Kanamycin Sulfate.

Dosage and Administration: *Intramuscularly* or *intravenously*. The recommended dosage for adults, children, and older infants with normal renal function is 15 mg/kg/day divided into 2 or 3 equal doses administered at equally-divided intervals. For newborn infants, the recommended initial loading dose is 10 mg/kg of body weight, followed with a dosage of 7.5 mg/kg every 12 hours. The usual duration of treatment is 7 to 10 days. *The total daily dose by all routes of administration should not exceed 15 mg/kg/day.*

Availability:
AMIKIN™ Injection in vials of 100 and 500 mg and 1 gm and in disposable syringes of 500 mg.
(Bristol)

AMINOCAPROIC ACID

Chemical Name: 6-Aminohexanoic acid.

Description: Aminocaproic acid is a synthetic monoaminocarboxylic acid which acts by inhibiting fibrinolysis. It occurs as a white to pale yellow powder freely soluble in water and slightly soluble in alcohol. The drug is discolored in the presence of aldehydes and aldehydic sugars.

The fibrinolysis-inhibitory effects appear to act principally via inhibition of plasminogen activator substances and, to a lesser degree, through antiplasmin activity. The drug is absorbed rapidly following oral administration and peak plasma levels are obtained in approximately 2 hours after a single dose. Whether administered orally or intravenously, a major portion of the drug is recovered unmetabolized in the urine. Its renal clearance is high, about 75% of the creatinine clearance. After prolonged administration, the drug is distributed throughout both the extravascular and intravascular compartments of the body and readily penetrates human red blood and other tissue cells.

Indications: Recommended for use, in many instances, in the treatment of excessive bleeding resulting from systemic and urinary fibrinolysis; in life-threatening situations, however, fresh whole blood transfusions, fibrinogen infusions and other emergency measures may be required. Specificity of action is inherent in its ability to inhibit both plasminogen activators and, to a lesser degree, plasmin activity. Systemic hyperfibrinolysis frequently may be associated with surgical complications following cardiac surgery, with or without cardiac bypass procedures, and portacaval shunt; hematologic disorders such as aplastic anemia, abruptio placentae, hepatic cirrhosis, neoplastic disease such as carcinoma of the prostate, lung, stomach and cervix.

Urinary fibrinolysis, usually a normal physiologic phenomenon, frequently may be associated with life-threatening complications following severe trauma, anoxia and shock. Symptomatic of such complications is surgical hematuria (following prostatectomy and nephrectomy) or nonsurgical hematuria (accompanying polycystic or neoplastic diseases of the genitourinary system).

Contraindications: A recognized, active intravascular clotting process.

Warnings: Since the effect of the drug on the fetus and transplacental pervasion is unknown, its use during the first and second trimesters of pregnancy should be confined to instances where the need outweighs possible hazards.

Precautions: The drug should be used only in dire emergencies where hemorrhage results from an overactivity of fibrinolysin. It should NOT be used without a definite diagnosis and/or laboratory findings indicative of hyperfibrinolysis; neither should it be used in patients with cardiac, hepatic or renal diseases without exercising due caution. The physician should be aware that this drug may possess the potential hazard of causing endocardial hemorrhage and myocardial fat degeneration. Rapid intravenous administration should be avoided since this may induce hypotension, bradycardia and/or arrhythmia.

Adverse Reactions: Occasionally, nausea, cramps, diarrhea, dizziness, tinnitus, malaise, conjunctival suffusion, stuffed nose, headache and skin rash have been reported. Rarely has it been necessary to discontinue medication or reduce dosage because of one or more of these effects. One fatality due to the development of cardiac and hepatic lesions was reported. Thrombophlebitis, a possibility with all intravenous therapy, should be avoided by paying strict attention to the proper insertion of the needle and the fixing of its position.

Dosage and Administration: The use of this drug should be accompanied by tests designed to determine the degree of fibrinolysis present. An initial priming dose of 5 gm (orally or IV) followed by 1 to 1.25 gm every hour thereafter should achieve and sustain plasma levels of 0.13 mg/ml of the drug. This is the concentration apparently necessary to inhibit systemic hyperfibrinolysis. A dosage of 30 gm/day should not be exceeded. *Orally. Acute bleeding syndromes:* Suggested dosage is 5 gm during the first hour followed by 1 gm every hour for about 8 hours or until the bleeding has been controlled. *Intravenously.* May be given by infusion, employing as the vehicle either water for injection, normal saline, 5% dextrose or Ringer's solution. The possibility of hypotension, bradycardia and/or arrhythmia may be avoided by refraining from rapid intravenous administration of the undiluted solution. *Acute bleeding syndromes:* Suggested dosage is 4 to 5 gm (16 to 20 ml) by infusion, during the first hour, followed by an infusion at the rate of 1 gm (4 ml) every hour for about 8 hours or until the bleeding has been controlled.

Availability:

AMICAR®: **(Lederle)**

Intravenous Solution, 250 mg/ml in vials of 20 ml.

Syrup, 250 mg/ml in bottles of 1 pint.

Tablets, 500 mg (scored, white) in bottles of 100.

AMINOPHYLLINE

Chemical Name: Theophylline ethylenediamine.

Description: Aminophylline is generally described as a double salt composed of theophylline and ethylenediamine, but is probably better represented as a salt of theophylline, e.g., aminophylline contains not less than 84% and not more than 86% of anhydrous theophylline (C_7H_8-

N_4O_2), and not less than 14% and not more than 15% of ethylenediamine ($C_2H_8N_2$), both calculated on the anhydrous basis. Aminophylline occurs as white or slightly yellowish granules or powder and has a slight ammoniacal odor and a bitter taste. It is soluble in water and insoluble in alcohol.

Aminophylline is a xanthine derivative with pharmacological effects on various structures. It is a CNS stimulant and has a specific use as a respiratory stimulant. Aminophylline has important actions on the circulatory system and all parts of the circulatory system are affected in some way. The direct myocardial action of aminophylline causes an increase in cardiac output which is not due to a more rapid cardiac rate for it may occur in the absence of tachycardia. There is an accompanying decrease in the venous filling pressure of the heart. In heart failure, the combination of cardiac stimulation and lowering of venous pressure leads to a marked increase in cardiac output which occurs almost immediately.

Experimentally, it can be demonstrated that aminophylline dilates coronary arteries and increases coronary blood flow. While prompt relief of pain has occasionally been observed to follow the administration of this drug in cardiac infarction, this apparently beneficial effect is rare and there is always danger that the stimulating action of the drug will harm a heart handicapped by a reduced blood supply. Aminophylline causes a marked increase in cerebral vascular resistance with an accompanying decrease in cerebral blood flow. The effects of aminophylline on the systemic blood pressure are unpredictable. The actions which would favor an increase in blood pressure are central vasomotor and direct myocardial stimulation. Conversely, the factors favoring a decrease in blood pressure are central vagal stimulation and peripheral vasodilation. The end result of the opposing action on blood pressure is not striking but a slight elevation usually occurs, mainly as a result of the increase in cardiac output in spite of peripheral vasodilation.

The smooth muscle of bronchi is relaxed by aminophylline, probably by a prostaglandin action, and this action makes it of great value in the treatment of asthma. It is particularly useful in patients refractory to epinephrine. Aminophylline is a diuretic, but its action is short in duration. The diuretic action is due mainly to the hemodynamic actions which result in an increased cardiac output, renal blood flow and glomerular filtration rate. However, aminophylline is capable of depressing the renal tubular reabsorptive transport of electrolytes.

Indications: Symptomatic relief of pulmonary emphysema, bronchial asthma, status asthmaticus, Cheyne-Stokes respiration, bronchitis and other pulmonary diseases associated with bronchospasm. Due to erratic absorption, orally administered aminophylline usually is not very effective clinically. In combination with ephedrine and a barbiturate, however, it often provides relief for less severe chronic asthma. The drug is used in acute pulmonary edema only if edema is accompanied by elevated blood pressure; it is contraindicated in hypotension. It may be of value in angina pectoris or coronary thrombosis, but results have been variable and unpredictable and the value of the drug in these conditions has not been established.

Contraindications: Hypotension, in the presence of coronary artery disease or angina pectoris when myocardial stimulation would be harmful, and in patients with peptic ulcer.

Warnings: Overdosage may result in peripheral vascular collapse and acute toxicity. The addition of a barbiturate may make the combination habit-forming. Patients should be cautioned that the compounds containing barbiturates can cause drowsiness which may impair their ability to perform potentially hazardous tasks such as driving a car or operating machinery.

Precautions: Cautious use is advised in patients who are overstimulated by ephedrine or other sympathomimetic drugs and in those with poor renal function, severe cardiac disease, hypertension, or hyperthyroidism. The ethylenediamine component can result in sensitivity reactions and contact dermatitis. Metabolism of aminophylline may be impaired in patients with severe pulmonary, renal or hepatic disease. Because too rapid intravenous administration may be associated with a transitory lowering of blood pressure, aminophylline should be injected slowly at rates approximating 1 ml/minute and used with considerable caution in the early stages of coronary occlusion. Rectal administration may cause local irritation. Intramuscular injection may be painful. It should not be administered concomitantly with other xanthine preparations.

Adverse Reactions: Nausea, vomiting, abdominal cramps, anorexia, reactivation of peptic ulcer, and intestinal bleeding may occur. Headache, nervousness, insomnia, skin rash, palpitation, dizziness or lightheadedness also may occur. Large doses may produce anxiety, excitement, confusion, accelerated or slow pulse, elevated blood pressure and deep respiration, all possible signs of overdosage. Large doses may also produce CNS irritability, increased reflex irritation of peripheral muscles and marked diuresis. ECG changes, shortened prothrombin and clotting times and transient proteinuria, albuminuria, and leukocytosis have occurred. Rapid intravenous injection may produce headache, flushing, palpitations, dizziness, fall in blood pressure or precordial pain. **Note:** Fatalities due to overdosage of aminophylline have been reported.

Dosage and Administration: *Orally,* 200 to 300 mg 3 or 4 times daily. *Intramuscularly,* 500 mg (2 ml) as required. *Intravenously,* 250 mg in 10 or 20 ml of diluent injected slowly as required. *Rectally,* one 250- or 500-mg suppository once or twice daily or 3 to 5 ml of solution as required. The frequency of dosage should be established by the physician. The 125-mg suppository may be used in patients weighing at least 30 lbs. For children, the doses are proportionately smaller and should be determined according to the child's age and weight. Extreme caution is required in infants weighing less than 25 lbs. Dosage always should be adjusted according to the individual's requirements.

Availability:

Aminophylline

Injection: Ampuls of 2 ml (500 mg) for IM use, 10 ml (250 mg) and 20 ml (500 mg) for IV use. **(Abbott, Searle and others)**

Suppositories: 100, 125, 250 and 500 mg in cartons of 12 and 25. **(Searle, Wyeth and others)**

Tablets: 100 and 200 mg in bottles of 100 and 1000. **(Searle, ICN and others)**

AMINODUR® Dura-tabs® Tablets, 300 mg in bottles of 100 and 250. **(Cooper)**

RECTALAD®-AMINOPHYLLINE Rectal Solution, 300 mg in disposable rectal applicators of 3 ml; 450 mg in disposable rectal applicators of 4.5 ml. **(Wallace)**

SOMOPHYLLIN®: **(Fisons)**

Oral Liquid (sugar and alcohol free), 105 mg/5 ml (equiv. to 90 mg theophylline base) in bottles of 240 ml.

Rectal Solution, 300 mg/5 ml (equiv. to 255 mg theophylline base) in bottles of 90 and 150 ml with accompanying Rectal Ject syringe.

w/Amobarbital

Pulvules®, 100 mg w/Amytal®, 32 mg in bottles of 100. **(Lilly)**

Combinations

AMODRINE® Tablets, 100 mg with racephedrine hydrochloride, 25 mg and phenobarbital, 8 mg in bottles of 100 and 500. **(Searle)**

AMINOSALICYLIC ACID

Chemical Name: *Para*-aminosalicylic acid.

Description: Aminosalicylic acid is used in the form of the acid, sodium, potassium and calcium salts. The acid occurs as a white, crystalline powder slightly soluble in water and soluble in alcohol. The salts are white to cream colored crystals freely soluble in water and vary from slightly soluble to sparingly soluble in alcohol.

Aqueous solutions of aminosalicylic acid are very unstable since decarboxylation with the formation of meta-aminophenol occurs. Decomposition occurs if the crystalline acid is exposed to heat, air, or moisture. Under no circumstances should a solution of aminosalicylic acid be used if its color is darker than that of a freshly prepared solution. Although it is closely related chemically to salicylic acid, the amino group greatly alters its systemic and bacteriostatic effects. It differs pharmacologically from the salicylates in that it is neither analgesic nor antipyretic and has no direct effect on the respiratory center.

The compound has a bacteriostatic effect on the organism *Mycobacterium tuberculosis* and inhibits the onset of bacterial resistance to streptomycin and isoniazid. The precise mechanism by which it inhibits growth of the tuberculous organism has not been established. However, this effect is increased by the addition of either streptomycin or isoniazid.

Aminosalicylic acid and its salts are readily and almost completely absorbed from the gastrointestinal tract. Following oral administration of a 4-gm dose of the acid, maximal plasma concentration of about 75 mcg/ml is attained within 1½ to 2 hours. Absorption of the sodium salt is even more rapid.

The drug diffuses into most tissues and fluids and reaches levels in pleural fluid equal to those in the circulation; however, it does not appear in the cerebrospinal fluid in significant amounts. The drug has a half-life of approximately 1 hour and negligible amounts are detected in the blood within 4 to 5 hours after administration of a conventional dose; over 80% is excreted by the kidney in approximately 10 hours with more than 50% in the acetylated form. Since the free acid is relatively insoluble and the acetylated form even more so, the urine should be kept neutral or alkaline during treatment in order to prevent crystalluria. The sodium salt reduces significantly the risk of this complication. Probenecid has been shown to decrease the renal excretion of aminosalicylic acid; blood levels are about doubled when this agent is employed.

Indications: Treatment of pulmonary and extrapulmonary tuberculosis when it is administered with streptomycin, isoniazid, or both. **Note:** Aminosalicylic acid should not be used as the sole therapeutic agent in the treatment of tuberculosis.

Contraindications: Severe hypersensitivity to aminosalicylic acid and its congeners. The sodium and calcium salts may be contraindicated in patients with certain conditions.

Precautions: If symptoms of hypersensitivity develop, therapy should be discontinued. The drug should be used cautiously in patients with impaired renal function, decreased hepatic function, or gastric ulcer. The clinician should bear in mind that since the drug decreases the rate of acetylation of isoniazid, the plasma levels of isoniazid are thereby increased. Patients who are being treated with anticoagulants may require an adjustment of the anticoagulant dosage. Crystalluria due to aminosalicylic acid may be prevented by maintaining the urine at a neutral or alkaline pH. This compound and its salts deteriorate rapidly in contact with water, heat, and sunlight. A brownish or purplish color of the powder or tablets, and especially of a solution made with them, is indicative of such deterioration. If this is evident, the drug should be discarded.

Adverse Reactions: The most commonly noted is *gastrointestinal intolerance* manifested by nausea, vomiting, diarrhea, and abdominal pain. Others noted were *hypersensitivity reactions* (fever, skin eruptions of various types, an infectious mononucleosis-like syndrome, leukopenia, agranulocytosis, thrombocytopenia, hemolytic anemia, jaundice, hepatitis, encephalopathy, Loffler's syndrome, and vasculitis); *endocrine reactions* (goiter with or without myxedema), and *homeostatic reactions* (hypokalemia and acidosis).

Dosage and Administration: *Orally.* The adult dose of aminosalicylic acid is 10 to 12 gm daily, ranging from 8 to 15 gm daily, either as a single dose or in 2 or 3 divided doses. The pediatric dosage is 200 to 300 mg/kg/day in a single dose or in 3 or 4 divided doses. Gastrointestinal disturbances may be minimized by taking the drug with meals or with aluminum hydroxide gel.

Availability:

Aminosalicylic Acid

Enseals® Tablets, 500 mg in bottles of 500. **(Lilly)**

Tablets, 500 mg in bottles of 100 and 1000. **(Various Mfrs.)**

Calcium Aminosalicylate

PARASAL® CALCIUM: **(Panray)**

Powder in bottles of 1 lb.

Tablets, 500 mg in bottles of 1000.

Sodium Aminosalicylate

PARASAL® SODIUM: **(Panray)**

Crystals in cartons of 100 × 4.18 gm packets.

Powder in bottles of 1 lb.

Powder (lyophilized) in vials of 50 ml.

Tablets, 500 mg and 1 gm in bottles of 1000.

AMITRIPTYLINE HYDROCHLORIDE

Chemical Name: 10,11-Dihydro-*N,N*-dimethyl-5*H*-dibenzo[a,d]cycloheptene-Δ^5,γ-propylamine hydrochloride.

Description: Amitriptyline hydrochloride, a tricyclic compound, is a derivative of benzocycloheptadiene. Its chemical structure is similar to that of imipramine except for the substitution of C for N in the cycloheptene ring. Amitriptyline occurs as a white, crystalline powder that is readily soluble in water and very soluble in alcohol.

Amitriptyline is not a monoamine oxidase inhibitor nor does it act primarily by stimulation of the central nervous system. Although the manner in which it exerts its antidepressant action has not been clarified, it appears to inhibit the passage of norepinephrine into the adrenergic neurons. Pharmacologically, this action enhances and prolongs sympathetic activity, and this may account for the drug's antidepressant activity.

Following oral administration, amitriptyline is rapidly absorbed and metabolized. Plasma levels were found to be practically negligible, although significant amounts appeared in the urine within 4 to 6 hours and approximately 1/2 to 1/3 of the drug was excreted within 24 hours. Amitriptyline is detoxified in the liver where it is metabolized by N-demethylation to nortriptyline, which is further demethylated. Virtually the entire dose was found to be excreted as conjugates of glucuronide or sulfate, with little unchanged drug appearing in the urine.

Indications: Treatment of endogenous depression, and in depression accompanied by anxiety. A combination of amitriptyline with a phenothiazine tranquilizer is indicated for the treatment of patients with moderate to severe anxiety and/or agitation and depressed mood; patients with depression in whom anxiety and/or agitation are severe; patients with depression and anxiety in association with chronic physical disease; schizophrenics with associative depressive symptoms.

Contraindications: In patients who have shown prior hypersensitivity to amitriptyline. Concomitant administration with MAO inhibitors is also contraindicated. A medication-free period of at least 2 weeks should be observed when transferring patients from MAO inhibitors to amitriptyline to avoid a hyperpyretic crisis, severe convulsions, and death from occurring. This drug should not be given to patients during the acute recovery phase following myocardial infarction.

Warnings: Amitriptyline may block the antihypertensive action of guanethidine and similarly acting compounds. Since paralytic ileus may occur when the drug is used in combination with anticholinergic-type drugs, close supervision and careful adjustment of dosage is essential. It should be used with caution in patients with impaired liver function, in those who are hyperthyroid or who are receiving thyroid medication, in those with a history of seizures, and, because of its atropine-like action, in patients with a history of urinary retention, angle-closure glaucoma (even average doses may precipitate an attack), or increased intraocular pressure. Close supervision of patients with cardiovascular complications is advised since amitriptyline has been reported to produce cardiac arrhythmias and sinus tachycardia and to prolong the conduction time. Myocardial infarction and stroke may also occur. Patients on amitriptyline therapy should be cautioned against performing hazardous tasks because of the possibility of impaired judgment or diminished reflexes. Safe use of amitriptyline during pregnancy and lactation has not been established; therefore, in administering the drug to pregnant patients, nursing mothers, or to women who may become pregnant, the potential benefits must be weighed against the possible hazards to mother and child. Amitriptyline is not recommended for use in children under 12 years of age.

Precautions: Since amitriptyline may precipitate or aggravate psychotic manifestations in schizophrenic patients, a reduction of the dose or the concomitant administration with a major tranquilizer such as perphenazine is advised. The possibility of suicide in seriously depressed patients is an inherent factor of the illness and might remain a real danger until a significant remission has been obtained. Such patients should be closely supervised throughout therapy. Amitriptyline may potentiate the response to alcohol and other CNS depressants, and may increase the hazards of electroconvulsive therapy. Transient delirium has been reported in patients who were treated with 1 gm of ethchlorvynol (a hypnotic) and 75 to 150 gm of amitriptyline. Changes in blood sugar levels have also been noted. If possible, therapy with this drug should be discontinued several days before elective surgery.

Adverse Reactions: The following reactions have been noted with tricyclic compounds in general and may occur with the use of amitriptyline. *Cardiovascular:* Hypotension or hypertension, tachycardia, palpitation, myocardial infarction, arrhythmias, heart block, stroke. *CNS and Neuromuscular:* Confusional states; disturbed concentration; disorientation; delusions; hallucinations; excitement; anxiety; restlessness; insomnia; nightmares; numbness, tingling and paresthesias of the extremities; peripheral neuropathy; incoordination; ataxia; tremors; seizures; alteration in EEG patterns; extrapyramidal symptoms; tinnitus. *Anticholinergic:* Dry mouth, blurred vision, disturbance of accommodation, constipation, paralytic ileus, urinary retention, dilatation of urinary tract. *Allergic:* Skin rash, pruritus, urticaria, photosensitization, edema of face and tongue. *Hematologic:* Bone marrow depression including agranulocytosis, leukopenia, eosinophilia, purpura, thrombocytopenia. *Gastrointestinal:* Nausea, epigastric distress, vomiting, anorexia, stomatitis, peculiar taste, diarrhea, parotid swelling, black tongue, rarely hepatitis (including altered liver function and jaundice). *Endocrine:* Testicular swelling and gynecomastia in the male, breast enlargement and galactorrhea in the female, increased or decreased libido, elevation and lowering of blood sugar levels. *Other:* Dizziness, weakness, fatigue, headache, weight gain or loss, heartburn, increased perspiration, urinary frequency, mydriasis, drowsiness, jaundice, alopecia. *Withdrawal Symptoms:* Abrupt cessation of treatment after prolonged administration may produce nausea, headache, and malaise. These are not indicative of addiction. Overdosage may exacerbate these reactions, especially those of the central nervous and cardiovascular systems. Physostigmine, 1 to 3 mg intravenously, has been reported to counteract these adverse effects. Because physostigmine is rapidly metabolized, dosage should be repeated as required, particularly if life-threatening signs such as arrhythmias, convulsions, and deep coma recur or persist after the initial dose of physostigmine. All the standard measures should be employed to reverse any unfavorable or acute reaction. *For data on the component drug, see individual monograph.*

Dosage and Administration: *Orally.* Dosage should be initiated at a low level and increased gradually, noting carefully the clinical response and any evidence of intolerance. *For adults*—initially, 25 mg 3 times daily; if necessary, may be increased to 150 mg daily. Hospitalized patients may require 100 mg daily initially; the dose may then be increased to as much as 300 mg daily. *For adolescent and elderly patients*—10 mg 3 times daily with 20 mg at bedtime is usually satisfactory. The usual maintenance dose is 25 mg 2 to 4 times daily. In some patients, 10 mg 4 times daily is sufficient. When satisfactory improvement has been reached, dosage should be reduced to the lowest amount that will maintain relief of symptoms. *Intramuscularly.* Initially, 20 to 30 mg (2 to 3 ml) 4 times daily. The tablets should replace the injection as soon as possible.

Availability:

Amitriptyline Hydrochloride

AMITID Tablets, 10, 25 and 50 mg in bottles of 100 and 1000; 75 and 100 mg in bottles of 100. **(Squibb)**

AMITRIL® Tablets, 10, 25, 50, 75 and 100 mg in bottles of 100 and 1000; 150 mg in bottles of 100. **(Warner-Chilcott)**

AMITRIPTYLINE HYDROCHLORIDE Tablets, 10, 25 and 50 mg in bottles of 100 and 1000; 75 and 100 mg in bottles of 100. **(Lederle)**

AMITRIPTYLINE HYDROCHLORIDE Tablets, 10, 25, 50, 75, 100 and 150 mg in bottles of 100 and 1000 and in unit-dose packages of 100. **(Philips Roxane)**

ELAVIL®: **(Merck Sharp & Dohme)**

Injection, 10 mg/ml in rubber-capped vials of 10 ml.

Tablets, 10 and 25 mg in bottles of 100, 1000 and 5000; 50 mg in bottles of 100 and 1000; 75 and 100 mg in bottles of 100; 150 mg in bottles of 30 and 100. All potencies are available in single-unit packages of 100.

ENDEP® Tablets, 10, 25, 50, 75, 100 and 150 mg in bottles of 100 and 500; the 10, 25 and 50 mg tablets in Prescription Pak®s (unit-dose) packages of 60; the 75, 100 and 150 mg tablets in Prescription Paks of 30. The Prescription Paks are available in single units or in trays of 10. All potencies are available in Tel-E-Dose® (unit-dose) packages of 100. **(Roche)**

SK-AMITRIPTYLINE™ Tablets, 10, 25 and 50 mg in bottles of 100 and 1000; 75, 100 and 150 mg in bottles of 100. **(Smith Kline & French)**

w/Perphenazine

ETRAFON®: **(Schering)**

Tablets, '2-10', 10 mg w/perphenazine, 2 mg in bottles of 60, 100, 250 and 500 and in unit-dose packages of 100.

Tablets, **(A)** '4-10', 10 mg w/perphenazine, 4 mg in bottles of 100 and 500 and in unit-dose packages of 100.
Tablets, '2-25', 25 mg w/perphenazine, 2 mg in bottles of 100 and 500 and in unit-dose packages of 100.
Tablets, **(Forte)** '4-25', 25 mg w/perphenazine, 4 mg in bottles of 100 and 500 and in unit-dose packages of 100.
TRIAVIL®: **(Merck Sharp & Dohme)**
Tablets, '2-10', 10 mg w/perphenazine, 2 mg in bottles of 100 and 500 and in single-unit packages of 100.
Tablets, '4-10', 10 mg w/perphenazine, 4 mg in bottles of 100 and 500 and in single-unit packages of 100.
Tablets, '2-25', 25 mg w/perphenazine, 2 mg in bottles of 100 and 500 and in single-unit packages of 100.
Tablets, '4-25', 25 mg w/perphenazine, 4 mg in bottles of 100 and 500 and in single-unit packages of 100.
Tablets, '4-50', 50 mg w/perphenazine, 4 mg in bottles of 60 and 100 and in single-unit packages of 100.

AMOBARBITAL (C-II)

Chemical Name: 5-Ethyl-5-isopentylbarbituric acid.

Description: Amobarbital is a moderately rapid-acting sedative and hypnotic, with a duration of effect of about 8 to 11 hours and a half-life ranging from 14 to 42 hours. Its action is comparable to but of longer duration than that of secobarbital or pentobarbital. It occurs as an odorless, white, crystalline powder with a bitter taste; it is slightly soluble in water and freely soluble in alcohol.

Indications: *Orally,* for the relief of anxiety and tension or as a hypnotic for preanesthetic medication. *Parenterally,* for the control of convulsive seizures due to chorea, eclampsia, meningitis, tetanus, and for the control of reactions associated with poisoning from such drugs as strychnine or picrotoxin. It may also be used for the management of catatonic and negativistic reactions, manic reactions, and epileptiform seizures. It has been found useful in narcoanalysis and narcotherapy, and as a diagnostic aid in schizophrenia.

Contraindications: In patients with a history of porphyria, and in the presence of uncontrolled pain because of the possibility of inducing excitement. It is also contraindicated in patients with severely impaired liver function, and in those hypersensitive to barbituric acid derivatives.

Warnings: May be habit-forming. The rate of intravenous administration must be carefully regulated and should not exceed 1 ml/minute since a too rapid rate or relative overdosage may cause apnea or hypotension. Respiratory depression is more likely to develop when amobarbital is given concurrently with other CNS depressants. Only a clear solution may be injected, and no more than 30 minutes should elapse from the time the ampul is opened and the solution is injected. The sedative effect represents a hazard in ambulatory patients whose activities require alertness and motor coordination.

Precautions: Cautious use in patients with decreased liver function is advised. Dosage and rate of administration should be selected with utmost care in patients with hypertension, hypotension, or with pulmonary or cardiovascular disorders. Pulmonary edema may complicate long periods of unconsciousness. As with any drug, routine caution should be exercised when prescribing for pregnant patients.

Adverse Reactions: Idiosyncrasy, in the form of excitement, hangover, or pain may be experienced. Hypersensitivity reactions occur in some patients, especially in those with asthma, urticaria, or angioneurotic edema. The additive action of this agent when used concomitantly with other CNS depressants such as alcohol or opiates can result in fatality. Symptoms of overdosage include respiratory depression, reduction in superficial and deep reflexes, constriction or dilation of the pupils, decreased urine formation, reduced body temperature, and coma. Gastric lavage, administration of intravenous fluids, and maintenance of blood pressure, body temperature, and adequate respiratory exchange are the usual remedial measures.

Dosage and Administration: *Orally, intramuscularly* or *intravenously.* The average intramuscular dose ranges from 65 mg to 0.5 gm but should not exceed 0.5 gm, and the maximum intravenous dose is 1 gm. No more than 5 ml should be injected at any one site. *For daytime sedation,* the usual adult dosage is 30 to 50 mg 2 or 3 times daily; however, the dose may range from 15 to 120 mg 2 to 4 times daily. *For hypnosis,* the usual adult dose is 100 to 200 mg. *For insomnia,* 65 to 200 mg at bedtime. *For preanesthetic sedation,* 200 mg 1 or 2 hours before surgery. *For labor pain,* the initial dose is 200 to 400 mg; may be repeated at intervals of 1 to 3 hours to a total dose of not more than 1 gm.

Availability:
Ⓒ AMYTAL®: **(Lilly)**
Elixir, 8.8 mg/ml in pints and gallons.
Tablets, 15, 50 and 100 mg in bottles of 100 and 500; 30 mg in bottles of 100, 1000 and 5000.
Ⓒ AMYTAL® SODIUM: **(Lilly)**
Capsules (Pulvules®), 65 mg in bottles of 100, 500 and 5000; 200 mg in bottles of 100 and 500, and in 10 strips of 10 individually labeled blisters each containing 1 capsule.
Sterile Ampoules, U.S.P., 65 mg (dry powder) in packages of 6.
Sterile Ampoules, U.S.P., 125 mg (dry powder) in packages of 6 and 100.
Sterile Ampoules, U.S.P., 250 mg (dry powder) in cartons of 6 and 25 and in cartons of 10 with sterile water for injection.
Sterile Ampoules, U.S.P., 500 mg (dry powder) in cartons of 6 and 25 and in cartons of 10 with sterile water for injection.

AMODIAQUINE HYDROCHLORIDE

Chemical Name: 4-(7-Chloro-4-quinolylamino)-α-(diethylamino)-*o*-cresol dihydrochloride.

Description: Closely related to chloroquine, amodiaquine hydrochloride occurs as a bitter tasting, yellow, crystalline powder soluble in water and sparingly soluble in alcohol. The precise mechanism of antimalarial activity of the 4-aminoquinolines has not been determined. It has been postulated that this activity is based on the ability of these drugs to form complexes with deoxyribonucleic acid. However, the antimalarial activity of this drug appears to be limited to the erythrocytic stages, and is useful in benign tertian and quartan malaria with significant effect in malignant tertian malaria. Amodiaquine interrupts erythrocytic schizogony of the malarial parasites and in this manner is effective in terminating an acute attack. In suppressive treatment, the erythrocytic stage of development is inhibited, thereby the infected individual is kept free of the clinical manifestations of the disease. Infection is not prevented, however, and exo-erythrocytic stages will persist.

Indications: As suppressive treatment and for treatment of acute attacks of malaria due to *Plasmodium vivax, P. malariae, P. ovale,* and susceptible strains of *P. falciparum.* Adequate dosage results in prompt disappearance of plasmodia from the blood stream and clinical recovery from an acute attack. It is not effective against chloroquine-resistant strains of *P. falciparum.*

Contraindications: In the presence of retinal or visual field changes attributable to 4-aminoquinoline compounds, and in patients with known hypersensitivity to these compounds. However, exceptions should be considered in specific circumstances such as in the treatment of acute malarial attacks that are caused by strains of plasmodia susceptible only to these compounds.

Warnings: Since fatalities have been reported when amodiaquine was used for prolonged periods, it is thus not recommended except in a weekly dosage regimen for suppressive therapy of malaria. Cautious use is advised in patients with hepatic disease because of the high concentrations that occur in the liver. Children are especially susceptible to the 4-aminoquinoline compounds; therefore, patients should be cautioned to keep these drugs out of the reach of children. Use of amodiaquine in patients with psoriasis or porphyria may precipitate a severe attack of this condition. Therefore, the drug should not be used in these conditions unless in the judgment of the physician the clinical benefits outweigh the possible hazards. Use during pregnancy should be limited to the treatment of malaria.

Precautions: Use in patients with severe gastrointestinal, neurological, or blood disorders warrants extreme caution. Ophthalmological examinations should be performed prior to and during administration of amodiaquine to detect any eye abnormalities that may develop especially during prolonged use. The drug should not be given together with gold compounds, phenylbutazone or other agents known to cause dermatitis.

Adverse Reactions: Toxic manifestations following short-term use of the drug are rare but include agranulocytosis, nausea, vomiting, diarrhea, fatigue, lassitude, and vertigo. Symptoms involving the gastrointestinal system may be minimized by administering the drug with meals. Leukopenia, pancytopenia and fatal agranulocytosis has been noted in both short- and long-term therapy. Pigmentation of the palate, nailbeds and skin, pleomorphic skin eruptions have occurred but they were readily reversible on withdrawal of the drug. Other complications noted were corneal opacities, keratopathy, retinopathy, toxic psychosis, ototoxicity, toxic hepatitis, neuromyopathy, and polyneuritis. Since absorption of amodiaquine is very rapid and may occur within 30 minutes, symptoms of accidental overdosage manifested by headache, visual disturbances, cardiovascular collapse and convulsion followed by a sudden respiratory and cardiac arrest may occur within this time interval. Treatment is symptomatic and must be prompt, consisting of either inducing emesis or employing gastric lavage. Convulsions due to cerebral stimulation may be controlled by cautious use of an ultra-short acting barbiturate, and should be accomplished before using gastric lavage. When due to anoxia, supportive measures should be employed (oxygen, artificial respiration or vasopressors). After the disappearance of acute symptoms, the patient should be closely observed for at least 6 hours. Fluids may be forced and sufficient ammonium chloride may be administered for a few days in divided doses to acidify the urine and thus promote urinary excretion.

Dosage and Administration: *Orally. Treatment of malaria:* Adults, initially 600 mg followed by 300 mg 6 hours later and 300 mg at 24 and 48 hours. Children, 10 mg/kg of body weight divided into 3 doses at 12-hour intervals. *For suppressive treatment of malaria:* Adults, a single dose of 300 to 600 mg and children, 5 mg/kg (as the base) should be administered every week, preferably on the same day of each week.

Availability:
CAMOQUIN® Hydrochloride Tablets, 200 mg in bottles of 36. **(Parke-Davis)**

AMPHETAMINE Ⓒ

Chemical Name: *dl*-α-Methylphenethylamine.

Description: Amphetamine is a potent sympathomimetic agent and central nervous system stimulant. Physiologic response to the drug is manifested by a decrease in appetite, most likely by stimulation of the cerebral cortex, and an increase in alertness and in motor and psychial activity, coincidental with a decrease in fatigue accompanied by insomnia which may result in depression. The anorectic effect usually diminishes after a few weeks. Its cardiovascular effects have been found to be of a much longer duration than that of epinephrine. However, in contrast to epinephrine, amphetamine does not appear to modify carbohydrate utilization, to increase the blood level of glucose or lactate, or to alter the respiratory quotient. Peripheral effects include elevation of systolic and diastolic blood pressure and weak bronchodilator and respiratory stimulant action.

Amphetamines have a significant potential for abuse. In view of their limited short-term anorectic effect and rapid development of tolerance, they should be used with extreme caution and only for limited periods of time in weight reduction programs.

Indications: Treatment of narcolepsy, minimal brain dysfunction in children manifested by hyperkinetic behavior disorders, and for exogenous obesity as a short-term adjunct (a few weeks) in a regimen of weight reduction based on caloric restriction.

Contraindications: Advanced arteriosclerosis, symptomatic cardiovascular disease, moderate to severe hypertension, hyperthyroidism, known hypersensitivity or idiosyncrasy to the sympathomimetic amines, agitated states, patients with a history of drug abuse. If given during or within 14 days following the administration of monoamine oxidase inhibitors, a hypertensive crisis may result.

Warnings: Tolerance to the anorectic effect usually develops within a few weeks. When this occurs, the recommended dose should not be exceeded in an attempt to increase the effect; rather, the drug should be discontinued. Patients should be cautioned that amphetamines may mask extreme fatigue which can impair their ability to perform potentially hazardous activities (e.g., operating machinery or vehicles). Amphetamines have a significant potential for abuse. Tolerance and extreme psychological dependence have occurred; patients have been known to increase the dosage above that recommended. Should this become evident, the medication should be discontinued. Abrupt cessation following prolonged high dosage administration results in extreme fatigue and mental depression; changes have also been noted on the sleep EEG.

Manifestations of chronic intoxication with amphetamines include severe dermatoses, marked insomnia, irritability, hyperactivity, and personality changes. The most severe manifestation of chronic intoxication is psychosis, often clinically indistinguishable from schizophrenia. Safe use during pregnancy has not been established. Therefore, use of amphetamines by women who are or who may become pregnant and especially those in the first trimester of pregnancy, requires that the potential benefit be weighed against the possible hazard to mother and infant. Amphetamines are not recommended for use as anorectic agents in children under 12 years of age or in hyperkinetic behavior disorders in children under 3 years of age.

Precautions: Should be used sparingly in patients with mild hypertension. It should be considered that the insulin requirements in diabetes mellitus may be altered in association with the use of amphetamines and the concomitant dietary regimen. Amphetamines may also decrease the hypotensive effect of guanethidine. The smallest quantity feasible should be prescribed or dispensed at one time in order to minimize the possibility of overdosage.

Adverse Reactions: *Cardiovascular:* Palpitation, tachycardia, elevation of blood pressure. *Central Nervous System:* Overstimulation, restlessness, dizziness, insomnia, euphoria, dysphoria, tremor, headache; rarely, psychotic episodes at recommended doses. *Gastrointestinal:* Dryness of the mouth, unpleasant taste, diarrhea, other gastrointestinal disturbances. Anorexia and weight loss may occur as undesirable effects when amphetamines are used for other than the anorectic effect. *Allergic:* Urticaria. *Endocrine:* Impotence, changes in libido. Manifestations of acute overdosage may include restlessness, agitation, tremors, confusion, assaultiveness, hallucinations, hyperreflexia, muscle twitching, rapid respiration, and panic states. Fatigue and depression usually follow CNS stimulation. Cardiovascular effects may include arrhythmias, palpitations, hypertension or hypotension and circulatory collapse. Gastrointestinal symptoms are characterized by nausea, vomiting, diarrhea, and abdominal cramps. Fatal intoxication usually terminates in convulsions and coma. Management of acute intoxication is largely symptomatic and includes induction of emesis or gastric lavage, maintenance of adequate circulation and respiratory exchange. The patient should be protected against self-injury and disturbing external stimulation.

Dosage and Administration: *Orally.* Amphetamines should be administered at the lowest effective dosage, and dosage should be individually adjusted. It is advisable to begin treatment with a test dose of 5 mg and to increase the amount progressively until optimal dosage has been determined. *For narcolepsy*—adults, 5 to 60 mg daily; children 6 to 12 years of age, initially, 5 mg daily; may be raised in increments of 5 mg at weekly intervals until optimal response is obtained; children 12 years of age or older, 10 mg daily; may be raised in increments of 10 mg at weekly intervals until optimal response is obtained. *For minimal brain dysfunction in children*—5 to 40 mg or more daily; children 3 to 5 years of age, initially 2.5 mg daily; may be raised in increments of 2.5 mg weekly until optimal response is obtained. The first dose should be given upon awakening and additional doses at intervals of 4 to 6 hours. *For exogenous obesity*—5 to 10 mg 3 times daily, administered 30 to 60 minutes before each meal or 1 or 2 Spansules (long-acting form) in the morning.

Availability:

Ⓒ**II** **Amphetamine Hydrochloride**

Tablets, 5, 10 and 15 mg in bottles of 1000. **(Various Mfrs.)**

Ⓒ **Amphetamine Sulfate**
Tablets, 5, 10 and 15 mg in bottles of 1000. **(Various Mfrs.)**
Ⓒ BENZEDRINE®: **(Smith Kline & French)**
Spansules® (Capsules), 15 mg in bottles of 50.
Tablets, 5 and 10 mg in bottles of 100.

AMPHOTERICIN B

Description: Amphotericin B is an antifungal antibiotic produced from *Streptomyces nodosus.* It has a potency of not less than 0.75 mg of amphotericin B/mg, calculated on the anhydrous basis; amphotericin A may also be present. Amphotericin B occurs as a yellow or orange powder insoluble in water and in alcohol and soluble in propylene glycol. The preparation for intravenous injection containing 50 mg of the antibiotic also contains 41 mg of sodium desoxycholate as a solubilizing agent, and suitable buffering agents. The dry form is stable for 2 years when stored at 15° C. and protected from light. Solutions are stable for 24 hours at room temperature and for 1 week when stored at 4° C.

Amphotericin B is fungistatic rather than fungicidal in concentrations obtainable in body fluids. It probably acts by binding to sterols in the fungus cell membrane with a resultant change in membrane premeability which allows leakage of intracellular components. Mammalian cell membranes also contain sterols and it has been suggested that the damage to human cells (toxicity) and damage to fungal cells (antibiotic effect) may share common mechanisms. This drug is active against the fungi responsible for the deep mycoses; it is ineffective against bacteria, viruses and protozoa. Clinically, it is of value in curing or arresting cryptococcosis (torulosis), mucormycosis (phycomycosis), disseminated North American blastomycosis, disseminated moniliasis, and histoplasmosis, disseminated cryptococcosis and cryptococcic meningitis, and disseminated and meningeal coccidioidomycosis. Although poorly absorbed from the gastrointestinal tract, amphotericin B is active against species of *Candida* in the intestine and small doses may be used orally to treat monilial overgrowth resulting from oral antibiotic therapy (e.g., tetracycline). An oral dose of 3 gm daily produces blood levels ranging from less than 0.12 to about 0.5 mcg/ml. Extremely low levels of the drug can be detected in the spinal fluid. Following intravenous infusion, the drug is excreted slowly by the kidneys and demonstrable blood levels persist for 18 hours or longer. The cumulative urinary output over a 7-day period amounts to approximately 40% of the amount of drug infused. Acquired resistance in vivo has not been reported thus far.

Indications: *Topically,* the drug is used in the treatment of cutaneous and mucocutaneous monilial infections, including intertrigo, interdigital lesions, "diaper rash" and perleche, caused by *C. albicans.* Infections of the scalp and paronychia and onychomycosis due to *Candida albicans* may respond to treatment; however, relapses occur frequently when the drug is discontinued. In monilial infections complicated by concurrent dermatophyte or bacterial infection, supplemental topical and/or systemic antiinfective therapy is indicated. *Intravenously,* the drug is indicated for the treatment of cryptococcosis (torulosis); North American blastomycosis; and the disseminated forms of moniliasis, coccidioidomycosis, and histoplasmosis; mucormycosis (phycomycosis) caused by species of the genera Mucor, Rhizopus, Absidia, Entomophthora, and Basidiobolus; sporotrichosis *(Sporotrichum schenckii);* aspergillosis *(Aspergillus fumigatus).* May be helpful in the treatment of American mucocutaneous leishmaniasis, but it is not the drug of choice for primary therapy.

Contraindications: In patients known to be hypersensitive to the drug unless, in the opinion of the physician, the condition requiring treatment is life-threatening and amenable only to amphotericin B therapy.

Warnings: Amphotericin B injection should be used *primarily* for the treatment of patients with progressive and potentially fatal fungal infections. It is not intended for the treatment of common clinically inapparent forms of fungal disease which show only positive skin or serologic tests. Safe use during pregnancy has not been established; therefore, it should be used in pregnant patients only if the possible benefits to be gained outweigh the potential risks involved.

Precautions: When administered parenterally at therapeutic dosage levels, reactions are quite common, some of which are potentially dangerous. For this reason, amphotericin B should be used parenterally only in hospitalized patients or those under close medical supervision, and should be reserved for those patients in whom a diagnosis of the progressive, potentially serious forms of susceptible mycotic infections has been established, preferably by positive culture or histologic study. Periodic urinalyses, blood urea nitrogen (BUN) or nonprotein nitrogen (NPN) determinations are advisable during therapy. Patients taking the drug for prolonged periods should have liver, kidney and bone-marrow studies done at appropriate intervals. Weekly hemograms and serum potassium determinations are also advisable. Low serum magnesium levels have been noted during treatment with this drug. Whenever the medication is interrupted for a period longer than 7 days, therapy should be resumed by starting with the lowest dosage level (0.25 mg/kg of body weight) and increased gradually. Renal dysfunction is usually reversible on interruption of therapy, but serious and permanent renal damage has been reported in patients given large doses for prolonged periods; this possibility has been reported to increase when the total dosage exceeds 5 gm. Special care is required if amphotericin B is given concomitantly with corticosteroids, other nephrotoxic antibiotics and antineoplastic agents.

Adverse Reactions: Fever (perhaps with chills), headache, anorexia, weight loss, nausea, vomiting and malaise are the most frequently encountered side effects with intravenous therapy. Muscle and/or joint pain may occur. Dyspepsia or cramping epigastric pains and diarrhea may occur. Local venous pain is common, and phlebitis or thrombophlebitis, normochromic normocystic anemia, and hypokalemia occur frequently. Reactions occurring less frequently or rarely are anuria (oliguria); cardiovascular toxicity including arrhythmias, ventricular fibrillation, cardiac arrest, hypertension, and hypotension, coagulation defects, thrombocytopenia; leukopenia; agranulocytosis; eosinophilia; leukocytosis; melena or hemorrhagic gastroenteritis; maculopapular rash; hearing loss; tinnitus; transient vertigo; blurred vision or diplopia; peripheral neuropathy; convulsions and other neurologic symptoms; pruritus (without rash); anaphylactoid reactions, acute liver failure, and azotemia. If severe reactions occur, therapy should be discontinued for about 15 minutes; if the reaction recurs, therapy should be stopped and resumed at a lower dosage the next day. No evidence of any systemic toxicity or adverse reactions has been observed following topical application. If local intolerance occurs, when used topically, the drug should be discontinued. Dermatologic preparations do not stain the skin, but they may stain nail lesions. Fabric discoloration may be removed by washing with soap and water.

Dosage and Administration: *Topically.* Apply liberally 2 to 4 times daily. Duration of therapy depends upon the patient's response. Amphotericin B is prepared for parenteral use by reconstitution with 5% dextrose injection; sodium chloride solutions should not be used, since they cause precipitation of the antibiotic from solution. Since tolerance to amphotericin B varies, dosage must be adjusted to the specific requirements of each patient and administered *intravenously* in strict accordance with the directions in the package literature. Initially, a dose of 0.25 mg/kg of body weight is given and then increased gradually as tolerance permits. The injection should be administered by *slow* intravenous infusion over a period of 6 hours. Total daily dosage may range up to 1 mg/kg of body weight; alternate day dosage may range up to 1.5 mg/kg of body weight. *Under no circumstances should the dosage exceed 1.5 mg/kg/day.* The optimal dose is not known. Several months of therapy are usually necessary since a shorter period of therapy may produce an inadequate response and may lead to a relapse.

Availability:

FUNGIZONE®: **(Squibb)**

Cream, 3% in tubes of 20 gm.

Intravenous in vials of 50 mg.

Lotion, 3% in plastic-squeeze bottles of 30 ml.

Ointment, 3% in tubes of 20 gm.

For Tissue Culture (for laboratory use only), 50 mg/20-ml vial.

AMPICILLIN: see The Penicillins

ANILERIDINE Ⓒ

Chemical Name: 1-(*p*-Aminophenethyl)-4-phenylisonipecotic acid ethyl ester.

Description: Anileridine is a synthetic analgesic agent that is closely related to meperidine in chemical structure; a phenethyl group replaces the methyl group in the meperidine molecule. It occurs as a white, crystalline substance that is freely soluble in water and very soluble in alcohol.

Anileridine's chief pharmacologic action is exerted on the CNS. When administered either orally or parenterally in doses of 30 to 60 mg, it appears to possess significant pain-relieving capacity. Onset of action occurs within 15 minutes and persists for about 2 to 3 hours. Respiratory depression, when it occurs, is of shorter duration than that seen with morphine or meperidine when equivalent analgesic doses are administered. Anileridine is absorbed by all routes of administration. It is metabolized chiefly in the liver; only small amounts are excreted in the urine.

Indications: For relief of moderate to severe pain. Also indicated parenterally for preoperative medication, for support of anesthesia, for obstetrical analgesia, and for relief of anxiety in patients with dyspnea associated with acute ventricular failure and pulmonary edema.

Contraindications: In the presence of respiratory depression, and should be used with considerable caution, if at all, when respiratory failure is a possibility, as in head injury or brain tumor. Also contraindicated in patients with known hypersensitivity to anileridine. It should not be given to patients who are 12 years of age and under because clinical experience in this age group is limited.

Warnings: Since the addiction liability of anileridine is similar to that of morphine, and therefore has the potential for abuse, the drug should not be administered unnecessarily or for prolonged periods. As with other narcotic analgesics, anileridine should be used with extreme caution in patients with severe hepatic insufficiency, severe CNS depression or in coma, in those with head injuries, and in conditions in which intracranial pressure is increased. Utmost caution is also indicated in the presence of myxedema, Addison's disease, acute alcoholism, delirium tremens, convulsive disorders, and in patients taking MAO inhibitors. Safe use during pregnancy has not been established with regard to the possibility of adverse effects upon fetal development. Therefore, anileridine should be used in pregnant patients and in women of childbearing age only when in the judgment of the physician the potential benefits outweigh the possible hazards. The sudden intravenous injection of a dose greater than 10 mg may result in severe respiratory depression, apnea, hypotension and cardiac arrest. Therefore, anileridine should not be administered by direct intravenous injection, except in extreme emergencies when time or lack of facilities will not permit the use of a diluted preparation.

Precautions: Respiratory arrest and, to a lesser extent, circulatory depression are the chief hazards attending the use of anileridine. These effects are most likely to occur in elderly and debilitated patients and in those suffering from conditions accompanied by hypoxia or hypercapnia when even moderate therapeutic doses may dangerously decrease pulmonary ventilation. It should be given very cautiously to patients in shock, since the depressant effect upon respiration may act indirectly to further reduce the circulating blood volume, cardiac output, and blood pressure. If deep respiratory depression and circulatory collapse appear to be imminent, the administration of nalorphine or levallorphan may assist in counteracting these effects. Concomitant use with other narcotic, sedative, phenothiazines or anesthetic agents may enhance respiratory and circulatory depression.

Adverse Reactions: Reactions have been few and mild to date. However, elderly patients may experience respiratory and circulatory depression. Reactions may include vomiting, nausea, dry mouth, slight transient hypotension, bradycardia, dizziness, perspiration, a feeling of warmth, visual difficulty, itching, euphoria, restlessness, nervousness and excitement. A suitable narcotic antagonist such as nalorphine should be readily available to counteract toxic effects.

Dosage and Administration: *Orally* and *parenterally*. The recommended oral dose in adults is 25 to 50 mg, repeated every 4 to 6 hours if necessary. Up to 50 mg or more frequent doses may be desirable for more severe pain but neither is advised for ambulatory patients outside of home or hospital. For subcutaneous and intramuscular injection, 25 or 50 mg may be given to adults every 4 to 6 hours; 75 to 100 mg may be necessary for very severe pain. The preoperative dose for adults is 50 to 75 mg. For intravenous use in support of anesthesia, 50 to 100 mg should be added to 500 ml of 5% dextrose in water and administered by slow drip. During and directly following such use, provisions for oxygen administration and controlled respiration should be immediately available. As obstetric analgesia, 50 mg is given intramuscularly or subcutaneously every 3 or 4 hours, if necessary, for a total amount of 100 to 200 mg. For rapid action, 10 mg in dilution may be given intravenously slowly, at the same time that 40 mg is injected intramuscularly or subcutaneously. Direct intravenous injection of undiluted solution should not be employed except in grave emergency when lack of time or facilities precludes dilution of the drug.

Availability:
Ⓒ LERITINE®: **(Merck Sharp & Dohme)**
Injection, 25 mg/ml in ampuls of 1 and 2 ml in cartons of 25; and in vials of 30 ml.
Tablets, 25 mg in bottles of 100 and 500.

ANISINDIONE

Chemical Name: 2-(*p*-Methoxyphenyl)-1,3-indandione.

Description: A synthetic, anticoagulant drug, pharmacologically and structurally related to phenindione. Orally effective, it may be used for either short-or long-term therapy. Anisindione does not act in vitro but only in vivo as an antagonist to vitamin K to which it is structurally similar. It inhibits the synthesis of prothrombin with the prothrombin time serving as a guide to its anticoagulant activity.

The drug is well absorbed from the gastrointestinal tract. Following an oral dose, the prothrombin response is detected within 6 hours; however, it may take from 1 to 5 days to reach maximal response. Cumulative effects have not been reported, and upon withdrawal of the drug, the prothrombin time usually returns to normal within 1 to 3 days.

It is excreted mainly by the kidneys. In the liver it suppresses the synthesis of at least 4 clotting factors: factor II (prothrombin), factor VII (proconvertin), factor IX (Christmas), and factor X (Stuart-Prower).

Indications: Prophylaxis and treatment of venous thrombosis and its extension, the treatment of atrial fibrillation and embolization, and in the prophylaxis and treatment of pulmonary embolism. May also be useful as an adjunct in the treatment of coronary occlusion.

Contraindications: Hemophilia, thrombocytopenic purpura, leukemia with pronounced bleeding tendency, open wounds or ulcerations (particularly of the gastrointestinal tract), impaired hepatic or renal function, severe hypertension, acute nephritis, or subacute bacterial endocarditis.

Warnings: Although generally well tolerated, severe reactions (agranulocytosis, jaundice, and nephropathy) have occurred with other indandione derivatives and therefore may occur with anisindione. Treatment with this drug should be discontinued promptly if fever or skin rash occurs, because these reactions may signal the development of a severe complication. Since oral anticoagulants pass through the placental barrier, their use during pregnancy has been attended with increased risk to the fetus. They also pass into the mother's milk and cause hypoprothrombinemia in the nursing infant.

Precautions: The use of this drug should be controlled by dosage regulation based on periodic prothrombin-time determinations. Particular caution should be exercised in patients in whom even slight bleeding might be dangerous, such as those recovering from surgery of the eye, brain or spinal cord, or from cerebrovascular accidents involving bleeding. Caution should also be exercised in the treatment of women during menstruation. The presence of drainage tubes in any orifice or wound also necessitates utmost care in the use of anticoagulants. If hemorrhage occurs, treatment with anisindione should be discontinued. If necessary, a vitamin K_1 preparation should be administered. In an emergency, this treatment may be combined with transfusions of plasma or fresh (not stored), whole, citrated blood. In some patients with alkaline urine, the urine color may change to orange during anisindione treatment. This color reaction is due to the presence of catabolites of this drug in alkaline solution, not hematuria.

Anticoagulant activity may be exaggerated (prothrombin time prolonged) by concurrent administration of drugs such as sulfonamides, chloramphenicol, tetracyclines, neomycin and possibly other antibiotics, phenylbutazone, oxyphenbutazone, phenyramidol, phenytoin pyrazoline drugs, salicylates (aspirin in excess of 1 gm daily), quinidine, quinine, reserpine, dextrothyroxine, indomethacin, clofibrate, heparin, methylthiouracil, anabolic steroids, ACTH, and methylphenidate. Anticoagulant activity may be reduced (that is, larger amounts of anticoagulant may be needed) due to concurrent administration of alcohol, barbiturates, glutethimide, meprobamate, griseofulvin, ethchlorvynol, diazepam, vitamin K, haloperidol, and antihistamines. Frequent monitoring of the prothrombin time is suggested when chloral hydrate is administered to patients receiving this drug. Significant bleeding from the gastrointestinal or urinary tracts during anticoagulant therapy may indicate an occult lesion. Resistance to anticoagulant therapy, by contrast, may indicate underlying carcinoma of the lung, pancreas, or other viscera. Some studies have suggested that an increase in the incidence of postinfarction hemopericardium has occurred with the use of anticoagulants.

For complete information on potential drug interactions, see monograph on Diphenadione.

Adverse Reactions: Dermatitis has been the only adverse reaction reported to date. The following adverse reactions have been reported with other indandione derivatives and therefore may also occur with anisindione. These are agranulocytosis, jaundice, nephropathy, diarrhea, urticaria, and fever.

Dosage and Administration: *Orally.* Initial dosage is 300 mg the first day, 200 mg the second day and 100 mg the third day. Maintenance dosage is variable and will depend upon patient responsiveness; 75 to 100 mg is commonly used but it may vary from 25 to 250 mg daily. The amount administered should be that which maintains prothrombin time determinations at 2 to 2½ times the normal value.

Availability:
MIRADON® Tablets, 50 mg in bottles of 100. **(Schering)**

ANISOTROPINE METHYLBROMIDE

Chemical Name: 2-Propyl pentanoyl tropinium methylbromide.

Description: A quaternary ammonium anticholinergic agent structurally related to homatropine methylbromide, anisotropine methylbromide occurs as a white, crystalline powder soluble in water and freely soluble in alcohol. Its stability in both alkaline and acid solutions minimizes its inactivation.

In common with other parasympatholytic drugs, anisotropine produces effects which are qualitatively similar to those of atropine. It inhibits the motility of the gastrointestinal and urinary tracts and diminishes the volume of perspiration, saliva, and gastric and pancreatic secretions.

Both in vitro and oral in vivo data in mice and rats indicate that anisotropine is at least 2 or 3 times as potent as homatropine methylbromide in antispasmodic action while it is less than two-thirds as active in mydriatic effect. It has less than one-fiftieth of the mydriatic activity of atropine sulfate. In inhibition of salivary flow, anisotropine is one-fifth as active as homatropine methylbromide and only one-hundredth as active as atropine sulfate. This pharmacologic profile is consistent with relative specificity of action on the gastrointestinal smooth muscle and the lesser tendency to produce side effects.

Indications: Adjunctive therapy in the treatment of peptic ulcer. May also be useful in the irritable bowel syndrome (irritable colon, spastic colon, mucous colitis, acute enterocolitis, and functional gastrointestinal disorders); and in neurogenic bowel disturbances (including the splenic flexure syndrome and neurogenic colon). Formulated with phenobarbital to reduce the psychogenic component, and to allay the anxiety resulting from these somatic symptoms.

Important Note: As with all anticholinergic-antispasmodic agents, it should be understood that, at the present time, there is a lack of agreement as to their value in the treatment of gastric ulcer. It has not been shown conclusively whether or not these drugs aid in the healing of peptic ulcer, decrease the rate of recurrences or prevent complication.

Contraindications: Glaucoma, obstructive uropathy (bladder neck obstruction due to prostatic hypertrophy); obstructive disease of the gastrointestinal tract (achalasia, paralytic ileus, pyloroduodenal stenosis, pyloric obstruction); intestinal atony of the elderly or debilitated patient; unstable cardiovascular status in acute hemorrhage; severe ulcerative colitis; toxic megacolon complicating ulcerative colitis; and myasthenia gravis. Anisotropine methylbromide with phenobarbital is contraindicated in intermittent porphyria, and in those patients sensitive to phenobarbital.

Warnings: Safe use of these preparations during pregnancy or lactation, or in women of childbearing age has not been established; therefore, use of the drug in such patients requires that the potential benefits of the drug be weighed against its possible hazards to the mother and child. Since the drug inhibits the production of sweat, heat prostration accompanied by fever and heat stroke may occur in the presence of high environmental temperature. Diarrhea may be an early symptom of incomplete intestinal obstruction, especially in patients with ileostomy or colostomy. In this instance treatment with this drug would be inappropriate and possibly harmful. Since drowsiness and blurred vision may occur, patients should be cautioned to avoid activities requiring alertness, judgment or physical coordination. Phenobarbital may decrease the prothrombin time response to oral anticoagulants. More frequent monitoring of prothrombin time responses is indicated whenever phenobarbital is initiated or discontinued, and the dosage of anticoagulants should be adjusted accordingly. *Phenobarbital may be habit-forming* and should not be administered to individuals known to be addiction prone or to those with a history of physical and/or psychological dependence upon habit-forming drugs.

Precautions: Use with caution in patients with autonomic neuropathy, hyperthyroidism, coronary heart disease, congestive heart failure, cardiac arrhythmias, hypertension, nonobstructing prostatic hypertrophy, early evidence of ileus as in peritonitis, and in those with advanced hepatic and renal diseases. While anisotropine methylbromide alone or with phenobarbital has been used without ill effects in patients with known cardiovascular disease, any tachycardia existing before administration should be examined before giving these drugs. Caution should be observed in those patients with gastric ulcer since anticholinergic drugs *may* produce the complication of delayed gastric emptying (antral stasis), and may also aggravate hiatal hernia associated with reflux esophagitis. Large doses of anisotropine may suppress intestinal motility to the point of producing a paralytic ileus, and may precipitate or aggravate the serious complication of toxic megacolon. Caution is particularly urged when concomitant administration of anticholinergic or other drugs might lead to enhanced anticholinergic effects.

Adverse Reactions: Anticholinergics produce certain effects which may be physiologic or toxic depending upon the individual patient's response. While serious side effects due to atropinism have not been noted, anisotropine may rarely produce the following adverse reactions, which are common to all anticholinergics: mydriasis; dilatation of the pupil; cycloplegia; blurred vision; increased intraocular tension; xerostomia; loss of taste; headaches; nervousness; drowsiness; weakness; dizziness; insomnia; nausea; vomiting; impotence, urinary hesitancy and retention; tachycardia, palpitations; suppression of lactation; constipation; bloated feeling; severe allergic reaction or drug idiosyncrasies including anaphylaxis, urticaria and other dermal manifestations; some degree of mental confusion and/or excitement, especially in elderly patients. A curare-like action may occur with overdosage. Severe symptoms require prompt treatment with gastric lavage and other measures to limit intestinal absorption. Parenteral physostigmine may be necessary to counteract severe intoxication. Additionally, symptomatic therapy, including oxygen, sedatives, and control of hyperthermia may be required. In some individuals phenobarbital may produce excitement rather than a sedative effect, as well as musculoskeletal pain. Some patients may acquire a sensitivity to barbiturates.

Dosage and Administration: *Orally*, 1 tablet 3 times daily.

Availability:
VALPIN® Tablets, 50 mg in bottles of 100 and 1000. **(Endo)**
VALPIN®-PB Tablets, 50 mg with phenobarbital, 15 mg in bottles of 100 and 1000. **(Endo)**

ANTIHEMOPHILIC FACTOR, HUMAN

Description: Plasma from freshly drawn blood, rapidly processed to retain antihemophilic factor and other labile clotting factors; also contains relatively small amounts of fibrinogen and other plasma proteins. Must be stored at a temperature of 2 to 8 degrees centigrade. May also be obtained from frozen venous plasma found nonreactive for hepatitis B surface antigen. Must be kept frozen. Following injection, antihemophilic factor (human) accelerates the abnormally slow clotting time of hemophiliacs, which is due to a deficiency of factor VIII.

Indications: To control bleeding in classical hemophilia. It is not indicated for the management of bleeding in patients with Von Willebrand's disease.

Warnings: As with many human blood derivatives, the physician must evaluate the risk that serum hepatitis may follow its use. Use of more than 7 to 8 ml/lb body weight in 24 hours may cause a relative anemia which should be corrected with fresh whole blood. A transient hypervolemic state may result when large amounts of plasma are infused. This condition may be avoided by slow administration, perhaps following removal of some of the patient's plasma, as by plasmapheresis. Repeated use of this product may produce hypersensitivity, characterized by chills, fever, or urticaria. Acute reactions such as erythema, hives, and backache occur infrequently and usually will disappear within 15 to 20 minutes.

Dosage and Administration: *Intravenously.* Dosage must be individualized according to the weight of the patient, the severity of the bleeding or the blood condition or both, the source of the bleeding, the presence of inhibitors, and other factors as determined by the physician. *In hemophilia,* a single injection usually maintains normal clotting time for several hours, often for 1 to 2 days. Repeat dose as indicated by patient's clotting time; repeated injections do not reduce effectiveness. This preparation should be administered within 2 hours after reconstitution.

Availability:
FACTORATE Concentrate (lyophilized) of human antihemophilic factor (Factors VIII, AHF, AHG) in single-dose vials of 25 ml with diluent and administration set. **(Armour)**
HEMOFIL Concentrate (freeze-dried) of human antihemophilic factor (Factors VIII, AHF, AHG) in vials of 10 ml (250 units) and 30 ml (800 and 1000 units). **(Hyland)**
HUMAFAC® Concentrate (lyophilized, freeze-dried) of human antihemophilic factor (Factors VIII, AHF, AHG) in single-dose vials with 6-ml diluent. **(Parke-Davis)**
KOATE Concentrate (freeze-dried) of human antihemophilic factor (factors VIII, AHF, AHG) in vials of 10, 20 and 40 ml with diluent and filter needle. **(Cutter)**

ANTIRABIES SERUM

Description: A hyperimmune and purified preparation of *horse* origin which delays virus propagation, thus allowing more time for vaccine to induce antibodies to the virus.

Indications: Adjunct to the prophylactic treatment of all individuals who have been exposed to rabies infection, particularly those who have been exposed through bites about the head or neck. This serum is not a substitute for vaccine prophylaxis after exposure to rabies virus, but is offered as an additional protection.

Contraindications: Before administering full calculated dosage, sensitivity of the patient should be determined by means of one of the tests described in the product literature. A positive reaction to either test indicates a dangerous degree of sensitivity and is a strong contraindication to injection of this serum.

Precautions: The patient's blood should be typed as soon as possible, since the hemolysins present in the venom soon alter the blood protein structure, thus preventing accurate cross-matching. Broad spectrum antibiotics and appropriate tetanus prophylaxis are indicated. If opiates or barbiturates are considered necessary, these drugs should be used in small doses, and with caution. The parenteral administration of any biological agent should be accompanied by every known precaution for the prevention and arrest of allergic and unfavorable reactions. It is advised that before initiating therapy a careful history of the patient should be taken for past evidence of asthma, angioneurotic edema or other allergies including sensitivity to horse serum. A familial history of connective tissue disease may require special consideration. Sensitivity reactions may be of two types: (1) Immediate shock-like reactions manifested by itching, sneezing, coughing and asthmatic breathing. Generalized urticaria and marked hypotension may occur within minutes. Epinephrine administration is the treatment of choice. (2) Development of serum sickness within 6 to 12 days, even in those without a prior history of sensitivity. Common symptoms are skin eruption, itching, lymphadenopathy, and arthralgia. In severe cases, fever, abdominal pain, malaise, and headache may be noted.

Dosage and Administration: *Intramuscularly,* in a single dose of not less than 1000 units (one vial)/40 lb of body weight. Up to 1/2 of the total dose should be infiltrated into the tissue around the wound.

Patient's Weight	*Dosage Recommended*
Up to 40 lb	1000 units
40 to 80 lb	2000 units
80 to 120 lb	3000 units
120 to 160 lb	4000 units
160 to 200 lb	5000 units
Over 200 lb	6000 units

If the interval between exposure and treatment is greater than 24 hours, or if there are severe wounds about the head and neck, 2 or 3 times the recommended amount should be administered. The serum should be administered *only once.* Although it is usually given in conjunction with rabies vaccine, it should not be given in the same syringe, nor into the same site, since this might result in vaccine neutralization.

Availability:
ANTIRABIES SERUM in vials containing 1000 units. **(Lederle)**

ANTIVENIN (SNAKE)

Description: A hyperimmune *horse* serum containing protective substances against the venoms of all rattlesnakes and moccasins (North American and tropical); the fer-de-lance and similar species; bushmaster.

Indications: Treatment of poisoning by all crotaline snakes throughout the world.

Precautions: Preliminary skin and conjunctival test for sensitivity to horse serum is advisable. The patient's blood should be typed as early as possible, since the hemolysins present in the venom soon alter the blood protein structure, thus preventing accurate cross-matching. Broad-spectrum antibiotics and appropriate tetanus prophylaxis are indicated. If opiates or barbiturates are considered necessary, these drugs should be used in small doses, and with caution. Before use of this product, the physician should be familiar with the package direction circular, and the pertinent published medical literature concerning the use of this serum.

Adverse Reactions: Systemic reactions begin within the first 30 minutes after administration. Early or immediate reactions may include anaphylactic shock; itching; apprehension; urticaria; edema of face, tongue and throat; cough, dyspnea, cyanosis, vomiting and collapse in varying degrees of severity. Such an alarming type of reaction, which on rare occasions may be fatal, may occur in naturally sensitive individuals or in those whose sensitivity has been created by previous administration of horse serums. Appropriate therapeutic agents such as epinephrine 1:1000, oxygen, tourniquet, injectable antihistamines and adrenal corticosteroids should be available for immediate use. Serum sickness may occur within 6 to 24 days, but usually within 8 to 12 days, after administration of antiserum. Accelerated serum reactions may occur in sensitive persons within a period of 2 to 5 days, or in some patients, within a few minutes. Occurrence of this accelerated serum sickness serves as a warning that future injections of equine antiserum may prove dangerous.

Dosage and Administration: *Intramuscularly, subcutaneously* or, in grave cases, *intravenously* or *intraperitoneally.* Initial dose is 15 to 75 ml (1 to 5 vials), depending upon the size of the snake, the lapse of time between the bite and specific treatment, and the size and condition of the patient. The smaller the body of the patient, the larger the initial dose required. Usually, about half is administered subcutaneously or intramuscularly at various points around the limb, above the level of swelling, the rest higher on the bitten limb, or elsewhere as indicated. Repeat injections of 15 ml (1 vial) every ½ to 2 hours if pain and active swelling persist.

Availability:
ANTIVENIN (Crotalidae) Polyvalent, Equine Origin: Combination package consisting of 1 vacuum vial to yield 10 ml of serum, 1 disposable syringe containing 10 ml of bacteriostatic water for injection, U.S.P., 1 applicator vial of tincture of iodine, and 1 vial of 1 ml of normal horse serum as sensitivity testing material. **(Wyeth)**

ANTIVENIN (SPIDER)

Synonym: Black widow spider antivenin.

Description: Prepared by immunizing horses against the bite of black widow spider. The package contains one Vacule vial representing not less than 6000 antivenin units. Also included is one 1-ml vial of normal horse serum (diluted 1:10), as test and desensitizing material.

Indications: Specific treatment of the effect of the venom from bites of the black widow spider. Local treatment of the site of the bite is of no value, and nothing is gained by applying a tourniquet or by attempting to remove venom from the site of the bite by incision and suction.

Precautions: It is important that an intradermal skin test for serum hypersensitivity be made because some patients may be hypersensitive to equine serum and serious sickness and even death could result from the use of serum in a sensitive patient. Inject into (not under) the skin not more than 0.02 ml of the test material (1:10 dilution of normal horse serum in physiologic saline). Evaluate result in 10 minutes. A positive reaction is an urticarial wheal surrounded by a zone of erythema. *Desensitization should be attempted only when the administration of antivenin is considered necessary to save life.* The technique may be chosen from among those in standard texts. Epinephrine must be available in case of untoward reaction.

Dosage and Administration: *Intramuscularly.* The lyophilized material should be reconstituted by adding 2.5 ml pyrogen-free, sterile water for injection contained in the accompanying vial. As soon as a diagnosis of arachnidism due to the black widow spider is made, the patient should receive the contents of one restored Vacule vial (2.5 ml) of Lyovac antivenin (latrodectus mactans). May be given intravenously in 10 to 50 ml of saline solution over a 15-minute period. It is the preferred route in severe cases, or when the patient is under 12 years of age, or in shock. It is seldom necessary to administer more than 1 dose of 2.5 ml.

Availability:
ANTIVENIN (Latrodectus Mactans) in vials to yield 2.5 ml of restored serum.
(Merck Sharp & Dohme)

ANUGESIC

Description: Each gm of ointment and each suppository contains:

	Ointment	*Suppository*
Bismuth subgallate	22.5 mg	61.0 mg
Bismuth resorcin compound	17.5 mg	47.0 mg
Benzyl benzoate	12.0 mg	32.4 mg
Peruvian balsam	18.0 mg	48.6 mg
Zinc oxide	107.5 mg	300.0 mg
Pramoxine hydrochloride	10.0 mg	25.0 mg

Indications: To relieve the discomfort and pain associated with hemorrhoids, pruritus ani, proctitis, cryptitis, fissures and fistulas. Also used to relieve the localized pain following anorectal surgery. Pramoxine, an analgesic, is nonsensitizing and can be used with minimal risk of sensitization.

Contraindications: Hypersensitivity or idiosyncrasy to any of the components.

Precautions: Symptomatic relief should not delay definitive diagnosis or treatment.

Adverse Reactions: Occasionally, patients may experience burning upon application, especially if the skin is broken. If irritation or sensitivity is suspected, treatment should be discontinued.

Dosage and Administration: *Topically,* ointment is applied externally and internally (with applicator) every 3 to 4 hours. *Rectally,* 1 suppository is inserted every 3 to 4 hours. Dosage may be increased to every 2 hours if symptoms are severe.

Availability:
ANUGESIC® (OTC): **(Warner-Chilcott)**
Ointment in tubes of 30 gm with plastic applicator.
Suppositories (foil-wrapped) in cartons of 12.

ANUSOL-HC

Description: Each gm of cream and each individually foil-wrapped suppository contains:

	Cream	*Suppository*
Hydrocortisone acetate	5 mg	10 mg
Bismuth subgallate	22.5 mg	2.25%
Bismuth resorcin compound	17.5 mg	1.75%
Peruvian balsam (medicinal)	18 mg	1.8%
Zinc oxide	110 mg	11%
Benzyl benzoate	12 mg	1.2%

Indications: Relief of pain, itching and associated discomforts of acute and chronic proctitis and hemorrhoids, papillitis, cryptitis, and fissures, pruritus ani and incomplete fistulas, especially in the presence of severe inflammation. Also useful in relieving localized pain following anorectal surgery. The hydrocortisone component helps to alleviate hyperemia and swelling.

Contraindications: In patients with a history of sensitivity to any of the components. Topical corticosteroids should not be employed in tuberculous, fungal, and most viral lesions of the skin, including herpes, vaccinia and varicella.

Warnings: Safe use of topical steroids during pregnancy has not been established; therefore, they should not be used unnecessarily on extended areas, in large amounts, or for prolonged periods of time.

Precautions: Symptomatic relief should not delay definitive diagnosis or treatment. When there is bacterial skin infection, topical corticosteroids should be used only with appropriate concomitant antimicrobial therapy. Prolonged and excessive use might produce systemic effects.

Dosage and Administration: *Topically.* Apply cream to the interior surfaces of the anus 3 or 4 times daily for 3 to 6 days or until inflammation subsides. *Rectally,* 1 suppository in the morning and 1 at bedtime for 3 to 6 days or as directed.

Availability:
ANUSOL-HC®: **(Warner-Chilcott)**
Cream in tubes of 30 gm with plastic applicator.
Suppositories (foil-wrapped) in cartons of 12.

A.P.C. with CODEINE Ⓒ III

Description: Each capsule or tablet contains aspirin, approximately 230 mg; phenacetin, 150 mg and caffeine, 30 mg. In addition it contains either 7.5 mg (No. 1), 15 mg (No. 2), 30 mg (No. 3) or 60 mg (No. 4) of codeine (phosphate or sulfate).

Indications: An analgesic, antipyretic and antirheumatic for use in varying degrees of pain, from moderate trauma to severe pain, including that of neoplastic disease; for pain associated with upper respiratory infections.

Contraindications: Known hypersensitivity or idiosyncrasy to any of the components, and in the presence of blood dyscrasias.

Warnings: Codeine may be habit-forming. The recommended dose should not be exceeded nor should the drug be taken regularly for longer than 10 days unless directed by the physician. As with other opiate analgesics the usual precautions should be observed, especially in regard to psychic and physical dependence and tolerance. Because the drug is subject to abuse, its use should be carefully monitored. Patients should be warned about the possibility of dizziness or drowsiness, which may impair their ability to drive an automobile or safely perform potentially dangerous tasks. Concurrent use with alcohol or other CNS depressant drug (narcotic analgesic, general anesthetics, phenothiazines, other tranquilizers, sedative-hypnotics), requires that the dose of one or both agents be reduced. When intended for use in pregnant patients, the clinical benefits versus the hazards to the unborn child should be considered.

Precautions: Special attention is required in the presence of head injury, other intracranial lesion, a preexisting increase in intracranial pressure, or acute abdominal conditions, in elderly or debilitated patients and in those with severe impairment of hepatic or renal function, hypothyroidism, Addison's disease, prostatic hypertrophy or urethral stricture. Salicylates should be given with caution to patients with known allergies, peptic ulcer, nasal polyps and asthma. Phenacetin should not be taken repeatedly by persons with anemia or with cardiac, pulmonary or hepatic disease. Prolonged and excessive use of phenacetin-containing products may damage the kidneys or aggravate renal disease. Caffeine should not be given to persons extremely sensitive to CNS stimulants. In the presence of asthma or pulmonary emphysema, the indiscriminate use of codeine may, due to its drying action upon the mucosa of the respiratory tract, precipitate severe respiratory insufficiency resulting from increased viscosity of the bronchial secretions and suppression of the cough reflex.

Adverse Reactions: Some patients are unable to take salicylates without developing nausea and vomiting. Hypersensitivity may be manifested by a skin rash or even by an anaphylactic reaction (idiosyncrasy). With these exceptions, most reactions occur after large doses. They include headache, vertigo, mental confusion, tinnitus, drowsiness, sweating, thirst, nausea and vomiting. Reactions stemming from phenacetin usually are the result of overdosage and may include cyanosis, acute hemolytic anemia, skin lesions and fever. Reactions associated with caffeine, almost always the result of overdosage, include insomnia, restlessness, excitement, diuresis, tachycardia and extrasystoles.

Dosage and Administration: *Orally,* 1 or 2 capsules or tablets every 4 to 6 hours, repeated as required.

Availability:

C-III ANEXSIA® with CODEINE Tablets w/codeine sulfate, 32 mg in bottles of 100 and 1000. **(Beecham)**

C-III ANEXSIA®-D Tablets w/hydrocodone bitartrate, 7 mg in bottles of 100 and 1000. **(Beecham)**

C-III A.P.C. with CODEINE Tablets (codeine phosphate, 15 and 30 mg) in bottles of 1000. **(Lederle)**

C-III A.P.C. with CODEINE PHOSPHATE Tablets (codeine phosphate, 15, 30 and 60 mg) in Redipak (unit-dose) cartons of 25. **(Wyeth)**

C-III A.S.A.® and CODEINE COMPOUND: **(Lilly)**

Pulvules® No. 2 (codeine phosphate, 15 mg) in bottles of 100 and 500; No. 3 (codeine phosphate, 30 mg) in bottles of 100, 500 and in 10 strips of 10 individually labeled blisters each containing 1 pulvule; No. 4 (codeine phosphate, 60 mg) in bottles of 100 and 1000.

Tablets No. 2 (codeine phosphate, 15 mg) and No. 3 (codeine phosphate, 30 mg) in bottles of 100 and 500.

Ⓒ ASPIRIN COMPOUND with CODEINE PHOSPHATE Tablets No. 2 (codeine phosphate, 15 mg) and No. 3 (codeine phosphate, 30 mg) in bottles of 1000 and in unit-dose packages of 100. **(Parke-Davis)**

Ⓒ EMPIRIN® COMPOUND with CODEINE PHOSPHATE Tablets No. 1 (codeine phosphate, 7.5 mg) in bottles of 100 and 500; No. 2 (codeine phosphate, 15 mg), No. 3 (codeine phosphate, 30 mg) and No. 4 (codeine phosphate, 60 mg) in bottles of 100, 500 and 1000 and in Dispenserpak®s of 25. **(Burroughs Wellcome)**

Ⓒ P-A-C® COMPOUND with CODEINE SULFATE: **(Upjohn)**
Capsules (codeine sulfate, 30 mg) in bottles of 1000.
Tablets (codeine sulfate, 15 and 30 mg) in bottles of 100 and 1000.

APOMORPHINE HYDROCHLORIDE Ⓒ

Description: Apomorphine hydrochloride, an alkaloid produced synthetically from morphine, retains the centrally stimulant action of the parent compound, but not the depressant action which is significantly reduced. It occurs as an odorless, white or greyish-white, crystalline substance or as a white powder that is sparingly soluble in water and in alcohol. Amorphine induces emesis through its direct action on the chemoreceptor trigger zone of the medulla oblongata. Following subcutaneous administration, emesis occurs within 10 to 15 minutes and is preceded by nausea and vomiting.

Indications: To induce emesis.

Contraindications: Apomorphine should not be given to patients in shock (as from corrosive poisoning), or to those who are narcotized from an overdose of CNS depressant drugs such as alcohol, barbituates, opiates, etc., since severe depression, and even death, may occur.

Precautions: Due caution is required when treating children, debilitated individuals, those with cardiac decompensation, or with a predisposition to nausea and vomiting.

Adverse Reactions: Euphoria, tachypnea, restlessness, tremors, and peripheral vascular collapse. Excessive doses may cause violent emesis, cardiac depression, and death.

Dosage and Administration: *Subcutaneously.* The dose ranges from 2 to 10 mg, but the usual adult dose is 5 mg. Because of its dangerous central depressant action, the emetic dose should not be repeated if vomiting does not occur after the first dose.

Availability:
Ⓒ APOMORPHINE HYDROCHLORIDE Tablets (hypodermic), 6 mg in bottles of 100. **(Lilly)**

APROBARBITAL Ⓒ

Chemical Name: 5-Allyl-5-isopropylbarbituric acid.

Description: Classified as an intermediate-acting barbiturate, aprobarbital occurs as a bitter, white, crystalline powder very slightly soluble in water and soluble in alcohol.

Indications: For sedation and induction of sleep in all conditions requiring a sedative-hypnotic.

Warnings: Aprobarbital may be habit-forming.

Precautions: The usual precautions regarding the use of barbiturates should be observed.

Dosage and Administration: *Orally.* The recommended sedative dosage for adults is 1 teaspoonful 3 times daily. The adult hypnotic dose is usually 1 to 2 teaspoonsful (2 to 4 teaspoonsful for pronounced insomnia) before retiring. Dosage for children has not been established but, as for adults, the smallest effective dose should be used.

Availability:
Ⓒ ALURATE® Elixir (red), 40 mg/5 ml in pints and gallons; Elixir Verdum (green), 40 mg/5 ml in bottles of 1 pint. **(Roche)**

ARGININE HYDROCHLORIDE

Description: Arginine hydrochloride, the monohydrochloride salt of the amino acid L-arginine, occurs as a white, crystalline powder that is freely soluble in water. Each 100 ml of the hypertonic solution contains 10 gm of L-arginine in sterile water for injection; also contains 47.5 mEq of chloride ion. The drug acts as a stimulus to the pituitary gland to secrete growth hormone, which is measured in the plasma by radioimmunoassay.

Indications: As a diagnostic aid for measurement of pituitary reserve of human growth hormone. It is especially useful in such conditions as panhypopituitarism, pituitary dwarfism, chromophobe adenoma, postsurgical craniopharyngioma, hypophysectomy, pituitary trauma, acromegaly, gigantism and other problems of growth and stature. It can also be used to confirm a negative response to the insulin hypoglycemia test for deficiency of pituitary reserve for HGH following a 1-day waiting period.

Contraindications: Patients with highly allergic tendencies.

Warnings: Because of its hypertonicity, the solution should always be administered *intravenously.* A suitable antihistaminic should be readily available in the event that an allergic reaction occurs.

Precautions: The clinician should be aware that inadequate dosing or a prolonged infusion rate may diminish the stimulus to the pituitary and nullify the test. Also, that the rate of false positive responses has been reported to be approximately 32% and of false negative responses about 27%.

Adverse Reactions: Rapid infusion may cause flushing, nausea or vomiting. Local irritation at the injection site has been noted.

Dosage and Administration: *Intravenously.* The usual dose for adults is 300 ml, and for children, 5 ml/kg of body weight. If the patient does not respond, the test may be repeated the following day. The physician is urged to read carefully the package literature for additional information on procedures and clinical conditions.

Availability:
R-GENE™-10 Solution, 10% in Saftiflask (500-ml glass container containing 300 ml of solution) with administration set. **(Cutter)**

ASBRON G

Description: Each tablet and each tablespoonful (15 ml) of elixir contain theophylline sodium glycinate, 300 mg (equiv. to 150 mg theophylline) and guaifenesin, 100 mg. The elixir supplies the active ingredients in a solution containing 15% alcohol. The formulations provide the combined action of a bronchodilator and an expectorant which helps to liquefy tenacious mucus thereby increasing the fluidity of the inflammatory exudate.

Indications: Symptomatic relief of acute bronchial asthma and for reversible bronchospasm associated with chronic bronchitis and emphysema.

Contraindications: Hypersensitivity to any of the components. Xanthines generally should not be used in patients with peptic ulcer.

Warnings: Cautious use is required in the presence of hypertension, hyperthyroidism or cardiovascular disease.

Precautions: Because the serum half-life varies greatly from patient to patient, the dosage must be individualized. When possible, serum theophylline levels should be measured in order to assist in titration of dosage. It must be taken into account that the action of theophylline can be inhibited by acidifying agents and enhanced by alkalinizing agents.

Adverse Reactions: Large doses may produce reactions such as nervousness, agitation, headache, palpitations, tachycardia, nausea and vomiting. Theophylline has been known to cause cardiac arrhythmias and ventricular ectopic beats.

Dosage and Administration: *Orally,* 3 or 4 times daily. Adults, 1 or 2 tablets or tablespoonsful. Children 6 to 12 years, 2 to 3 teaspoonsful; 3 to 6 years, 1 to ½ teaspoonsful; 1 to 3 years, ½ to 1 teaspoonful. In severe attacks, higher dosage may be indicated the first day, after which dosage is adjusted on an individual basis. Administration after meals may reduce the incidence of unfavorable reactions.

Availability:
ASBRON G®: **(Dorsey)**
Elixir in bottles of 1 pint.
Inlay Tabs® in bottles of 100.

ASCODEEN-30 Ⓒ

Description: Each tablet contains 30 mg of codeine phosphate and 325 mg of aspirin.

Indications: For relief of virtually all moderate to severe pain, of acute or chronic nature, including: pain following surgery or trauma, involutional pain, earache, migraine, muscular pain, dysmenorrhea, pain and cough associated with upper respiratory tract infections and pain of neoplastic disease which does not require morphine or its equivalent. When severe pain of arthritis is not relieved by non-narcotic analgesics, this preparation usually provides relief.

Warnings: Codeine phosphate may be habit-forming.

Precautions: Salicylates should be given with caution to patients with known allergies, peptic ulcer, nasal polyps and asthma. Codeine possesses many of the disadvantages of morphine including respiratory depression, especially when given in large doses. Dependence liability of codeine however is less than that with morphine or meperidine, and physical dependence occurs only rarely.

Adverse Reactions: Some individuals are unable to take salicylates without developing gastrointestinal disturbances manifested by dyspepsia, nausea, vomiting and occult gastrointestinal bleeding. Codeine usually produces nausea, vomiting, constipation, and drowsiness. The sedative effect may be a hazard in ambulatory patients whose activities require alertness and motor coordination.

Dosage and Administration: *Orally,* 1 or 2 tablets 3 times daily, as required.

Availability:
Ⓒ ASCODEEN-30® Tablets in bottles of 100 and 1000 and in Dispenserpak®s of 25 in cartons of 40. **(Burroughs Wellcome)**

ASCORBIC ACID

Description: Ascorbic acid is a water-soluble, antiscorbutic vitamin. It occurs as white or slightly yellow crystals or powder that is unstable and gradually darkens on exposure to light. Body storage of ascorbic acid is limited.

Indications: Prevention and treatment of scurvy. Symptoms of mild deficiency may include faulty bone and tooth development, gingivitis, bleeding gums, and loosened teeth. Febrile states, chronic illness, and infection may increase the need for ascorbic acid. Premature and immature infants require relatively large amounts of the vitamin.

Contraindications: None known.

Precautions: Too-rapid intravenous administration should be avoided. As ascorbic acid has on occasion been used as a specific antidote for symptoms resulting from interaction between ethanol and disulfiram, it may be expected that the concurrent administration of ascorbic acid will interfere with the effectiveness of disulfiram given to patients for encouraging abstention from alcoholic beverages.

Adverse Reactions: Transient mild soreness may occur at the site of intramuscular or subcutaneous injection. When the intravenous administration is given too rapidly, the patient may experience temporary faintness or dizziness.

Dosage and Administration: *Intramuscularly, intravenously* or *subcutaneously.* The average therapeutic dose for adults is 300 mg to 1 gm daily while the protective dose is 70 to 150 mg daily. However, as much as 6 gm has been administered parenterally to normal adults without evidence of toxicity. The average therapeutic dose for infants is 100 to 300 mg daily while the protective dose is 30 mg daily. Premature infants require 75 to 100 mg daily.

Availability:
ASCORBIC ACID
Injection, 250 mg/ml in ampuls of 2 ml. **(Parke-Davis)**
Injection, 50 mg/ml in ampuls of 10 ml; 250 mg/ml in ampuls of 2 ml. **(Various Mfrs.)**
CENOLATE® Injection, 500 mg/ml in ampuls of 1 and 2 ml. **(Abbott)**
CEVALIN® Injection, 50 mg/ml in ampuls of 2 ml; 500 mg/ml in ampuls of 1 ml; 100 mg/ml in ampuls of 10 ml. **(Lilly)**

ASCRIPTIN with CODEINE Ⓒ III

Description: Each No. 2 tablet contains codeine phosphate, 16.2 mg; aspirin, 325 mg and magnesium-aluminum hydrochloride, 150 mg. Each No. 3 tablet contains codeine phosphate, 32.4 mg; aspirin, 325 mg and magnesium-aluminum hydrochloride, 150 mg.

Indications: An analgesic for the relief of pain of all degrees of severity up to that which requires morphine.

Warnings: Codeine phosphate may be habit-forming.

Adverse Reactions: Nausea, constipation and drowsiness may occur.

Dosage and Administration: *Orally,* 2 (No. 2) tablets or 1 or 2 (No. 3) tablets every 3 or 4 hours when necessary.

Availability:
Ⓒ III ASCRIPTIN® with CODEINE Tablets (No. 2 & No. 3) in bottles of 100. **(Rorer)**

ASPARAGINASE

Chemical Name: L-Asparagine amidohydrolase, type EC-2.

Description: An antineoplastic agent primarily employed in the treatment of acute lymphocytic leukemia, asparaginase is an enzyme isolated from cultures of the microorganism *Escherichia coli.* It occurs as a white crystalline powder that is freely soluble in water and practically insoluble in organic solvents (methanol, acetone, ether, and chloroform). Its therapeutic value is dependent upon the distinct, biochemical difference between certain tumor cells and normal cells. Because malignant cells, unlike normal cells, are incapable of synthesizing asparagine, an amino acid essential for cell replication, they are dependent on exogenous (circulating) asparagine for their survival. By increasing the rate of hydrolysis of asparagine to aspartic acid and ammonia, asparaginase deprives the tumor cells of this important element thus causing cell destruction without similarly damaging normal tissue. Because plasma concentrations are dose-dependent, cumulative effects can be expected on repeated administration. The plasma half-life has been found to range from 8 to 30 hours and does not appear to be influenced by the amount of drug received, the age, sex or surface area of the patient, hepatic or renal function or type or extent of the disease. This enzyme is apparently distributed into various body tissues, has been detected in thoracic and cervical lymph while less than 1% of the concurrent plasma levels appear in the cerebrospinal fluid and only trace amounts are recoverable from the urine.

Experiments with animals have shown that the drug is capable of inducing embryotoxic and teratogenic effects, and of causing immunosuppressive effects. Asparaginase's activity is expressed in terms of international units, and its specific activity is at least 225 IU/mg of protein. Each vial of the commercial product contains 10,000 IU of asparaginase and 80 mg of mannitol. The drug should be administered only by or under the supervision of a qualified clinician who is experienced in cancer chemotherapy. Because of the possibility of serious toxic reactions, including anaphylaxis and sudden death, it is essential that all patients be hospitalized during treatment.

Results of acute toxicity studies in animals have shown a reduction in the serum levels of total protein and albumin with loss of body weight at the highest dose and anorexia, emesis, and diarrhea at all dosage levels. BSP retention and fatty changes in the liver were noted in some of the animals. A single intravenous dose of 1000 IU/kg injected into the rabbit produced hypocalcemia associated with necrosis of the parathyroid cells. Convulsions and death occurred in about one-third of the animals. Postmortem studies revealed small thymic and lymph node hemorrhages and necrosis of the germinal centers in the lymph nodes and spleen. The intravenous administration of calcium gluconate apparently alleviates or prevents these harmful effects. Tissue culture and animal studies also indicate that asparaginase can diminish or abolish the effect of methotrexate on malignant cells, and that this effect generally persists as long as plasma asparagine levels are suppressed.

Indications: Treatment of acute lymphocytic leukemia. Favorable results can be expected when used primarily in combination with other chemotherapeutic agents for the induction of remissions of the disease in children. Unless combination therapy is deemed inappropriate, asparaginase should not be used as the sole induction agent, nor should it be employed for maintainance therapy in this parameter.

Contraindications: In patients who have undergone a previous anaphylactic reaction to its effects and in those with pancreatitis or with a history of this complication since drug-induced hemorrhagic pancreatitis, in some instances fatal, has been reported.

Warnings: Since asparaginase is a relatively large, foreign protein, it is antigenic, and can therefore produce hypersensitivity responses ranging from mild allergic reactions to anaphylaxis and death. These effects may be observed during the primary course of therapy in hospitalized patients under appropriate observation. Unfortunately, the intradermal skin test is not completely reliable in detecting patient sensitivity. Those undergoing induction therapy must be carefully monitored and the therapeutic regimen adjusted according to response and toxicity. Anaphylactic reactions require the immediate availability and use of epinephrine, oxygen, and intravenous steroids. Retreatment generally provokes an increased risk of allergic complications. Patients with known hypersensitivity to asparaginase (positive intradermal test) or those who have previously been treated with this drug should be successfully desensitized before therapy is instituted. Because asparaginase has an adverse effect on liver function in the majority of patients, it may therefore increase preexisting liver impairment caused by prior therapy or by the underlying disorder. Intravenous administration immediately prior to or simultaneously with a course of vincristine and prednisone may be associated with increased toxicity; also the possibility exists that asparaginase may increase the toxicity of other medications.

Precautions: A significant fall in circulating lymphoblasts, and normal or below normal leukocyte counts are noted frequently, particularly within the first several days after commencing therapy. This may be accompanied by a marked rise in serum uric acid; therefore, the possible development of uric acid nephropathy should be borne in mind. It is advised that appropriate preventive measures including allopurinol, increased fluid intake, and alkalization of the urine be included in the regimen. As a guide to the effects of treatment, the patient's peripheral blood cell count and bone marrow response should be monitored regularly, as well as blood sugar levels in order to detect an approaching hyperglycemic condition. Frequent serum amylase determinations should be obtained to detect early evidence of pancreatitis; if pancreatitis develops, therapy should be discontinued and should not be reinstituted. Because of its immunosuppressive activity, patients may be predisposed to infection. Toxic reactions to the drug have been reported to be greater in adults than in children.

Adverse Reactions: Allergic reactions, including skin rashes, urticaria, arthralgia, respiratory distress, and acute anaphylaxis have been reported. Acute reactions have occurred in the absence of a positive skin test and during continued maintenance of therapeutic serum levels of asparaginase. Fatal hyperthermia, and pancreatitis, sometimes fulminant, have been reported. Occasionally, hyperglycemia with glucosuria and polyuria has been noted. Serum and urine acetone usually have been absent or negligible in these patients; this syndrome thus resembles the hyperosmolar, nonketotic hyperglycemia induced by a variety of other agents. This complication usually responds to withdrawal of asparaginase, judicious use of intravenous fluid, and insulin, but may be fatal on occasion. In addition to hypofibrinogenemia, depression of various other clotting factors has been reported. Most marked has been a decrease in the plasma levels of factors V and VIII with a variable decrease in factors VII and IX. A decrease in circulating platelets has occurred in low incidence which, together with the increased levels of fibrin degradation products in the serum, may indicate development of a consumption coagulopathy. Bleeding has been a problem in only a few patients with demonstrable coagulopathy; however, fatal bleeding associated with low fibrinogen levels has been reported. Increased fibrinolytic activity, apparently compensatory in nature, also has occurred.

Some patients have shown CNS effects consisting of depression, somnolence, fatigue, coma, confusion, agitation, and hallucinations varying from mild to severe. Rarely, a Parkinson-like syndrome has occurred with tremor and progressive increase in muscular tone. These side effects usually have reversed spontaneously after treatment was discontinued. Therapy with asparaginase is associated with an increase in blood ammonia during the conversion of asparagine to aspartic acid and ammonia by the enzyme. No definite correlation exists between the degree of elevation of blood ammonia levels and the appearance of CNS changes. Chills, fever, nausea, vomiting, anorexia, abdominal cramps, weight loss, headache, and irritability may occur and are usually mild. Azotemia, usually prerenal, occurs frequently. Acute renal shutdown and fatal renal insufficiency have been reported during treatment. Proteinuria has occurred infrequently.

A variety of liver function abnormalities have been reported, including elevations of SGOT, SGPT, alkaline phosphatase, bilirubin (direct and indirect), and depression of serum albumin, cholesterol (total and esters), and plasma fibrinogen. Increases and decreases of total lipids have occurred. Marked hypoalbuminemia associated with peripheral edema has been reported. However, these abnormalities usually are reversible on discontinuance of therapy and some reversal may occur during the course of therapy. Fatty changes in the liver have been documented by biopsy. Malabsorption syndrome, transient bone marrow depression (rare), and marked leukopenia have also been reported.

Dosage and Administration: *Intramuscularly or intravenously by infusion.* An intradermal skin test should be performed prior to the initial administration of asparaginase and when the drug is given after an interval of a week or more has elapsed between doses. The skin test solution may be prepared by reconstituting the contents of a 10,000 IU vial with 5 ml of diluent. From this solution (2000 IU/ml) withdraw 0.1 ml and inject it into another vial containing 9.9 ml of diluent, yielding a skin test solution of approximately 20 IU/ml. Use 0.1 ml of this solution for the skin test. The skin test site should be observed for at least 1 hour for the appearance of a wheal or erythema either of which indicates a positive reaction. Patients who are positive reactors to the skin test or those requiring retreatment who may have acquired a hypersensitivity to the drug should be desensitized. One reported schedule begins with a total of 1 IU given *intravenously,* doubling the dose every 10 minutes until the accumulated total amount given equals the planned doses for that day. When the drug is intended for intramuscular administration the 10,000 unit vial should be reconstituted by adding 2 ml of sodium chloride solution for injection. The resulting solution should be used within 8 hours and only if it is clear. The volume of a single injection site should be limited to 2 ml, if more than 2 ml is to be administered 2 injection sites should be used. When intended for intravenous use, the 10,000 unit vial should be reconstituted with 5 ml of Sterile Water for Injection or with Sodium Chloride Injection. Ordinary shaking during reconstitution does not inactivate the enzyme, and as long as the solution remains clear, it may be used for direct intravenous administration within an 8-hour period following restoration. The intravenous administration should be given over a period of not less than 30 minutes through the side arm of an already running infusion of Sodium Chloride Injection or Dextrose Injection, 5% (D_5W). For administration by infusion, solutions should be diluted with isotonic solution, Sodium Chloride Injection or Dextrose Injection, 5%. Intravenous administration rarely causes phlebitis.

The suggested dosage for the induction of remissions in acute lymphoblastic leukemia in adults and children is 200 IU/kg daily *intravenously* for 28 days. Remissions obtained with this regimen generally last from 1 to 3 months. Higher daily doses of 1000 IU/kg for periods up to, but not exceeding, 10 days have been employed as a method of avoiding anaphylactic reaction which ordinarily appears only after the 10th day of therapy. Combined therapy has been recommended for the induction of remission of the disease in children. The physician is advised to consult the package literature for the proposed combination regimens.

Availability:
ELSPAR® Injection in vials of 10 ml containing 10,000 units. **(Merck Sharp & Dohme)**

ATROPINE

Description: Atropine is an alkaloid usually obtained from such botanical sources as *Atropa belladonna, Datura stramonium* and *Hyoscyamus niger,* or is produced synthetically. It occurs as white crystals, usually needle-like, or as a white, crystalline powder slightly soluble in water and freely soluble in alcohol. Although atropine is sometimes used as the pure alkaloid, it most often is used as the sulfate or, less frequently, as the tannate. The sulfate occurs as colorless crystals, or white, crystalline powder very soluble in water and freely soluble in alcohol. Atropine tannate is about half as potent as the sulfate, 1 mg of the tannate being equivalent to 0.5 mg of the sulfate.

Atropine inhibits the structures innervated by postganglionic parasympathetic nerves; stimulates higher cerebral centers and medulla; controls smooth-muscle spasm; inhibits the secretions of the salivary, respiratory tract, sweat and other glands; accelerates heart action by blocking vagal impulses; and in ophthalmology, produces mydriasis and cycloplegia.

Indications: Symptomatic treatment of postencephalitic parkinsonism and paralysis agitans; cardiospasm and pylorospasm, hyperirritability of the gastrointestinal tract; suppresses excessive salivation and bronchial secretions; relieves muscarine-like symptoms and some CNS manifestations due to poisoning by parathion-type insecticides (containing organic phosphate cholinesterase inhibitors); as an anhidrotic; in syncope due to carotid sinus hypersensitivity or heart block. It is used for its spasmolytic effect in the eye to produce dilatation and cycloplegia prior to retinoscopy, and for the treatment of uveitis, iridocyclitis and keratitis.

Contraindications: Glaucoma, asthma, organic pyloric stenosis and adhesions between iris and lens of the eye.

Warnings: Atropine should be used with caution in prostatism, urinary retention, in elderly patients and in children under 6 years of age. If eye pain occurs, the drug should be discontinued since this may indicate undiagnosed glaucoma. Patients should be cautioned not to exceed the prescribed dose, to decrease the dose if dryness of the mouth occurs and to discontinue use if rapid pulse, blurring of vision or dizziness occurs. Frequent or prolonged use of atropine should be avoided. Prolonged use in the eye may cause local irritation, hyperemia, edema, follicular conjunctivitis or dermatitis. Excessive use in children and certain susceptible individuals may produce general toxic symptoms.

Precautions: Use with caution in patients over 40 years of age, especially when used in the eye, because of the danger of precipitating incipient glaucoma; and in patients with prostatic hypertrophy or cardiac disease.

Adverse Reactions: Average doses may produce blurred vision, dry nose and mouth, flushing, bradycardia, mydriasis, conjunctivitis, swelling of the eyelid, and urinary retention. Larger doses may produce, in addition, tachycardia, tachypnea, scarlatiniform rash, disturbances of speech, difficulty in swallowing, headache, and restlessness with asthenia. Toxic doses may produce in addition delirium, stupor, fever, coma and respiratory failure. Death, although rarely occurring, is usually due to paralysis of the medullary centers.

Antidote: Pilocarpine hydrochloride, 5 mg until mouth becomes moist again. Barbiturates may be used cautiously to combat delirium. Adequate fluid intake is important. Respiratory failure should be treated with oxygen, carbon dioxide inhalation and artificial respiration if necessary. Vasopressor agents may be necessary in the event of circulatory collapse.

Dosage and Administration: *Orally.* Adults, usually 0.32 to 0.65 mg; in parkinsonism, this may be increased gradually to several milligrams daily if tolerated. *Intramuscularly.* Adults, 0.4 to 0.6 mg and children, 0.01 mg/kg of body weight ½ to 1 hour prior to surgery; 0.8 mg in poisoning due to parathion-type insecticides, followed in 30 minutes with 2 mg at hourly intervals until signs of atropinization are observed. Up to 2 or 3 times this dose may be required in severe cases. Removing contaminated clothing, washing the skin, and instituting artificial respiration and supportive measures are also indicated. *Subcutaneously.* Adults, 0.5 mg and children, 0.01 mg/kg of body weight every 4 to 6 hours. In *ophthalmology,* the usual dose to produce cycloplegia is 1 drop of a 1% solution of atropine sulfate instilled into each eye 3 times daily for 3 days prior to examination. For iritis, a 1% solution or ointment is used 2 or 3 times daily or as needed to keep the pupil dilated and the ciliary body relaxed.

Availability:

Atropine Sulfate

ATROPINE SULFATE Injection, 0.1 mg/ml in Abboject® (disposable syringes) of 5 and 10 ml. **(Abbott)**

ATROPINE SULFATE: **(Allergan)**
Ophthalmic Ointment, 0.5 and 1% in tubes of 3.5 gm.
Ophthalmic Solution, 1 and 2% in dropper bottles of 15 ml.

ATROPINE SULFATE Injection, 0.4 mg/0.5 ml in ampuls of 0.5 ml; 0.5 mg/ml in multiple-dose vials of 20 ml. **(Burroughs Wellcome)**

ATROPINE SULFATE: **(Lilly)**
Hypodermic Tablets, 0.3, 0.4 and 0.6 mg in bottles of 100.
Injection, 0.4 mg/ml in ampuls of 20 ml.
Ophthalmic Ointment, 1% in tubes of 3.5 gm.
Tablets, 0.4 mg in bottles of 100.

ATROPINE SULFATE Injection, 1 mg/ml in ampuls of 1 ml. **(Wyeth)**

ATROPISOL: **(Smith, Miller & Patch)**
Ophthalmic Ointment, 0.5% in tubes of 3.5 gm.
Ophthalmic Solution, 1% in dropper bottles of 5 and 15 ml; 0.5, 1 and 2% in Dropperettes applicators of 1 ml in cartons of 10.

Isopto® ATROPINE Ophthalmic Solution, 0.5 and 3% in Drop-Tainer® bottles of 5 ml; 1% in Drop-Tainer bottles of 5 and 15 ml. **(Alcon)**

AUROTHIOGLUCOSE

Chemical Name: (D-Glucosylthio) gold.

Description: Aurothioglucose occurs as a yellow, odorless powder that is freely soluble in water and practically insoluble in organic solvents. It differs from other gold compounds in that it contains the aurothio group in lieu of the hydroxyl group at C-1 of the pyranose form of glucose.The compound contains approximately 50% gold. It is available as a sterile suspension of aurothioglucose in a suitable vegetable oil to promote slow absorption and prolonged effects.

Although its precise mode of action has not been determined, the predominant action appears to be a suppressive effect on the synovitis of active rheumatoid disease. The greatest benefit appears to occur when the disease is in the early active stage, since in the late stages when cartilage and bone damage have occurred, gold can only check the progression of rheumatoid arthritis and thus prevent further structural damage to joints. It cannot repair damage caused by previously active disease. Appreciable amounts are found in the liver, spleen, kidneys, and skin from which it is slowly eliminated, principally by the kidneys, but also in the feces probably due to biliary secretion. Studies with pregnant rats and rabbits have shown the drug to be teratogenic.

Indications: Treatment of active adult or juvenile rheumatoid arthritis.

Contraindications: In severe uncontrolled diabetes, severe debilitation, pregnancy, renal and active hepatic disease or a history of infectious hepatitis, marked hypertension, heart failure, in patients with a history of agranulocytosis, and hemorrhagic diathesis, in those with blood dyscrasias and in those patients who have recently had radiation treatment. The concomitant use of antimalarials, immunosuppressants, phenylbutazone, or oxyphenbutazone is contraindicated because of their potential to cause blood dyscrasias.

Warnings: Since gold therapy is potentially toxic, patients should be thoroughly informed about this drug. Severe reactions may respond to chelating agents such as dimercaprol. Treatment with this agent should be initiated at the first sign of a serious adverse reaction to gold therapy. Frequent urinalyses and complete blood counts including platelet estimation (every 2 weeks) are advised throughout therapy and the patient must be carefully observed for toxic symptoms especially those of dermatitis, stomatitis, and jaundice. Weekly inquiry regarding rash, pruritus, stomatitis, and metallic taste is indicated.

Adverse Reactions: A variety of adverse reactions may occur at anytime during therapy or up to many months after discontinuance of treatment, but mostly they tend to occur during the second and third month, after the amount injected has reached 250 to 500 mg. Dermatitis (ranging from erythema to exfoliative dermatitis, which can lead to alopecia and shedding of nails) is the most common reaction. Any eruption, especially if pruritic, may signify the early development of a skin reaction. Also reported were lesions of the mucous membranes such as stomatitis, colitis, pharyngitis, tracheitis, vaginitis and inflammation of the upper respiratory tract; therefore, careful oral hygiene is important. Conjunctivitis was rarely observed. Effects on the kidneys range from proteinuria to the nephrotic syndrome. Hematologic reactions such as granulocytopenia, agranulocytosis, thrombocytopenia with or without purpura, leukemia, eosinophilia, panmyelopathy, hemorrhagic diathesis, hypoplastic and aplastic anemia have been reported. These hematologic disorders may occur separately or in combination. Anaphylactic or "Nitritoid-type" reactions such as flushing, syncope, dizziness and sweating are most frequently reported. Other symptoms that may occur include nausea, vomiting, malaise and weakness. More severe, but less common effects include anaphylactic shock, bradycardia, thickening of the tongue, difficulty in swallowing and breathing, angioneurotic edema; if these occur treatment should be discontinued at once. Gastrointestinal reactions such as nausea, vomiting, colic, anorexia, abdominal cramps, diarrhea, ulcerative enterocolitis, as well as headache have rarely been reported, and may or may not be drug-induced. There have been rare reports of reactions involving the eye such as iritis, corneal ulcers, and gold deposits in ocular tissue. Hepatitis with jaundice, toxic hepatitis, acute yellow atrophy, encephalitis, immunological destruction of the synovia, EEG abnormalities, peripheral neuritis, gold bronchitis, pulmonary injury manifested by interstitial pneumonitis and fibrosis, and partial or complete hair loss have also been reported. Sometimes arthralgia occurs for a day or two after an injection, but this reaction usually subsides after the first few injections. In the presence of mild reactions, it is usually sufficient to discontinue therapy for a short period, and then to resume treatment with smaller doses. When severe reactions occur, treatment should be discontinued immediately.

Dosage and Administration: *Intramuscularly* only. Adults, the drug is administered at weekly intervals: 10 mg the first week, 25 mg the second and third weeks, 50 mg the fourth week and thereafter until 0.8 to 1 gm has been administered. If the patient has improved and no toxic symptoms have developed, a dose of 50 mg may be given at 3- to 4-week intervals. Some clinicians advocate therapy until a specific total amount has been administered; others recommend continuing therapy as long as the activity of the condition is under good control. A weekly dose of more than 50 mg is usually unnecessary and contraindicated. Children 6 to 12 years of age, 1/4 the adult dose, governed chiefly by body weight.

Availability:
SOLGANAL® Injection, 50 mg/ml suspended in oil in multiple-dose vials of 10 ml. **(Schering)**

AVC

Description: Contains:

	Cream	*Suppositories*
Aminacrine hydrochloride	0.2%	14 mg
Sulfanilamide	15%	1.05 gm
Allantoin	2%	140 mg

With lactose and buffered with lactic acid to about pH 4.5.

Aminacrine is a highly ionized acridine derivative. It possesses a wide range of bactericidal activity that includes many gram-positive and gram-negative organisms, as well as trichomonads and fungi. It is thought to act by interfering or competing with certain hydrogen ions in microbial enzyme systems; thus the growth of invading organisms is inhibited. Sulfonamide is believed to block certain metabolic processes essential for the growth of susceptible bacteria.

Indications: Treatment of trichomoniasis, vulvovaginal candidiasis, and vaginitis due to *Hemophilus vaginalis* and other susceptible bacteria.

Contraindications: Known hypersensitivity to sulfonamides.

Precautions: Those usually associated with sulfonamides. Patients should be observed for the appearance of a skin rash or other evidence of systemic toxicity, and should these develop, the medication should be withdrawn. This recommendation also applies to any evidence of a local reaction such as a burning sensation or increased discomfort.

Adverse Reactions: Those usually associated with sulfonamides apply.

Dosage and Administration: One applicatorful or 1 suppository *intravaginally* 1 or 2 times daily. Adequate control or eradication of Candida and trichomonads usually requires prolonged treatment. Since exacerbation of the infection may occur during menstruation, it is advisable to continue the applications for a minimum of 1 month, or through 1 complete menstrual cycle.

Availability:
AVC™: **(Merrell-National)**
Cream in tubes of 120 gm with applicator and in unit-dose tubes of 7.5 gm in packages of 24.
Suppositories in cartons of 16 with applicator.

AVC with DIENESTROL

Description: Contains:

	Cream	*Suppositories*
Dienestrol	0.01%	0.7 mg
Aminacrine hydrochloride	0.2%	14 mg
Sulfanilamide	15%	1.05 gm
Allantoin	2%	140 mg

Buffered with lactic acid to about pH 4.5.

Indications: Dienestrol, a synthetic estrogen, has been added to the AVC formulation (without dienestrol) to stimulate the restoration of normal vaginal epithelium to its premenopausal state. This decreases its susceptibility to trauma and to infection, and aids in the eradication of any preexisting infection. Recommended for the treatment of postmenopausal and senile vulvovaginitis, atrophic vaginitis, pruritus vulvae caused by atrophic changes in the vulval epithelium, and dyspareunia associated with an atrophic vaginal epithelium. May also be effective in the treatment of trichomoniasis, vulvovaginal candidiasis, and vaginitis due to *Hemophilus vaginalis* or other susceptible bacteria.

Contraindications: Known hypersensitivity to sulfonamides or to any of the other ingredients. Additional contraindications to the use of this preparation are known or suspected carcinoma of the breast, except those cases of progressing disease not amenable to surgery or irradiation occurring in women who are at least 5 years postmenopausal; known or suspected estrogen dependent neoplasia, such as carcinoma of the endometrium; precarcinomatus lesions of the vagina or vulva; undiagnosed abnormal genital bleeding or a bloody discharge; thrombophlebitis, thromboembolic disorders, thrombosis or patients with a past history of these conditions; and during pregnancy, especially the first 12 weeks.

Warnings: A statistically significant association has been reported between maternal ingestion of diethylstilbestrol, or a closely related congener, during early pregnancy and the occurrence of vaginal adenocarcinoma in the postpubertal stage of the offspring. It is therefore recommended that periodic examinations of such patients be undertaken. The drug should be immediately withdrawn at the earliest manifestation of thrombotic disorders (thrombophlebitis, cerebrovascular complications, pulmonary embolism and retinal thrombosis); if there is a sudden onset of proptosis, diplopia or migraine, if examination reveals papilledema or retinal vascular lesions, or if hypercalcemia develops in patients with metastatic breast cancer, since this indicates progression of bone metastasis. Estrogens are excreted in the mother's milk; therefore, the estrogenic effect on the nursing infant should be taken into consideration when this product is prescribed for lactating women.

Precautions: Treatment should be discontinued if either local or systemic manifestations of sulfonamide toxicity or sensitivity occur; however, withdrawal of therapy should be gradual rather than spontaneous because of the possibility of endometrial withdrawal bleeding. When used in atrophic lesions of the vulvae, or in atrophic vaginitis with bleeding or a bloody discharge in menopausal or postmenopausal patients, careful diagnostic measures must be instituted to eliminate the possibility of a serious neoplastic disease. Patients highly responsive to estrogenic therapy may experience abnormal or excessive uterine bleeding, mastodynia, edema and other estrogen-induced undesirable effects. Estrogens should be used with considerable care in patients with epilepsy, migraine, asthma, cardiac or renal disease (because of possible retention of salt and water); in those with preexisting uterine fibromyomata (since they may increase in size); those with an established familial history of cancer, recurrent chronic cystic mastitis, or abnormal mammograms; diabetic patients (because of a decrease in glucose tolerance); and in those with renal insufficiency. Estrogens have been associated with a two to threefold increase in the risk of developing surgically confirmed gallbladder disease, particularly in postmenopausal women, and may also be responsible for the development of hepatic adenomas; rupture of these tumors can result in abdominal pain and tenderness, abdominal mass, hypovolemic shock, and possibly death. Also, high doses of estrogens have been reported to increase blood pressure; therefore, routine monitoring of the patient is essential. Patients with a history of psychic depression should be carefully observed and the drug discontinued if the depression recurs to a serious degree. Because of the effects of estrogens on epiphyseal closure, it should be used judiciously in young patients in whom bone growth is incomplete. Estrogens induce changes in menopausal vaginal epithelium, uterine endothelium and breast tissue and these changes should be considered when specimens are sent for pathology examination. A pretreatment physical examination should include breast and pelvic organs as well as a Papanicolaou smear. Large doses of estrogen may result in urinary stress incontinance in nonpregnant women and prolonged high doses may suppress ovulation as a consequence of its inhibitory effect on anterior pituitary function; this should be considered when treating patients in whom fertility is desired. Since certain endocrine and liver function tests may give abnormal results during estrogen intake, it is recommended that the tests be repeated two months after withdrawal of the drug.

Adverse Reactions: Absorption of considerable quantities of dienestrol may result in breast tenderness and enlargement, and worsening of menstrual irregularity. It may also cause serious bleeding in women sterilized because of endometriosis, in whom remaining foci of endometrium could be activated. Therapy should be discontinued if local reactions such as increased discomfort or a burning sensation are noted. Additional adverse reactions that may occur with the use of estrogens are nausea, vomiting, anorexia, gastrointestinal symptoms such as abdominal cramps or bloating, edema, breakthrough bleeding, spotting or withdrawal bleeding, increase or decrease in body weight, increase in cervical mucus, allergic rash, loss of libido, aggravation of migraine headaches, hepatic cutaneous porphyria becoming manifest, cholestatic jaundice, rise in blood pressure in susceptible individuals, mental depression, cystitis-like syndrome, alopecia, erythema nodosum, erythema multiform, hemorrhagic eruption, premenstrual-like syndrome, changes in libido, nervousness, dizziness, fatigue, backache, headache, possible decrease in lactation when given immediately postpartum, irritability, and malaise.

Dosage and Administration: *Intravaginally,* 1 applicatorful or 1 suppository inserted into the vaginal vault once or twice daily. A douche with a suitable cleansing solution may be advisable prior to insertion. The control or elimination of trichomonads or monilia usually requires treatment for at least 4 weeks or longer.

Availability:
AVC™ with DIENESTROL: **(Merrell-National)**
Cream in tubes of 120 gm with applicator.
Suppositories in cartons of 16 with applicator.

AXOTAL

Description: Each tablet contains:

Phenobarbital	15 mg
Phenacetin	120 mg
Aspirin	250 mg

Indications: To help relieve the fever, minor aches and pains which may occur in patients with upper respiratory infections. It may be useful in those patients who may experience insomnia due to such discomforts; in neuralgia, headache and toothache.

Contraindications: Patients with impaired renal function or those patients with an idiosyncrasy to barbiturates or salicylates. It is also contraindicated in patients with persistent anemia or hepatic disease.

Warnings: Phenobarbital may be habit-forming. Patients receiving these drugs should be cautioned against hazardous occupations requiring complete alertness such as operating machinery or a motor vehicle.

Adverse Reactions: Untoward reactions such as excitement may occur in patients sensitive to barbiturates. Phenacetin and aspirin, in excessive dosage, may cause nausea, vomiting and/or diarrhea.

Dosage and Administration: *Orally.* Adults, 1 or 2 tablets every 2 or 3 hours depending upon the severity of pain.

Availability:
AXOTAL Tablets in bottles of 100 and 1000. **(Warren-Teed)**

AZATADINE MALEATE

Chemical Name: 6,11-Dihydro-11-(1-methyl-4-piperidylidene)-5H-benzo [5,6] cyclohepta [1,2-6] pyridine maleate (1:2).

Description: Azatadine provides the advantages of antihistaminic action at a low dose, combined with long-acting properties. Chemically related to cyproheptadine, the drug also provides antiserotonin, anticholinergic and sedative effects. Its action is exerted directly on those peripheral effector cells which respond to histamine, thereby competitively antagonizing the effects of histamine at receptor sites.

Indications: Recommended for the treatment of perennial and seasonal allergic rhinitis and chronic urticaria.

Contraindications: Patients hypersensitive to the drug or to related compounds, newborn or premature infants, nursing mothers, concomitant use with monoamine oxidase inhibitors (MAOI), and patients with lower respiratory tract symptoms (including asthma). It is not intended for use in children under 12 years of age.

Warnings: Patients should be well-informed that antihistamines often cause drowsiness, and produce additive effects with other CNS depressants including alcohol. Because of its anticholinergic activity, azatadine should be used with considerable care in patients with narrow-angle glaucoma, stenosing peptic ulcer, pyloroduodenal obstruction, symptomatic prostatic hypertrophy, and bladder neck obstruction. Hallucinations, convulsions, and possibly death may occur in infants and children receiving excessive doses. Histamine antagonizing agents occasionally may produce signs and symptoms of excitation in children, and are more likely to cause dizziness, sedation, and hypotension in geriatric patients. Safe use during pregnancy or lactation has not been established; therefore, the expected benefits must be weighed against the potential hazards.

Precautions: Since the drug demonstrates an atropine-like action, it should be used with utmost care in patients with increased intraocular pressure, hyperthyroidism, cardiovascular disease, hypertension, or with a history of bronchial asthma.

Adverse Reactions: The most frequent untoward effects with azatadine are sedation, sleepiness, dizziness, disturbed coordination, epigastric distress, and thickening of bronchial secretions. General adverse reactions include urticaria, drug rash, anaphylactic shock, photosensitivity, excessive perspiration, chills, dryness of mouth, nose and throat. Cardiovascular side effects may include hypotension, headache, palpitations, tachycardia, and extrasystoles. Those involving the hematologic system are usually hemolytic anemia, thrombocytopenia, and agranulocytosis. Other CNS manifestations are fatigue, confusion, restlessness, excitation, nervousness, tremor, irritability, insomnia, euphoria, paresthesias, blurred vision, diplopia, vertigo, tinnitus, acute labyrinthitis, hysteria, neuritis, and convulsions. Gastrointestinal side effects may also include anorexia, nausea, vomiting, diarrhea, and constipation. Genitourinary tract symptoms include urinary frequency, difficult urination, urinary retention, and early menses. Respiratory side effects produce tightness of chest and wheezing, and nasal stuffiness. Reactions due to overdosage vary from CNS depression to stimulation. Atropine-like signs and symptoms include dry mouth; fixed, dilated pupils; flushing; and gastrointestinal symptoms. Since there is no specific therapy to counteract acute overdosage, general symptomatic and supportive measures should be instituted promptly and maintained for as long as required.

Dosage and Administration: *Orally.* The usual dosage is 1 or 2 tablets twice daily.

Availability:
OPTIMINE® Tablets, 1 mg in bottles of 100. **(Schering)**

AZATHIOPRINE

Chemical Name: 6-[(1-Methyl-4-nitroimidazo-5-yl)thio]purine.

Description: Azathioprine is an imidazolyl derivative of, and similar in action to, mercaptopurine. Like its parent compound mercaptopurine, azathioprine is an antimetabolite, interfering with purine metabolism at the enzyme level. The drug is split extensively to 6-mercaptopurine, which is then subject to catabolic destruction to form a variety of oxidized and methylated derivatives, among which 6-thiouric acid, formed by the oxidation of mercaptopurine by xanthine oxidase, predominates. The fate of the nitromethylimidazole portion of azathioprine is not completely understood. Small amounts of the compound are also cleaved to give 1-methyl-4-nitro-5-thioimidazole. The proportions of the different metabolites vary from individual to individual depending upon the relative amounts of the catabolic enzymes available. Azathioprine occurs as a light-sensitive, yellow powder insoluble in water and in alcohol. The drug is stable in neutral or acid solutions, but is split to mercaptopurine by alkalies.

Following oral administration, the drug is readily absorbed from the gastrointestinal tract. Blood levels are extremely low (below 1 mcg/ml); however, because purine antagonists rapidly enter into anabolic and catabolic pathways of purines, this blood level measurement actually represents several compounds and the significance of blood level is questionable. Both azathioprine and mercaptopurine show moderate binding (about 30%) to serum proteins, but both appear to be dialyzable. Although elimination of azathioprine is mainly by metabolic destruction, small amounts of unchanged drug and mercaptopurine are eliminated by the kidney, and the biological effectiveness and toxicity may therefore be increased as much as two-fold in the anuric patient. Its immunosuppressive properties have been found useful in patients who have received organ transplants. Approximately 80% of all transplants in which azathioprine was administered were functioning 3 months after the transplant operation and about 55% after 2 years. May be used alone or in conjunction with other immunosuppressive agents such as corticosteroids, and other cytotoxic agents.

The maximum effectiveness of azathioprine occurs when it is administered during the induction period of the antibody response, starting either at the time of antigenic stimulation or within 2 days thereafter. The effects of the drug and its active metabolite, mercaptopurine, may not appear until several days after therapy has been initiated and may persist for several days after clearance of the compounds is completed.

Indications: As an adjunct for the prevention of rejection in renal homotransplantation. Other uses remain investigational.

Contraindications: Known hypersensitivity to the drug.

Warnings: Azathioprine is a potent drug capable of producing severe and irreversible bone marrow depression. Complete blood counts, including platelets, should be performed at least weekly, and more frequently during the initial stage of therapy and when high doses are used. A persistent decrease or a rapid fall in the leukocyte count calls for a decrease in dosage or a temporary withdrawal of the drug. In the presence of severe and unremitting rejection, it is probably preferable to allow the kidney transplant to be rejected rather than increase the drug to very toxic dosage levels in an attempt to prevent rejection. The patient may then be maintained by dialysis until another kidney becomes available. Infection is always a constant hazard of the therapeutic regimen used for the prevention of rejection. There have been reports of fungal, protozoal, viral and uncommon bacterial infections, some of which have been fatal. If intercurrent infection develops, it should be treated appropriately and consideration should be given to the possibility of reducing the dosage of azathioprine, corticosteroids and/or ancillary drugs. In a few cases lymphomas have been known to occur. Persistent negative nitrogen balance has been observed in some patients on continuous therapy with azathioprine and corticosteroids; if this occurs, dosage should be reduced. If there is evidence of toxic hepatitis or biliary stasis, consideration should be given to withholding the drug.

Drugs of this type are potentially teratogenic; the benefits and risks must be weighed before use in women of childbearing potential.

Precautions: Cadaveric kidneys frequently develop a tubular necrosis with delayed onset of adequate function, and clearance of azathioprine and its metabolites may be impaired; dosage therefore should be reduced appropriately. Patients taking allopurinol and azathioprine concomitantly require a reduction in dosage of the latter to approximately 1/3 to 1/4 its usual dosage.

Adverse Reactions: The chief toxic effect is hematologic, manifested by leukopenia, anemia, thrombocytopenia and bleeding. Oral lesions, skin rashes, drug fever, alopecia, pancreatitis, arthralgia and steatorrhea are not generally seen, but may occur. Nausea, vomiting, diarrhea and anorexia sometimes occur, especially at higher dosages. Jaundice has been observed in some patients, suggesting liver damage or biliary stasis; this has been characterized by extremely high alkaline phosphatase levels with slightly elevated bilirubin.

Dosage and Administration: The dosage which will be tolerated or will be effective will vary from patient to patient and, therefore, careful management is necessary to obtain the optimum therapeutic effect without incurring toxicity. Caution must be exercised to avoid toxicity, the chief manifestation of which is bone marrow depression, resulting most commonly in leukopenia and less often in thrombocytopenia and bleeding. **Since this drug may have a delayed action, it is important to reduce dosage or withdraw the drug temporarily at the first sign of an abnormally large fall in the leukocyte count and/or other evidence of persistent depression of the bone marrow.** Patients with impaired renal function may have slower elimination of the drug with a consequent greater cumulative effect; therefore, the dosage should be reduced appropriately.

The usual initial dosage is approximately 3 to 5 mg/kg/day, *orally* or *intravenously.* Adjunctive therapy of various types has generally been used in suppressing rejection of renal homografts and this may add to the toxic potential of the regimen. Dosage must be adjusted to attempt to provide satisfactory maintenance of the homograft without producing toxic effects; it may be possible to reduce the maintenance dosage to 1 to 2 mg/kg/day.

Availability:
IMURAN®: **(Burroughs Wellcome)**
Injection (as sodium salt), 100 mg in vials of 20 ml.
Tablets, 50 mg in bottles of 100.

AZOTREX

Description: Induces high initial tetracycline levels in the blood plus high tetracycline and sulfonamide levels in the urine. Provides systemic and local antibacterial action, plus analgesia, in acute and chronic urinary tract infections due to organisms sensitive to tetracycline or sulfamethizole.

Each capsule contains tetracycline phosphate complex equivalent to 125 mg tetracycline hydrochloride; sulfamethizole, 250 mg and phenazopyridine hydrochloride, 50 mg.

Indications: For mixed infections in which the causative organisms are more sensitive to the combination than to either antibacterial agent alone. It is indicated in the treatment of cystitis, urethritis, pyelonephritis, ureteritis, and prostatitis due to bacterial infection, prior to and following genitourinary surgery and instrumentation, and as a prophylactic agent in patients with urethrostomies and cord bladders. May be particularly useful in the geriatric patient when exacerbations of infection occur in such conditions as cystocele, prostatitis and nonspecific urethritis.

Contraindications: Hypersensitivity to any of the components; in premature infants, neonates, pregnant patients at term; patients with chronic glomerulonephritis, uremia, severe hepatitis, hepatic or renal failure, or severe pyelitis of pregnancy.

Warnings: Hypersensitive patients may develop a photodynamic reaction precipitated by direct exposure to natural or artificial sunlight during the use of tetracyclines. For further details, see the general statement on the Tetracyclines.

Precautions: The use of tetracycline during the period of tooth development (last trimester of pregnancy, neonatal period and early childhood) may cause discoloration of the teeth. Patients should be told that phenazopyridine, an azo dye, will impart an orange-red color to the urine. Refer to the general statement on the Tetracyclines for comprehensive details.

Adverse Reactions: As with all sulfonamides, the following reactions may occur: nausea, vomiting, diarrhea, hepatitis, pancreatitis, blood dyscrasias, neuropathy, drug fever, skin rash, infection of the conjunctiva and sclera, petechiae, purpura, hematuria and crystalluria. The reactions associated with tetracycline (e.g., glossitis, stomatitis, proctitis and vaginitis) may occur. Dosage should be decreased or the drug withdrawn depending upon the severity of the reaction.

See monographs on Tetracycline, Sulfonamides and Phenazopyridine Hydrochloride for complete details.

Dosage and Administration: *Orally,* 1 or 2 capsules 4 times daily. Higher doses may be used in severe infections. For maximal benefit the drug should be taken on an empty stomach. Calcium, in particular, interferes with the absorption of tetracycline. Infections due to beta-hemolytic streptococci require at least 10 days of treatment in order to prevent the occurrence of rheumatic fever or glomerulonephritis. In acute uncomplicated urinary tract infections, therapy should be continued until the urine specimens become sterile, i.e., 7 to 14 days.

Availability:
AZOTREX® Capsules in bottles of 100. **(Bristol)**

BACITRACIN

Description: Bacitracin is a polypeptide antibiotic produced by the growth of a gram-positive, spore-forming organism belonging to the *licheniformis* group of *Bacillus subtilis.* It has a potency of not less than 40 units of bacitracin activity/mg, except that when intended for parenteral use its potency is not less than 50 units/mg. It is active against a wide variety of gram-positive organisms, including streptococci; staphylococci and pneumococci; anaerobic cocci and clostridia of the gas gangrene group; corynebacteria; *Treponema pallidum; Treponema vincenti;* and certain gram-negative cocci, including gonococci and meningococci. It is ineffective against most gram-negative bacilli. However, because of the high rate of nephrotoxic reactions, only staphylococcal infections qualify for consideration in the use of bacitracin systemically.

Absorption of bacitracin following intramuscular injection is rapid and complete. A dose of 200 or 300 mg/kg every 6 hours gives serum levels of 0.2 to 2 mcg/ml in individuals with normal renal function. The drug is excreted slowly by glomerular filtration. It is widely distributed in all body organs and is demonstrable in ascitic and pleural fluids after intramuscular injection. Bacitracin does not appear to be absorbed when used topically.

Indications: Intramuscularly in the treatment of infants with staphylococcal pneumonia and empyema caused by bacitracin-sensitive organisms resistant to penicillin and other antibiotics; and by local injection into circumscribed areas of infection, such as furuncles, carbuncles, or abscesses. Bacitracin is also employed locally by topical application in the treatment of susceptible infections of the skin, the eye, and the nose and throat, and in surgical infections of soft tissues and bone, as well as prophylactically in burns.

Contraindications: This drug is contraindicated in those individuals with a history of previous hypersensitivity or toxic reaction to bacitracin.

Warnings: Bacitracin in parenteral (intramuscular) therapy may cause renal failure due to tubular and glomerular necrosis. Its use should be restricted to infants with staphylococcal pneumonia and empyema when due to organisms shown to be susceptible to bacitracin. It should be used only where adequate laboratory facilities are available and when constant supervision of the patient is possible. Renal function should be carefully determined prior to and daily during therapy. The recommended daily dose should not be exceeded and fluid intake and urinary output maintained at proper levels to avoid kidney toxicity. If renal toxicity occurs the drug should be discontinued. The concurrent use of other nephrotoxic drugs, particularly streptomycin, kanamycin, polymyxin B, polymyxin E (colistin), neomycin, and viomycin, should be avoided.

Precautions: The use of antibiotics, including bacitracin, may result in an overgrowth of nonsusceptible organisms, particularly monilia. Constant observation of the patient is essential. If new infections caused by nonsusceptible bacteria or fungi appear during therapy, appropriate measures should be taken. Adequate fluid intake should be maintained *orally,* or if necessary, by parenteral method.

Adverse Reactions: The intramuscular use of bacitracin often is complicated by the occurrence of a reversible depression of renal tubular and glomerular function with manifestations of albuminuria, cylinduria, azotemia, and rising blood levels of the antibiotic without any increase in dosage. Other reactions noted include nausea, vomiting, skin rash, and painful induration at the site of injection. Patients receiving bacitracin should be observed carefully for evidence of renal damage. Urinalysis and blood chemistry should precede initiation of treatment.

Following topical application, bacitracin is poorly absorbed and toxic reactions are therefore not expected. However, signs of nephrotoxicity should be looked for and treated appropriately whenever large surface areas are treated topically. Also, if signs of irritation and sensitivity (itching, burning or inflammation) occur, the drug should be discontinued.

Dosage and Administration: *Intramuscularly. For infants under 2500 gm,* 900 units/kg/day divided into 2 or 3 doses. *For infants over 2500 gm,* 1000 units/kg/day divided into 2 or 3 doses. The drug should be administered in the upper outer quadrant of the buttocks, alternating right and left and avoiding multiple injections in the same region because of the transient pain following administration. *Topically.* The ointments may be applied 1 or more times daily as prescribed by the physician.

Availability:
BACIGUENT®: **(Upjohn)**
Ointment, 500 units/gm in tubes of 15, 30 and 120 gm.
Ophthalmic Ointment, 500 units/gm in tubes of 3.5 gm with applicator tip.
BACIMYCIN® Ointment, 500 units/gm with neomycin sulfate, 0.5% in tubes of 15 gm. **(Merrell-National)**
BACITRACIN Ointment, 500 units/gm in tubes of 15 and 30 gm. **(Pfipharmecs)**
BACITRACIN: **(Lilly)**
Ointment, 500 units/gm in tubes of 15, 30 and 120 gm.
Ophthalmic Ointment, 500 units/gm in tubes of 3.5 gm.
BACITRACIN Sterile Powder in vials of 50,000 units. **(Pfizer)**
BACITRACIN Sterile Powder in vials of 10,000 and 50,000 units. **(Upjohn)**

BACLOFEN

Chemical Name: 4-Amino-3-(*p*-chlorophenyl) butyric acid.

Description: Baclofen is a skeletal muscle relaxant drug designated primarily for the relief of the signs and symptoms of spasticity resulting from multiple sclerosis. Additionally, it may provide some beneficial effects in spinal cord injuries and other spinal cord disorders. The drug apparently achieves its antispastic action by inhibiting both monosynaptic and polysynaptic reflexes at the spinal cord level, possibly by hyperpolarization of afferent terminals, although actions at supraspinal sites may also occur and contribute to its clinical effect. Consequently, exaggerated motor impulses are inhibited, thus abolishing the hyperreflexic action of spasticity. An analog of gamma aminobutyric acid, it occurs as a white to off-white crystalline substance that is slightly soluble in water and poorly soluble in organic solvents. Molecular weight of the compound has been reported to be 213.67.

Although the drug has demonstrated rapid and extensive absorption and elimination, clinical observations have found a relatively large variation in these parameters among patients. Also, absorption tends to be dose-related in that it appears to be reduced with increasing amounts of the drug. Baclofen is excreted primarily by the kidneys in unchanged form.

Indications: Alleviation of the signs and symptoms of spasticity resulting from multiple sclerosis, particularly flexor spasms and concomitant pain, clonus, and muscular rigidity. The drug may also be of some value in patients with spinal cord injuries and other spinal cord diseases, but it is not indicated in skeletal muscle spasm resulting from rheumatic disorders. Since effective use in stroke, cerebral palsy, and Parkinson's disease has not been established, it is therefore not recommended for use in these conditions.

Contraindications: Hypersensitivity to the compound.

Warnings: Because hallucinations have occurred upon abrupt withdrawal of the drug, the dose should be reduced slowly when discontinuation of treatment is anticipated. Caution should be exercised in patients with impaired kidney function, and it should be given to pregnant patients only if the benefit clearly justifies the risk to the fetus.

Precautions: The use of baclofen in children under 12 years of age is not recommended. Because of the possibility of sedation, patients should be cautioned regarding the operation of automobiles or other dangerous machinery, and activities made hazardous due to decreased alertness. They should also be cautioned that the CNS effects of the drug may be additive to those of alcohol and other CNS depressants. Baclofen should be used with caution in patients in whom spasticity is utilized to sustain an upright posture and balance in locomotion or whenever spasticity is utilized to obtain increased function. In patients with epilepsy, the clinical state and EEG should be monitored at regular intervals, since deterioration in seizure control and EEG have been reported. Lactating women should be cautioned not to nurse their infants while taking this drug. A dose-related increase in the incidence of ovarian cysts and a less marked increase in enlarged and/or hemorrhagic adrenal glands were observed in female rats treated chronically with baclofen; however, the relevance of these findings to humans is not known.

Adverse Reactions: The most commonly observed adverse reactions to baclofen include transient drowsiness with an incidence of 10 to 63%; dizziness, 5 to 15%; weakness, 5 to 15%; and fatigue, 2 to 4%. Other reported reactions include *neuropsychiatric symptoms* manifested by confusion, 1 to 11%; headache, 4 to 8%; insomnia, 2 to 7%; and rarely, euphoria, excitement, depression, hallucinations, paresthesia, muscle pain, tinnitus, slurred speech, coordination disorders, tremor, rigidity, dystonia, ataxia, blurred vision, nystagmus, strabismus, miosis, mydriasis, diplopia, dysarthria, and epileptic seizures. Those involving the *cardiovascular system* include hypotension, 0 to 9%; and rare occurrences of dyspnea, palpitation, chest pain, and syncope; the *gastrointestinal system* include nausea, 4 to 12%; constipation, 2 to 6%; and rarely, dry mouth, anorexia, taste disorder, abdominal pain, vomiting, diarrhea, and positive test for occult blood in stool; the *genitourinary system* include urinary frequency, 2 to 6%; and rarely, enuresis, urinary retention, dysuria, impotence, inability to ejaculate, nocturia, and hematuria; *miscellaneous symptoms* include rash, pruritus, ankle edema, excessive perspiration, weight gain, and nasal congestion. The following laboratory tests have been found to be abnormal in a few patients and include increased SGOT, elevated alkaline phosphatase, and elevation of blood sugar. The signs and symptoms of overdosage include vomiting, muscular hypotonia, drowsiness, accommodation disorders, coma, respiratory depression, and seizures.

Dosage and Administration: *Orally.* Although optimal dosage requires individualized titration, most patients take between 40 and 80 mg daily. Therapy should be initiated at a low dosage and increased gradually until optimum effect is achieved. The recommended initial dosage is 5 mg tid for 3 days, 10 mg tid for 3 days, 15 mg tid for 3 days, and 20 mg tid for 3 days. Thereafter, additional increases may be necessary but the total daily dose should not exceed 80 mg daily (20 mg qid).

Availability:
LIORESAL® Tablets, 10 mg in bottles of 100. **(Geigy)**

BARBIDONNA

Description: Each tablet contains:

Phenobarbital	16 mg
Hyoscyamine sulfate	0.1286 mg
Atropine sulfate	0.025 mg
Scopolamine hydrobromide	0.0074 mg

Barbidonna No. 2 tablets have the same composition as the above, but with 32 mg of phenobarbital.

Each teaspoonful of elixir contains:

Phenobarbital	21.6 mg
Hyoscyamine sulfate	0.174 mg
Atropine sulfate	0.034 mg
Scopolamine hydrobromide	0.010 mg
Alcohol	15%

Indications: Antispasmodic and sedative for the treatment of peptic ulcer, gastroenteritis, ulcerative or spastic colitis, pylorospasm, gastritis, dyspepsia, spastic constipation and other conditions attributable to smooth muscle spasm of the digestive tract. May also be used for ureteral spasm, nocturnal enuresis, dysmenorrhea, renal colic, biliary spasms due to cholecystitis and cholelithiasis, and for motion sickness.

Contraindications: Glaucoma, impaired renal or hepatic function, and idiosyncrasy to barbiturates or belladonna.

Warnings: Phenobarbital may be habit-forming; therefore, the usual precautions pertaining to the use of barbiturates should be observed.

Precautions: Caution should be exercised in those patients with increased intraocular pressure, obstructive uropathy or intermittent porphyria.

Adverse Reactions: Dryness of mouth and skin, blurred vision, urinary retention, tachycardia or flushing of the skin may occur with high doses.

Dosage and Administration: *Orally.* Adults, 1 or 2 tablets or teaspoonsful of elixir 3 to 4 times daily. Children, 1/4 to 1 teaspoonful 3 or 4 times daily.

Availability:
BARBIDONNA® **(Mallinckrodt)**
Elixir (light orange-colored, apricot-flavored) in bottles of 1 pint.
Tablets (white) and No. 2 (light brown) in bottles of 100 and 500.

BCG VACCINE

Description: The vaccine is a dry, standardized preparation of BCG bacillus prepared from a Glaxo substrain of a Danish strain of BCG bacillus that is dispersed in Sauton's medium with Triton® and cultured for 14 days at 37° C. The organisms are harvested by centrifugation and freeze-dried from a suitable concentration of a dextran-glucose medium and Triton.

Indications: Prophylaxis of tuberculosis. It has been suggested that the following should be considered likely candidates for immunization:

1. Recipients should have negative tuberculin skin tests and who are repeatedly exposed to persistently untreated or ineffectively treated sputum-positive cases of pulmonary tuberculosis.
2. Individuals or groups living in communities where an excessive rate of new infections can be demonstrated and the usual surveillance and treatment programs have failed or have been shown not to be applicable.
3. Individuals involved in situations or environments (hospitals, institutions, public health service, etc.) in which the risk of tuberculosis is increased.

All authorities agree that BCG vaccine should not be considered a substitute for established programs of control, case-finding measures and proper treatment.

Contraindications: In tuberculin-positive individuals, and in those with recent smallpox vaccination, and in burn patients. In addition, the vaccine probably should not be given to patients on chronic corticosteroid therapy or to those with hypogammaglobulinemia or any other disorder in which the natural immunologic capacity of the host may have been adversely affected by disease processes. Although chronic diseases involving the skin are not contraindications, individuals with such conditions should be vaccinated in a healthy area of skin. BCG vaccine will not be effective if given during isoniazid (INH) administration, because the drug inhibits multiplication of BCG.

Precautions: Vaccinations must not be undertaken without prior determination that the patient is nonreactive to tuberculin skin tests. The individual to be vaccinated should first be tested with the more dilute solutions of O.T. (Old Tuberculin) or P.P.D. (Purified Protein Derivative). If this test is negative, the patient should be retested with the more concentrated solutions to insure as far as possible that sensitivity to tuberculosis does not exist. These tests should be performed within the 6-week period preceding vaccination. The protection from tuberculosis afforded by BCG vaccination is only relative and is not permanent or entirely predictable. If the tuberculin test again becomes negative and the risk of infection continues, BCG vaccination may need to be repeated. Although no harmful effects on the fetus have been observed with this vaccine, it is prudent to refrain from vaccination during pregnancy unless there is excessive risk of unavoidable exposure to infectious tuberculosis.

Adverse Reactions: Occasionally, a lymphangitis with regional adenitis from the site of injection has been observed. If the injection has been too deep, there may be ulceration at the vaccination site. An intense ulcerative lesion may also be produced if the vaccine is administered to a tuberculin-positive subject. This generally appears earlier than the normal papule observed following vaccination of the tuberculin-negative subject. Autoinoculation ulcers are seen occasionally. Abscesses in the skin at the site of inoculation may occur from secondary infection. Rarely, abscesses may develop in the regional lymph nodes draining the site of the BCG vaccination.

Granulomas, appearing approximately 4 to 6 weeks following the vaccination, have been reported at the site of the injection. They may result from application of irritating dressings to a normal BCG reaction or may occur occasionally as an idiosyncrasy. Such granulomas may persist for variable periods of time and may have a keloid scar after final healing. Rarely, persistent lupus reactions of the skin that required treatment have been reported. For these, isoniazid in a daily dose of 4 mg/kg of body weight has been recommended. One case of histiocytoma at the vaccination site required excision. Transient urticaria of the limbs and trunk has been observed following BCG vaccination, and one instance of erythema nodosum occurred in a large series of vaccinees in England.

Dosage and Administration: After the vaccine has been prepared, the immunizing dose of 0.1 ml is given by *intradermal* injection. Following reconstitution, the ampul should be used immediately, and any material remaining in the ampul should be discarded. **Note:** Do not expose the vial to sunlight.

Availability:
BCG VACCINE (Dry Powder) in ampules of 1 ml (10 doses). **(Lilly)**

BECLOMETHASONE DIPROPIONATE: see The Adrenal Corticosteroids

BELLADENAL

Description: Each tablet and Spacetab contains Bellafoline®, 0.25 mg and phenobarbital, 50 mg. Bellafoline consists of the levorotatory alkaloids of belladonna, as malates.

The levorotatory alkaloids of belladonna (Bellafoline) provide the antispasmodic-anticholinergic action of belladonna with only minimal central side effects. One Belladenal tablet has the antispasmodic-anticholinergic action of 27 minims of tincture belladonna.

Indications: To relieve pain and control hypersecretion and hypermotility in conditions such as peptic ulcer, acute enterocolitis, irritable colon, spastic colon and mucous colitis.

Contraindications: Glaucoma, elevated intraocular pressure, advanced hepatic or renal disease, and hypersensitivity to any of the components.

Warnings: Phenobarbital may be habit-forming.

Precautions: Caution is advised in elderly patients.

Adverse Reactions: Urinary retention, blurred vision, dry mouth, flushing or drowsiness may occur. The sedative effect represents a hazard in ambulatory patients whose activities require alertness and motor coordination.

Dosage and Administration: *Tablets:* Adults, 2 to 4 tablets daily in divided doses. Children, 1/4 to 1/2 tablet 1 to 4 times daily, according to age. *Spacetabs:* Adults, 1 tablet in the morning and 1 at night.

Availability:
BELLADENAL® Tablets (white) in bottles of 100. **(Sandoz)**
BELLADENAL-S™ Spacetabs (salmon pink, emerald green and white) in bottles of 100. **(Sandoz)**

BELLADONNA ALKALOIDS

Description: The principal alkaloids of belladonna most frequently used therapeutically are atropine, scopolamine, hyoscyamine and hyoscine. They usually are employed collectively in a specific, fixed ratio combined with a barbiturate to provide both prompt peripheral antispasmodic action and smooth central sedation. Through the synergism of the individual alkaloids, greater efficacy is achieved with smaller doses and consequently a minimum of side effects.

Indications: Because of their antispasmodic-anticholinergic and mild sedative properties, the alkaloids in combination with a barbiturate may be useful as adjunctive therapy in the treatment of peptic ulcer, irritable bowel syndrome (irritable colon, spastic colon, mucous colitis) and acute enterocolitis. However, one should bear in mind that there is no conclusive evidence as to whether or not anticholinergic drugs aid in the healing of peptic ulcer, decrease the rate of recurrences or prevent complications.

Contraindications: Glaucoma, advanced hepatic or renal disease, and in patients hypersensitive to any of the components. Barbiturates are contraindicated in patients with porphyria.

Warnings: Barbiturates may be habit-forming.

Precautions: Caution is advisable when given to patients with incipient glaucoma, bladder neck obstruction, urinary bladder atony or prostatic hypertrophy. Prolonged use of barbiturates may result in habituation. Patients should be advised not to engage in activities requiring alertness or motor coordination.

Adverse Reactions: Blurred vision, dry mouth, constipation, photophobia, vertigo, tachycardia, difficult urination, urinary retention, drowsiness, flushing of the skin, and dry skin may occur at higher dosage levels; rarely at the usual dosage level.

For the contraindications, warnings, precautions, and adverse reactions attributable to any of the components in combination with Belladonna Alkaloids, their individual monographs should be consulted.

Dosage and Administration: *Orally:* Adults, 1 or 2 tablets, capsules, or teaspoonsful of a liquid preparation 3 or 4 times daily according to condition and severity of symptoms. One or 2 extended-release forms morning and night for sustained around the clock effects, or 1 repeat-action tablet 3 times daily. Children, ½ to 1 teaspoonful of a liquid preparation 3 or 4 times daily as indicated. Infants, a proportionate amount of a liquid preparation 30 minutes prior to or with each feeding, increasing if necessary.

Availability:
BELAP®: **(Lemmon)**
Elixir (per 5 ml) contains 0.045 ml of belladonna leaf fluidextract with 16.2 mg of phenobarbital and 22% alcohol in bottles of 1 pint and 1 gallon.
SE Tablets, 10.8 mg of belladonna extract in bottles of 100 and 1000.
Tablets, 10.8 mg of belladonna extract with 16.2 mg of phenobarbital in bottles of 100, 1000 and 5000.
BELLADONNA: **(Lilly)**
Ointment, 0.125% in tubes of 30 gm.
Powdered Extract in packages of 30 gm.
Tablets (powdered extract), 15 mg (equiv. to 0.187 mg total alkaloids) in bottles of 100.
Tincture (alcohol, 67%) in bottles of 120 ml and 1 pint.
BELLADONNA and PHENOBARBITAL Tablets, 8 mg with phenobarbital, 15 mg in bottles of 100 and 1000; Ⓒ-IV 4 and 8 mg with phenobarbital, 15 and 30 mg respectively in bottles of 100 and 1000. **(Lilly)**
BELLADONNA Tincture, 27 to 33 mg/100 ml in bottles of 1 gallon. **(Parke-Davis)**
BUTIBEL®: **(McNeil)**
Elixir (per 5 ml) and *tablets* contain 15 mg each of sodium butabarbital and belladonna extract in bottles of 100 and 1000 tablets in pints of elixir.
BUTIBEL-ZYME® Tablets contain the equivalent of one Butibel tablet; 10 mg of proteolytic enzyme; 20 mg of amylolytic enzyme; 5 mg of cellulolytic enzyme; 100 mg of lipolytic enzyme; and 30 mg of iron ox bile (45% cholic acid) in bottles of 100 and 500.
Ⓒ-IV CHARDONNA®-2 Tablets (belladonna extract, 15 mg; phenobarbital, 15 mg and activated charcoal, 11.2 mg) in bottles of 100. **(Rorer)**
DONNATAL®: **(Robins)**
Capsules, Tablets and *Elixir* (per 5 ml) contain hyoscyamine sulfate, 0.1037 mg; atropine sulfate, 0.0194 mg; hyoscine hydrobromide, 0.0065 mg and phenobarbital, 16.2 mg. Elixir in 120 ml, pints and gallons and in Dis-Co-Paks® of 5 ml. Capsules and Tablets in bottles of 100 and 1000. Tablets in Dis-Co-Paks of 1000.
Extentabs® contain the equivalent of 3 Donnatal tablets, the release of the ingredients controlled to provide the effects of 1 Donnatal tablet uniformly sustained for 10 to 12 hours. Bottles of 100 and 500.
DONNATAL No. 2 Tablets contain the equivalent of 1 Donnatal tablet, but with 32 mg of phenobarbital. Bottles of 100 and 1000.
KINESED® Tablets contain hyoscyamine sulfate, 0.1 mg; atropine sulfate 0.02 mg; scopolamine hydrochloride, 0.007 mg and phenobarbital, 16 mg in bottles of 100 and 500. **(Stuart)**
PRYDON® Spansule® Capsules, 0.4 and 0.8 mg of belladonna alkaloids in bottles of 50. **(Smith Kline & French)**

BELLAFOLINE

Description: A stable preparation of the pure levorotatory alkaloids of belladonna which are twice as active therapeutically, on a weight basis, as atropine. When used in doses of the same order of therapeutic potency, toxicity is about ½ that of atropine.

Indications: Whenever belladonna is indicated, particularly in spastic conditions of smooth muscle and excessive secretion: digestive tract (spasm, peptic ulcer, pylorospasm, spastic colitis, intestinal and biliary colics); genitourinary tract (dysmenorrhea, renal colic, nocturia, enuresis); respiratory tract (hypersecretion); and the nervous system (vagal inhibition, postencephalitic parkinsonism, motion sickness).

Contraindications: Hypersensitivity, glaucoma, increased intraocular pressure, advanced hepatic or renal disease.

Precautions: Caution is advised in geriatric patients.

Adverse Reactions: Urinary retention, blurred vision, dry mouth or flushing may occur.

Dosage and Administration: *Orally.* Adults, 1 or 2 tablets 3 times daily. Children over 6 years of age, 1/2 to 1 tablet 3 times daily according to age. *Subcutaneously.* Adults *only,* 0.25 to 1 ml once or twice daily.

Availability:
BELLAFOLINE®: **(Sandoz)**
Injection, 0.5 mg/ml in ampuls of 1 ml.
Tablets, 0.25 mg (white, grooved) in bottles of 100.

BELLERGAL

Description: The combined action of the three components exerts an inhibitory influence on all divisions of the autonomic nervous system. Contains in each:

	Tablet	*Spacetab*
Phenobarbital	20 mg	40 mg
Ergotamine tartrate	0.3 mg	0.6 mg
l-belladonna alkaloids (as maleates)	0.1 mg	0.2 mg

Indications: The management of disorders characterized by nervous tension and exaggerated autonomic response: Menopausal disorders with hot flushes, sweats, restlessness and insomnia; cardiovascular disorders with palpitation, tachycardia, chest oppression and vasomotor disturbances; gastrointestinal disorders with hypermotility, hypersecretion, "nervous stomach," and alternatively diarrhea and constipation; genitourinary disorders such as uterine cramps, etc.; premenstrual tension; and interval treatment of recurrent, throbbing headache.

Contraindications: Peripheral vascular disease, coronary heart disease, hypertension, impaired hepatic or renal function, intermittent porphyria, sepsis, third trimester of pregnancy, glaucoma, and hypersensitivity to any component.

Warnings: Phenobarbital may be habit-forming.

Precautions: Caution should be exercised if large or prolonged dosage is contemplated, and consideration should be given to the possibility of peripheral vascular complications in patients highly sensitive to ergot.

Adverse Reactions: Blurred vision, dry mouth, flushing and drowsiness.

Dosage and Administration: *Orally.* Usually, 1 tablet in the morning, 1 tablet at noon and 2 tablets at bedtime. In resistant cases, begin with 6 tablets daily, then reduce gradually at weekly intervals according to response. The Spacetabs should be given in the morning and in the evening (2 per day).

Availability:
BELLERGAL® Tablets (flesh pink, sugar coated) in bottles of 100 and 1000. **(Dorsey)**
BELLERGAL-S™ Spacetabs® (dark green, orange and light lemon yellow) in bottles of 100. **(Dorsey)**

BENACTYZINE HYDROCHLORIDE

Chemical Name: 2-Diethylaminoethyl benzilate hydrochloride.

Description: Benactyzine hydrochloride is a potent cholinergic blocking agent chemically related to adiphenine. Its action closely resembles those of atropine and scopolamine. It occurs as a white, crystalline substance that is freely soluble in water.

Benactyzine appears to act predominantly on the CNS, and has been employed to manage mild psychoneurotic disorders. However, it does not appear to relieve psychotic symptoms. It also possesses a spasmolytic effect approximately 1/2 that of papaverine; a quinidine-like effect on the heart about 3 times that of quinidine; a slight antihistaminic effect, and a local anesthetic action.

Studies with mice have revealed that benactyzine potentiates the anesthetic effect of some barbiturates and of alcohol. Following administration, the drug is readily metabolized in the body and about 87% of the drug is excreted in the urine within 24 hours.

Indications: Benactyzine is combined with meprobamate for the treatment of psychoneurotic disorders manifested by anxiety reaction, or those of a mild depressive character associated with anxiety, insomnia, agitation, and rumination.

Contraindications: In patients with glaucoma, acute intermittent porphyria, and in those who are hypersensitive to benactyzine or to the component drug.

Warnings: See monograph on Meprobamate.

Precautions: Patients receiving this drug should be cautioned not to engage in activities requiring alertness or skill. In some patients, the neurotic condition is intensified by a sense of depersonalization and unreality and by an inability to concentrate. Patients may also experience a feeling of excessive muscular relaxation, which may be accompanied by clumsiness and paresthesias of the limbs. The drug is not intended for use in children and if considered for administration to pregnant women, the possibility of risk to the fetus must be weighed against the anticipated benefits.

Adverse Reactions: Benactyzine in high dosage may produce dizziness, blocking of thought processes, a sense of depersonalization, aggravation of anxiety, or disturbance of sleep patterns, and a subjective feeling of muscle relaxation. There may also be anticholinergic effects such as blurred vision, dryness of mouth, or failure of visual accommodation. Other reported side effects have included gastric distress, allergic response, ataxia, and euphoria. For additional reactions attributable to its component, see monograph on Meprobamate.

Dosage and Administration: *Orally.* The suggested initial dosage for adults is 1 tablet 3 or 4 times daily, increased gradually, in the absence of a favorable response, to 6 tablets daily. The dosage is then reduced gradually to maintenance levels upon establishment of relief. Dosages of more than 6 tablets daily are not recommended. The drug should be given after meals to minimize or obviate the occurrence of systemic side effects or nausea and vomiting.

Availability:

ⒸⅣ DEPROL® Tablets (benactyzine, 1 mg and meprobamate, 400 mg) in bottles of 100 and 500 and in unit-dose packages of 1000. **(Wallace)**

BENAT with B-12

Description: Each ml contains:

Liver injection, crude*	0.5 ml
Cyanocobalamin	30 μg
Niacinamide	50 mg
Thiamine hydrochloride	10 mg
Riboflavin	2 mg
Pyridoxine hydrochloride	1 mg
D-Pantothenyl alcohol	1 mg
Benzyl alcohol, 4% and phenol, 0.5%.	

*The vitamin B-12 activity is equivalent to 1 mcg of cyanocobalamin.

Indications: The parenteral treatment of pernicious anemia and other types of macrocytic anemia, especially when liver extract factors other than cyanocobalamin are desired. Because this product also contains other B-complex vitamins, it is a valuable adjunct in the high-vitamin regimen which has proved so useful in the treatment of Laennec's cirrhosis. It is also of value in treating the neuritis and psychosis that accompany chronic alcoholism. It frequently is beneficial in the treatment of the neuritis seen in pregnancy, and for conditions associated with inadequate intake, altered absorption or increased requirements for these vitamin B factors.

Contraindications: In patients with a history of sensitivity reactions to injections of thiamine or crude liver extract.

Precautions: Not to be injected intravenously. Intramuscular administration should be preceded by every known precaution for the prevention and arrest of allergic and other untoward reactions. A careful history should review possible sensitivity. A separate heat-sterilized syringe and needle should be used for each patient to prevent the transmission of homologous serum hepatitis and other infections from one patient to another.

Adverse Reactions: Although rare, thiamine, when given parenterally, may act as an anaphylactogen thereby inducing an unusual or exaggerated reaction. Also patients susceptible to the effects of niacinamide may experience flushing, itching or burning of the skin.

Dosage and Administration: *Intramuscularly* only. Uncomplicated pernicious anemia, fish-tapeworm anemia and macrocytic anemia following gastrectomy: 0.5 to 1 ml daily for 1 week, then twice weekly until remission is complete. Maintenance dosage should not be less than 0.5 ml every 2 weeks. Pernicious anemia with neurologic complications: 1 ml daily for 1 week, then once or twice weekly until remission is complete. Maintenance dosage should not be less than 1 ml every 2 weeks. Sprue and megaloblastic anemia of pregnancy and infancy: 0.5 to 1 ml once or twice weekly as indicated. Vitamin B complex deficiencies: a course of 5 to 10 ml or more in divided doses as indicated.

Availability:
BENAT™ with B-12 Injection in vials of 10 ml. **(Merrell-National)**

BENDECTIN

Description: Each specially-coated tablet contains 10 mg each of doxylamine succinate and pyridoxine hydrochloride.

The formulation provides the action of two unrelated compounds, each having a different type of effect: the antihistamine is related chemically to other drugs used to control nausea and motion sickness; pyridoxine corrects vitamin B deficiency that may occur during pregnancy. The antiemetic action of this product is delayed by a special coating that permits the nighttime dose to be effective in the morning hours, when the patient needs it most.

Indications: Nausea and vomiting of pregnancy.

Contraindications: A hypersensitivity or idiosyncratic reaction to doxylamine succinate.

Precautions: Because of potential drowsiness, this preparation should be given with caution to patients who must drive automobiles or operate machinery. Although studies with pregnant rats and rabbits given up to 90 times the maximal clinical dose showed no evidence of drug-induced fetal abnormalities, its use during pregnancy, particularly during the first trimester, should be undertaken only when therapeutically essential.

Adverse Reactions: Those that may occur are attributable to the individual components. In particularly sensitive patients, *doxylamine succinate* may cause drowsiness, vertigo, nervousness, epigastric pain, headache, palpitation, diarrhea, disorientation or irritability. *Pyridoxine* is a vitamin that is generally recognized as having no adverse effects.

Dosage and Administration: *Orally,* 2 tablets at bedtime. In severe cases or when nausea occurs during the day, 1 additional tablet in the morning and another in midafternoon.

Availability:
BENDECTIN® Tablets in bottles of 100. **(Merrell-National)**

BENDROFLUMETHIAZIDE: see The Thiazide Diuretics

BENOXINATE HYDROCHLORIDE

Chemical Name: 2-Diethylaminoethyl 4-amino-3-butoxybenzoate hydrochloride.

Description: Benoxinate is chemically related to procaine and occurs as odorless, white crystals or as a crystalline powder very soluble in water and in chloroform, soluble in alcohol, and insoluble in ether. Aqueous solutions have a pH of about 5 and are stable to heat, light and air. It has local anesthetic and slightly bacteriostatic properties. Its onset of action is quite rapid, usually within 1 minute; its duration of action is relatively short.

Indications: As a topical anesthetic for ophthalmic use in tonometry and gonioscopy; for the removal of foreign bodies and sutures; or for short operative procedures on the cornea or conjunctiva.

Contraindications: In patients with known hypersensitivity to benoxinate.

Warnings: Prolonged use is not recommended since it may produce permanent corneal opacification with accompanying visual loss. Use of the drops should be discontinued if signs of sensitivity develop.

Precautions: The solution should be used cautiously and sparingly in patients with known allergies, cardiac disease or hyperthyroidism; also prolonged use may delay wound healing. Systemic toxicity manifested by CNS stimulation followed by depression occurs infrequently.

Adverse Reactions: Temporary stinging, burning, and conjunctival redness may occur occasionally.

Dosage and Administration: *Topically only,* by instillation into the eye(s). For removal of foreign bodies and sutures, and for tonometry, a single instillation of 1 to 2 drops prior to the procedure. For ophthalmic anesthesia, 3 instillations of 2 drops at 90-second intervals.

Availability:
DORSACAINE® Ophthalmic Solution, 0.4% in plastic dropper bottles of 15 ml with dropper tips. **(Dorsey)**

BENZENE HEXACHLORIDE, GAMMA

Chemical Name: 1,2,3,4,5,6-Hexachlorocyclohexane.

Description: Gamma benzene hexachloride is the gamma isomer of hexachlorocyclohexane and occurs as a white, crystalline powder practically insoluble in water, slightly soluble in ethylene glycol and has a slight musty odor. The compound is a member of the large class of synthetic chlorinated hydrocarbon insecticides of which chlorophenothane (DDT) is the prototype. It is highly toxic being readily absorbed through the chitinous exoskeletal membrane causing fatal convulsions similar to those produced by DDT, but with a more rapid onset of action. Most patients experience effective relief from itching within 24 hours.

Indications: The cream and lotion are indicated for the treatment of scabies and all forms of pediculosis. The shampoo is indicated *only* for the treatment of *Pediculus capitis* (head louse) and *Phthirus pubis* (crab louse), and their ova. **Note:** The shampoo is intended for the treatment of pediculosis and should *not* be used as a routine shampoo. For other ectoparasitic infestations, such as scabies, the cream or lotion is recommended.

Contraindications: In individuals hypersensitive to benzene hexachloride or to any of the components of the product.

Warnings: The lipoid solvents enhance the percutaneous absorption of gamma benzene hexachloride. Prolonged or repeated applications should be avoided, and because of its possible toxic effect on the CNS, it should be employed with special care, particularly in infants, children, and pregnant patients. Specific antiinfective measures should be instituted where secondary infection is present. Precautions should be taken to prevent contact with the eyes or mucous membranes. The development of irritation or sensitivity requires prompt discontinuation of the product.

Precautions: If ingested accidentally, prompt gastric lavage is indicated. Saline cathartics, rather than oil laxatives, should be given for intestinal evacuation. If CNS stimulation occurs, phenobarbital or pentobarbital may be given. Intravenous calcium gluconate may be used in conjunction with the barbiturates. Epinephrine should not be used because ventricular fibrillation may result. May be absorbed through the skin.

Adverse Reactions: Eczematous eruptions have been reported. Preliminary patch tests should be performed whenever hypersensitivity is suspected.

Dosage and Administration: *Topically.* For *scabies,* the initial therapy consists of bathing with warm water followed by the application of the cream or lotion in a thin layer over the entire skin surface, left on for 8 to 12 hours and then washed thoroughly. If necessary, a second or third application may be made at weekly intervals. Freshly laundered or dry-cleaned clothing should be worn. For *pediculosis,* the cream or lotion is applied in a thin layer to hairy infested areas and adjacent areas and left on for 12 hours and then washed thoroughly; the patient dressed in freshly laundered or dry-cleaned clothing and treatment repeated in 7 days if necessary. The shampoo is applied after wetting the hair thoroughly with warm water. Pour 2 tablespoonsful (30 ml) of shampoo onto the affected area and adjacent hairy areas and rub well into the hair and scalp. Rub vigorously for at least 4 minutes making certain to cover all hairy areas, then rinse thoroughly and rub with a dry towel, and finally, comb with a fine-tooth comb to remove any remaining nit shells. A second application is seldom needed; if necessary, however, treatment should be repeated at weekly intervals.

Availability:
GAMENE®: **(Barnes-Hind)**
Lotion, 1% in bottles of 60 ml and 1 pint.
Shampoo, 1% in bottles of 60 ml and 1 pint.
KWELL® **(Reed & Carnrick)**
Cream, 1% in tubes of 60 gm and in jars of 480 gm.
Lotion, 1% in bottles of 60 ml, 1 pint and 1 gallon.
Shampoo, 1% in bottles of 60 ml, 1 pint and 1 gallon.

BENZONATATE

Chemical Name: 2,5,8,11,14,17,20,23,26-Nonaoxaoctacosan-28-yl p-(butylamino) benzoate.

Description: Benzonatate occurs as a viscous, pale yellow liquid having a faint characteristic odor. Chemically related to tetracaine, it exhibits a local anesthetic action when applied topically.

It is a non-narcotic antitussive agent which acts peripherally by anesthetizing the stretch receptors located in the respiratory passages, lungs, and pleura by diminishing their activity and thereby reducing the cough reflex at its source. It acts rapidly, within 15 to 20 minutes, and the effect persists for 3 to 8 hours. It decreases cough frequency without interfering with productivity or expectoration. Benzonatate has no inhibitory effect on the respiratory center in recommended dosage.

Indications: Symptomatic relief of cough.

Contraindications: Hypersensitivity to the drug or to related compounds.

Warnings: The safe use of benzonatate in pregnant women or during lactation has not been established; therefore, the benefits to be obtained must be weighed against the potential hazards to the mother and child.

Precautions: The perles should be swallowed without chewing in order to avoid temporary local anesthesia of the oral mucosa.

Adverse Reactions: Sedation, headache, mild dizziness, pruritus and skin eruptions, nasal congestion, constipation, nausea, gastrointestinal upset, sensation of burning in the eyes, a vague "chilly" sensation, numbness in the chest, and hypersensitivity have been reported. If the perles are chewed or dissolved in the mouth, oropharyngeal anesthesia will develop rapidly. The resultant stimulation of the CNS may cause restlessness and tremors which may proceed to clonic convulsions followed by profound CNS depression.

Dosage and Administration: *Orally.* Adults and children over 10 years of age, the usual dose is 1 perle 3 times daily as required. If necessary, up to 6 perles daily may be given.

Availability:
TESSALON® Perles, 100 mg (yellow) in bottles of 100. **(Endo)**

BENZPHETAMINE HYDROCHLORIDE Ⓒ III

Chemical Name: d-*N*-Benzyl-*N*,α-dimethylphenethylamine hydrochloride.

Description: Benzphetamine is an amphetamine congener and occurs as a white, crystalline powder soluble in water and in alcohol. Readily absorbed from the gastrointestinal tract, its effects persist for about 4 hours after oral administration.

As a sympathomimetic compound, it exhibits a marked anorexigenic action, an action which is selective in that vasopressor and cardiac effects are minimal. In recommended dosages, there has been relatively little effect on the CNS. Although the mechanism by which appetite is depressed is not quite clear, it probably acts centrally rather than by sympathomimetic action on the gastrointestinal tract. While appetite is depressed, normal food appreciation is unaffected, permitting the obese patient to reduce caloric intake while retaining appetite appeasement.

Indications: The control of simple exogenous obesity as a short-term (i.e., a few weeks) adjunct in a regimen of weight reduction based on caloric restriction.

Contraindications: In patients with advanced arteriosclerosis, symptomatic cardiovascular disease, moderate to severe hypertension, hyperthyroidism, known hypersensitivity or idiosyncrasy to sympathomimetic amines, and agitated states, and in patients with a history of drug abuse. Hypertensive crises have resulted when sympathomimetic amines have been used concomitantly or within 14 days following use of monamine oxidase inhibitors. Benzphetamine should not be used concomitantly with other CNS stimulants.

Warnings: Tolerance to sympathomimetic anorexiants usually develops in a few weeks. Should this occur with benzphetamine, the recommended dose should not be exceeded in an attempt to maintain the anorectic effect. Because of its effect on the central nervous system, benzphetamine may impair the ability of the patient to engage in potentially hazardous activities such as operating machinery or driving a motor vehicle; the patient should therefore be cautioned accordingly. Extreme psychological dependence has occurred with sympathomimetic anorexiants; therefore, the physician should be aware that it may occur with benzphetamine hydrochloride.

Patients have been known to increase the dosage of drugs of this type above that recommended. Abrupt cessation following prolonged high dosage administration results in extreme fatigue and mental depression as well as prolonged changes noted on the EEG. Manifestations of chronic intoxication with agents of this class include severe dermatoses, marked insomnia, irritability, hyperactivity and personality changes. The most severe manifestation of chronic intoxication is psychosis, often clinically indistinguishable from schizophrenia. Safe use during pregnancy has not been established. Therefore, use of benzphetamine by women who are or who may become pregnant, and especially those in the first trimester of pregnancy, requires that the potential benefit be weighed against the possible hazard to mother and infant. Use of benzphetamine hydrochloride is not recommended in children under 12 years of age.

Precautions: Insulin requirements in diabetes mellitus may be altered in association with use of anorexigenic drugs and the concomitant dietary restrictions. Psychological disturbances have been reported in patients who receive an anorectic agent together with a restrictive dietary regimen.

Adverse Reactions: The following have been associated with the use of benzphetamine: Overstimulation, restlessness, dizziness, insomnia, gastrointestinal disturbances, nausea, diarrhea, palpitation, tachycardia, elevation of blood pressure, tremor, sweating, headache, dryness of the mouth or unpleasant taste, urticaria and other allergic reactions involving the skin, changes in libido; rarely, psychotic episodes at recommended dosage; depression following withdrawal of drug. Management of overdosage is mainly symptomatic and includes sedation with a barbiturate. If hypertension is severe, the use of a nitrite or rapidly acting alpha receptor blocking agent should be considered. Experience with hemodialysis or peritoneal dialysis is inadequate to permit recommendation at the present time.

Dosage and Administration: *Orally.* A dosage of 25 to 50 mg 1 to 3 times daily is suggested. Dosage should be adjusted to the response of the patient. Treatment should begin with 25 to 50 mg once daily with a subsequent increase in individual dose or frequency according to response. A single dose is preferably given in midmorning or midafternoon, according to the patient's eating habits. In an occasional patient, it may be desirable to avoid late afternoon administration.

Availability:
Ⓒ DIDREX™ Tablets, 25 mg (press-coated, unscored) in bottles of 100; 50 mg (press-coated, scored) in bottles of 100 and 500. **(Upjohn)**

BENZQUINAMIDE

Chemical Name: *N, N*-Diethyl-1, 3, 4, 6, 7, 11*β*-hexahydro-2-hydroxy-9, 10-dimethoxy-2*H*-benzo (a) quinolizine-3-carboxamide acetate hydrochloride.

Description: Benzquinamide, an antiemetic agent, is a nonamine-depleting benzoquinolizine derivative. It is structurally related to reserpine and tetrabenazine to some extent, but is chemically unrelated to the phenothiazines and to other antiemetic agents. Results of studies with animals revealed that the drug produces antiemetic, antihistaminic, mild anticholinergic and sedative activity. Although its mechanism of action has not been established, it has been shown to suppress apomorphine-induced vomiting. Following parenteral administration, the onset of action usually occurs within 15 minutes. Its plasma half-life is about 40 minutes and approximately 58% is bound to plasma proteins. More than 95% of the drug is excreted within 72 hours in both urine and feces. Although no teratogenic effects were observed in reproduction studies in chick embryos, mice, rats and rabbits, the susceptibility of the human offspring to the drug is not known.

Indications: Prevention and treatment of nausea and vomiting associated with anesthesia and surgery.

Contraindications: Hypersensitivity to the drug.

Warnings: Safe use in pregnant women has not been established. Intramuscular administration is the preferred route since a sudden increase in blood pressure and transient arrhythmias (premature ventricular and auricular contractions) have been reported following intravenous administration of benzquinamide. The intravenous route should be restricted to patients who do not have cardiovascular disorders and who are not receiving preanesthetic and/or concomitant cardiovascular drugs. It is not recommended for use in children since proper dosage in this age group has not been established.

Precautions: Benzquinamide may mask the signs of overdosage of toxic drugs, and may obscure the presence of such conditions as intestinal obstruction or brain tumor.

Adverse Reactions: The most common reaction reported was drowsiness. One case of a pronounced allergic reaction characterized by pyrexia and urticaria has been noted. Other complications reported were dryness of mouth, shivering, sweating, hiccoughs, flushing, salivation, blurred vision; hypertension, hypotension, dizziness, atrial fibrillation, premature auricular and ventricular contractions; insomnia, restlessness, headache, excitement, nervousness; anorexia, nausea; muscle twitching, shaking and/or tremors, feeling of weakness; hives and/or rash; fatigue, chills and fever.

Dosage and Administration: *Intramuscularly* or *intravenously*. Initially, 50 mg intramuscularly, repeated in 1 hour with subsequent doses every 3 to 4 hours as indicated. Injection should be made deeply within a large muscle mass, preferably the deltoid area, but only if well developed. Inadvertant intravascular injection should be avoided. The intravenous dose is 25 mg administered slowly (1 ml/½ to 1 min); subsequent doses should be given intramuscularly. Intravenous administration in elderly or debilitated patients should be given with extreme care and in the lower dose range.

Availability:

Benzquinamide Hydrochloride

EMETE-CON® Injection, 25 mg/ml (equivalent) in vials of 2 ml in packages of 10. **(Roerig)**

BENZTHIAZIDE: see The Thiazide Diuretics

BENZTROPINE MESYLATE

Chemical Name: 3-(Diphenylmethoxy) tropane methanesulfonate.

Description: Structurally, benztropine mesylate resembles atropine and diphenhydramine, exhibiting anticholinergic, antihistaminic and local anesthetic properties. It occurs as a white, odorless, crystalline powder very soluble in water and freely soluble in alcohol.

The anticholinergic effect of benztropine is about equal to that of atropine; its antihistaminic activity is similar to that of pyrilamine maleate. The effects of the drug are cumulative and may not become evident until 2 or 3 days following administration.

Indications: As an adjunct in the treatment of all forms of parkinsonism (postencephalitic, arteriosclerotic, and idiopathic). Benztropine has also been found useful in the control of extrapyramidal disorders (except tardive dyskinesia) due to CNS drugs such as reserpine and phenothiazines.

Contraindications: Because of its atropine-like side effects, this drug is contraindicated in children under 3 years of age, and should be used with caution in older children.

Warnings: Safe use during pregnancy has not been established. The antihistaminic property may cause sedation. Patients receiving the drug should be cautioned against driving a car, or operating machinery or apparatus requiring alertness or skill. Fatal paralytic ileus has occurred in patients receiving combinations of drugs with anticholinergic properties; therefore, patients receiving phenothiazines and/or tricyclic antidepressants in addition to benztropine should be advised to report promptly any gastrointestinal complaints.

Precautions: Since the drug has cumulative action, continued supervision is advisable. Patients with a tendency to tachycardia or those with prostatic hypertrophy should be closely observed during treatment. Dysuria may occur, but rarely becomes a problem. Large doses of the drug may cause complaints of weakness and inability to move particular muscle groups. Mental confusion and excitement may occur with large doses, or in susceptible patients. Visual hallucinations have been reported occasionally. Furthermore, in the treatment of side effects of phenothiazine derivatives and reserpine in patients with a mental disorder, occasionally there may be intensification of mental symptoms. In such cases, at times, increased doses of antiparkinsonian drugs can precipitate a toxic psychosis. These patients should be kept under careful observation, especially at the beginning of treatment or if dosage is increased. Permanent extrapyramidal symptoms, such as tardive dyskinesia, have been described with prolonged phenothiazine therapy. The masking action of benztropine on the possible development of these symptoms has not been investigated.

Since benztropine contains structural features of atropine, it may produce anhidrosis which can be severe and can lead to fatal hyperthermia. For this reason, it should be given with caution during hot weather, especially to the old, the chronically ill, the alcoholic, those who have CNS disease and those who do manual labor in a hot environment. Anhidrosis may be anticipated to occur more readily when some disturbance of sweating already exists. If there is evidence of anhidrosis, dosage should be decreased at the discretion of the physician so that the ability to maintain body heat equilibrium by perspiration is not impaired. The physician should be aware of the possible occurrence of glaucoma. Although the drug does not appear to have any adverse effect on simple glaucoma, it probably should not be used in angle-closure glaucoma.

Adverse Reactions: Side effects may be anticholinergic or antihistaminic in nature. Dry mouth, blurred vision, nausea and nervousness may develop. Adjustment of dosage or time of administration sometimes helps to control these reactions. If dry mouth is so severe that there is difficulty in swallowing or speaking, or loss of appetite and weight, reduce dosage, or discontinue temporarily. Vomiting occurs infrequently. Nausea unaccompanied by vomiting usually can be disregarded. Slight reduction in dosage may control the nausea and still give sufficient relief of symptoms. Vomiting may be controlled by temporary discontinuation, followed by resumption at a lower dosage. Other side effects include constipation, numbness of the fingers, listlessness and depression. Occasionally, an allergic reaction, e.g., skin rash, develops. Sometimes this can be controlled by reducing dosage, but occasionally medication has to be discontinued.

Dosage and Administration: *Orally* or *parenterally.* The tablets should be used when the patient is able to take oral medication. Because of the drug's cumulative action, therapy should be initiated with a low dose, increased gradually in increments of 0.5 mg at intervals of 5 or 6 days to the smallest amount necessary for optimal relief, up to a maximum of 6 mg daily. In arteriosclerotic, idiopathic and postencephalitic parkinsonism, the usual daily dosage is 1 to 2 mg *orally* or *parenterally.* May be used concomitantly with levodopa or with carbidopa-levodopa combination in which case periodic dosage adjustment of each may be required in order to maintain optimal response. In arteriosclerotic and idiopathic parkinsonism, therapy may be initiated with a single daily dose of 0.5 to 1 mg at bedtime. In some patients, this will be adequate; in others, 4 to 6 mg daily may be required. In postencephalitic parkinsonism, therapy may be initiated in most patients with 2 mg daily in 1 or more doses. When treating drug-induced parkinsonism, the recommended dosage is 1 to 4 mg once or twice daily, orally or parenterally. In acute dystonic reactions, 1 or 2 ml of the injection quickly relieves the condition. After that, 1 to 2 mg orally twice daily usually prevents a recurrence. For more detailed prescribing information, the physician is urged to study the package literature.

Availability:
COGENTIN®: **(Merck Sharp & Dohme)**
Injection, 1 mg/ml in ampuls of 2 ml in cartons of 6.
Tablets, 0.5 and 1 mg in bottles of 100; 2 mg in bottles of 100 and 1000; 1 and 2 mg in single-unit packages of 100.

BENZYLPENICILLOYL POLYLYSINE

Description: A skin-test antigen used for detecting allergic hypersensitivity to penicillin. It has been observed that virtually everybody who receives penicillin develops specific antibodies to the drug as measured by hemagglutination studies. Also, numerous investigators have reported that individuals who have previously received penicillin therapy may have positive skin reactions to this agent as well as to a number of nonbenzylpenicilloyl haptenes. However, it must be kept in mind that there is a high degree of cross-reactivity between all penicillins as well as some cross-allerginicity between penicillins and cephalosporins. The drug reacts specifically with benzylpenicilloyl skin-sensitizing antibodies (reagins: IgE class) to initiate release of chemical mediators that produce an immediate wheal and flare reaction at the skin-test site. Clinical experience has shown that less than 5% of the patients will develop an allergic reaction to penicillin following a negative response to the test as compared with more than 20% following a positive response. Nevertheless, consideration should be given to the fact that no reagent, test or combination of tests will competely assure that a reaction to penicillin therapy will not occur. The drug is a derivative of poly-l-lysine where the epsilon amino groups are substituted with benzylpenicilloyl groups (50 to 70%) forming benzylpenicilloyl alpha amide. To date, the development of systemic allergic reactions to the test itself has been rare (0.4 to 0.7/1000 tests).

Indications: Useful as an adjunct in assessing the risk of administering penicillin (benzylpenicillin or penicillin G) when it is the preferred drug of choice in patients who have previously received penicillin or who have a history of hypersensitivity to penicillin.

Contraindications: Patients who previously have shown either a systemic or marked local reaction to this antigen, or those known to be extremely sensitive to penicillin.

Warnings: Present data are insufficient to assess the potential hazard of sensitization to penicillin from repeated skin testing with this antigen. A systemic allergic reaction usually can be avoided by first applying the scratch test, and if negative, then the intradermal test. Until further clinical studies assure its safe use during pregnancy, the hazards of skin testing in pregnant women should be weighed against the risk of penicillin therapy without skin testing.

Precautions: Little or no data are available in the following situations for determining the clinical value of this test as a means of estimating the risk of penicillin therapy: Adult patients with no prior history of penicillin hypersensitivity; pediatric patients; cases where exposure to penicillin is suspected as a cause of a drug reaction; patients who are undergoing routine allergy evaluation; patients receiving semisynthetic or cephalosporin-derived antibiotics; or those who responded negatively to the skin test. If penicillin is the absolute drug of choice in a life-threatening situation, successful desensitization with therapeutic penicillin may be possible irrespective of a positive skin test and/or a positive history of hypersensitivity to penicillin.

Adverse Reactions: Occasionally, an intense local inflammatory response may develop at the skin-test site; rarely, systemic reactions (e.g., generalized erythema, pruritus, angioneurotic edema, urticaria, dyspnea and/or hypotension) which are usually of short duration and can be controlled.

Dosage and Administration: Scratch-test method: Using a 20-gauge needle make a light scratch (3 to 5 mm) sufficient to produce a nonbleeding surface on the inner volar aspect of the arm. If bleeding occurs, another site should be chosen. Then apply a small drop of the solution to the scratch and rub gently with an applicator, toothpick, or the side of the needle. During the next 15 minutes, the test site should be observed for the development of a wheal, erythema and itching, after which time the solution is wiped off. A positive reaction usually occurs within 10 minutes and consists of the appearance of a pale wheal, usually with pseudopods, surrounding the scratch site, and varying in diameter from 5 to 15 mm or more. The wheal may be accompanied by variable degrees of itching and erythema. As soon as a positive response occurs, the solution should be wiped off immediately. If no wheal occurs or a wheal of less than 5 mm appears with little or no erythema and no itching, the intradermal test may be performed. **Intradermal-test method:** Prepare a sterile skin test area on the upper, outer arm, sufficiently below the deltoid muscle to permit proximal application of a tourniquet later. Inject an amount of the solution (between 0.01 and 0.02 ml), sufficient to raise the smallest possible perceptible wheal, below the skin surface. Using a separate syringe and needle, inject an equal amount of saline solution as a control at least 1½ inches away from the test site. Most skin reactions will develop within 5 to 15 minutes. If the response is negative there will be no increase in the size of the original bleb and/or no greater reaction than that of the control site. If the response is ambiguous the wheal will be only slightly larger than the initial bleb with or without erythema, and will be larger than that of the control site. If the response is positive there will be itching and a marked increase in the size of the original bleb; the wheal may exceed 20 mm in diameter and exhibit pseudopods. The control site should be completely reactionless. If it exhibits a wheal greater than 2 to 3 mm in diameter, the test should be repeated, and if the same reaction is observed, a physician experienced in allergy skin testing should be consulted.

Availability:
PRE PEN® Solution in single-dose ampuls of 0.25 ml in cartons of 5. **(Kremers-Urban)**

BETA-CAROTENE

Description: Beta-carotene, a hydrocarbon compound ($C_{40}H_{56}$), is a carotenoid pigment that occurs naturally in most plants containing chlorophyll and in green and yellow vegetables. Trans-beta-carotene is a red, crystalline substance that is practically insoluble in water and moderately soluble in ether and oils. The commercial product is a synthetic formulation of pure beta-carotene.

Although its precise mode of action has not been established, the drug has been found effective in reducing photosensitivity in patients with erythropoietic protoporphyria. In a clinical study with 74 patients who were given beta-carotene in oral doses ranging from 15 to 300 mg daily for varying periods of up to 25 consecutive weeks, it was found that tolerance to sunlight was increased in 49 of 53 patients exposed to natural sunlight and in 20 of 21 patients exposed to artificial sunlight. Also observed was that 46 of the 53 patients and 11 of the 21 patients showed a threefold or better response. Of the 46 patients 10 were able to remain in the sun all day without experiencing discomfort or developing skin lesions, and some were able to develop a suntan. The protective effect was found not to be total since photosensivity reactions occurred, but these were reported to be less severe and to disappear more rapidly.

Although beta-carotene is an important precursor of vitamin A, levels of the vitamin did not appear to rise above normal when blood levels of carotene were markedly elevated. An accumulation of the drug in the body may cause the skin to develop a slightly yellow color; however, this is not observed in the sclera in contrast to patients with icterus. Several weeks of therapy are necessary to accumulate enough beta-carotene in the skin to exert its protective effect. Patients should therefore be instructed not to increase their exposure to sunlight until they appear carotenemic which is first manifested as yellowness of the palms of the hands and the soles of the feet.

Indications: To ameliorate photosensitivity in patients with erythropoietic protoporphyria.

Contraindications: Patients with known hypersensitivity to the drug.

Warnings: Since beta-carotene is not effective as a sunscreen in normal individuals, it should not be used for this purpose. Safe use in the recommended dosage range in women who are or who may become pregnant has not been established; hence, it should be given only when the potential benefits have been weighed against the possible hazards to the mother and fetus.

Precautions: Caution should be exercised in patients with impaired renal or hepatic function. Patients should be forewarned that their skin may appear slightly yellow while receiving beta-carotene therapy. Since the drug will fulfill normal vitamin A requirements, additional vitamin A should not be prescribed.

Adverse Reactions: Patients may experience loose stools. This reaction tends to be sporadic and may not require discontinuance of the medication.

Dosage and Administration: *Orally* either as a single daily dose or in divided doses preferably with meals. The usual dosage is 30 to 300 mg (1 to 10 capsules) daily. Children under 14 years of age, the usual dosage is 30 to 150 mg (1 to 5 capsules) daily. The capsules may be opened and the contents mixed in orange or tomato juice.

Availability:
SOLATENE® Capsules, 30 mg (blue and green) in bottles of 100. **(Roche)**

BETAMETHASONE: see The Adrenal Corticosteroids.

BETAZOLE HYDROCHLORIDE

Chemical Name: 3-(2-Aminoethyl)pyrazole dihydrochloride.

Description: An analog of histamine, betazole occurs as a white, crystalline, nearly odorless powder soluble in water and practically insoluble in chloroform.

In the recommended dosage, betazole stimulates gastric secretion to an extent equal to that obtained with the usual dosage of histamine, but because of its minimal effects on other organs, evokes less severe side effects. Betazole is believed to have most of the actions of histamine, but in varying degrees. In appropriate doses, its effect on the gastric secretion of acid and pepsin is the same as that of histamine. In clinical studies with ordinary doses, no significant change in blood pressure and only a minimal increase in pulse rate have been observed, indicating that its vasodepressor response is infinitely less than that of histamine. Betazole does not cause contraction of the guinea pig ileum, as does histamine.

Indications: The clinical testing of gastric secretion. Its effect in other conditions in which histamine is used clinically, as in suspected pheochromocytoma, histamine cephalalgia, and cerebral ischemia, has not been tested.

Warnings: Patients with an allergic diathesis may react severely to betazole; therefore, the drug should be used with caution in patients with moderate to severe allergic conditions. Safe use of this drug during pregnancy has not been confirmed; therefore, the potential hazards must be weighed against the anticipated benefits.

Precautions: Weakness and syncope may occur. Overdosage may produce hypotension, acute asthma, and urticaria.

Adverse Reactions: The most commonly observed reaction is flushing of the face accompanied by a sense of warmth. Headache and urticaria may also occur.

Dosage and Administration: *Intramuscularly* or *subcutaneously.* The dosage to be used for fractional gastric analyses may be calculated on the basis of 0.5 mg/kg of body weight. If a simplified procedure is desired, a fixed amount of 50 mg may be given to all adults of nearly average weight. Although this provides a slightly higher dosage on a weight basis for most patients, the side effects will not be significantly greater. As much as 200 mg have been given without apparent harm, but have produced a higher incidence and increased severity of side effects. Until further studies have been made, oral administration of betazole is not recommended for routine use. For data on the technique of fractional gastric analysis and the interpretation of results, see the package literature.

Availability:
HISTALOG™ Injection, 50 mg/ml in ampuls of 1 ml in packages of 6. **(Lilly)**

BETHANECHOL CHLORIDE

Chemical Name: (2-Hydroxypropyl)trimethylammonium chloride carbamate.

Description: Bethanechol chloride occurs as colorless or white crystals or as a white, crystalline powder, usually having a slight amine-like odor. It is freely soluble in water and in alcohol and insoluble in chloroform and in ether.

Bethanechol is a synthetic cholinergic drug closely related to, but differing from, acetylcholine in that it exhibits little if any ganglionic stimulating action and is not destroyed by cholinesterase; therefore, it has a more prolonged and predictable effect. It is similar in action to methacholine chloride but is less toxic and also less active. In therapeutic doses, it has little or no effect on the heart rate, blood pressure or peripheral circulation of normal subjects. It increases peristalsis and stimulates micturition and defecation.

Indications: As a parasympathomimetic in the treatment of acute postoperative and postpartum nonobstructive (functional) urinary retention and for neurogenic atony of the urinary bladder with retention.

Contraindications: Hyperthyroidism, pregnancy, peptic ulcer, latent or active bronchial asthma, pronounced bradycardia or hypotension, vasomotor instability, coronary artery disease, epilepsy, and parkinsonism. Bethanechol should not be employed when the strength or integrity of the gastrointestinal or bladder wall is in question, or in the presence of mechanical obstruction; when increased muscular activity of the gastrointestinal tract or urinary bladder might prove harmful, as following recent urinary bladder surgery, gastrointestinal resection and anastomosis, or when there is possible gastrointestinal obstruction; in bladder neck obstruction, spastic gastrointestinal disturbances, acute inflammatory lesions of the gastrointestinal tract, or peritonitis; or in marked vagotonia.

Warnings: *Bethanechol chloride should never be administered either intravenously or intramuscularly.* Violent symptoms of cholinergic over-stimulation, such as circulatory collapse, fall in blood pressure, abdominal cramps, bloody diarrhea, shock, or sudden cardiac arrest are likely to occur. Although rare, these same symptoms have occurred after subcutaneous injection, and may occur in cases of hypersensitivity or overdosage.

Precautions: When administering bethanechol chloride subcutaneously, a hypodermic syringe containing atropine sulfate should be readily available for immediate use. Special care is required if this drug is administered to patients receiving ganglionic blocking agents because a critical fall in blood pressure may occur; however, severe abdominal symptoms usually appear before such a fall in blood pressure is experienced. Also, the cholinergic effects may be inhibited by such drugs as quinidine or procainamide or may be increased by cholinergic drugs, particularly cholinesterase inhibitors. In the presence of urinary retention, if the sphincter fails to relax as bethanechol contracts the bladder, urine may be forced up the ureter into the kidney pelvis. If bacteria is present in the urine, this may cause a reflux infection.

Adverse Reactions: Untoward reactions are rare following oral therapeutic doses of bethanechol chloride. Those that may occur are usually the result of overdosage and may be expressed by abdominal discomfort, salivation, flushing of the skin, sweating, nausea, vomiting, asthmatic attacks, substernal pressure or pain, myocardial hypoxia, transient syncope with cardiac arrest, transient complete heart block, dyspnea, orthostatic hypotension, and involuntary defecation and urinary urgency. Short periods of atrial fibrillation have been observed in hyperthyroid individuals following the administration of cholinergic drugs. If necessary, the action of the drug can be promptly abolished by the subcutaneous or intravenous injection, of 0.6 mg or more of atropine sulfate for adults.

Dosage and Administration: *Orally.* The usual dosage ranges from 10 to 30 mg 3 or 4 times daily. The minimum effective dose is determined by giving 5 to 10 mg initially and repeating the same amount at hourly intervals up to a maximum of 30 mg or until a satisfactory response is obtained; the effect of the drug is apparent within 30 to 90 minutes and lasts about 1 hour. *Subcutaneously,* the smallest amount that will produce a satisfactory response. This is established by injecting 2.5 mg initially and repeating at intervals of 15 to 30 minutes thereafter as a second, third or fourth dose if a satisfactory response is not obtained and if no disturbing side effects appear. The aggregate amount may be repeated as a single dose 3 or 4 times daily if required.

Availability:
DUVOID® Tablets, 10, 25 and 50 mg in bottles of 100 and in single-unit packages of 100. **(Norwich-Eaton)**
MYOTONACHOL™ Tablets, 5, 10 and 25 mg in bottles of 100; 10 and 25 mg in unit-dose packages of 100. **(Glenwood)**
URECHOLINE®: **(Merck Sharp & Dohme)**
Injection, 5 mg/ml in ampuls of 1 ml.
Tablets, 5, 10 and 25 mg in bottles of 100 and in single-unit packages of 100.

BIOZYME

Description: Each gm of ointment contains neomycin palmitate equivalent to 3.5 mg of neomycin and trypsin-chymotrypsin concentrate, 10,000 units. The primary action of the enzymatic concentrate is to digest necrotic tissue, pyogenic membranes and crusts, thereby cleansing wounds and removing foul odors thus allowing for maximum neomycin-antiinfective activity. The enzymes are a concentrate derived from mammalian pancreas and are measured in terms of proteolytic activity. A specially prepared water-washable ointment base has been employed to provide optimal release of medicaments with ease of application. The base is nonirritating, nontoxic and nonallergenic.

Indications: In skin conditions infected with neomycin-susceptible organisms where the debriding-cleansing action of enzymes is indicated, such as abscesses and furuncles (open or incised), infected burns, pyodermas such as folliculitis and impetigo, infected skin ulcers such as arteriosclerotic, decubitus, diabetic, stasis, traumatic, varicose, etc.

Contraindications: Local application is contraindicated in those patients known to be hypersensitive to any of the components.

Warnings: Prolonged use of antibiotics may result in the overgrowth of nonsusceptible organisms. If superinfection occurs, the drug should be discontinued and appropriate therapy instituted. Clinical evidence suggests an increasing prevalence of individuals sensitive to neomycin.

Precautions: Because of the potential hazards of nephrotoxicity and ototoxicity, prolonged use or applications of large amounts of this product should be avoided in the treatment of skin infections following extensive burns, trophic ulceration, and other conditions in which systemic absorption of neomycin is possible. As with any drug, the usual precautions should be observed when prescribed for pregnant patients.

Adverse Reactions: Although generally well tolerated, an itching or stinging sensation is sometimes experienced with the first few applications. Hypersensitivity or allergic reactions are seen occasionally. The proteolytic action can be halted by removing the ointment and irrigating with water.

Dosage and Administration: *Topically.* The ointment is applied directly to the lesions 1 to 3 times daily and covered with gauze. **Note:** Not for ophthalmic use.

Availability:
BIOZYME® Ointment in tubes of 15 and 30 gm. **(Armour)**

BIPERIDEN

Chemical Name: α-5-Norbornen-2-yl-α-phenyl-1-piperidinepropanol.

Description: A synthetic anticholinergic agent structurally and pharmacologically related to trihexyphenidyl, procyclidine and cycrimine. The hydrochloride occurs as a white, crystalline powder slightly soluble in water and in alcohol.

Its atropine-like action on parasympathetic-innervated peripheral structures is similar to that of other parasympatholytic agents of the trihexyphenidyl group. Studies in experimental animals have shown that in addition to its spasmolytic, antisecretory and mydriatic effects, it has a nicotinolytic potency about 6 times that of atropine and 5 times that of trihexyphenidyl on a weight basis.

Indications: As an adjunct in the treatment of postencephalitic, idiopathic and arteriosclerotic types of Parkinson's disease; drug-induced parkinsonism and/or drug-induced dyskinetic disturbances of the extrapyramidal system during treatment with the phenothiazines or reserpine known to produce parkinsonian symptoms.

Contraindications: Hypersensitivity to biperiden.

Warnings: Highly susceptible patients may experience mental confusion, euphoria, agitation and disturbed behavior. Safe use during pregnancy has not been established.

Precautions: Although no prohibitive rise in intraocular pressure has been noted following parenteral or oral administration, caution should be exercised in patients with manifest glaucoma. Patients with prostatism or cardiac arrhythmia should be given this drug with caution.

Adverse Reactions: Principally those of anticholinergic agents such as dry mouth, blurred vision, and, occasionally, drowsiness, disorientation or euphoria, effects which usually can be minimized or eliminated completely by a reduction of the oral dosage or by slow parenteral administration. Gastric irritation can be avoided by administering the drug during or after meals. A decrease in urinary flow has been noted in a few patients. Mild, transient, postural hypotension may follow parenteral administration. No local tissue reaction has been reported when administered intramuscularly. Symptoms of overdosage resemble those of atropine toxicity and would necessitate the same supportive therapy.

Dosage and Administration: To achieve the therapeutic goal, doses must be individually and gradually adjusted. *Orally:* In Parkinson's disease, the average dosage is 2 mg 3 or 4 times daily. In drug-induced extrapyramidal disorders, the average dosage is 2 mg 1 to 3 times daily. *Parenterally:* In drug-induced extrapyramidal disorders, the average dosage is 2 mg *intramuscularly* or *intravenously*, repeated every half hour until symptoms have abated. No more than 4 consecutive doses should be given in a 24-hour period. Intravenous and intramuscular routes of administration appear equally rapid in onset and as effective in action. Initial parenteral treatment can be followed by oral treatment when desired. The drug does not produce any gross disorganization of cerebral electrical activity.

Availability:
AKINETON®: **(Knoll)**
Injection, 5 mg/ml (as lactate) in ampuls of 1 ml in cartons of 10.
Tablets, 2 mg (as hydrochloride) in bottles of 100 and 1000.

BIPHETAMINE Ⓒ

Description: Capsules containing equal parts of dextroamphetamine and racemic amphetamine as cation exchange resin complexes of sulfonated polystyrene. Three potencies: '7½' capsule contains 3.75 mg of each of the two amphetamines; '12½' capsule contains 6.25 mg of each of the two amphetamines and '20' contains 10 mg each. Amphetamines are sympathomimetic amines with CNS stimulant activity. Peripheral actions include elevation of systolic and diastolic blood pressures and weak bronchodilator and respiratory stimulant action. The anorectic effect diminishes after a few weeks.

Indications: Exogenous obesity, as a short term (a few weeks) adjunct in a regimen of weight reduction based on caloric restriction.

Contraindications: Advanced arteriosclerosis, symptomatic cardiovascular disease, moderate to severe hypertension, hyperthyroidism, known hypersensitivity or idiosyncrasy to the sympathomimetic amines, glaucoma, agitated states, patients with a history of drug abuse. During or within 14 days following the administration of monoamine oxidase inhibitors, hypertensive crisis may result.

Warnings: Amphetamines have a significant potential for abuse. In view of their limited short-term anorectic effect and rapid development of tolerance, they should be used with extreme caution and only for limited periods of time in weight reduction programs. Tolerance to the anorectic effect usually develops within a few weeks. When this occurs, the recommended dose should not be exceeded in an attempt to increase the effect; rather, the drug should be discontinued. Amphetamines may impair the ability of the patient to engage in potentially hazardous activities such as operating machinery or driving a motor vehicle; therefore, the patient should be cautioned accordingly. Abrupt cessation following prolonged high dosage administration results in extreme fatigue and mental depression; changes are also noted in the sleep EEG. Manifestations of chronic intoxication with amphetamines include severe dermatoses, marked insomnia, irritability, hyperactivity, and personality changes. The most severe manifestation of chronic intoxication is psychosis, often clinically indistinguishable from schizophrenia. Safe use during pregnancy has not been established. Use of amphetamines by women who are or who may become pregnant, and especially those in the first trimester of pregnancy, requires that the potential benefit be weighed against the possible hazard to mother and infant. Amphetamines are not recommended for use as anorectic agents in children under 12 years of age.

Precautions: Caution is to be exercised in prescribing amphetamines for patients with even mild hypertension. Insulin requirements in diabetes mellitus may be altered in association with the use of amphetamines and the concomitant dietary regimen. Amphetamines may decrease the hypotensive effect of guanethidine. The least amount feasible should be prescribed or dispensed at one time in order to minimize the possibility of overdosage.

Adverse Reactions: *Cardiovascular:* Palpitation, tachycardia, elevation of blood pressure. *Central nervous system:* Overstimulation, restlessness, dizziness, insomnia, euphoria, dysphoria, tremor, headache; rarely, psychotic episodes at recommended doses. *Gastrointestinal:* Dryness of the mouth, unpleasant taste, diarrhea, other gastrointestinal disturbances. Anorexia and weight loss may occur as undesirable effects when amphetamines are used for other than the anorectic effect. *Allergic:* Urticaria. *Endocrine:* Impotence, changes in libido. Refer to monograph on Amphetamine for symptoms and management of overdosage.

Dosage and Administration: *Orally,* 1 capsule daily 10 to 14 hours before retiring. The potency best suited to patient's requirement should be used.

Availability:
Ⓒ BIPHETAMINE® Capsules, '7½' (white), '12½' (black and white) and '20' (black) in bottles of 100. **(Pennwalt)**

BISACODYL TANNEX

Chemical Name: 4,4′-(Diacetoxydiphenyl)-(pyridyl-2)-methane complexed with tannic acid.

Description: Bisacodyl is a tasteless, crystalline substance practically insoluble in water and alkaline solutions but soluble in acids, alcohol, acetone, propylene gylcol and other organic solvents. Bisacodyl complexed with tannic acid occurs as a fluffy, light tan powder that is readily soluble in water. The addition of tannic acid serves not only to solubilize bisacodyl but also to inhibit secretion of mucus in the walls of the large intestine.

Bisacodyl tannex is a nonabsorbable colonic evacuant. Its primary effect is upon the colon; it appears to initiate reflex peristalsis by stimulating the nerve endings in the mucosa.

Indications: Preparation of patients for radiologic examinations of the colon, sigmoidoscopy and proctologic examinations.

Contraindications: In patients under 10 years of age, and in those individuals with known or suspected extensive ulcerative lesions of the colon.

Warnings: Safe use during pregnancy has not been established; therefore, bisacodyl tannex should not be given to women of childbearing potential, particularly to those in the first trimester of pregnancy, except where the potential benefits outweigh the possible adverse effects upon fetal development.

Precautions: Since tannic acid is hepatotoxic if absorbed in sufficient quantity, it should be used with considerable care in a regimen where multiple enemas have been administered.

Adverse Reactions: Cramping, weakness, nausea, and fainting.

Dosage and Administration: *Rectally* as an enema. **Cleansing enema:** Prepare by dissolving the contents of 1 packet (2.5 gm) in 1 liter of lukewarm water and administer. **Barium enema:** Prepare by dissolving the contents of 1 or 2 packets in 1 liter of a barium suspension and administer. The total concentration of bisacodyl tannex should *never* exceed 0.5% (2 packets/liter). **Note:** the total dosage for any one complete colonic examination, including the cleansing enema, should not exceed 7.5 gm (3 packets), and no more than 10 gm (4 packets) should be administered to any individual within a 72-hour period.

Availability:
CLYSODRAST® Packet contains 1.5 mg of bisacodyl complexed with 2.5 gm of tannic acid in cartons of 25 and 50 packets. **(Barnes-Hind)**

BISHYDROXYCOUMARIN

Chemical Name: 3,3′-Methylenebis(4-hydroxycoumarin).

Description: Bishydroxycoumarin is an orally effective anticoagulant which decreases the prothrombin concentration of the blood. It occurs as a white or creamy white, crystalline powder, having a faint, pleasant odor and a slightly bitter taste. It is practically insoluble in water, in alcohol, and in ether; slightly soluble in chloroform; readily soluble in solutions of fixed alkali hydroxides.

After a latent period of 12 to 24 hours, the prothrombin time slowly increases to a maximum in 36 to 48 hours, remaining effective for 5 to 6 days after cessation of therapy. The drug inhibits the formation of prothrombin in the liver. The concentration of prothrombin in the blood is thus reduced, and the prothrombin time is increased. The drug also interferes with the synthesis of factors VII, IX and X by the liver. It has been postulated that bishydroxycoumarin competes with vitamin K for an enzyme essential for prothrombin synthesis.

Indications: Prophylaxis and treatment of venous thrombosis and its extension, the treatment of atrial fibrillation with embolization, the prophylaxis and treatment of pulmonary embolism, and as an adjunct in the treatment of coronary occlusion.

Contraindications: In patients who are bleeding or who have hemorrhagic tendencies, open wounds, visceral carcinoma, ulcerations of the gastrointestinal tract, subacute bacterial endocarditis, severe liver or kidney disease, or severe uncontrolled hypertension. It is also contraindicated in patients who have had recent operations on the eye, brain or spinal cord, or who are deficient in vitamin K.

Warnings: Bishydroxycoumarin is a potent drug. Its effects tend to be cumulative and prolonged, and severe hemorrhage may result from overdosage. At the earliest signs of bleeding, the drug should be withdrawn. Also, patients vary in their response. Dosage can be controlled only by periodic determination of prothrombin time, since determinations of clotting and bleeding times are of no value for measuring the effects of this drug. Utmost caution should be exercised in the presence of diverticulitis, colitis, mild or moderate uncontrolled hypertension, mild or moderate liver or kidney disease, patients undergoing regional or lumbar block anesthesia or those with indwelling drainage catheters. When heparin sodium, which prolongs the one-stage prothrombin time, is given with bishydroxycoumarin, a period of at least 5 hours after the last intravenous dose and 24 hours after the last subcutaneous dose of heparin sodium should elapse in order to obtain a valid prothrombin time. Since the drug passes the placental barrier, fetal hemorrhage may occur and cause fetal death *in utero*. Also, congential malformations have been reported to occur in children born to mothers who received oral anticoagulants during pregnancy. These included nasal hypoplasia and other abnormalities consistent with a diagnosis of chondrodysplasia punctata. A casual relationship with oral anticoagulant therapy has not been established but is strongly suggested. Therefore, the physician should carefully consider these possible events in the fetus before prescribing the drug for women of childbearing potential. Bishydroxycoumarin is secreted in the maternal milk; therefore it should be administered to pregnant patients or to lactating mothers only when the risk of withholding the drug is weighed against the potential hazards entailed in administering it. Since the drug appears in mother's milk, the nursing infant should be closely observed for evidence of unexpected bleeding.

Precautions: The anticoagulant activity of the drug may be altered by any changes in the intake of vitamin K, fat or leafy green vegetables; vitamin K deficiency of the newborn; fever, alcoholism; vitamin C deficiency; roentgenographic therapy; or diarrhea which causes increased loss of vitamin K in the stool and/or decreased absorption from the intestine. Care in patient selection is desirable to ensure cooperation, particularly from alcoholic, emotionally unstable, psychotic, or senile patients. The drug should be used judiciously in patients with active tuberculosis, severe diabetes, a history of ulcerative disease of the gastrointestinal tract; and during menstruation and the postpartum period. Bleeding during oral anticoagulant therapy may not always correlate with prothrombin time. Since patients with congestive heart failure frequently become more sensitive to the drug, an appropriate reduction in dosage may be necessary in such cases. It is of utmost importance that no other drug be administered with bishydroxycoumarin without full appreciation of its potential for interacting with it, thereby increasing or decreasing its anticoagulant effect. Fatalities have been reported from interactions affecting the metabolism of coumarin anticoagulants or their binding to plasma proteins. Drugs which stimulate metabolic degradation of this anticoagulant include phenobarbital as well as other barbiturates, glutethimide, meprobamate, rifampin, ethchlorvynol, and griseofulvin. In addition, oral contraceptives, ACTH, and adrenocorticosteroids have been reported to reduce the response to coumarin anticoagulants. Patients receiving these drugs may require larger doses of bishydroxycoumarin to achieve an optimal anticoagulant effect. When these drugs are discontinued, it may be necessary to reduce the dose of bishydroxycoumarin. Such drugs as phenylbutazone, oxyphenbutazone, diazoxide, chloral hydrate, and mefenamic, ethacrynic, and nalidixic acids increase the quantity of free drug available by displacing bishydroxycoumarin from protein binding sites. Quinine, quinidine, and salicylates in large doses depress prothrombin formation in the liver, and thus may increase the patient's sensitivity to bishydroxycoumarin and cause hemorrhage. Broad-spectrum antibiotics, which suppress the organisms comprising the normal bacterial flora of the intestine and reduce production of vitamin K, may increase anticoagulant activity, but this is usually not observed unless there is a dietary deficiency of vitamin K. Other drugs which have been reported to cause an exaggerated response and a prolonged prothrombin time are methylthiouracil, propylthiouracil, phenyramidol, disulfiram, dextrothyroxine, clofibrate, glucagon, chloramphenicol, nortriptyline, and various anabolic steroids. Bishydroxycoumarin has been reported to inhibit the enzymatic degradation of phenytoin in the liver thus leading to increased serum levels and prolonged half-life of phenytoin which could result in drug intoxication. Conversely, phenytoin stimulates bishydroxycoumarin metabolism, thereby decreasing serum levels of the anticoagulant and thus increasing the plasma prothrombin-proconvertin concentrations. The coumarin anticoagulants also are known to potentiate the hypoglycemic effect of tolbutamide by inhibiting its degradation in the liver. They have also been shown to elevate the serum levels of chlorpropamide and phenobarbital. Therefore, with the addition or withdrawal of any of these drugs, there is the danger of either inadequate anticoagulant response to bishydroxycoumarin or bleeding. In such cases, the dosage of this drug should be carefully regulated or its use discontinued.

Adverse Reactions: Doses in excess of those recommended may cause bleeding or hemorrhaging. The occurrence of significant gastrointestinal or urinary tract bleeding during therapy may indicate the presence of an underlying occult lesion. Paralytic ileus and intestinal obstruction have been reported from submucosal or intramural hemorrhage. Excessive uterine bleeding has occurred but menstrual flow is usually normal. Nonhemorrhagic adverse reactions, which have been reported with coumarin anticoagulants, include dermatitis, urticaria, alopecia, fever, nausea, vomiting, cramps, diarrhea, and leukopenia. Hemorrhagic necrosis (bleeding into the skin and subcutaneous tissue with necrosis, vasculitis, and thrombosis) of the female breast and other areas has also been reported. Adrenal hemorrhage with resultant acute adrenal insufficiency has occurred; therefore, anticoagulant therapy should be discontinued in patients who develop signs and symptoms compatible with acute adrenal hemorrhage or insufficiency. Plasma cortisol levels should be measured immediately, and vigorous therapy with intravenous corticosteroids should be instituted promptly. Initiation of therapy should not depend upon laboratory confirmation of the diagnosis, since any delay in an acute situation may result in the patient's death. Overdosage may cause an overly-prolonged prothrombin time or minor hemorrhage which usually responds satisfactorily to withdrawal of the drug alone, but whole blood transfusions may be needed in some cases. If prothrombin activity falls below 15% of normal or if hemorrhaging occurs, the drug should be withdrawn temporarily. If warranted by the clinical situation, phytonadione (vitamin K_1) may be administered by slow intravenous injection in doses of 1 to 5 mg in cases of mild overdosage and 20 to 40 mg in cases of severe overdosage. Such use of vitamin K complicates subsequent anticoagulant therapy; therefore, caution must be observed in determining the need for this vitamin. A hypercoagulable state has been reported to occur following the rapid reversal of a prolonged prothrombin time.

Dosage and Administration: *Orally.* Dosage must be individualized and adjusted according to prothrombin time. The usual aim of therapy is to reduce prothrombin activity to 20 to 30% of normal. However, a range of 15 to 35% of normal is almost as satisfactory and may be more practical in some instances. The following schedule serves only as a guide. The average dosage the first day for adults with normal prothrombin activity is 200 to 300 mg, followed on subsequent days by 25 to 200 mg if the prothrombin activity is 25% or more. The drug should not be given on any day when the prothrombin activity is less than 25%. *Combined use with heparin:* Because bishydroxycoumarin has a slow onset of action, heparin should be used when a rapid anticoagulant effect is desired. Both drugs can be given together at the start of therapy, and heparin may be continued for 24 to 72 hours or until a satisfactory effect from bishydroxycoumarin is obtained as determined by prothrombin-time studies.

Availability:
DICUMAROL Tablets, 25 and 50 mg bottles of 100 and 1000; 100 mg in bottles of 100. **(Abbott)**
DICUMAROL Capsules (Pulvules®), 25 and 50 mg in bottles of 100. **(Lilly)**

BLEOMYCIN SULFATE

Description: Bleomycin sulfate is composed of basic cytotoxic glycopeptide antibiotics isolated from a strain of *Streptomyces verticillus*. It is highly soluble in water.

Although the precise mechanism of action of this drug has not been established, available evidence indicates that the primary mode of action appears to be the inhibition of DNA synthesis with some evidence of lesser inhibition of RNA and protein synthesis.

When administered to mice, high concentrations of bleomycin are found in the skin, lungs, kidneys, peritoneum, and in the lymphatic glands. The drug has shown a strong affinity for tumor cells in the skin and lungs in contrast to the lack of the drug's affinity for such cells in hematopoietic tissue. This selective affinity for different sites and cell types affords a better understanding of the drug's therapeutic benefits and toxic potential. The toxicity of bleomycin appears to be dose-related with a striking increase in symptoms when the total dose is more than 400 units. Approximately 60 to 70% of the clinical dose is recovered in the urine as active bleomycin.

Indications: Palliative treatment and/or adjuvant agent to other approved chemotherapeutic agents in selected tumors. It has been found useful in the management of squamous cell carcinoma of the head and neck involving the mouth, tongue, tonsil, nasopharynx, oropharynx, sinus, palate, lip, buccal mucosa, gingiva and epiglottis; skin; larynx and paralarynx; penis; cervix, and vulva. The response is poorer in patients with head and neck cancer which has been irradiated prior to treatment with this drug. Also for the management of lymphomas such as Hodgkin's, reticulum cell sarcoma, and lymphosarcoma. Most of the patients with Hodgkin's disease had the disseminated type (stage IV) that was no longer responsive to bone marrow-depressant agents. Bleomycin is also indicated for testicular carcinoma such as embryonal cell, choriocarcinoma and teratocarcinoma. Studies have revealed that the use of vinblastine sulfate with bleomycin increases the response rate of testicular tumors.

Contraindications: Patients with a prior hypersensitivity reaction to the drug.

Warnings: A total dose of more than 400 units should be given with extreme caution. Bleomycin should be administered under the supervision of a qualified physician experienced in the use of cancer chemotherapeutic agents. Since facilities for necessary laboratory studies must be available, hospitalization of patients is recommended. The physician should be aware that pulmonary fibrosis is the most serious toxic reaction to bleomycin; also, he must consider carefully not only the possible therapeutic benefits but also the potential toxic reactions to this drug (see Adverse Reactions). A hypersensitivity reaction similar to anaphylaxis, and which may result in death, occurred in 1% of the patients, particularly in those patients with lymphoma. This occurs only after the first or second dose and the symptoms may appear immediately or may be delayed for several hours. These consist of hypotension, fever, chills, mental confusion, and wheezing. Treatment is symptomatic and may include such measures as volume expansion, pressor agents, antihistamines, and corticosteroids. Safe use of bleomycin in pregnant women has not been established; therefore, the therapeutic benefits to the patient must be weighed against the potential hazards to the embryo or fetus.

Precautions: Extreme caution is necessary in patients with significant impairment of renal or hepatic function or compromised pulmonary function due to disease other than malignancy. To monitor the onset of pulmonary toxicity, roentgenograms of the chest should be taken every 1 to 2 weeks. If pulmonary changes are noted, treatment should be discontinued until it can be determined whether or not the cause is drug-related. Pneumonitis due to the drug should be treated with corticosteroids in an effort to prevent progression to pulmonary fibrosis, and infectious pneumonitis should be treated with appropriate antibiotic therapy.

Adverse Reactions: The most frequent complication noted has been skin changes that occurred in approximately 52.3% of the patients. These have consisted of vesiculations, alopecia, hyperpigmentation, redness, hyperkeratosis, nail changes, rash, tenderness, pruritus, striae, and stomatitis. In only 2% of treated patients was it necessary to discontinue bleomycin therapy because of skin toxicity. This complication was a relatively late manifestation developing usually in the 2nd or 3rd week of therapy after 150 to 200 units of the drug had been given and, in general, was related to total cumulative dose.

Pulmonary toxicity is potentially the most serious side effect, and occurs in about 10% of the patients treated. The most frequent manifestation is pneumonitis occasionally progressing to pulmonary fibrosis which may result in death. Approximately 1% of patients treated died of pulmonary fibrosis. An analysis of the data revealed that pulmonary toxicity is usually both dose- and age-related, being more common in patients over 70 years of age who received more than 400 units total dose. However, this complication is unpredictable and has been seen occasionally in young patients receiving low doses. The identification of patients with pulmonary toxicity due to bleomycin has been extremely difficult due to the lack of specificity of (1) the clinical syndrome; (2) the roentgenographic changes; and (3) the tissue changes seen on examination of biopsy and autopsy specimens.

In some patients drug-induced pneumonitis apparently produces dyspnea and fine rales that appear to be no different from those produced by infectious pneumonias or from the signs and symptoms produced by primary or metastatic lung disease. Also, x-ray shows that this complication produces patchy opacities, usually of the lower lung fields, that appear the same as those observed in infectious bronchopneumonia or lung metastases. The microscopic tissue changes due to toxicity with this drug are frequently present as bronchiolar squamous metaplasia, reactive macrophages, atypical alveolar epithelial cells, fibrinous edema, and interstitial fibrosis. The acute stage may involve capillary changes and subsequent fibrinous exudation into alveoli, thus producing a change similar to hyaline-membrane formation and progressing to a diffuse interstitial fibrosis resembling the Hamman-Rich syndrome. These findings are nonspecific and are similar to the changes produced in radiation pneumonitis, pneumocystic pneumonitis and, at times, reaction to long-standing malignant pulmonary disease.

Serial pulmonary function tests in 156 patients receiving bleomycin therapy revealed some demonstrable alteration in approximately 20% of the patients. The most common changes were a decrease in total lung volume and in vital capacity. However, no predictive correlation between these changes and the development of pulmonary fibrosis could be ascertained. The most frequently observed reactions were fever, chills, nausea, and vomiting. Renal, hepatic and CNS toxicity may also occur; therefore, these systems should be monitored. Infrequently reported were pain at the tumor site, phlebitis, and other local reactions. There has been no evidence of bone marrow or immunological depression thus far. Anorexia and weight loss are common and may persist long after termination of this medication. Since these signs and symptoms occur with malignancy, it may be difficult to determine whether or not they are drug-induced.

Dosage and Administration: *Intramuscularly, intravenously, or subcutaneously.* The usual dosage schedule is 0.25 to 0.5 units/kg of body weight once or twice weekly. After a 50% clinical response, the maintenance dose is 1 unit daily or 5 units weekly, given either *intravenously* or *intramuscularly.* Because of the possibility of an anaphylactic reaction, all patients with lymphoma should receive 2 units or less for the first 2 doses. If no acute reaction occurs, the regular dosage schedule should be followed. Improvement of Hodgkin's disease and testicular carcinoma usually occurs within 2 weeks. If no improvement is seen by this time, the chances of improvement are very low. Squamous cell cancers respond more slowly, sometimes requiring as long as 3 weeks before improvement is noted.

Availability:
BLENOXANE® Injection in ampuls of 15 units. **(Bristol)**

BOTULISM ANTITOXIN, BIVALENT

Description: Botulism antitoxin is a sterile solution of the refined and concentrated proteins, chiefly globulins, containing antitoxic antibodies obtained from the blood serum or plasma of healthy horses that have been immunized against the toxins produced by both the type A and type B strains of *Clostridium botulinum.* It contains not more than 20% solids, and contains a suitable preservative.

Indications: Treatment of all cases of toxemia in which the toxin is known or suspected to be produced by *Cl. botulinum,* type A or B.

Warnings: The parenteral administration of any biologic product should be governed by every known precaution for the prevention and arrest of allergic and other untoward reactions. A careful history should review possible sensitivity of the patient to the type of protein to be injected.

Precautions: Immediate reactions may occur during, or immediately after injection, if the patient is sensitive to the protein material contained in this serum. To avoid such possible reactions, certain precautions are necessary. In addition to a careful history to determine whether or not a patient may be subject to asthma, angioneurotic edema or other allergy, or whether the individual has received an injection of serum more than 7 days previously, every patient should be tested for sensitivity to horse serum before injecting this antiserum. Testing may be done intradermally or conjunctivally. The latter test should be used if there is danger of a severe systemic reaction to the intradermal test dose or it may be used instead.

Adverse Reactions: Serum sickness may occur approximately 5 to 13 days after administration of this antitoxin to patients who have shown no evidence of sensitivity to the antitoxin. The most prominent manifestations of serum sickness are urticaria, fever, arthralgias and pruritus. An antihistaminic drug will usually give substantial relief.

Dosage and Administration: Before administering any antitoxin, the patient must be tested for possible allergic reactions. See "Precautions." A dosage of 10,000 units of each type of antitoxin (contents of 1 vial) should be injected *intravenously* as early as possible. This dose should be repeated at intervals of 4 hours until the toxic condition is alleviated. The intravenous route, rather than the intramuscular route, is advocated because the seriousness of the intoxication necessitates rapid neutralization of the toxin. The antitoxin is diluted 1:10, preferably with 10% glucose; 5% glucose or normal saline may be used. The first 10 ml (1 ml antitoxin) is injected very slowly over a period of 5 minutes. After an interval of 15 minutes, the remainder may be injected more rapidly. A syringe filled with 1 ml of epinephrine hydrochloride solution (1:1000) should be readily available, and used at once if respiratory difficulty or other signs of allergic reactions occur.

Availability:
BOTULISM ANTITOXIN, BIVALENT (equine origin, globulin-modified) in vials of 10,000 units each of types A and B. **(Lederle)**

BRETYLIUM TOSYLATE

Chemical Name: o-Bromobenzyl ethyldimethylammonium p-toluene sulfonate.

Description: Bretylium, an adrenergic neuronal blocking agent, is a bromobenzyl quaternary ammonium compound with antiarrhythmic properties. It has been found to be most useful in the treatment of refractory ventricular arrhythmias, particularly ventricular fibrillation and tachycardia. It has a positive inotropic effect and normally augments cardiac output. It occurs as a white, bitter-tasting, crystalline powder that is freely soluble in water and in alcohol.

Although the mechanisms of the antifibrillatory and antiarrhythmic actions have not been clearly defined, the following electrophysiologic actions have been demonstrated in animal experiments: (1) An increase in ventricular fibrillation threshold. (2) An increase in action potential duration and effective refractory period without changes in heart rate. (3) Little effect on the rate of rise or amplitude of the cardiac action potential (Phase 0) or in resting membrane potential (Phase 4) in normal myocardium. However, when cell injury slows the rate of rise, decreases amplitude, and lowers resting membrane potential, bretylium restores these parameters toward normal. (4) An increase in impulse formation and spontaneous firing rate of pacemaker tissue as well as increased ventricular induction velocity. The restoration of injured myocardial cell electrophysiology toward normal, as well as the increase of the action potential duration and effective refractory period without changing their ratio to each other may be important factors in suppressing reentry of aberrant impulses and decreasing induced dispersion of local excitable states.

The drug appears to act by depressing adrenergic transmitter release, since it is taken up by adrenergic nerve terminals in the heart and subsequently prevents the release of norepinephrine. It has been found to induce a chemical sympathectomy-like state which resembles a surgical sympathectomy. The relationship of adrenergic blockade to the antifibrillatory and antiarrhythmic actions of bretylium is not clear. In a study in patients with frequent ventricular premature beats, peak plasma concentration and peak hypotensive effects were observed within 1 hour following intramuscular administration of the drug, presumably reflecting adrenergic neuronal blockade. However, suppression of premature ventricular beats was not maximal until 6 to 9 hours later when mean plasma concentration had declined to less than $^1/_2$ of peak level. This suggests that a slower mechanism, other than neuronal blockade, is involved in suppression of the arrhythmia. On the other hand, antifibrillatory effects generally occurred within minutes following intravenous administration suggesting that the effect on the myocardium may occur quite rapidly. Suppression of ventricular tachycardia and other ventricular arrhythmias develops more slowly, usually 20 minutes to 2 hours after parenteral administration. Following intravenous administration of 5 mg/kg of body weight to patients with acute myocardial infarction, there was a mild increase in arterial pressure, followed by a modest decrease, remaining within normal limits throughout. Pulmonary artery pressure, pulmonary capillary wedge pressure, right atrial pressure, cardiac index, stroke volume index, and stroke work index were not significantly changed. These hemodynamic effects were not correlated with antiarrhythmic activity.

Bretylium appears to be eliminated intact by the kidney, since no metabolites have, as yet, been identified. Approximately 70 to 80% of an intramuscular dose is excreted in the urine during the first 24 hours, with an additional 10% excreted over the next 3 days. Estimates of the terminal half-life have varied from about 5 to approximately 10 hours, but may range from 4 to 17 hours.

Indications: Treatment of life-threatening ventricular arrhythmias, principally ventricular fibrillation and tachycardia. It is designed for use in situations where present antiarrhythmic therapy does not produce the desired results, and only when the patient's progress can be constantly monitored.

Contraindications: There are no contraindications to use in the treatment of ventricular fibrillation or life-threatening refractory ventricular arrhythmias.

Warnings: Administration of bretylium regularly results in postural hypotension, and may occur at doses lower than those needed to suppress arrhythmias; therefore, patients should be kept supine until tolerance to the hypotensive effect develops. Patients exhibiting a fall in supine systolic pressure below 25 mm Hg may be given an infusion of dopamine or norepinephrine. Since the pressor effects of catecholamines are enhanced by bretylium, they should be administered in dilute solutions, and the blood pressure should be monitored closely. Volume expansion with blood or plasma and correction of dehydration should be initiated where appropriate. Due to the initial release of norepinephrine from adrenergic postganglionic nerve terminals, transient hypertension or increased frequency of premature ventricular contractions and other arrhythmias may occur. Simultaneous initiation of therapy with a digitalis glycoside and bretylium should be avoided since the presence of norepinephrine may aggravate digitalis toxicity. Patients with fixed cardiac output, such as severe aortic stenosis or severe pulmonary hypertension should not be given the drug because severe hypotension may result from a fall in peripheral resistance without a compensatory increase in cardiac output. However, if the arrhythmia is severe, the drug may be used but vasoconstrictive catecholamines should be given promptly if severe hypotension occurs. When considered for use in pregnant women, the therapeutic benefits must outweigh the potential risk to the fetus. Use in children is not recommended until safe and effective use and proper dosage have been determined.

Precautions: When intended for intravenous use the drug should be diluted in amounts of 1 part of bretylium to 4 parts of Dextrose Injection or normal saline solution, and the solution should be infused over a period of more than 8 minutes, since rapid administration may cause severe nausea and vomiting. However, when treating life-threatening ventricular fibrillation, the drug should be given as rapidly as possible and may be administered without dilution. When injected intramuscularly, no more than 5 ml should be injected at any one site because repeated intramuscular injection into the same site may cause atrophy and necrosis of muscle tissue, fibrosis, vascular degeneration and inflammatory responses. Dosage should be reduced in patients with impaired kidney function.

Adverse Reactions: Supine and postural hypotension have been the most frequently reported adverse reaction. Nausea and vomiting occurred in about 3% of patients, primarily when the drug was administered rapidly by the intravenous route. Vertigo, dizziness, lightheadedness and syncope, which sometimes accompanied postural hypotension, were reported in about 0.7% of patients. A few individuals experienced bradycardia, increased frequency of premature ventricular contractions, transitory hypertension, initial increase in arrhythmias, precipitation of anginal attacks, and sensation of substernal pressure. Renal dysfunction, diarrhea, abdominal pain, hiccups, erythematous macular rash, flushing, hyperthermia, confusion, paranoid psychosis, emotional lability, lethargy, generalized tenderness, anxiety, shortness of breath, diaphoresis, nasal stuffiness, and mild conjunctivitis have also been reported, but their relationship to the drug has not been established.

Dosage and Administration: *Intramuscularly* or *intravenously. For life-threatening ventricular fibrillation,* a dosage of 5 mg/kg of body weight of undiluted solution should be administered by rapid intravenous injection. Supplementary cardiopulmonary resuscitative procedures, including electrical cardioversion, should be employed prior to and following the injection. If ventricular fibrillation persists, the dosage may be increased to 10 mg/kg and repeated at 15- to 30-minute intervals until a total dose of no more than 30 mg/kg has been given. For other ventricular arrhythmias, a dosage of 5 to 10 mg/kg of body weight of diluted solution by intravenous infusion over a period extending beyond 8 minutes. A second dose may be given in 1 to 2 hours if the arrhythmia persists. *Intramuscularly.* A dosage of 5 to 10 mg/kg of body weight of the undiluted solution should be injected, and may be repeated in 1 to 2 hours if the results are not satisfactory. For maintenance, the same dosage may be repeated every 6 to 8 hours. For additional dosage information, refer to the package literature.

Availability:
BRETYLOL Solution, 50 mg/ml in vials of 10 ml. **(Arnar-Stone)**

BROMELAINS

Description: Bromelains is a concentrate of proteolytic enzymes obtained from the stem of the pineapple plant, *Ananus sativus.* It occurs as a buff-colored powder slightly soluble in water and insoluble in alcohol.

Its potency is expressed in units which are based on the amount of enzyme required to hydrolyze a standard casein substrate under specified conditions. It is also assayed biologically in rats in which edema has been induced by egg white. Proteolytic enzymes generally supplement and augment standard therapeutic procedures; they reduce inflammation and edema, ease pain, speed healing and tissue repair.

While the mode of action of proteolytic enzymes has not been fully established, it seems most probable that depolymerization of fibrin and permeability modifications of venules and lymphatics underlie the action.

Indications: As adjunctive therapy to supplement and augment standard therapeutic procedures for reduction of inflammation and edema in postoperative tissue reactions (for example, following episiotomy) and in accidental trauma.

Contraindications: Contraindicated in patients known to be hypersensitive to the drug or to pineapple or its products.

Warnings: Safe use of this drug during pregnancy has not been established. Due to limited clinical experience, the use of this drug in children 12 years of age and under is not recommended.

Precautions: Caution is essential in patients with abnormalities of the blood clotting mechanism, such as hemophilia, or in those with severe hepatic or renal disease. Patients on anticoagulant therapy should be observed carefully because of possible potentiation of the anticoagulant effect by bromelains.

Adverse Reactions: While seldom observed, sensitivity manifested by urticaria or skin rash has occurred. There has been no report of anaphylactoid reaction. One case of hypofibrinogenemia and several cases of menorrhagia and metrorrhagia possibly related to the drug have been reported. Nausea, vomiting or diarrhea have rarely been reported. Adverse reactions are usually reversible upon discontinuation of the drug.

Dosage and Administration: *Orally.* The usual dosage initially 100,000 units 4 times daily. For maintenance, 100,000 units twice daily, or 50,000 units 4 times daily.

Availability:
ANANASE®/-100 Tablets (yellow, enteric coated), 50,000 and 100,000 Rorer units in bottles of 100 and 500. **(Rorer)**
(One Rorer unit of protease activity is defined as that amount of enzyme which will so hydrolyze a standardized casein substrate at pH 7 and 25° C as to cause an increase in absorbence at 280 mu of 1×10^{-5}/minute of reaction time.)

BROMOCRIPTINE MESYLATE

Chemical Name: 2-Bromo-α-ergocriptine mesylate.

Description: A semisynthetic, brominated ergot alkaloid, bromocriptine is a dopamine-receptor agonist capable of directly activating postsynaptic dopaminergic receptors in the same manner as does endogenous dopamine. This compound is largely devoid of any of the pharmacologic properties generally associated with ergot alkaloids such as uterotonic, vasoconstrictive or pressor effects. A nonhormonal, nonestrogenic agent, it inhibits the secretion of prolactin with little or no effect on other pituitary hormones with the exception of growth hormone in which it lowers elevated levels in patients with acromegaly. The drug's therapeutic benefits derive from its ability to stimulate dopamine receptors located on the prolactin secreting cells of the anterior pituitary, thereby significantly inhibiting prolactin release which consequently leads to a reduction in abnormally high plasma levels of prolactin. This occurs because dopamine is a major prolactin inhibitory factor. It is therefore primarily useful in treating hyperprolactinemia and its accompanying amenorrhea and galactorrhea due to causes which may disrupt the hypothalamic-pituitary relationship. Treatment with bromocriptine may effectively lower prolactin levels in patients with pituitary tumors, but this does not obviate the necessity for radiotherapy or surgical intervention where appropriate. Effective relief of breast pain and congestion as well as the restoration of normal ovulatory menstrual cycles has been reported in a significant number of patients. Maximum reduction of prolactin levels generally occurred within the first 4 weeks of therapy, and reduced levels were obtained throughout the entire course of treatment.

Approximately 28% of a 2.5-mg oral dose was found to be absorbed from the gastrointestinal tract reaching blood levels in the range of approximately 2 to 3 ng/ml and plasma levels in the range of about 4 to 6 ng/ml, indicating that the red blood cells do not incorporate appreciable amounts of the drug or its metabolites. In vitro experiments showed that 90 to 96% of the drug binds to plasma proteins. Completely metabolized prior to excretion, it is eliminated chiefly in the bile with only minor amounts (2.5 to 5.5%) appearing in the urine. Almost all of the administered dose was excreted in the feces within 5 days. Various clinical and laboratory studies suggest that the drug may have abortient possibilities and may provoke developmental defects in the unborn child, but it appears that additional studies will be needed to establish a definite causal relationship to bromocriptine.

Indications: For short-term treatment of amenorrhea and galactorrhea associated with hyperprolactinemia due to varied etiologies, excluding demonstrable pituitary tumors. It is not indicated in patients with normal prolactin levels or in the management of infertility.

Contraindications: Unusual sensitivity to ergot alkaloids, and during pregnancy until safe use has been established.

Warnings: Complete evaluation of the sella-turcica in patients with pituitary tumors (Forbes-Albright syndrome) is advised before initiating drug therapy. The occurrence of pregnancy warrants immediate withdrawal of the medication. Bromocriptine is not recommended for use in children under 15 years of age until safe and effective use and proper dosage have been established.

Precautions: Since infertility may be reversed by restoration of normal menses and ovulation, women who might possibly conceive should be firmly advised to use contraceptive measures, other than the oral contraceptives, throughout the course of treatment. However, the possibility exists that patients may not respond to this recommendation, and since pregnancy may occur prior to reinitiation of menses, a pregnancy test should be performed at least every 4 weeks during the amenorrheic period, and once menses has been reestablished, then every time the patient misses a menstrual period. Knowledge concerning the drug's safe and effective use in long-term continuous dosage or in repeated courses is still incomplete. Amenorrhea and galactorrhea have been reported to recur in the range of 70 to 80% following the initial therapy.

Adverse Rections: The incidence of adverse effects is quite high (68%) but these are generally mild to moderate in degree, and may be ameliorated by temporarily reducing the dosage to one-half tablet 2 or 3 times daily. Nevertheless, therapy had to be discontinued in approximately 6% of patients. The following occurred in decreasing order of frequency: nausea, 51%; headache, 18%; dizziness, 16%; fatigue, 8%; abdominal cramps, 7%; lightheadedness, 6%;

vomiting and/or nasal congestion, 5%; and constipation and/or diarrhea, 3%. In addition, a slight hypotensive effect may accompany treatment.

Dosage and Administration: *Orally.* The therapeutic dosage is 1 tablet 2 or 3 times daily with meals. It is recommended that treatment be initiated with 1 tablet once daily with the evening meal for 3 days, then increased to 1 tablet twice daily with the morning and evening meal on the following day. Duration of treatment should not exceed 6 months.

Availability:
PARLODEL® Tablets, 2.5 mg in packages of 30. **(Sandoz)**

BROMODIPHENHYDRAMINE

Chemical Name: 2-(*p*-Bromo-α-phenylbenzyloxy)-*N, N*-dimethylethylamine.

Description: Bromodiphenhydramine hydrochloride is an antihistaminic agent. Drugs of this type antagonize in varying degrees most, but not all, of the pharmacological effects of histamine by acting as H_1-receptor antagonists. Because they do not block the release of histamine, they offer only palliative relief of allergic disorders.

Indications: Perennial and seasonal allergic rhinitis (hay fever); vasomotor rhinitis; allergic conjunctivitis due to inhalant allergens and foods; mild, uncomplicated allergic skin manifestations of urticaria and angioedema; amelioration and prevention of allergic reactions to blood or plasma in patients with any known history of such reactions; dermographism; as therapy for anaphylactic reactions adjunctive to epinephrine and other standard measures after the acute manifestations have been controlled; for mild, local allergic reactions to insect bites; physical allergy; for minor drug and serum reactions characterized by pruritus.

Contraindications: This drug should not be used in premature or newborn infants, and should not be administered to patients with hypersensitivity to the drug or to those with asthmatic attack, narrow-angle glaucoma, prostatic hypertrophy, stenosing peptic ulcer, pyloroduodenal obstruction, bladder-neck obstruction. Preparations containing bromodiphenhydramine should not be given to patients receiving monoamine oxidase inhibitors.

Warnings: Overdosage or accidental ingestion of large quantities of antihistamines may produce convulsions or death, especially in infants and children. As in the case of other preparations containing CNS depressant drugs, patients receiving bromodiphenhydramine should be cautioned about probable additive effects with alcohol and other CNS depressants (hypnotics, sedatives, and tranquilizers). Patients who become drowsy should be cautioned against engaging in activities requiring alertness or skill, such as driving a car or operating heavy machinery or appliances. Although there is no evidence that the use of this agent is detrimental to the mother or fetus, the use of any drug during pregnancy or lactation should be carefully assessed. As with all anticholinergics an inhibitory effect on lactation may occur.

Precautions: Bromodiphenhydramine has an atropine-like action which should be considered when prescribing this drug. Use with caution in patients with a history of asthma.

Adverse Reactions: Drug-induced side effects may include drowsiness, confusion, nervousness, restlessness, nausea, vomiting, diarrhea, blurring of vision, diplopia, difficulty in urination, constipation, tightness of the chest and wheezing, thickening of bronchial secretions, dryness of mouth, nose and throat, tingling, heaviness and weakness of hands, nasal stuffiness, vertigo, palpitation, headache, insomnia, urticaria, drug rash, photosensitivity, hemolytic anemia, hypotension, epigastric distress, anaphylactic shock.

Dosage and Administration: *Orally.* Adults, usually 25 mg 3 times daily for control of symptoms. Some patients may require up to 150 mg daily.

Availibility:
AMBODRYL® HYDROCHLORIDE: **(Parke-Davis)**
Elixir, 12.5 mg/5 ml in bottles of 1 pint. Contains 14% alcohol.
Kapseals® (Capsules), 25 mg in bottles of 100.

BROMPHENIRAMINE MALEATE

Chemical Name: 2-{*p*-Bromo-α-[2-(dimethylamino)ethyl]benzyl}pyridine bimaleate.

DEXBROMPHENIRAMINE MALEATE

Chemical Name: *d*-2-[4-Bromo-α-(2-dimethylaminoethyl)benzyl]pyridine maleate.

Description: Brompheniramine is an antihistamine which differs from chlorpheniramine only in that the former has a bromine atom substituted for the chlorine atom of the latter compound. The discovery of the racemic nature of brompheniramine led to recent resolution of the compound into its optical isomers. Subsequent pharmacologic studies have shown that the antihistaminic activity of the racemic substance resides almost exclusively in the *dextro* isomer.

Dexbrompheniramine, the dextrorotatory isomer, is approximately twice as potent as racemic brompheniramine; however, both drugs generally share the actions and uses of other antihistamines.

Indications: Symptomatic treatment of seasonal and perennial allergic rhinitis; vasomotor rhinitis, and allergic conjunctivitis due to inhalant allergens and foods; mild uncomplicated allergic skin manifestations of urticaria and angioedema; for the amelioration of allergic reactions to blood or plasma or to insect bites; dermographism; and as an adjunctive measure for anaphylactic reactions, after the acute manifestations have been controlled. Preparations containing pseudoephedrine are recommended for the relief of symptoms associated with upper respiratory mucosal congestion as in seasonal and perennial nasal allergies, acute rhinitis and rhinosinusitis, and blockage of the eustachian tubes.

Contraindications: Hypersensitivity to antihistamines; in newborn or premature infants; in nursing mothers; in the treatment of lower respiratory tract disorders including asthma; in patients receiving MAO inhibitors because the drugs intensify and prolong the anticholinergic effects of antihistamines. Should be used with utmost caution, if at all, in patients with narrow-angle glaucoma, stenosing peptic ulcer, prostatic hypertrophy, bladder neck obstruction, or pyloroduodenal obstruction. Pseudoephedrine-containing preparations are contraindicated in children under 12 years of age, in pregnant women or nursing mothers, and in patients with severe hypertension and coronary artery disease. Hypersensitivity to the component drug.

Warnings: Dosage should be carefully regulated when administering antihistamines to infants and young children since large doses may result in hallucinations, convulsions, and even death. Until further clinical experience is gained, safe use in pregnant women has not been confirmed. It is well to bear in mind that these drugs may have additive effects with alcohol and other CNS depressants such as hypnotics, sedatives, tranquilizers, antianxiety agents, etc. Patients taking antihistaminic agents should be cautioned not to engage in activities requiring alertness or skill such as driving a car or operating machinery. Dizziness, sedation, and hypotension are more likely to occur in elderly patients.

Precautions: Since these drugs possess an atropine-like action, routine caution is advised when prescribing to patients with a history of bronchial asthma, increased intraocular pressure, hyperthyroidism, cardiovascular disease, or hypertension.

Adverse Reactions: The physician should be alert to the possibility of any of the adverse reactions which have been observed with sympathomimetic and antihistaminic drugs such as sedation, sleepiness, dryness of mouth, nose and throat, thickening of bronchial secretions, dizziness, epigastric distress, disturbed coördination, fatigue, confusion, restlessness, excitation, nervousness, tremor, irritability, hysteria, neuritis, convulsions, insomnia, euphoria, anorexia, nausea, vomiting, diarrhea, constipation, hypotension, tightness of chest and wheezing, urticaria, drug rash, anaphylactic shock, blurred vision, diplopia, vertigo, tinnitus, headache, palpitation, tachycardia, nasal stuffiness, urinary frequency, difficult urination, urinary retention, early menses, photosensitivity, hemolytic anemia, thrombocytopenia and agranulocytosis. For additional adverse reactions, see monograph on Pseudoephedrine.

Dosage and Administration: *Orally.* The usual dosage for adults is 4 to 8 mg 3 or 4 times daily. The extended-release dosage forms may be given in a dosage of 8 or 12 mg 2 or 3 times daily. Children over 6 years of age, 4 mg 3 or 4 times daily. The extended-release dosage form may be given in a dosage of 8 or 12 mg every 12 hours, or 1 or 2 teaspoonsful of elixir 3 or 4 times daily. Children under 6 years of age, 0.2 mg/lb of body weight/24 hours (equivalent to 1 teaspoonful of elixir/10 lb/24 hours). For infants, 0.5 to 1 mg 4 times daily. The combination product should not be given to children under 12 years of age. *Parenterally.* The physician is urged to study carefully the package literature for complete directions. Usually 5 to 20 mg twice daily should be adequate. Dosage should not exceed 40 mg/day. For *intravenous* administration, brompheniramine may be added to normal saline or 5% glucose or fresh whole blood, and injected slowly while the patient is in a recumbent position.

Availability:

Brompheniramine Maleate

DIMETANE®: **(Robins)**

Elixir, 2 mg/5 ml in pints and gallons.
Extentabs, 8 and 12 mg in bottles of 100 and 500.
Injectable (DIMETANE-10), 10 mg/ml in ampuls of 1 ml.
Tablets, 4 mg in bottles of 100 and 500.

Dexbrompheniramine Maleate w/Pseudoephedrine Sulfate

DISOPHROL®: **(Schering)**

Chronotab® *Tablets* (sustained-action), 6 mg with pseudoephedrine sulfate, 120 mg in bottles of 100.
Tablets (scored), 2 mg with pseudoephedrine sulfate, 60 mg in bottles of 100.
DRIXORAL® Tablets (sustained-action), 6 mg with pseudoephedrine sulfate, 120 mg in bottles of 100. **(Schering)**

BRONDECON

Description: Brondecon is a combination of oxtriphylline and guaifenesin, and is available in 2 dosage forms: tablets containing 200 mg of oxtriphylline and 100 mg of guaifenesin, and an elixir each 5-ml teaspoonful of which contains 100 mg of oxtriphylline and 50 mg of guaifenesin. Alcohol, 20%.

Oxtriphylline, the choline salt of theophylline, is a xanthine bronchodilating agent. Compared with aminophylline, oxtriphylline is less irritating to the gastric mucosa, better absorbed from the gastrointestinal tract, more stable and more soluble. Guaifenesin tends to increase the secretion and decrease the viscosity of fluids of the respiratory tract. These physiologic fluids help to lubricate the inflamed mucous membranes of the bronchi and also help the patient to expel viscid mucus thus making the cough more productive.

Indications: An adjunct in the management of bronchitis, bronchial asthma, asthmatic bronchitis, pulmonary emphysema and similar chronic obstructive lung disease. It is indicated when both relaxation of bronchospasm and expectorant action are desirable.

Precautions: Concurrent use of other xanthine preparations may lead to adverse reactions, particularly CNS stimulation in children.

Adverse Reactions: Gastric distress and, occasionally, palpitation and CNS stimulation have been reported.

Dosage and Administration: *Orally.* Dosage should be individualized according to the severity of the condition and the response of the patient. The usual dosage for patients over 12 years of age is 1 tablet or 2 teaspoonsful of elixir 4 times daily. Children from 2 to 12 years, 1 teaspoonful/60 lb of body weight 4 times daily.

Availability:

BRONDECON®: **(Warner-Chilcott)**

Elixir (dark red, cherry-flavored) in bottles of 240 ml and 1 pint.
Tablets (salmon-pink, uncoated) in bottles of 100.

BRONKEPHRINE

Description: Bronkephrine is designated generically as ethylnorepinephrine hydrochloride and chemically as α-(1-aminopropyl)-3,4-dihydroxybenzyl alcohol hydrochloride. Ethylnorepinephrine is a synthetic sympathomimetic amine, largely *beta*-active in effect. Its bronchodilating properties closely simulate those of epinephrine but without significant pressor effects. It may be safer than epinephrine for hypertensive patients and severely ill patients in whom such effects are undesirable. It is particularly adapted for use in children because of its lack of adverse effects, especially CNS excitation. It may also be of value in diabetic asthmatics due to its lack of glycogenolytic activity.

Indications: Relief of bronchospasm in bronchial asthma.

Contraindications: Idiosyncrasy to sympathomimetic drugs.

Precautions: Should be used with caution in patients with cardiovascular disease, a history of stroke or coronary artery disease. It is a potent drug and may cause toxic symptoms through idiosyncratic response or overdosage. As with all parenteral medications, care should be exercised in the anatomical selection of injection sites to avoid inadvertent intravascular or intraneural injection.

Adverse Reactions: The drug is generally well tolerated. It may, however, increase or decrease blood pressure, increase the pulse rate, and may produce palpitation, headache, dizziness or nausea.

Dosage and Administration: The usual dosage for adults is 0.5 to 1 ml *subcutaneously* or *intramuscularly*. Depending on severity of the asthmatic attack, smaller doses (0.3 to 0.5 ml) may suffice. Dosage in children varies according to age and weight; usually 0.1 to 0.5 ml is sufficient.

Availability:
BRONKEPHRINE® Injection, 2 mg/ml in ampuls of 1 ml in cartons of 5 and 25. **(Breon)**

BRONKOLIXIR
BRONKOTABS

Description: Each 5 ml of elixir or each tablet contains:

	Bronkolixir	*Bronkotabs*
Ephedrine sulfate	12 mg	24 mg
Guaifenesin	50 mg	100 mg
Theophylline	15 mg	100 mg
Phenobarbital	4 mg	8 mg

The Bronkotabs-Hafs contain the same ingredients as the Bronkotabs but in 1/2 the amount.

Indications: To prevent or relieve symptoms of bronchial asthma, asthmatic bronchitis, chronic bronchitis with emphysema, and emphysematous bronchospasm. Provides bronchodilatation, decongestion, promotes the removal of tenacious mucus, and aids in reducing local bronchial edema. Also serves as a mild sedative to allay anxiety and tension.

Warnings: Phenobarbital may be habit-forming. Epinephrine may cause urinary retention, especially in the presence of partial obstruction, as in prostatism.

Precautions: Frequent or prolonged use may cause nervousness, restlessness, or sleeplessness. Use with caution if hypertension, heart disease, diabetes, or hyperthyroidism is present. Since drowsiness may occur, patients should be cautioned to refrain from engaging in activities requiring alertness or skill.

Dosage and Administration: *Orally.* Adults, 2 teaspoonsful of elixir every 3 or 4 hours (4 times) daily, or 1 tablet every 3 or 4 hours daily. Children 6 years of age and over, 1/2 the adult dosage; under 6 years of age, as directed by the physician.

Availability:
BRONKOLIXIR® in bottles of 1 pint. **(Breon)**
BRONKOTABS® in bottles of 100 and 1000; (Bronkotabs-Hafs) in bottles of 50. **(Breon)**

BUCLIZINE HYDROCHLORIDE

Chemical Name: 1-(p-tert-Butylbenzyl)-4-(p-chloro-α-phenylbenzyl) piperazine hydrochloride.

Description: Buclizine is a tranquilizing agent with pharmacological actions similar to those of hydroxyzine to which it is closely related chemically. It possesses antiemetic and antihistaminic actions in addition to its CNS depressant effects. Doses in excess of the clinical therapeutic range induced fetal abnormalities in pregnant rats.

Indications: Management of nausea, vomiting, and dizziness associated with motion sickness or which may occur in a variety of conditions such as labyrinthitis and Meniere's syndrome.

Contraindications: Known hypersensitivity to the drug, and during early pregnancy.

Warnings: Since drowsiness may occur, especially during the early period of dosage adjustment, patients should be cautioned not to engage in activities requiring alertness or physical coordination. Safe and effective dosage in children has not been established.

Adverse Reactions: Generally, drowsiness, dryness of mouth, headache, and jitteriness may occasionally be encountered.

Dosage and Administration: *Orally.* Since the tablet melts in the mouth, it may be chewed or swallowed whole without water. Adults, usually 1 tablet is enough to prevent nausea in mild conditions. In severe cases, 3 tablets daily may be taken. The usual maintenance dosage is 1 tablet twice daily. In the prevention of motion sickness, 1 tablet at least ½ hour before beginning travel usually suffices. For extended travel, a second tablet may be taken 4 to 6 hours later.

Availability:
BUCLADIN™-S SOFTAB® Tablets, 50 mg in bottles of 100. **(Stuart)**

BUPIVACAINE HYDROCHLORIDE

Chemical Name: 1-Butyl-2′, 6′-pipecoloxylidide hydrochloride.

Description: Bupivacaine is a local anesthetic agent that is chemically and pharmacologically allied to the aminoacyl local anesthetics. It is a homologue of mepivacaine and is chemically related to lidocaine. All 3 of these anesthetics contain an amide linkage between the aromatic nucleus and the amino or piperidine group. They differ in this respect from the procaine-type local anesthetics which have an ester linkage. Bupivacaine occurs as a white, crystalline powder that is freely soluble in 95% alcohol, soluble in water, and slightly soluble in chloroform or acetone. Solutions of the anesthetic may be reautoclaved if they do **not** contain epinephrine.

Bupivacaine stabilizes the neuronal membrane and prevents initiation and transmission of nerve impulses, thereby effecting local anesthetic action. It has been reported that anesthesia is maintained 2 to 3 times longer with bupivacaine than with either lidocaine or mepivacaine, and approximately 20% longer than with tetracaine. Following administration for caudal, epidural, or peripheral nerve block in patients, the onset of action is rapid and peak levels are attained within 30 to 45 minutes. The effect may last for a few hours followed by a decline to insignificant levels within 3 to 6 hours. The addition of epinephrine (1:200,000) may prolong the action. Because of its amide structure, the drug is not hydrolyzed by plasma esterases into inactive compounds. It has been noted that when bupivacaine is administered in the recommended dose and concentration, irritation or tissue damage rarely occurs nor does it cause methemoglobinemia.

Studies with various animals showed that bupivacaine produced no significant pathologic changes, except for dose-related inflammatory reactions in the muscle tissue at the injection site; also, no immediate or delayed allergic responses, and no evidence of drug-induced teratogenic effects. Subcutaneous doses appeared to be rapidly absorbed and transported to various organs. The drug appears in the urine conjugated with glucuronic acid.

Indications: Bupivacaine is indicated to produce local anesthesia by infiltration injection, peripheral nerve block, sympathetic, caudal or epidural block.

Contraindications: Known hypersensitivity to the amide group of local anesthetics or to methylparaben which is added to the multiple-dose vial. Although not particularly contraindicated, bupivacaine is not recommended for use in children under 12 years of age.

Warnings: Resuscitative equipment and drugs should be readily available when a local anesthetic agent is used. Safe use in pregnant women, other than those in labor, has not been established. In obstetrics, if vasopressor drugs are used during caudal analgesia, either to correct hypotension or to add to the local anesthetic solution, the obstetrician should be cautioned that if an oxytocic drug is also employed, severe persistent hypertension may occur. Solutions containing a vasoconstrictor, particularly epinephrine or norepinephrine, should be used with considerable caution in patients receiving MAO inhibitors or antidepressants of the triptyline or imipramine types, in order to avoid precipitating a severe, prolonged hypertensive state.

Precautions: The usual precautions observed with all local anesthetics also apply to bupivacaine. Systemic absorption from the tissues may be minimized by giving the lowest dosage possible to achieve effective anesthesia, and the actual amount to be administered should be determined in advance. Tolerance varies with the status of the patient; debilitated, elderly patients and acutely ill patients should be given reduced doses commensurate with age and physical condition. Local anesthetics containing epinephrine or other vasoconstrictors should be used with extreme care in areas with limited blood supply, in the presence of diseases that may adversely affect the patient's cardiovascular system, or in patients with peripheral vascular problems, and also should not be used during or following the administration of chloroform, halothane, cyclopropane, trichlorethylene, or other related agents, since such concomitant use may produce serious cardiac arrhythmias. Caution is advised in the administration of additional doses to patients with severe liver disease. Fetal bradycardia and depression at birth and perinatal death have been associated with the use of amide-type local anesthetics; therefore, until further clinical experience is gained, paracervical block with this anesthetic is not recommended. Added risk appears to be present in prematurity, toxemia of pregnancy, and fetal distress.

Adverse Reactions: Toxic reactions are usually due to high plasma levels resulting from excessive dosage, inadvertent intravascular injection, slow metabolic degradation, or may result from hypersensitivity, idiosyncrasy, or diminished tolerance on the part of the patient. Such reactions are systemic in nature and involve the CNS and/or the cardiovascular system. The CNS reactions are characterized by excitation or depression or both. The first manifestation may be nervousness, dizziness, blurred vision, or tremors, followed by drowsiness, convulsions, unconsciousness, and possibly respiratory arrest. The excitatory reactions may be very brief or may not occur at all, in which case the first manifestations of toxicity may be drowsiness, sometimes merging into unconsciousness and respiratory arrest. Other CNS reactions may be nausea, vomiting, chills, constriction of the pupils, or tinnitus. Cardiovascular manifestations may include depression of the myocardium, blood pressure changes (usually hypotension), and cardiac arrest. Allergic reactions characterized by cutaneous lesions, urticaria, and edema have been reported. The detection of sensitivity by skin testing is of doubtful value. Reactions following epidural or caudal anesthesia also may include high or total spinal block; urinary retention, fecal incontinence; loss of perineal sensation and sexual function; persistent analgesia, paresthesia, and paralysis of the lower extremities; headache and backache; and slowing of labor and increased incidence of forceps delivery. If a reaction does occur, prompt action should be taken and the institution of the necessary means to reverse respiratory depression, combat convulsions and to counteract hypotension should be employed.

Dosage and Administration: *Parenterally.* The lowest dosage needed to provide effective anesthesia should be administered. In recommended doses, bupivacaine produces complete sensory blockade, but the effect on motor function differs among the 3 concentrations. For caudal, epidural or peripheral nerve block the 0.25 and 0.5% solutions are used in operations in which complete muscle relaxation is not essential or when other means of providing muscle relaxation is used concurrently. They also do not provide complete motor blockade. The

0.75% solution produces complete motor blockade and is most useful in abdominal operations requiring complete muscle relaxation. With continuous (intermittent) techniques, repeat doses will increase the degree of motor blockade, but in most situations a single dose is usually sufficient. When bupivacaine is employed with epinephrine (1:200,000) a single dose of up to 225 mg may be used and when used alone up to 175 mg is usually sufficient. These doses may be repeated every 3 hours. A total daily dose of 400 mg may be given but this dose should not be exceeded within a 24-hour period.

Availability:
MARCAINE®: **(Breon)**
with or without epinephrine bitartrate (1:200,000)
Solution, 0.25% in single-dose ampuls and in multiple-dose vials of 50 ml; 0.5% in single-dose ampuls of 30 ml and in multiple-dose vials of 50 ml; 0.75% in single-dose ampuls of 30 ml.

BUSULFAN

Chemical Name: 1,4-Butanediol dimethanesulfonate.

Description: Busulfan is classified as a "polyfunctional alkylating agent." The basic reaction of the alkylating agents is the replacement of the hydrogen in a reacting chemical with an alkyl group. Despite its poor solubility, busulfan is adequately absorbed from the gastrointestinal tract.

The rather selective action of busulfan on myeloid elements led to the use of the drug in patients with chronic granulocytic leukemia. At low doses it selectively depresses granulocytopoiesis. As the dosage is raised, platelets and erythroid elements may be eliminated and eventually a pancytopenia results. Cytotoxic action does not appear to extend to either the lymphoid tissues or the gastrointestinal epithelium. Busulfan enters the fetal circulation via the placenta.

The most favorable effects in cases of chronic myelocytic leukemia are a rise in the hemoglobin level, a decrease in leukocyte count, a selective reduction or even disappearance of immature myeloid cells from the blood, normalization of the bone marrow cellularity, a diminution in the size of the enlarged spleen, and pronounced subjective improvement. This reduction in morbidity is frequently associated with a prolonged survival. The drug is of no value in chronic lymphocytic leukemia, acute leukemia or in the "blastic crisis" of chronic granulocytic leukemia.

Busulfan given to rats in the diet in an amount equivalent to about 0.5 mg/kg of final body weight/day slowed weight gain and produced bone marrow depression, pancytopenia and cataracts after about 10 weeks. In rats, the estimated litter LD-50 for busulfan given intraperitoneally was found to be 34 mg/kg. A single intraperitoneal injection of 10 to 15 mg/kg of busulfan in oil to pregnant rats was definitely teratogenic. When the drug was administered on day 13, 14 or 15 of gestation in a dose of 10 mg/kg, the progeny were permanently sterile.

Indications: In therapeutic doses, for the control of symptoms of chronic myelocytic leukemia. It is not a cure, but life expectancy may be prolonged. The drug has been found useful in patients who no longer respond to radiation therapy or to previously used chemotherapeutic agents. However, patients untreated by any other means also usually respond well initially. In appropriate doses, the drug depresses myelopoiesis, but has little effect on the lymphocytes.

Contraindications: Busulfan should not be given to patients who have received other similar chemotherapeutic agents or radiation therapy in the recent past, or if the neutrophil or platelet counts are depressed.

Warnings: If possible, the use of busulfan in pregnant women should be deferred until after the first trimester. The benefits of the use of this drug later in pregnancy should be weighed against the considered risks. Safe use during lactation has not been established.

Precautions: *Because busulfan is a potent cytotoxic drug,* its use should be restricted to patients who are situated where facilities are available for *complete blood counts at weekly, or more frequent, intervals* and for other laboratory studies which may be deemed necessary. The most careful clinical and hematological supervision is essential for early detection and prompt management of toxic effects.

Adverse Reactions: The chief toxic effect is a dosage-related myelosuppression which may cause thrombocytopenia (hemorrhage) and eventually lead to pancytopenia. Rapid destruction of granulocytes may be accompanied by hyperuricemia and uric acid nephropathy. This complication may now be avoided by using allopurinol. Other complications of therapy include nausea, vomiting, diarrhea, cheilosis, glossitis, impotence, sterility, amenorrhea, gynecomastia, generalized skin pigmentation, anhidrosis, alopecia and interstitial pulmonary fibrosis. The melanoderma accompanied at times with digestive troubles, fatigue, muscular weakness and weight loss may simulate adrenocortical insufficiency.

Dosage and Administration: *Orally.* Usual dosage is 4 to 8 mg daily depending upon the total leukocyte count and the severity of the disease. Therapy is continued until the leukocyte count falls below 10,000/cu mm. During remission the patient is examined at monthly intervals and treatment is resumed when the leukocyte count reaches 50,000/cu mm. When remission is shorter than 3 months, maintenance therapy of 1 to 3 mg daily may be advisable in order to keep the hematological status under control and to prevent a rapid relapse. *Careful individual control is very important.*

Availability:
MYLERAN® Tablets, 2 mg (scored) in bottles of 25. **(Burroughs Wellcome)**

BUTABARBITAL SODIUM Ⓒ III

Chemical Name: 5-*sec*-Butyl-5-ethylbarbiturate sodium.

Description: Butabarbital sodium is classified as an intermediate-acting barbiturate. It occurs as a bitter, white powder freely soluble in water and in alcohol. Aqueous solutions are unstable, but stable solutions may be prepared with propylene glycol.

Average oral doses of 15 to 30 mg produce a mild sedative effect within 30 minutes that persists for about 5 to 6 hours. Larger doses have been useful as a hypnotic for bedtime use, or as a preoperative sedative.

Indications: Sedative and hypnotic.

Contraindications: In patients with known hypersensitivity or idiosyncrasy to barbiturates, in those with a history of manifest or latent porphyria or marked impairment of liver function, or with respiratory disease where dyspnea or obstruction is evident. It is also contraindicated in patients known to be addiction-prone. Barbiturates should not be administered in the presence of uncontrolled pain because a paradoxical excitement may be manifested. Butabarbital, however, is not contraindicated in the presence of kidney disease.

Warnings: May be habit-forming.

Precautions: Since the drug is probably detoxified in the liver, it should be used with caution in the presence of moderate to severe hepatic disease. Evidence has been produced that barbiturates stimulate hepatic microsomal enzymes and therefore may increase the metabolism of some drugs, including the coumarin anticoagulants. Also, since the systemic effects of exogenous or endogenous hydrocortisone may be diminished, the drug should be administered with special care to patients with borderline hypoadrenal function, whether of pituitary or primary adrenal origin. Patients should be cautioned about the combined effects of alcohol and other CNS depressant drugs. Susceptible individuals may develop a psychological dependence on butabarbital, and may subsequently increase the dosage beyond that prescribed by the physician. In such cases, an abrupt discontinuance of this drug may precipitate typical withdrawal symptoms, including convulsions. Therefore, the drug should be withdrawn gradually from any patient known to be taking excessive dosages for prolonged periods. As with other sedatives and hypnotics, elderly or debilitated patients may react to barbiturates with marked excitement or depression. Particular care is advised in patients with elevated intraocular pressure, prostatic hypertrophy, severe anemia, congestive heart failure, fever, neuroses, hyperthyroidism, diabetes mellitus, or any condition in which respiratory depression may be characteristic. Barbiturates readily cross the placental barrier; also small amounts have been found in the milk of nursing mothers.

Adverse Reactions: Those occurring usually include slight hangover, drowsiness, lethargy, headache, skin eruptions, nausea and vomiting. Drowsiness at daytime sedative dose levels rarely occurs. However, should drowsiness occur, the patient should be cautioned not to engage in activities requiring alertness and skill such as driving a motor vehicle or operating machinery. Hypersensitivity reactions may occur, especially in those individuals with asthma, urticaria, angioneurotic edema, or similar conditions. Manifestations of overdosage are usually extensions of the pharmacologic effects of the drug, primarily CNS depression. Treatment should be initiated by gastric lavage or inducing emesis, followed by maintenance of an open airway. Fluid therapy should be instituted to counteract shock and if renal failure occurs or if the patient does not respond to treatment, extracorporeal hemodialysis or peritoneal dialysis should be carried out.

Dosage and Administration: *Orally.* As a daytime sedative: adults, 15 to 30 mg 3 or 4 times daily. Children, 7.5 to 30 mg daily, depending upon age, weight and the degree of sedation desired. As a hypnotic: adults, 50 to 100 mg. Children, dose to be determined by the physician according to age and weight.

Availability:
C-III BUTISOL SODIUM®: **(McNeil)**
Capsules (BUTICAPS®): 15 mg (lavender and white), 30 mg (green and white), 50 mg (orange and white) and 100 mg (pink and white) in bottles of 100.
Elixir, 30 mg/5 ml (green) in pints and gallons. Alcohol, 7%.
Tablets: 15 mg (lavender, scored) and 30 mg (green, scored) in bottles of 100, 1000, 5000; 50 mg (orange, scored) and 100 mg (pink, scored) in bottles of 100 and 1000.

BUTAPERAZINE MALEATE: see The Phenothiazines

BUTIGETIC

Description: Each tablet contains:

Acetaminophen	200 mg
Phenacetin	150 mg
Caffeine, anhydrous	30 mg
Sodium butabarbital	15 mg

Indications: Specifically for the relief of tension headache caused by anxiety or sustained muscular tension. Also useful in other painful conditions such as dysmenorrhea, premenstrual tension, arthritic and rheumatic conditions involving musculoskeletal pain, myalgia, neuralgia, postoperative pain, dental pain, pain accompanying upper respiratory infections and otitis media.

Contraindications: In patients with known hypersensitivity or idiosyncrasy to any of the components. Barbiturates are contraindicated in patients with a history of manifest or latent porphyria or marked impairment of liver function, or in those with respiratory disease where dyspnea or obstruction is evident. They are also contraindicated in patients who are known to be addiction-prone.

Warnings: Sodium butabarbital may be habit-forming.

Precautions: Since sodium butabarbital is probably detoxified in the liver, it should be used with caution in patients with moderate to severe hepatic disease. Evidence has been produced that barbiturates stimulate hepatic microsomal enzymes and therefore may increase the metabolism of some drugs, including the coumarin anticoagulants. Also, susceptible individuals may develop a psychological dependence on butabarbital. Elderly or debilitated patients may react to barbiturates, as they do with other sedatives and hypnotics, with marked excitement or depression. Since phenacetin in large amounts may be harmful to the kidneys, dosage recommendation should not be exceeded. Also, large doses of phenacetin may cause methemoglobinemia; however, this is rarely clinically significant when used in therapeutic amounts for a limited time.

Adverse Reactions: This product seldom produces untoward reactions. Side effects have been rare with sodium butabarbital; drowsiness at a dosage level of 15 to 30 mg occurs rarely. Skin rashes, "hangover," and systemic disturbances often accompanying tranquilizer therapy are seldom seen. Rarely has acetaminophen produced any side effects such as gastric discomfort; it is usually well tolerated by patients sensitive to aspirin.

Dosage and Administration: *Orally.* The usual dosage for adults is 2 tablets 3 or 4 times daily.

Availability:
BUTIGETIC® Tablets in bottles of 100 and 1000. **(McNeil)**

BUTORPHANOL TARTRATE

Chemical Name: Levo-N-Cyclobutylmethyl-6-10$\alpha\beta$-dihydroxy-1,2,3,9,10,10a-hexahydro-(4H)-10,4a-Iminoethanophenanthrone.

Description: Butorphanol, a nonopiate, synthetic analgesic with narcotic agonist-antagonist capability, is a member of the phenanthrene group of compounds. Duration of analgesic activity (3 to 4 hours) is approximately equivalent to that of morphine, and its antinarcotic activity virtually corresponds to that of nalorphine, is 30 times that of pentazocine and 1/40 that of naloxone as measured by the antagonism of morphine analgesic in the rattail Flick test. Moreover, in equipotent doses of 2 mg of butorphanol or 10 mg of morphine, both drugs produce about the same degree of respiratory depression. However, the magnitude of butorphanol-induced respiratory depression, unlike that of morphine, does not appreciably increase with higher doses, but duration corresponds to the amount administered and is apparently dose-related. Any respiratory depression that may occur is reversible by naloxone which is a specific antagonist. It occurs as a white, crystalline substance that is very soluble in aqueous solutions; molecular weight has been found to be 477.56.

The specific mechanism by which the drug exerts its effect is not known, but it is felt that the antinarcotic analgesics exert their analgesic effect by means of a CNS mechanism. Currently, it is believed that the site of action is subcortical, probably focusing their pharmacologic activity on the limbic system. Analgesic effect appears in less than 30 minutes following intramuscular injection, attaining maximum in about 1 hour. The effect occurs very rapidly following intravenous administration, reaching peak limits within 30 minutes. The intravenous administration of butorphanol produces the same hemodynamic changes as those reported for pentazocine. These changes include increased pulmonary artery and wedge pressure, left ventricular end-diastolic pressure, systemic arterial pressure, and pulmonary vascular resistance. Although not as pronounced as those following pentazocine administration, they nevertheless increase the work of the heart, especially in the pulmonary circuit.

Results of reproduction studies in rats, mice, and rabbits have revealed no evidence of impaired fertility or harm to the fetus.

Indications: Relief of moderate to severe pain.

Contraindications: Known hypersensitivity to the drug.

Warnings: Butorphanol is not recommended for patients who are physically dependent on narcotics, and should be used with special care in those who have recently received substantial amounts of such medication. Detoxification of these patients prior to its use is advised. Emotionally unstable individuals, and those with a history of or a tendency to drug misuse should be closely supervised, particularly if long-term therapy is being considered. It is important that the dose and frequency of administration not be increased, and that the drug be used only for the relief of pain rather than in anticipation of pain. Butorphanol, like other potent analgesics, may increase cerebrospinal fluid pressure, thereby producing effects which may obscure the clinical course of patients with head injury. In such patients, it must be used with extreme caution and only if its use is deemed essential. Use in patients with acute myocardial infarction, ventricular dysfunction or coronary insufficiency should be limited to those who are hypersensitive to morphine or meperidine.

Precautions: Special care and low dosage are advised in patients with respiratory depression, severely limited respiratory reserve, bronchial asthma, obstructive respiratory conditions, or cyanosis, and in those with renal or hepatic dysfunction. Safe use prior to bilary tract surgery, during pregnancy, labor or parturition has not been established. The drug is not recommended for use in nursing mothers or in children under 18 years of age.

Adverse Reactions: The most frequently reported complaints were sedation, nausea, and diaphoresis. Less frequently reported were headache, vertigo, floating feeling, dizziness, lethargy, confusion, and lightheadedness. Rarely reported were nervousness, unusual dreams, agitation, euphoria, hallucinations; flushing of the skin and a feeling of warmth, dry mouth, and sensitivity to cold; palpitations, and increase or decrease in blood pressure; vomiting; slowing of respiration, and shallow breathing; skin rash or hives; diplopia or blurred vision. Overdosage may produce some degree of respiratory depression and variable cardiovascular and CNS effects. The immediate treatment of suspected overdosage is intravenous naloxone. The respiratory and cardiovascular status of the patients should be evaluated and appropriate supportive measures instituted, such as oxygen, intravenous fluids, vasopressors, and assisted or controlled respiration.

Dosage and Administration: *Intramuscularly* or *intravenously*. The usual recommended *intramuscular* dose is 2 mg, but may range from 1 to 4 mg. Clinical experience with single doses of more than 4 mg is limited. The usual recommended *intravenous* dose is 1 mg, but may range from 0.5 to 2 mg. Doses may be repeated every 3 to 4 hours if necessary.

Availability:
STADOL® Injection, 1 mg/ml (equiv. to 0.68 mg base) in vials of 1 ml; 2 mg/ml in vials of 1, 2 and 10 ml. **(Bristol)**

CAFFEINE AND SODIUM BENZOATE

Description: Caffeine and sodium benzoate is a mixture of approximately 50% each of anhydrous caffeine and anhydrous sodium benzoate. It occurs as a white, odorless powder, having a slightly bitter taste, is freely soluble in water, sparingly soluble in alcohol and slightly soluble in chloroform. A portion of the caffeine usually separates on standing.

The mixture is similar to caffeine itself in its physiologic effects and therapeutic use in that it is a potent stimulant of the CNS.

Indications: Because of its stimulating effect on the CNS, the drug is useful as a respiratory stimulant, particularly in the nonspecific treatment of respiratory depression due to poisoning from morphine or alcohol. It has also been used to stimulate respiration in cases of electric shock and to relieve the headache caused by spinal puncture.

Warnings: Caffeine and sodium benzoate injection should be administered slowly using a small-gauge needle.

Precautions: Too-vigorous treatment with the drug can produce further depression in the already depressed patient; therefore, a single dose should not exceed 1 gm. Care must be exercised in the intravenous administration of this drug in patients with myocardial damage.

Adverse Reactions: Side effects produced by caffeine include nausea, insomnia, restlessness, excitement, tinnitus, scintillating scotoma, muscular tremor, tachycardia, extrasystoles and diuresis. Short-acting barbiturates, such as pentobarbital sodium, may be used to counteract these effects on the CNS.

Dosage and Administration: *Parenterally*. For CNS stimulation, the usual dosage is 500 mg in 2 ml of solution, administered *intramuscularly* as necessary. It may be given *intravenously* in emergency situations of respiratory failure.

Availability:
CAFFEINE AND SODIUM BENZOATE Injection, 500 mg in ampuls of 2 ml. **(Lilly)**

CALCIDRINE Ⓒ

Description: Each 5 ml (teaspoonful) contains codeine, 8.4 mg; calcium iodide (anhydrous), 152 mg and alcohol, 6% in a palatable, aromatic syrup.

Indications: Symptomatic relief of coughs due to colds, bronchitis or allergy.

Contraindications: Prolonged use is contraindicated during pregnancy since iodides readily cross the placenta and may produce goiter with hypothyroidism and resultant acute respiratory distress in the newborn. Also contraindicated in patients with known hypersensitivity to iodides or to any of the components.

Warnings: Codeine may be habit-forming.

Precautions: Routine precautions should be followed in patients with hypertension, heart disease, diabetes, or thyroid disease, and in those with marked sensitivity to any of the components. Symptoms of hypothyroidism and iodism can occur with long-term administration. When cough persists or accompanies a high fever, the underlying cause and the need for other medication should be reevaluated.

Adverse Reactions: Those that may occur consist of nausea, vomiting, constipation, and iodism generally manifested by metallic taste, acneform skin lesions, irritation of mucous membrane, swelling of salivary glands, and gastric distress. These complications promptly subside upon discontinuation of the drug. Prolonged use of iodides may lead to severe and sometimes fatal skin eruptions (ioderma) although this phenomenon occurs rarely.

Dosage and Administration: *Orally.* The usual dosage for adults and children over 10 years of age is 1 to 2 teaspoonsful every 4 hours, for children 6 to 10 years of age, 1 teaspoonful every 4 hours and for children 2 to 6 years of age, ½ teaspoonful every 4 hours.

Availability:
Ⓒ CALCIDRINE® Syrup in bottles of 120 ml and in pints and gallons. **(Abbott)**

CALCITONIN (SALMON)

Description: Calcitonin is a hormonal agent that controls blood calcium and bone metabolism by directly inhibiting osteoclastic bone resorption thus reducing the concentration of calcium in the serum. Its primary therapeutic application is in the treatment of Paget's disease of the bone; however, the precise biochemical mechanism involved is not completely understood. The drug is a synthetic polypeptide of 32 amino acids structured in the same linear sequence that is found in calcitonin of salmon origin. Activity is stated in MRC (Medical Research Council) units.

Following a single injection, a marked decrease in the rate of bone resorption occurs, but with prolonged use of the drug there is a persistent, smaller decrease in this rate. It apparently is due to a decrease not only in the number of osteoclasts but also in their resorptive capacity. Decreased osteocytic resorption may also be involved. There is some evidence that bone formation may be augmented by calcitonin through increased osteoblastic activity.

The effectiveness of the drug has been demonstrated principally in patients with moderate to severe Paget's disease. Approximately ⅔ of the patients show a decreased rate of bone turnover with a resultant fall in serum alkaline phosphatase and in the excretion of urinary hydroxyproline. These biochemical changes appear to correspond to changes toward more normal bone as evidenced by radiologic regression of pagetic lesions. Well-documented instances of reversal of neurologic impairment have occurred, including improvement in hearing and other neurologic functions; and also decreases in abnormally elevated cardiac output due to extensive Paget's disease. At present, clinical experiences are not adequate to predict the likelihood of improvement of any given neurologic lesion, although hearing loss appears to improve in 5% of the patients.

Initially, some patients experience a good response to calcitonin but later relapse to the pretreatment state. It has been suggested that the loss of therapeutic effects may be due to the formation of neutralizing antibodies to the drug or to the development of secondary hyperparathyroidism, or to some other cause. Although the parathyroid hormone levels do appear to rise transiently during each hypocalcemic response to this hormone, most investigators have been unable to demonstrate persistent hypersecretion of parathyroid hormone in patients treated for prolonged periods. After 2 to 18 months of therapy, circulating antibodies have been reported in about ½ of the patients, but in many cases treatment remained effective. Patients producing high antibody titers usually become drug-resistant and will relapse.

Calcitonin is rapidly metabolized in the kidney to inactive metabolites; little urinary excretion of intact drug is believed to occur.

Indications: Treatment of symptomatic Paget's disease of the bone.

Contraindications: Hypersensitivity to the drug or to its gelatin diluent.

Warnings: Safe use of calcitonin during pregnancy has not been established. Studies with two species of pregnant animals have revealed decreases in fetal birth weight. Therefore, the use of this drug in women who are or who may become pregnant requires that the potential benefit be weighed against the possible risk to the fetus.

Precautions: Because of the protein nature of calcitonin and its gelatin diluent, the possible occurrence of a systemic allergic reaction should be kept in mind. Skin testing should be considered prior to treatment of patients suspected of being sensitive to these two proteins. Hypocalcemic tetany under special circumstances may occur although no cases have, as yet, been reported. Nevertheless, provisions for parenteral calcium administration should be available during the first several administrations of this drug. Patients on prolonged therapy should be periodically examined for any abnormalities of urine sediment. Until further clinical experience has been gained, the use of this drug in pediatric patients should be limited to investigational purposes only.

Adverse Reactions: Nausea with or without vomiting has been noted in about 10% of the patients. It is most evident when treatment is first initiated and tends to decrease or disappear with continued administration. Local inflammatory reactions at the site of subcutaneous or intramuscular injection have also been noted in about 10% of the patients. Facial flushing occurred in about 2% of the patients.

Dosage and Administration: *Intramuscularly* or *subcutaneously*. The recommended initial dose is 100 MRC units daily. Some patients may be maintained on 50 MRC units daily or every other day. When self-administered by the patient, subcutaneous injection is the preferred method. In patients who relapse, a dosage of more than 100 MRC units daily does not usually appear to evoke an improved response. Drug effect should be monitored by periodic measurement of serum alkaline phosphatase and 24-hour urinary hydroxyproline (if available) and evaluation of symptoms. If a decrease toward normal of the biochemical abnormalities occurs, it is usually seen within the first few months. Bone pain may also decrease during this period. Improvement of neurologic lesions often requires more than 1 year of treatment. **Important Note:** When reconstituted, the solution should be used within 1 week and should be stored in the refrigerator when not in use.

Availability:
CALCIMAR® Powder (lyophilized) in vials of 400 MRC units with a vial of 20 mg of hydrolyzed gelatin. **(Armour)**

CALCITRIOL

Chemical Name: 9,10-Seco(5Z,7E)-5,7,10(19)-cholestatriene-1α,3β-triol.

Description: Calcitriol is the *synthetic* form of the natural, metabolically active hormone of vitamin D-3. It has been found to be particularly useful in the management of hypocalcemia in patients undergoing chronic renal dialysis. It occurs as a colorless, crystalline substance that is relatively insoluble in water and soluble in organic solvents.

It is now known that vitamin D-3 must be metabolically activated in the liver and kidney before it can be fully active on its target tissues. When ingested, it is enzymatically metabolized in the liver to 25-hydroxy-vitamin D-3, a compound that is subsequently hydroxylated in the kidney to calcitriol, the active form of vitamin D-3. Patients without kidneys or with nonfunctional kidneys are therefore unable to achieve this final step.

The two known sites of action of calcitriol are the intestine and bone, but additional evidence suggests that it also acts on the kidney and the parathyroid gland. It is the most active form of vitamin D-3 in stimulating intestinal calcium transport. Studies with acutely uremic rats have shown that the drug stimulates the intestinal absorption of calcium. Consequently, it has been suggested that since a vitamin D-resistant state exists in patients with uremia, it is probably because the kidney cannot adequately convert the precursors to calcitriol.

Following oral administration of a radioactive, titrated dose, the drug was found to be rapidly absorbed from the intestine, to reach peak levels in the serum after 4 hours, and to remain pharmacologically active for 3 to 5 days. Evidence is available that vitamin D metabolites are transported in the blood bound to specific plasma proteins.

Additional studies will be necessary to determine a potential carcinogenic, mutagenic, or antifertility activity since the drug has been found to be teratogenic in rabbits given doses 4 to 15 times that recommended for clinical use.

Indications: Management of hypocalcemia in patients undergoing chronic renal dialysis. In studies to date, it has been shown to reduce elevated parathyroid hormone levels in some of these patients.

Contraindications: Calcitriol should not be given to patients with hypercalcemia or with evidence of vitamin D toxicity.

Warnings: It has been suggested that vitamin D and its derivatives be withheld during treatment, and to avoid concomitant use of calcitriol with magnesium-containing antacids because such use may lead to the development of hypermagnesemia. It is advised to use aluminum carbonate or hydroxide gel in order to control serum phosphate levels in patients undergoing dialysis. Progressive hypercalcemia due to overdosage of vitamin D and its derivatives may be so severe as to require emergency attention, and it should be kept in mind that chronic hypercalcemia can lead to generalized vascular calcification, nephrocalcinosis and other soft tissue calcification. The serum calcium times phosphate (Ca x P) product should not be allowed to exceed 70. Radiographic evaluation of suspect anatomical regions may be useful in the early detection of this condition.

Precautions: Since excessive dosage of the drug may induce hypercalcemia and in some instances hypercalciuria, serum calcium levels should be determined twice weekly, particularly during the initial phase of dosage adjustment. A fall in serum alkaline phosphatase usually precedes the appearance of high calcium blood levels and may therefore be an indication of impending hypercalcemia. Should this condition develop, therapy must be discontinued immediately. The drug should be given cautiously to patients taking digitalis because elevated serum calcium in such patients may precipitate cardiac arrhythmias. The patient and the parents or spouse should be informed about compliance with dosage instructions, adherence to instructions regarding diet and calcium supplementation and avoidance of the use of unapproved nonprescription drugs. Patients should also be informed about the symptoms of hypercalcemia. Serum calcium, phosphorus, magnesium and alkaline phosphatase and 24-hour urinary calcium and phosphorus levels should be determined periodically. Simultaneous use with cholestyramine may impair intestinal absorption of calcitriol. Safe use in pregnant and lactating women has not been established; nursing should not be attempted while the patient is taking the drug. Until safe and effective use and proper dosage have been determined, the drug is not recommended for use in children.

Adverse Reactions: Since calcitriol is believed to be the active hormone which exerts vitamin D activity in the body, complications are generally similar to those encountered with excessive vitamin D intake. The early signs and symptoms of hypercalcemia include weakness, headache, somnolence, nausea, vomiting, dry mouth, constipation, muscle pain, bone pain, and metallic taste. These may later be followed by polyuria, polydipsia, anorexia, weight loss, nocturia, conjunctivitis (calcific), pancreatitis, photophobia, rhinorrhea, pruritus, hyperthermia, decreased libido, elevated BUN, albuminuria, hypercholesterolemia, elevated SGOT and SGPT, ectopic calcification, hypertension, cardiac arrhythmias, and rarely, overt psychosis. Overdosage may cause hypercalcemia, hypercalciuria, and hyperphosphatemia. In the event of hypercalcemia, the drug and all calcium supplements should be withdrawn and the patient placed on a low calcium diet. When serum calcium levels have returned to within normal limits, the drug may be reintroduced at a reduction of 0.25 mcg/day of the previous dose.

Dosage and Administration: *Orally.* The recommended initial dose is 0.25 mcg daily; may be increased in increments of 0.25 mcg/day at intervals of 2 to 4 weeks until the desired response is achieved. Therapy should be supplemented with an adequate daily intake of calcium.

Availability:
ROCALTROL® Capsules, 0.25 mcg (light orange) in bottles of 30 and 100. **(Roche)**

CALCIUM DISODIUM EDETATE

Chemical Name: Calcium disodium ethylenediaminetetraacetate.

Description: Calcium disodium edetate, the calcium chelate of disodium edetate, is a mixture of the dihydrate and trihydrate of calcium (ethylenedinitrilo) tetraacetate and occurs as a white, crystalline powder or as granules freely soluble in water.

Edetate combines with metallic ions that have a greater affinity for it than has calcium to form stable, nonionized, water-soluble complexes or chelates that are readily eliminated unchanged in the urine within about 6 hours following intravenous administration. Its value in the treatment of lead poisoning is due primarily to the ability of lead to displace calcium from the chelate. It appears to be less effective in combining with nonionized organic lead compounds such as tetraethyl lead. Acting as a chelating agent, this compound can dissolve readily such ordinarily insoluble salts as calcium oxalate, barium sulfate and lead phosphate in the neutral and alkaline pH ranges. This "solubilizing" property accounts for the value of the agent as a means for mobilizing heavy metals from the body. Only 5 to 10% of an oral dose is absorbed from the gastrointestinal tract. With the increased excretion of lead in the urine there is a concomitant decrease in blood lead levels and in urine coproporphyrin.

Indications: *Parenterally,* it may be used to reduce blood and depot lead in acute or chronic lead poisoning, lead encephalopathy, and prophylactically against symptomatic exacerbations in chronic lead poisoning; also worthy of trial in poisoning by other heavy metals; and it has potential value in the removal of radioactive and nuclear fission products such as plutonium and yttrium, etc. *Orally,* it is used as a follow-up to parenteral therapy and to increase the excretion of lead in asymptomatic patients who present laboratory evidence of lead accumulation. It is *not* recommended for use in acute lead poisoning. Its effectiveness by the oral route has not been established, and there may be potentially harmful effects from oral administration in the acute stages. The drug should be used intravenously in acute lead poisoning when the patient is symptomatic.

Contraindications: Severe renal disease. It should be used with caution in tuberculosis—active or healed—and in the presence of renal disease. The drug should not be given orally if lead may be present in the gastrointestinal tract and the patient has signs or symptoms of lead poisoning.

Warnings: Overdosage of calcium disodium edetate is capable of producing toxic and potentially fatal effects. The dosage schedule should be followed; at no time should the recommended daily dosage be exceeded. The customary precautions should be exercised when intended for use in pregnant patients.

Precautions: Occasionally, acute renal tubular necrosis may result from very large doses of this drug, and fatalities, although rare, have been reported. It is suggested that routine urinalysis be done daily during each course of therapy. The presence of large renal epithelial cells, and increasing numbers of red blood cells in the urinary sediment or increased proteinuria calls for immediate discontinuation of therapy. Evidence of renal impairment should be looked for by periodic measurement of BUN, serum creatinine, and phosphorus levels. The patient should also be monitored for irregularities of cardiac rhythm.

Adverse Reactions: Administered orally, the drug may act as a mild gastrointestinal irritant in some individuals, resulting in diarrhea, abdominal cramps and vomiting. Other side effects reported in a relatively small percentage of patients were leg and other muscle cramps, weakness, malaise, and albumin or red cells in the urine. These are not considered serious if detected early. Excessive doses may result in renal toxicity.

Dosage and Administration: The drug is most effective when administered *intravenously*. The usual method of administration is as follows: The contents of a 5-ml ampul is diluted with 250 to 500 ml of normal saline solution or sterile 5% dextrose solution suitable for intravenous injection. This diluted solution is administered by intravenous drip over a period of 1 hour; such doses may be given twice daily for periods up to 5 days. Therapy should then be interrupted for 2 days, and followed by an additional 5 days of therapy, if indicated. For children, the dosage should not exceed 0.5 gm/30 lb of body weight, given twice daily (total, 1 gm/30 lb/day). This is equivalent to 35 mg/kg twice daily. In mild cases, a dose of 50 mg/kg/day should not be exceeded. For young children, the total daily dose may be given in divided doses every 8 to 12 hours for 3 to 5 days. A second course may be given after a drug-free period of 4 or more days. The **intramuscular route** is advised for children since extravasation at the intravenous injection site presents a special hazard. Clinical experience to date does not suggest that larger daily doses will prove more effective. *Orally*, the average adult dosage is 8 tablets (4 gm)/day, in divided doses. For children, the dosage should be adjusted on the basis of 1 gm/35 lb/day, in divided doses.

Availability:
CALCIUM DISODIUM VERSENATE®: **(Riker)**
Injection, 1 gm/5 ml in ampuls of 5 ml.
Tablets, 500 mg in bottles of 250.

CALCIUM GLUCEPTATE
CALCIUM GLUCONATE

Description: Calcium gluceptate is the calcium salt of *d*-glucoheptonic acid. Calcium gluconate is the normal calcium salt of gluconic acid with 1 molecule of water, and occurs as white, crystalline, odorless, tasteless granules or powder sparingly soluble in water and insoluble in alcohol and many other organic solvents. It contains 9% calcium ion.

Calcium is necessary for the proper functioning of nerves and muscles, for blood clotting, for normal cardiac function and for the maintenance of the body skeleton. It is readily absorbed in the upper part of the intestine; the acidic reaction increases the solubility of calcium and thus promotes its absorption.

Indications: Treatment of hypocalcemia in those conditions requiring a prompt increase in blood plasma calcium levels, such as neonatal tetany and tetany due to parathyroid deficiency, vitamin D deficiency, and alkalosis. It is also indicated for the prevention of hypocalcemia during exchange transfusions.

Precautions: Because of its additive effect, calcium should be administered only with considerable care to patients receiving digitalis glycosides. Intramuscular administration to infants and young children should be used only in emergencies when technical difficulty makes intravenous injection impossible.

Adverse Reactions: Following intramuscular administration, mild local reactions may occur; severe inflammatory reactions have not been observed. Rapid intravenous administration may cause the patient to complain of tingling sensations, a calcium taste, a sense of oppression or "heat waves."

Dosage and Administration: To supplement the normal calcium intake of the body, the average adult requires approximately 1 gm of calcium daily, while the pregnant or lactating woman requires 1.5 to 2 gm daily. Children require from 1 to 1.4 gm daily. For the treatment of hypocalcemic tetany, calcium gluconate in the form of a 10% solution is injected *intravenously* slowly in doses of 5 to 20 ml at a rate not to exceed 2 ml/minute. Calcium gluconate may also be administered *intramuscularly* to adults although some tissue irritation may result; the solution should *never* be injected intramuscularly in children. Calcium salts are better utilized when administered about one hour after meals. For mild or latent hypocalcemic tetany, calcium gluconate may be taken orally. Calcium gluceptate may be given *intramuscularly* in doses of 2 to 5 ml. When 5 ml are administered, the dose should be injected in the gluteal region, or in infants, in the lateral thigh. During exchange transfusions in newborns, the usual dose is 0.5 ml after every 100 ml of blood exchanged.

Availability:
CALCIUM GLUCEPTATE Injection in ampuls of 5 ml and in Abboject® (disposable syringes) of 5 ml. Each ml represents 18 mg of elemental calcium (0.9 mEq), as *d*-glucoheptonic acid, and is equivalent in calcium content to 2 ml of a 10% calcium gluconate solution. **(Abbott)**
CALCIUM GLUCEPTATE Injection in ampuls of 5 ml. Each ml represents 18 mg of calcium (0.9 mEq), as *d*-glucoheptonic acid, and is equivalent in calcium content to 2 ml of 10% calcium gluconate solution. **(Lilly)**
CALCIUM GLUCONATE Injection, 10% in ampuls of 10 ml. **(Parke-Davis, Upjohn and others)**

CALCIUM LEUCOVORIN

Chemical Name: *N*-{*p*–{[(2-Amino-5-formyl-5,6,7,8-tetrahydro-4-hydroxyl-6-pteridinyl) methyl]-amino}benzoyl}glutamic acid, calcium salt.

Description: Calcium leucovorin is the calcium salt of a folic acid metabolite, and occurs as an odorless, yellowish, microcrystalline powder very soluble in water and practically insoluble in alcohol. Leucovorin, or folinic acid, is a growth factor utilized by the bacterial species *Leuconostoc citrovorum* and is therefore referred to as citrovorum factor, although it is not identical to the citrovorum factor obtained from the liver.

As the formyl derivative and active form of folic acid, leucovorin's activity in the treatment of megaloblastic anemias is comparable to that of folic acid. However, leucovorin is superior to folic acid as an antidote in instances of overdosage of folic acid antagonists. This is probably due to the fact that folic acid antagonists interfere with the conversion of folic acid to leucovorin, but do not interfere with the action of leucovorin itself.

Indications: Calcium leucovorin is useful in diminishing the toxicity and reversing the action of an inadvertently administered overdosage of a folic acid antagonist such as aminopterin and methotrexate. Leucovorin has also demonstrated its effectiveness in producing amelioration of the blood picture in a number of megaloblastic anemias such as those encountered in infancy, pregnancy, sprue and nutritional deficiency.

Warnings: Calcium leucovorin is *not* the proper therapy for pernicious anemia and other megaloblastic anemias secondary to lack of vitamin B-12. A hematologic remission may occur while the neurologic manifestations remain progressive. In the treatment of overdosage of folic acid antagonists leucovorin must be administered within 1 hour, if possible, and is usually ineffective if administered after a delay of 4 hours.

Precautions: Although no adverse reactions have been reported with the dosages recommended, the administration of leucovorin should be accompanied by every known precaution for the prevention and arrest of untoward reactions.

Adverse Reactions: Allergic sensitization has been reported following both oral and parenteral administration of folic acid.

Dosage and Administration: *Intramuscularly. For the treatment of megaloblastic anemia,* there is no evidence that doses greater than 1 mg daily have greater efficacy than those of 1 mg. Additionally, loss of folate in the urine becomes roughly logarithmic as the amount administered exceeds 1 mg. *For the treatment of overdosage of folic acid antagonists,* to be given in amounts equal to the weight of the antagonist administered.

Availability:
CALCIUM LEUCOVORIN Injection in ampuls of 3 mg and in vials of 50 mg. **(Lederle)**

CALDECORT

Description: Each gm contains the antifungal agent, calcium undecylenate, 3% and the adrenal corticosteroid, hydrocortisone acetate, 1% in a water-washable ointment base. This product provides antiinflammatory, antipruritic, antifungal and vasoconstrictive activity.

Indications: Treatment of contact and atopic dermatitis, and skin conditions complicated by fungal and bacterial infections when due to susceptible organisms.

Contraindications: Hypersensitivity to any component. Preparations containing a corticosteroid with or without a fungistatic agent are contraindicated in tuberculosis of the skin, or viral lesions such as herpes simplex, vaccinia or varicella.

Precautions: Existing or superimposed infections unresponsive to therapy with this product require initiation of appropriate therapy and identification of the infecting organism and its sensitivity to therapy. If signs of hypersensitivity or irritation occur, this preparation should be discontinued. When extensive areas are treated, the possibility of systemic absorption of the steroid exists and suitable precautions should be taken. The ointment is intended for topical use only; it should not be used in or near the eyes, nor should it be used needlessly during pregnancy on extended areas in large amounts or for prolonged periods.

Adverse Reactions: Application of the ointment to excoriated areas may be followed by a slight, transient stinging due to calcium undecylenate. Idiosyncratic reactions to any of the components may occur on rare occasions, in which case this preparation should be discontinued. When steroid-containing preparations are used for prolonged periods in intertriginous areas or under occlusive dressings, striae may occur; also, miliaria, folliculitis and pyoderma may develop. Other local adverse reactions which may occur with or without occlusive dressing include burning sensations, itching, irritation, dryness, secondary infection, atrophy of the skin, acneform eruption, and hypopigmentation.

Dosage and Administration: *Topically.* Apply a small amount to affected area 2 or 3 times daily, or as directed by the physician.

Availability:
CALDECORT® Topical Ointment in tubes of 7 and 28 gm. **(Pennwalt)**

CALUSTERONE

Chemical Name: 7*β*, 17*α*-Dimethyl-17-*β*-hydroxyandrost-4-en-3-one; or 7*β*, 17-dimethyltestosterone.

Description: Calusterone is a synthetic androgenic steroid that is chemically related to testosterone. The biochemical activity by which it produces its therapeutic effects in the treatment of breast cancer has not been determined. Calusterone has been found to be effective in approximately 25% of patients with advanced or disseminated mammary cancer according to the following criteria: (1) a measurable decrease in size of all demonstrable tumor masses; (2) a decrease in the size of more than 50% of nonosseous lesions with all bone lesions remaining static; or (3) an improvement of more than 50% of total lesions while the remainder were static.

Results of teratology studies performed in rabbits and rats suggest that the drug produces litters exhibiting signs of immaturity at birth as compared to control litters.

Indications: Calusterone is recommended *only* for the palliative treatment of advanced inoperable or metastatic carcinoma of the breast in postmenopausal women when hormonal therapy is indicated. It may also be used in women who were diagnosed as having had disseminated breast carcinoma when premenopausal and in whom ovarian function has been subsequently terminated.

Contraindications: Carcinoma of the male breast and in premenopausal women.

Warnings: Safe use of calusterone has not been established with regard to adverse effects upon fetal development, and since the drug is intended for use only in postmenopausal women, it should not be used during pregnancy.

Precautions: In general, the usual precautions pertaining to the use of androgens should also apply to calusterone, although the androgenic effects noted appear to be of low incidence and are generally mild. Routine determinations of plasma calcium levels should be performed, since hypercalcemia may develop, particularly during periods of active remission of body metastases. If hypercalcemia occurs, appropriate measures should be instituted. Occasionally, a drug-related edema (usually mild) may be seen; however, patients with significant edema may require diuretics prior to and during treatment with this steroid. Objective evidence of tumor progression should be evaluated periodically by physical examination, x-rays of known or suspected metastasis, and determinations of serum calcium and alkaline phosphatase levels. The latter determination may reflect improvement in bony lesions if there is a slight to moderate rise after initiation of treatment, or it may be indicative of extensive hepatic metastases if the level is markedly elevated.

Since calusterone may increase the patient's sensitivity to oral anticoagulants, the dosage of the anticoagulant may require reduction in order to maintain a satisfactory therapeutic hypoprothrombinemia. Mild increases in BSP retention have been noted in a few patients, and increases in SGOT to abnormal levels were apparent in about 20% of the patients. Many of these patients had progressive disease with liver involvement. Few showed the concomitant increases in serum bilirubin and alkaline phosphatase that might suggest a drug-related excretory dysfunction. Although cholestatic jaundice has rarely been reported, it is advisable to perform liver function tests during treatment with this drug. There are no reports in the use of calusterone in carcinoma of the breast during pregnancy or in carcinoma of the breast in males with or without associated carcinoma of the prostate.

Adverse Reactions: Androgen-related side effects such as mild or moderate deepening of the voice, acne, and growth of facial hair are seen in about 20 to 25% of the patients. Other side effects, such as edema or clitoral enlargement, are uncommon and are usually mild. Hypercalcemia was noted in a few cases but it usually accompanied progression of the disease. Libido is rarely affected. Increases in nausea and vomiting, noted in about 5 to 10% of patients, were usually mild or moderate and controllable, but a few cases of severe vomiting required discontinuation of the drug. Brief periods of intensely increased pain have been reported in a few patients experiencing osseous flares. Other signs and symptoms that have been reported in association with the use of this drug have been related to the underlying disease state.

Dosage and Administration: *Orally.* The usual dose is 200 mg daily administered in 4 equally divided doses. Doses of 150 to 300 mg daily have been used successfully. In order to evaluate the response, therapy should be continued for a minimum of 3 months, unless there is active progression of the disease. Therapy with this drug should not replace supportive measures such as transfusion, antibacterial therapy or corticosteroids.

Availability:
METHOSARB® Tablets, 50 mg in bottles of 120. **(Upjohn)**

CANDICIDIN

Description: Candicidin is a polyene antifungal antibiotic derived from a soil actinomycete similar to *Streptomyces griseus,* and occurs as a greenish-brown powder partially soluble in water and in alcohol. It closely resembles amphotericin B both chemically and in its spectrum of activity. Although amphoteric, candicidin loses its potency in solutions sufficiently acidic or basic to cause the formation of soluble salts.

Its exact mode of action is not known. In vitro, the drug has demonstrated activity against a broad spectrum of fungi including *Candida albicans.* It is both fungistatic and fungicidal. It is ineffective against bacteria, viruses and protozoa.

Indications: The topical treatment of vaginal moniliasis caused by *C. albicans* and other species of Candida. The vaginal tablets are particularly suited for the gravid patient.

Contraindications: In patients hypersensitive to any component. During pregnancy, the use of the ointment applicator may be contraindicated; the tablet inserter should be used only on the advice of a physician. It may be preferable to insert the tablet manually.

Precautions: To avoid reinfection, it is recommended that the patient abstain from sexual intercourse, or that the husband wear a condom.

Adverse Reactions: Rare instances of sensitization or temporary irritation have been reported.

Dosage and Administration: *Topically.* One applicatorful of the ointment or 1 vaginal tablet is inserted high in the vagina twice daily, morning and at bedtime, for 14 days. Treatment may be repeated if symptoms persist or reappear.

Availability:
CANDEPTIN®: **(Schmid)**
Vaginal Ointment, 0.6 mg/gm (3 mg/5-gm applicatorful) in tubes of 75 gm with applicator in cartons of 2.
Vaginal Tablets, 3 mg in cartons of 28 individually foil-wrapped tablets with inserter.
VANOBID: **(Merrell-National)**
Vaginal Ointment, 3 mg/5 gm (applicatorful) in tubes of 75 gm with applicator in cartons of 2.
Vaginal Tablets, 3 mg in cartons of 28 individually foil-wrapped tablets with inserter.

CAPREOMYCIN SULFATE

Description: Capreomycin sulfate is a polypeptide antibiotic isolated from *Streptomyces capreolus.* It is a complex of 4 microbiologically active components which have been characterized in part; however, the complete structural determination has not been established. Capreomycin is supplied as the disulfate salt and occurs as a white, amorphous powder soluble in water. Aqueous solutions are almost colorless.

Absorption from the gastrointestinal tract is not significant. Following a single intramuscular injection of 1 gm in normal individuals, peak blood levels were reached in 1 to 2 hours, with average peak levels at 28 and 32 mcg/ml respectively. Low serum concentrations were present at 24 hours. About 52% of the drug is excreted unchanged in the urine within 12 hours; urine concentrations averaged 1.68 mg/ml during the 6 hours following a 1-gm dose. Injections of 1 gm of capreomycin daily for 30 days or more produced no significant accumulation in patients with normal renal function, but patients with impaired renal function showed high serum concentrations 24 hours after administration.

Capreomycin is active against human strains of *Mycobacterium tuberculosis.* The susceptibility of strains of *M. tuberculosis* in vitro varies with the media and techniques employed.

In addition to renal and eighth-cranial-nerve toxicity demonstrated in animal toxicologic studies, 2 dogs developed cataracts while receiving doses of 62 mg/kg and 100 mg/kg of capreomycin for prolonged periods. Teratologic studies showed a low incidence of "wavy ribs" in rats receiving 50 mg/kg or more daily.

Cross-resistance between capreomycin and viomycin is common. Also, varying degrees of cross-resistance between capreomycin and kanamycin and neomycin have been reported. Cross-resistance has not been observed between capreomycin and isoniazid, aminosalicylic acid, cycloserine, streptomycin, ethionamide or ethambutol.

Indications: As adjunctive measure with other antituberculous agents in the treatment of pulmonary infections caused by susceptible strains of *M. tuberculosis.* It is recommended for use in patients where primary agents, such as isoniazid, streptomycin and aminosalicylic acid cannot be used because of toxicity or the development of resistant organisms.

Contraindications: Hypersensitivity to capreomycin.

Warnings: The use of capreomycin in patients with renal insufficiency or preexisting auditory nerve impairment must be undertaken with considerable caution, and the risk of additional eighth-nerve impairment or renal injury should be weighed against the benefits to be derived from therapy. Since the toxic manifestations of capreomycin are similar to those of streptomycin and viomycin, simultaneous administration of these agents with capreomycin is not recommended. Due caution is also advised when the drug is used with nontuberculous agents (polymyxin, colistin sulfate, gentamicin, kanamycin, and neomycin) possessing ototoxic or nephrotoxic potential. Safe use in pregnant women and in infants and children has not been determined.

Precautions: Audiometric determinations should be carried out before capreomycin therapy is initiated and should be repeated at frequent intervals during the period of treatment. Renal function should be evaluated regularly in patients with known or suspected renal impairment, since renal injury, with tubular necrosis, elevation of BUN and NPN, and the development of an abnormal urinary sediment, has been noted. The appearance of casts, red cells and white cells in the urine has been observed in a high percentage of patients receiving prolonged therapy. Since hypokalemia may occur during therapy with this drug, serum potassium levels should be determined frequently. A partial peripheral neuromuscular block was produced by large intravenous doses of capreomycin. This action was enhanced by ether anesthesia and was antagonized by neostigmine. Patients subject to allergy, particularly to antibiotics, should be carefully observed.

Adverse Reactions: Noted were impaired renal and liver function; auditory dysfunction, tinnitus and vertigo; leukocytosis and leukopenia; urticaria and maculopapular skin rashes associated in some cases with febrile reactions; pain, induration, and sterile abscesses, as well as excessive bleeding at the injection site.

Dosage and Administration: *Intramuscularly.* The usual dose is 1 gm daily (not to exceed 20 mg/kg/day) for 2 to 4 months followed by 1 gm 2 or 3 times a week. The dose should be injected into a large muscle mass. To be administered in combination with at least one other antituberculous agent but probably not with streptomycin or viomycin. **Note:** Therapy for tuberculosis should be maintained for 18 to 24 months.

Availability:
CAPASTAT® Injection, 1 gm (equiv. to capreomycin activity) in ampuls of 5 ml. **(Lilly)**

CARBACHOL

Chemical Name: Choline chloride carbamate.

Description: Carbachol is a choline ester which is pharmacologically similar to acetylcholine. It occurs as white, or faintly yellow crystals or crystalline powder freely soluble in water and sparingly soluble in alcohol; practically insoluble in chloroform and in ether. Solutions are neutral to litmus.

Because of its stability, it is the most potent of the choline-like parasympathomimetic drugs and possesses a powerful miotic action. Following intracameral injection, prompt, complete miosis occurs which persists for 15 hours. It also produces spasm of accommodation. In simple aqueous solution, the drug does not penetrate the cornea readily. However, penetration occurs readily when it is applied in a vehicle containing a wetting agent such as benzalkonium chloride. A 1.5% solution [carbachol] in a suitable wetting agent exerts an action both more pronounced and more prolonged than that of a 2% solution of pilocarpine nitrate.

Indications: The reduction of intraocular pressure in open-angle or narrow-angle glaucoma. May be used in eyes that have become irritated by or resistant to pilocarpine. An 0.01% solution is used for the production of pupillary miosis during surgery.

Contraindications: In the presence of corneal abrasion because of the danger of increased absorption; in cases where pupillary constriction is undesirable, such as in acute iritis, and in patients with known hypersensitivity to the drug.

Precautions: Carbachol is for topical ophthalmic use only to reduce intraocular tension in glaucoma simplex and for obtaining pupillary miosis during surgery. It should not be used orally or parenterally because death from overdosage may result. If systemic effects occur after topical application in the eye or accidental intake, atropine sulfate in a dose (for adults) of 0.4 to 0.6 mg or more should be administered parenterally (intravenously if necessary). A proportionately smaller amount should be given to children. The possibility of atropinization with large doses of atropine, particularly in sensitive individuals, should be considered. Carbachol should be used with caution if the epithelial barrier of the conjunctiva and cornea has been reduced by topical anesthetics, tonometry or trauma; or if the patient is asthmatic. Cautious use is also recommended in the presence of acute cardiac failure, peptic ulcer, hyperthyroidism, gastrointestinal spasm, urinary tract obstruction, and parkinsonism. Dosage should be individualized to avoid aching of the eye and frontal headache caused by intense constriction of the iris sphincter and ciliary-muscle spasm.

Adverse Reactions: Slight hyperemia during the first few days of treatment, also aching of the eye(s) and headache which usually subsides after a few days. Lens opacities following the use of this drug have been reported, but as yet a causal relationship has not been established.

Dosage and Administration: *Topically. In primary open-angle glaucoma,* 1 or 2 drops of a 0.75 to 3% solution are instilled into each eye every 4 to 8 hours. *In acute primary angle-closure glaucoma prior to surgery,* initially, 1 or 2 drops of a 1.5% solution are instilled into the affected eye(s) every minute for 5 minutes; then 1 or 2 drops every 5 minutes for 25 minutes, followed by 1 or 2 drops 3 or 4 times an hour until the angle opens. To avoid a bilateral attack, 3 drops may be instilled into the unaffected eye every 8 hours. *Intracameral.* Instill 0.4 to 0.5 ml of an 0.01% solution into the anterior chamber of the eye.

Availability:
Isopto® CARBACHOL Solutions, 0.75, 1.5, and 3% in Drop-Tainer bottles of 15 and 30 ml; 2.25% in Drop-Tainer bottles of 15 ml. **(Alcon)**
MIOSTAT® Solution, 0.01% in vials of 1.5 ml in packages of 6. **(Wyeth)**
MISTURA C Solution, 3% in mist-dispensing bottles of 15 ml. **(Lederle)**

CARBAMAZEPINE

Chemical Name: 5H-dibenz[b,f]azepine-5-carboxamide.

Description: Carbamazepine is an iminostilbene derivative structurally and pharmacologically related to the tricyclic antidepressants; its nucleus is identical to some of these compounds, but differs in that it contains a carbamate side chain. It occurs as a white, crystalline powder insoluble in water and soluble in propylene glycol. Molecular weight is 236.23.

Pharmacologically, carbamazepine appears to be qualitatively similar to phenytoin. It apparently relieves the pain of trigeminal neuralgia by reducing nervous impulses at the synaptic junction within the trigeminal nucleus. The drug appears to be well absorbed from the gastrointestinal tract and is metabolized in the liver. Experimental data indicate that the serum half-life of carbamazepine exceeds 14 hours but does not appear to extend beyond 29 hours. It is highly bound to plasma proteins and tissues. The initial relief of pain is usually experienced within 24 to 48 hours and can often be maintained with reduced dosages or intermittent courses of therapy.

Indications: Treatment of pain associated with true trigeminal neuralgia (tic douloureux). With the exception of glossopharyngeal neuralgia, results in other facial neuralgias have been equivocal. **Important Note:** Carbamazepine should not be considered a simple analgesic and should never be given casually for the relief of trivial facial aches or pains. It is also indicated in the management of psychomotor (temporal lobe) and grand mal epilepsy, in secondary or partial epilepsy with complex symptomatology or other secondarily generalized seizures either alone or in combination with other antiepileptic medication. *It is not effective in petit mal epilepsy.* The drug should be reserved for those patients whose seizures have not been satisfactorily controlled by or who are refractory to other anticonvulsant drugs.

Contraindications: Patients with a history of bone marrow depression and/or hypersensitivity to the drug, in those known to be sensitive to tricyclic compounds such as amitriptyline, desipramine, imipramine, etc. Theoretically, *carbamazepine should not be used concomitantly with MAO inhibitors.* When it seems desirable to prescribe carbamazepine to patients taking MAO inhibitors, the latter should be discontinued for at least 14 days, as the clinical situation permits. The initial dosage of carbamazepine in these situations should be low, with gradual increments given under close observation.

Warnings: Following administration of carbamazepine, deaths from aplastic anemia have been reported. Agranulocytosis, thrombocyctopenia and transitory leukopenia also have been observed. Before initiating therapy, a complete blood count, including an estimate of platelets, should be performed and, if abnormal, the drug should not be used. Patients should be made aware of the early toxic signs and symptoms of a potential hematologic problem (e.g., fever, sore throat, ulcers in the mouth, easy bruising, petechial or purpuric hemorrhage), and they should be advised to discontinue the drug and to report to the physician immediately if any such signs or symptoms appear. These blood tests should be done at weekly intervals during the first month of therapy, every 2 weeks during the second and third months, and at monthly intervals thereafter for as long as the patient is taking the drug. Where feasible, carbamazepine should not be used in conjunction with any potent drug which may increase the possibility of toxic reactions. The drug should not be given to nursing mothers, and to pregnant women during the first trimester, and thereafter only to patients in whom the clinical situation justifies the potential risk. There have been reports that the use of anticonvulsant drugs in pregnant epileptic patients is suspected of producing birth defects in the unborn child, but the situation is complicated because other drugs or the illness itself may contribute to the effect. Nevertheless, patients in whom the drug is administered to prevent major seizures should continue to receive such therapy in order to avoid the consequence of status epilepticus with its attendant hypoxia and threat to life. Because of the drug's mild anticholinergic activity, patients with increased intraocular pressure should be closely observed during therapy and, because of the drug's relationship to other tricyclic compounds, the possibility of activation of a latent psychosis and, in elderly patients, of confusion or agitation, should be borne in mind. Since dizziness and drowsiness may occur, patients should be cautioned about the hazards of operating machinery or engaging in activities that require alertness or skill.

Precautions: The drug should be used with caution in patients with a history of coronary artery disease, organic heart disease and congestive failure. Patients with a history of liver disease should be fully evaluated before considering treatment with carbamazepine. Baseline evaluations of the liver should be obtained prior to therapy and reviewed at regular intervals. The benefit-risk ratio should be carefully weighed in this class of patient, and the drug discontinued immediately if there is evidence of aggravated liver dysfunction or active liver disease. Complete urinalysis and blood urea nitrogen should be done on patients treated with this drug, because of observed renal dysfunction. A trend toward a decrease in white blood cells should suggest a reduction in dosage and more frequent laboratory and clinical evaluations. If this trend persists, the drug should be discontinued. Evidence is lacking that carbamazepine produces changes in the cornea, lens or retina. However, it should be recognized that phenothiazines and related drugs have demonstrated the ability to cause changes in the eye. On this basis, slit-lamp, funduscopic and tonometric examinations are recommended periodically for patients taking this medication.

Adverse Reactions: If adverse reactions are of such severity that the medication must be withdrawn, the physician must take into consideration that abrupt discontinuation of any anticonvulsant in a responsive epileptic patient may lead to seizures and possibly status epilepticus with its attendant life-threatening hazards. Those most frequently observed, particularly during the initial phases of therapy, are dizziness, drowsiness, unsteadiness on the feet, nausea and vomiting. Initiating therapy at a low dosage level usually will minimize the possibility of these reactions.

Genitourinary complications include urinary frequency, acute urinary retention, and oliguria with elevated blood pressure, and impotence. While albuminuria, glycosuria, elevated BUN and microscopic deposits in the urine have also been reported, only infrequently was it considered likely that carbamazepine was responsible for the changes.

Hematopoietic complications include aplastic anemia, leukopenia, agranulocytosis, eosinophilia, leukocytosis, thrombocytopenia, and purpura.

Hepatic disorders involve abnormalities in liver function tests and cholestatic and hepatocellular jaundice.

Neurologic and sensory reactions reported include dizziness, drowsiness, disturbances of coordination, confusion, headache, fatigue, blurred vision, visual hallucinations, transient diplopia and oculomotor disturbances, speech disturbances, and involuntary abnormal movements. Peripheral neuritis and paresthesias, depression with agitation, talkativeness, nystagmus, tinnitus, and hyperacusis also have been reported. There have been reports of associated paralysis and other symptoms of cerebral arterial insufficiency but the exact relationship of these reactions to carbamazepine has not been established.

Dermatologic manifestations include pruritic and erythematous rashes, urticaria, Stevens-Johnson syndrome, photosensitivity reactions, alterations in skin pigmentation, exfoliative dermatitis, alopecia, diaphoresis, erythema multiforme and nodosum, and aggravation of disseminated lupus erythematosus. In certain cases, it may be necessary to discontinue therapy.

Digestive disorders include nausea, vomiting, gastric distress and abdominal pain, diarrhea, constipation, anorexia, and dryness of the mouth and pharynx, including glossitis and stomatitis.

Cardiovascular complications including left ventricular failure, aggravation of hypertension, hypotension, syncope and collapse, edema, and aggravation of coronary artery disease have been reported. Some of these have resulted in fatalities. Congestive heart failure and recurrent thrombophlebitis in patients with a prior history of thrombophlebitic episodes have also been reported. It may be well to bear in mind that although no causal relationship to carbamazepine has been established, other cardiovascular complications including myocardial infarction and arrhythmias have been associated with other tricyclic compounds.

Other reactions reported include fever and chills, adenopathy or lymphadenopathy, aching joints and muscles, leg cramps, and conjunctivitis.

The gravity and severity of the adverse reactions should govern the necessity to discontinue therapy and to institute other measures appropriate to the patient's response.

Dosage and Administration: *Orally. For trigeminal neuralgia,* initially, 100 mg twice daily the first day, always with meals if possible. Thereafter, the dosage should be increased gradually in increments of 100 mg every 12 hours until pain is no longer manifest. The dose necessary to relieve pain may vary from 200 mg to 1.2 gm in a 24-hour period. Initial control of pain can be maintained in most patients with a dosage of 400 to 800 mg daily. However, some patients may be maintained on as little as 200 mg daily, while others may require as much as 1.2 gm daily. At least once every 3 months throughout the treatment period, attempts should be made to reduce the dosage to the minimum effective level or even to discontinue the drug. *For epilepsy,* a low initial daily dosage with gradual increments is recommended. The dosage for adults and children over 12 years of age is 200 mg twice daily the 1st day, followed by daily increases of up to 200 mg divided into 3 or 4 doses/day until the optimal therapeutic response is obtained. Generally, the daily dosage should not exceed 1.2 gm in patients over 15 years of age and 1 gm in children 12 to 15 years of age, but dosages up to 1.6 gm have been given in rare instances. For most adults, the maintenance dosage is 800 mg to 1.2 gm daily.

Availability:
TEGRETOL® Tablets, 200 mg (round, white, single-scored) in bottles of 100 and 1000 and in unit-dose packages of 100. **(Geigy)**

CARBARSONE

Chemical Name: *p*-Ureidobenzenearsonic acid.

Description: Carbarsone is a pentavalent organic arsenical containing about 29% arsenic and occurs as a white, crystalline, odorless solid practically insoluble in water, and soluble in carbonate or bicarbonate solutions. It is readily absorbed from the gastrointestinal tract, but because of its slow urinary excretion, interrupted therapy is necessary to avoid cumulative poisoning.

Indications: Treatment of intestinal amebiasis; effective against the trophozoite form of *Entamoeba histolytica* in the lumen and shallow ulcers of the colon.

Contraindications: Should not be used initially when amebic hepatitis of any degree may be present, when there is any other liver or kidney disease, in the presence of contracted visual or color fields, or when the patient is hypersensitive or intolerant to organic or inorganic arsenic given systemically or applied topically.

Precautions: To avoid cumulative poisoning, it is mandatory that the recommended daily dosage not be exceeded, that a course of treatment be no longer than 10 days, and that a rest period of at least 10 days be allowed before another course of treatment is started. The drug should be discontinued immediately if there is any evidence of intolerance or toxicity manifested by increased severity of existing gastrointestinal symptoms, development of nausea, vomiting, abdominal pain or cramps, or diarrhea when these symptoms have previously been absent; urinary symptoms; dermatitis or other skin lesions suggesting sensitivity to arsenic; any central or peripheral nervous-system changes; or any of the signs or symptoms mentioned under Adverse Reactions. Since the drug accumulates in the tissues and is eliminated slowly, the patient should be instructed to report any unusual signs or symptoms for a given period after treatment has been discontinued.

Adverse Reactions: Signs of toxicity are sore throat, edema, splenomegaly, icterus, pruritus, skin eruptions, gastrointestinal irritation, hepatitis, neuritis, papillitis with retinal edema, and visual disturbances. Fatalities from exfoliative dermatitis and liver necrosis and from hemorrhagic encephalitis are on record. If it is warranted, untoward reactions to carbarsone may be treated with the specific antiarsenical, dimercaprol (BAL). Overdosage is manifested by nausea, vomiting, abdominal pain, diarrhea, shock, coma, convulsions, ulceration of mucous membranes and skin, and kidney damage. Unexplained fatalities have been reported with therapeutic doses. Treatment includes administering dimercaprol, 3 to 4 mg/kg of body weight every 6 hours for the first 2 days and then twice daily for a total of 10 days. General management should be symptomatic and supportive and may include gastric lavage, administration of oxygen and intravenous fluids, and maintenance of body temperature.

Dosage and Administration: *Orally.* Adults, usually 250 mg 2 or 3 times daily for 10 days, followed by additional courses of treatment as indicated after a drug-free interval of 10 to 14 days. Children, the average total dose is about 75 mg/kg of body weight. The following schedule will be effective: ages 2 to 4 years, 66 mg 3 times daily in milk or orange juice; ages 5 to 8 years, 100 mg 3 times daily; ages 9 to 12 years, 132 mg 3 times daily; and from puberty on to young adulthood, 166 mg 3 times daily. This schedule for all age groups is to be carried out for a period of 10 days. The package literature should be consulted for specific details.

Availability:
CARBARSONE Capsules (Pulvules®), 250 mg in bottles of 20. **(Lilly)**

CARBAZOCHROME SALICYLATE

Description: A complex of adrenochrome monosemicarbazome and sodium salicylate, it occurs as an orange-red, odorless powder soluble in alcohol and in water; it has a salty, sweetish taste.

Carbazochrome may decrease excessive capillary permeability for a variable length of time. It appears to have no effect upon cardiovascular dynamics or any of the blood components associated with the clotting mechanism.

Indications: For conditions characterized by increased capillary permeability and associated capillary oozing.

Contraindications: In patients hypersensitive to salicylates and to any component of this drug. *It should not be given intravenously.*

Warnings: The parenteral form of this drug should be administered *intramuscularly* only. In cases of persistent bleeding, hematological evaluation is advised. Carbazochrome is ineffective in massive hemorrhage or arterial bleeding. Safe use during pregnancy has not been established; therefore it should not be used in women of childbearing potential, and particularly during the first trimester of pregnancy, unless in the judgment of the physician, the potential benefits outweigh the possible hazards to the fetus.

Precautions: Caution should be exercised in patients with known allergy or drug sensitivity. Since antihistamines tend to inhibit the action of carbazochrome, they should be discontinued 48 hours prior to the use of this drug. Sensitivity to salicylates may develop with repeated use.

Adverse Reactions: Intramuscular administration may produce a stinging sensation.

Dosage and Administration: *Intramuscularly.* The dose of carbazochrome salicylate often is expressed in terms of the adrenochrome semicarbazone content: 26 mg of the former represents 1 mg of the latter. *Preoperatively as a prophylactic.* Adults and children over 12 years of age, 10 mg the night before operation; 10 mg with on-call medication. Children under 12 years of age, 5 mg. *Postoperatively.* Carbazochrome may be administered either *orally* or *intramus-*

cularly. Adults and children over 12 years of age, 5 mg every 2 hours as indicated. If not used preoperatively, 10 mg every 2 hours as necessary. Children under 12 years, 5 mg.

Availability:
ADRENOSEM®: **(Beecham)**
Injection, 5 mg/ml in ampuls of 1 and 2 ml.
Syrup, 2.5 mg/5 ml in bottles of 120 ml.
Tablets, 2.5 mg (sugar-coated, yellow) in bottles of 50.

CARBENICILLIN: see The Penicillins

CARBIDOPA: see Levodopa

CARBINOXAMINE MALEATE

Chemical Name: 2-[*p*-Chloro-α-(2-dimethylaminoethoxy)benzyl]pyridine bimaleate.

Description: Carbinoxamine maleate is an antihistamine, occurring as a white, odorless, crystalline powder very soluble in water, freely soluble in alcohol and in chloroform, and very slightly soluble in ether. It differs structurally from chlorpheniramine maleate in that a dimethylaminoethoxy group replaces a dimethylamino*ethyl* group [of chlorpheniramine maleate].

Carbinoxamine is a potent antihistamine with a low incidence of drowsiness, and comparatively weak anticholinergic effect. The clinical response persists for about 4 to 6 hours; the repeat-action forms persist for about 8 to 12 hours.

Indications: Symptomatic treatment of allergic disorders such as seasonal and perennial allergic rhinitis, vasomotor rhinitis, allergic conjunctivitis due to inhalant allergens and foods, mild uncomplicated allergic skin manifestations of urticaria and angioedema. It is also useful for the amelioration of the severity of allergic reactions to blood or plasma in patients with a known history of such reactions. A combination with antitussives and expectorants is useful for the treatment of cough associated with the common cold and other respiratory infections such as bronchitis and tracheitis, and for the relief of symptoms associated with allergic disorders. Another combination, containing an analgesic-antipyretic and a nasal decongestant, is indicated for the relief of nasal congestion, fever, and pain associated with the common cold, sinusitis and allergic or vasomotor rhinitis.

Contraindications: In patients hypersensitive to carbinoxamine maleate or to any of the components formulated with it.

Precautions: As with any antihistaminic preparation, an occasional patient may experience some drowsiness, in which case the patient should refrain from engaging in any activity requiring alertness or skill. Safe use during pregnancy has not been established.

Adverse Reactions: Rarely encountered were dizziness, drowsiness, nausea, and dryness of the mouth.

For additional information, see monographs on Dextromethorphan Hydrobromide and Pseudoephedrine Hydrochloride.

Dosage and Administration: *Orally.* Dosage for carbinoxamine maleate should be based on the severity of the condition and the response of the patient. Dosage ranges from 4 mg/day to 24 mg daily in divided doses. The dosage for children should be reduced proportionately. The usual dosage for the expectorant is 1 teaspoonful every 3 hours for adults, and ½ to 1 teaspoonful every 3 hours for children 6 years of age and older. The usual adult dosage for the decongestant-analgesic is 2 tablets 3 or 4 times daily or 2 teaspoonsful of elixir every 4 hours. Children 1 to 6 years of age, ½ to 1 teaspoonful every 4 hours; children 6 years of age and older, 1 to 2 teaspoonsful every 4 hours.

Availability:

Carbinoxamine Maleate

CLISTIN®: **(McNeil)**

Elixir, 4 mg/5 ml (dark red) in bottles of 1 pint and 1 gallon. Contains 7% alcohol.

Tablets, 4 mg (pink) in bottles of 100 and 1000.

Repeat-Action Tablets (CLISTIN R-A), 8 mg (orange) and 12 mg (yellow) in bottles of 100 and 500.

Combinations

CLISTIN Expectorant Syrup (yellow, fruit-flavored) in pints. Each 5-ml teaspoonful contains carbinoxamine maleate, 2 mg; ammonium chloride, 120 mg; sodium citrate (hydrous), 120 mg; potassium guaiacolsulfonate, 60 mg and benzyl alcohol, 0.3% (v/v).

CLISTIN-D:

Tablets (light-yellow, scored) in bottles of 100. Each tablet contains carbinoxamine maleate, 2 mg; acetaminophen, 300 mg and phenylephrine hydrochloride, 10 mg.

RONDEC D,S,T and C™: **(Ross)**

Drops in dropper bottles of 20 ml. Each dropperful (1 ml) contains carbinoxamine maleate, 2 mg and pseudoephedrine hydrochloride, 25 mg.

Syrup in bottles of 120 ml and 1 pint. Each 5-ml teaspoonful contains carbinoxamine maleate, 4 mg and pseudoephedrine hydrochloride, 60 mg.

Tablets with Filmtab® and *Chewable Tablets* in bottles of 60 and 100, respectively. Each tablet is equivalent in content to 1 teaspoonful of Rondec Syrup. *Tablets* are also available in bottles of 500.

RONDEC-DM™: **(Ross)**

Oral Drops in dropper bottles of 20 ml. Each dropperful (1 ml) contains carbinoxamine maleate, 2 mg; pseudoephedrine hydrochloride, 25 mg and dextromethorphan hydrobromide, 4 mg. Contains less than 0.6% alcohol.

Syrup in bottles of 120 ml and 1 pint. Each teaspoonful (5 ml) contains carbinoxamine maleate, 4 mg; pseudoephedrine hydrochloride, 60 mg and dextromethorphan hydrobromide, 15 mg. Contains less than 0.6% alcohol.

CARISOPRODOL

Chemical Name: *N*-Isopropyl-2-methyl-2-propyl-1,3-propanediol dicarbamate.

Description: Carisoprodol differs structurally from meprobamate in that an isopropyl group has been substituted for a hydrogen at one of the nitrogen atoms. It occurs as a white, crystalline powder slightly soluble in water and has a bitter taste.

Following oral administration, the drug is rapidly absorbed from the gastrointestinal tract; its effects are noted within 30 minutes and persist for 4 to 6 hours. The liver is the major site of its metabolic degradation and only small amounts are excreted unchanged in the urine. The mechanism of action by which it relieves pain and spasm differs from that of morphine and its derivatives, salicylates and other currently used analgesics. The drug apparently modifies perception of pain centrally without affecting peripheral pain reflexes or withdrawal reflexes. In addition, it relaxes abnormal tension of skeletal muscles by a potent selective blocking action on the interneurons in the descending reticular formation and spinal cord.

Indications: Symptomatic relief in conditions characterized by skeletal muscle spasm and mild to moderate pain. Its use should be accompanied by rest, physical therapy and other appropriate measures that have been proved beneficial in treating the discomfort associated with acute, painful musculoskeletal conditions. Other drugs may be added, such as phenacetin, codeine, caffeine, to enhance the analgesic action of carisoprodol.

Contraindications: Patients who have had allergic or idiosyncratic reactions to it or to related compounds such as meprobamate or mebutamate and also in patients who have acute intermittent porphyria or in whom such condition is suspected.

Warnings: The patient should be cautioned that carisoprodol may impair the mental and/or physical abilities required for the performance of hazardous tasks such as driving a motor vehicle or operating machinery. The drug should be used with caution in addiction-prone individuals. Withdrawal symptoms including abdominal cramps, insomnia, chilliness, headache, and nausea have occurred following abrupt cessation of higher than recommended dosage. There have been rare instances of psychological dependence. On very rare occasions, the first dose has been followed by idiosyncratic symptoms appearing within minutes or hours. Symptoms reported include extreme weakness, transient quadriplegia, dizziness, ataxia, temporary loss of vision, diplopia, mydriasis, dysarthria, agitation, euphoria, confusion, and disorientation. Symptoms usually subside over the course of the next several hours. Supportive and symptomatic therapy, including hospitalization, may be necessary. Safe use in pregnant women has not been established. Therefore, the expected benefits must be weighed against the potential hazards. In lactating mothers receiving carisoprodol, the concentration in breast milk is 2 to 4 times that of maternal plasma. This factor should be taken into account when use of the drug is contemplated in nursing mothers. This drug is not recommended for use in children under 12 years of age. Since the effects of carisoprodol and alcohol or other CNS depressants may be additive, appropriate caution should be exercised.

Precautions: Caution should be exercised in patients with compromised liver or kidney function.

Adverse Reactions: *CNS reactions:* Drowsiness and other CNS effects may require dosage reduction. Other adverse reactions include dizziness, vertigo, ataxia, tremor, agitation, irritability, headache, depressive reactions, syncope and insomnia. *Allergic or idiosyncratic reactions:* Such complications occasionally develop and are usually seen within the period of the first to fourth dose in patients having had no previous contact with the drug. Skin rash, erythema multiforme, pruritus, eosinophilia, and fixed drug eruption with cross reaction to meprobamate have been reported. Severe reactions have been manifested by asthmatic episodes, fever, weakness, dizziness, angioneurotic edema, smarting eyes, hypotension, and anaphylactoid shock. If such reactions do occur, discontinue the drug and initiate appropriate symptomatic therapy, utilizing epinephrine, antihistamines, and possibly corticosteroids. In evaluating possible allergic reactions, also consider allergy to excipients. *Cardiovascular reactions:* Tachycardia, postural hypotension, and facial flushing have been reported. *Gastrointestinal reactions:* Nausea, vomiting, hiccup, and epigastric distress have also been noted. *Hematologic reactions:* Leukopenia, for which other drugs or viral infection may have been responsible, and pancytopenia, attributed to phenylbutazone, have been reported. No serious blood dyscrasias have been attributed to carisoprodol. Overdosage has produced stupor, coma, shock, respiratory depression and, rarely, fatality. Reactions to **phenacetin** have been rare with short-term use of recommended doses. Prolonged overdosage may produce kidney changes, dyspnea, cyanosis due to sulfhemoglobinemia and methemoglobinemia, hemolytic anemia, skin rash, anorexia, subnormal temperature, insomnia, headache, mental disturbances and tolerance. Reactions to **caffeine** are almost always the result of overdosage, and may consist of nausea, nervousness, insomnia, diuresis, restlessness, tolerance, tinnitus, tremors, scintillating scotomas, tachycardia and cardiac arrhythmias. Reactions to **codeine** may be nausea, vomiting, constipation and miosis.

Dosage and Administration: *Orally.* Pediatric use is not recommended. The average dosage for adults is 350 mg of carisoprodol 3 times daily and at bedtime. The usual dosage for adults and children over 5 years of age of the compound product (with or without codeine) is 1 or 2 tablets 3 times daily and at bedtime. Usage in children under 5 years of age is not recommended.

Availability:

Carisoprodol

RELA® Tablets, 350 mg (pink, coated) in bottles of 100. **(Schering)**

SOMA® Tablets, 350 mg (white) in bottles of 100 and 500 and in unit-dose packages of 500. **(Wallace)**

Combinations

SOMA® Compound Tablets in bottles of 100 and 500 and in unit-dose packages of 500 and 1000. Each tablet contains carisoprodol, 200 mg; phenacetin, 160 mg and caffeine, 32 mg.

C-III SOMA Compound with CODEINE in bottles of 100 tablets (capsule-shaped). Each tablet contains in addition to above, codeine phosphate, 16 mg.

CARMUSTINE (BCNU)

Chemical Name: 1,3-bis(2-Chloroethyl)-1-nitrosourea.

Description: Carmustine, a nitrosourea chemotherapeutic agent, is used primarily in the treatment of brain tumors and Hodgkin's disease and in combination with prednisone in the treatment of multiple myeloma. Experimental data suggest that the drug alkylates DNA and RNA and inhibits several enzymes by carbomoylation of amino acids in proteins. It occurs as a white, lyophilized powder that is very soluble in alcohol and lipids and poorly soluble in water. Molecular weight has been reported to be 214.06.

When administered intravenously, carmustine is rapidly degraded, with no intact drug detectable after 15 minutes. However, in studies with C^{14}-labeled drug, prolonged levels of the isotope were observed in the plasma and tissue, probably representing radioactive fragments of the parent compound. It has been proposed that the antineoplastic and toxic activities of the drug may be due to its metabolites. Within 96 hours the major portion of the drug (60 to 70%) is excreted in the urine and 10% as respiratory carbon dioxide; the fate of the remainder is undetermined.

Because of its high lipid solubility and relative lack of ionization at a physiological pH, carmustine effectively crosses the blood brain barrier and the level of a radio-labeled dose in the cerebral spinal fluid is 50% or greater than that present in the plasma. Animal studies have revealed that the drug can cause embryotoxic, teratogenic and carcinogenic effects.

Indications: Palliative therapy in brain tumors (glioblastoma, brainstem glioma, medullablastoma, astrocytoma, ependymona, and metastatic brain tumors); in multiple myeloma in combination with prednisone; and in Hodgkin's disease or non-Hodgkin's lymphoma as secondary therapy in combination with other approved drugs in patients who relapse while being treated with, or who fail to respond to, primary therapy.

Contraindications: Patients with known hypersensitivity to carmustine, those with decreased circulating platelets, leukocytes, or erythrocytes due to previous chemotherapy or to other etiologies.

Warnings: Safe use during pregnancy has not been established; therefore, the benefits to be gained versus the risk of toxicity must be carefully considered.

Precautions: Because of the potential severity of reactions to carmustine, the drug should be administered only by clinicians experienced in the use of antineoplastic chemotherapy. The main serious toxic effect is delayed bone marrow depression. Complete blood counts should be conducted frequently for at least 6 weeks following administration of the drug, and repeat doses should not be given more frequently than every 6 weeks. The bone marrow toxicity is cumulative, and therefore dosage adjustment must be considered on the basis of the nadir of the blood cell count from the prior dose. Additionally, liver function tests should also be conducted.

Adverse Reactions: The most frequent and most serious toxicity is delayed myelosuppression. It usually occurs 4 to 6 weeks after administration and is dose-related. Platelet nadirs occur at 4 to 5 weeks; leukocyte nadirs occur at 5 to 6 weeks post therapy. Thrombocytopenia is generally more severe than leukopenia; however, both are dose-limiting responses. Anemia also occurs but is generally less severe. Nausea and vomiting may occur within 2 hours, and may persist for 4 to 6 hours. Prior administration of antiemetics is effective in diminishing and sometimes preventing this reaction. When high doses are employed, a reversible type of hepatic toxicity manifested by increased levels of transaminase, alkaline phosphatase and bilirubin has been reported in a small percentage of patients. Burning at the site of injection is common but true thrombosis is rare. Rapid transfusion may produce intensive flushing of the skin and suffusion of the conjunctiva within 2 hours and may last for about 4 hours.

Dosage and Administration: *Intravenously* by slow infusion over a period of 1 to 2 hours. For adults and children with normal bone marrow function, 200 mg/m² every 6 weeks. This may be given as a single dose or divided into daily injections such as 100 mg/m² on 2 successive days. When combined with other myelosuppressive drugs or given to patients in whom bone marrow reserve is depleted, the dose of carmustine should be individualized and adjusted appropriately. Subsequent doses should be based on the hematologic response of the patient to the preceding dose.

Availability:
BiCNU™ Injection in vials of 100 mg with 3-ml vial of diluent. **(Bristol)**

CARPHENAZINE MALEATE: see The Phenothiazines

CEBENASE

Description: Each tablet contains:

Intrinase® (vitamin B-12 with intrinsic factor concentrate)	1/6 unit
Ascorbic acid (as sodium ascorbate)	150 mg
Thiamine mononitrate	10 mg
Riboflavin	10 mg
Pyridoxine hydrochloride	2.5 mg
Calcium pantothenate	10 mg
Niacinamide	75 mg

Indications: Therapeutic amounts of water-soluble vitamins are supplied for use in the prevention and treatment of vitamin B and C deficiencies, and during the acute phase of a major illness or injury when the patient's vitamin requirements are increased. The intrinsic factor concentrate augments vitamin B-12 absorption. The presence of anemia requires specific therapy.

Contraindications: Hypersensitivity to any of the components.

Warnings: Not all patients with pernicious anemia show a satisfactory response to oral vitamin B-12-intrinsic factor preparations. Some patients who respond well initially appear to become refractory to intrinsic factor after varying periods of oral therapy. Periodic examinations and laboratory studies are essential and recommended. Failure of response, or an inadequate response, is an indication for parenteral vitamin B-12, recognized as the treatment of choice for pernicious anemia.

Dosage and Administration: *Orally.* The usual adult dosage is 1 tablet daily; may be increased depending on the clinical status of the patient.

Availability:
CEBENASE® Tablets (tan-colored, coated) in bottles of 50 and 500. **(Upjohn)**

CEFADROXIL MONOHYDRATE: see The Cephalosporins

CEFAMANDOLE NAFATE: see The Cephalosporins

CEFAZOLIN SODIUM: see The Cephalosporins

CEFOL

Description: Each tablet contains:

Thiamine mononitrate	15 mg
Riboflavin	10 mg
Pyridoxine hydrochloride	5 mg
Niacinamide	100 mg
Calcium pantothenate	20 mg

Ascorbic acid (as sodium ascorbate) .... 750 mg
Folic acid .... 500 μg
Cyanocobalamin (vitamin B-12) .... 6 μg
Vitamin E (as d-α tocopheryl acid succinate) .... 30 IU

Indications: Prevention and treatment of vitamin B and folate deficiency states due to diminishing utilization or intake of these vitamins or to increased vitamin requirements.

Warnings: Folic acid alone is not recommended in the treatment of pernicious anemia and other megaloblastic anemias where vitamin B-12 is deficient.

Precautions: Folic acid may obscure pernicious anemia in that the peripheral blood picture may revert to normal while the neurological manifestations progress.

Adverse Reactions: Allergic sensitization has been reported following both oral and parenteral administration of folic acid.

Dosage and Administration. *Orally.* The usual adult dosage is 1 tablet daily.

Availability:
CEFOL® Filmtabs in bottles of 100. **(Abbott)**

CELLULOSE, OXIDIZED

Description: Oxidized cellulose is an absorbable hemostatic agent prepared from cellulose by a special process that converts it into cellulosic acid (polyanhydroglucuronic acid). Oxidation of cellulose by nitrogen dioxide is controlled to yield an absorbable product of known acidity, and which is soluble in alkali. It appears in the form of surgical gauze or cotton that may vary from off-white to dusty-yellow in color, and which is somewhat more friable than the parent material. It does not enter into the normal physiologic clotting mechanism but, when applied to the bleeding area, it promotes clotting by a reaction between cellulosic acid and hemoglobin, thus forming an artificial clot. Since the cellulose swells on contact with blood, the resultant pressure adds to the hemostatic action. The cellulose is converted into a dark, reddish-brown or almost black, tenacious, adhesive mass which conforms and adheres readily to the bleeding surface. Twenty-four to 48 hours after application, it forms a gelatinous mass that can be removed without causing additional bleeding. If left in situ, absorption occurs between the 2nd and 7th day, depending on the size of the implant, the adequacy of the blood supply, and the degree of chemical degradation of the material. However, it may take 6 weeks or longer for complete absorbtion of large amounts of blood-soaked gauze.

Indications: For the control of capillary, venous, and small arterial hemorrhage when conventional methods are impractical or ineffective. Also indicated for use in oral surgery and exodontia.

Contraindications: This product should not be used for packing or implantation in fractures or laminectomies because it interferes with bone regeneration and can cause cyst formation. It is not recommended for use in hemorrhages from large arteries; on non-hemorrhagic serous-oozing surfaces; as a cover in vascular surgery; around the optic nerve or chiasm; or for application as a wadding or packing for hemostatic purposes.

Warnings: Oxidized cellulose is supplied sterile and *should not be autoclaved.* It should not be implanted in contaminated or infected wounds, nor should it be used as a substitute for careful surgery and the proper use of sutures and ligatures. The hemostatic action of this agent is greatest when it is applied dry and therefore should not be moistened with water or saline solution. It should not be impregnated with antiinfective or with buffering agents or with other hemostatic agents such as thrombin. Thrombin would be inactivated by the low pH of this agent. Although the gauze may be left in situ when necessary, it is advisable to remove it once hemostasis is achieved.

Precautions: Excess amounts should be removed prior to surgical closure to minimize the possibility of foreign-body reaction and to facilitate absorption. It should be packed loosely against bleeding surfaces. Wadding or packing tightly should be avoided, especially within the bony enclosure of the CNS and within other relatively rigid cavities where the extra pressure induced by the swelling mass of cellulose may interfere with normal function and may even cause necrosis. It should be used sparingly in open reduction of fractures and in cancellous bone. In urological procedures minimal amounts of the cellulose gauze should be employed and the patient should be observed carefully in the event that a portion of the cellulose becomes dislodged and plugs the urethra or ureter, or a catheter. It should not be used in sites of infection or following silver nitrate or other escharotic chemical agents. When used in large open wounds, it should be placed so as not to overlap the skin edges. It should also be removed from open wounds by forceps or by irrigation with sterile water or saline solution after bleeding has stopped.

Adverse Reactions: Those usually noted include foreign-body reactions with or without infection; necrosis of nasal mucous membrane or perforation of nasal septum due to tight packing; intestinal obstruction due to transmigration of a bolus of cellulose from the gallbladder to the terminal ileum or due to adhesions in a loop of denuded intestine to which this agent has been applied; urethral obstruction following retropubic prostatectomy and the introduction of cellulose within enucleated prostatic capsule. Headache, stinging sensations, and burning have been reported; sneezing in cases of epistaxis has been noted.

Dosage and Administration: *Topically,* to wounds at the operative site. The minimal amount required to control hemorrhage should be used and should be held firmly against the tissues until hemostasis is obtained.

Availability:
OXYCEL®. **(Parke-Davis)**
Pads (gauze type) 3 inches × 3 inches, 8 ply in packages of 10.
Pledgets (cotton type) 2 inches × 1 inch × 1 inch in packages of 10.
Strips (gauze type) 5 inches × 1/2 inch, 4 ply in individual packages; 18 inches × 2 inches, 4 ply in packages of 10; 36 inches × 1/2 inch, 4 ply in individual packages.

CEPHALEXIN MONOHYDRATE: see The Cephalosporins

CEPHALOGLYCIN: see The Cephalosporins

CEPHALORIDINE: see The Cephalosporins

THE CEPHALOSPORINS

Description: The cephalosporins are semisynthetic, broad-spectrum bactericidal antibiotics partly derived from the fungus *Cephalosporium acremonium* which produces cephalosporin C from which the cephalosporanic nucleus (7-aminocephalosporanic acid) is formed. The nucleus has 2 sites for substitution in the 3- and 7-position from which a series of semisynthetic derivatives are prepared. They are closely related chemically to the penicillins in that they contain a β-lactam ring as part of their nucleus and appear to be quantitatively and qualitatively similar in their mechanism of action to that of these agents. The cephalosporins interfere with the synthesis of the bacterial cell wall by inactivating the enzyme transpeptidase, thereby preventing a cross-linkage of peptidoglycan chains. This results in an accumulation of nucleotides in the cell and the appearance of morphologically abnormal organisms.

The cephalosporins are indicated in the treatment of infections caused by both gram-positive and gram-negative microorganisms sensitive to their action. They are active against *Proteus mirabilis, E. coli, H. influenzae,* and *Enterobacter* (Klebsiella) organisms, but not against the *Aerobacter* species, many strains of enterococci, indole-positive strains of *Proteus*, or virtually any strains of *Pseudomonas*.

Indications: Treatment of infections caused by sensitive gram-negative and gram-positive organisms, especially those of the respiratory tract caused by *Streptococcus (Diplococcus) pneumoniae* and group A *beta* hemolytic streptococci (follicular tonsillitis, bronchopneumonia, pneumonia, empyema, lung abscess); those of the genitourinary tract caused by *E. coli, P. mirabilis* and the *Klebsiella* species (acute and chronic pyelonephritis, cystitis, asymptomatic bacteriuria, and urethritis in the male), and skin and soft tissue infections (furunculosis, abscesses, infected burns, postoperative wound infections, infected descubitus ulcers, carbuncles, wound infections with cellulitis, symbiotic gangrene, pyoderma caused by pathogenic strains of coagulase-positive staphylococci). Also indicated in the treatment of *Hemophilus influenzae,* bacterial enteritis due to *Salmonella* strains of *Shigella,* and *Staphylococcus aureus* (penicillin-sensitive and penicillin-resistant), acute and chronic osteomyelitis, septic arthritis caused by staphylococci, streptococci and *Neisseria gonorrhoeae,* bacterial endocarditis, subacute bacterial endocarditis, septicemia due to susceptible bacteria, peritonitis, septic abortion and meningitis due to susceptible bacteria. They are indicated in the treatment of gonorrhea when penicillin is not considered the drug of choice. Data are presently insufficient to establish their efficacy in the prevention of rheumatic fever, even though cephapirin will eradicate group A streptococci from the nasopharnyx. However, penicillin is usually the drug of choice for the treatment and prevention of group A beta hemolytic streptococcal infection including prophylaxis of rheumatic fever. Therapy with a cephalosporin should ordinarily not be initiated until culture and sensitivity tests show that the organism is susceptible, and the patient's renal status has been determined.

Contraindications: In patients hypersensitive to the cephalosporin C group of antibiotics.

Warnings: Cephalosporin derivatives should be used with extreme caution in patients sensitive to penicillin since there is clinical and laboratory evidence of partial cross-allergenicity of these two agents. Instances of patients who have had severe reactions to both drugs, including death from anaphylaxis, have been reported. Patients with demonstrable allergies, particularly to drugs, should receive these agents cautiously and only when absolutely necessary. Epinephrine, oxygen, intravenous steroids, and airway management, including intubation should be readily available in the event of an acute reaction. Safe use during pregnancy and in premature infants or infants under 1 month of age has not been established. The most serious complication produced by cephaloridine is renal tubular necrosis; renal impairment has also been attributed to cephalothin, but the incidence is not as pronounced as with cephaloridine. Therefore, renal status should be determined prior to and during therapy with these drugs. Patients with known or suspected impairment of renal function should be under close clinical observation for changes in renal function. Cephaloridine should not be used in patients with azotemia. Some azotemic patients have been found to develop positive direct Coombs' test during therapy, although there has not been definite evidence of hemolytic anemia from the use of these drugs. In cases in which renal impairment is present, the drug should be used with caution and the dose reduced. The appearance of casts in the urine, proteinuria, falling urinary output, or a rising BUN or serum creatinine may indicate impairment of renal function. Routine precaution should be followed when these drugs are given concurrently with other antibiotics having nephrotoxic potential. The results of experimental studies in animals suggest that the concomitant use of potent diuretics, such as furosemide or ethacrynic acid, may increase the risk of renal toxicity.

Precautions: Prolonged use of any antibiotic may result in the overgrowth of nonsusceptible organisms. If superinfection occurs during therapy, the drug should be withdrawn and appropriate countermeasures instituted. A false-positive reaction for glycosuria may occur with Benedict's or Fehling's solution and with Clinitest® tablets but not with Tes-Tape®.

Adverse Reactions: Anorexia, dyspepsia, abdominal pain, nausea, vomiting, and diarrhea. Diarrhea, ranging from soft stools to frequent bowel movements, has been the reaction most frequently noted to date. Although diarrhea sufficiently severe to justify cessation of therapy occurred in a small percentage of patients, it apparently is not so much related to dosage as it is to a previous history of gastrointestinal disturbances due to other antibiotics. However, reducing the dosage or withdrawing the drug for 1 or 2 days when possible has alleviated the diarrhea in some instances, thereby permitting therapy to be continued. Hypersensitivity reactions attended by maculopapular rash, urticaria, anogenital pruritus, those resembling serum-sickness, and anaphylaxis have been noted. Eosinophilia and drug fever were more likely to occur in patients with a history of allergy to drugs, particularly to penicillin. Rare instances of neutropenia, leukopenia, thrombocytopenia, and anemia were reported. Some individuals, particularly those with azotemia, have developed a positive direct and indirect Coombs' test during therapy with some of the cephalosporins. Transient rise in SGPT, SGOT, alkaline phosphatase, and bilirubin levels and elevation in BUN (frequently occurs in patients over 50 years of age) have also been observed without clinical evidence of renal or hepatic impairment. Other complications which developed were genital moniliasis, vaginitis and vaginal discharge, oral candidiasis (oral thrush), malaise, fever, chills, dizziness or vertigo, fatigue, headache, pain at the injection site after intramuscular administration, some with induration, and phlebitis at the site of injection.

The preceding discussed briefly the physiologic, clinical and therapeutic similarities of the cephalosporins as a group. The individual monographs which follow review specifically each of the following cephalosporins:

Cefadroxil Monohydrate
Cefamandole Nafate
Cefazolin Sodium
Cephalexin Monohydrate
Cephaloglycin
Cephaloridine
Cephalothin Sodium
Cephapirin Sodium
Cephradine

CEFADROXIL MONOHYDRATE

Chemical Name: 7-[[D-2-Amino-2-(4-hydroxyphenyl)acetyl]amino]-3-methyl-8-oxo-5-thia-1-azabicyclo[4.2.0]oct-2-ene-2-carboxylic acid monohydrate.

Description: Cefadroxil monohydrate is an acid-stable, semisynthetic cephalosporin antibiotic intended for oral use only. In common with other members of this group, its bactericidal action appears to be due to interference with cell-wall synthesis. It possesses an antimicrobial spectrum similar to that of other cephalosporins, but cefadroxil's duration of action has been reported to be significantly prolonged. Many pathogens that infect the urinary tract such as *Escherichia coli, Klebsiella* species and *Proteus mirabilis* readily respond to its action; however, it is not effective against *Pseudomonas* and *Herella* species, and most strains of enterococci (*Streptococcus faecalis* and *S. faecium*), *Enterobacter, Pr. morganii* and *Pr. vulgaris*. It occurs as a white to yellowish-white, crystalline powder that is soluble in water.

The drug is rapidly absorbed from the gastrointestinal tract producing peak serum levels of approximately 16 and 28 mcg/ml following oral doses of 0.5 and 1 gm respectively. These decline gradually with only measurable levels obtainable at 12 hours. Over 90% of the drug is excreted unchanged in the urine within 8 hours. Urine concentrations are dose-related, and a peak level of approximately 1800 mcg/ml is usually attained following a single dose of 0.5 gm. The urine antibiotic concentration was found to be maintained well above the MIC of all typical urinary pathogens for 12 hours and, in most instances, for 18 hours.

Indications: Treatment of urinary tract infections caused by *E. coli, Pr. mirabilis,* and *Klebsiella* species.

For contraindications, warnings and precautions, see general statement.

Adverse Reactions: The most frequent untoward effect is nausea, which occasionally is severe enough to warrant discontinuing the medication. Administration with food generally decreases this complication while not appreciably affecting absorption of the antibiotic. Diarrhea and dysuria also have been observed. Allergies in the form of rash, urticaria, and angioedema have occurred, but these usually subsided upon withdrawal of the drug. Other reactions have included genital pruritus and/or moniliasis; vaginitis; and moderate, transient neutropenia.

Dosage and Administration: *Orally.* The usual adult dosage is 2 capsules twice daily for patients with normal renal function or for those with only mild renal insufficiency (creatinine clearance of over 50 ml/minute). The usual daily dose may be given every 12 hours if the creatinine clearance is 25 to 50 ml/minute; every 24 hours if 10 to 25 ml/minute, and every 36 hours if 0 to 10 ml/minute. Cefadroxil may be taken without regard to meals. Safe use and proper dosage have not been established for patients in the pediatric age group.

Availability:
DURICEF® Capsules, 500 mg in bottles of 24 and 100. **(Mead Johnson)**

CEFAMANDOLE NAFATE

Chemical Name: 7-D-Mandelamido-3-[[(1-methyl-1*H*-tetrazol-5-yl-thio-]methyl]-3-cephem-4-carboxylic acid formate sodium.

Description: Cefamandole nafate is a semisynthetic, bactericidal, cephalosporin antibiotic designed for parenteral administration. Its broad-spectrum activity is directed against many strains of gram-positive and gram-negative organisms. Susceptible strains generally include *Staphylococcus aureus,* including penicillinase and nonpenicillinase producing strains, *Staphylococcus epidermidis, Beta-hemolytic* and other streptococci, *Streptococcus pneumoniae, Escherichia coli, Klebsiella* species, *Enterobacter* species (initially-susceptible organisms may become resistant during therapy), *Haemophilus influenzae, Pr. mirabilis, Pr. rettgeri, Pr. morganii,* some strains of *Pr. vulgaris, Peptococcus* and *Peptostreptococcus* species, gram-positive bacilli (including *Clostridium* species) and gram-negative bacilli (including *Bacteroides* and *Fusobacterium* species). However, most strains of enterococci *(Streptococcus faecalis)* and some strains of *Pr. vulgaris* are resistant to its antibacterial effects. Those uniformly resistant to cephalosporins in general include most strains of *Bacteroides fragilis, Serratia, Pseudomonas, Acinetobacter calcoaceticus* (formerly *Mima* and *Herellea* species).

Following dilution, cefamandole nafate is rapidly hydrolyzed to cefamandole, and both compounds have microbiologic activity in vivo. Each gm of the drug contains approximately 77 mg (3.3 mEq) of sodium. The normal pH range of freshly prepared solutions is between 6 to 8.5.

The intramuscular administration of 0.5 or 1 gm produced peak plasma concentrations of 13 and 25 mcg/ml respectively within 1/2 to 2 hours, and the intravenous administration of 1, 2 and 3 gm produced peak plasma concentrations of 139, 240 and 533 mcg/ml respectively in 10 minutes, declining to 0.8, 2.2, and 2.9 mcg/ml respectively in 4 hours. Intravenous doses of 4 gm every 6 hours produced no evidence of accumulation of the drug in the serum. The half-life is 60 minutes after an intramuscular injection and 32 minutes after an intravenous injection. Approximately 65 to 85% is excreted by the kidneys over an 8-hour period resulting in high urinary concentrations. Following intramuscular doses of 0.5 and 1 gm, urinary concentrations average 254 and 1357 mcg/ml respectively, while intravenous doses of 1 and 2 gm produced urinary levels averaging 750 and 1380 mcg/ml respectively. The antibiotic reaches therapeutic levels in pleural and joint fluids, in bile and in bone tissue.

Susceptible strains may be determined by employing the Bauer-Kirby-Sherris-Turck method. A disc containing 30 mcg of cefamandole should give a zone of 18 mm or greater when tested against a cefamandole-susceptible bacterial strain, and a zone of 15 to 17 mm with an organism of intermediate susceptibility. Resistant organisms produce zones of 14 mm or less, indicating that other therapy should be selected. Probenecid has been reported to slow tubular excretion thereby raising and prolonging the serum concentration of the drug.

Indications: Treatment of susceptible infections of the lower respiratory tract, including pneumonia; urinary tract infections; septicemia; skin and soft tissue infections; peritonitis; and pelvic (nongonococcal) inflammatory diseases in the female.

For contraindications, warnings and precautions, see general statement.

Adverse Reactions: Side effects observed in patients are generally mild in nature, and include hypersensitivity reactions manifested by maculopapular rash, urticaria, eosinophilia, and drug fever; hematological reactions by neutropenia, thrombocytopenia, and a positive direct Coombs' test. Other reactions noted include transient increases in SGOT, SGPT, and alkaline phosphatase levels; decreased creatinine clearance in patients with prior renal impairment; transitory elevations of BUN; infrequent pain on intramuscular injection, and rare instances of thrombophlebitis.

Dosage and Administration: The physician is urged to read carefully the package literature for proper methods of dilution, storage, etc. Cefamandole may be administered *intravenously* or by deep *intramuscular* injection into a large muscle mass such as the gluteal muscle or the lateral aspect of the thigh. The usual adult dosage ranges from 0.5 to 1 gm every 4 to 8 hours. Soft skin infections and uncomplicated pneumonia may be treated adequately with 0.5 gm every 8 hours. For urinary tract infections, a dosage of 0.5 to 1 gm every 8 hours may be needed. More severe infections may be treated with 1 gm every 4 to 6 hours. Doses up to 2 gm every 4 hours may be needed in life-threatening infections. In infants and children, a daily total dosage of 50 to 100 mg/kg of body weight, in equally divided doses every 4 to 8 hours has been found to be effective in mild to moderately severe infections. A daily total dosage of 150 mg/kg of body weight (not to exceed the maximum adult dose) may be needed for more serious infections. Treatment should be continued for a minimum of 48 to 72 hours after the patient becomes asymtomatic or after evidence of bacterial eradication has been obtained. A minimum of 10 days is recommended in infections caused by group A beta-hemolytic streptococci in order to guard against the risk of rheumatic fever or glomerulonephritis. If combination therapy with an aminoglycoside is indicated, each drug should be added to a separate syringe and administered in different sites. The aminoglycoside should *never* be mixed with cefamandole in the same intravenous container. The intravenous route may be preferable for patients with bacterial septicemia, localized parenchymal abscesses, peritonitis or other severe or life-threatening infections when they may be poor risks because of lowered resistance. In those with normal renal function, the intravenous dosage for such infections is 3 to 12 gm daily. For intermittent administration, a solution of cefamandole, 1 gm/10 ml, is injected slowly directly into a vein over a period of 3 to 5 minutes or it may be given through the tubing of a running infusion. A continuous intravenous infusion may be obtained by diluting 1 gm with 10 ml of diluent and adding an appropriate quantity of this solution to an IV bottle. Cefamandole is compatible with sterile distilled water, normal saline or dextrose solutions. When renal function is impaired, a reduced dosage must be employed and the serum levels closely monitored. Continued dosage schedule should be determined by the degree of renal impairment, severity of the infection and susceptibility of the causative organism.

Availability:
MANDOLE® Dry Powder in vials of 0.5, 1 and 2 gm. **(Lilly)**

CEFAZOLIN SODIUM

Chemical Name: 3-{[(5-methyl-1, 3, 4-thiadiazol-2-yl)-thio]methyl}-7-[2-(1*H*-tetrazol-1-yl) acetamido]-3-cephem-4-carboxylic acid sodium.

Description: Cefazolin sodium is a semisynthetic, bactericidal, cephalosporin antibiotic. The bactericidal action appears to be due to the inactivation of the bacterial enzyme transpeptidase thus hindering cell-wall synthesis. The normal pH range for optimum chemical stability for reconstituted cefazolin is between 5 and 7. In more acidic or alkaline media, it is hydrolyzed to products that possess little or no antibacterial activity. Each gm of the drug contains 46 mg (2 mEq) of sodium.

The intramuscular administration of 250 or 500 mg produced peak plasma concentrations of approximately 17 and 37 mcg/ml respectively in 1 hour and measurable amounts were obtainable 6 to 8 hours after injection. Normal adults receiving constant intravenous infusion with dosages of 3.5 mg/kg of body weight for 1 hour (approx. 250 mg) and 1.5 mg/kg the next 2 hours (approx. 100 mg) showed a steady serum level at the third hour of about 28 mcg/ml. Controlled studies on adult normal volunteers who received 1 gm 4 times daily for 10 days indicated no clinically significant changes in CBC, SGOT, SGPT, bilirubin, alkaline phosphatase, BUN and creatinine levels, and urinalysis.

The drug is excreted in unchanged form in the urine; 60% within the first 6 hours and 70 to 80% within 24 hours with peak urine concentrations of approximately 2400 mcg/ml and 4000 mcg/ml respectively following 500 mg and 1 gm intramuscular dose. In three separate studies, the serum half-life of the drug when administered intramuscularly was reported to be 1.8 to 2.2 hours in patients with normal renal function, as compared with 1.2 to 1.5 hours for cephaloridine and 0.5 hours for cephalothin. Bile and synovial fluid levels are about 1/2 that of serum concentration. About 86% of cefazolin is bound to plasma protein. Studies of cord blood showed prompt transfer of the drug across the placenta; and it was found to be present in very low concentrations in the milk of lactating mothers. Probenecid has been reported to slow tubular excretion thereby raising and prolonging the serum concentration of the drug.

Most strains of Enterobacter cloacae and indole positive Proteus (*P. vulgaris, P. morganii, P. rettgeri)* are resistant. Methicillin-resistant staphylococci, serratia, pseudomonas, mima, herellea species are almost uniformly resistant to cefazolin.

Indications: Cefazolin is indicated in the treatment of infections such as respiratory tract, genitourinary tract and skin and soft tissue infections, bone and joint infections, septicemia, and endocarditis caused by both gram-positive and gram-negative microorganisms sensitive to its action. These include *Escherichia coli, Proteus mirabilis, Klebsiella* species, some strains of enterobacter and enterococci, *Staphylococcus aureus* (penicillin-sensitive and penicillin-resistant), group A beta-hemolytic streptococci and other strains of streptococci and *Streptococcus (Diplococcus) pneumoniae.* **Note:** The organism should be cultured and its susceptibility to cefazolin should be established. Data are presently insufficient to establish that cefazolin will prevent rheumatic fever even though it will eradicate group A streptococci from the nasopharynx.

For contraindications, warnings and precautions, see general statement.

Adverse Reactions: The following complications have been reported: Hypersensitivity reactions manifested by drug fever, skin rash, vulvar pruritus, and eosinophilia have occurred. Other reactions noted included neutropenia, leukopenia, thrombocythemia, positive direct and indirect Coombs' test; also a transient rise in SGOT, SGPT, BUN and alkaline phosphatase levels have been observed without clinical evidence of renal or hepatic impairment. Other reactions reported were nausea, anorexia, vomiting, diarrhea, oral candidiasis (oral thrush); pain at the injection site after intramuscular administration, some with induration, and phlebitis at the site of injection, as well as genital and anal pruritus, genital moniliasis, and vaginitis.

Dosage and Administration: The clinician is urged to read carefully the package literature for proper methods of storage, dilution, etc. Cefazolin may be administered *intravenously* or by deep *intramuscular* injection into a large muscle mass such as the gluteal muscle or the lateral aspect of the thigh. **Adults:** The usual dosage for mild gram-positive infections is 250 to 500 mg every 8 hours and for acute uncomplicated urinary tract infections 1 gm every 12 hours. For moderate or severe infections, the usual dosage is 500 mg to 1 gm every 6 to 8 hours. For pneumococcal pneumonia, the usual dosage is 500 mg every 12 hours. For serious infections such as endocarditis and septicemia, a dosage of 6 to 12 gm daily has been administered. Patients with reduced renal function should receive the following dosage adjustments: For mild to moderate renal impairment (creatinine clearance of 40 to 60 ml/min) 60% of the normal daily dose and for moderate renal impairment (creatinine clearance of 20 to 40 ml/min) 25% of the normal daily dosage. These are given in divided doses every 12 hours. For marked impairment (creatinine clearance of 5 to 20 ml/min) 10% of the normal daily dose given every 24 hours should be adequate. All dosage recommendations apply after an initial loading dose of 500 mg. **Children:** A total daily dosage of 25 to 50 mg/kg (approx. 10 to 20 mg/lb) of body weight divided into 3 or 4 equal doses is effective for most mild to moderately severe infections, and for severe infections the dosage may be increased to 100 mg/kg (45 mg/lb) of body weight. Until further clinical experience is gained, the drug is not recommended for use in premature infants and in infants under 1 month of age.

Availability:
ANCEF® Dry Powder in vials of 250 and 500 mg and 1 gm and in piggyback vials of 500 mg, 1, 5 and 10 gm. **(Smith Kline & French)**
KEFZOL® Dry Powder in ampuls of 250 and 500 mg and 1 and 10 gm. **(Lilly)**

CEPHALEXIN MONOHYDRATE

Chemical Name: 7-(D-α-amino-α-phenylactamido)-3-methyl-3-cephem-4-carboxylic acid, monohydrate.

Description: Cephalexin monohydrate is an acid-stable, semi-synthetic, oral, cephalosporin antibiotic. The bactericidal action of the drug appears to be due to its interference with cellwall synthesis. However, most strains of enterococci *(Streptococcus faecalis)* and a few strains of staphylococci are resistant to cephalexin. It is also not active against many strains of *Enterobacter* species, *Pr. morganii*, and *Pr. vulgaris* and shows no activity against *Pseudomonas* or *Herellea* species. In-vitro tests reveal that staphylococci exhibit cross-resistance between cephalexin and the methicillin-type antibiotics.

The oral administration of 250 or 500 mg or 1 gm produced a peak plasma concentration of approximately 9, 18 and 32 mcg/ml respectively in 1 hour and measurable amounts were obtainable 6 hours after administration. Over 90% of the drug was excreted unchanged in the urine within 8 hours with peak urine concentration of about 1 mg/ml following a 250-mg dose, 2.2 mg/ml following a 500-mg dose and 5 mg/ml following a 1-gm dose.

Indications: Treatment of respiratory tract infections caused by *Streptococcus (Diplococcus) pneumoniae* and group A beta-hemolytic streptococci; staphylococci-induced infections of the skin and soft tissues; otitis media due to *Diplococcus pneumoniae, H. influenzae*, staphylococci, streptococci, and *N. catarrhalis;* osteomyelitis caused by staphylococci and/or *Pr. mirabilis;* and genitourinary tract infections including acute prostatitis caused by *Esch. coli, Pr. mirabilis* and *Klebsiella* species. Its efficacy in the prevention of rheumatic fever has not been established; however, penicillin is usually the drug of choice for the treatment and prevention of streptococcus infection including prophylaxis of rheumatic fever.

For contraindications, warnings, and precautions, see general statement.

Adverse Reactions: The most frequent side effect has been diarrhea, but this was rarely severe enough to warrant cessation of therapy; nausea, vomiting, dyspepsia, and abdominal pain have also been encountered. Other reactions included allergies in the form of rash, urticaria, and angioedema which usually subsided upon discontinuation of the drug; genital and anal pruritus, genital moniliasis, vaginitis and vaginal discharge; dizziness, fatigue, and headache; eosinophilia, neutropenia and slight elevations of SGOT and SGPT.

Dosage and Administration: *Orally.* The adult dosage ranges from 1 to 4 gm daily in divided doses. The usual adult dose is 250 mg every 6 hours. For more severe infections or those caused by less susceptible organisms, larger doses may be needed. If daily doses of more than 4 gm are required, parenteral cephalosporins, in appropriate dosage, should be administered. The recommended daily dosage for children is 25 to 50 mg/kg of body weight divided into 4 doses; dosage may be doubled for severe infections. Otitis media generally requires from 75 to 100 mg/kg of body weight divided into 4 doses. Culture and susceptibility tests should be initiated prior to, and during, therapy. If given for the treatment of beta-hemolytic streptococcal infections, the drug should be administered for at least 10 days in therapeutic dosages.

Availability:
KEFLEX®: **(Lilly)**
Oral Suspension, 125 mg/5 ml (equivalent) in bottles of 60, 100 and 200 ml and in Identi-Dose® (unit-dose) of 5 ml; 250 mg/5 ml in bottles of 100 and 200 ml and in Identi-Dose (unit-dose) of 5 ml.
Pediatric Drops, 100 mg/ml (5 mg/drop) (equivalent) in bottles of 10 ml with calibrated dropper.
Pulvules (capsules), 250 and 500 mg (equivalent) in bottles of 24 and 100 and in Identi-Dose (unit-dose) in packages of 100.
Tablets, 1 gm in bottles of 24 and in unit-dose packages of 100.

CEPHALOGLYCIN

Chemical Name: 7-(D-α-Aminophenylacetamido)cephalosporanic acid, zwitterion form.

Description: Cephaloglycin is a phenylglycine analogue of the antibiotic, cephalosporin C. The bactericidal activity of the cephalosporins is said to stem from their ability to inhibit the synthesis of protein in the bacterial cell wall. Food has no significant effect on the total amount of drug absorbed, although the excretion of peak urinary levels, which may exceed 1.3 mg/ml following an oral dose of 500 mg, may be delayed. Cephaloglycin is excreted in the urine almost entirely as the active metabolite, desacetylcephaloglycin.

Indications: Treatment of acute and chronic infections of the urinary tract, including cystitis, pyelitis, pyelonephritis and "asymptomatic bacteriuria," when caused by susceptible strains of *E. coli, Klebsiella-Aerobacter,* some species of *Proteus, staphylococci* and *enterococci.*

For contraindications, warnings, precautions, see general statement.

Adverse Reactions: Nausea, vomiting and diarrhea. Diarrhea, ranging from soft stools to frequent bowel movements, has been the reaction most frequently noted to date. Although diarrhea sufficiently severe to justify cessation of therapy occurred in a small percentage of patients, it apparently is not as much related to dosage as it is to a previous history of gastrointestinal disturbances due to other antibiotics. However, reducing the dosage or withdrawing the drug for 1 or 2 days when possible has alleviated the diarrhea in some instances permitting therapy to be continued. An allergic reaction as manifested by skin rash, urticaria, angioedema or exfoliative dermatitis has occurred in about 3% of patients, a situation readily controlled by discontinuing therapy. Other reactions reported include monilial vaginitis, malaise, fever, chills, headache and dizziness or vertigo. Eosinophilia has been reported infrequently. No consistent alteration in the hematocrit level, WBC count, urinalysis, BUN or SGOT could be attributed to cephaloglycin.

Dosage and Administration: *Orally,* before, during or after meals. Adults: 250 or 500 mg 4 times daily, depending upon the severity of the urinary infection. If larger doses are deemed necessary, initial therapy with the injectable cephalosporins should be considered. Children: 25 to 50 mg/kg/day is suggested. Any infection unresponsive to treatment indicates the need for further study of the susceptibility of the offending organism, a thorough investigation of the urinary tract or both. Not recommended for use in premature infants and in infants under 1 month of age.

Availability:
KAFOCIN® Pulvules (Capsules), 250 mg in bottles of 100 and in Identi-Dose® (unit-dose packages) of 100. **(Lilly)**

CEPHALORIDINE

Chemical Name: 7-(Thiophene-2-acetamido)-3-(1-pyridylmethyl)-3-cephem-4-carboxylic acid betaine.

Description: Cephaloridine, a semisynthetic derivative of the antibiotic cephalosporin C, is produced by the organism *Cephalosporium acremonium.* It is structurally similar to sodium cephalothin, differing only in the substitution of a pyridine group for the acetoxy group in position 3 of the cephalosporanic acid nucleus and in zwitterion formation, thus making it unnecessary to solubilize the drug in the form of a sodium salt. Therefore, cephaloridine contains neither inorganic anions nor cations. The drug occurs as a white, crystalline powder very soluble in water, forming aqueous solutions with a pH of 4.5 to 5.

The mechanism of action of cephaloridine may be similar to that of sodium cephalothin and the penicillins; cephaloridine appears to inhibit mucopeptide synthesis in the bacterial cell wall. The drug is both bactericidal and bacteriostatic. Peak serum concentrations of 7 and 14 mcg/ml following an intramuscular dose of 250 and 500 mg respectively are generally reached within ½ to 1 hour with detectable amounts being present in serum after 12 hours. The drug is excreted unchanged in the urine; approximately 65 to 75% of an administered dose is excreted during a 24-hour period following administration, most of which occurs within the first 6 hours.

Indications: Treatment of serious infections of the respiratory tract, genitourinary tract (including gonorrheal urethritis in the male), bones and joints, bloodstream, soft tissue, and skin due to susceptible strains of *beta*-hemolytic and other streptococci (many strains of enterococci such as *Streptococcus faecalis* are relatively resistant); staphylococci, both coagulase-negative and coagulase-positive (some strains of staphylococci are resistant to cephaloridine); pneumococci; gonococci; *Haemophilus influenzae; E. coli* and other coliform bacteria;

Klebsiella, Proteus mirabilis and *Treponema pallidum*. It is indicated in the treatment of gonorrhea when penicillin is not considered to be the drug of choice, and in early syphilis when penicillin is contraindicated. The drug should not be used until culture and sensitivity tests show that the organism is susceptible and the patient's renal status has been determined. For this reason, the drug normally should not be used to initiate therapy.

For contraindications, warnings and precautions, see general statement.

Adverse Reactions: Reactions have been reported as having occurred in a small percentage of patients. They include nausea, vomiting, maculopapular and erythematous rashes, urticaria, anaphylaxis, drug fever and eosinophilia have been reported. Hypersensitivity reactions are more likely to occur in patients with a history of allergy, particularly to penicillin. Other unfavorable responses included neutropenia and leukopenia. Some individuals have developed positive direct Coombs' test during therapy. Transient elevations of transaminase and alkaline phosphatase levels, pain at the site of intramuscular injection, and phlebitis at the site of intravenous injection. Severe, acute renal failure had occurred in a few patients, some of which proved fatal. The possibility of renal failure seems to be greater in seriously ill patients given cephaloridine in doses in excess of those recommended. Postmortem examination of affected patients revealed the presence of acute tubular necrosis.

Dosage and Administration: The clinician is urged to read carefully the package literature for proper methods of storage, dilution, etc. Cephaloridine usually is injected *intramuscularly* into a large muscle mass such as the gluteal muscle or the lateral aspect of the thigh. The usual adult dosage for infections of moderate severity is 500 mg to 1 gm 3 times daily. Milder and more susceptible infections have been treated with 250 to 500 mg 2 or 3 times daily. More severe infections may be treated with 500 mg to 1 gm 4 times daily. A single dose of 2 gm is recommended for the treatment of acute gonorrhea and doses of 0.5 to 1 gm daily for 10 to 14 days for early syphilis. In children, a daily total of 30 to 50 mg/kg (15 to 25 mg/lb) of body weight, in divided doses, has been found effective in mild to moderately severe infections. A daily total dosage of 100 mg/kg (50 mg/lb) of body weight (not to exceed doses recommended for adults) may be needed for very severe infections. It is not recommended for use in premature infants and in infants under 1 month of age until further studies establish its safe use in patients of this age group. *Intravenous* administration may be indicated when the infection seems overwhelming or when it is extremely serious (such as bacteremia). Total daily dosages are the same as those for intramuscular injection. For very susceptible organisms, 500 mg to 1.5 gm/day may be sufficient; for less susceptible organisms and for serious infections, 2 to 4 gm/day may be needed. If very high intermittent levels of antibiotic are desired, 500 mg or 1 gm of cephaloridine dissolved respectively in 5 or 10 ml of diluent may be injected slowly (over a period of 3 or 4 minutes 3 or 4 times daily) directly into a vein or into the tubing of a running infusion. A continuous infusion may be obtained by adding the total daily dosage to the daily volume of fluid being administered intravenously. Cephaloridine is compatible with distilled water, normal saline, or dextrose solutions. In the case of infections due to beta-hemolytic streptococci, antibiotic therapy should be continued for at least 10 days.

Availability:
LORIDINE® Injection (dry powder), 0.5 and 1 gm in vials of 10 ml. **(Lilly)**

CEPHALOTHIN SODIUM

Chemical Name: 7-(Thiophene-2-acetamido) cephalosporanic acid sodium.

Description: Sodium cephalothin, a broad-spectrum bactericidal antibiotic, is obtained by the interaction between thiophene-2-acetic acid and 7-aminocephalosporanic acid. The cephalosporanic acid nucleus is obtained from cephalosporin C, which is produced by the fungus *Cephalosporium*. It is structurally similar to cephaloridine and to the penicillins. It occurs as a cream-colored, crystalline powder freely soluble in water, forming aqueous solutions with a pH of 5.2. Solutions of the drug are incompatible with compounds of high molecular weight or with alkaline earth metals or with solutions having a pH below 4 or above 7.

The mechanism by which it acts may be similar to that of penicillin and of cephaloridine; it apparently inhibits mucopeptide synthesis in the bacterial cell wall. The drug is bactericidal as well as bacteriostatic. Purified penicillinase has little activity against cephalothin. Peak serum concentrations are generally reached within 1/2 to 1 hour following intramuscular injection, and within 15 to 30 minutes following intravenous injection; detectable amounts being present in the serum of patients with normal renal function by the fourth hour. The drug is excreted in the urine, unchanged and as the desacetyl metabolite, most of which occurs within 6 hours.

Susceptible strains may be determined by employing the Bauer-Kirby-Sherris-Turck method. A disc containing 30 mcg of cephalothin should give a zone of over 17 mm when tested against a cephalothin-susceptible bacterial strain, and a zone of over 14 mm with an organism of intermediate susceptibility. Probenecid has been reported to slow tubular excretion thereby raising and prolonging the serum concentration of the drug.

Indications: Treatment of infections caused by sensitive gram-negative and gram-positive organisms, such as follicular tonsillitis, bronchopneumonia, pneumonia, empyema, lung abscess, acute and chronic pyelonephritis, cystitis, asymptomatic bacteriuria, furunculosis, abscesses, infected burns, postoperative wound infections, infected decubitus ulcers, carbuncles, wound infection with cellulitis, symbiotic gangrene, pyodermas caused by pathogenic strains of coagulase-positive staphylococci, group A *beta*-hemolytic streptococci and gram-negative organisms, bacterial enteritis due to *Salmonella,* strains of *Shigella,* and *Staphylococcus aureus,* acute and chronic osteomyelitis, septic arthritis caused by staphylococci, streptococci and *Neisseria gonorrhoeae,* bacterial endocarditis, subacute bacterial endocarditis, septicemia due to susceptible bacteria, peritonitis, septic abortion, and meningitis due to susceptible bacteria. Before initiating treatment for any infection, the offending organism should be cultured and its susceptibility to cephalothin should be firmly established.

For contraindications, warnings and precautions, see general statement.

Adverse Reactions: *Hypersensitivity*—Maculopapular rash, urticaria, reactions resembling serum sickness, and anaphylaxis have been reported. Eosinophilia and drug fever have been reported as associated with other allergic reactions. These reactions are most likely to occur in patients with a history of allergy, particularly to penicillin. *Blood*—Neutropenia, thrombocytopenia, and hemolytic anemia have been reported. Some individuals, particularly those with azotemia, have developed positive direct Coombs' tests during cephalothin therapy. *Liver*—Transient rise in SGOT has been reported. *Kidney*—Rise in BUN and decrease in creatinine clearance have been observed; however, some patients with elevated BUN at the beginning of cephalothin therapy have had values return to normal during therapy. *Local Reactions*—Pain, induration, tenderness, and elevation of temperature have been reported following repeated intramuscular injections. Thrombophlebitis has occurred and is usually associated with daily doses of over 6 gm given by infusion for more than three days.

Dosage and Administration: The clinician is urged to read carefully the package literature for the proper methods of preparing solutions, etc. Cephalothin may be given *intravenously* or by deep *intramuscular* injection into a large muscle mass to minimize pain and induration. The usual dosage for adults is 500 mg to 1 gm every 4 to 6 hours, increased if necessary in severe infections by giving the injections every 4 hours or, when the desired response is not obtained, by raising the dose to 1 gm. In life-threatening infections, doses up to 2 gm every 4 hours may be required. When renal function is reduced, an intravenous loading dose of 1 to 2 gm may be given. Continued dosage schedule should be determined by the degree of renal impairment, severity of infection and susceptibility of the causative organism. In infants and children, the dosage should be proportionately less in accordance with age, weight and severity of infection. Daily administration of 100 mg/kg (80 to 160 mg/kg) in divided doses has been found effective in most infections caused by susceptible organisms. For bacteremia, septicemia, or other severe or life-threatening infections in severely debilitated patients, the intravenous dosage is 4 to 12 gm daily. For intermittent administration, a solution of cephalothin, 1 gm/10 ml, is injected slowly directly into a vein over a period of 3 to 5 minutes or it may be given through the tubing of a running infusion. In *peritoneal dialysis* procedures, cephalothin has been added to dialysis fluid in concentrations of up to 6 mg/100 ml and instilled into the peritoneal space throughout an entire dialysis (16 to 30 hours). Careful assay procedures have shown that 44% of the administered drug was absorbed into the bloodstream. Serum levels of 10 mcg/ml were reported, with no evidence of accumulation and no untoward local or systemic reactions.

Availability:
KEFLIN® Injection (dry powder), 1 gm in ampuls of 10 and 100 ml; 2 gm in ampuls of 20 and 100 ml; 4 gm in ampuls of 50 ml and 20 gm in ampuls of 200 ml. **(Lilly)**

CEPHAPIRIN SODIUM

Chemical Name: 7-[α-(4-Pyridylthio)-acetamide-]-cephalosporanic acid sodium.

Description: Sodium cephapirin is a broad-spectrum cephalosporin antibiotic that is intended for parenteral use. In common with other cephalosporins its bactericidal action appears to be due to interference with cell-wall synthesis. In vitro studies reveal that it is active against streptococcal organisms including *Beta-hemolytic streptococci*, staphylococcal coagulase-positive and coagulase-negative strains, and penicillinase and nonpenicillinase producing strains, pneumococci, *Haemophilus influenzae, Proteus mirabilis, Escherichia coli*, and the *Klebsiella* species. However, many strains of enterococci such as *Streptococcus faecalis* and some strains of staphylococci are resistant to cephapirin. It is also not active against most strains of the *Enterobacter* species and the indole-positive Proteus *(P. vulgaris, P. morganii*, and *P. rettgeri)*. Methicillin-resistant staphylococci, *Serratia, Pseudomonas, Mima* and the *Herellea* species are almost uniformly resistant to this antibiotic.

Intramuscular administration of 0.5 and 1 gm produced peak plasma concentrations of approximately 9 and 16.4 mcg/ml respectively in 30 minutes and measurable amounts were obtainable 6 hours after injection. Intravenous administration of a 0.5-, 1-, and 2-gm dose produced peak plasma concentrations of approximately 35, 67, and 129 mcg/ml respectively at 5 minutes, and measurable amounts were detected 3 hours later. Each 500-mg dose contains 1.07 mEq of sodium.

Between 44 and 50% of cephapirin is bound to plasma proteins; its average half-life in patients with normal renal function is about 36 minutes. Approximately 70% of the drug is excreted unchanged and as the active desacetyl metabolite, most of which occurs within 6 hours.

Indications: Treatment of susceptible infections of the respiratory and urinary tracts, skin and soft tissue infections and bacteremia including endocarditis and osteomyelitis. Cephapirin is effective in the eradication of streptococci from the nasopharynx; however, data establishing its effectiveness in the subsequent prevention of rheumatic fever are not available. Parenteral benzathine penicillin is considered to be the drug of choice in the treatment and prevention of streptococcal infections, including the prophylaxis of rheumatic fever. **Note:** Before initiating treatment for any infection, the offending organism should be cultured and its susceptibility to cephapirin should be firmly established.

For contraindications, warnings and precautions, see general statement.

Adverse Reactions: Hypersensitivity reactions manifested by maculopapular rash, urticaria, those resembling serum-sickness, and anaphylaxis have been reported. Eosinophilia and drug fever were more likely to occur in patients with a history of allergy to drugs, particularly to penicillin. Rare instances of neutropenia, leukopenia, and anemia were reported. Some individuals, particularly those with azotemia, have developed positive direct Coombs' test during therapy with other cephalosporins. Elevations in SGPT or SGOT, alkaline phosphatase, bilirubin, and rises in BUN (frequency increases in patients over 50 years of age) have also been noted.

Dosage and Administration: The clinician is urged to read carefully the package literature for proper methods of storage, dilution, etc. Cephapirin may be administered *intravenously* or by deep *intramuscular* injection into a large muscle mass such as the gluteal muscle or the lateral aspect of the thigh. The 1-gm vial should be reconstituted with 2 ml of Sterile Water for Injection; each 1.2 ml contains 500 mg of the drug. The intravenous route may be preferable for patients with bacteremia, septicemia, or other severe or life-threatening infections. Adults: The usual dosage is 6 to 8 gm daily for several days, then depending on the clinical response and laboratory findings, the dosage may gradually be reduced. Up to 12 gm daily may be used for infections that have been refractory to previous forms of treatment. *For intermittent intravenous* injections, the contents of the 1- or 2-gm vial should be diluted with 10 ml or more of diluent and administered slowly over a 3- to 5-minute period, or may be given with intravenous infusion. *For continuous intravenous infusion,* the choice of diluent and volume should be dictated by the fluid and electrolyte management of the patient.

Availability:
CEFADYL® Dry Powder in vials of 1 and 2 gm and in piggyback vials of 1, 2, 4 and 20 gm.
(Bristol)

CEPHRADINE

Chemical Name: 7-[D-2-amino-2-(1,4-cyclohexadien-1-yl) acetamido]-3-methyl-8-oxo-5-thia-1-azabicyclo [4.2.0.]-oct-2-ene-2-carboxylic acid.

Description: Cephradine is an acid-stable, semi-synthetic, cephalosporin antibiotic that is intended for both oral and parenteral use. The bactericidal action appears to be due to the interference with cell-wall synthesis. However, some strains of enterococci *(Streptococcus faecalis)* are resistant to cephradine. It is not active against most strains of *Enterobacter* species, *Pr. morganii,* and *Pr. vulgaris* and shows no activity against *Pseudomonas* or *Herellea* species. In vitro tests reveal that staphylococci exhibit cross-resistance between cephradine and methicillin-type antibiotics.

In the fasting state, oral administration of 250 and 500 mg produced peak plasma levels of approximately 9 and 16.5 mcg/ml respectively within 1 hour. Over 90% of the drug was excreted unchanged in the urine within 6 hours with peak concentration of about 1.6 mg/ml following a 250-mg dose and 3.2 mg/ml following a 500-mg dose. The presence of food in the gastrointestinal tract delays the absorption of cephradine but does not affect the total amount of drug absorbed.

The intravenous administration of 1 gm produced peak serum concentrations of approximately 86 mcg/ml in 5 minutes and measurable amounts were obtainable in patients with normal kidney function 4 hours after the injection. Intramuscular administration generally produced peak serum concentrations within ½ to 1 hour and measurable amounts were obtainable 6 hours after injection.

Indications: Treatment of respiratory tract infections caused by organisms of group A beta-hemolytic streptococci and *Streptococcus (Diplococcus) pneumoniae;* staphylococci-induced infections of the skin and soft tissues; otitis media caused by group A beta-hemolytic streptococci, *Streptococcus (Diplococcus) pneumoniae, Haemophilus influenzae,* and staphylococci, and genitourinary tract infections including prostatitis caused by *Escherichia coli, Pr. Mirabilis* and *Klebsiella* species. Since its efficacy in the prevention of rheumatic fever has not been established, penicillin is usually the drug of choice for the treatment and prevention of streptococcus infections including the prophylaxis of rheumatic fever. Cephradine is generally effective in the eradication of streptococci from the nasopharynx. **Note:** Culture and susceptibility tests should be initiated prior to and during therapy. Renal function studies should be performed when indicated.

For contraindications, warnings and precautions, see general statement.

Adverse Reactions: As with other cephalosporins, unfavorable reactions are limited essentially to gastrointestinal disturbances and to hypersensitivity phenomena. The latter are more likely to occur in individuals who have previously demonstrated hypersensitivity and those with a history of allergy, including asthma, hay fever, or urticaria. Side effects which have been reported include glossitis, nausea, vomiting, diarrhea or loose stools, abdominal pain and heartburn; mild urticaria or skin rash, pruritus, joint pains; mild, transient eosinophilia, leukopenia and neutropenia; transient mild rise of SGOT, SGPT, and total bilirubin have been observed with no evidence of hepatocellular damage; transitory rises in BUN which may or may not be accompanied by a rise in serum creatinine. Other adverse reactions have included dizziness, feeling of tightness in the chest, and candidal vaginitis.

Dosage and Administration: *Orally.* The adult dosage ranges from 1 to 4 gm daily in divided doses. The usual adult dosage is 250 mg 4 times daily for mild infections, and 500 mg 4 times daily for acute infections; severe and chronic infections may require up to, but should not exceed, 4 gm daily. The usual dosage for children is 25 to 50 mg/kg/day in 4 equally divided doses. For otitis media due to *H. influenzae,* doses from 75 to 100 mg/kg/day in 4 equally divided doses are recommended. Therapy should be continued for a minimum of 48 to 72 hours after the patient becomes asymptomatic or evidence of bacterial eradication has been obtained. In infections caused by group A beta-hemolytic streptococci, a minimum of 10 days of treatment is advised to guard against the risk of rheumatic fever or glomerulonephritis. In the treatment of urinary tract infection, frequent bacteriologic and clinical appraisal is necessary during therapy and may be required for several months following withdrawal of the drug. Doses smaller than those recommended are not advised. A modified dosage schedule is necessary for patients with impaired renal function. The following dosage schedule based on the creatinine clearance/minute is recommended as a guideline. The adult initial loading dose is 750 mg and a maintenance dosage of 250 or 500 mg is given at the suggested time intervals. If creatinine clearance is greater than 20 ml/minute, the dose is 500 mg and the time interval is 6 hours; 5 to 20 ml/minute, the dose is 250 mg and the time interval is 6 hours; and less than 5 ml/minute, the dose is 250 mg and the time interval is 12 hours. Children may require dosage modification proportional to their weight and severity of the infection.

Cephradine may be administered *intravenously* or by deep *intramuscular* injection into a large muscle mass such as the gluteal muscle or the lateral aspect of the thigh. The adult daily dose ranges from 2 to 4 gm administered in 4 equally divided doses. The usual dosage is 500 mg 4 times daily for mild infections and every 4 hours for severe infections. The total daily dose may be increased up to, but should not exceed, 8 gm. The dosage for infants and children should be regulated by the age and weight of the patient and by the severity of the infection being treated. The usual daily dose ranges from 50 to 100 mg/kg of body weight administered in 4 equally divided doses. Doses as high as 300 mg/kg/day have been found effective and safe in severely ill infants and children. The maximal daily pediatric dose should not exceed the amount recommended for adults. Cephradine is compatible with sterile water, 5% dextrose, normal saline or M/6 sodium lactate solution. **Note:** Do not use Lactated Ringer's solution. The clinician is urged to read carefully the package literature for proper methods of storage, dilution, etc.

Availability:
ANSPOR®: **(Smith Kline & French)**
Capsules, 250 mg in bottles of 100; 500 mg in bottles of 20 and 100. Both potencies are available in single-unit packages of 100.
Powder for Oral Suspension, 125 and 250 mg/5 ml in bottles of 100 ml.
VELOSEF®: **(Squibb)**
Capsules, 250 and 500 mg in bottles of 24 and 100.
Powder for Injection in vials of 250 mg and 0.5 and 1 gm and in infusion bottles of 2 and 4 gm.
Powder for Oral Suspension, 125 and 250 mg/5 ml in bottles of 100 ml.

CERUMENEX

Description: A solution containing 10% triethanolamine polypeptide oleate-condensate in propylene glycol with chlorobutanol, 0.5%. This preparation emulsifies ear wax.

Indications: For removal of impacted and excessive wax (cerumen) from the ear.

Contraindications: In patients with a previous unfavorable response to the drug, and with positive reaction to the patch test. Relatively contraindicated in patients with known or suspected perforated eardrum or otitis media.

Precautions: Considerable caution should be exercised when used in patients with demonstrable dermatologic idiosyncrasies or with a history of allergic reaction in general. A skin patch test with the solution will establish sensitivity to one of the components. Patients should be cautioned not to use the drops more frequently than as directed by the physician, nor should they attempt to remove ear wax by mechanical means. The drops should not remain in situ for longer than 15 to 30 minutes. The use of this medication should be avoided in the presence of underlying disease of the middle ear, and should be used with caution in certain types of external otitis. In the event of a reaction, patients should be advised to discontinue the medication and to consult their physician promptly.

Adverse Reactions: Although the incidence has been low, a small number of local skin reactions have been observed, manifested as localized dermatitis ranging from very mild erythema and pruritus of the external canal to a severe eczematoid reaction involving the external ear and periauricular tissue, generally lasting 2 to 10 days.

Dosage and Administration: *Locally.* The ear canal is filled with the solution, a cotton plug is inserted and allowed to remain 15 to 30 minutes, and then the ear is flushed gently or washed with a soft-rubber ear syringe (avoid excessive pressure) using lukewarm water. Procedure may be repeated if necessary. Undue exposure to large skin areas should be avoided.

Availability:
CERUMENEX® Drops in bottles of 8 and 15 ml with blunt-end dropper. **(Purdue Frederick)**

CHLOPHEDIANOL HYDROCHLORIDE

Chemical Name: 2-Chloro-α-(2-dimethylaminoethyl)benzhydrol hydrochloride.

Description: Chlophedianol is structurally related to chlorpheniramine and to diphenhydramine and occurs as a white, crystalline powder insoluble in water, but soluble in alcohol.

The drug is cited as having a cough suppressant potency comparable to that of the narcotics, but with a slower onset of peak effect and a longer duration of action. The drug apparently depresses the cough reflex, presumably by selectively depressing the CNS. Tolerance or addiction has not been observed.

Indications: Management of acute cough associated with upper respiratory infection, the common cold, influenza, pneumonia, bronchitis, tracheitis, laryngitis, croup, pertussis and pleurisy.

Contraindications: None known.

Warnings: It has not been established that the drug is safe to use during pregnancy or in infants. Not recommended for children under 2 years of age.

Precautions: Should be used judiciously in sedated or debilitated patients. Patients with a productive cough should not have their cough reflex severely inhibited since this may lead to retention of secretions. Since chlophedianol acts centrally, it should be used with caution in patients taking drugs that depress or stimulate the CNS.

Adverse Reactions: Centrally acting drugs occasionally may evoke excitation, hyperirritability and nightmares, usually disappearing within a few hours after withdrawal of therapy. Hallucinations developed in a few patients who had been taking the drug in large or even excessive amounts in the presence of existing stimulation. When the drug was discontinued, the patients recovered rapidly within a few hours. Hypersensitivity reactions and urticaria have been infrequent. Because of its mild anticholinergic properties, large doses of chlophedianol produced dry mouth, vertigo, visual disturbances, nausea, vomiting and drowsiness.

Dosage and Administration: *Orally.* Adults, 1 or 2 teaspoonsful 3 or 4 times daily. Children 6 to 12 years of age, 1/2 to 1 teaspoonful 3 or 4 times daily. Children 2 to 6 years of age, 1/2 teaspoonful 3 or 4 times daily.

Availability:
ULO® Syrup, 25 mg/5 ml in bottles of 360 ml. **(Riker)**

CHLORAL HYDRATE Ⓒ IV

Chemical Name: 2,2,2-Trichloro-1,1-ethanediol.

Description: Chloral hydrate is a hypnotic drug that is useful in the treatment of insomnia, and as a pre- and/or postoperative sedative. It occurs as colorless or white, volatile, hygroscopic crystals very soluble in water and in olive oil and freely soluble in alcohol. It has an aromatic, pungent odor and a slightly bitter, caustic taste.

Chloral hydrate is also available as chloral betaine, a chloral hydrate-betaine hydrate adduct, and occurs as a white, crystalline complex which releases chloral hydrate immediately upon solution.

The mechanism by which chloral hydrate acts is not known, but its effects on the CNS resemble those of the hydrocarbon anesthetics. It is readily absorbed from the gastrointestinal tract following oral administration and in doses used for hypnosis, produces mild cerebral depression and quiet, deep sleep with little or no hangover; blood pressure and respiration are depressed only slightly more than in normal sleep and reflexes are not significantly depressed, so that the patient can be awakened and completely aroused. It is rapidly reduced in the body to the principal pharmacologically active metabolite trichloroethanol which possesses a half-life of 8 to 10 hours, and is distributed through all the tissues. It appears in breast milk and crosses the placental barrier.

Some of the drug is oxidized to trichloroacetic acid in the liver and kidneys, and is then excreted in the urine and bile together with trichloroethanol in free or conjugated form.

Indications: For nocturnal sedation in all types of patients and especially for the ill, the young and the elderly patient. When combined with barbiturates, it is a useful hypnotic and sedative during the first stage of labor. In postoperative care and control of pain, it is a valuable adjunct to opiates and analgesics. The tranquilizing and calming effects of phenyltoloxamine help the patient to relax, lessen inner tension and improve the ability to sleep.

Contraindications: In patients who have previously exhibited an idiosyncrasy or hypersensitivity to the drug, in those with gastritis, hepatic or renal impairment, or with severe heart disease, and in lactating women.

Warnings: Chloral hydrate may be habit-forming. Long-term use of larger than the usual therapeutic doses may result in psychic and physical dependence; therefore, caution must be exercised when administering this drug to patients susceptible to drug abuse. Sudden withdrawal may result in delirium. The drug may alter the effectiveness of coumarin-type anticoagulants. The prothrombin time of patients receiving chloral hydrate with concurrent anticoagulant therapy should therefore be continually monitored. This is particularly important when chloral hydrate is withdrawn, as alteration of prothrombin time may occur even in the patient whose schedule had previously been relatively stable. The drug may produce a hemodynamic reaction manifested by vasodilation, diaphoresis, flushing, hypertension, and tachycardia in patients receiving intravenous furosemide preceded by oral chloral hydrate. Caution is essential when combining this drug with other CNS depressants. Chloral hydrate may interfere with the copper sulfate test for glycosuria. Suspected glycosuria should be confirmed by a glucose oxidase test when the patient is receiving this hypnotic.

Precautions: Although therapeutic doses have had no harmful effect, large doses should not be used in patients with cardiac decompensation since it may depress the heart. When prescribed for pregnant patients, the physician should carefully consider the benefits versus the risk to the fetus. Since alertness, judgment and physical coordination may be impaired, use cautiously in patients who must drive a vehicle or operate dangerous machinery. Long-term chronic administration should be accompanied by periodic blood studies.

Adverse Reactions: With the exception of gastric symptoms (gastric upset, epigastric irritation, nausea and vomiting) which may occur in some patients there have been few unfavorable effects. These may include headache, hangover, drowsiness, staggering gait, ataxia, unpleasant taste, ketonuria, relative eosinophilia, urticaria, lightheadedness, vertigo, nightmares, malaise, and reduction in total white blood cell count. Excitement and delirium are rarely encountered and tolerance and addiction are uncommon. Accidental overdosage should be treated by gastric lavage. Phenyltoloxamine has a low incidence of side effects and, in particular, no toxic effect upon the liver, kidneys or blood-forming organs.

Dosage and Administration: *Orally.* The usual *hypnotic* dose for adults is 500 mg to 1 gm taken 15 to 30 minutes before bedtime or 30 minutes before surgery. The usual *sedative* dose is 250 mg 3 times daily after meals. Single doses or daily dosage generally should not exceed 2 gm. For children, the usual *hypnotic* dosage is 50 mg/kg of body weight; the maximal single dose is 1 gm. The *sedative* dosage is ½ the hypnotic dosage. With phenyltoloxamine, the recommended dosage is 1 or 2 capsules at bedtime. The dosage of chloral betaine is 1 or 2 tablets taken 15 to 30 minutes before bedtime or 60 to 90 minutes before surgery. When administered orally, each dose should be taken with a full glass of liquid.

Availability:

Ⓒ **Chloral Hydrate**

Syrup, 250 mg/5 ml in Abbo-Pac® (unit-dose) packages of 5 and 10 ml. **(Abbott)**
Capsules, 500 mg in bottles of 100. **(ICN)**
Capsules, 500 mg in bottles of 30, 100 and 500. **(Lederle)**
Syrup, 500 mg/5 ml in bottles of 1 pint and 1 gallon. **(Lederle)**
Capsules, 500 mg in bottles of 100 and in unit-dose packages of 100 (10 × 10). **(Parke-Davis)**
Capsules, 500 mg in bottles of 100 and in unit-dose packages of 100 (10 × 10). **(Philips Roxane)**
Syrup, 0.5 and 1 gm/10 ml in unit-dose (Patient Cup) of 10 ml in cartons of 10. **(Philips Roxane)**
Capsules, 500 mg in Redipak® (unit-dose) containers of 25. **(Wyeth)**

Ⓒ KESSODRATE®: **(McKesson)**
Capsules, 250 and 500 mg in bottles of 100 and in unit-dose cartons of 100.
Syrup, 500 mg/5 ml in bottles of 1 pint and 1 gallon.

Ⓒ NOCTEC®: **(Squibb)**
Capsules, 250 and 500 mg in bottles of 100 and in Unimatics® of 25 and 100 unit-dose capsules.
Syrup, 500 mg/5 ml (orange-flavored) in bottles of 1 pint and 1 gallon and in Unimatics of 5 ml in cartons of 25.

Ⓒ SK-CHLORAL HYDRATE™ Capsules, 500 mg in bottles of 100. **(Smith Kline & French)**
Ⓒ SOMNOS® Elixir, 267 mg/5 ml in bottles of 1 pint. **(Merck Sharp & Dohme)**

w/Phenyltoloxamine

Ⓒ LORYL® Capsules, 337.5 mg with phenyltoloxamine citrate, 37.5 mg in bottles of 50 soft-gelatin capsules. **(Kremers-Urban)**

Chloral Betaine

Ⓒ BETA-CHLOR® Tablets, 870 mg equivalent to 500 mg of chloral hydrate in bottles of 100. **(Mead Johnson)**

CHLORAMBUCIL

Chemical Name: *p*-(Di-2-chloroethyl)aminophenyl butyric acid.

Description: Chlorambucil is a derivative of nitrogen mustard. It acts mainly on the lymphoid tissues in contrast to busulfan which affects primarily the myeloid structures.

Indications: Produces remissions in chronic lymphocytic leukemia and in malignant lymphomas including lymphosarcoma, giant follicular lymphoma and Hodgkin's disease.

Contraindications: Should not be administered within 4 weeks of a full course of radiation therapy or treatment with another chemotherapeutic agent that depresses bone marrow function.

Precautions: Chlorambucil is a potent drug causing bone marrow depression characterized by leukopenia, thrombocytopenia, and anemia. To avoid irreversible damage, hemoglobulin determinations, total and differential leukocyte counts and platelet counts should be performed on a weekly schedule. During the initial 3 to 6 weeks of therapy, it is also recommended that white blood cell counts be made 3 to 4 days after each of the weekly complete blood counts. The drug should be discontinued or the dosage reduced upon evidence of abnormal depression of the bone marrow. Many patients develop a slowly progressive lymphopenia that reverses rapidly to normal levels upon completion of drug therapy. After the third week of therapy, most patients have some degree of neutropenia that may persist for as long as 10 days after the last dose. A severe neutropenia usually occurs in patients who have received a total dosage of 6.5 mg/kg of body weight (about 450 mg) or more in one course; as the total dose approaches this amount, there is a serious risk that irreversible bone marrow damage may occur. When the bone marrow has been infiltrated with lymphomatous tissue or is in a hypoplastic condition as indicated by persistently low neutrophil and platelet counts or peripheral lymphocytosis, the dosage of chlorambucil should not exceed 0.1 mg/kg of body weight. When cytotoxic drugs are used during pregnancy, the possible adverse effects on the fetus should be kept in mind. It is therefore advisable to delay treatment with this drug until after the first trimester of pregnancy.

Adverse Reactions: Apart from the depressant action on the bone marrow, adverse effects rarely occur with therapeutic doses. Gastric discomfort may occasionally be observed especially with large dosages.

Dosage and Administration: *Orally.* To initiate therapy or for short courses of treatment, the usual dosage is 0.1 to 0.2 mg/kg of body weight daily for 3 to 6 weeks as required. This usually amounts to 4 to 10 mg daily for the average patient. The entire daily dosage may be taken at one time. Patients with Hodgkin's disease usually require 0.2 mg/kg daily. If maintenance dosage is used, it should not exceed 0.1 mg/kg daily and may well be as low as 0.03 mg/kg daily. Ordinarily, it is 2 to 4 mg daily or less, depending upon the response of the patient.

Availability:
LEUKERAN® Tablets, 2 mg (sugar coated) in bottles of 50. **(Burroughs Wellcome)**

CHLORAMPHENICOL

Chemical Name: D(-)-*threo*-2,2-Dichloro-*N*-[β-hydroxy-α-(hydroxymethyl)-*p*-nitrophenethyl] acetamide.

Description: Chloroamphenicol is a bacteriostatic antibiotic formerly isolated from *Streptomyces venezuelae,* but is now produced synthetically. It occurs as fine, white to grayish white or yellowish white, needle-like crystals or elongated plates slightly soluble in water and freely soluble in alcohol, in propylene glycol, acetone and in ethyl acetate. The *palmitate ester* is insoluble in water and sparingly soluble in alcohol; the *sodium succinate ester* is freely soluble in water and in alcohol. Action of chloramphenicol is due to inhibition of protein synthesis by interfering with the transfer of activated amino acids from soluble RNA to ribosomes.

Although relatively insoluble in water, free chloramphenicol is absorbed rapidly from the intestinal tract, peak blood levels appearing within 2 hours and detectable levels persisting for about 8 hours. It is excreted in the urine for the most part as conjugated glucuronide metabolites. It enters cerebrospinal fluid and measurable levels are detectable in pleural and in ascitic fluids, in saliva, milk and in the aqueous and vitreous humors. Transport across the placental barrier occurs with somewhat lower concentrations in cord blood of newborn infants than in maternal blood. Studies have shown that chloramphenicol is not absorbed in measurable amounts by topical application to the eye.

Administered orally, the *palmitate ester* is hydrolyzed by the pancreatic and intestinal lipases in the upper intestinal tract to release active chloramphenicol. Although absorption is thus somewhat slower than that after ingestion of the free antibiotic, blood levels persist for longer periods. Similarly, the *sodium succinate ester* is hydrolyzed by tissue enzymes to the free antibiotic producing demonstrable blood levels for about 8 hours after intravenous injection. Intravenous administration should be replaced by oral administration as soon as feasible.

Chloramphenicol is well distributed in body tissues, diffusing into both extracellular and intracellular fluid. The mechanism by which it exerts its bacteriostatic effect is by interfering with or inhibiting protein synthesis in intact cells and cell-free systems.

Indications: Chloramphenicol is clinically useful, but should be reserved for *only* those serious infections caused by susceptible organisms for which less potentially hazardous therapeutic agents are ineffective or contraindicated. Chloramphenicol may be chosen to initiate therapy on the clinical impression that one of the conditions mentioned below is believed to be present; in vitro sensitivity tests should be performed concurrently so that the drug may be discontinued as soon as possible if less potentially dangerous agents are indicated by these tests. The decision to continue with chloramphenicol rather than with another antibiotic, when both are suggested by in vitro studies to be effective against a specific pathogen, should be based upon the severity of the infection, the susceptibility of the organism to the various antimicrobial drugs, and upon the efficacy of the various drugs in the infection.

Chloramphenicol is recommended for use *only* in (1) acute infections caused by *Salmonella typhi* (not for routine use in typhoid "carrier state"); (2) serious infections caused by susceptible strains in accordance with the concepts outlined above: *Salmonella* species; *H. influenzae* (specifically meningeal infections); rickettsia; lymphogranuloma-psittacosis group; various gram-negative bacteria causing bacteremia, meningitis or other serious gram-negative infections; other susceptible organisms which have been demonstrated to be resistant to all other appropriate antimicrobial agents; and (3) cystic fibrosis regimens.

Chloramphenicol is also useful in the treatment of superficial infections of the eye and ear due to susceptible organisms including gram-negative and gram-positive organisms, as well as certain rickettsia; it is also effective in certain viral-like infections.

In *dermatology,* chloramphenicol is effective against certain protozoa, rickettsia and viral-like infections as well as against many gram-positive and gram-negative organisms. It is useful in the treatment of superficial pyodermas, impetigo, acute folliculitis, seborrhea-like streptodermatitis, and infectious eczematoid dermatitis.

Prior to treatment with this antibiotic, bacteriologic studies should be performed to determine the causative organisms and their sensitivity to chloramphenicol.

Contraindications: In patients with a history of previous hypersensitivity and/or toxic reaction to chloramphenicol. It must not be used in the treatment of trivial infections or where it is not indicated, as in colds, influenza, or infections of the throat where other antibiotics are effective; nor should it be used prophylactically to prevent bacterial infection.

Warnings: Serious and fatal blood dyscrasias, such as aplastic anemia, hypoplastic anemia, thrombocytopenia and granulocytopenia, have occurred following therapy with chloramphenicol. In addition, there have been reports of aplastic anemia attributed to chloramphenicol which later terminated in leukemia. Blood dyscrasias have occurred after short-term and long-term therapy with the drug.

It is essential that adequate blood studies be carried out during therapy with chloramphenicol. While these studies may detect early peripheral blood changes (e.g., leukopenia, reticulocytopenia or granulocytopenia) before they become irreversible, they [blood studies] cannot be relied on to detect bone marrow depression before the development of aplastic anemia. To facilitate appropriate studies and observation during therapy, it is advisable to hospitalize the patient. Ophthalmic ointments may retard corneal healing.

Precautions: Repeated courses of the drug should be avoided if at all possible. Treatment should not be continued longer than necessary when a cure is in sight with little or no risk of a relapse. Concurrent therapy with other drugs that may cause bone marrow depression should be avoided. Excessive blood levels may result from administration of the drug in recommended doses to patients with impaired hepatic or renal function, including infants in whom excessive blood levels may result from immature hepatic metabolic processes. Dosage should be adjusted accordingly or, preferably, the blood concentration should be determined at appropriate intervals. Whether chloramphenicol is safe to use during pregnancy has not been established. Since the drug readily crosses the placental barrier, caution is particularly important during pregnancy at term or during labor because of the potential toxic effects on the fetus. Caution should also be exercised when treating premature and full-term infants to avoid "gray syndrome" toxicity (see "Adverse Reactions"). Serum drug levels should be followed carefully during therapy in the neonate. Toxic effects on the nursing infant, too, are a possibility; therefore caution should be used during the lactation period. The use of any antibiotic may result in the overgrowth of nonsusceptible organisms, including fungi. If infections caused by nonsusceptible organisms appear during therapy, proper countermeasures should be taken.

Adverse Reactions: *Blood dyscrasias:* Reversible and irreversible types of bone marrow depression, aplastic and hypoplastic anemia, thrombocytopenia, granulocytopenia, pancytopenia, paroxysmal nocturnal hemoglobinuria, and drug-induced aplastic anemia subsequently terminating in leukemia. *Gastrointestinal Reactions:* Nausea, vomiting, glossitis and stomatitis, diarrhea and enterocolitis may occur in low incidence. *Neurotoxic Reactions:* Headache, mild depression, mental confusion and delirium, optic and peripheral neuritis following long-term therapy in which case the drug should be withdrawn promptly. *Hypersensitivity Reactions:* Fever, macular and vesicular rashes, angioedema, urticaria and anaphylaxis may occur. Herxheimer reactions have occurred during therapy for typhoid fever. *"Gray*

Syndrome:" Toxic reactions including fatalties have occurred in the premature and in the newborn infant; the signs and symptoms have been referred to as the "gray syndrome." One case has been reported in an infant born to a mother taking chloramphenicol during labor; one case has been reported in a 3-month infant. The following summarizes the clinical and laboratory studies made on these patients: (1) in most cases, therapy with chloramphenicol had been instituted within the first 48 hours of life; (2) symptoms first appeared after 3 or 4 days of continued treatment with high doses of chloramphenicol; (3) symptoms appeared in the following order: abdominal distention with or without emesis; progressive pallid cyanosis; vasomotor collapse, frequently accompanied by irregular respiration; death within a few hours of onset of these symptoms; (4) the progression of symptoms from onset to exitus was accelerated with higher dosage schedules; (5) preliminary blood serum level studies revealed unusually high concentrations of chloramphenicol (over 90 mcg/ml after repeated doses); and (6) termination of therapy upon early evidence of the associated symptomatology frequently reversed the process with complete recovery. May cause stinging when used in the eyes.

Dosage and Administration: Administration of 50 mg/kg/day, *orally* or *intravenously,* in divided doses at intervals of 6 hours, will produce blood levels of a magnitude to which most susceptible organisms will respond. Except in certain circumstances (e.g., premature and newborn infants and patients with impaired hepatic or renal function) lower doses may not achieve these levels. *Adults:* 50 mg/kg/day in divided doses at intervals of 6 hours, increased, if necessary, to 100 mg/kg/day to inhibit moderately resistant organism. But these high doses should be reduced as soon as possible. *Children:* Dosage is the same as for adults. Severe infections (e.g., bacteremia or meningitis), especially when adequate cerebrospinal fluid concentrations are desired, may require up to 100 mg/kg/day; however, it is recommended that dosage be reduced to 50 mg/kg/day as soon as possible. *Newborn infants:* A total of 25 mg/kg/day usually is sufficient to control most infections for which the drug is indicated. In severe infections and after the first 2 weeks of life, full-term infants may receive as much as 50 mg/kg/day in divided doses at intervals of 6 hours. These dosage recommendations are extremely important because blood levels in all premature infants and full-term infants under 2 weeks of age differ from those of other infants. This difference is due to variations in the maturity of the metabolic functions of the liver and the kidneys. When these functions are immature (or seriously impaired in adults), high concentrations which are found tend to increase with succeeding doses. *Infants and children with immature metabolic processes:* a dosage of 25 mg/kg/day usually produces therapeutic levels of the drug in the blood. In this group particularly, concentration of the drug in the blood should be followed carefully by microtechniques. *Locally.* For use in the eye, an ophthalmic preparation may be applied to the conjunctival sac every 3 hours or more often if required, day and night for the first 48 hours. For use in the ear, 2 or 3 drops of the otic preparation are instilled 2 to 3 times daily. *Topically.* The topical cream may be applied 3 or 4 times daily after cleansing the affected area. Treatment should be continued for at least 48 hours after the affected area has been restored to normal.

Availability:

CHLOROMYCETIN®: **(Parke-Davis)**

Capsules, 50 and 100 mg in bottles of 100.

Cream, 1% in tubes of 30 gm.

Kapseals® (white capsules with gray band), 250 mg in bottles of 16 and 100 and in unit-dose cartons of 100 (10 × 10).

Ophthalmic in vials of 25 mg with dropper and 15-ml bottles of sterile distilled water.

Ophthalmic Ointment, 1% in tubes of 3.5 gm.

Oral Suspension (as palmitate), 150 mg/5 ml in bottles of 60 ml.

Otic, 0.5% in dropper bottles of 15 ml.

Sodium Succinate in Steri-Vials® of 1 gm.

Solution, 500 mg in ampuls of 2 ml (NOT for pediatric use).

CHLOROMYCETIN-HYDROCORTISONE Ophthalmic, 12.5 mg with hydrocortisone acetate, 25 mg in dropper bottles of 5 ml. **(Parke-Davis)**

CHLOROMYXIN™ Ophthalmic Ointment, 1% with polymyxin B sulfate, 5000 units/gm in tubes of 3.5 gm. **(Parke-Davis)**

CHLOROPTIC®: **(Allergan)**

S.O.P.® Ophthalmic Ointment (sterile), 10 mg/gm in tubes of 3.5 gm.

Ophthalmic Solution, 0.5% in plastic dropper bottles of 7.5 ml.

CHLOROPTIC-P® S.O.P.® Ophthalmic Ointment, 1% with prednisolone alcohol, 0.5% in tubes of 3.5 gm. **(Allergan)**
ECONOCHLOR: **(Alcon)**
Ophthalmic Ointment, 1% in tubes of 3.5 gm.
Ophthalmic Solution, 0.5% in Drop-Tainer® dispensers of 15 ml.
OPHTHOCHLOR® Ophthalmic Solution, 5 mg/ml in dropper bottles of 15 ml. **(Parke-Davis)**
OPHTHOCORT® Ophthalmic Ointment, 1% with hydrocortisone acetate, 0.5% and polymyxin B sulfate, 5000 units/gm in tubes of 3.5 gm. **(Parke-Davis)**

CHLORCYCLIZINE + HYDROCORTISONE

Description: Chlorcyclizine hydrochloride is an antihistamine which is related structurally to cyclizine and meclizine. It is designated chemically as 1-(*p*-Chloro-α-phenylbenzyl)-4-methylpiperazine hydrochloride and occurs as a white, crystalline powder freely soluble in water and soluble in alcohol.

A combination with hydrocortisone acetate provides antiinflammatory, antipruritic and anesthetic properties. It blocks the actions of histamine, antagonizes allergic manifestations and anesthetizes free nerve endings that mediate pain, itch and touch. The combination provides, by different mechanisms, dual and additive effects to combat antigen-antibody reaction and histamine effect such as inflammation, itching, whealing, and pain. Available in a bland, nongreasy, nonocclusive, water-washable cream that has a pH of about 4.5. The cream contains chlorcyclizine hydrochloride, 2% and hydrocortisone acetate, 0.5% in a base consisting of liquid petrolatum, white petrolatum, purified water, emulsifying wax, and is preserved with methylparaben.

Indications: Treatment of itching, painful skin eruptions and dermatoses including allergic, nuchal and nummular eczema; anogenital pruritus; atopic, lichenoid, seborrheic and contact dermatitis including poison oak, poison ivy and poison sumac; intertrigo; localized neurodermatitis; sunburn and insect bites.

Contraindications: As with other topical preparations containing hydrocortisone the cream should not be used in bacterial infection of the skin without concomitant antibacterial therapy; tuberculosis of the skin; viral infections including varicella, dendritic keratitis of the eye and herpes simplex of the adjacent skin. Not for ophthalmic use.

Dosage and Administration: *Topically.* May be applied 2 to 5 times daily. If condition of the skin will permit, the cream should be rubbed in well.

Availability:
MANTADIL® Cream in tubes of 15 gm. **(Burroughs Wellcome)**

CHLORDANTOIN

Chemical Name: 5-(1-Ethylamyl)-3-(trichloromethylthio)hydantoin.

Description: Chlordantoin, a synthetic mercaptan derivative, occurs as a white, crystalline powder practically insoluble in water and soluble in alcohol. Preparations are stable, odorless and nonstaining.

The drug is active against various fungi, including *Candida albicans,* but is not effective against *Trichomonas vaginalis;* it also possesses some antibacterial activity. The halogenated portion of the molecule is said to promote penetration of the fatty barrier of the infecting organism. It is unaffected by vaginal fluid and is safe to use during pregnancy.

Indications: May be useful in the treatment of vulvovaginal candidiasis.

Contraindications: None known.

Precautions: Although instances reportedly have been rare, use of the cream should be discontinued when sensitization and irritation do occur.

Dosage and Administration: *Intravaginally,* 1 applicatorful twice daily for 14 days. A course of therapy may be repeated if necessary.

Availability:
SPOROSTACIN® Cream, 1% with benzalkonium chloride, 0.05% in tubes of 95 gm with measured-dose applicator. **(Ortho)**

CHLORDIAZEPOXIDE Ⓒ

Chemical Name: 7-Chloro-2-methylamino-5-phenyl-3*H*-1,4-benzodiazepine-4-oxide hydrochloride.

Description: Chlordiazepoxide hydrochloride is a benzodiazepine derivative used primarily in the treatment of anxiety and alcoholism. It is related both pharmacologically and chemically to diazepam and oxazepam. The chemical is a colorless, crystalline substance which is soluble in water and unstable in solution.

The preparation is well absorbed following oral administration, 2 to 4 hours being required to reach peak blood levels although it can be detected in the blood within 1 hour. Significant pharmacologic effects are noted within 15 to 30 minutes if the preparation is administered in therapeutic dosage intramuscularly; within 3 to 30 minutes if administered intravenously. The half-life of the drug following oral administration is approximately 24 hours. Clinically, the activity of the base of chlordiazepoxide and its hydrochloride salt are indistinguishable, and they may be used interchangeably on a milligram-for-milligram basis.

The drug is excreted in the urine both as a conjugate and in unchanged form, and this excretion continues for a number of days after the last dose so that a cumulative effect may be noted. The drug readily crosses the placental barrier.

Extensive studies in animals suggest that chlordiazepoxide acts by depressing the limbic system of the brain which is believed to be involved in emotional reactions. There is also evidence of depression of the brain stem reticular formation, the cerebral cortex and the reflex arcs of the spinal cord. It is claimed to produce muscle relaxation by a central action although objective electromyelographic data in humans are not available. Unlike the phenothiazines and the rauwolfia compounds, an anticonvulsant effect has not been demonstrated in animals.

Indications: For the relief of anxiety and tension, withdrawal symptoms of acute alcoholism, preoperative apprehension and anxiety; and as an adjunct in the treatment of various disease states in which anxiety and tension are significant components of the clinical profile. The physician is urged to periodically reassess the usefulness of the drug when administered for periods continuing beyond 4 months. A combination with the atropine-like anticholinergic, clidinium bromide, is recommended for the relief of hypersecretion, hypermotility and anxiety and tension states associated with organic or functional gastrointestinal disorders, and adjunctively in the management of peptic ulcer, gastritis, duodenitis, irritable bowel syndrome, spastic colitis and mild ulcerative colitis.

Contraindications: Hypersensitivity to the drug(s). The preparation containing clidinium bromide is contraindicated in patients with glaucoma, prostatic hypertrophy and benign bladder neck obstruction.

Warnings: As in the case of other centrally acting drugs, patients should be cautioned about possible potentiating effects of alcohol and other CNS depressants, and about engaging in hazardous occupations requiring alertness. Although incidents have been rare, care must nevertheless be exercised when giving the drug to addiction-prone persons or to those whose history suggests they may increase the dosage on their own initiative. Withdrawal symptoms following discontinuance of the drug have been reported; the symptoms, including convulsions, are similar to those seen with barbiturates. Results of studies with animals revealed an increased risk of congenital anomalies, particularly during the first trimester of pregnancy; therefore, the use of any drug during pregnancy, the lactation period, or in women in childbearing age requires that the potential benefit of the drug be weighed against its possible hazards to the mother and child. Anticholinergic drugs may have an inhibiting effect on lactation. The physician is urged to read carefully the package literature for the management of overdosage.

Precautions: To preclude the development of ataxia, oversedation or confusion, not more than 10 mg/day initially should be given to elderly or debilitated patients, and may then be increased gradually as needed and tolerated. Patients receiving parenteral therapy should be carefully observed and kept in bed for about 3 hours. Ambulatory patients should not be permitted to operate a motor vehicle following an injection. In general, concomitant administration of chlordiazepoxide or its hydrochloride salt and other psychotropic agents or MAO inhibitors is not recommended. The usual precautions in treating patients with impaired renal or hepatic function should be observed. Psychiatric patients and hyperactively aggressive children should be observed for such paradoxical reactions as excitement, stimulation and acute rage. Caution should be exercised when treating anxiety states where there is any evidence of impending depression, since suicidal tendencies may be present requiring protective measures. It should be borne in mind that the concomitant administration of chlordiazepoxide and oral anticoagulants may have variable effects on blood coagulation.

Adverse Reactions: Most commonly seen reactions, particularly in the elderly and debilitated, are drowsiness, ataxia and confusion. Syncope, hypotension, tachycardia, skin eruptions, edema, minor menstrual irregularities, nausea, constipation, extrapyramidal symptoms, blurred vision, increased and decreased libido, hypotension associated with spinal anesthesia, pain following intramuscular injection, changes in electrocardiographic patterns, and blood dyscrasias including agranulocytosis, jaundice and hepatic dysfunction have been observed infrequently and are generally controlled with reduction of dosage. When therapy is prolonged, periodic blood counts and liver function tests are advisable. Adverse effects reported with the use of clidinium bromide are those typical of anticholinergic agents, e.g., dry mouth, blurred vision, urinary hesitancy and constipation.

Dosage and Administration: *Orally.* Because of the wide range of clinical indications, the optimal dosage varies with the diagnosis and response of the patient. The dosage, therefore, should be individualized for maximal beneficial effects. The usual dosage for adults ranges from 5 to 25 mg 3 or 4 times daily, and for elderly or debilitated patients, 5 mg 2 to 4 times daily. In acute agitation, alone or associated with chronic alcoholism and alcohol withdrawal (including delirium tremens), the suggested initial dose is 50 to 100 mg, to be followed by repeated doses as needed until agitation is controlled—up to 300 mg daily. Dosage should then be reduced to maintenance levels. Children 6 years of age and older, usually 5 mg 2 to 4 times daily, increased in some children to 10 mg 2 or 3 times daily. *Intramuscularly or intravenously.* Intravenous administration of a solution prepared with the intramuscular diluent is not recommended. Solutions prepared with normal saline or sterile water for injection should not be given intramuscularly because of pain on injection. In most cases, intramuscular injection is preferred and should be given slowly and injected deep into the upper outer quadrant of the gluteus muscle. Intravenous administration is suggested when, in the judgment of the physician, a rapid action is mandatory. Dosage should be tailored to the diagnosis and response of the patient. While 300 mg may be given during a 6-hour period, this dose should not be exceeded in any 24-hour period. The usual adult dosage for *alcoholism* is 50 to 100 mg IM or IV initially, repeated in 2 to 4 hours if necessary. In *acute or severe anxiety and tension states,* 50 to 100 mg IM or IV initially followed by 25 to 50 mg 3 or 4 times daily if necessary. *For preoperative apprehension,* 50 to 100 mg IM 1 hour before surgery. Lower doses (usually 25 to 50 mg) should be used for elderly or debilitated patients, and for children 12 years of age and older. In most cases, acute symptoms may be controlled rapidly by parenteral administration so that subsequent treatment, if necessary, may be given orally.

Availability:

Chlordiazepoxide

C-IV LIBRITABS® Tablets: 5, 10 and 25 mg in bottles of 100 and 500. **(Roche)**

Chlordiazepoxide Hydrochloride

C-IV *Capsules,* 5, 10 and 25 mg in bottles of 100 and 500. **(Lederle)**

C-IV *Capsules,* 5, 10 and 25 mg in bottles of 500 and in unit-dose cartons of 100. **(Parke-Davis)**

C-IV *Capsules,* 5, 10 and 25 mg in bottles of 100 and 500. **(Squibb)**

C-IV A-POXIDE™ Capsules, 5 and 10 mg in bottles of 500; 25 mg in bottles of 100. **(Abbott)**

C-IV LIBRIUM®: **(Roche)**

Capsules, 5 mg (green & yellow), 10 mg (green & black) and 25 mg (green & white) in bottles of 100 and 500, in Tel-E-Dose® (single-dose) packages of 100, in Reverse Number packs of 25 and in Prescription Paks of 50.

For Injection (dry powder), 100 mg in ampuls of 5 ml and ampuls of 2 ml (containing special intramuscular diluent).

C-IV SK-LYGEN® Capsules, 5, 10 and 25 mg in bottles of 100 and 500 and in unit dose cartons of 100. **(Smith Kline & French)**

w/Amitriptyline Hydrochloride

Ⓒ LIMBITROL® Tablets, 5 and 10 mg with amitriptyline hydrochloride, 12.5 and 25 mg, respectively in bottles of 100 and 500 and in Tel-E-Dose® (unit-dose) packages of 100.
(Roche)

w/Clidinium Bromide

LIBRAX® Capsules (green), 5 mg with clidinium bromide, 2.5 mg in bottles of 100 and 500 and in Prescription Paks of 50 and Tel-E-Dose® packages of 100. **(Roche)**

CHLORMEZANONE

Chemical Name: 2-(*p*-Chlorophenyl) tetrahydro-3-methyl-4*H*-1,3-thiazin-4-one 1,1-dioxide.

Description: Chlormezanone is a substituted metathiazanone and occurs as a white, tasteless, crystalline powder slightly soluble in water and in alcohol.

A CNS depressant agent that improves the emotional state by quieting the patient without impairing clarity of consciousness. The relief of symptoms is usually apparent within 15 to 30 minutes and may continue for up to 6 hours or longer.

Indications: Treatment of mild anxiety and tension states.

Contraindications: Previous history of hypersensitivity to chlormezanone.

Warnings: If drowsiness occurs, the dosage should be reduced and the patient cautioned not to operate a motor vehicle or other dangerous machinery. Since safe use has not been established, use of the drug during pregnancy, lactation, and in women in childbearing potential requires that the therapeutic benefit of the drug be weighed against its possible hazards to the mother and fetus.

Adverse Reactions: Reported reactions include drug rash, dizziness, flushing, nausea, drowsiness, depression, edema, inability to void, and weakness. Therapy should be discontinued or modified as the case demands. Cholestatic jaundice has occurred rarely and was reversible when the drug was discontinued.

Dosage and Administration: *Orally.* The usual adult dosage is 200 mg 3 or 4 times daily; however, 100 mg may be adequate for some patients. Children 5 to 12 years of age, 50 to 100 mg 3 or 4 times daily.

Availability:

TRANCOPAL® Caplets® 100 mg (scored, peach) in bottles of 100; 200 mg (scored, green) in bottles of 100 and 1000. **(Breon)**

CHLOROPROCAINE HYDROCHLORIDE

Chemical Name: 2-(Diethylamino)ethyl 2-chloro-4-aminobenzoate hydrochloride.

Description: Chloroprocaine hydrochloride, a local anesthetic of the benzoic acid ester type, differs structurally from procaine hydrochloride only in the presence of a chlorine atom on the benzene ring. It occurs as a white, crystalline powder soluble in water and sparingly or slightly soluble in alcohol. On a weight basis, chloroprocaine is about twice as potent as procaine. The drug is hydrolyzed in plasma more rapidly than is procaine, and its onset and duration of action are somewhat shorter.

In common with other local anesthetics, chloroprocaine appears to block the initiation and transmission of nerve impulses by stabilizing nerve membrane potential or by elevating the threshold of excitability through chemical combination with polar groups in the lipoprotein film of the nerve membrane. Local anesthetics may also interfere with oxidative processes within the nerve.

The onset of action occurs within 6 to 12 minutes and the duration of anesthesia lasts for 30 to 60 minutes depending upon the amount used.

Indications: The solution *with preservative* is indicated for infiltration and regional nerve blocks. *It is not to be used for caudal or epidural anesthesia.* The solution *without preservative* is indicated for the production of caudal (sacral) and epidural (peridural) nerve blocks. May also be used for infiltration and regional nerve blocks.

Contraindications: In patients hypersensitive to chloroprocaine hydrochloride. Although disease of the CNS is generally considered a contraindication to caudal or epidural nerve block, it is not a contraindication to peripheral nerve block. Pathologic changes of the vertebral column may make epidural puncture impossible or inadvisable.

Warnings: Resuscitative equipment and drugs should be immediately available when chloroprocaine is administered. Solutions containing preservatives should not be used for caudal or epidural anesthesia. Equipment and drugs necessary for the treatment of inadvertent intravascular, intrathecal, or excessive dosage should be readily available. Safe use during pregnancy has not been established with respect to adverse effects upon fetal development. Therefore, it should not be used in women of childbearing potential unless in the judgment of the physician the potential benefits outweigh the unknown hazards. When chloroprocaine is employed in obstetrics, the obstetrician should be aware that some oxytoxic drugs, when used either to correct hypotension or added to the local anesthetic solution, may cause severe persistent hypertension and even rupture of a cerebral blood vessel may occur during the post partum period. Also solutions containing vasoconstrictors, particularly epinephrine and norepinephrine, should be used with extreme caution in patients receiving antidepressant drugs such as MAO inhibitors, and tricyclic compounds since a severe prolonged hypertension may be experienced.

Precautions: The safety and effectiveness of chloroprocaine depends upon proper dosage, correct technique, adequate precautions and readiness for emergencies. The lowest dosage that results in effective anesthesia should be used to avoid high plasma levels and serious undesirable systemic side effects. Debilitated, elderly, or acutely ill patients, and children should be given reduced doses commensurate with their age and physical status. Solutions containing vasoconstrictors should be used cautiously in the presence of disease which may adversely affect the patient's cardiovascular system. The physician should carefully evaluate the benefits versus the risks in such instances as during labor (paracervical block) when fetal distress is anticipated or when toxemia, prematurity, diabetes or other condition which may cause fetal distress is present; when solutions containing epinephrine are intended for areas with limited blood supply (ear, nose, digits, etc.) since use in these areas may be followed by ischemia which may progress to gangrene, or when solutions containing a vasopressor are employed during or following the administration of chloroform, halothane, cyclopropane, trichloroethylene, or other related agents since serious cardiac arrhythmias may occur. Chloroprocaine should be used cautiously in patients with known drug allergies or sensitivities. As with all local anesthetics, care should be exercised to prevent accidental intravascular injection; this is particularly important when performing a regional nerve block, since blood vessels frequently are in close proximity to the nerve or ganglion to be anesthetized. Although the drug is well tolerated, hypersensitivity to the drug can be determined by the usual intradermal skin test. If the skin test is negative, a small test dose of chloroprocaine should precede the administration of a full dose. In the event of overdosage, the rapid appearance of symptoms including nausea, vomiting, talkativeness, syncope and convulsions requires prompt treatment with oxygen, artificial respiration and if convulsions occur, intravenous administration of a short-acting barbiturate.

Adverse Reactions: Adverse reactions result from high plasma levels due to rapid absorption, inadvertent intravascular injection or excessive dosage. Hypersensitivity, idiosyncrasy, or diminished tolerance are other causes of reactions. Reactions due to overdosage (high plasma levels) are systemic and involve the central nervous system and the cardiovascular system. Reactions involving the CNS are characterized by excitation and/or depression. Nervousness, dizziness, blurred vision or tremors may occur followed by drowsiness, convulsions, unconsciousness and possibly respiratory arrest. Since excitement may be transient or absent, the first manifestations may be drowsiness merging into unconsciousness and respiratory arrest. Reactions involving the cardiovascular system include depression of the myocardium, hypotension, bradycardia and even cardiac arrest. Allergic reactions are characterized by cutaneous lesions, urticaria, edema and other manifestations of allergy.

Treatment of toxic manifestations consists of maintaining an airway, and supporting ventilation using oxygen and assisted or controlled respiration. Supportive treatment of the cardio vascular system consists of using vasopressors, preferably those that stimulate the myocardium such as ephedrine, metaraminol, etc., and intravenous fluids. Convulsions may be controlled by the intravenous administration (in small increments) of an ultrashort or short-acting barbiturate, or a short-acting muscle relaxant.

Dosage and Administration: *Parenterally* for infiltration anesthesia and regional nerve blocks. The recommended maximal single dose is 1000 mg and 800 mg respectively with or without epinephrine. Fractional doses of 300 to 600 mg may be given at intervals of 50 minutes. For caudal anesthesia, the initial dose is 15 to 25 ml of a 2 or 3% solution; repeated at intervals of 40 to 60 minutes. For epidural anesthesia in the cervical or thoraxic region, 1.5 to 2 ml for each segment. In the lumbar or sacral region, 2 to 2.5 ml for each segment. The usual total volume is from 15 to 25 ml. Repeated doses of 2 to 6 ml less than the original dose may be given at intervals of 40 to 50 minutes. For detailed information, the physician is urged to study carefully the package literature.

Availability:
NESACAINE® Solution (with preservative), 1 and 2% in multiple-dose vials of 30 ml in cartons of 12. **(Pennwalt)**
NESACAINE-CE® Solution (without preservative), 2 and 3% in single-dose vials of 30 ml in cartons of 12. **(Pennwalt)**

CHLOROQUINE

Chemical Name: 7-Chloro-4-(4-diethylamino-1-methylbutylamino)quinoline.

Description: Chloroquine is a 4-aminoquinoline derivative closely related to amodiaquine and hydroxychloroquine. It resembles quinacrine in that it possesses the same alkyl side chain, but differs only in having a quinoline instead of an acridine nucleus and in lacking the methoxy radical. It has been found to possess three times the activity of quinacrine when assessed against standardized strains of *Plasmodium vivax* and *P. falciparum*. The hydrochloride and phosphates salts of chloroquine are white, crystalline substances freely soluble in water and practically insoluble in alcohol. Chloroquine is readily absorbed from the gastrointestinal tract and about 25% of the daily dose is excreted in the urine. Urine excretion is decreased by alkalinization and increased by acidification. It can be found deposited in the tissues particularly in the liver, spleen, kidney, lung, skin, and leukocytes.

Chloroquine has been found to be highly active against the erythrocytic forms of *P. vivax* and *malariae* and most strains of *P. falciparum* but not the gametocytes of *P. falciparum*. The precise mechanism of action of the drug is not known. It does not prevent relapses in patients with vivax or malariae malaria because it is not effective against exoerythrocytic forms of the parasite, nor will it prevent vivax or malariae infection when administered as a prophylactic. It is highly effective as a suppressive agent in patients with vivax or malariae malaria, in terminating acute attacks, and significantly lengthening the interval between treatment and relapse. In patients with falciparum malaria, chloroquine abolishes the acute attack and effects complete cure of the infection, unless due to a resistant strain of *P. falciparum*. In vitro studies with trophozoites of *Entamoeba histolytica* have demonstrated that chloroquine phosphate also possesses amebicidal activity comparable to that of emetine.

Chloroquine phosphate with primaquine phosphate produced antimalarial activity against all stages of human-malaria parasites, except for certain strains of *P. falciparum* which are resistant to chloroquine.

Carefully controlled clinical studies have found that the weekly administration of 300 mg of chloroquine base and 45 mg of primaquine base (administered as the phosphate salts) proved highly effective as a prophylactic against severe *P. vivax* infections with the Chesson strain and did not produce clinical hemolysis even among primaquine-sensitive American Negro adult volunteers. A weekly dose of primaquine phosphate equivalent to 45 mg primaquine base cured 90% of the infections. These studies suggest that the toxicity of primaquine phosphate, in regard to the production of hemolysis, is markedly diminished when administered in weekly doses. In a double-blind study with 24 Caucasian male adults who received the two drugs once a week for 15 weeks, it was concluded that there was no effect on vision, time of useful consciousness, or psychomotor performance. No deleterious synergistic effect of the two drugs was noted.

Indications: Treatment of extraintestinal amebiasis and of acute attacks of malaria due to *P. vivax, P. malariae, P. ovale,* and susceptible strains of *P. falciparum.* Chloroquine phosphate with primaquine phosphate is intended solely for use in the prophylaxis of malaria, regardless of the species, in all areas where this disease is endemic.

Contraindications: Use of this drug is contraindicated in the presence of retinal or visual field changes either attributable to 4-aminoquinoline compounds or to any other etiology, and in patients with known hypersensitivity to 4-aminoquinoline compounds. However, in the treatment of acute attacks of malaria caused by susceptible strains of plasmodia, the physician may elect to use this drug after carefully weighing the possible benefits and risks to the patient. Chloroquine with primaquine is contraindicated in acutely ill patients suffering from systemic disease manifested by a tendency to granulocytopenia, such as rheumatoid arthritis and lupus erythematosus. The drug is also contraindicated in those patients receiving concurrently other potentially hemolytic drugs or depressants of myeloid elements of the bone marrow. Because quinacrine hydrochloride appears to potentiate the toxicity of antimalarial compounds which are structurally related to primaquine, the use of quinacrine in patients receiving primaquine is contraindicated. Similarly, primaquine should not be administered to patients who have received quinacrine recently, as toxicity is increased.

Warnings: In recent years it has been found that certain strains of *P. falciparum* have become resistant to 4-aminoquinoline compounds (including chloroquine and hydroxychloroquine) as shown by the fact that normally adequate doses have failed to prevent or cure clinical malaria or parasitemia. Treatment with quinine or other specific forms of therapy is therefore advised for patients infected with a resistant strain of parasites. Irreversible retinal damage has been observed in some patients who had received long-term or high dosage 4-aminoquinoline therapy. Retinopathy has been reported to be dose-related. Children are especially sensitive to these compounds, since a number of fatalities have been reported following the accidental ingestion of chloroquine, sometimes in relatively small doses (0.75 or 1 gm in one 3-year-old child). Patients should be strongly warned to keep these drugs out of the reach of children. When prolonged therapy with any antimalarial compound is contemplated, initial (base line) and periodic ophthalmologic examinations (including visual acuity, slitlamp, funduscopic, and visual field tests) should be performed. If there is any indication (past or present) of abnormality in the visual acuity, visual field, or retinal macular areas (such as pigmentary changes, loss of foveal reflex), or any visual symptoms (such as light flashes and streaks) which are not fully explainable by difficulties of accommodation or corneal opacities, the drug should be discontinued immediately and the patient closely observed for possible progression. Retinal changes (and visual disturbances) may progress even after cessation of therapy. Use of chloroquine phosphate in patients with psoriasis may precipitate a severe attack of psoriasis. When used in patients with porphyria the condition may be exacerbated. The drug should not be used in these conditions unless in the judgment of the physician the benefit to the patient outweighs the possible hazard.

Hemolytic reactions (moderate to severe) may occur, even after a weekly dose of chloroquine with primaquine, in glucose-6-phosphate dehydrogenase (G-6-PD) deficient Caucasians (particularly in Sardinians and in individuals with a family or personal history of favism). Dark-skinned persons (Negroes, for example) have a great tendency to develop hemolytic anemia (due to congenital deficiency of erythrocytic glucose-6-phosphate dehydrogenase) while receiving primaquine and related drugs. The drug should be discontinued immediately if marked darkening of the urine, sudden decrease in hemoglobin concentration or leukocyte count, or skin reaction occurs. Safe use during pregnancy has not been established. Therefore, use of chloroquine during pregnancy should be avoided except when in the judgment of the physician the benefit outweighs the possible hazard. It should be noted that radioactively tagged chloroquine administered intravenously to pregnant pigmented CBA mice passed rapidly across the placenta, accumulated selectively in the melanin structures of the fetal eyes and was retained in the ocular tissues for five months after the drug had been eliminated from the rest of the body.

Precautions: Since the drug is known to concentrate in the liver, it should be used with caution in patients with hepatic disease or alcoholism or in conjunction with known hepatotoxic drugs. If any severe blood disorder appears which is not attributable to the disease under treatment, discontinuance of the drug should be considered. The drug should be administered with caution to patients having G-6-PD (glucose-6-phosphate dehydrogenase) deficiency. Chloroquine phosphate with primaquine phosphate is intended for malaria prophylaxis only; it should not be used for the treatment of clinical malaria. The recommended dosage (1 tablet weekly, on the same day each week) should not be exceeded. The drug should not be taken more often than once every seven days to minimize danger of toxicity. If the combination is prescribed for an individual who has shown a previous idiosyncrasy to either chloroquine or primaquine (as manifested by dermatitis, hemolytic anemia, methemoglobinemia, or leukopenia), or an individual with nicotinamide adenine dinucleotide (NADH) methemoglobin reductase deficiency, the person should be observed closely for tolerance. Since anemia, methemoglobinemia, and leukopenia have been observed following administration of large doses of primaquine phosphate, it is advisable to make periodic blood examinations (particularly blood cell counts and hemoglobin determinations) during prolonged therapy. In areas with endemic falciparum malaria due to strains that are resistant to the 4-aminoquinolines (chloroquine, amodiaquine, hydroxychloroquine), chemoprophylaxis with this combination alone may not be effective.

Adverse Reactions: In adults, adverse reactions are unlikely when therapeutic doses are given parenterally. Should a toxic dose be given inadvertently, respiratory depression or shock with hypotension may result. In infants and children, adverse reactions (convulsions and deaths) have been reported after parenteral administration of an overdose of chloroquine. In oral doses adequate for the treatment of an acute malarial attack, mild and transient headache, pruritus, psychic stimulation, pleomorphic skin eruptions, have been observed. None of these manifestations has been constitutionally serious and all have been readily reversible on withdrawal of the drug. *Gastrointestinal reactions:* anorexia, nausea, vomiting, epigastric distress, and abdominal cramps. *Hematologic reactions:* leukopenia, hemolytic anemia in glucose-6-phosphate dehydrogenase (G-6-PD) deficient individuals, methemoglobinemia in nicotinamide adenine dinucleotide (NADH) methemoglobin reductase deficient individuals. *Cardiovascular effects,* such as hypotension and electrocardiographic changes (particularly inversion or depression of the T-wave, widening of the QRS complex), have rarely been noted in patients receiving usual antimalarial doses of the drug. In a study of chronic toxicity of chloroquine phosphate employing a dosage of 800 mg once a week, one patient in 31 after 8 months developed a lichen planus-like eruption which subsided 10 days after discontinuation of the drug. A few cases of a nerve type of deafness, neuromyopathy, blood dyscrasias, and skin and mucosal pigmentary changes have been noted on prolonged therapy. *Visual disturbances,* consisting of blurring of vision or difficulty in focusing or accommodation, have occasionally been noted when chloroquine has been employed for malaria. These symptoms are reversible and disappear on discontinuation of therapy. Other types of visual disturbances (reversible corneal changes) and ocular complications including retinal changes (narrowing of the arterioles, macular lesions, pallor of the optic disc, optic atrophy, and patchy retinal pigmentation) have been reported during the use of chloroquine for long-term therapy usually in daily doses exceeding 250 mg of chloroquine phosphate. These changes have not been reported with the use of chloroquine with primaquine for malaria prophylaxis.

For additional data, see monograph on Hydroxychloroquine Sulfate.

Dosage and Administration: *Orally,* before or after meals. For *suppressive therapy* in adults and children over 8 years of age, a dose of 500 mg taken on exactly the same day each week is recommended. Children, 62 to 125 mg depending on age. For *treatment of an acute attack* in adults, 1 gm initially followed by 500 mg after 6 to 8 hours and a single dose of 500 mg on each of 2 consecutive days. Infants up to 1 year, 125 mg initially followed by 3 doses of 125 mg at intervals of 6 or 8 hours. Children 2 to 5 years, 500 mg initially and 250 mg 8 hours later. Children 6 to 10 years, 500 mg initially plus 2 doses of 250 mg at 8-hour intervals. Children 11 to 15 years, 750 mg initially followed by 250 mg 8 hours later and 250 mg 24 hours later. For *extraintestinal amebiasis* in adults, 1 gm daily for 2 days followed by 500 mg daily for at least 2 to 3 weeks. Treatment is usually combined with an effective intestinal amebicide.

Chloroquine-primaquine dosage for adults is 1 tablet taken the same day each week, starting at least 1 day before entering a malarious area. This schedule (1 tablet weekly) should be continued for 6 weeks after leaving the endemic area. Children, suggested dosage, based on body weight, may be seen in the package literature.

Parenterally, the dihydrochloride salt should be used only in critically ill patients and/or when oral medication is not feasible. *Malaria:* An initial dose of 4 or 5 ml (160 to 200 mg base) may be injected *intramuscularly* and repeated in 6 hours if necessary. The total parenteral dosage in the first 24 hours should not exceed 800 mg of chloroquine base. Treatment by mouth should be started as soon as practicable and continued until a course of approximately 1.5 gm of base in 3 days is completed. *Extraintestinal Amebiasis:* In adults not able to tolerate oral therapy, from 4 to 5 ml may be injected daily for 10 to 12 days. Oral administration should be substituted or resumed as soon as possible.

Availability:
ARALEN® Phosphate Tablets, 500 mg (equiv. to 300 mg base) in bottles of 25. **(Winthrop)**
ARALEN® Hydrochloride Injection, 50 mg/ml (equiv. to 40 mg base) in ampuls of 5 ml. **(Winthrop)**
ARALEN® Phosphate with PRIMAQUINE Phosphate Tablets in bottles of 100. Each tablet contains chloroquine phosphate, 500 mg (equiv. to 300 mg base) and primaquine phosphate 79 mg (equiv. to 45 mg base). **(Winthrop)**

CHLOROTHIAZIDE: see The Thiazide Diuretics

CHLOROTRIANISENE: see The Estrogens

CHLOROXINE

Chemical Name: 5,7-Dichloro-8-hydroxyquinoline.

Description: Chloroxine is a synthetic antibacterial agent structurally similar to a number of substituted 8-hydroxyquinoline compounds. It is used primarily as a shampoo to combat dandruff and seborrheic dermatitis of the scalp. The commercial product contains 2% of the active ingredient in a cream base consisting of sodium nonoxynol-1 sulfate, PEG-6 lauramide, corn starch, coceth-6, sodium lauryl sulfoacetate, dioctyl sodium sulfosuccinate, magnesium aluminum silicate, PEG-14M, EDTA and citric acid. pH is 6.7.

Indications: Treatment of dandruff and mild to moderately severe seborrheic dermatitis of the scalp.

Contraindications: Hypersensitivity to hydroxyquinolines, EDTA or to any of the components, and acutely inflamed (exudative) lesions of the scalp.

Precautions: Care should be exercised to avoid contact with the eyes. **Note:** For external use only.

Adverse Reactions: Irritation and burning of the scalp and adjacent areas have been reported. Allergic-type skin eruptions may occur, and if the drug enters the eyes, a chemical conjunctivitis may result. Also reported were a slight yellow tint to white or grey hair, dryness of the scalp and increased itching.

Dosage and Administration: *Topically.* Apply to the wet scalp and massage thoroughly, carefully avoiding contact with the eyes. Lather should remain on the scalp for approximately 3 minutes, then rinsed. The application should be repeated and the scalp rinsed thoroughly. Two treatments a week are usually sufficient.

Availability:
CAPITROL Cream Shampoo, 2% (20 mg/gm) in plastic tubes of 85 gm. **(Westwood)**

CHLORPHENESIN CARBAMATE

Chemical Name: 3-(*p*-Chlorophenoxy)-2-hydroxypropyl carbamate.

Description: Chlorphenesin carbamate, a skeletal muscle relaxant of the propanediol series, is structurally and pharmacologically related to mephenesin carbamate and to methocarbamol. It occurs as a white to off-white, crystalline powder almost insoluble in cold water and readily soluble in alcohol and in acetone.

Animal studies suggested that the drug possesses selective internuncial blocking action (depression of spinal cord polysynaptic potential and unchanged or augmental monosynaptic potentials). Chlorphenesin effectively antagonized the convulsions produced by strychnine and supramaximal electroshock; however, it was ineffective in preventing or decreasing the intensity of pentylenetetrazol convulsions.

Following oral administration, the drug is rapidly absorbed from the gastrointestinal tract, and maximal serum concentrations are reached in 1 to 3 hours. The drug is partly metabolized in the liver and excreted in the urine primarily in the form of the glucuronide conjugate, but with traces of phenolic and acidic metabolites. Chlorphenesin appears to exert its relaxant effect on skeletal muscles by depressing polysynaptic pathways at both the spinal and supraspinal levels and not by a direct effect on the muscle itself.

Indications: For the relief of discomfort associated with acute, painful musculoskeletal conditions as an adjunct to physiotherapy, rest and other beneficial measures.

Contraindications: Not recommended in pediatric patients; or in patients hypersensitive to the drug.

Warnings: Safe use of chlorphenesin in pregnant women has not been established; therefore, its use during pregnancy or lactation, or in women of childbearing potential is not advised, unless, in the opinion of the physician, the potential benefits outweigh the potential hazards to mother and fetus. Since chlorphenesin may impair mental and/or physical abilities, patients should be cautioned not to engage in activities requiring alertness or skill.

Precautions: Safe use of chlorphenesin for periods exceeding 8 weeks has not been established. It is recommended that liver function studies as well as blood counts be performed on all patients taking this drug, especially those with preexisting liver disease or impaired hepatic function.

Adverse Reactions: Those noted were *Hematopoietic reactions:* rare cases of leukopenia, thrombocytopenia, agranulocytosis and pancytopenia. *Hypersensitivity reactions:* anaphylactoid and drug fever have been observed occasionally. The possibility of other allergic phenomena should be considered; however, such reactions are an indication for discontinuing the medication. Drowsiness, dizziness, confusion, nausea and epigastric distress have been infrequently reported. While not established as drug related, two instances of gastrointestinal bleeding have been reported. Occasionally paradoxical stimulation, insomnia, increased nervousness and headache have been noted. Reduction in dose will usually control these symptoms. Measures to counteract overdosage include gastric lavage or saline catharsis.

Dosage and Administration: *Orally.* Initially, 2 tablets 3 times daily is recommended until the desired therapeutic effect is obtained. For maintenance, dosage may then be reduced to 1 tablet 4 times daily, or less as required.

Availability:
MAOLATE® Tablets, 400 mg in bottles of 50 and 500 and in unit-dose (foil-strips) packages of 100. **(Upjohn)**

CHLORPHENIRAMINE MALEATE
DEXCHLORPHENIRAMINE MALEATE

Chemical Name: *dl*-2-*p*-Chloro-α-[2-(dimethylamino)ethyl] benzyl pyridine bimaleate.

Description: Chlorpheniramine, an antihistamine of the propylamino type (alkylamine), differs from its parent compound, pheniramine, in that a chlorine atom is present in the *para* position on the benzene ring of its nucleus, whereas the structure of pheniramine is nonhalogenated (neither chlorine nor bromine is present). Chlorpheniramine maleate occurs as a white, crystalline powder freely soluble in water and in alcohol.

Dexchlorpheniramine, the *dextro* isomer, is about twice as potent as racemic chlorpheniramine, and shares with chlorpheniramine its actions, uses and cautions. Following oral administration, both drugs are well absorbed from the gastrointestinal tract; their effects are discernible within 20 to 60 minutes and persist for about 4 hours. Chlorpheniramine is detoxified by the liver, probably by hydroxylation followed by conjugation with glucuronic acid; the metabolites are excreted in the urine.

Indications: Both chlorpheniramine and its *dextro* isomer are capable of antagonizing many of the characteristic effects of histamine, and when taken *orally,* are used for the symptomatic relief of some of the manifestations of allergic states, such as hay fever and perennial allergic rhinitis, vasomotor rhinitis, allergic conjunctivitis due to inhalant allergens and foods; mild, uncomplicated allergic skin manifestations of urticaria and angioedema; and dermographism, and for the temporary relief of the distressing symptoms accompanying the common cold, sinusitis, and sneezing. *Parenterally:* Therapeutically, in relatively severe conditions; when a more rapid response is desired than is obtainable orally; when an allergic condition fails to respond to oral medication; or when oral medication is contraindicated. Prophylactically, for transfusion reactions, drug reactions, adjunctively in desensitization procedures, reduction in incidence and severity of sequelae following oral surgery, and conjunctively with epinephrine and supportive measures in anaphylactic reactions. With expectorants, antitussives and decongestants, for symptomatic relief in allergic disorders of the respiratory tract, and selected cases of asthma.

Contraindications: In newborn or premature infants, nursing mothers, in the treatment of lower respiratory tract symptoms, in patients hypersensitive to the drugs, in the presence of asthmatic attack, and in patients receiving MAO inhibitors.

Warnings: Codeine may be habit-forming. Patients should be informed that the concomitant use of alcohol or other CNS depressant agents may have an additive effect. The use of these drugs during pregnancy should be carefully considered. Infants and children are particularly sensitive to these drugs and excessive dosage may lead to convulsions and/or death. Considerable caution is advised in patients with narrow angle glaucoma, stenosing peptic ulcer, pyloroduodenal obstruction, symptomatic prostatic hypertrophy, and bladder neck obstruction. Dosage should be carefully regulated for elderly patients since they are more likely to experience dizziness, sedation, and hypotension.

Precautions: Until their response to antihistamines has been determined, patients who may experience blurred vision, drowsiness or dizziness should be cautioned not to engage in operations requiring alertness. Chlorpheniramine has an atropine-like action and should be used with caution in patients who may have increased intraocular pressure, hyperthyroidism, cardiovascular disease, hypertension or in those with a history of bronchial asthma. Sympathomimetic drugs such as phenylephrine hydrochloride should also be used with due caution in patients with cardiovascular disease, hypertension, thyrotoxicosis, or diabetes mellitus. Although *d*-isoephedrine [in expectorant mixtures] causes virtually no pressor effect, it should be used with special care in patients with hypertension.

Adverse Reactions: Slight to moderate drowsiness occurs relatively infrequently with chlorpheniramine. Other possible reactions include urticaria, drug rash, anaphylactic shock, photosensitivity, excessive perspiration, chills, dryness of mouth, nose, and throat; headache, palpitations, tachycardia, extrasystols; hemolytic anemia, thrombocytopenia, agranulocytosis; sedation, dizziness, disturbed coordination, fatigue, confusion, restlessness, excitation, nervousness, tremor, irritability, insomnia, euphoria, paresthesias, blurred vision, diplopia, vertigo, tinnitus, acute labyrinthitis, hysteria, neuritis, convulsions; epigastric distress, anorexia, nausea, vomiting, diarrhea, constipation; urinary frequency, difficult urination, urinary retention, early menses; thickening of the bronchial secretions, tightness of chest and wheezing, and nasal stuffiness, and very rarely dermatitis. Transitory stinging or a burning sensation at the injection site usually persists no longer than 5 minutes. Sweating, pallor, weak pulse, and transitory hypotension, also occur rarely with the parenteral formulations and usually subside within an hour without specific treatment, in which case the drug should be discontinued. For reactions to other components, see their respective monographs.

Dosage and Administration: The package literature should be consulted for more detailed information. *Orally.* Adults, usually 2 or 4 mg 3 or 4 times daily. Repeat-action formulations, 8 mg at bedtime or every 8 to 10 hours during the day; or 12 mg in the morning and again at bedtime. In sustained-release formulations, 1 capsule every 12 hours for adults and children 12 years of age or over. One to 2 teaspoonsful of an expectorant preparation 3 or 4 times daily usually will be adequate. Children, dosage is proportionately smaller according to age, weight and response. As with all potent medications, dosage must be individualized and adjusted according to the condition being treated and the response obtained. *Parenterally.* The injection, 100 mg/ml is intended for intramuscular or subcutaneous use only and should not be used when intravenous administration is indicated. Intradermal administration is not recommended. The injection, 10 mg/ml, for intravenous use, is indicated for the prophylaxis of transfusion reactions; maximal daily dosage is 40 mg. The dosage for intramuscular or subcutaneous injection ranges from 5 to 20 mg depending upon the indication for such use.

Availability:

Chlorpheniramine Maleate

Capsules, 12 mg in bottles of 1000. **(Elder)**

Capsules (timed-release), 4 mg in bottles of 100 and 1000; 8 and 12 mg in bottles of 1000. **(ICN)**

Capsules (timed-disintegration), 4, 8 and 12 mg in bottles of 1000. **(Lederle)**

Syrup, 2 mg/5 ml in bottles of 120 ml and 1 pint. **(Lederle)**

ALLERBID: **(Amfre-Grant)**

Tablets, 4 mg in bottles of 100 and 1000.

Tymcaps (Capsules), 8 and 12 mg in bottles of 50.

ANTAGONATE® Tablets, 4 mg in bottles of 100. **(Dome)**

CHLOR-TRIMETON®: **(Schering)**

Expectorant (OTC) in bottles of 1 pint. Each 5 ml contains chlorpheniramine maleate, 2 mg; phenylephrine hydrochloride, 10 mg; ammonium chloride, 100 mg; sodium citrate, 50 mg; guaifenesin, 50 mg and alcohol, 1%.

Ⓒ *Expectorant with Codeine* in bottles of 1 pint. Each 5 ml contains, in addition to the above, 10 mg of codeine phosphate and 5.25% alcohol.

Injection, 10 mg/ml in ampuls of 1 ml; 100 mg/ml in multiple-dose vials of 2 ml.

Repetabs® Tablets, 8 and 12 mg in bottles of 100 and 1000 and canisters of 5000.

Syrup (OTC), 2 mg/5 ml in gallons and in "Split" pints of 120 ml (4 x 120 ml).

Tablets (OTC), 4 mg in bottles of 48, 100 and 1000 and canisters of 5000 and in unit-dose packages of 24 in cartons of 12 units.

DECONAMINE: **(Cooper)**

Elixir in bottles of 1 pint. Each 5 ml contains chlorpheniramine maleate, 2 mg, d-pseudoephedrine hydrochloride, 30 mg and alcohol, 15%.

SR Capsules (sustained-release), 8 mg with d-pseudoephedrine hydrochloride, 120 mg in bottles of 30, 100 and 500.

Tablets, 4 mg with d-pseudoephedrine hydrochloride, 60 mg in bottles of 30, 100 and 500.

HISTASPAN® Capsules, 8 and 12 mg in sustained-release micro-dialysis cells in bottles of 100 and 1000. **(USV)**

ISOCLOR®: **(Arnar-Stone)**

Liquid, 2 mg/5 ml with pseudoephedrine hydrochloride, 12.5 mg/5 ml in bottles of 1 pint and 1 gallon.

Tablets, 4 mg with pseudoephedrine hydrochloride, 25 mg in bottles of 100.

Timesules (sustained-action), 10 mg with pseudoephedrine hydrochloride, 65 mg in bottles of 100 and 500.

Ⓒ ISOCLOR EXPECTORANT in bottles of 1 pint and 1 gallon. Each 5 ml contains chlorpheniramine maleate, 2 mg; pseudoephedrine hydrochloride, 12.5 mg; guaifenesin, 83.3 mg and codeine phosphate, 10 mg. **(Arnar-Stone)**

TELDRIN® Spansule® Capsules, 8 and 12 mg in bottles of 50 and 500 and in single-unit packages of 100. **(Smith Kline & French)**

w/Methoxyphenamine Hydrochloride

PYRROXATE®: **(Upjohn)**

Capsules, 2 mg with methoxyphenamine hydrochloride, 25 mg and APC compound in bottles of 30 and 500.

Tablets, 2 mg with methoxyphenamine hydrochloride, 25 mg and APC compound in Dispenser packages of 600 tablets and drums of 5000 tablets.

Ⓒ PYRROXATE w/Codeine Phosphate Capsules, 2 mg with codeine phosphate, 15 mg; methoxyphenamine hydrochloride, 25 mg and APC compound in bottles of 100.

w/Phenylephrine

DEMAZIN®: **(Schering)**

Repetabs® (OTC), *Tablets,* 4 mg with phenylephrine, 20 mg in bottles of 100 and 1000 and in unit-dose cartons of 24 (3 × 8).

Syrup, (OTC), 1 mg/5 ml with phenylephrine hydrochloride, 2.5 mg/5 ml and alcohol, 7.5% in bottles of 120 ml and 1 gallon.

HISTABID® Durabid® (long-acting capsules), 8 mg with phenylephrine hydrochloride, 15 mg and phenylpropanolamine hydrochloride, 35 mg in bottles of 100 and 500. **(Meyer)**

HISTASPAN-D® Capsules, 8 mg with phenylephrine hydrochloride, 20 mg and methscopolamine nitrate, 2.5 mg in sustained-release micro-dialysis cells in bottles of 100 and 1000. **(USV)**

HISTASPAN®-PLUS Capsules, 8 mg with phenylephrine hydrochloride, 20 mg in sustained-release micro-dialysis cells in bottles of 100. **(USV)**

NOVAHISTINE®: **(Dow)**

Ⓒ *DH Liquid* in bottles of 120 ml, 1 pint and 1 gallon. Each 5 ml contains chlorpheniramine maleate, 2 mg with phenylephrine hydrochloride, 18.75 mg; codeine phosphate, 10 mg and alcohol, 5%.

Elixir in bottles of 120 and 240 ml. Each 5 ml contains chlorpheniramine maleate, 2 mg with phenylpropanolamine hydrochloride, 18.75 mg and alcohol, 5%.

LP Tablets, 4 mg with phenylephrine hydrochloride, 20 mg in bottles of 100.

SINUSULE® Capsules (timed-release), 8 mg with phenylephrine hydrochloride, 20 mg and methscopolamine nitrate, 2.5 mg in bottles of 50. **(ICN)**

U.R.I.™ Capsules (timed-release), 8 mg with phenylephrine hydrochloride, 15 mg and phenylpropanolamine hydrochloride, 25 mg in bottles of 50 and 1000. **(ICN)**

Dexchlorpheniramine Maleate

POLARAMINE®: **(Schering)**

Expectorant in bottles of 1 pint. Each 5 ml contains dexchlorpheniramine maleate, 2 mg; *d*-isoephedrine sulfate, 20 mg, guaifenesin, 100 mg and alcohol, 7.2%.

Repetabs® Tablets, 4 mg in bottles of 100; 6 mg in bottles of 100 and 1000.

Syrup, 2 mg/5 ml in bottles of 1 pint.

Tablets, 2 mg in bottles of 100.

CHLORPHENOXAMINE HYDROCHLORIDE

Chemical Name: 2-[(*p*-Chloro-α-methyl-α-phenylbenzyl)oxy]-N,N-dimethylethylamine hydrochloride.

Description: Chlorphenoxamine, a diphenhydramine derivative possessing antihistaminic and anticholinergic properties, differs structurally from diphenhydramine in that a chlorine atom is present in the *para* position on one of the benzene rings and that a methyl group is present on the first carbon atom in the chain. Chlorphenoxamine occurs as a white, crystalline powder soluble in water.

The precise mode of action in relieving muscle rigidity is obscure, but available data suggest that its beneficial effects are due largely to a depressant action on the motor nerve centers of the brain stem and spinal cord. Although it does not appear to act peripherally upon the voluntary muscle or myoneural junction, it does exhibit an atropine-like action on parasympathetic-innervated peripheral structures including smooth muscle. When taken orally, the drug is rapidly absorbed from the gastrointestinal tract, begins to exert its effect in about 30 minutes; the antispasmodic effect usually persists for 4 to 6 hours.

Indications: The symptomatic treatment of all types of Parkinson's disease (postencephalitic, arteriosclerotic, idiopathic). It is especially useful when rigidity and impairment of muscle contraction are primary complaints.

Contraindications: Myasthenia gravis.

Precautions: Because the drug has some peripheral anticholinergic properties, consideration should be given to the possibility that intraocular pressure may be increased and that glaucoma may become aggravated. The drug should be given with caution to patients with tachycardia, signs of urinary retention, prostatic hypertrophy, stenosing peptic ulcers, duodenal or pyloric obstruction, or cardiospasm with megaesophagus. Although potentiation of barbiturates has not been reported in clinical use, the drug should be used with caution if the patient is also taking a barbiturate. The sedative effect manifested by drowsiness and/or dizziness represents a hazard in ambulatory patients whose activities require alertness and motor coordination.

Adverse Reactions: The need to discontinue therapy, because of serious reactions, occurs only rarely. Reported reactions, such as indigestion, drowsiness, dizziness, dry mouth, anorexia, nausea, occur in about 20% of patients. Other reactions reported include vomiting, burning sensation in the mouth, nervousness, numbness of the hand, excessive sweating, fullness of the stomach, blurred vision, confusion, mental dullness, tiredness or weakness, swelling of the feet and urinary retention. Increased tolerance may develop after continuous therapy over a period of several months.

Dosage and Administration: *Orally.* Initially, 50 mg 3 times daily; some patients may require up to 100 mg 4 times daily. Patients should be maintained on therapy that is giving them a measure of relief, adding chlorphenoxamine to the therapeutic regimen. With this regimen, it is sometimes possible to reduce the dose of a potentially more toxic drug. Ideally, a therapeutic regimen should be established that will provide the greatest measure of relief with minimal undesirable side effects.

Availability:
PHENOXENE® Tablets (amber-colored, coated), 50 mg in bottles of 100. **(Dow)**

CHLORPHENTERMINE HYDROCHLORIDE (C-III)

Chemical Name: 4-Chloro-α, α-dimethylphenethylamine hydrochloride.

Description: Chlorphentermine hydrochloride, a congener of amphetamine is a sympathomimetic amine. It occurs as a white to off-white powder freely soluble in water and in alcohol.

The pattern of action is not precisely known. This appetite-suppressing amine has a central stimulant action as well as peripheral effects. The anorectic effect diminishes after several weeks.

Following oral administration, the drug appears to be readily absorbed from the gastrointestinal tract, reaches peak blood levels in 2 to 4 hours, and is excreted primarily in the urine.

Indications: Management of exogenous obesity, as a short term (several weeks) adjunct in a regimen of weight reduction based upon caloric restriction.

Contraindications: Glaucoma, hyperthyroidism, hypersensitivity to sympathomimetic amines, and agitated states; in patients with a history of drug abuse or symptomatic cardiovascular disease such as advanced arteriosclerosis or moderate to severe hypertension. It is also contraindicated during or within 14 days following administration of MAO inhibitors, since a hypertensive crisis may occur.

Warnings: The possibility of tolerance and psychological dependence should be kept in mind, and when weight loss is unsatisfactory, the recommended dosage should not be increased; it is advised that the drug be withdrawn. Because of possible drowsiness or overstimulation, patients should be cautioned not to engage in activities requiring alertness or skill such as driving a motor vehicle or performing tasks requiring precision or critical judgment. The physician should be aware that pulmonary hypertension may result with the use of this drug. Safe use during pregnancy has not been established. The use of chlorphentermine by women who are or may become pregnant, and especially those in the first trimester of pregnancy, requires that the potential benefit be weighed against the possible hazard to the mother and fetus. Use of the drug during lactation is not recommended. Also, it is not recommended for use in children under 12 years of age.

Precautions: Use with caution when obesity complicates the management of patients with mild to moderate cardiovascular disease or diabetes mellitus, and only when dietary restriction alone has been unsuccessful in achieving desired weight reduction. Frequent monitoring of blood pressure is advised for patients with hypertension. Insulin requirements may be altered and psychologic disturbance may result in association with the use of chlorphentermine and the concomitant dietary regimen.

Adverse Reactions: *CNS*—drowsiness and sedation or overstimulation and restlessness, insomnia, dizziness, headache, euphoria, dysphoria, and tremor may occur. Psychotic episodes, although rare, have been noted even at recommended doses. *Cardiovascular*—tachycardia, palpitation, and elevation of blood pressure which rarely occurs and is usually not serious. *Gastrointestinal*—nausea and vomiting, diarrhea, abdominal cramps, unpleasant taste, and constipation. *Endocrine*—changes in libido and impotence. *Autonomic*—dryness of mouth, sweating and mydriasis. *Allergic*—urticaria. *Genitourinary*—diuresis and, rarely, difficulty in initiating micturition. Acute intoxication is manifested by restlessness, confusion, assaultiveness, hallucinations, panic states, and hyperpyrexia. Fatigue and depression usually follow CNS stimulation. Fatal poisoning usually terminates in convulsions and coma. Management of overdosage is largely symptomatic and supportive and often includes sedation with a barbiturate. If hypertension is marked, the use of a nitrate or rapid-acting alpha receptor blocking agent should be considered. Experience with hemodialysis or peritoneal dialysis has not been adequate to suggest its use at this time.

Dosage and Administration: *Orally.* The daily dosage for adults should be 1 tablet (65 mg), taken after breakfast.

Availability:
Ⓒ III PRE-SATE® Tablets, 65 mg in bottles of 100 and 1000. **(Warner-Chilcott)**

CHLORPROMAZINE HYDROCHLORIDE: see The Phenothiazines

CHLORPROPAMIDE

Chemical Name: 1-[(*p*-Chlorophenyl)sulfonyl]-3-propylurea.

Description: Chlorpropamide, a sulfonylurea compound, is structurally and pharmacologically related to tolbutamide, acetohexamide and tolazamide; potency is estimated to be 6 times that of tolbutamide which may be due to chlorpropamide's longer half-life (slower excretion and absence of significant deactivation). Its chemical similarity to the sulfonamides does not imply any antibacterial activity. Chlorpropamide appears to act initially by stimulating the synthesis and release of endogenous insulin from the islet tissue of the pancreas. The insulin thus released appears to act chiefly in the liver to decrease the output of hepatic glucose. It occurs as a white, crystalline powder practically insoluble in water and soluble in alcohol.

Following oral administration, the drug is readily absorbed from the gastrointestinal tract, exerts a hypoglycemic effect in normal humans within 1 hour, reaches a peak effect in 3 to 6 hours and persists for at least 24 hours. The drug is slowly excreted in the urine (80 to 90% of a single oral dose is excreted within 96 hours), primarily unchanged; very small amounts may be metabolized to p-chlorobenzenesulfonamide. Chlorpropamide is intended to supplement, not replace, dietary regulation of diabetes. Its precise mechanism of action is not understood. It is an oral hypoglycemic agent; *not* an oral insulin.

Indications: Primarily in uncomplicated, stable, mild or moderately severe nonketotic, maturity-onset type of diabetes mellitus, which cannot be controlled completely by diet alone. The drug often can be used successfully, instead of insulin, in this type of patient. It also may prove effective in controlling certain patients who have shown an inadequate response or true primary or secondary failure with other sulfonylurea agents. In patients requiring high doses or frequent administration of another oral hypoglycemic agent, control may be facilitated through its use.

Contraindications: Juvenile or growth-onset diabetes; severe or unstable "brittle" diabetes; diabetes complicated by ketosis and acidosis, diabetic coma, major surgical procedures, severe infection, or trauma, during pregnancy, seriously impaired hepatic, renal or thyroid function. Serious consideration should be given to the potential hazards of its use in women of childbearing potential.

Warnings: The severity of the diabetes, the nature of the complications, and availability of laboratory facilities determine whether or not therapy with chlorpropamide can be continued or should be withdrawn while insulin is being used.

Precautions: Animal studies suggest that chlorpropamide may prolong the action of barbiturates, and cause an exaggerated hypoglycemic effect in adrenalectomized animals. For these reasons, the drug should be given with caution to patients taking barbiturates and to patients with Addison's disease. In some patients, a disulfiram-like reaction may be provoked by alcohol. If it occurs, hypoglycemia may be prolonged. The physician should see the patient at least once weekly during the initial 6-week period of therapy, after which the patient should be seen as often as is necessary to maintain careful management. Since not all diabetic patients are suitable candidates for chlorpropamide, it is essential that the physician become thoroughly familiar with the specific indications for the drug, the limits of its application, and the criteria for the selection of patients. Therapy with chlorpropamide does not alleviate the necessity for standard dietary regulation.

Caution should be exercised when antibacterial sulfonamides, phenylbutazone, oxyphenbutazone, salicylates, probenecid, bishydroxycoumarin, or MAO inhibitors are administered concomitantly with chlorpropamide, as hypoglycemia resulting from either potentiation or accumulation of sulfonylureas has been reported.

Adverse Reactions: Most reactions have been dose-related, transient, and have responded to dosage reduction or withdrawal of the drug. However, some reactions associated with hypersensitivity may be severe and death has been reported in rare instances. Certain idiosyncratic or hypersensitivity reactions which have occurred occasionally may include cholangiolitic jaundice, skin eruptions rarely progressing to erythema multiforme and exfoliative dermatitis, and probably depression of formed blood elements. These have been mild and readily reversible on withdrawal of the drug, while the more severe manifestations may require other measures, including corticosteroids. Skin rash may be a manifestation of sensitivity, or it may occur in association with jaundice. Incipient jaundice constitutes an indication for withdrawal of the drug. Low grade fever and eosinophilia also may occur in association with, or preceding the development of, clinical jaundice. Rarely, severe diarrhea sometimes accompanied by bleeding in the lower bowel, and due to nonspecific proctocolitis, has been associated with other hypersensitivity manifestations, particularly jaundice, skin rash, or both. Reversible, benign leukopenia, thrombocytopenia and mild anemia have occurred occasionally. Mild leukopenia, not associated with a shift in the differential count, may be transient and frequently reverts to normal even while the drug is continued. Clinically insignificant lymphocytosis, and rare cases of aplastic anemia and agranulocytosis have been reported.

Dose-related reactions generally are transient and not serious and would include anorexia, nausea, vomiting and epigastric discomfort as evidence of gastrointestinal intolerance, and various vague neurologic symptoms, particularly weakness and paresthesias. Hypoglycemia, although not a true side effect, but rather an exaggeration of the expected therapeutic action, is usually the result of dosage in excess of the patient's immediate requirements. Since the development of hypoglycemia is a function of many factors including diet, this effect is at times seen in patients on the usual recommended dosage. It is readily controlled by administration of glucose. Its occurrence is an obvious indication for immediate reevaluation and adjustment of the insulin or chlorpropamide dosage. Because of its prolonged hypoglycemic action, patients who become hypoglycemic during therapy with chlorpropamide require close supervision for at least 3 to 5 days, during which time frequent feedings or glucose administration is essential. The anorectic patient or profoundly hypoglycemic patient should be hospitalized. Rare cases of phototoxic reactions have been reported.

Dosage and Administration: *Orally.* The total daily dosage is generally taken at a single time each morning with breakfast. Occasional cases of gastrointestinal intolerance may be relieved by dividing the daily dosage. A loading or priming dose is not necessary and should not be used. Dosage, initially, may range from 100 to 250 mg daily, with or without insulin, depending upon the type of diabetes and the age of the patient. Dosage may subsequently be adjusted upward or downward by increments of not more than 50 to 125 mg at intervals of 3 to 5 days to obtain optimal control. More frequent adjustments are usually undesirable. Most moderately severe, middle-aged, stable diabetic patients are controlled by about 250 mg daily, while milder diabetics do well on daily doses of 100 mg or less. Many of the more severe diabetics may require 500 mg daily for adequate control. Patients who do not respond completely to 500 mg daily will usually not respond to higher doses. Maintenance doses above 750 mg daily should be avoided.

Availability:
DIABINESE® Tablets, 100 mg in bottles of 100 and 500 and in unit-dose packages of 100; 250 mg in bottles of 100, 250 and 1000 and in unit-dose packages of 100. **(Pfizer)**

CHLORPROTHIXENE

Chemical Name: 2-Chloro-*N,N*-dimethylthioxanthene-Δ⁹,-γ-propylamine.

Description: Chlorprothixene is structurally and pharmacologically related to chlorpromazine and thiothixene. Although its chemical structure resembles the phenothiazines, the variation in the central ring may account for the differences in clinical activity; however, the tranquilizing effects of the former parallel those of the latter. It occurs as a yellow, crystalline powder slightly soluble in water and soluble in alcohol. Following oral administration, the drug is partially absorbed from the gastrointestinal tract. Following intramuscular administration, its effects are apparent within 10 to 30 minutes. It is metabolized, presumably in the liver, to chlorprothixene sulfoxide; free chlorprothixene and its sulfoxide metabolites are excreted in the urine and stools. In addition to its psychotherapeutic properties, the drug also possesses sympatholytic, parasympatholytic and spasmolytic properties.

Indications: To modify the symptoms of acute and chronic psychotic disorders. It is of no value in the management of behavioral disorders in patients with mental retardation.

Contraindications: Circulatory collapse, comatose states due to CNS depressants (alcohol, hypnotics, opiates, etc.) and known hypersensitivity to chlorprothixene.

Warnings: Since the safety of the drug during pregnancy or lactation has not yet been established, its use in women of childbearing age requires that the potential benefits of the drug be weighed against its possible hazards to mother and child. Patients taking CNS-acting drugs, including chlorprothixene, should be cautioned not to engage in hazardous occupations requiring complete alertness, such as driving a motor vehicle or operating machinery. These same patients should also be cautioned about the possible potentiating effects of alcoholic beverages and other CNS depressants. The safety and efficacy of chlorprothixene have not been established for oral administration in children under 6 years of age or for parenteral use in those under 12 years of age.

Precautions: Seldom has it been necessary to discontinue chlorprothixene because of toxic effects. However, because of its structural similarity to the phenothiazines, all of the known serious side effects or toxicity associated with the phenothiazines should be considered when patients receive this agent. Chlorprothixene should be used with caution in patients who are exposed to extreme heat or phosphorous insecticides, and in those receiving barbiturates or narcotics because of the additional depressant effects on the CNS. The dosage of the narcotic or barbiturates should be reduced when administered concomitantly with chlorprothixene. Caution is also advised in patients who are receiving atropine or related drugs, or who have a history of epilepsy, ulcer condition, cardiovascular disease, or respiratory impairment such as acute pulmonary infections, or chronic respiratory disorders manifested by severe asthma or emphysema. When necessary, chlorprothixene may be used concomitantly with anticonvulsant drugs. However, use of this drug may lower the convulsive threshold; therefore, adequate dosage of the anticonvulsant should be maintained. Simultaneous use with other psychotropic agents may augment or interfere with the absorption, metabolism or therapeutic activity of these drugs and vice versa. Also, the concurrent use of chlorprothixene with electroconvulsive therapy should be reserved for those patients for whom it is essential, since the hazards may be increased. The appearance of signs of blood dyscrasias requires immediate discontinuance of the drug and the institution of appropriate therapy. The possibility of liver damage, variations in thyroid function, pigmentary retinopathy, lenticular or corneal deposits and development of irreversible dyskinesias should be considered when patients are on prolonged therapy. When used in the treatment of agitated states accompanying depression, the usual precautions indicated for such patients are necessary, particularly the recognition that a suicidal tendency may be present and protective measures necessary. Gastritis, nausea and vomiting, dizziness and tremulousness have been reported following abrupt cessation of high-dose therapy.

Adverse Reactions: Death may occur due to cardiac arrest, or to asphyxia due to failure of the cough reflex; jaundice; hematological disorders may include agranulocytosis, eosinophilia, leukopenia, hemolytic anemia, thrombocytopenic purpura and pancytopenia. Most cases of agranulocytosis have occurred between the 4th and 10th weeks of therapy. Patients should be observed closely during that period for the sudden appearance of sore throat or other signs of infection. If white blood count and differential show significant cellular depression, the drug should be discontinued and appropriate therapy initiated. Cardiovascular involvement may be manifested by postural hypotension, tachycardia (especially with a sudden marked increase in dosage), bradycardia, cardiac arrest, faintness and dizziness. Occasionally, the hypotensive effect may produce a shock-like condition. In the event a vasoconstrictor is required, levarterenol and phenylephrine are the most suitable. Other pressor agents, including epinephrine, should not be used, as a paradoxical further lowering of the blood pressure may ensue. ECG changes, nonspecific, usually reversible, have been observed in some patients. Their relationship to myocardial damage has not been confirmed. Extrapyramidal reactions, which are usually dose-related, may be manifested by pseudoparkinsonism, akathisia (motor restlessness), and dystonias (spasms of the neck muscles, extensor rigidity of back muscles, carpopedal spasm, eyes rolled back, convulsions, trismus and swallowing difficulties). These symptoms usually subsided within 48 hours after discontinuance of medication. Hyperreflexia may occur in the newborn when the drug is administered during pregnancy. Other reactions that may occur include paradoxical exacerbation of psychotic symptoms, cerebral edema, abnormality of cerebrospinal fluid proteins, convulsive seizures—particularly in patients with ECG abnormalities or a history of such disorders, hyperpyrexia, urticaria, itching, erythema, photosensitivity (avoid undue exposure to sunlight), eczema, rarely exfoliative dermatitis, contact dermatitis, asthma, laryngeal edema, angioneurotic edema, anaphylactoid reaction; lactation and moderate breast engorgement in females and gynecomastia in males on large doses, changes in libido, false-positive pregnancy tests, amenorrhea, hyperglycemia, hypoglycemia, glycosuria, dry mouth, nasal congestion, constipation, adynamic ileus, miosis, mydriasis, urinary retention, enlargement of the parotid gland, increases in appetite and weight, and peripheral edema. Another complication reported was systemic lupus erythematosus-like syndrome. After prolonged administration of high doses, pigmentation of the skin has occurred chiefly in the exposed areas, especially in females on large doses. Ocular changes consisting of deposition of fine particulate matter in the cornea and lens, progressing in more severe cases to star-shaped lenticular opacities, epithelial keratopathies, and pigmentary retinopathy may occur.

Tardive dyskinesia may appear in some patients on long-term therapy or may occur after therapy with chlorprothixene has been discontinued. The risk appears to be greater in elderly patients on high-dose therapy, especially female patients. The symptoms are persistent and in some patients appear to be irreversible. The syndrome is characterized by rhythmical involuntary movements of the tongue, face, mouth or jaw (e.g., protrusion of the tongue, puffing of cheeks, puckering of mouth, chewing movements). These may also be accompanied by involuntary movements of the extremities. There is no known treatment for this condition; antiparkinsonism agents usually do not alleviate the symptoms. It is advised that this drug be discontinued if the above phenomenon appears. The syndrome may be masked if treatment is reinstituted or the dosage is increased, or if another drug is substituted. It has been suggested that fine vermicular movements of the tongue may be an early sign of the syndrome, and that the full-blown syndrome may not develop if medication is withdrawn when lingual vermiculation appears. Elderly patients (female patients especially) and probably all patients over 50 years of age should be carefully observed.

Overdosage in the range of 2.5 to 4 gm or above can be fatal. Drowsiness, coma, respiratory depression, hypotension (which may appear after a delay of several hours and may persist for 2 or 3 days), tachycardia, pyrexia, and constricted pupils are the overt manifestations. Convulsions, hyperactivity and hematuria may be seen in the recovery period. Treatment is essentially symptomatic and involves gastric lavage, supportive measures and maintenance of an adequate airway.

Dosage and Administration: Dosage should be adjusted according to diagnosis and severity of the condition. In general, small doses should be used initially, and increased to the optimal effective level as rapidly as possible based on the therapeutic response of the patient. In psychotic states, the average daily *oral* dosage is 25 to 50 mg 3 or 4 times daily (up to 600 mg). Dosages exceeding 600 mg daily are rarely required. Children over 6 years of age, 10 to 25 mg 3 or 4 times daily. For debilitated or elderly patients, 10 to 25 mg 3 or 4 times daily. When a rapid and potent calming action is desired, as in agitated states associated with psychoses, the average daily dosage is 25 to 50 mg *intramuscularly* 3 or 4 times daily. Since postural hypotension may occur in some patients, injection should be given with the patient seated or recumbent. If hypotension does occur, the patient should be observed until symptoms of weakness or dizziness pass. As soon as the acutely agitated patient is brought under control, oral medication should be instituted. The change-over should be made gradually, with oral and parenteral doses being given alternately on the same day, then oral doses only, adjusted to the required maintenance level. Use of the parenteral form of this drug in children is not currently recommended. The physician is urged to read carefully the package literature for the management of overdosage.

Availability:
TARACTAN®: **(Roche)**
Concentrate, 100 mg/5 ml (fruit-flavored) in bottles of 1 pint.
Injection, 25 mg/2 ml in ampuls of 2 ml in cartons of 10.
Tablets, 10, 25, 50 and 100 mg in bottles of 100 and 500.

CHLORTETRACYCLINE HYDROCHLORIDE

Chemical Name: 7-Chloro-4-dimethylamino-1,4,4α,5,5α,6,11,12α-octahydro-3,6,10,12,12α-pentahydroxy-6-methyl-1,11-dioxo-2-naphthacenecarboxamide hydrochloride.

Description: Chlortetracycline hydrochloride is the salt of an antibiotic derived from *Streptomyces aureofaciens* and occurs as a yellow, odorless, bitter, crystalline powder sparingly soluble in water and slightly soluble in alcohol. It is soluble in solutions of alkali hydroxides and carbonates.

The mechanism by which it acts remains obscure; it has been postulated, however, that it may interfere with the synthesis of bacterial proteins or with cellular oxidative metabolism. Readily absorbed and bound to plasma proteins in varying degrees, it is concentrated by the liver in the bile and excreted in the urine and feces at high concentrations and in a biologically active form. Chemically, microbiologically, pharmacologically and therapeutically, chlortetracycline is closely similar to other tetracyclines.

Indications: Primarily for the treatment of gram-negative bacillary infections, rickettsial diseases, gram-positive infections resistant to penicillin, and susceptible bacterial infection in patients hypersensitive to other antibiotics. The **Topical Ointment** is indicated for the treatment of superficial pyogenic infections of the skin. It is effective against both gram-negative bacteria (*coli-aerogenes* group) and gram-positive cocci (streptococci, staphylococci and pneumococci). The **Ophthalmic** preparation is indicated for use in the treatment of susceptible ocular infections caused by staphylococci, pneumococci, *H. influenzae, diplobacillus* of Morax-Axenfeld, the Friedlander bacillus, streptococci, *A. aerogenes, P. vulgaris* and *morganii, E. coli, Alcaligenes faecalis, Ps. pyocyanea* and in the treatment of trachoma (in conjunction with oral therapy).

Contraindications: In individuals with a history of hypersensitivity to the antibiotic.

Precautions: The use of antibiotics occasionally may result in the overgrowth of nonsusceptible organisms necessitating constant observation of the patient. If therapy is ineffective, or if new infections due to nonsusceptible organisms appear during therapy, appropriate measures should be taken.

Dosage and Administration: *Topical Ointment,* in the treatment of local skin infections, is applied directly to the involved area, preferably on sterile gauze, one or more times daily as the condition warrants. In severe local infections, topical application should be supplemented by oral administration. *Ophthalmic ointment* is applied to the infected eye every 2 hours or more often as the condition and response indicate. Severe or stubborn infections may require treatment for many days or oral administration in addition to local treatment. Mild infections may respond in as little as 48 hours.

Availability:
AUREOMYCIN®: **(Lederle)**
Ophthalmic Ointment (sterile or non-sterile), 1% in tubes of 3.5 gm.
Topical Ointment, 3% in tubes of 15, 20 (Display Paks) and 30 gm.

CHLORTHALIDONE

Chemical Name: 2-Chloro-5-(1-hydroxy-3-oxo-1-isoindolinyl)benzenesulfonamide.

Description: Chlorthalidone is a nonmercurial, sulfonamide diuretic that, although not a thiazide, resembles the pharmacologic action of thiazide diuretics both qualitatively and quantitatively. It differs from other sulfonamide diuretics in that a double ring system is incorporated into its chemical structure. It occurs as a white, crystalline powder sparingly soluble in water.

The drug causes sodium and chloride to be excreted in approximately equal amounts, presumably by inhibiting their reabsorption in the cortical diluting segment of the ascending limb of Henle's loop of the nephron. Following oral administration, diuresis occurs within 2 hours and, because of its low solubility and resultant slow absorption from the gastrointestinal tract, continues for up to 72 hours. It has been suggested that the drug's initial antihypertensive action is due to a reduction of plasma volume following diuresis. The drug is excreted in the urine, unchanged, and does not accumulate in the body.

Indications: Management of moderate to more severe forms of hypertension and in the control of hypertension of pregnancy either alone or in conjunction with other antihypertensive drugs, and as adjunctive therapy in edema associated with congestive heart failure, hepatic cirrhosis, corticosteroid, and estrogen therapy. Has also been found useful in edema due to various forms of renal dysfunction such as the nephrotic syndrome, acute glomerulonephritis, and chronic renal failure, and in severe edema when due to pregnancy. The fixed combination drug is not indicated for initial therapy of hypertension since this condition requires that therapy be titrated to the individual patient. However, if the fixed combination represents the dosage so determined, its use may be more convenient in patient management.

Contraindications: Hypersensitivity to the drug; anuria. The routine use of diuretics in an otherwise healthy pregnant woman with or without mild edema is contraindicated and possibly hazardous. (Reserpine is contraindicated in patients with mental depression.)

Warnings: Caution is advised in patients with severe renal disease since the drug may precipitate azotemia, and the possibility of electrolyte imbalance should be kept in mind, particularly in cirrhotic patients. Caution is also advised in patients with impaired hepatic function or progressive liver disease since minor alterations of fluid and electrolyte balance may precipitate hepatic coma. Therapy with chlorthalidone should always be initiated cautiously in patients who have undergone sympathectomy and in those receiving other antihypertensive drugs, ganglionic or peripheral adrenergic blocking agents, or curare. Careful and continous supervision of patients on such regimens is essential, and the dosage of these drugs should be reduced by 50%. Sensitivity reactions may occur in patients with a history of allergy or bronchial asthma, and in susceptible patients bronchial asthma may occur. The combination with reserpine should not be given to patients with preexisting mental depression, and if drug-induced, treatment should be suspended (the possibility of suicide should be kept in mind). Also electroconvulsive therapy should be deferred while the patient is taking this drug since severe and fatal reactions have been known to occur; a lapse of at least 7 days from the time of drug withdrawal and the initiation of electroconvulsive therapy should take place. Peptic ulcer may be precipitated or activated in susceptible patients. For additional warnings, see monograph on reserpine. Since chlorthalidone may cross the placental barrier and appear in cord blood, it should be used with caution in pregnant women and nursing mothers. The drug may cause fetal or neonatal jaundice, thrombocytopenia and possibly other adverse reactions which have occurred in the adult. Also, increased respiratory secretions, nasal congestion, cyanosis and anorexia may occur in infants born to mothers treated with this drug. When used in women of childbearing age, the potential benefits of the drug should be weighed against possible hazards to the fetus.

Precautions: Periodic determinations of serum electrolytes to detect possible electrolyte imbalance should be performed at appropriate intervals, since without due care use of the drug may lead to hyponatremia, hypochloremic alkalosis, and hypokalemia. Serum and urine electrolyte determinations are particularly important when the patient is vomiting excessively or receiving parenteral fluids. Digitalis may also influence serum electrolytes. Warning signs irrespective of the cause include dryness of mouth, thirst, weakness, lethargy, drowsiness, restlessness, muscle pains or cramps, muscular fatigue, hypotension, oliguria, tachycardia, and nausea and vomiting. Emphasis should be focused on hypokalemia, especially when the drug is used in patients with cirrhosis or in those taking adrenal corticosteroids or ACTH. Digitalis may exaggerate the metabolic effects of hypokalemia especially with reference to myocardial activity. Hypochloremic alkalosis often precedes other signs of severe potassium deficiency. If potassium depletion occurs during therapy, the drug should be discontinued and potassium supplementation instituted, either as oral or parenteral potassium chloride or foods high in potassium content. Since some patients receiving rauwolfia preparations have experienced hypotension when undergoing surgery, it is therefore advised to discontinue drug therapy about 2 weeks prior to elective surgical procedures. Emergency surgery may be carried out by using, if necessary, anticholinergic or adrenergic drugs to prevent vagocirculatory responses; other supportive measures may be employed as indicated. Because renal function may deteriorate, blood urea nitrogen levels should be determined periodically. The drug should be discontinued when the BUN is rising and when hepatic dysfunction has been aggravated. Insulin requirement in diabetic patients may be altered, and latent diabetes mellitus may become manifest during therapy. Also, this drug and related compounds may decrease arterial responsiveness to norepinephrine, may increase responsiveness to tubocurarine, and may decrease serum PBI levels without signs of thyroid disturbance. Because reserpine increases gastrointestinal motility and secretion, the combination product should be used cautiously in patients with ulcerative colitis or gallstones where biliary colic may be precipitated. For complete information on reserpine therapy, see specific monograph.

Adverse Reactions: Reactions which may be seen in various degrees of frequency are nausea, gastric irritation, anorexia, vomiting, diarrhea, constipation, weakness, dizziness, vertigo, restlessness, headache, transient myopia, impotence, dysuria, skin rashes, urticaria, purpura, decreased glucose tolerance, hyperuricemia, necrotizing angiitis, Lyell's syndrome (toxic epidermal necrolysis), aplastic anemia, thrombocytopenia, leukopenia, agranulocytosis, possible pancreatitis, jaundice, xanthopsia, paresthesia and photosensitization. Symptoms of accidental overdosage include nausea, weakness, dizziness, and electrolyte imbalance. In the absence of a specific antidote, gastric lavage followed by supportive treatment is recommended. When necessary, this may consist of dextrose, saline and potassium administered intravenously with caution.

Dosage and Administration: *Orally.* Initially, 50 or 100 mg daily. Because of the drug's prolonged duration of action, therapy may also be initiated in most cases with a dosage of 100 mg 3 times a week, on alternate days; some patients may require 150 or 200 mg at these intervals. Occasionally, a daily dosage of 200 mg may be necessary, but dosage beyond this level usually does not evoke a greater response. Divided doses are unnecessary; a single dose in the morning with food is recommended. Maintenance doses often may be lower than the initial doses and should be tailored to the needs of the patient.

Availability:
HYGROTON® Tablets, 25 mg (peach color) in bottles of 100 and 1000; 50 mg (aqua-color) and 100 mg (white, scored) in bottles of 100 and 1000, in Compliance Paks® (single dose) of 28 in packages of 6 and in Strip-Dispenser packages of 100. **(USV)**
REGROTON® Tablets (pink, scored), 50 mg with reserpine, 0.25 mg in bottles of 100 and 1000. **(USV)**
DEMI-REGROTON™ Tablets (white, round) contain 1/2 the amounts in bottles of 100. **(USV)**

CHLORZOXAZONE

Chemical Name: 5-Chloro-2-benzoxazolol.

Description: Chlorzoxazone is a metabolite of zoxazolamine, and occurs as a white, crystalline powder very slightly soluble in water.

Chlorzoxazone is a centrally-acting skeletal muscle relaxant. Data available from animal experiments as well as clinical studies indicate that the drug acts primarily at the level of the spinal cord and subcortical areas of the brain where it inhibits multisynaptic reflex arcs involved in producing and maintaining skeletal muscle spasm of varied etiology. It has no direct effect on the muscle itself. The clinical result is a reduction of the skeletal muscle spasm with relief of pain and increased mobility of the involved muscles. Blood levels can be detected in patients during the 1st hour after administration; peak levels are attained in the 3rd and 4th hours. Chlorzoxazone is rapidly metabolized and is excreted in the urine, primarily in a conjugated form as the glucuronide. Less than 1% of a dose is excreted unchanged in the urine in 24 hours.

Indications: As an adjunct to rest, physical therapy and other measures for the relief of discomfort associated with acute painful musculoskeletal conditions. Chlorzoxazone may be given in conjunction with acetaminophen in those conditions where the pain is severe.

Contraindications: Hypersensitivity to either component.

Warnings: Safe use during pregnancy has not been established. Therefore, it should be used in women of childbearing potential only when, in the judgment of the physician, the potential benefits outweigh the possible adverse effects on the fetus.

Precautions: Caution is advisable in patients with a known allergy or with a history of allergic reactions to drugs. If signs suggesting a sensitivity reaction such as urticaria, redness or itching of the skin or any signs or symptoms suggestive of liver dysfunction develop, the drug should be discontinued.

Adverse Reactions: Occasionally, drowsiness, dizziness, lightheadedness, malaise, overstimulation, and gastrointestinal disturbances with bleeding on rare occasions. Rarely, allergic-type skin rashes, petechiae, ecchymoses, angioneurotic edema, anaphylactic reactions, discolored urine resulting from a phenolic metabolite of chlorzoxazone, and liver damage. In some patients, the liver damage was reversible upon discontinuance of therapy, and in others, a causal relationship to the drug had not been established.

Dosage and Administration: *Orally.* Adults, 1 or 2 tablets 3 or 4 times daily, depending upon severity of muscle spasm—increased to 3 tablets 3 or 4 times daily if necessary and reduced as improvement is seen. Children, usually ½ to 2 tablets 3 or 4 times daily according to age and weight. The tablets may be crushed and mixed with food or a suitable vehicle for administration to children. The usual adult dosage for chlorzoxazone-acetaminophen is 2 tablets 4 times daily.

Availability:

Chlorzoxazone

PARAFLEX® Tablets, 250 mg (scored, orange) in bottles of 100 and 1000. **(McNeil)**

w/Acetaminophen

PARAFON FORTE® Tablets, 250 mg with acetaminophen, 300 mg in bottles of 100 and 500, in Dispenser Packs of 250 and in unit-dose packages of 200. **(McNeil)**

CHOLERA VACCINE

Description: Cholera Vaccine is a sterile suspension, in isotonic sodium chloride solution or other suitable diluent, of killed cholera vibrios *(Vibrio comma)* organisms. It is prepared from equal portions of suspensions of cholera vibrios of the Inaba and Ogawa strains. The Inaba strain used has an antigenic value not less than that of N.I.H. Inaba strain 35-A-3, and the Ogawa strain has an antigenic value not less than that of N.I.H. Ogawa strain 41. At the time of manufacture, the vaccine contains in each ml about 8 billion cholera organisms, and a suitable preservative.

Indications: Active immunization against cholera. Since it is impossible to confer immunity in the face of massive exposure to cholera organisms, booster injections may be required every 6 months to maintain an effective immunity.

Contraindications: The same as for other immunizing biologicals. The vaccine should not be given during an acute illness, during convalescence from surgery or trauma, or in other conditions that would depress the immune response. The concomitant administration of cholera vaccine and adrenocorticotropin and adrenal corticosteroids is not recommended.

Precautions: Cholera vaccine is not recommended for treatment of an established cholera infection whether manifested by clinical disease or a carrier state, since it apparently does not prevent development of a carrier state. Injection should be made either deeply subcutaneously or intramuscularly, *never* intravenously. The parenteral administration of any biological product should be provided with every known precaution for the prevention and arrest of allergic and other untoward reactions. A careful history of the patient is essential to determine whether any possible sensitivity to the vaccine such as anaphylaxis, rash, fever, etc. exists.

Adverse Reactions: Erythema, swelling, tenderness at the injection site, malaise and low-grade fever may begin soon after injection or they may be delayed for 3 to 10 days. The symptoms usually subside within 24 to 48 hours. Although evidence of serious major reactions is lacking, postvaccinal neurologic disorders have been reported following the injection of almost all biological products; they are extremely uncommon but they may be serious. The possibility of their occurrence must be appreciated by those responsible for immunization against infectious disease.

Dosage and Administration: *Subcutaneously* or *intramuscularly.* Adults and children 10 years of age and older, 0.5 ml followed in 7 to 10 days by another injection of 1 ml. Booster doses of 1 ml should be given every 6 months for as long as protection is desired. For children, 3 injections at intervals of 7 to 10 days are recommended as follows:

	1st dose	*2nd dose*	*3rd dose*
6 months to 4 years of age	0.1 ml	0.3 ml	0.3 ml
5 to 9 years of age	0.3 ml	0.5 ml	0.3 ml

Booster injections of 0.3 to 0.5 ml, according to the child's age, should be given every 6 months. Each dose should be given in a site not previously used for a vaccine or toxoid. A separate heat-sterilized syringe and needle should be used for each patient to prevent transmission of homologous serum hepatitis virus and other infectious agents from one individual to another.

Availability:
CHOLERA VACCINE in vials of 1.5 ml. **(Lederle and Lilly)**
CHOLERA VACCINE in vials of 1.5 and 20 ml. **(Wyeth)**

CHOLESTYRAMINE RESIN

Description: Cholestyramine is the chloride salt of a basic anion exchange resin which has an affinity for sodium chloride and a particularly strong affinity for acidic materials such as bile acids. It occurs as a white to off-white powder insoluble in water and has an amine-like odor.

During normal digestion, bile acids are secreted by the liver and gallbladder into the intestine where fat and lipid materials present in food are emulsified, thus facilitating absorption. A major portion of the bile acid secreted is also reabsorbed from the intestinal tract. When cholestyramine is administered, it absorbs and combines with the bile acids in the intestine to form an insoluble complex thus causing the enterohepatic cycle to be partially disrupted by the fecal excretion of increased amounts of bile acids. Cholesterol is the major, if not the sole, precursor of bile acids which are formed by the oxidation of cholesterol. The increased fecal loss of bile acids, mentioned earlier, ultimately leads to reduced levels of serum bile acids and increased oxidation of cholesterol, thereby increasing the rate of LDL removal; nonetheless, the serum triglyceride levels may increase or remain unchanged in cholestryamine-treated patients. However, no conclusive reports are available to establish whether or not drug-induced lowering of serum cholesterol or other lipid levels has a detrimental, a beneficial or no effect on the morbidity or mortality due to atherosclerosis or coronary heart failure.

In patients with partial biliary obstruction, the reduction of serum bile acid levels by cholestyramine is thought to reduce excess bile acids deposited in the dermal tissues by promoting their fecal excretion. The prompt and continuing relief from severe and persistent pruritus afforded most of these patients may be due to this mobilization.

Indications: To reduce serum cholesterol concentrations, particularly type II hyperlipoproteinemia as an adjunct to dietary control, and for the relief of pruritus associated with partial biliary obstruction.

Contraindications: In patients with *complete* biliary obstruction, since it is thought that cholestyramine is not effective where bile is not secreted into the intestine, and in those with prior hypersensitivity to the drug.

Warnings: The resin should not be taken in the dry form; it should always be mixed with water or other fluids before administration. Large doses may interfere with normal fat digestion. To prevent nutritional deficiencies of the fat-soluble vitamins in those patients taking the resin for prolonged periods, the diet should be supplemented with vitamins A, D and K. Whether cholestyramine is safe to use during pregnancy has not been established. The use of any drug by pregnant or lactating women or by women of childbearing age requires that the potential benefits of the drug outweigh the possible hazards to the mother and child. Since cholestyramine is an anion exchange resin, the drug may have a strong affinity for acidic substances and may also absorb to some extent substances that are neutral or basic in nature. Therefore, this resin may delay or reduce the absorption of concomitant oral medication such as phenylbutazone, warfarin, chlorothiazide, as well as tetracycline, phenobarbital, thyroid and thyroxine preparations, and digitalis. Discontinuance of the cholestyramine resin could pose a hazard to health if a potentially toxic drug such as digitalis has been titrated to a maintenance level while the patient was taking this drug. Furthermore, the dosage of anticoagulants given concomitantly should be closely monitored.

Precautions: If the resin is to be taken for a prolonged period, fat-soluble vitamins A and D should be taken daily in water-miscible form; they may be given parenterally if preferred. Prolonged use may increase bleeding tendencies due to hypoprothrombinemia associated with vitamin K deficiency. Parenteral vitamin K will reverse the trend promptly; oral vitamin K will prevent recurrences. If given concomitantly with cholestyramine, chlorothiazide, phenylbutazone or warfarin, these latter drugs should be taken 1 hour before meals. It may be wise for patients taking other drugs to take them ½ to 1 hour before taking this resin. Since the resin is a chloride, it is possible, theoretically, that prolonged use may lead to hyperchloremic acidosis. Currently, there is no rationale for the use of cholestyramine in the relief of pruritus associated with other disease processes. Periodic measurements of serum triglyceride levels are recommended to ensure that significant changes have not occurred. Because of reduced absorption of folic acid, a deficiency in this vitamin is a possibility.

Adverse Reactions: The most common adverse reactions are confined to the gastrointestinal tract. Constipation is the major single complication which can at times be severe and is occasionally accompanied by fecal impaction and/or hemorrhoids (with or without bleeding). This usually occurs with doses in excess of 24 gm/day and in patients over 60 years of age. However, most instances of constipation are mild and transient in nature and can readily be controlled with standard treatment. Some patients require a temporary decrease in dosage or discontinuation of therapy. Less frequently reported are abdominal discomfort (abdominal pain and distension), flatulence, nausea, vomiting, diarrhea, heartburn, anorexia, feeling of indigestion, and steatorrhea. Bleeding tendencies due to hypothrombinemia (vitamin K deficiency) as well as deficiencies of vitamin A (one case of night blindness reported) and vitamin D have been noted. Other reported reactions included rash and irritation of the skin, tongue and perianal area; hyperchloremic acidosis in children, and osteoporosis. A ten-month old baby with biliary atresia developed acute intestinal sepsis and died after having been given a dosage of 9 gm/day for 3 days. Occasionally, calcified material has been observed in the biliary tract, including calcification of the gallbladder. One patient experienced biliary colic on each of three occasions on which the drug was taken, and another patient was found to have "pasty mass" in the transverse colon on x-ray. Other events, not necessarily drug-related, include rectal bleeding, black stools, hemorrhoidal bleeding, bleeding from known duodenal ulcer, dysphagia, hiccups, ulcer attack, sour taste, pancreatitis, rectal pain, and diverticulitis; decreased prothrombin time, ecchymosis, anemia; claudication, xanthomas of hands and fingers, angina, arteritis, thrombophlebitis, myocardial ischemia, increased postprandial angina, chest pains; urticaria, asthma, wheezing, shortness of breath; backache, muscle and joint pains, arthritis; headache, anxiety, vertigo, dizziness, fatigue, tinnitus, syncope, drowsiness, femoral nerve pain, paresthesia; arcus juvenilis, uveitis; hematuria, dysuria, urine with burnt odor, diuresis; weight loss or gain, increased libido, swollen glands, edema, and dental bleeding.

Dosage and Administration: *Orally.* The recommended initial adult dose is 1 packet or 1 scoopful (containing 4 gm of cholestyramine resin in 9 gm of the drug) 3 times daily before meals. Dosage may then be adjusted as required to meet the patient's clinical situation; however, the total daily dosage should not exceed 24 gm. The usual maintenance dosage is 4 gm 3 or 4 times daily before meals and at bedtime. The dosage for infants and children has not been established. **Important Note:** The powder should always be mixed with water or other fluids before ingesting.

Availability:
QUESTRAN® Powder in packets of 4 gm; cartons of 50 packets and in containers of 378 gm.
(Mead Johnson)

CHOLINE MAGNESIUM TRISALICYLATE

Description: A new form of salicylate possessing effective antiarthritic properties. Choline magnesium trisalicylate (CMT) provides antiinflammatory, analgesic and antipyretic activity similar to that of aspirin, but with more rapid absorption and greater gastric tolerance. The drug has been reported to promote satisfactory relief of the signs and symptoms of rheumatoid arthritis, osteoarthritis and other arthritic conditions. The compound is composed of 293 mg of choline salicylate and 362 mg of magnesium salicylate to provide 500 mg of nonacetylated salicylate, and is freely soluble in water.

Although the mechanism of the antiinflammatory effect is not known, the drug has been found to be effective in the treatment of rheumatoid arthritis as judged by a decrease in pain, joint swelling and tenderness and duration of morning stiffness. Unlike aspirin, CMT does not inhibit blood platelet aggregation or serotonin release, nor does it cause any significant increase in fecal blood loss as demonstrated by radioactive chromium of red blood cells. Results of comparative studies with indomethacin indicate that it is as effective as indomethacin in the treatment of osteoarthritis, but exhibits less serious adverse effects, and no observable stomach mucosal irritation as determined by endoscopic examination.

Readily absorbed from the gastrointestinal tract, it reaches maximum blood levels within 2 hours. At recommended doses, a therapeutic range of 5 to 30 mg/100 ml is achieved, and a steady state condition is generally attained after 4 or 5 doses. Since it has the advantage of a long half-life of from 9 to 17 hours, adequate plasma salicylate levels are maintained on a twice-a-day regimen. CMT is primarily excreted by the kidneys chiefly as glycine and glucuronide conjugates.

Indications: Relief of the signs and symptoms of rheumatoid arthritis, osteoarthritis and other arthritic conditions. May be used as the sole therapeutic agent or in combination with gold salts. Safe and effective use in patients in the acute stages of the disease (incapacitated, bedridden, or confined to a wheel chair) has not been established.

Contraindications: Unusual sensitivity to salicylates.

Precautions: Routine caution is required in patients with chronic renal insufficiency, or with active erosive gastritis, or peptic ulcer, and in those requiring anticoagulant medications (coumarin, heparin or indandione preparations). Moreover, gastrointestinal ulceration may be increased when the drug is taken with steroids, the butazone-type agents, or with alcohol. The usual care should be exercised when administering CMT during pregnancy. Since high doses of salicylates may inhibit prostaglandin synthetase, the use of this drug is not recommended prior to parturition. Data are not sufficient to justify use in children under 12 years of age.

Adverse Reactions: CMT is generally well tolerated at recommended dosage levels; however, large doses or prolonged therapy may cause salicylism. Tinnitus is the initial most common sign of salicylate intoxication, and indicates the need for a reduction of dosage.

Dosage and Administration: *Orally* on a twice-a-day schedule. The recommended daily dose for *rheumatoid arthritis and severe arthritic conditions* is 4 to 6 tablets, and for *osteoarthritis and mild to moderate arthritic conditions* is 2 to 4 tablets in equally divided doses. If the physician prefers, 1 or 2 tablets 3 times daily may be administered.

Availability:
TRILISATE™ Tablets, 500 mg in bottles of 100. **(Purdue Frederick)**

CHORIONIC GONADOTROPIN

Description: Chorionic gonadotropin is the water-soluble, anterior pituitary-like hormone isolated from the urine of gravid women. It occurs as a highly purified crystalline material, standardized in international units (IU or in equipotent U.S.P. units); one IU is equal to the gonadotropic activity of 0.1 mg of the Standard Preparation of the World Health Organization.

In the male, it is given in an attempt to stimulate the interstitial cells of the testes (cells of Leydig) to produce androgen. The response may be considered similar to the effect produced by the interstitial cell-stimulating hormone (ICSH) from the anterior lobe of the pituitary. Chorionic gonadotropin is likely to be of benefit in all conditions directly related to insufficient secretion of androgen provided the interstitial cells of the testes are capable of stimulation.

In the female, it is given in an attempt to stimulate the corpus luteum of the ovary to produce progesterone. The response may be considered similar to the effect produced during the normal menstrual cycle when luteinizing hormone participates with follicle stimulating hormone in the development and maturation of the normal ovarian follicle, and the midcycle LH surge triggers ovulation. Chorionic gonadotropin can substitute for LH in this function.

Indications: Treatment of prepubertal cryptorchidism in the absence of anatomical lesions, and in selected cases of male hypogonadism secondary to pituitary failure. It is also employed to induce ovulation and pregnancy in the anovulatory, infertile woman in whom the cause of anovulation is secondary and not due to primary ovarian failure, and who has been appropriately pretreated with menotropins. Use of this agent as an aid to weight reduction is unjustified because there is no substantial evidence of effectiveness or safety.

Contraindications: Precocious puberty, prostatic carcinoma or other androgen-dependent neoplasia, and prior allergic reaction to chorionic gonadotropin.

Warnings: Chorionic gonadotropin is indicated for intramuscular injection and *should not* be administered intravenously.

Precautions: Boys should be observed carefully for signs of premature sexual development, in which case the drug should be withdrawn. However, a reduced dosage regimen may be resumed after regression of undue development in those cases in which therapy is believed warranted. Since androgens may cause fluid retention, the drug should be used with caution in patients with epilepsy, migraine, asthma, cardiac or renal disease. The development of edema has been reported in instances where a high dosage regimen was being used. This is usually regarded as a manifestation of salt and water retention attributable to androgen secretion resulting from stimulation of the testicular cells of Leydig. Dosage should be reduced considerably in such cases. Induction of controlled ovulation should not be attempted without full knowledge of the precautionary measures (see package literature) required to achieve the desired effect and obviate the potential development of ovarian hyperstimulation, such as polycystic ovaries, rupture, multiple pregnancies. For additional data, see monograph on Menotropins.

Adverse Reactions: Complications noted were headache, irritability, restlessness, depression, tiredness, edema, precocious puberty, gynecomastia, and pain at the injection site.

Dosage and Administration: *Intramuscularly.* In cryptorchidism, therapy is usually instituted between the ages of 4 and 9. The following dosage regimens are recommended and the one selected should depend upon the age and weight of the patient, the condition to be corrected and the expected clinical response. Dosage may be 4000 units 3 times a week for 3 weeks; 5000 units every second day for 4 injections; 15 injections of 500 to 1000 units over a period of 6 weeks, or 500 units 3 times a week for 4 to 6 weeks. This last regimen may be repeated after an interval of 1 month giving 1000 units/injection. In hypogonadism, the dosage regimen may be 500 to 1000 units 3 times a week for 3 weeks followed by the same dose 2 times a week for 3 weeks; 1000 to 2000 units 3 times a week or 4000 units 3 times a week for 6 to 9 months, following which the dosage may be reduced to 2000 units 3 times a week for an additional 3 months. In induction of ovulation and pregnancy, the dose is 5000 to 10,000 units 1 day following the last dose of menotropins.

Availability:
ANTUITRIN-S® (dry powder) in Steri-Vials® of 5000 U.S.P. units with 10-ml vials of sterile diluent. **(Parke-Davis)**
A.P.L.® (dry powder) in Secules® of 5000, 10,000 and 20,000 U.S.P. units with 10-ml vial of diluent. **(Ayerst)**
CHORIONIC GONADOTROPIN (dry powder) in vials of 10,000 units with 10-ml vials of diluent. **(Amfre-Grant)**
FOLLUTEIN® (dry powder) in vials of 10,000 U.S.P. units with 10-ml vials of diluent. **(Squibb)**
PREGNYL® (dry powder) in vials of 10,000 U.S.P. units with 10-ml vials of diluent. **(Organon)**

CHYMOTRYPSIN

Description: Chymotrypsin is one of the proteolytic enzymes obtained from the mammalian pancreas. It occurs as a mixture of chymotrypsins, of which *alpha* chymotrypsin is the most stable and diffusible. Chymotrypsin occurs as a white to yellowish white, odorless, crystalline or amorphous powder slightly soluble in water. It is assayed for potency on the basis of its proteolytic activity; the potency of commercial preparations is expressed in units. Calculated on the dry basis, each milligram contains not less than 1000 N.F. units.

The exact mechanism by which it clears the inflammatory process is not known. It has been suggested that the enzyme reduces or removes the fibrin-like material blocking the capillaries and the lymphatics of the involved area of inflammation, thus releasing the products of congestion so that the healing process is accelerated.

Indications: As adjunctive aid in conditions in which inflammation, edema and pain prolong the clinical course as in episiotomy. May be useful in reducing moderate to severe inflammation associated with accidental or surgical trauma when used to supplement and augment other methods of therapy such as immobilization, elevation, compresses, and chemotherapy. *Alpha* chymotrypsin is indicated specifically in ophthalmic surgery where dissection of the lens zonule facilitates intracapsular cataract extraction with less trauma to the eye. Dilute solutions of the enzyme dissolve the delicate filaments or zonules which hold the lens, obviating extracapsular extraction of the lens. Zonulysis is usually effected in about 2 minutes with a 1:5000 solution, and in about 4 minutes with a 1:10,000 solution.

Contraindications: In patients hypersensitive to this or other enzymes, in the presence of severe generalized or localized infection or known disorders of blood coagulation. Nor is chymotrypsin recommended for use in children under 6 years of age, because death has occurred due to anaphylactic shock. The *alpha* form of chymotrypsin is contraindicated in the presence of high vitreous pressure or gaping incisional wounds and in congenital cataracts. Use in patients under 20 years of age is not recommended because of the danger of loss of vitreous humor.

Warnings: The safe use of enzymes during pregnancy has not been established. Although serious and even fatal anaphylactic reactions have occurred, current data seem to indicate that these reactions are rare provided necessary precautions are taken. The usual remedial agents such as epinephrine, corticosteroids, antihistamines, aminophylline, etc. should be readily available in case of untoward reactions following injection.

Precautions: Since chymotrypsin is a foreign protein, sensitivity may develop from repeated injections; this is characterized by local edema, erythema, or urticaria at the site of injection, and possible anaphylactic shock. In patients with known or suspected allergies, scratch tests are advisable prior to the parenteral administration of this drug. Every patient should be observed for 30 minutes after an injection. Chymotrypsin preparations should be given with caution to patients with severe renal or hepatic disease, septicemia, hepatic disease, severe generalized or localized infection, or known disorders of blood coagulation. Patients taking anticoagulants concomitantly should be observed carefully. An appropriate antibiotic should be used concomitantly in accidental injury or in surgery where infection is present or suspected.

Adverse Reactions: Some of the most common reactions to chymotrypsin are allergic and sensitivity reactions such as exanthemas, pruritus, angioedema and anaphylactic shock; increased intraocular pressure following uncomplicated intracapsular cataract extraction;

pain and swelling at the site of injection; nausea; vomiting and diarrhea. The following have been reported following the use of *alpha* chymotrypsin in ophthalmic surgery: moderate uveitis, corneal edema, corneal striation, transient increases in intraocular tension. After complicated surgery on the eye, transient postoperative glaucoma has been reported. This glaucoma is self-limited, apparently requires no treatment and thus far has caused no known structural or functional damage to any aphakic eye in which there was no other major postoperative complication. An occasional patient may experience gastrointestinal upset following oral administration. Hematuria, mild skin rash, urticaria or itching has been reported in rare instances. Withdrawal of therapy is recommended in such cases.

Dosage and Administration: *Intramuscularly,* 0.5 to 1 ml once or twice daily depending upon the severity of the condition; frequency of injections may be decreased as the course of the disease is altered. In some of the chronic or recurrent conditions, 0.5 to 1 ml may be injected once or twice weekly. *Alpha* chymotrypsin is used by *irrigation* of the posterior chamber [eye] according to directions in the package literature. *Orally,* usually 1 or 2 tablets 4 times daily initially then 1 tablet 3 or 4 times daily for maintenance and prophylaxis. The tablets may be taken before meals and at bedtime. Treatment should begin as soon as possible after injury occurs.

Availability:

AlphaChymotrypsin

ALPHA CHYMAR® Dry Powder for Ophthalmic Use, 750 units (lyophilized) with 10-ml vial of diluent. **(Armour)**

AVAZYME®/-100 Tablets (enteric-coated), 50,000 and 100,000 units in bottles of 48 and 250. **(Wallace)**

CATARASE® Dry Powder For Ophthalmic Use, 150 units/ml in 2-Chamber Univials of 2 ml containing the enzyme in the lower chamber and the sterile diluent in the upper chamber. **(Smith, Miller & Patch)**

ZOLYSE® Dry Powder for Ophthalmic Use, 750 units (lyophilized) with 10-ml vial of Balanced Salt Solution (BSS®) diluent. **(Alcon)**

w/Trypsin

CHYMORAL® Tablets (red) in bottles of 48. Contains 50,000 units of trypsin and chymotrypsin in a ratio of 6:1. **(Armour)**

CHYMORAL®-100 Tablets (red-orange) in bottles of 48 and 250. Contains 100,000 units of trypsin and chymotrypsin in a ratio of 6:1. **(Armour)**

ORENZYME®: **(Merrell-National)**

Bitabs (enteric-coated, yellow) in bottles of 100. Each double-strength tablet contains chymotrypsin, 8000 units and trypsin, 100,000 units; equivalent in tryptic activity to 40 mg of trypsin, N.F.

Tablets (enteric-coated, red) in bottles of 48 and 500. Contains trypsin 50,000 units and chymotrypsin, 4000; equivalent in tryptic activity to 20 mg of trypsin, N.F.

CIMETIDINE

Chemical Name: N''-Cyano-N-methyl-N'-[2][(5-methyl-1H imidazole-4-yl)thio]-ethylguanidine.

Description: Cimetidine is a synthetic histamine H_2-receptor antagonist that provides effective treatment of peptic ulcer through the suppression of gastric acid secretion. Unlike the anticholinergic agents, the drug offers a more physiologic attack on peptic ulcers by significantly blocking the reception of gastric histamine at the histamine H_2 receptors of the parietal cells. It not only inhibits both daytime and nocturnal basal gastric secretion but also inhibits gastric acid output stimulated by food, histamine, pentagastrin, caffeine, and insulin. Preliminary clinical studies have demonstrated that the drug provides a consistent effect of diminishing ulcer pain and promoting healing.

Cimetidine is rapidly absorbed following oral administration with peak activity occurring in approximately 1 hour and persisting for about 4 hours. The drug has a half-life of 2 hours, and is excreted primarily by the kidney. The effects of a 300-mg dose taken orally were studied in patients with active duodenal ulcers. The drug significantly lowered acid output and increased intragastric pH. The degree and duration of inhibition of acid secretion appeared to correlate with blood cimetidine levels. Studies to date do not provide evidence for the safe use of cimetadine in uncomplicated duodenal ulcer for periods of more than 8 weeks.

Indications: Short-term (up to 8 weeks) treatment of duodenal ulcer and for the treatment of pathological hypersecretory conditions such as Zollinger-Ellison syndrome, systemic mastocytosis, and multiple endocrine adenomas. Concomitant antacids should be given as needed for the relief of pain.

Contraindications: None known.

Precautions: Safe use in pregnant patients, or in women of childbearing potential has not been established; therefore, the drug should not be given to these patients unless, in the judgment of the physician, the anticipated benefits outweigh the potential risks to the fetus. Moreover, safe and effective use in children under 16 years of age has not been confirmed. Although there is at present no evidence that the drug is secreted in the milk of lactating women, it is nevertheless advised that such women refrain from nursing their infants.

Adverse Reactions: Mild and transient diarrhea, muscular pain, dizziness, and rash have been reported in about 1% of patients. Mild gynecomastia has also been reported in a few patients treated for one month or longer. In patients being treated for pathological hypersecretory states, this problem occurred in about 4% of cases while in all others the incidence was about 0.3%. No evidence of drug-induced endocrine dysfunction was found, and the condition remained unchanged or returned to normal with continuing treatment. A few instances of neutropenia were also noted. Regularly observed were small increases in plasma creatinine levels which did not progress with continued therapy and disappeared at the termination of treatment. Some increases in serum transaminase were also observed.

Dosage and Administration: *Orally* or *intravenously by slow infusion.* The recommended oral dosage is 300 mg 4 times daily with meals and at bedtime. The recommended intravenous dosage is 300 mg every 6 hours. Patients with severely impaired renal function should be limited to 300 mg every 12 hours whether administered orally or intravenously.

Availability:
TAGAMET®: **(Smith Kline & French)**
Injection, 300 mg in single-dose vials of 2 ml in packages of 10.
Tablets, 300 mg (pale green) in bottles of 100.

CLEMASTINE FUMARATE

Chemical Name: 2-[2-[1-(4-Chlorophenyl)-1-phenylethoxy]ethyl]-1-methylpyrrolidine hydrogen fumarate.

Description: An antihistaminic compound with antipruritic activity.

Indications: Symptomatic relief of seasonal allergic rhinitis (sneezing, rhinorrhea, pruritus, lacrimation); relief of mild, uncomplicated allergic skin manifestations of urticaria and angioedema.

Contraindications: Hypersensitivity to the drug or to other antihistamines of similar chemical structure; nursing mothers; lower respiratory tract symptoms including asthma; concomitant therapy with monoamine oxidase inhibitors (MAOI), since a prolonged and intensified anticholinergic effect of the antihistamine may result.

Warnings: Antihistamines should be used with considerable caution in patients with narrow angle glaucoma, stenosing peptic ulcer, pyloroduodenal obstruction, symptomatic prostatic hypertrophy, and bladder neck obstruction. It is not recommended for use in children under 12 years of age, nor in pregnant women until there is adequate experience to determine safe use. Alcohol, hypnotics, sedatives, tranquilizers, and other CNS depressant drugs may have an additive effect when used with clemastine and should therefore be prescribed with caution. Since drowsiness may occur, sensitive patients should be cautioned not to engage in activities requiring alertness and skill until their response to the drug has been established. Elderly patients are more likely to experience dizziness, sedation, and hypotension.

Precautions: Routine caution is essential in patients with a history of bronchial asthma, increased intraocular pressure, hyperthyroidism, cardiovascular disease, and hypertension.

Adverse Reactions: Transient drowsiness occurs relatively frequently and may require discontinuation of therapy. The most frequent complications involve the CNS and include sedation, sleepiness, dizziness, disturbed coordination, and fatigue. Those that occur less frequently are confusion, restlessness, excitation, nervousness, tremor, irritability, insomnia, euphoria, paresthesias, blurred vision, diplopia, vertigo, tinnitus, acute labyrinthitis, hysteria, neuritis, and convulsions. *Cardiovascular effects* are manifested by hypotension, headache, palpitation, tachycardia, and extrasystoles; *hematologic effects* by hemolytic anemia, thrombocytopenia, and agranulocytosis; *gastrointestinal effects* by epigastric distress, anorexia, nausea, vomiting, diarrhea, and constipation; *genitourinary effects* by urinary frequency, difficult urination, urinary retention, and early menses; *respiratory effects* by thickening of bronchial secretions, tightness of chest and wheezing, and nasal stuffiness; *miscellaneous effects* by urticaria, drug rash, anaphylactic shock, photosensitivity, excessive perspiration, chills, dryness of mouth, nose and throat. Reactions to overdosage may vary from CNS depression to stimulation, although children are more prone to stimulation. Atropine-like signs and symptoms are dry mouth; fixed, dilated pupils; flushing; and gastrointestinal symptoms. If vomiting has not occurred spontaneously, emesis should be induced by having the patient drink a glass of water or milk. Precautions against aspiration must be taken, especially in infants and children. If vomiting is unsuccessful, gastric lavage is indicated within 3 hours after ingestion and even later if large amounts of milk or cream were given beforehand. Isotonic saline is the lavage solution of choice, and saline cathartics, which draw water into the bowels are valuable for their action in rapid dilution of bowel content. Stimulants should not be used, but vasopressors may be employed to treat hypotension.

Dosage and Administration: *Orally.* The maximum recommended dosage is 1 tablet 3 times daily. Many patients respond favorably to a single tablet dose, which may be repeated as required, but not to exceed 3 tablets daily.

Availability:
TAVIST® Tablets, 2.68 mg in bottles of 100. **(Dorsey)**

CLIDINIUM BROMIDE

Chemical Name: 3-Hydroxy-1-methylquinuclidinium bromide benzilate.

Description: Clidinium bromide is a synthetic quaternary ammonium compound with anticholinergic and antispasmodic activity. It occurs as a white or nearly white, crystalline substance that is soluble in water. Its molecular weight is 432.36.

Clidinium has been found to inhibit gastrointestinal motility and to diminish gastric acid secretion. Its anticholinergic activity approximates that of atropine sulfate and propantheline bromide.

Indications: Adjunctive therapy in the treatment of peptic ulcer. It does not heal the ulcer, decrease the rate of recurrence or prevent complications.

Contraindications: Known hypersensitivity to the drug or to other anticholinergic agents; glaucoma; obstructive uropathy (e.g., bladder neck obstruction due to prostatic hypertrophy); obstructive disease of the gastrointestinal tract (as in achalasia, pyloroduodenal stenosis, etc.); obstructive or paralytic ileus; intestinal atony of the elderly or debilitated patient; severe ulcerative colitis; toxic megacolon complicating ulcerative colitis; unstable cardiovascular status in acute hemorrhage; and myasthenia gravis.

Warnings: Since drowsiness and blurred vision may occur, patients should be cautioned not to engage in hazardous occupations requiring alertness or skill. Decreased sweating may occur, which in high environmental temperature may lead to heat prostration. Diarrhea may be an early symptom of incomplete intestinal obstruction especially in patients with ileostomy or colostomy. In this instance treatment with clidinium would be inappropriate and possibly harmful. Overdosage may result in a curare-like action manifested by neuromuscular blockade which can result in muscular weakness and possible paralysis. The use of this drug in pregnant women or in women of childbearing potential requires that the therapeutic benefits be weighed against the possible hazards to the mother and fetus. As with all anticholinergic drugs, clidinium may inhibit secretion of milk in lactating women; therefore, it is generally recomended that nursing should not be undertaken nor should the drug be used by nursing mothers. Safe and effective use in children has not been established.

Precautions: Cautious use is advised in the elderly patient and in individuals with autonomic neuropathy, hepatic or renal disease, hyperthyroidism, coronary heart disease, congestive heart failure, cardiac arrhythmias, tachycardia, hypertension, and prostatic hypertrophy. Utmost caution is recommended in the presence of ulcerative colitis since large doses may suppress intestinal motility to the point of producing a paralytic ileus, and which may then precipitate or aggravate the serious complication of toxic megacolon. Clidinium may exacerbate hiatal hernia associated with reflux esophagitis.

Adverse Reactions: The most frequently reported side effects are dry mouth, blurred vision, urinary hesitancy, and constipation. Other reported reactions include decreased sweating, urinary retention, tachycardia, palpitations, mydriasis, cycloplegia, increased ocular tension, loss of taste, headaches, nervousness, mental confusion, drowsiness, weakness, dizziness, insomnia, nausea, vomiting, bloated feeling, impotence, suppression of lactation, and severe allergic reactions or drug idiosyncrasies including anaphylaxis, urticaria, and other dermal manifestations. An intensification of these reactions and a curare-like action usually occur with overdosage. Treatment generally consists of gastric lavage; maintenance of adequate airway, using artificial respiration if necessary; administration of intravenous fluids, and if fever is present, alcohol sponging or ice packs.

Dosage and Administration: *Orally.* The usual dosage is 2.5 to 5 mg 3 or 4 times daily before meals and at bedtime. Dosage in excess of 20 mg daily is usually not required to obtain maximal effectiveness. The recommended dosage for the aged or debilitated patient is 2.5 mg 3 times daily before meals.

Availability:
QUARZAN® Capsules, 2.5 mg (green and red) and 5 mg (green and gray) in bottles of 100 and 500 and in Prescription Paks® of 50. **(Roche)**

CLINDAMYCIN

Chemical Name: Methyl 7(S)-chloro-6,7,8-trideoxy-6-trans-(1-methyl-4-propyl-L-2-pyrrolidine-carboxamido)-1-thio-L-*threo*-α-galacto-octopyranoside.

Description: Clindamycin is an antibiotic produced synthetically by replacing the 7(R)-hydroxyl group of the parent compound, lincomycin, with a 7-chloro group. Isolated as the hydrochloride hydrate salt, it occurs as a white, crystalline substance soluble in water, but insoluble in most organic solvents.

Clindamycin is said to act by inhibiting the synthesis of protein in the bacterial cell. Depending upon the sensitivity of the organism and concentration of the antibiotic, clindamycin may be either bactericidal or bacteriostatic. Following oral administration of 150 mg, the drug is rapidly and virtually completely (90%) absorbed, reaching peak serum levels within 45 minutes and persisting in diminishing concentrations for up to 6 hours. The drug is widely distributed in body fluids and tissues, including bones. About 10% of the drug's bioactivity is excreted in the urine, 3.6% in the feces, and the remainder is excreted as bioinactive metabolites.

Cross resistance has not been reported except with lincomycin. Penicillinase-producing and methicillin-resistant staphylococci usually are susceptible to clindamycin, whereas some staphylococci originally resistant to erythromycin have demonstrated resistance.

Indications: Infections caused by susceptible gram-positive pathogens, particularly streptococci, pneumococci and staphylococci, including infections of the upper and lower respiratory tract, skin and soft tissue. May be used as adjunctive therapy in dental infections.

Contraindications: Patients hypersensitive to either clindamycin or lincomycin.

Warnings: Instances of severe and persistent diarrhea with accompanying severe abdominal cramps have been reported and have at times necessitated withdrawal of the drug. The diarrhea has been occasionally associated with blood and mucus in the stools and can result in acute colitis which may have a fatal outcome. Moderate to severe cases of diarrhea should be promptly treated with fluid, electrolyte and protein supplementation as indicated. Antiperistaltic agents such as opiates, meperidine, and diphenoxylate with atropine may prolong and/or worsen the condition. Systemic corticoids and corticoid retention enemas may help to relieve the colitis. A careful inquiry should be made concerning the patient's previous sensitivities to drugs and other allergens. Safe use of clindamycin during pregnancy has not been confirmed. Considerable caution is advised when administering to newborns and infants, and appropriate monitoring of organ system functions is a necessary requirement. It is not indicated for the treatment of meningitis since the drug does not adequately diffuse into the cerebrospinal fluid.

Precautions: The drug should not be used concomitantly with erythromycin because of possible antagonism. It should be used with caution in atopic individuals. When therapy is prolonged, liver function studies and blood counts should be performed periodically. The serum half-life in patients with impaired renal function is about twice that in normal patients; hemodialysis and peritoneal dialysis do not remove the drug effectively from the blood. It is essential, therefore, to determine periodically the serum levels of clindamycin in patients with severe renal insufficiency, and to reduce the dose proportionately. The use of antibiotics occasionally results in the overgrowth of nonsusceptible organisms, particularly yeasts. If superinfection occurs, appropriate countermeasures should be instituted. Clindamycin has been shown to have neuromuscular blocking properties that may enhance the action of the other neuromuscular blocking agents. Therefore, it should be used with caution in patients receiving such drugs.

Adverse Reactions: Abdominal pain, nausea, vomiting and diarrhea occasionally with bloody stools have been reported; the occurrence of colitis demands immediate withdrawal of the drug. **Important note:** The physician should be aware that diarrhea has been observed to begin up to several weeks following cessation of therapy. Transient granulocytopenia and eosinophilia have also been reported; no causal relationship has been established. Maculopapular rash and urticaria have been observed during therapy with this agent. Generalized mild to moderate morbilliform-like skin rashes are the most frequently reported of all adverse reactions. Rare instances of erythema multiforme, some resembling Stevens-Johnson syndrome, have been associated with clindamycin. A few cases of anaphylactoid reaction have also been noted. If a hypersensitivity reaction occurs, the drug should be discontinued. The usual agents (epinephrine, corticosteroids, and antihistamines) should be readily available for emergency treatment of serious reactions. Jaundice, and transient and reversible abnormalities in liver function values (elevated alkaline phosphatase and serum transaminases) have been noted in a few instances. The significance of these changes in relation to drug therapy is not known.

Dosage and Administration: *Orally.* Adults: mild to moderately severe infections, 150 to 300 mg every 6 hours. Severe infections, 300 to 450 mg every 6 hours. Children: mild to moderately severe infections, 8 to 16 mg/kg/day divided into 3 or 4 equal doses. Severe infections, 16 to 20 mg/kg/day divided into 3 or 4 equal doses. Treatment of beta-hemolytic streptococcal infections should be continued for at least 10 days to minimize the likelihood of rheumatic fever or glomerulonephritis. Concomitant administration with food does not adversely affect absorption of the drug. *Intravenously* or *intramuscularly.* Adults: mild infections or infections due to highly susceptible pathogens, 0.6 gm daily in 2 equal doses. Moderately severe infections, 0.6 to 1.2 gm and severe infections, 1.2 to 2.7 gm daily in 2, 3 or 4 equal doses. **Note:** For more serious infections, these doses may be increased. In life-threatening situations, doses up to 4.8 gm may be given *intravenously.* Children over 1 month of age: mild infections or infections due to highly susceptible pathogens, 10 to 15 mg/kg/day. Moderately severe infections, 15 to 25 mg/kg/day. Severe infections, 25 to 40 mg/kg/day. Children's doses are given in 3 or 4 equal doses. **Note:** in severe infections it is recommended that children be given no less than 300 mg daily regardless of body weight. The dose may also be determined on the basis of square meters of body surface. Consult package literature for dilution and infusion rates.

Availability:

CLEOCIN® Capsules, 75 and 150 mg (as hydrochloride hydrate) in bottles of 16 and 100 and in Blister Pack (unit-dose) packages of 100. **(Upjohn)**

CLEOCIN PEDIATRIC™ Granules for Oral Solution, 75 mg/5 ml (as palmitate hydrochloride) in bottles of 100 and 200 ml. **(Upjohn)**
CLEOCIN® PHOSPHATE Injection, 150 mg/ml (as phosphate) in ampuls of 2 and 4 ml. **(Upjohn)**

CLOFIBRATE

Chemical Name: Ethyl 2-(*p*-Chlorophenoxy)-2-methylpropionate.

Description: Clofibrate is a colorless to pale yellow, oily liquid insoluble in water and soluble in alcohol and in other commonly used solvents.

Following oral administration of effective doses (25 mg/kg), clofibrate is uniformly absorbed from the gastrointestinal tract; serum levels are measurable within 3 to 24 hours. It is rapidly hydrolyzed by serum enzymes to the free acid which is extensively bound to plasma proteins, and is cleared from plasma within 10 to 14 hours. The estimate of clearance rate is confirmed by measurement of the rate of its appearance in the urine as the glucuronide conjugate. The precise mechanism by which clofibrate reduces serum lipid levels has not been clearly defined. However, it appears to have a greater depressant effect on the very low density lipoproteins (S_f 20-400) rich in triglycerides than on the low density lipoproteins (S_f 0-20) rich in cholesterol. Animal studies suggest that clofibrate interrupts cholesterol biosynthesis prior to mevalonate formation. At the present time it has not been established whether or not the drug-induced lowering of serum cholesterol or lipid levels has any effect, determinal, beneficial or none at all, on the morbidity or mortality due to atherosclerosis or coronary heart disease.

Indications: As adjunctive therapy to diet and other measures for the reduction of serum lipids in patients with hypercholesterolemia, hypertriglyceridemia or both. It is also indicated for the treatment of patients with xanthoma tuberosum associated with hyperlipidemia; the skin lesions frequently have regressed as a result of therapy with clofibrate.

Contraindications: Pregnancy, lactation, significant renal or hepatic dysfunction, primary biliary cirrhosis since it may raise the existing elevated cholesterol, and in children.

Warnings: In patients taking anticoagulants concomitantly, the dosage of the anticoagulant should be reduced sufficiently (usually ⅓ to ½) so that prothrombin time can be maintained at the desired level in order to prevent bleeding complications. Frequent laboratory studies are advisable until it has been established that prothrombin times have been stabilized. Strict birth control procedures must be exercised by women of childbearing potential. In patients who plan to become pregnant, clofibrate should be withdrawn several months before conception. Because of the possibility of pregnancy occurring despite birth control precautions in patients taking this drug, the possible benefits should be weighed against the potential harm to the fetus.

Precautions: Attempts should first be made to control serum lipids with appropriate dietary regimens, weight loss in obesity, control of diabetes mellitus, etc. Because the drug may necessarily be given for prolonged periods, adequate baseline studies should be performed to determine whether the patient has significantly elevated serum lipid levels. Serum cholesterol and triglyceride levels should be determined frequently during the first few months of therapy and periodically thereafter. If response is inadequate after 3 months, the drug should be discontinued. However, in the presence of xanthoma tuberosum, the drug should be continued for periods up to 1 year provided the size and/or number of the xanthomata has been reduced. During the early stages of therapy, serum transaminase should be determined; mild transient increases, noted in some patients, are the result of the metabolic effects of the drug. However, if abnormalities are rising steadily or are excessive, the drug should be withdrawn immediately since this may indicate hepatic involvement. It has been advised that the drug be used with utmost care in patients with a history of jaundice or hepatic disorders. Clofibrate may produce "flu-like" symptoms characterized by muscular aching, soreness and cramping; may reactivate peptic ulcer, and may also cause various cardiac arrhythmias. Since anemia, and more frequently leukopenia, have been observed, complete blood studies should be performed periodically.

Adverse Reactions: Of the pertinent reactions, the most common is nausea. Less frequently encountered were such gastrointestinal reactions as vomiting, loose stools, dyspepsia, flatulence, and abdominal distress. Less frequently reported were headache, dizziness, and fatigue; muscle cramping, aching, and weakness; skin rash, urticaria, and pruritus. Occasionally encountered were dry, brittle hair and alopecia. Cardiac arrhythmias, both swelling and phlebitis at the site of xanthomas, dry skin, diarrhea, bloating, stomatitis and gastritis, impotence and decreased libido, dysuria, hematuria, proteinuria, decreased urine output, leukopenia, potentiation of anticoagulant effect, anemia, eosinophilia, "flu-like" symptoms, arthralgia, fatigue, weakness, drowsiness, weight gain, polyphagia, abnormal liver function tests as evidenced by increased transaminase (SGOT and SGPT), BSP retention, increased thymol turbitity, proteinuria and increased creatine phosphokinase. Reported adverse reactions whose direct relationship to the drug have not been established are peptic ulcer (caution is advised to avoid reactivation), gastrointestinal hemorrhage, rheumatoid arthritis, tremors, increased perspiration, systemic lupus erythematosus, blurred vision, gynecomastia, and thrombocytopenic purpura.

Dosage and Administration: *Orally.* For adults only. One capsule (500 mg) 4 times daily is the recommended dosage.

Availability:
ATROMID-S® Capsules, 500 mg in bottles of 100. **(Ayerst)**

CLOMIPHENE CITRATE

Chemical Name: 2-[*p*-(2-Chloro,1,2-diphenylvinyl)phenoxy]triethylamine citrate.

Description: Clomiphene citrate, a nonsteroidal triarylethylene compound, is structurally related to the estrogen, chlorotrianisene, and to the antilipemic agent, triparanol (MER-29), which is no longer marketed in the United States. Clomiphene citrate occurs as a white to pale yellow, crystalline powder sparingly soluble in water and in alcohol.

The drug is both estrogenic and anti-estrogenic, is neither progestational, androgenic nor anti-androgenic, and apparently does not interfere with pituitary-adrenal or pituitary-thyroid functions. The precise mechanism by which it induces ovulation in anovulatory patients has not been determined. The ovulatory response to the drug seems to be mediated through increased output of pituitary gonadotropins which stimulate the maturation and endocrine activity of the ovarian follicle and the subsequent development and function of the corpus luteum. The role of the pituitary is indicated by increased urinary excretion of gonadotropins and the response of the ovaries, as manifested by increased urinary excretion of estrogen. Following oral administration, the drug is readily absorbed, and is excreted chiefly in the feces.

Indications: To induce ovulation in selected anovulatory women who wish to become pregnant. Best results are obtained in those women whose anterior pituitary, adrenal, ovarian and thyroid glands are functioning adequately. Although better results are usually achieved in patients with adequate estrogen levels, a reduced estrogen level does not always rule out successful therapy.

Contraindications: During pregnancy; in patients with liver disease or a history of liver dysfunction; in those with abnormal bleeding of undetermined origin.

Warnings: Visual symptoms may occur during therapy that increase the hazards of driving a motor vehicle or operating machinery, in which case the drug should be withdrawn and a complete ophthalmologic evaluation should be performed.

Precautions: Diagnostic procedures and complete pelvic examinations are mandatory when an ovarian cyst, endometrial carcinoma or abnormal bleeding is suspected. At recommended dosage, abnormal ovarian enlargement is infrequent, although the usual cyclic variation in ovarian size may be exaggerated. Similarly, cyclic ovarian pain may be accentuated. With higher or prolonged dosage, more frequent ovarian enlargement and cyst formation (usually luteal) may occur and the luteal phase of the cycle may be prolonged. Rare instances of massive ovarian enlargement are on record. Abnormal ovarian enlargement usually regresses spontaneously, and, while laparotomy was performed on several such patients, investigators believe most of these patients should have been treated conservatively. Therefore, to minimize the hazard, the lowest dose consistent with expectation of good results should be administered.

Adverse Reactions: The more common side effects include hot flushes, abdominal discomfort (distension, bloating, pain or soreness), ovarian enlargement, and visual blurring. The vasomotor symptoms resembling menopausal hot flushes are not usually severe and disappear promptly after treatment is discontinued. Abdominal symptoms may be most often related to ovulatory or premenstrual phenomena, or to ovarian enlargement. Visual symptoms (see Warning for further recommendations), described usually as "blurring" or spots or flashes, disappear within a few days or weeks after the drug is discontinued. Other reported visual disorders were diplopia, scotomata, after-images, and photophobia. Infrequently reported symptoms during therapy have included nausea or vomiting, increased nervous tension, depression, fatigue, dizziness, or lightheadedness, insomnia, headache, breast soreness, heavier menses, weight gain, increased urinary frequency or volume, increased appetite, constipation, diarrhea, ascites, urticaria or allergic dermatitis, and moderate, reversible hair loss. Clomiphene citrate has not been reported to cause significant abnormality in the hematologic or renal systems, in protein bound iodine, or in serum cholesterol. Sulfobromophthalein retention of greater than 5% has been reported in 32 of 141 patients in whom it was measured, including 5 of 43 patients who received approximately the dose of clomiphene citrate now recommended. Retention was usually minimal unless associated with prolonged continuous clomiphene administration or with apparently unrelated liver disease. In some patients, preexisting sulfobromophthalein retention decreased even though clomiphene therapy was continued. Other liver function tests were usually normal. One patient developed jaundice on the nineteenth day of treatment (50 mg/day); liver biopsy revealed bile stasis without evidence of hepatitis. Birth defects in the neonate were also observed; some infants were born to mothers who had taken this drug for 6 weeks following conception. Other reported events that occurred during therapy, but whether or not drug-related has not been confirmed, include posterior capsulary cataract, detachment of the posterior vitreous, spasm of retinal arteriole, thrombosis of temporal arteries of retina, and hydatiform mole.

Dosage and Administration: *Orally.* Patients should be chosen for clomiphene therapy only after careful diagnostic evaluation by physicians experienced in the management of gynecologic or endocrine disorders. The recommended initial dosage is 50 mg daily for 5 days. If ovulation has not occurred, a second course of therapy consisting of 100 mg daily (in a single dose) for 5 days can be given 30 days following the completion of the previous course. The daily dosage should never exceed 100 mg, nor should the course of therapy extend beyond 5 days. A maximum of 3 courses is recommended, particularly for those women who have shown no response. Treatment may be started at any time so long as the patient has had no recent uterine bleeding. If progestin-induced bleeding is planned, or if spontaneous uterine bleeding occurs prior to therapy, the regimen of 50 mg daily for 5 days should be started on or about the 5th day of the cycle. Patients should be advised of the potential for a multiple pregnancy, which is possible with clomiphene citrate.

Availability:
CLOMID® Tablets, 50 mg in cartons of 30. **(Merrell-National)**

CLONAZEPAM

Chemical Name: 5-(2-Chlorophenyl)-1, 3-dihydro-7-nitro-2H-1, 4-benzodiazepin-2-one.

Description: A benzodiazepine derivative, clonazepam is a synthetic, oral anticonvulsant agent for use in the symptomatic treatment of certain epileptic seizures. It has been found helpful in patients with absence seizures (petit mal) who have failed to respond to succinimides. It occurs as a light yellow, crystalline powder, and has a molecular weight of 315.7.

The drug has been shown to antagonize convulsions induced by pentylenetetrazol or eletrical stimulation in rodents, and also those induced by photic stimulation in susceptible baboons. It produces a taming effect in aggressive primates, as well as some muscle weakness and hypnotic effects. Clinical studies have shown that the drug is capable of suppressing the spike and wave discharge in absent seziures (petit mal) and of decreasing the frequency, amplitude, duration and spread of discharge in minor motor seizures.

Following a single oral dose, maximal blood levels appear, in most instances, within 1 to 2 hours. The half-life of unmetabolized drug varies from about 18 to 50 hours. It is eliminated chiefly by the kidney and appears in the urine as unchanged drug and metabolites. In general, the biotransformation of clonazepam appears to follow 2 pathways: oxidative hydroxylation at the C-3 position and reduction of the 7-nitro function to form 7-amino and/or 7-acetyl-amino derivatives.

Recent reports strongly suggest an association between the use of anticonvulsant drugs and an increased incidence of birth defects in the offspring. Laboratory studies with pregnant rabbits receiving clonazepam orally have demonstrated the occurrence of malformations in some of the developing fetuses at doses of 0.2 and 5 mg/kg/day. However, the effects of this drug in pregnant women and in nursing infants are still unknown. It is important to note that anticonvulsant medications should not be discontinued in pregnant patients in whom the drug is administered to prevent seizures because of the strong possibility of precipitating status epilepticus with its attendant hypoxia and threat to life.

Up to 30% of patients have shown a loss of anticonvulsant activity, often within 3 months of administration. In some cases dosage adjustment may reestablish efficacy.

Indications: Prophylactic management of Lennox-Gastaut syndrome (petit mal variant) and akinetic and myoclonic seizures either alone or as adjunctive therapy.

Contraindications: Patients with a history of sensitivity to benzodiazepines, significant liver disease, acute narrow-angle glaucoma, and in open-angle glaucoma unless patients are receiving appropriate therapy.

Warnings: Because of its depressant effect on the CNS, all patients receiving clonazepam should avoid undertaking activities that require alertness, judgment, and physical coordination such as operating machinery or driving a car, especially during the early period of dosage adjustment. They should also be warned about the concomitant use of alcohol, since the effects may be additive. If the drug is considered for administration to pregnant women or to those of childbearing potential, the possibility of risk to the fetus must be weighed against the expected therapeutic benefits. Because of the possibility that adverse effects on physical and mental development could become apparent only after many years, a benefit versus risk consideration of the long-term use of this drug is important in pediatric patients. Withdrawal symptoms (similar to those noted with barbiturates and alcohol) have occurred following abrupt discontinuance of this drug (convulsions, tremor, abdominal and muscle cramps, vomiting and sweating). Addiction-prone individuals should be under careful supervision when receiving clonazepam because of the predisposition of such patients to habituation and dependence.

Precautions: When used in patients in whom mixed types of seizures are present, the drug may increase or precipitate the onset of generalized tonic-clonic seizures (grand mal). This reaction may require an increase in their dosage or the addition of appropriate anticonvulsants. Because of the toxic nature of this drug, periodic blood counts and liver function tests are advisable. The usual precautions in treating patients with impaired renal function should be observed. The abrupt withdrawal of therapy, particularly in those patients on long-term, high-dose schedules, may precipitate status epilepticus. Therefore, when the drug is to be discontinued, the dosage should be reduced gradually, and the simultaneous substitution of another anticonvulsant may be essential. Particular care is required in patients with chronic respiratory disease because clonazepam increases salivation, and may also cause respiratory depression. Because of the CNS-depressant action of this drug, its effects may be potentiated by alcohol, narcotics, barbiturates, nonbarbiturate hypnotics, antianxiety agents, the phenothiazines, thioxanthene and butyrophenone classes of antipsychotic agents, MAO inhibitors, and the tricyclic antidepressants, and by other anticonvulsant drugs.

Adverse Reactions: Most frequently reported were drowsiness (50%), ataxia (30%), and behavioral problems (25%). Other reactions that may occur can be classified as follows: *Neurologic:* abnormal eye movements, aphonia, choreiform movements, coma, diplopia, dysarthria, dysdiadochokinesis, "glassy-eyed" appearance, headache, hemiparesis, hypotonia, nystagmus, respiratory depression, slurred speech, tremor, vertigo. *Psychiatric:* confusion, depression, forgetfulness, hallucinations, hysteria, increased libido, insomina, psychosis, suicidal tendencies (the behavior effects are more likely to occur in patients with a history of psychiatric disturbances). *Respiratory:* chest congestion, rhinorrhea, shortness of breath, hypersecretion in upper respiratory passages. *Cardiovascular:* palpitations. *Dermatologic:* hair loss, hirsutism, skin rash, ankle and facial edema. *Gastrointestinal:* anorexia, coated tongue, constipation, diarrhea, dry mouth, encopresis, gastritis, hepatomegaly, increased appetite, nausea, sore gums. *Genitourinary:* dysuria, enuresis, nocturia, urinary retention. *Musculoskeletal:* muscle weakness, pains. *Miscellaneous:* dehydration, general deterioration, fever, lymphadenopathy, weight loss or gain. *Hematopoietic:* anemia, leukopenia, thrombocytopenia, eosinophilia. *Hepatic:* transient elevations of serum transaminases and alkaline phosphatase. Overdosage is manifested by somnolence, confusion, coma and diminished reflexes. Treatment includes monitoring of respiration, pulse rate and blood pressure, general supportive measures and immediate gastric lavage. Intravenous fluids should be administered and an adequate airway maintained. Hypotension may be combated by the use of levarterenol or metaraminol, and CNS depression by methylphenidate or caffeine and sodium benzoate. Dialysis is of no known value.

Dosage and Administration: *Orally.* Adults: The suggested initial dose should not exceed 1.5 mg daily divided into 3 doses. Dosage may be increased in increments of 0.5 to 1 mg every 3 days until seizures are adequately controlled or until side effects preclude any further increase. Maintenance dosage must be individualized for each patient. The maximal recommended daily dose is 20 mg. Infants and children up to 10 years of age or 30 kg of body weight: The suggested initial dose ranges from 0.01 to 0.03 mg/kg of body weight daily, but should not exceed 0.05 mg/kg daily, divided into 2 or 3 doses. Dosage should be increased by no more than 0.25 to 0.5 mg every 3 days until a daily maintenance dose of 0.1 to 0.2 mg/kg of body weight has been reached. Whenever possible, the daily dose should be divided into 3 equal doses. If doses are not equally divided, the largest dose should be given before retiring.

Availability:
CLONOPIN® Tablets (scored), 0.5 mg (orange), 1 mg (blue) and 2 mg (white) in Prescription Paks® (unit-dose) packages of 100. **(Roche)**

CLONIDINE HYDROCHLORIDE

Chemical Name: 2-(2, 6-Dichlorophenylamino)-2-imidazoline hydrochloride.

Description: Clonidine, an antihypertensive agent, is an imidazoline derivative. It occurs as an odorless, bitter, white crystalline powder that is soluble in water and alcohol. It possesses a molecular weight of 266.57.

The most important pharmacologic effect of clonidine is on systemic blood pressure. It has been reported to significantly lower systolic and diastolic blood pressure in both recumbent and standing positions. It acts centrally to reduce sympathetic activity by inhibiting the vasomotor and cardio-acceleratory centers as a result of central alpha-adrenergic stimulations. Initially, the drug stimulates the alpha-adrenergic receptors in the peripheral vascular smooth muscle thus producing transient vasoconstriction. There is evidence that clonidine reduces plasma renin activity and catecholamine and aldosterone excretion.

Following oral administration, blood pressure declines within 1/2 to 1 hour and reaches maximal effect within 2 to 4 hours; the antihypertensive action usually lasts for 6 to 8 hours. Peak plasma level of the drug occurs in approximately 3 to 5 hours with a plasma half-life of 12 to 16 hours. It is excreted primarily in the urine as unchanged drug and metabolites. The simultaneous use of a diuretic tends to enhance the therapeutic activity of clonidine. The preparation combining clonidine with clorthalidone has been found to consistently produce greater reduction in blood pressure than can be achieved with either drug alone. Also, the combination provides a stable dosage level of clonidine which can maintain effective antihypertensive control in patients who develop severe postural hypotension or who are otherwise refractory to treatment with the usual sympathetic blocking agents.

Studies with albino rats that were given the drug for 6 months or longer disclosed a dose-dependent increase in the incidence and severity of spontaneously occurring retinal degeneration. Further studies with dogs and monkeys revealed that clonidine was concentrated in the choroid of the eye. In clinical studies with 908 patients, no drug-related abnormal ophthomologic findings were recorded with the exception of some dryness of the eyes.

Indications: Treatment of hypertension. The fixed combination of clonidine and chlorthalidone is not recommended for initial therapy unless it represents the dose that is clinically effective for the patient.

Contraindications: Hypersensitivity to clonidine and chlorthalidone. Chlorthalidone is also contraindicated in patients with severe renal or hepatic disease.

Warnings: In some patients tolerance may develop which may necessitate reevaluation of therapy. Since reproduction studies in 3 animal species reflected no teratogenicity but some embryotoxicity, the safe use of this drug in pregnant patients or in women of childbearing potential has not been confirmed; due consideration should be given to the possible risks to the mother and fetus. No clinical data are available on the usefulness of this drug in pediatric patients.

Precautions: It is advisable that when therapy with clonidine is being discontinued the dose should be reduced gradually over a period of 2 to 4 days in order to avoid a possible rapid rise in blood pressure and associated subjective symptoms such as nervousness, agitation, and headache. Patients should be cautioned not to discontinue therapy without first consulting the physician. The occurrence of an excessive rise in blood pressure upon interruption of therapy can be reversed by reinstituting clonidine therapy or by intravenous phentolamine. The sedative activity of the drug represents a hazard in ambulatory patients whose activities require alertness and motor coordination. Clonidine should be used with caution in patients with severe coronary insufficiency, recent myocardial infarction, cerebrovascular disease or chronic renal failure. Patients requiring long-term therapy should receive periodic eye examinations. The monograph on chlorthalidone should be consulted for additional precautions.

Adverse Reactions: Those most commonly found were dryness of mouth (about 40%), drowsiness (about 35%), and sedation (about 8%). Other reported reactions include constipation, dizziness, headache, and fatigue. Generally, these effects tend to diminish with continued therapy. Those rarely encountered were anorexia, malaise, nausea, vomiting, parotid pain, mild transient abnormalities in liver function tests. There has been one report of possible drug-induced hepatitis without icterus and hyperbilirubinemia. Also noted were weight gain, transient elevation of blood glucose or serum creatine phosphokinase, gynecomastia; congestive heart failure, Raynaud's phenomenon, and electrocardiographic abnormalities manifested as Wenckebach's phenomenon or ventricular trigeminy; vivid dreams or nightmares, insomnia, other behavioral changes, nervousness, restlessness, anxiety, and mental depression; rash, angioneurotic edema, hives, urticaria, thinning of the hair, pruritus not associated with a rash; impotence, and urinary retention; increased sensitivity to alcohol, dryness, itching or burning of the eyes, dryness of the nasal mucosa, pallor, or a weakly positive Coombs' test. The monograph on chlorthalidone should be consulted for additional adverse reactions. Overdosage is usually manifested by profound hypotension, weakness, somnolence, diminished or absent reflexes, and vomiting. Gastric lavage and the administration of an analeptic and vasopressor may be instituted. Tolazoline in intravenous doses of 10 mg at 30-minute intervals will usually abolish all the undesirable effects of overdosage.

Dosage and Administration: *Orally.* The usual initial oral dosage is 1 tablet (0.1 mg) twice daily. Daily increments of 0.1 or 0.2 mg may be made until the desired response is achieved. Maintenance dosage may vary from 0.2 to 0.8 mg daily given in divided doses. Studies have indicated that 2.4 mg is the maximum effective daily dose. Chlorthalidone: The usual initial dose is 50 mg daily which may be administered in divided doses. The fixed combination drug may be given if the amount therein corresponds to that determined for the individual patient. Initially, 1 tablet twice daily, increased gradually to 3 or 4 times daily; up to a maximum of 8 tablets daily.

Availability:
CATAPRES® Tablets, 0.1 and 0.2 mg in bottles of 100 and 1000. **(Boehringer Ingelheim)**
with Chlorthalidone
COMBIPRES® Tablets, 0.1 and 0.2 mg with chlorthalidone, 15 mg in bottles of 100.
(Boehringer Ingelheim)

CLORAZEPATE DIPOTASSIUM/MONOPOTASSIUM Ⓒ IV

Chemical Name: 7-Chloro-2, 3-dihydro-2, 2-dihydroxy-5-phenyl-1*H*-1, 4-benzodiazepine-3-carboxylic acid dipotassium.

Description: Clorazepate dipotassium is a CNS depressant agent that possesses the pharmacological characteristics of the benzodiazepines. It occurs as a fine, light yellow, practically odorless powder that is very soluble in water and insoluble in the common organic solvents. When administered orally, the primary metabolite, nordiazepam, usually reaches peak serum levels in approximately 1 hour and the antianxiety action may persist for about 24 hours. The serum half-life is approximately 2 days. The drug is detoxified in the liver and is excreted primarily in the urine.

Indications: Symptomatic relief of anxiety associated with neurosis or in psychoneurotic reactions in which anxiety is the predominant feature, and as an adjunct in disease states in which anxiety is manifested. Also indicated for the symptomatic relief of acute alcohol withdrawal. It is not recommended for patients with depressive neuroses or psychotic reactions, or in patients under 18 years of age.

Contraindications: Hypersensitivity to clorazepate; in acute narrow angle glaucoma; in lactating patients.

Warnings: Patients should be cautioned about the possible potentiating effects of alcohol and other CNS depressant drugs, and about engaging in hazardous occupations requiring alertness or skill. Symptoms of nervousness, insomnia, irritability, diarrhea, muscle aches, and memory impairment have followed abrupt withdrawal after prolonged use of high dosages.

Precautions: Protective measures may be required when giving the drug to addiction-prone individuals, or to those predisposed to severe depressions or suicidal tendencies; the least amount feasible should be available to the patient. The usual precautions in treating patients with impaired renal or hepatic function should also be observed. In elderly or debilitated patients, the initial dose should be small and increments should be made gradually in accordance with the response of the patient in order to preclude ataxia or excessive sedation. The usual considerations should be exercised when giving any drug to pregnant patients or to women of childbearing potential.

Adverse Reactions: The most frequently reported was drowsiness. Less commonly reported were dizziness, various gastrointestinal symptoms, nervousness, blurred vision, dry mouth, headache, mental confusion, insomnia, transient skin rashes, fatigue, ataxia, genitourinary symptoms, irritability, diplopia, depression, slurred speech, abnormal liver and kidney function, a decrease in hematocrit and in systolic blood pressure. If clorazepate is used to treat anxiety associated with somatic disorders, careful attention must be paid to possible drug interaction with concomitant medication. The management of overdosage is essentially the same as that of other CNS depressant agents. See monograph on Ethchlorvynol.

Dosage and Administration: *Orally* in divided doses. *For anxiolytic activity,* the usual daily dose of **clorazepate dipotassium** is 30 mg; the dose should be adjusted gradually within the range of 15 to 60 mg daily in accordance with the response of the patient. In elderly or debilitated patients, the recommended initial dose is 7.5 to 15 mg daily. The *SD* tablets should not be used to initiate therapy, but can be administered after the patient has been stabilized on a dose of 7.5 mg 3 times daily. The usual dose is 1 SD tablet daily. *For acute alcohol withdrawal,* 30 mg initially followed by 30 to 60 mg for the first day; 45 to 90 mg for the second day; 22.5 to 45 mg for the third day and 15 to 30 mg for the fourth day. Thereafter, the daily dose should be gradually reduced to 7.5 to 15 mg. The drug should be discontinued as soon as the patient's condition is stabilized.

For anxiolytic activity, the usual daily dose of **clorazepate monopotassium** is 26 mg; the dose should then be adjusted gradually within the range of 13 to 52 mg daily in accordance with the response of the patient. May also be administered as a single daily dose of 13 mg at bedtime, with subsequent adjustment according to the clinical response. In elderly or debilitated patients, the recommended initial dose is 6.5 to 13 mg daily. *For acute alcohol withdrawal,* 26 mg initially followed by 26 to 52 mg for the first day; 39 to 78 mg for the second day;

19.5 to 39 mg for the third day and 13 to 26 mg for the fourth day. Thereafter, the daily dose should be gradually reduced to 6.5 to 13 mg. The maximum recommended total daily dose is 78 mg. The drug should be discontinued as soon as the patient's condition is stabilized.

Availability:

Clorazepate Dipotassium

Ⓒ TRANXENE®: **(Abbott)**

Capsules, 3.75 and 7.5 mg in bottles of 100 and 500 and in Abbo-Pac® (unit-dose) packages of 100; 15 mg in bottles of 100 and in Abbo-Pac® (unit dose) packages of 100.

SD (single-dose) Tablets, 11.25 mg (half strength) and 22.5 mg in bottles of 30 and 100.

Clorazepate Monopotassium

Ⓒ AZENE™ Capsules, 3.25 and 6.5 mg in bottles of 100 and 500; 13 mg in bottles of 100. **(Endo)**

CLORTERMINE HYDROCHLORIDE Ⓒ

Chemical Name: *o*-Chloro-α, α-dimethylphenylethylamine hydrochloride.

Description: Clortermine is an anorexigenic-sympathomimetic amine that differs from other compounds of the phenylethylamine group in that it has a chlorine atom in the *ortho* position of its chemical structure. Pharmacologically, the anorexiant activity of clortermine is similar to that of the amphetamines. This anorectic effect usually diminishes after a few weeks. Qualitatively, it exhibits the same clinical effects on the CNS (stimulation) and the cardiovascular system (elevation of blood pressure) as do the amphetamines.

Reproduction studies with animals that were given doses in excess of the usual clinical dose exhibited no interference with the course of pregnancy; however, slight delays in skeletal ossification of fetuses occurred in some animals. There was a 20% reduction in conception rate when rats of both sexes were fed approximately 16 to 19 times the usual clinical dose.

Indications: Clortermine is indicated for the management of exogenous obesity as a short-term (a few weeks) adjunctive measure in a regimen of weight reduction based on caloric restriction.

Contraindications: Hyperthyroidism; known hypersensitivity, or idiosyncrasy to clortermine or to the sympathomimetic amines; glaucoma; agitated states; during or within 14 days following the administration of monoamine oxidase inhibitors (hypertensive crises may result); and patients with a history of drug abuse.

Warnings: When tolerance to the anorectic effect develops, the recommended dose should not be exceeded in an attempt to increase the effect; rather, the drug should be discontinued. Patients should be cautioned that clortermine may impair their ability to engage in potentially hazardous activities such as operating machinery or driving a motor vehicle. The possibility that this drug may produce physical and psychological dependence should be considered when evaluating the desirability of including the drug in the weight reduction programs of individual patients. Abuse of amphetamine-type drugs may result in intense psychological dependence and severe social dysfunction. There are reports of patients who have increased the dosage to many times that recommended. Abrupt withdrawal of the drug following prolonged high dosage administration results in extreme fatigue and mental depression accompanied by abnormal sleep EEG. Manifestations of chronic intoxication include severe dermatoses, marked insomnia, irritability, hyperreactivity, personality changes, and psychosis often indistinguishable from schizophrenia. Safe use during pregnancy requires that the potential benefit be weighed against the possible hazard to the mother and fetus. Clortermine is *not* recommended for use in children under 12 years of age.

Precautions: Although the drug may be used with caution in patients with mild hypertension (blood pressure should be monitored), it should be given with considerable caution, if at all, to patients with severe hypertension or in the presence of symptomatic cardiovascular disease including arrhythmias. Insulin requirements in diabetes mellitus may be altered in association with the use of clortermine and the concomitant dietary regimen. It may also decrease the hypotensive effect of guanethidine. In order to minimize the possibility of overdosage, the smallest amount feasible should be prescribed or dispensed at one time.

Adverse Reactions: The usual untoward reactions observed with the amphetamines have been noted with clortermine. These include: *Cardiovascular* reactions: palpitation, tachycardia, and elevation of blood pressure. *CNS* reactions: overstimulation, restlessness, dizziness, insomnia, euphoria, dysphoria, tremor, headaches, and rarely, psychotic episodes at recommended doses. *Gastrointestinal* reactions: dryness of the mouth, unpleasant taste, diarrhea, constipation, and other gastrointestinal disturbances. *Allergic* reaction: urticaria. *Endocrine* reactions: impotence and changes in libido.

Manifestations of acute overdosage with anorectic agents of this type may include restlessness, agitation, tremor, confusion, assaultiveness, hallucinations, hyperreflexia, and muscle twitching. Fatigue and depression usually follow CNS stimulation. Cardiovascular effects may include arrhythmias, palpitations, hypertension or hypotension and circulatory collapse. Gastrointestinal symptoms include nausea, vomiting, diarrhea, and abdominal cramps. Fatal intoxication usually terminates in convulsions and coma. Management of acute intoxication is largely symptomatic and includes induction of emesis or gastric lavage, maintenance of adequate circulation and respiratory exchange. The patient should be protected against self-injury and disturbing external stimulation. The effectiveness of peritoneal dialysis or extracorporeal hemodialysis for anorectic agents of this type has not been established. Although severe hypertensive reactions to clortermine have not been observed, should these occur, the intravenous administration of phentolamine may be employed.

Dosage and Administration: *Orally.* Adults and children 12 years of age and over, 1 tablet daily at mid-morning.

Availability:
Ⓒ III VORANIL® Tablets, 50 mg (pale yellow) in bottles of 100. **(USV)**

CLOTRIMAZOLE

Chemical Name: 1-(o-Chloro-α, α-diphenylbenzyl) imidazole.

Description: Clotrimazole is a synthetic, organic antifungal agent intended for the topical treatment of fungal infections of the skin. Because of its fungistatic action, it is especially useful in the treatment of pathogenic dermatophytoses, yeasts, and *Malassezia furfur.* It occurs as a white, crystalline powder that is practically insoluble in water and soluble in most organic solvents. Its molecular weight is 344.8 and the pH is approximately 6. It is chemically related to miconazole in that both compounds contain the imidazole ring and the chlorinated phenol group; however, it differs significantly from miconazole in that it does not contain the ether oxygen. It also differs from other synthetic antifungal agents due to a quarternary substitution at the carbon atom.

In vitro studies show that it possesses fungicidal action against Trichophyton, Epidermophyton, Microsporum, and Candida species. Clinical trials have shown the drug to be well-tolerated, and no systemic adverse effects have been recorded following topical application to intact or diseased skin. Improvement, with relief of pruritus, usually occurs within the first week of therapy. No resistance to the drug has developed during successive passages of *Candida albicans* and *Trichophyton mentagrophytes,* and it has not been found to be inactivated either by washing or by any topical preparation.

Indications: Treatment of skin infections caused by tinea pedis, tinea cruris, and tinea corposis due to *Trichophyton rubrum, Trichophyton mentagrophytes, Epidermophyton floccosum* and *Microsporum canis;* candidiasis due to *Candida albicans;* and tinea versicolor due to *Malassezia furfur.* Also indicated for the treatment of vulvovaginal candidiasis (moniliasis).

Contraindications: Known hypersensitivity to any of the components.

Warnings: Not for ophthalmic use.

Precautions: Discontinue use upon the appearance of any symptoms suggesting sensitivity or irritation and institute the appropriate treatment. May be used during the first trimester of pregnancy only when it is deemed essential to the welfare of the patient.

Adverse Reactions: Those reported include erythema, stinging, blistering, peeling, edema, pruritus, urticaria, and general irritation of the skin. Rare instances of mild burning, skin rash, lower abdominal cramps, slight urinary frequency, and burning or irritation in the sexual partner have been reported following vaginal application; however, these occurrences do not warrant discontinuation of therapy.

Dosage and Administration: *Topically.* Gently massage into the affected and surrounding areas twice daily (morning and evening). If, after 4 weeks of treatment, no clinical improvement is noted, the diagnosis should be reevaluated. *Intravaginally.* Insert 1 tablet high into the vaginal vault once daily at bedtime for 7 days.

Availability:
LOTRIMIN®: **(Schering)**
Cream, 1% in a vanishing cream base in tubes of 15 and 30 gm.
Solution, 1% in plastic bottles of 10 and 30 ml.
GYNE-LOTRIMIN® Vaginal Tablets, 100 mg in cartons of 7 individually foil-wrapped tablets. **(Schering)**

CLOXACILLIN: see The Penicillins

COBRA VENOM SOLUTION

Description: A solution of a highly purified fraction of cobra venom in which the neurotoxic principle has been concentrated to more than twice its original potency, and from which most hemotoxic and proteolytic constituents have been removed. The solution is standardized in terms of mouse units; each ml of the solution provides 50 mouse units. One mouse unit has been defined by the Division of Biological Standards of the NIH (National Institutes of Health) as that quantity of venom extract that will kill a 20-gram mouse in 24 hours.

Indications: As an analgesic for use in intractable pain, especially that due to malignant disease. The action of the extract is cumulative. A series of 14 to 30 daily injections ordinarily are necessary to establish the full analgesic effect, after which the frequency of injections may often be reduced, depending upon the patient's condition and response.

Contraindications: None known.

Precautions: The solution should not be used if a precipitate occurs. The same precautions should be taken as with other proteinaceous substances, because occasional sensitivity reactions may occur. Epinephrine, antihistamines, and facilities for supportive treatment of possible allergic or anaphylactic reactions should be readily available. When an allergic reaction is noted, therapy may be reestablished by using reduced doses.

Adverse Reactions: Tenderness and erythema at the site of subcutaneous injection.

Dosage and Administration: *Subcutaneously* or *intramuscularly.* Injections are usually started when 15 mg of codeine is necessary to control the pain. When the full effect of this preparation is established, opiates may be discontinued in most cases, or greatly reduced in others, until the terminal stages. The first injection is usually 0.1 ml to determine the patient's reaction. This is followed by 0.5 ml the second day and 1 ml the third day. Daily injections of 1 to 3 ml are continued until relief of pain is noticeable, after which dosage may be reduced to 1 injection every other day or every third day.

Availability:
COBROXIN® Injection, 50 mouse units/ml in ampuls of 1 ml in cartons of 10 and 25 ampuls. **(Hynson, Westcott & Dunning)**

COCCIDIOIDIN

Description: Coccidioidin is a sterile, standardized liquid concentrate obtained from a culture of 10 selected strains of *Coccidioides immitis,* grown on a synthetic medium. Potency is standardized with a reference standard of the NIH of the U.S. Public Health Service.

Indications: As an aid in the diagnosis of coccidioidomycosis and to differentiate suspected coccidioidomycosis from blastomycosis, histoplasmosis or tuberculosis. A history of having been in some areas of the western or southwestern parts of the United States, together with clinical findings and a positive reaction to the skin test, are important factors in establishing a diagnosis.

Precautions: Precautions usually observed when using other biologicals should be followed with this preparation. Excessive dosage may produce severe erythema and induration followed by necrosis and ulceration. If too high a concentration is used, systemic reactions may occur, and erythema nodosum precipitated in those patients with recently acquired infection.

Dosage and Administration: The usual dose is 0.1 ml of a 1:100 dilution injected *intradermally* with a new or dichromate-washed tuberculin syringe. The reaction may be read after 24 hours; another reading at 48 hours is recommended to avoid false negative results. A positive reaction consists of an area of induration 5 mm or greater in diameter.

Availability:
COCCIDIOIDIN Liquid (U.S.P.), 1:100 dilution in vials of 1 ml (10 tests). Dilutions of 1:10 are prepared upon request. **(Cutter)**

CODEINE (C-II)

Chemical Name: Morphine 3-menthyl ether.

Description: A narcotic analgesic and antitussive agent that resembles morphine in pharmacologic properties, but because its action is much weaker, it is less apt to cause nausea, vomiting, constipation, miosis, or respiratory and cortical depression. Average doses are sedative and analgesic, and have a suppressing effect on the cough reflex, but larger amounts (in excess of 60 mg) may cause restlessness and hyperexcitability. On a weight basis, codeine is approximately 1/6 as analgesic as morphine, and if 60 mg of the drug fails to relieve pain, larger doses are unlikely to be effective. Codeine is usually prepared from morphine by methylation, i.e., by replacing the hydroxyl group with a methoxy group at the C-3 position on the morphine nucleus. *Codeine Phosphate* occurs as an odorless, white, crystalline powder that is freely soluble in water and slightly soluble in alcohol. *Codeine Sulfate* occurs as white crystals that are sparingly soluble in water and very slightly soluble in alcohol. Due to its greater solubility, codeine phosphate is most often used in cough mixtures. Because its dependency liability is considerably less than that of morphine, tolerance to codeine is difficult to develop, but cases of addiction have been reported. The drug is biodegraded in the liver, and appears in the urine as free and bound drug and as metabolites. When injected subcutaneously, peak analgesic action is reached within 30 to 60 minutes, and the effect usually persists for 3 to 4 hours.

Indications: For the relief of mild to moderate pain which does not respond to a nonaddictive analgesic. May also be used for its antitussive action.

Contraindications: Patients who are hypersensitive to codeine.

Warnings: May be habit-forming.

Precautions: Because of its drying action on the respiratory mucosa, the indiscriminate use of codeine may precipitate severe respiratory insufficiency resulting from increased viscosity of the bronchial secretions and suppression of the cough reflex. The CNS-depressant effects of codeine may be enhanced by such drugs as the phenothiazines, the MAO inhibitors, and the tricyclic antidepressants, and may be additive when used with other CNS depressants. Since drowsiness and dizziness are a possibility, patients should be advised to use special care when undertaking activities requiring alertnesss and physical coordination.

Adverse Reactions: Average or usual doses may cause nausea, vomiting, dizziness, and drowsiness. Excessive doses may, in addition, produce exhilaration, convulsions, narcosis, respiratory depression, hypotension, miosis, and tachycardia.

Dosage and Administration: *Orally, subcutaneously, intramuscularly.* For analgesic action:

The average adult dosage is 30 mg every 4 hours; however, the dose may range from 15 to 60 mg. Children, 3 mg/kg of body weight daily divided into 6 doses. For antitussive action: The usual daily oral dosage for adults is 5 to 10 mg every 3 or 4 hours, and for children, 1 to 1.5 mg/kg of body weight divided into 6 doses.

Availability:

Ⓒ **Codeine Phosphate**

Injection, 15, 30 and 60 mg in ampuls of 1 ml. **(Knoll)**
Hypodermic Tablets (soluble), 15, 30 and 60 mg in bottles of 100 and 500. **(Lilly)**
Injection, 30 mg/ml in multiple-dose vials of 20 ml. **(Lilly)**
Injection, 30 mg/ml in Steri-Dose® (unit-dose) syringes of 1 ml. **(Parke-Davis)**
Injection, 30 and 60 mg in Carpujects® (half-filled syringes) of 2 ml. **(Winthrop)**
Injection, 30 and 60 mg/ml in Tubex® syringes of 1 ml. **(Wyeth)**

Ⓒ **Codeine Sulfate**

Hypodermic Tablets (soluble), 15, 30 and 60 mg in bottles of 100 and 500. **(Lilly)**
Oral Tablets, 30 mg in bottles of 100 and 1000. **(ICN)**
Oral Tablets, 30 and 60 mg in bottles of 100. **(Knoll)**
Oral Tablets, 15, 30 and 60 mg in bottles of 100 and 1000; 30 mg tablets are also available in blister pack (unit-dose) cartons of 100 (10 x 10). **(Lilly)**
Oral Tablets, 15, 30 and 60 mg in Redipak® cartons of 25. **(Wyeth)**

COLCHICINE

Description: Colchicine is an alkaloid obtained from *Colchicum autumnale.* It occurs as pale yellow, amorphous scales or powder soluble in water and freely soluble in alcohol and in chloroform.

Although its exact mechanism of action is not completely known, it has been found to involve a reduction in lactic acid production by leukocytes, which results in a decrease in urate deposition, and also a reduction in phagocytosis, with abatement of the inflammatory response. When it is used early and in adequate dosage in acute gout, the response is usually prompt and effective. It does not prevent recurrences and may not be successful in every instance. It has no effect on uric acid metabolism or serum uric acid levels.

Colchicine has been reported to arrest cell division in animals and plants, to cause teratogenic effects in certain species of animals, and to adversely affect spermatogensis. Reversible azoospermia has been reported in one patient.

Indications: Acute attacks of gouty arthritis. It is also recommended for regular use between attacks as a prophylactic measure, and may be effective in aborting an attack when taken at the first sign of articular discomfort. Intravenous administration may be desirable when a rapid response is sought or when gastrointestinal disturbances interfere with oral administration.

Contraindications: In patients with gout who have serious gastrointestinal, renal or cardiac disorders.

Precautions: Considerable caution should be exercised when administering colchicine to aged and debilitated patients, especially those with renal, gastrointestinal, or heart disease. Reduction of dosage is indicated if weakness, anorexia, nausea, vomiting, or diarrhea appears. Parenteral colchicine *must be given intravenously.* Severe local irritation occurs if administered subcutaneously or intramuscularly.

Adverse Reactions: *Oral:* Full doses produce nausea, vomiting or diarrhea; these usually do not occur following intravenous administration unless the dosage exceeds those recommended. However, it is generally necessary to reach full dosage levels for an adequate therapeutic effect. Antidiarrheal agents may be given either concurrently or when diarrhea develops. Since prolonged administration may cause bone-marrow depression, with agranulocytosis, thrombocytopenia, and aplastic anemia, repeated blood counts are advised. Peripheral neuritis and loss of body and scalp hair have also been reported.

Regardless of the route of administration, a latent period exists between the onset of toxic symptoms which are initially gastrointestinal and generally produce nausea, vomiting, abdominal pain, and severe and bloody diarrhea owing to hemorrhagic gastroenteritis. Burning sensations in the throat, stomach, and skin may also occur. Extensive vascular damage may result in shock. Hematuria and oliguria which may occur are evidence of kidney damage. Muscular weakness is marked and an ascending paralysis of the CNS may develop. Fatalities, the result of respiratory depression, have been reported after an 8-mg dose, but larger amounts need not be fatal. Thrombophlebitis occurs rarely at the site of injection. In the event of acute overdosage, hemodialysis or peritoneal dialysis, in addition to gastric lavage, may be employed. Respiratory assistance should be instituted to assure proper oxygenation and ventilation. Atropine and morphine may be administered to relieve abdominal pain.

Dosage and Administration: *Orally:* Therapy should be intiated at the first warning of an acute attack; a delay of a few hours impairs the drug's efficacy. For acute attacks of gouty arthritis, initially 0.5 mg granule or 0.6 mg tablet followed by 0.5 or 0.6 mg every hour; alternately, twice this amount may be given every 2 hours until articular symptoms subside or gastrointestinal distress occurs. If the intravenous route is used to complement the oral administration, the oral form should be discontinued after about 4 mg has been administered. For prophylaxis, the dosage depends upon the severity of the condition, including the frequency of acute attacks. If the disorder is mild or moderate, 0.5 mg granule or 0.6 mg tablet is given up to 4 times weekly; if severe 0.5 or 0.6 mg is given 1 to 4 times daily. *Intravenously.* For acute attacks, initially 1 or 2 mg, followed by 0.5 mg every 3 to 6 hours until a satisfactory response is obtained. Generally, the total intravenous dosage for 1 complete course of treatment should not exceed 4 mg. Many patients can be transferred to a similar oral dosage. In the prophylactic or maintenance therapy of recurrent or chronic gouty arthritis, 0.5 to 1 mg may be given once or twice daily. In these cases, however, oral colchicine is preferable, usually in conjunction with a uricosuric agent.

Availability:
COLCHICINE:
Granules (sugar coated), 0.5 mg in bottles of 100. **(Abbott)**
Injection, 1 mg in ampuls of 2 ml. **(Lilly)**
Tablets, 0.6 mg in bottles of 100. **(Abbott)**
Tablets, 0.6 mg in bottles of 100 and 1000. **(Lilly)**

COLESTIPOL HYDROCHLORIDE

Description: Colestipol is the insoluble chloride salt of a basic anion exchange resin, prepared in the form of odorless and tasteless macromolecular beads that are hydrophilic and thus swell when placed in water or aqueous fluids. The drug acts as a bile acid sequestrant in that it absorbs and combines with bile acids in the intestine forming an insoluble complex that is excreted in the feces. This prevents their reabsorption from the intestine and reexcretion in the bile. Since cholesterol is the major and probably the sole precursor of bile acids, the reduced level of these acids stimulates the conversion of more cholesterol to bile acids in the liver, resulting in a decrease in circulating cholesterol. Even though colestipol induces an increase in the hepatic synthesis of cholesterol, serum cholesterol levels nonetheless fall. Therefore, the major effect of the drug in hypercholesterolemia is the increased removal rate of low density lipoproteins. However, serum triglyceride levels may increase or remain unchanged in colestipol-treated patients.

The decline in serum cholesterol levels is usually evident in about one month, but may rise with continued use of the drug. It is advised that serum levels be determined periodically to confirm that a favorable initial response is maintained. When the drug is discontinued, serum cholesterol levels usually return to pretreatment status within one month.

Indications: Recommended as an adjunctive therapy to diet for the reduction of elevated serum cholesterol in patients with primary hypercholesterolemia (elevated low density lipoproteins). There is as yet no clinical evidence that lowering lipid levels beneficially affects atherosclerosis including coronary heart disease.

Contraindications: Hypersensitivity to colestipol.

Warnings: The resin should not be taken in the dry form; it should always be mixed with water or other fluids before administration.

Precautions: Before instituting therapy with this drug, a vigorous attempt should be made to control serum cholesterol by an appropriate dietary and weight reduction program. Additionally, any underlying disorder that may contribute to the hypercholesterolemia should be corrected. To prevent nutritional deficiencies of the fat-soluble vitamins in those patients taking the resin for prolonged periods, the diet should be supplemented with vitamins A, D and K. Since long-term use may increase bleeding tendencies due to hypoprothrombinemia associated with vitamin K deficiency, parenteral vitamin K will reverse the trend promptly, and oral vitamin K will prevent recurrences. When the drug is given for extended periods of time, both cholesterol and triglyceride levels may rise to baseline values. The most common complaint of therapy is constipation which may aggravate preexisting hemorrhoids or may cause fecal impaction. Constipation may be especially troublesome in patients with symptomatic coronary artery disease and therefore this reaction should be avoided. Safe and effective use in children has not been established, and its use by pregnant or lactating women or by women of childbearing age requires that the potential benefits of the drug outweigh the possible hazards to the mother and fetus. Since colestipol is an anion exchange resin, it may have a strong affinity for anions other than the bile acids, and may consequently delay or reduce the absorption of concomitant oral medication such as thyroxine, aspirin, warfarin and nicotinic acid as well as tetracycline, phenobarbital, cortisone acetate, chlorpromazine, sulfadiazine, clofibrate, hydrochlorothiazide and digitalis. Discontinuance of the colestipol resin could pose a hazard to health if a potentially toxic drug that is significantly bound to the resin has been titrated to a maintenance level while the patient is taking this product.

Adverse Reactions: The most common adverse reactions are confined to the gastrointestinal tract. Constipation is the major single complication which can at times be severe and is occasionally accompanied by fecal impaction and/or homorrhoids. However, most instances of constipation are mild and transient in nature and can readily be controlled with standard treatment, although some patients require a temporary decrease in dosage or discontinuation of therapy. Less frequently reported are abdominal discomfort (abdominal pain and distension), belching, flatulence, nausea, vomiting, and diarrhea. Peptic ulceration, gastrointestinal irritation and bleeding, cholecystitis and cholelithiasis have been reported by fewer than one in 500 patients and are not necessarily drug-related. Urticaria and dermatitis were noted in fewer than one in 1000 patients. Asthma and wheezing were not reported in the colestipol studies but have been noted during treatment with other cholesterol-lowering agents. Other events, not necessarily drug-related, and rarely reported were muscle and joint pains, arthritis, headache, dizziness, anxiety, vertigo, drowsiness, anorexia, fatigue, weakness, and shortness of breath. Transient and modest elevations of serum glutamic oxaloacetic transaminase and of alkaline phosphatase were observed on a few occasions as were an increase in serum phosphorous and chloride, and a decrease in sodium and potassium.

Dosage and Administration: *Orally.* The recommended adult dosage is 15 to 30 gm daily divided into 2 to 4 doses. **Important Note:** The drug should always be mixed with water or other fluids before ingestion. Patients should take other drugs at least 1 hour before or 4 hours after ingestion of colestipol to minimize interference with their absorption.

Availability:
COLESTID® Powder in bottles of 500 gm and in packets of 5 gm in cartons of 30 packets.
(Upjohn)

COLISTIMETHATE SODIUM

Chemical Name: Sodium colistimethanesulfonate.

Description: Colistin base is a complex polypeptide antibiotic obtained from *Bacillus polymyxa.* Sodium colistimethate, the sodium salt of the methane sulfonate derivative of colistin, and colistin sulfate occur as white to slightly yellow, crystalline powders soluble in water.

Following intramuscular injection, the drug is rapidly absorbed, and reaches peak blood levels in 1 to 2 hours; higher serum levels were obtained at 10 minutes following intravenous administration. Serum concentration declined with a half-life of from 2 to 3 hours following either intravenous or intramuscular administration in adults and children including premature infants; only trace amounts were detected in 12 to 24 hours. Colistimethate may enter the cerebrospinal fluid and reach a concentration of approximately ½ the amount present in the plasma. Clinical studies have shown that sodium colistimethate is transferred across the placental barrier. Blood levels of about 1 mcg/ml were detected in the fetus following intravenous administration to the mother. Average urine levels ranged from about 270 mcg/ml at 2 hours to about 15 mcg/ml at 8 hours following intravenous injection and from about 200 to about 25 mcg/ml during a similar period following intramuscular injection. Clinically, it is bactericidal against most gram-negative organisms, including *Pseudomonas aeruginosa, E. coli, Aerobacter aerogenes, Klebsiella pneumoniae* and *Brucella.* Most strains of *Proteus,* however, are resistant to colistin. Its antibacterial activity is not hampered by serum, whole blood or other body fluids. Moreover, susceptible organisms do not develop resistance readily, and cross-resistance to broad-spectrum antibiotics has not been encountered.

In vitro studies have indicated that bacterial resistance to the drug and cross-resistance to polymyxin B can develop.

Indications: Treatment of severe, acute and resistant chronic urinary tract infections due to sensitive organisms; respiratory tract infections; surgical, wound, and burn infections; and septicemia due to susceptible organisms. It is particularly indicated when any of these infections is caused by sensitive strains of *Pseudomonas aeruginosa.* Colistin is used with neomycin and hydrocortisone in the treatment of acute and chronic external otitis and otitis media and fenestration cavities due to or complicated by bacterial and/or fungal infections caused by susceptible organisms; and in the prophylaxis of "swimmer's ear." Colistin sulfate is used alone in the treatment of acute bacterial diarrhea in infants and children when caused by susceptible gram-negative intestinal pathogens and in gastroenteritis due to Shigella organisms.

Contraindications: A history of sensitivity to any of the components. Hydrocortisone is contraindicated in tuberculous, fungal and most viral lesions, especially herpes simplex, vaccinia and varicella.

Warnings: Because of possible transient neurologic disturbances, patients should be cautioned not to drive a motor vehicle or operate machinery requiring alertness while receiving the drug. Overdosage can result in renal insufficiency, muscle weakness and apnea. When colistin sulfate alone is used, the possibility of renal involvement should be kept in mind, particularly if doses larger than those recommended are used or if the patient is already azotemic. Prolonged use of any antibiotic may suppress the intestinal bacterial flora. **Important Note:** In view of the evidence of possible embryotoxic and teratogenic effects in pregnant rabbits, caution should be exercised in the use of this drug in women of childbearing potential.

Precautions: When impaired renal function is suspect or a reality, the drug should be used with extreme caution, and the dosage reduced in proportion to the extent of the impairment. The decline in renal function in the elderly should be considered. Dosage in excess of renal excretory capacity will lead to high serum levels and can result in further impairment of renal function, initiating a cycle which, if not recognized, can lead to acute renal insufficiency, renal shutdown and further concentration of the antibiotic to toxic levels in the body. At this point, interference of nerve transmission at neuromuscular junctions may occur and result in muscle weakness and apnea. The drug should be discontinued immediately at the first signs of impaired renal function: diminishing urinary output, rising BUN and serum creatinine. If a life-threatening situation exists, therapy may be reinstated at a lower dosage after blood levels have fallen. Curariform relaxants should be used with extreme caution in patients receiving colistimethate sodium since their pharmacologic action also interferes with nerve transmission at neuromuscular junctions, and apnea (requiring artificial respiration) can result. Certain other antibiotics should not be given concomitantly except with the greatest caution, because they, too, interfere with the transmission of impulses at the neuromuscular junction. These antibiotics include kanamycin, streptomycin, dihydrostreptomycin, polymyxin, neomycin.

If sensitivity or irritation occurs as the result of use in the ear, the otic preparation should be discontinued promptly. Overgrowth of resistant organisms is possible. Use with care in patients with a perforated ear drum or with chronic otitis media because of the possibility of ototoxicity caused by neomycin. Current medical literature indicates an increase in the prevalence of individuals sensitive to neomycin. Some cases of mixed infection caused by *Proteus* and *Pseudomonas* have been reported in which a normally sensitive strain of *Pseudomonas* was not controlled by colistin sulfate. Patients with infections of this type should therefore be followed closely.

Adverse Reactions: Reactions reported include transient perioral paresthesia and tingling of the extremities, or of the tongue, vertigo, dizziness, slurred speech, drug fever, gastrointestinal upset, generalized itching or urticaria, local irritation and pain at the injection site, mild burning or painful sensation in the ear, and sensitivity reactions. Respiratory arrest has been reported following intramuscular administration of colistimethate sodium.

Dosage and Administration: *Intramuscularly* or *intravenously* in 2 to 4 divided doses ranging from 1.5 mg to 5 mg/kg/day. In most infections, an average dosage of 2.5 mg/kg/day in 2 to 4 divided doses has been effective; in the presence of bacteremia, septicemia or other serious infections, greater than average doses may be required. Maximal daily dosage should not exceed 5 mg/kg/day in patients with normal renal function, and the interval between injections should be increased in patients with impaired renal function. The intravenous dosage must be administered slowly over a period of 3 to 5 minutes or given by intravenous drip.

After the ear has been completely cleansed and dried, 4 drops of the *otic suspension* should be instilled into the canal, or applied to the surface of the affected ear, 3 or 4 times daily. Prophylactically, 4 drops before and after swimming. Until acute pain has subsided, it may be preferable or necessary in some patients to pack the ear with a cotton wick saturated with the suspension and kept wet at all times.

The usual dosage of the *oral suspension* is equivalent to 3 to 5 mg/kg/day of colistin base in 3 divided doses. For example, a 50-lb patient would receive 1 to 1½ teaspoonsful 3 times daily. Daily dosage should rarely exceed 7.5 mg/kg/day of colistin base.

Availability:
COLY-MYCIN®: **(Warner/Chilcott)**
M Parenteral (colistimethate sodium) in vials of 20 or 150 mg of colistin base.
S Otic Suspension in bottles of 5 and 10 ml, each ml of which contains colistin base, 3 mg; neomycin base, 3.3 mg; hydrocortisone acetate, 10 mg and thonzonium bromide, 0.5 mg.
S Oral Suspension (dry powder) in bottles of 300 mg of colistin base.

COLREX COMPOUND CAPSULES Ⓒ III
COLREX COMPOUND ELIXIR Ⓒ V

Description: Each capsule and each 5 ml (teaspoonful) of elixir contains:

	Capsule	*Elixir**
Codeine phosphate	16 mg	8 mg
Acetaminophen	300 mg	120 mg
Phenylephrine hydrochloride	10 mg	5 mg
Chlorpheniramine maleate	2 mg	1 mg
Ascorbic acid	100 mg	—
Alcohol (v/v)	—	9.5%

*Sugar free

Indications: As an adjunct for the temporary relief of cough, congestion, headache, and muscle soreness associated with common colds and upper respiratory tract infections.

Contraindications: Hypersensitivity to any of the components.

Warnings: Codeine phosphate may be habit-forming.

Precautions: Codeine may cause constipation, and an occasional patient may experience an idiosyncratic response to it. In the event of drowsiness, patients should be cautioned not to engage in activities requiring alertness or skill. Gastric disturbance may result from phenylephrine and, because of its sympathomimetic effect, it should be used with caution in patients with cardiovascular disease, thyrotoxicosis or diabetes.

Adverse Reactions: Those complications that may result from hypersensitivity to any of the components.

Dosage and Administration: *Orally.* Adults, 1 or 2 capsules or 2 to 4 teaspoonsful of elixir 3 or 4 times daily. Children 6 to 12 years of age, 1 capsule or 2 teaspoonsful of elixir 3 or 4 times daily. Children 2 to 6 years of age, 1 teaspoonful 3 to 4 times daily. The capsules are not recommended for children under 6 years of age.

Availability:
C-III COLREX COMPOUND CAPSULES™ in bottles of 100 and 1000. **(Rowell)**
C-V COLREX COMPOUND ELIXIR™ in bottles of 60 ml, 1 pint and 1 gallon. **(Rowell)**

COMBID

Description: Each capsule contains isopropamide, 5 mg as the iodide and prochlorperazine, 10 mg as the maleate, in sustained-release form. The formulation combines the tranquilizing and antiemetic actions of prochlorperazine with the anticholinergic action of isopropamide.

The drug acts by reducing gastric secretion, inhibiting spasm and motility, relieving anxiety and tension, and controlling nausea and vomiting.

Indications: May be helpful as adjunctive therapy in the treatment of peptic ulcer, functional gastrointestinal disorders, irritable or spastic colon, functional diarrhea, and mucous colitis.

Contraindications: Known hypersensitivity to any of the components; in the presence of existing drug-induced CNS depression; glaucoma; pyloric obstruction; prostatic hypertrophy; bladder-neck obstruction; obstructive intestinal lesions, or ileus or both; bone marrow depression; jaundice; hepatic disease, and blood disease. This combination should not be given to children under 12 years of age. Because of the antiemetic action of prochlorperazine, the drug should not be administered to patients in whom nausea and vomiting are believed to be a manifestation of intestinal obstruction or brain tumor.

Warnings: Cautious use is advised in patients with a history of jaundice, hepatic abnormality or blood dyscrasias. Concomitant use of CNS-depressant drugs may cause an additive effect. Patients should be cautioned about undertaking activities requiring alertness and skill. In women of childbearing age, pregnant women, and nursing mothers, the potential benefits of the drug must be weighed against the potential hazards to the mother and fetus. As with all anticholinergic drugs, an inhibiting effect on lactation may occur.

Precautions: Use cautiously in patients known to be sensitive to drugs, and in elderly people. Because the iodine in isopropamide may alter the results of PBI tests and will suppress I-^{131} uptake, it is therefore advised to discontinue the medication one week before undertaking such studies. Although rare, an iodide skin rash may occur.

Adverse Reactions: Reactions that may occur are those attributable to either component. See monographs on Isopropamide Iodide, and Prochlorperazine Maleate (The Phenothiazines).

Dosage and Administration: *Orally.* Adults and children over 12 years of age, 1 capsule every 12 hours. Some patients require only 1 capsule taken upon arising and an exceptional patient may require 2 capsules in the morning and 2 capsules at night. A therapeutic dose is released promptly and the remaining medication, released gradually, sustains the effect for prolonged periods.

Availability:
COMBID® Spansule® (Capsules) in bottles of 50 and 500 and in single-unit packages of 100.
(Smith Kline & French)

COPAVIN C-III

Description: Each pulvule or tablet contains codeine sulfate, 15 mg and papaverine hydrochloride, 15 mg.

Indications: Relief of general malaise and cough due to acute respiratory infections.

Contraindications: In patients addicted to analgesic-type drugs or in those hypersensitive to any of the components.

Warnings: Codeine sulfate may be habit-forming.

Precautions: Although this is a relatively innocuous drug, the monograph on the individual components should be consulted to anticipate or avert any possible event.

Adverse Reactions: Symptoms such as headache, dizziness, fainting, and nausea are encountered only infrequently. Constipation occurs in approximately 6% of patients treated. Overdosage may produce difficulty in hearing, dim vision, mental confusion, sweating, nausea and vomiting, increasing CNS depression, stupor, and coma. Death results from respiratory failure. A gross overdosage of papaverine can cause cardiac arrhythmia. Treatment includes administering narcotic antagonists to relieve respiratory depression; also gastric lavage, intravenous fluids and electrolytes, with cautious regard for the total amount of fluid and sodium given, and judicious use of 5% carbon dioxide and 95% oxygen.

Dosage and Administration: *Orally.* Adults, 1 pulvule after each meal and 2 pulvules at bedtime for a period of 3 days. Severe symptoms may require additional doses. Children of elementary school age, ½ the usual adult dose. Dosage should be adjusted according to weight.

Availability:
Ⓒ III COPAVIN® Pulvules® (Capsules) in bottles of 100. **(Lilly)**

CO-PYRONIL

Description: A combination of the long and short-acting antihistamines, pyrrobutamine phosphate and methapyrilene hydrochloride with the vasoconstrictor, cyclopentamine hydrochloride.

	Pulvules	*Pediatric Pulvules*	*Suspension 5 ml (teaspoonful)*
Pyrrobutamine phosphate	15 mg	7.5 mg	7.5 mg
Methapyrilene hydrochloride	25 mg	12.5 mg	12.5 mg
Cyclopentamine hydrochloride	12.5 mg	6.25 mg	6.25 mg

Indications: Seasonal and perennial allergic rhinitis, mild uncomplicated allergic skin manifestations of urticaria and angioedema, allergic conjunctivitis due to foods and inhalant allergens, gastrointestinal allergy, allergic headache, and chronic urticaria.

Contraindications: Patients allergic to antihistamines or to any of the components of this product; in newborn and premature infants; in nursing mothers; and in the presence of lower respiratory disease, including asthma. Also contraindicated in patients receiving MAO inhibitors, and in those with narrow-angle glaucoma, stenosing peptic ulcer, symptomatic prostatic hypertrophy, bladder neck obstruction, or pyloroduodenal obstruction.

Warnings: Overdosage of compounds containing antihistamines may cause hallucinations, convulsions, and death, particularly in infants and children. Since mental function may be impaired, patients should be cautioned not to engage in activities requiring alertness or skill such as driving a motor vehicle or operating machinery. Antihistaminics in the young child may produce a paradoxical stimulating effect. They may also add to the depressant effects of alcohol and other CNS depressants such as hypnotics, sedatives, tranquilizers, antianxiety agents, etc. There is, at present, insufficient information as to whether or not this drug may reduce fertility in men or women or have teratogenic or other adverse effects on the fetus.

Precautions: Since this drug has an atropine-like action, it should be used with caution in patients with a history of bronchial asthma, increased intraocular pressure, hyperthyroidism, cardiovascular-renal disease, hypertension, or diabetes. Sympathomimetics may cause urinary retention in patients with prostatism.

Adverse Reactions: The most frequent side effects encountered were sedation; sleepiness; dryness of mouth, nose, and throat; thickening of bronchial secretions; dizziness; epigastric distress; and disturbed coordination. Other adverse reactions that may occur are fatigue, confusion, restlessness, excitation, nervousness, insomnia, euphoria, anorexia, nausea, vomiting, diarrhea, constipation, hypotension, tightness of chest and wheezing, urticaria, drug rash, anaphylactic shock, blurred vision, diplopia, vertigo, tinnitus, headache, palpitation, tachycardia, nasal stuffiness, urinary frequency, difficult urination, urinary retention, photosensitivity, hemolytic anemia, leukopenia, and agranulocytosis. Individuals hypersensitive to sympathomimetics may experience nervousness and insomnia. Symptoms of overdosage include CNS depression, followed by stimulation and later by depression. CNS stimulation may progress to the point of convulsions, especially in children. Death results from respiratory arrest. There is no specific therapy. General management involves mechanical support of respiration which is safer and more effective than the use of respiratory stimulants. Convulsions may be treated with CNS depressants (short-acting barbiturates) in amounts just adequate to control convulsive seizures. Oversedation should be avoided.

Dosage and Administration: *Orally.* Pulvules and suspension. The usual adult dosage *for mild symptoms,* 1 pulvule or 2 teaspoonsful every 12 hours. *For moderate symptoms,* 1 pulvule or 2 teaspoonsful every 8 hours. *For severe symptoms,* 2 pulvules or 4 teaspoonsful every 8 hours or 1 pulvule or 2 teaspoonsful every 4 hours. Children 20 to 40 lbs of body weight: *For mild symptoms,* ½ teaspoonful every 12 hours. *For moderate symptoms,* ½ teaspoonful every 8 hours. *For severe symptoms,* ½ to 1 teaspoonful every 8 hours. Children 40 to 60 lbs of body weight: *For mild symptoms,* 1 pediatric pulvule or 1 teaspoonful every 12 hours. *For moderate symptoms,* 1 pediatric pulvule or 1 teaspoonful every 8 hours. *For severe symptoms,* 2 pediatric pulvules or 2 teaspoonsful every 8 hours.

Availability:
CO-PYRONIL®: **(Dista)**
Pulvules® and *Pediatric Pulvules* in bottles of 100; the pulvules are also available in bottles of 1000 and in individual-doses of 100.
Suspension in bottles of 1 pint.

CORIFORTE

Description: Each capsule containing chlorpheniramine maleate, 4 mg; salicylamide, 190 mg; phenacetin, 130 mg; caffeine, 30 mg and ascorbic acid, 50 mg provides antihistaminic, analgesic and antipyretic action.

Indications: For the relief of the early symptoms of the common cold, such as "running nose" and "watery eyes," and for the symptomatic relief of muscular aches and pains accompanying the common cold.

Contraindications: Hypersensitivity to any of the components.

Warnings: Phenacetin may damage the kidneys when used in large amounts or for prolonged periods of time. Safe use during pregnancy has not been established; should be used only when the potential benefits outweigh the possible risks.

Precautions: Since drowsiness may occur with chlorpheniramine maleate, patients should be cautioned not to engage in activities that require alertness or skill until their response has been determined. Caffeine should not be given to individuals who are extremely sensitive to its CNS-stimulating action.

Adverse Reactions: Slight to moderate drowsiness occurs infrequently. Other possible side effects include restlessness, dry mouth, dizziness, weakness, anorexia, nausea, headache, nervousness, polyuria, heartburn, diplopia, sweating, dysuria, and very rarely dermatitis and diuresis.

Dosage and Administration: *Orally.* For adults: 1 capsule every 4 to 6 hours as required, and continued for several days if necessary.

Availability:
CORIFORTE® Capsules (red and yellow) in bottles of 100. **(Schering)**

CORILIN INFANT LIQUID

Description: One ml of the buffered liquid contains chlorpheniramine maleate, 0.75 mg; sodium salicylate, 80 mg; glycine (aminoacetic acid), 25 mg, and alcohol less than 1% in a raspberry flavored vehicle. Combines analgesic, antipyretic and antihistaminic action to relieve symptoms of the common cold and to alleviate muscular aches and pains and reduce fever.

Indications: For the pediatric management of common cold symptoms, teething problems, postinoculation reactions and pruritic conditions.

Adverse Reactions: Slight to moderate drowsiness occurs relatively infrequently. Other possible side effects include restlessness, dry mouth, dizziness, weakness, anorexia, nausea, headache, nervousness, polyuria, heartburn, sweating, diplopia, dysuria, and very rarely dermatitis.

Dosage and Administration: *Orally* every 4 hours as required. Six months and under, 0.5 ml. Six months to 1 year, 1 ml. One year to 3 years, 2 ml. When used for postinoculation therapy, the first dose should be given at the time of inoculation. The liquid may be mixed with formulas, milk, tea, fruit juices, carbonated beverages, apple sauce, cereals, etc.

Availability:
CORILIN® INFANT LIQUID in bottles of 30 ml with calibrated dropper. **(Schering)**

COR-TAR-QUIN

Description: Microdispersed hydrocortisone alcohol: 0.25%, 0.5% or 1%; liquor carbonis detergens, 2% and diiodohydroxyquin, 1% in Acid Mantle® vehicle.

Indications: May be effective alone or as adjunctive therapy in the treatment of subacute and chronic lichenified eczemas, that are complicated by or threatened with invasion by bacteria, and in the management of skin disorders due to fungal infections such as moniliasis, tinea axillae, tinea corporis, and tinea palmaris.

Contraindications: Tuberculous lesions of the skin, acute herpes simplex, vaccinia, varicella, fungal lesions unresponsive to diiodohydroxyquin, and in those patients hypersensitive to any of the components.

Precautions: Safety and efficacy in fungal conditions other than those mentioned have not been established. Discontinue treatment if irritation or sensitivity occurs and/or infection persists. Systemic absorption is a possibility when extensive areas are treated. Although topical steriods reportedly have had no adverse effect, and although the safety of their use has not been established, care should be exercised when used during pregnancy. If a secondary skin infection does not respond to diiodohydroxyquin, discontinue use until the infection has been properly controlled by other measures. Treated areas should not be exposed to direct sunlight. Not for ophthalmic use. Hair or clothing may become stained.

Dosage and Administration: *Topically.* Apply 2 or 3 times daily. Applications may be reduced during maintenance therapy as required.

Availability:
COR-TAR-QUIN®: **(Dome)**
Creme, 0.25% in tubes of 30 gm and in Dispensajar®s of 120 gm; 0.5% in tubes of 15 gm and in Dispensajars of 30 gm and in jars of 120 gm; 1% in tubes of 15 and 30 gm.
Lotion, 0.25% in bottles of 120 ml; 0.5% in bottles of 15 and 30 ml.

CORTICOTROPIN

Description: Corticotropin Injection is a sterile preparation of the principle(s) derived from the anterior lobe of the pituitary gland of domestic mammals used for food, which exert a tropic influence on the adrenal cortex. It occurs as an odorless, colorless or light straw-colored liquid, or soluble amorphous solid obtained by drying the liquid from the frozen state. The injection is available also as a solution of corticotropin in partially hydrolyzed gelatin, or as a sterile suspension adsorbed on zinc hydroxide; these are specifically formulated to prolong the therapeutic effect by retarding absorption.

Corticotropin stimulates the functioning adrenal cortex to produce and secrete its entire spectrum of steroids, of which hydrocortisone is the principal component. In contrast, corticosteroids may depress adrenal cortical function and produce adrenal atrophy. Its direct action on the adrenal cortex provides the basis for the use of corticotropin in treating adrenal insufficiency produced by cortisone, hydrocortisone, prednisone and the other synthetic adrenocorticosteroids by direct stimulation of the atrophic adrenal glands.

Because of its rapid absorption and utilization, the therapeutic effects of corticotropin appear more promptly than do those of cortisone acetate.

Indications: As a diagnostic test to determine adrenocortical function. Since the physiologic and metabolic effects are due to the endogenous adrenal corticosteroids and since these effects generally are similar to those of cortisone, corticotropin is of value in the same disease conditions for which exogenous adrenal corticosteroids are indicated; however, corticotropin is not effective in Addison's disease or other conditions where the adrenals are not functioning (acute or chronic adrenal insufficiency).

Contraindications: In patients with scleroderma, osteoporosis, systemic fungal infections, ocular herpes simplex, recent surgery, history of or the presence of a peptic ulcer, congestive heart failure, hypertension, or sensitivity to proteins of animal origin. It is also contraindicated in the treatment of idiopathic thrombocytopenia purpura in adults and of conditions accompanied by primary adrenocortical insufficiency or adrenocortical hyperfunction. Intravenous administration is contraindicated except for diagnostic testing.

Warnings: Prolonged use of corticotropin may lead to irreversible side effects; may increase the risks of hypersensitivity reactions; may produce posterior subcapsular cataracts and glaucoma with possible damage to the optic nerve; and may necessitate the additional use of rapidly-acting corticosteroids before, during and after an unusual stressful event. The drug may suppress the signs and symptoms of chronic disease without altering the natural course of the disease; may mask the signs of infections, and new infections including those of the eye due to fungi or viruses may appear. Additionally, there may be decreased resistance and inability to localize infection. Corticotropin can cause elevation of blood pressure, promote salt and water retention, and increase the excretion of potassium and calcium. Patients should *not* be vaccinated against smallpox; other immunization procedures should be undertaken with caution, especially when high doses are administered because of the possible hazards of neurological complications and lack of antibody response. Since fetal abnormalities have been observed in experimental animals, use of this drug in pregnant women, nursing mothers, or in women of childbearing potential requires that the expected benefits be weighed against the possible hazards to the mother and embryo or fetus. Infants born to mothers who have received substantial doses of corticotropin during pregnancy should be carefully observed for signs of hypoadrenalism. Skin testing should be considered before treating hypersensitive patients. All patients should be observed for at least 15 minutes after administration. Epinephrine 1:1000 should be readily available for emergency treatment.

Precautions: Corticotropin should be given only with full knowledge of the characteristic activity of, and the varied responses to, the drug. If corticotropin is indicated in patients with latent tuberculosis or in those reacting to tuberculin, close observation is necessary as the disease may become active; during prolonged therapy, these patients should receive chemoprophylaxis. To avoid relative pituitary hypofunction or adrenocortical insufficiency, corticotropin therapy should be terminated gradually, particularly when patients are receiving large doses or have undergone prolonged treatment. Furthermore, if such patients are subjected to undue stress while being treated, or within one year after treatment has been terminated, hormone therapy should be augmented or reinstated and continued for the duration of the stress period and immediately following it. The effects of corticotropin may be enhanced in patients with hypothyroidism and in those with cirrhosis of the liver. The lowest possible dosage should be used to control the condition under treatment, and when reduction in dosage is possible the reduction should be gradual. Treatment of acute gouty arthritis should be limited to a few days, since rebound attacks may occur when corticotropin is discontinued;

therefore, conventional concomitant therapy should be administered during corticotropin treatment and for several days after it is discontinued. Psychic disorders ranging from euphoria, insomnia, mood swings, personality changes, and severe depression, to frank psychotic manifestations may appear; also, existing emotional instability or psychotic tendencies may be aggravated by this drug. In the presence of hypoprothrombinemia, aspirin should be used with caution in conjunction with corticotropin. The drug should be used cautiously in patients with diabetes mellitus, abscess, pyogenic infections, diverticulitis, renal insufficiency, and myasthenia gravis. Also, growth and development of infants and children on prolonged therapy should be carefully followed. Corticotropin should be administered for treatment only when the disease is intractable to more conventional therapy, and should be used as an adjunct and not as the sole therapy in the treatment of a disease.

Adverse Reactions: Reactions usually are reversible and disappear when the drug is discontinued. They usually are the same as those experienced with synthetic adrenal corticosteroids (see general statement on the Adrenal Corticosteroids).

Dosage and Administration: Because the adrenals vary in their sensitivity to stimulation by corticotropin, there can be no specifically uniform dose that would be effective in all individuals. The aim is to obtain a therapeutic effect with minimal dosage and with minimal or no metabolic alterations. A clinical response—the criterion of adequate dosage—may be seen within 2 weeks in most conditions. *Intramuscularly* Dosage usually is 20 U.S.P. units 4 times daily and ranges from 10 to 40 units/dose. The usual dosage for the repository injections initially is 40 units daily and ranges from 10 to 100 units. Maintenance dosage is 20 units 2 or 3 times weekly. Corticotropin injections may be used *intravenously* only for diagnostic testing of adrenocortical function. The IV dosage is 10 to 25 units of corticotropin injection or 40 to 80 units of repository injection in 500 ml of 5% glucose in water given as a continuous intravenous infusion over a period of 8 hours (once daily). Dosage for children should be reduced proportionately.

Availability:

Corticotropin Injection

ACTHAR® (lyophilized powder) in vials of 25 and 40 U.S.P. units. **(Armour)**

ACTH (dry powder) in Steri-Vials® of 25 and 40 U.S.P. units. **(Parke-Davis)**

Repository Corticotropin Injection

CORTICOTROPIN GEL 80 units/ml in Tubex® (disposable-syringes) of 1 ml. **(Wyeth)**

CORTROPHIN® GEL 40 units/ml in vials of 1 and 5 ml; 80 units/ml in vials of 5 ml. **(Organon)**

H.P. ACTHAR® GEL 40 and 80 units/ml in vials of 1 and 5 ml. **(Armour)**

Corticotropin Zinc Hydroxide Suspension

CORTROPHIN®-ZINC 40 units/ml (2 mg zinc) in vials of 5 ml. **(Organon)**

CORTISONE ACETATE: see The Adrenal Corticosteroids

CORTISPORIN

Description: A combination of two or more of the antibiotics, bacitracin, gramicidin, neomycin and polymyxin with hydrocortisone in a variety of dosage forms. It incorporates the antiallergic, antiinflammatory and antipruritic effects of hydrocortisone with the antibacterial action of the antibiotics. Active against most gram-positive organisms, including *Staphyloccus aureus* and many gram-negative organisms including *Pseudomonas aeruginosa*. It also provides symptomatic relief of edema, pain, and itching, by reducing erythema, edema and exudation.

Indications: General: For topical bacterial infections due to susceptible organisms, when the antipruritic, antiallergic and antiinflammatory effect of hydrocortisone is indicated as in burns, wounds, skin grafts; otitis externa; also in plastic, proctologic, gynecologic or general surgical procedures. Dermatologic: Atopic, contact, stasis and infectious eczematoid dermatitis; neurodermatitis, eczema; anogenital pruritus; and in impetigo and ecthyma. Ophthalmic: Nonpurulent bacterial, allergic, vernal and phlyctenular conjunctivitis; nonpurulent blepharitis and episcleritis, interstitial, sclerosing, postoperative, or acne rosacea keratitis, superficial chemical and thermal burns of the cornea. Otic: External otitis, infectious otitis media, and in infections of mastoidectomy and fenestration cavities.

Contraindications: Acute purulent conjunctivitis and blepharitis; tuberculous, fungal or viral lesions of the skin or eye including herpes simplex, vaccinia, varicella and dendritic keratitis, in conditions involving the posterior segment of the eye, and in the presence of perforated eardrum; also in patients hypersensitive to any of the ingredients. The cream is contraindicated for use in the eye.

Warnings: Because of the potential hazard of nephrotoxicity and ototoxicity due to the neomycin component, care should be exercised when using this drug in treating extensive burns, trophic ulceration and other extensive conditions where absorption of neomycin is possible. In burns where more than 20% of the body surface is affected, especially if the patient has impaired renal function or is receiving other aminoglycoside antibiotics concurrently, no more than 1 application/day is recommended.

Precautions: Prolonged use of antibiotics may result in overgrowth of nonsusceptible organisms, including fungi, in which case appropriate measures should be instituted. Use of antiinflammatory steroids on infected areas may encourage the spread of infection; therefore, therapy should be discontinued and appropriate antibacterial drugs used. During pregnancy, unnecessary use on extended areas, in large amounts or for prolonged periods of time should be avoided. It is advisable to check intraocular pressure frequently, since it may rise (resulting in glaucoma) with extended use of ophthalmic, topical steroids; also care should be taken in diseases causing thinning of the cornea as perforation may occur. Careful regulation of therapy is required in patients with perforated ear and/or long-standing chronic otitis media in order to prevent ototoxicity. Treatment should not exceed 10 days. The physician should bear in mind that, in the event supplementary treatment with another antibiotic is indicated, allergic cross reactions with kanamycin, paromomycin, streptomycin, and possibly gentamicin may occur.

Adverse Reactions: When steroid preparations are used for long periods of time in intertriginous areas or over extensive body areas, with or without occlusive nonpermeable dressings, striae may occur. There also exists the possibility of systemic side effects when steroid preparations are used over larger areas or for long periods of time. A possible allergic reaction to neomycin should also be kept in mind.

Dosage and Administration: *Topically.* Apply a thin film of ointment or cream 2 to 4 times daily. In chronic conditions, withdraw treatment by decreasing the frequency of application until a once a week regimen is reached. Ophthalmic Ointment: Initially, every 3 or 4 hours. Ophthalmic Suspension: One or 2 drops every 3 to 4 hours, or more frequently if necessary. Otic Solution: After gentle cleansing and drying of the ear canal, instill 4 drops 3 or 4 times daily, or saturate a wick placed in the external canal. If warm drops are preferred, avoid heating above body temperature. Potency of drug is not affected if a slight buff color develops. Patient should be told to avoid contaminating dropper and to shake bottle well before using.

Availability:

CORTISPORIN®: **(Burroughs Wellcome)**

Cream: Each gm contains polymyxin B sulfate, 10,000 units; neomycin sulfate, 5 mg (equivalent to 3.5 mg neomycin base); gramicidin, 0.25 mg, and hydrocortisone acetate, 5 mg (0.5%) in tubes of 7.5 gm.

Ointment: Each gram contains polymyxin B sulfate, 5000 units; zinc bacitracin, 400 units; neomycin sulfate, 5 mg (equivalent to 3.5 mg neomycin base), and hydrocortisone, 10 mg (1%) in tubes of 3.5 and 15 gm with applicator tip (3.5 gm tube for ophthalmic use only).

Ophthalmic Suspension (sterile): Each ml contains polymyxin B sulfate, 10,000 units; neomycin sulfate, 5 mg (equivalent to 3.5 mg neomycin base), hydrocortisone, 10 mg (1%) in dropper bottles of 5 ml.

Otic Solution (clear, sterile) and Suspension (sterile): Each ml contains polymyxin B sulfate, 10,000 units; neomycin sulfate, 5 mg (equivalent to 3.5 mg neomycin base), and hydrocortisone, 10 mg (1%) in dropper bottles of 10 ml.

CORYZTIME

Description: Each timed-release capsule contains phenylpropanolamine hydrochloride, 50 mg; chlorpheniramine maleate, 8 mg and atropine sulfate, 0.36 mg.

Indications: Relief of upper respiratory tract congestion and hypersecretion associated with the common cold, sinusitis, influenza, vasomotor rhinitis, hay fever, rose fever and other allergies.

Contraindications: Glaucoma, severe hypertension, prostatic hypertrophy and hypersensitivity to any of the components.

Precautions: Use with caution in elderly patients and in those with hypertension, cardiovascular disease, hyperthyroidism, diabetes, or prostatic hypertrophy. Should not be administered to children under 6 years of age unless directed by the physician. The medication should be discontinued if rapid pulse, dryness of the mouth, nose, throat, blurring of vision, pain in the eyes or dizziness occurs. Since drowsiness may occur, the patient should be instructed not to engage in activities requiring alertness or skill. On account of the possible vasopressor effects of phenylpropanolamine, special care is required when coadministered with MAO inhibitors, digitalis, ergot alkaloids, oxytocics, appetite suppressants or stimulants, and other vasopressor agents.

Adverse Reactions: Commonly noted were drowsiness and nervousness. Average or large doses may cause xerostomia, bradycardia, mydriasis, and blurred vision. Overdosage may result in tachycardia, delirium, fever, stupor, respiratory failure, and death.

Dosage and Administration: *Orally.* Adults and children over 6 years of age, 1 capsule every 12 hours.

Availability:
CORYZTIME Capsules in bottles of 100 and 1000. **(Elder)**

CROMOLYN SODIUM

Chemical Name: 1, 3-*bis* (2-Carboxychromon-5-yloxy)-2-hydroxypropane disodium.

Description: Cromolyn sodium is a bronchial asthma prophylactic agent. It occurs as a white or creamy-white, hydrated powder that is soluble in water (1 in 20). Solutions of the powder have a pH of 7. It possesses a slight odor and although it is tasteless at first, it leaves a slightly bitter after-taste. Its molecular weight is 512.

Cromolyn sodium is neither a bronchodilator, antihistaminic nor an antiinflammatory agent. Its action appears to be specific for the reaginic antigen/antibody reaction. It inhibits the degranulation of sensitized and nonsensitized mast cells following exposure to a variety of allergens. It also inhibits the release of mediators from nonimmunologically oriented systems such as dextran and phospholipase A. It has been found effective in the treatment of Ig-E-mediated (extrinsic) bronchial asthma apparently by blocking the release of histamine and SRS-A (the slow reacting substance of anaphylaxis) from sensitized lung tissue. No reports of resistance or tolerance to the drug are available.

Chronic toxicity studies in macaque monkeys revealed proliferative arterial lesions which appeared predominately in the medium sized arteries of the kidney causing eccentric thickening of the arterial wall. However, none of the animals developed the physical signs or symptoms usually associated with vascular and/or renal disease. Whether or not the occurrence of the lesions was due to the administration of cromolyn sodium has not been confirmed. Parenteral doses greater than 30 mg/kg of body weight produced degeneration of the renal tubular epithelium in the macaque monkey and in several rodent species studied. Also, reproduction studies performed in various species of animals, that were given high parenteral doses of the drug, showed adverse fetal effects such as increased resorptions and decreased fetal weight.

The drug is poorly absorbed from the gastrointestinal tract. After the medication is inhaled, approximately 8% of the total dose administered is absorbed from the lung; it is then rapidly excreted unchanged in the bile and urine. The remainder of the dose is deposited in the oropharynx, and is then swallowed and excreted in the alimentary tract. Following inhalation, response to the drug usually occurs within 2 to 4 weeks, and is manifested by a notable decrease in the severity of the clinical symptoms of asthma, or in the need for concomitant therapy, or both. Prolonged treatment is suggested only for those patients who show a significant initial clinical response.

Indications: As adjunctive agent in the management of patients with severe perennial bronchial asthma. Pulmonary function tests must show that these patients have a significant bronchodilator-reversible component to their airway obstruction. **Cromolyn sodium is not indicated for the treatment of an acute attack of asthma, especially status asthmaticus.**

Contraindications: In patients hypersensitive to the drug.

Warnings: Because of the possible event of proliferative arterial lesions in patients on long-term treatment, the physician should be well aware of the risks as well as the therapeutic effects of this drug. Cromolyn should be used with considerable care, if at all, in patients with impaired renal or hepatic function. Although eosinophilic pneumonia is rarely noted, if it occurs, the drug should be discontinued. Cromolyn sodium is not recommended for use in pregnant patients or in children under 5 years of age.

Precautions: Occasionally, patients may experience cough and/or bronchospasm following inhalation of the drug; this effect may necessitate discontinuation of the medication, despite prior bronchodilator administration. Symptoms of asthma may recur if the dosage is reduced below the recommended level, or if the drug is withdrawn.

Adverse Reactions: Instances of maculopapular rash and urticaria have been reported; these were promptly reversible upon withdrawal of therapy. Bronchospasm, transient coughing, nasal congestion, pharyngeal irritation, and wheezing have been frequently associated with the administration of cromolyn. Other symptoms which may develop include angioedema, dizziness, dysuria and urinary frequency, joint swelling and pain, lacrimation, nausea and headache, swelling of parotid glands, and rarely, laryngeal edema. In addition, the following have been reported as rare events, but their relationship to the drug has not been determined. These include anaphylaxis, anemia, exfoliative dermatitis, hemoptysis, hoarseness, myalgia, nephrosis, periarteritic vasculitis, pericarditis, peripheral neuritis, photodermatitis, polymyositis, esoinophilic pneumonia, and vertigo.

Dosage and Administration: *By inhalation.* The dose for adults and children 5 years of age and over is the contents of 1 capsule inhaled 4 times daily at regular intervals. Each patient should be carefully instructed in the use of the turbo-inhaler and should be carefully advised that the effect of therapy is dependent upon the administration of the drug at regular intervals. It should be emphasized to the patient that the capsules are not absorbed when swallowed and that the drug is not effective by that route of administration. Concomitant corticosteroids, as well as bronchodilators, should be continued following the use of cromolyn sodium. Whether or not clinical improvement is noted, a gradual tapering off of the corticosteroid should be attempted. It is important that the dose be reduced slowly, maintaining close supervision of the patient, to avoid an exacerbation of asthma and/or the incidence of adrenocortical insufficiency. However, a potentially critical degree of adrenal insufficiency may persist asymptomatically for some time even after gradual discontinuation of adrenocortical steroids. Therefore, if the patient is subjected to significant stress after corticosteroid treatment has been terminated, consideration should be given to reinstituting corticosteroid therapy. When inhalation of cromolyn is impaired, as may occur in severe exacerbation of asthma, a temporary increase in the amount of corticosteroids and/or other medications may be required. It is particularly important that considerable care be exercised if for any reason cromolyn is withdrawn in cases where its use has permitted a reduction in the maintenance dose of steroids. In such cases, continued close supervision of the patient is essential since there may be a sudden reappearance of severe manifestations of asthma which will require immediate therapy and possible reintroduction of the corticosteroid agent.

Availability:

AARANE® Capsules, 20 mg in strip-packages of 60 and 300. The Aarane inhaler is supplied in individual containers. **(Fisons)**

INTAL® Capsules, 20 mg in strip-packages of 60 and 120. The Spinhaler® (turbo-inhaler) is supplied in individual containers. **(Fisons)**

C-RON FA

Description: Each tablet contains ferrous fumarate, 200 mg (elemental iron, 66 mg); ascorbic acid, 600 mg and folic acid, 0.5 mg.

Indications: Treatment and prophylaxis of iron deficiency and megaloblastic anemias of pregnancy, especially during the third trimester. It is also useful in situations of which poor nutrition, multiple pregnancy and multiparity increase the need for folic acid.

Contraindications: *Folic acid:* Pernicious anemia, and anaphylactic sensitivity: *Iron therapy:* Hemachromatosis, iron storage disease or the potential for iron storage disease due to chronic hemolytic anemia (e.g., inherited anomalies of hemoglobin structure or synthesis and/or red cell enzyme deficiencies, etc.), pyridoxine responsive anemia, or cirrhosis of the liver.

Warnings: Patients with untreated pernicious anemia may show hematologic improvement with daily therapeutic doses of folic acid as low as 0.4 mg. In such cases, degenerative lesions of the spinal cord may progress irreversibly after 3 months, despite the absence of anemia. Pernicious anemia must be ruled out prior to folic acid therapy by means of a Schilling test and a vitamin B-12 blood level determination. Resistance to treatment may be due to depressed hematopoiesis, alcoholism, the presence of antimetabolic drugs, and to deficiencies of vitamins B-6, B-12, C and E. Iron deficiency anemia may be due to occult blood loss, the etiology of which should be determined and treated appropriately. Prolonged therapeutic use of iron salts may produce iron storage disease.

Precautions: Folic acid and vitamin B-12 microbiological blood assays are invalidated by the administration of most antibiotics, methotrexate, and pyrimethamine. Folic acid is not effective in reversing the toxic effects of methotrexate; folinic acid (5-formyltetrahydrofolic acid) is the drug of choice. Occult bleeding and/or iron therapy may produce black tarry stools.

Adverse Reactions: An occasional patient may experience mild gastric symptoms, which may be alleviated by taking the drug with meals. Sensitivity reactions to folic acid may occur on rare occasions.

Dosage and Administration: *Orally.* Treatment: 3 tablets daily. Prophylaxis: 1 tablet daily. Poor dietary habits should be corrected and a well-balanced diet prescribed.

Availability:
C-RON FA™ Tablets in bottles of 100 and 1000. **(Rowell)**

CROTAMITON

Chemical Name: *N*-Ethyl-*o*-crotonotoluidide.

Description: A bacteriostatic, nonirritating and nontoxic agent with a low index of sensitivity.

Indications: For the eradication of scabies and for the symptomatic treatment of most pruritic skin conditions.

Contraindications: In patients hypersensitive to crotamiton or those who manifest a primary irritation response.

Warnings: This agent should not be applied to acutely inflamed skin, raw, weeping surfaces, or in the eyes or mouth. Withhold use until acute inflammation has subsided.

Precautions: If severe irritation or sensitization develops, treatment should be discontinued and appropriate therapy instituted.

Adverse Reactions: Allergic sensitivity or primary irritation may occur.

Dosage and Administration: *Topically. Pruritus:* Massage gently into affected areas until medication is completely absorbed. Symptoms are alleviated promptly with sustained relief after each application. *Scabies:* Thoroughly massage the whole body except face and scalp paying particular attention to the sites of predilection. To assure complete eradication, a second application is advisable after an interval of 24 hours. Change of all bed linens and clothing should be made the next morning, followed by a cleansing bath 48 hours after the last application.

Availability:
EURAX® Cream, 10% in tubes of 60 gm. **(Geigy)**

CRYPTENAMINE

Description: Cryptenamine is the generic name for the ester alkaloids of *Veratrum viride* obtained by a selective, nonaqueous extraction process. The mixture of tannate salts of the alkaloids occurs as a tan, amorphous powder slightly soluble in water and soluble in alcohol. The mixture of acetate salts occurs as a white, amorphous powder more soluble in water than the tannates.

Following oral administration, effects may be seen within 2 hours and persist for 4 to 6 hours. Intravenously, the hypotensive response occurs within minutes and lasts about 1 to 3 hours. Intramuscularly, the onset of action varies from 1/2 to 1 1/2 hours, and the effects lasts for about 3 to 6 hours. The metabolic fate of veratrum alkaloids is uncertain, but they probably are degraded in the liver and excreted primarily in the feces.

The principal mechanism by which cryptenamine lowers blood pressure involves widespread arteriolar dilatation mediated centrally without peripheral adrenergic or ganglionic blockade. The increase in afferent impulses leads to a negative feed-back from the CNS, thereby decreasing sympathetic tone, increasing vagal tone, and reducing blood pressure. Both systolic and diastolic pressures are lowered and the heart is slowed. The hypotensive response to the drug may be potentiated by the addition of reserpine, sodium nitrate or other antihypertensive agents.

Indications: Treatment of mild, moderate and severe benign essential hypertension and in hypertensive cardiovascular disease. Parenterally in acute hypertensive episodes such as encephalopathy, preeclampsia, eclampsia, and preeclampsia with underlying essential hypertension. Parenteral administration is urgently indicated where subjective signs such as headache, blurred vision and epigastric pain are present. Dosage should be carefully titrated to the individual patient on account of the narrow margin between the therapeutic and toxic (emetic) dose. The addition of methyclothiazide potentiates the hypotensive effect of cryptenamine.

Contraindications: In patients with an idiosyncrasy to any of the components and in patients who recently have had a coronary artery occlusion or cerebral thrombosis. The monograph on methyclothiazide should be consulted for additional information.

Warnings: Since safe use has not been established, formulations of veratrum alkaloids should be used with caution during pregnancy, lactation, and in women of childbearing age; potential benefits to the mother should be weighed against the possible hazards to the child. Parenteral solutions may be administered undiluted when given intramuscularly; they *must* be diluted when given intravenously. The fixed combination drug is not recommended for initial therapy unless the amount therein corresponds to the dose that is clinically effective for the patient. Additionally, the concurrent use of this drug and a saluretic agent may have an additive effect that can result in a greater reduction in blood pressure than may be obtained with either drug alone. Therefore, the dose of both drugs should be reduced accordingly. The monograph on methyclothiazide should be consulted for additional information.

Precautions: Temporary reduction of dosage during excessively hot weather may be necessary. Use with caution in patients with angina pectoris, coronary thrombosis or cerebrovascular disease, history of bronchial asthma, renal insufficiency, or preexisting uremia, with a history of peptic ulcer or other gastrointestinal disorders. Caution must be exercised when this preparation is used in conjunction with surgery because of the possible additive hypotensive effects of anesthetic and preanesthetic agents. Concurrent administration with digitalis may lead to ectopic cardiac rhythms, and the bradycrotic effect of cryptenamine is additive to, but not synergistic with, that produced by morphine and related drugs. The monograph on methyclothiazide should be consulted for additional information.

Adverse Reactions: Those reported in patients treated with veratrum alkaloids include excessive hypotension, prostration, anorexia, nausea and vomiting, epigastric and substernal burning—which may be mistaken for angina pectoris—unpleasant taste, salivation, sweating, hiccough, blurring of vision, mental confusion, cardiac arrhythmias, bradycardia, and from excessive doses, bronchial constriction and respiratory depression. Since cryptenamine is a potent hypotensive and occasional bradycardic drug, overdosage may produce nausea and vomiting, excessive hypotension and prostration and, rarely, bronchoconstriction. If necessary, atropine sulfate, 0.5 to 1 mg, may be administered to reverse the bradycardic effect. In the event of excessive fall in blood pressure, vasopressors should be given subcutaneously, e.g., 30 to 50 mg of ephedrine sulfate or 5 mg of phenylephrine hydrochloride. The reaction, if left alone, will disappear gradually during the next 60 to 90 minutes. Other reactions that may occur usually are those attributable to any component formulated with the drug. The monograph on methyclothiazide should be consulted for additional information.

Dosage and Administration: Dosage is expressed either in terms of alkaloid, or as Carotid Sinus Reflex Units (C.S.R.U.). One milligram of cryptenamine is equivalent to 130 C.S.R. units. One unit is defined as the smallest dose of the drug/kilogram of body weight that will abolish the pressor response to the carotid sinus reflex resulting from occlusion of the carotid artery in dogs. *Orally,* the initial adult dosage usually is 2 mg twice daily, after breakfast and at bedtime. Dosage should be increased gradually, if necessary, on a day-to-day or week-to-week basis. When dosage is increased, the drug should be given in 3 divided doses; the additional dose should be taken in the early afternoon. Daily dosage should not exceed 12 mg. *Intramuscularly,* 1 mg (0.5 ml) is given, after which blood pressure and pulse rate are recorded every 15 to 30 minutes. In the absence of a hypotensive response after 1 hour, the dose may be increased by increments of 0.1 ml. If a response is indeed noted, dosage may be repeated as often as every hour if necessary or whenever the blood pressure exceeds the desired level (usually 140/90 to 160/100). *Intravenously,* 1 mg (0.5 ml) is diluted with 20 ml of sterile 5% glucose in water and infused at the rate of 1 ml/minute. The injection should be stopped as soon as the blood pressure falls 20 mm systolic or 10 mm diastolic. The package literature should be consulted for complete details.

Availability:

Cryptenamine Acetates

UNITENSEN® AQUEOUS, 2 mg/ml in ampuls of 2 ml in cartons of 5. **(Mallinckrodt)**

Cryptenamine Tannates

UNITENSEN® Tablets, 2 mg (white, scored) in bottles of 100 and 500. **(Mallinckrodt)**

Combinations w/Tannates

DIUTENSEN® Tablets (round, scored, mottled), 2 mg w/ 2.5 mg of methyclothiazide in bottles of 100 and 500. **(Mallinckrodt)**

CYANOCOBALAMIN

Synonym: Vitamin B-12.

Chemical Name: 5,6-Dimethyl-benzimidazolyl cyanocobamide.

Description: Cyanocobalamin is a cobalt-containing compound usually obtained from *Streptomyces griseus.* First isolated from commercial liver extracts, it is currently accepted as the erythrocyte-maturing factor of the liver. It occurs as dark red crystals or amorphous or crystalline red powder sparingly soluble in water and soluble in alcohol. The cobalt content is 4.34%.

Its hemopoietic activity appears to be identical with that of the antianemia factor of liver. When given in adequate individualized doses, it will produce a satisfactory clinical and hematologic response and prevent progression of the cord lesions of pernicious anemia (vitamin B-12 deficiency secondary to intrinsic factor deficiency) and certain other macrocytic anemias. Vitamin B-12 is also essential to growth, cell reproduction, and nucleoprotein and myelin synthesis.

Cyanocobalamin is quantitatively and rapidly absorbed from intramuscular and subcutaneous sites of injection. Peak plasma levels are attained within 1 hour following intramuscular injection. It is stored primarily in the liver with lesser amounts in other organs; excretion occurs mainly in the bile.

Indications: Treatment of all clinical conditions resulting from deficiency of vitamin B-12.

These include pernicious anemia with or without neurological manifestations; malabsorption syndromes; certain other macrocytic or megaloblastic anemias; hemorrhage; blindloop syndrome; infection due to the fish tapeworm, *Diphyllobothrium latum;* nutritional macrocytic anemias of infancy, pregnancy and chronic liver disease complicated by deficiency of vitamin B-12; malignancy; thyrotoxicosis; renal disorders, and as the flushing dose in the Schilling test.

Contraindications: Hypersensitivity to cobalt and/or vitamin B-12.

Warnings: Patients with early Leber's disease or those predisposed to optic nerve atrophy have been found to develop severe and sudden optic atrophy when given this drug.

Precautions: Care should be taken when administering folic acid in conjunction with vitamin B-12 in the treatment of pernicious anemia because such combined therapy may result in irreparable neurologic damage. Also, most antibiotics, methotrexate, and pyrimethamine nullify the diagnostic microbiological blood assays of folic acid and vitamin B-12, and colchicine, paraminosalicylic acid or excessive alcohol intake for more than 2 weeks may produce malabsorption of vitamin B-12. Because hypokalemia may occur at the beginning of therapy of severe megaloblastic conditions, serum potassium levels should be monitored in patients receiving cyanocobalamin.

Adverse Reactions: There is no evidence that cyanocobalamin itself is toxic, even in large doses. Allergic type reactions have been reported only rarely; it is not known whether these were related to the preservative, the drug, or neither. These include itching, transitory exanthema, feeling of swelling of the entire body, polycythemia vera, peripheral vascular thrombosis, pulmonary edema, congestive heart failure, and anaphylactic shock which has been reported to result in death in a few instances. The occurrence of a mild transient diarrhea following each injection in one patient and the occurrence of "tuberculin-type" reaction to a skin test of vitamin B-12 in a patient previously sensitized to cobalt have been reported. A few patients may experience mild pain following injection of cyanocobalamin.

Dosage and Administration: *Intramuscularly* or *subcutaneously.* Intravenous administration implies no particular advantage. Treatment with this vitamin should be sufficient to replenish and, when necessary, to maintain body stores. A variety of dosage regimens have been recommended by clinicians for the management of pernicious anemia and other macrocytic anemias. The initial dosage requirements vary with the individual patients. Doses of 100 mcg once or twice a week, continued until normal hemoglobin levels are obtained, are usually sufficient. In severe cases of pernicious anemia doses as high as 100 mcg daily may be required, particularly when neurological manifestations are present. When remission occurs, maintenance dosage should be determined individually on the basis of RBC count. Doses of 100 mcg every month or every other month are generally sufficient to maintain normal blood values. In nutritional megaloblastic anemias, a single initial dose of 15 mcg usually produced a favorable response. The suggested dose may be repeated every 2 weeks to prevent a relapse. In certain macrocytic anemias, concomitant therapy with folic acid may be required. In the Schilling test for pernicious anemia, the flushing dose is 1000 mcg.

Availability:

Cyanocobalamin Injection

Solution, 30, 100 and 1000 mcg/ml in vials of 10 and 30 ml. **(Various Mfrs.)**

Solution, 1000 mcg/ml in vials of 10 ml. **(Merrell-National)**

Solution, 100 and 1000 mcg/ml in (Tubex®) 1-ml disposable syringes with needle; 1000 mcg/ml is also available in half-filled disposable syringes of 2 ml. **(Wyeth)**

BERUBIGEN® Solution, 1000 mcg/ml in vials of 10 ml. **(Upjohn)**

BETALIN® 12 Solution, 100 mcg/ml in ampuls of 10 ml; 1000 mcg/ml in ampuls of 5 and 10 ml. **(Lilly)**

DEPINAR® Repository Solution, 500 mcg/ml in ampuls of 1 ml. **(Armour)**

DODEX® Solution, 1000 mcg/ml in ampuls of 1 ml and in vials of 10 ml. **(Organon)**

REDISOL® Solution, 100 and 1000 mcg/ml in vials of 10 ml. **(Merck Sharp & Dohme)**

RUBRAMIN PC® Solution, 100 mcg/ml in vials of 10 ml; 1000 mcg/ml in vials of 1 and 10 ml. Both potencies are also available in Unimatic® (single-dose) syringes of 1 ml. **(Squibb)**

SYTOBEX® Solution, 100 mcg/ml in Steri-Vials® of 10 ml; 1000 mcg/ml in ampuls of 1 ml, in

Steri-Vials® of 10 ml and in half-filled (Steri-Dose®) disposable syringes of 2 ml. **(Parke-Davis)**
VITAMIN-B-12 Solution, 1000 mcg/ml in vials of 30 ml. **(Amfre-Grant)**

CYCLANDELATE

Chemical Name: 3,3,5-Trimethylcyclohexyl mandelate.

Description: Cyclandelate is a spasmolytic and vasodilating drug that differs chemically from the majority of such agents in that it contains no nitrogen in its molecular structure. It occurs as a white, crystalline powder slightly soluble in water and soluble in alcohol and in other organic solvents. Its mechanism of action is similar to that of papaverine in that it acts directly on the vascular smooth musculature to produce a gradual and progressive relaxation that enhances the flow of peripheral and cerebral blood, resulting in an increase in peripheral circulation and a slight rise in skin temperature of the extremities.

Following oral administration, the effects are evident in about 15 minutes, reach a peak in about 1 to 1.5 hours, and persist for about 3 to 4 hours. The drug is musculotropic and does not stimulate or block adrenergic impulses significantly.

Indications: May be helpful when used adjunctively in the treatment of occlusive and vasospastic diseases of the vascular system associated with impaired circulation, such as intermittent claudication, arteriosclerosis obliterans, thrombophlebitis (to control associated vasospasm and muscular ischemia), nocturnal leg cramps, Raynaud's phenomenon, and for selected cases of ischemic cerebral vascular disease. It is important that the patient continue to observe established precautions such as proper care of feet, no smoking, etc.

Contraindications: Hypersensitivity to the drug.

Warnings: Because it is a vasodilator, the drug should be used with caution in patients with severe obliterative coronary artery or cerebral vascular disease because the vasodilatory effects of the drug in other parts of the body may compromise these other diseased areas. Although therapeutic doses have not prolonged bleeding time in patients, it has been reported in animals receiving very large doses. Therefore, the hazard of a prolonged bleeding time should be carefully considered when giving the drug to patients with active bleeding or a tendency to bleed. Since safe use of the drug has not been established, it should not be used during pregnancy or lactation or in women of childbearing age unless in the judgment of the physician its use is deemed essential to the welfare of the patient.

Precautions: Because of its vasodilating action, it should be used with caution in patients with glaucoma.

Adverse Reactions: Infrequently, mild gastrointestinal distress (heartburn, pain and eructation), usually relieved by administration with meals or with antacids. Mild flush, headache, weakness, or tachycardia may occur during the first weeks of administration.

Dosage and Administration: *Orally.* Initially, 300 to 400 mg 4 times daily before meals and at bedtime, decreased in decrements of 50 mg until a maintenance level is reached. The usual maintenance dosage is between 400 and 800 mg daily in 2 to 4 divided doses. The patient should be told that long-term therapy may be necessary, since short-term use is rarely beneficial, nor is it likely to be of any permanent value.

Availability:
CYCLOSPASMOL®: **(Ives)**
Capsules, 200 mg (blue) in bottles of 100, 500 and 1000; 400 mg (blue and red) in bottles of 60, 100 and 500.
Tablets, 100 mg (orange) in bottles of 100 and 500.

CYCLIZINE

Chemical Name: N-Benzhydryl-N′-methylpiperazine.

Description: An antihistaminic compound that is structurally and pharmacologically related to meclizine and chlorcyclizine. It occurs as a bitter, white, crystalline powder or as colorless crystals slightly soluble in water and in alcohol. Cyclizine lactate is freely soluble in water.

Cyclizine also exhibits CNS depressant, anticholinergic, antiemetic, antispasmodic and local anesthetic activity. It has a marked depressant effect on the labyrinthine-vestibular-cerebellar pathways. When measured against nystagmus produced by stimulation of the labyrinth, cyclizine appears to be more potent on a weight basis than meclizine, but its duration of action (4 to 6 hours) is not as prolonged as that of meclizine. Its metabolic fate in the body is not known. A review of available animal data reveals that the drug exerts a teratogenic response in the rat, mouse and rabbit.

Indications: The *tablets* are indicated for the prevention and treatment of motion sickness, and the *injection* may be of value for the control of postoperative nausea and vomiting.

Precautions: Since drowsiness may occur, this drug should be used with caution in those individuals whose activities require constant alertness, as in the operation of motor vehicles or machines.

Adverse Reactions: Serious consideration should be given to the potential hazards when prescribing this compound or its salts to pregnant women.

Dosage and Administration: *Intramuscularly.* Usual dose is 50 mg every 4 to 6 hours. For prophylaxis of postanesthetic vomiting 50 mg may be administered with preoperative medications or 20 to 30 minutes before the expected termination of surgery, and continued every 4 to 6 hours as needed. Children up to 6 years of age, 1/4 the adult dose; 6 to 10 years of age, 1/2 the adult dose. Accurate pediatric dosages have not been established.

Availability:
MAREZINE®: **(Burroughs Wellcome)**
Injection (as lactate), 50 mg/ml in ampuls of 1 ml.
Tablets (OTC) (as hydrochloride), 50 mg in bottles of 100 and 1000 and in cartons of 12.

CYCLOBENZAPRINE HYDROCHLORIDE

Chemical Name: 3-(5H-Dibenzo[a,d]cyclohepten-5-ylidene)-N,N-dimethyl-1-propanamine hydrochloride.

Description: Cyclobenzaprine, a tricyclic spasmolytic agent, has been found useful in alleviating the signs and symptoms of skeletal muscle spasm of local origin without interfering with muscle function. This effect is accomplished through its action within the CNS, primarily at the brain stem, and not to a direct action at the neuromuscular junction or on skeletal muscle. However, it is of no value in relieving muscle spasm due to CNS disorders nor will it relieve pain unrelated to spasm. Evidence suggests that the drug diminishes muscle hypertonia, and selectively influences both the alpha and gamma motor systems. The clinical response is a reduction of muscle spasm with relief of pain and tenderness and increased motility of the involved muscles. Comparable studies with diazepam showed that their therapeutic effectiveness in these parameters are similar. It occurs as a white, crystalline powder that is freely soluble in water and alcohol, sparingly soluble in isopropanol and insoluble in hydrocarbon solvents. Its molecular weight was reported to be 311.9.

Pharmacological studies in animals revealed a similarity between the effects of cyclobenzaprine and the structurally related tricyclic antidepressants, including reserpine antagonism, norepinephrine potentiation, potent peripheral and central anticholinergic effects, and sedation. The drug has been noted to cause a slight to moderate increase in heart rate in animals.

Cyclobenzaprine is almost completely absorbed from the gastrointestinal tract, reaching peak plasma levels within 3 to 8 hours. It is eliminated quite slowly with a half-life extending from 1 to 3 days. Highly bound to plasma proteins, the drug is extensively metabolized primarily to glucuronide-like conjugates, and is excreted chiefly by the kidneys.

Results of animal studies with pregnant mice and rabbits given oral doses of 20 mg/kg/day produced no evidence of external, visceral or skeletal abnormalities in the offspring.

Indications: As an adjunct to rest, physical therapy and other helpful measures for the relief of muscle spasm associated with acute, painful musculoskeletal conditions. Improvement is manifested by relief of muscle spasm and its characteristic signs and symptoms. Cyclobenzaprine has not been found effective in the treatment of muscle spasm associated with cerebral or spinal cord disease, or in children with cerebral palsy.

Contraindications: Hypersensitivity to the drug, during the acute recovery phase of myocardial infarction and patients with arrhythmias, heart block, conduction disturbances, or congestive heart failure, and those with hyperthyroidism. Concomitant administration with MAO inhibitors is also contraindicated. A medication-free period of at least 2 weeks should be observed when transferring patients from MAO inhibitors to cyclobenzaprine to avoid a hyperpyretic crisis, severe convulsions, and death from occurring.

Warnings: Use of the drug for periods longer than 2 or 3 weeks is not recommended. Because of its close relationship to the tricyclic antidepressant agents such as amitriptyline and imipramine, large doses of cyclobenzaprine have been associated with the more serious CNS reactions usually observed with these agents. It is advised that all the precautions attendant with the use of tricyclic antidepressants be observed with this drug. Close supervision of patients with cardiovascular complications is recommended since this drug has been reported to produce cardiac arrythmias and sinus tachycardia and to prolong the conduction time. Myocardial infarction and stroke may also occur. Since drowsiness is a frequent occurrence, patients should be cautioned against performing hazardous tasks because of the possibility of impaired judgment or diminished reflexes. Caution is essential when skeletal muscle relaxants and other CNS depressants (e.g., alcohol, sedative-hypnotics, etc.) are used concomitantly since their effects may be enhanced.

Precautions: Because of its atropine-like action, cyclobenzaprine should be used with caution in patients with a history of urinary retention, angle-closure glaucoma, increased intraocular pressure, and in patients taking anticholinergic medication. The physician should keep in mind that tricyclic compounds prevent the amine-uptake mechanism of guanethidine and similarly acting agents and thereby reduce their antihypertensive effect. Although hepatotoxic reactions were noted in studies with rats receiving high doses and prolonged administration of cyclobenzaprine, liver function abnormalities have not been observed in patients taking the recommended clinical regimen. Safe use during pregnancy has not been established; therefore, the anticipated benefits must be weighed against the possible hazards to the mother and fetus. Lactating women should be advised not to nurse their infants while taking this drug. Additionally, cyclobenzaprine is not recommended for children under 15 years of age until safe and effective use has been confirmed.

Adverse Reactions: Drowsiness, dizziness, and dry mouth are the most frequently encountered adverse reactions. Increased heart rate or tachycardia, weakness, dyspepsia, paresthesia, unpleasant taste, blurred vision, and insomnia are less frequently noted; and hyperhydrosis, myalgia, dyspnea, abdominal pain, constipation, coated tongue, tremors, dysarthria, euphoria, nervousness, disorientation, confusion, headache, urinary retention, decreased bladder tone, and ataxia are rarely noted. Other adverse reactions characteristic for all of the tricyclic compounds in general, and which may be associated with cyclobenzaprine include the following: *Cardiovascular effects:* Hypotension, hypertension, palpitation, myocardial infarction, arrhythmias, heart block, and stroke. *CNS and neuromuscular effects:* Confusional states, disturbed concentration, delusions, hallucinations, excitement, anxiety, restlessness, nightmares, paresthesias of the extremities, peripheral neuropathy, incoordination, seizures, EEG abnormalities, extrapyramidal symptoms, tinnitus, and a syndrome of inappropriate ADH (antidiuretic hormone) secretion. *Anticholinergic effects:* Disturbance of accommodation, paralytic ileus, and dilatation of the urinary tract. *Allergic reactions:* Skin rash, urticaria, photosensitization, and edema of the face and tongue. *Blood dyscrasias:* Bone marrow depression including agranulocytosis, leukopenia, eosinophilia, purpura, and thrombocytopenia. *Gastrointestinal effects:* Nausea, epigastric distress, vomiting, anorexia, stomatitis, diarrhea, parotid swelling, black tongue; rarely, hepatitis (including altered liver function and jaundice). *Endocrine effects:* Testicular swelling and gynecomastia in the male, breast enlargement with galactorrhea in the female, increased or decreased libido, and either hyperglycemia or hypoglycemia. *Miscellaneous reactions:* Fatigue, weight gain or loss, urinary frequency, mydriasis, jaundice, and alopecia. Abrupt cessation of treatment after prolonged administration may produce withdrawal symptoms such as nausea, headache, and malaise. Overdosage may cause temporary confusion, disturbed concentration, transient visual hallucinations, agitation, hyperactive reflexes, muscle rigidity, vomiting, or hyperpyrexia, in addition to those listed above. Based on the known pharmacologic actions of the drug, high doses may cause drowsiness, hypothermia, tachycardia and other cardiac rhythm abnormalities such as bundle branch block, ECG evidence of impaired conduction, and congestive heart failure. Other manifestations may include dilated pupils, convulsions, severe hypotension, stupor, and coma. Treatment is based on general symptomatic and supportive measures. Emesis and gastric lavage have been recommended. An ECG should be taken and close monitoring of cardiac function must be instituted if there is any evidence of dysrhythmia. Maintenance of an open airway, adequate fluid intake, and regulation of body temperature are necessary. Physostigmine (1 to 3 mg) can be helpful in controlling arrhythmias, convulsions, and deep coma; the course may have to be repeated because physostigmine has a short duration of action. Standard medical measures should be used to manage circulatory shock and metabolic acidosis. Cardiac arrhythmias may be treated with neostigmine, pyridostigmine, or propranolol. When signs of cardiac failure occur, the use of a short-acting digitalis preparation should be considered. Close monitoring of cardiac function for no less than 5 days is advisable. Dialysis is probably of no value because of low plasma concentration of the drug.

Dosage and Administration: *Orally.* The usual dosage is 10 mg 3 times daily, with a range of 20 to 40 mg daily in divided doses. Dosage should not exceed 60 mg daily. Use of cyclobenzaprine for periods longer than 2 or 3 weeks is not recommended.

Availability:
FLEXERIL™ Tablets, 10 mg (butterscotch yellow) in bottles of 100. **(Merck Sharp & Dohme)**

CYCLOMETHYCAINE SULFATE

Chemical Name: 3-(Methylpiperidino)-propyl-*p*-cyclohexyloxybenzoate sulfate.

Description: A local anesthetic agent belonging to the benzoic group of compounds, but it does not yield *p*-aminobenzoic acid upon hydrolysis.

Acts by blocking nerve impulses at the sensory nerve endings in the skin and mucous membranes. Relieves itching, burning and pain when applied to the mucous membranes of the rectum, vagina, urethra, nose and throat and other areas amenable to topical anesthesia. Exerts an anesthetic action on damaged skin areas within 5 to 10 minutes providing sustained relief. The drug does not penetrate the tympanic membrane and is of no value in the treatment of otitis media.

Indications: Symptomatic relief of abrasions; anal fissures, fistulas and ulcers, anal spasm associated with anal pain; burns of the skin or vagina; chafing; contact dermatitis; episiotomy wounds; fissured nipples; hemorrhoids; herpes zoster; insect bites; intertrigo; pruritus (including pruritus vulvae and ani); senile vaginitis; sunburn. The jelly form is useful as an anesthetic aid in bronchoscopy; cystoscopy; digital rectal examination in labor, examination of anus, rectum and prostate; passage of urethral sounds; sigmoidoscopy; tracheal intubation, and vaginal pain after plastic surgery.

Contraindications: Not to be used in patients with an idiosyncrasy or allergy to one or more of the ingredients. It is also contraindicated for use in the eyes. Local anesthetics should not be applied over extensive areas or for prolonged periods. Because its base contains petrolatum, the ointment is contraindicated in vesicular lesions.

Precautions: Prolonged or indefinite use of cyclomethycaine should be undertaken only if close observation of the patient can be maintained to detect possible development of an allergic reaction. Increase in redness, itching, papules, or vesicles suggests possible allergy. The medication should be discontinued if an allergic or unfavorable response occurs. Patients with a history of allergic asthma, rhinitis or urticaria may have an increased risk of such reactions. One probable anaphylactoid reaction was noted following the introduction of a suppository in a patient with a history of multiple allergies. No systemic toxicity has been noted. Urethral administration should be performed only by the physician or by those individuals under his direction. When used in urethral instillation, extreme caution must be exercised when injected into a traumatized urethra or under conditions in which injury may occur. Overdistention of the urethra by application of the jelly may produce trauma with stinging and burning and if the injury is extensive, these symptoms may recur when the anesthetic effect is dissipated.

Adverse Reactions: A transitory stinging and/or burning sensation may be experienced before onset of the anesthetic effect. In hypersensitive individuals contact dermatitis should be anticipated.

Dosage and Administration: *Topically.* A small quantity of cream or ointment should be applied as needed. Before using the jelly consult the package literature. One suppository placed low in the rectum provides relief for 4 to 8 hours.

Availability:
SURFACAINE®: **(Lilly)**
Cream, 0.5% in tubes of 30 gm and in jars of 1 lb.
Jelly, 0.75% in tubes of 3.5, 30 and 150 gm with urethral tip.
Ointment, 1% in tubes of 30 gm with rectal pipe and in jars of 1 lb.
Rectal or *Vaginal Suppositories,* 10 mg in cartons of 12.

CYCLOPENTOLATE

Chemical Name: 1-Hydroxy-α-phenylcyclopentaneacetic acid, 2-(dimethylamino) ethyl ester.

Description: Cyclopentolate is an anticholinergic agent that induces complete relaxation of the sphincter of the iris and the ciliary muscles. When applied topically to the eyes, it causes a rapid, intense cycloplegic and mydriatic effect that attains maximal degree in 30 to 60 minutes; recovery usually occurs in 3 to 6 hours. The cycloplegic effect also is readily achievable in patients who have dark pigmented irises.

Indications: To induce mydriasis and cycloplegia prior to diagnostic procedures. The addition of phenylephrine hydrochloride produces rapid and profound mydriasis in patients who are being prepared for funduscopic examination.

Contraindications: In the presence of narrow-angle glaucoma or excessive intraocular pressure.

Precautions: Tonometer readings should be scheduled before administering this agent to patients who are past middle age and in those individuals with increased intraocular pressure. To minimize systemic absorption, the lacrimal sac should be compressed for 1 or 2 minutes following instillation of the drops. Cyclopentolate with phenylephrine may adversely affect patients who have cardiovascular disease, hypertension, or hyperthyroidism.

Adverse Reactions: In rare instances, atropine-like symptoms have been reported with the 2% solution in young children. These included ataxia, incoherent speech, restlessness, hallucination, disorientation as to time and place, failure to recognize people and tachycardia.

Dosage and Administration: *Topically.* For cycloplegia in adult caucasians—2 drops of 0.5% solution in each eye (1 drop followed by a second drop 5 minutes later), or 1 drop of either a 1 or 2% solution. Although complete recovery usually occurs in 24 hours, 1 or 2 drops of a 1 to 2% solution of pilocarpine nitrate reduces recovery time to 3 to 6 hours in most instances. While no appreciable increase in intraocular tension has been reported, it is advisable to minimize any cycloplegia in older individuals in whom unrecognized preglaucomatous changes may be present, and in patients with shallow anterior chambers of the eyes. For cycloplegia in adult negroes, or those individuals with darkly pigmented eyes—the 2% solution is recommended. A 1% solution also has produced satisfactory results. Subsequent instillation of 2% pilocarpine nitrate reduces recovery time to 6 hours or less. For children, pretreatment on the day prior to examination usually is not necessary. One drop of 0.5, 1 or 2% solution is instilled in each eye at the time of refraction, followed 10 minutes later by a second application of 0.5 or 1% solution, if necessary. For mydriasis—1 or 2 drops of 0.5% solution or 1 drop of 1 or 2% solution every 6 to 8 hours to induce paralysis of the sphincter, thus inhibiting inflammatory spasm. The usual supportive measures should be administered. Cyclopentolate + phenylephrine: For funduscopy—1 drop in each eye.

Availability:

Cyclopentolate Hydrochloride

CYCLOGYL® Ophthalmic Solution, 0.5, 1 and 2% in Drop-Tainer® bottles of 2, 5 and 15 ml. **(Alcon)**

w/Phenylephrine Hydrochloride

CYCLOMYDRIL® Ophthalmic Solution, 0.2% with phenylephrine hydrochloride, 1% in Drop-Tainer® bottles of 2 and 5 ml. **(Alcon)**

CYCLOPHOSPHAMIDE

Chemical Name: 2-[Bis(2-chloroethyl)amino]tetrahydro-2*H*-1,3,2-oxazaphosphorine-2-oxide.

Description: A cytotoxic agent of the alkylating type, chemically related to the nitrogen mustards, it is a white, crystalline powder soluble in water, in physiological saline and in alcohol.

In suitable cases, the drug exerts a destructive effect on cancer cells that is reflected by subjective or objective improvement or by both. Evidence of improvement may include decrease in pain and other symptoms, increase in strength, improved appetite, and regression in size of neoplasm.

Cyclophosphamide interferes with the growth of susceptible neoplasms and, to some extent, certain normal tissues. However, its mechanism of action is not known. It is absorbed from the gastrointestinal tract and the injection sites. It is metabolized (the precise details are not fully known) and the drug and its metabolites are distributed throughout the body, including the brain. When administered intravenously, cyclophosphamide is reported to have a serum half-life of approximately 4 hours; however the drug or its metabolites or both may be detected in plasma for up to 72 hours. Cyclophosphamide and its metabolites are excreted by the kidneys, but the extent to which they are excreted by other routes is not known. Of 3 alkylating metabolites found in the urine, only 1 (nor-nitrogen mustard) has been positively identified.

Indications: For the palliative treatment of certain malignant neoplasms such as myeloproliferative and lymphoproliferative disorders. These include malignant lymphomas (Stages III and IV, Peter's Staging System): Hodgkin's disease, follicular lymphoma, lymphocytic lymphosarcoma, reticulum cell sarcoma, lymphoblastic lymphosarcoma, and Burkitt's lymphoma; multiple myeloma; leukemias such as chronic lymphocytic leukemia, chronic granulocytic leukemia (it is ineffective in acute blastic crises), acute myelogenous and monocytic leukemia, acute lymphoblastic (stem-cell) leukemia in children (cyclophosphamide given during remission is effective in prolonging its duration); mycosis fungoides (advanced disease); frequently responsive solid malignancies such as neuroblastoma (in patients with disseminated disease), adenocarcinoma of the ovary, retinoblastoma, and in infrequently responsive malignancies such as carcinoma of the breast, and malignant neoplasms of the lung.

Warnings: Since cyclophosphamide has been reported to be more toxic in adrenalectomized dogs, adjustment of the doses of both replacement steroids and cyclophosphamide may be necessary for the adrenalectomized patient. Chronic administration of high doses of phenobarbital has been reported to increase the metabolic rate and leukopenic activity of this drug. Therefore, the physician should be aware of possible combined drug actions. Since studies with mice and rats have revealed drug-induced oncogenic activity, the possibility of this reaction occurring in patients should be kept in mind. Experimental studies have indicated that cyclophosphamide can be teratogenic or cause fetal reabsorption in animals. Therefore, it should not be used during pregnancy, particularly in the first trimester, unless in the judgment of the physician, the potential benefits outweigh the possible risks. Since it is postulated that cyclophosphamide is excreted in breast milk, breast-feeding should be terminated prior to institution of therapy. Patients capable of conception should be advised of the drug's mutagenic potential.

Precautions: Cautious use is advised in the presence of leukopenia, thrombocytopenia, tumor cell infiltration of bone marrow, previous radiation therapy, or therapy with other cytotoxic agents, and impaired hepatic or renal function. Cyclophosphamide may interfere with normal healing of wounds. Because the drug may exert a suppressive action on immune mechanisms, the interruption or modification of dosage should be considered for patients who develop bacterial, fungal or viral infections, and in those patients receiving concomitant steroid therapy, and in those with a recent history of steroid therapy, since infections in some of these patients have been fatal. Varicella-zoster infections appear to be particularly dangerous under these circumstances.

Adverse Reactions: *Hematopoietic.* Leukopenia is an expected effect and is used ordinarily as a guide to therapy. Thrombocytopenia or anemia may occur in a few patients. These effects are almost always reversible when therapy is interrupted. *Gastrointestinal.* Anorexia, nausea, or vomiting are common and related to dose as well as individual susceptibility. There are isolated reports of hemorrhagic colitis, oral mucosal ulceration and jaundice occurring during therapy. *Genitourinary.* Sterile hemorrhagic cystitis can result from the administration of cyclophosphamide. This can be severe, even fatal, and is probably due to metabolites in the urine. Ample fluid intake and frequent voiding help to prevent the development of cystitis, but when it appears, it is usually necessary to interrupt therapy. A few cases of nephrotoxicity including hemorrhage and clot formation were reported. There is a possibility that gonadal suppression in either sex can occur. Fibrosis of the ovary, amenorrhea (possibly irreversible) and hot flushes can occur during therapy with cyclophosphamide. *Integument.* It is ordinarily advisable to inform patients in advance of possible alopecia, a frequent complication of therapy with this drug. Regrowth of hair can be expected although occasionally the new hair may be a different color or texture. The skin and fingernails may become darker during therapy. Nonspecific dermatitis has been noted. *Pulmonary.* Interstitial pulmonary fibrosis has been reported in patients receiving high doses of this drug over a prolonged period. *Secondary neoplasia.* Secondary malignancies, particularly urinary bladder, myeloproliferative, and lymphoproliferative malignancies should be anticipated since they have occurred in some patients. Those most susceptible are patients with primary myeloproliferative and lymphoproliferative malignancies and primary nonmalignant diseases in which immune processes are believed to be involved pathologically. In some instances, the secondary malignancy was detected up to several years after treatment with cyclophosphamide was discontinued. Secondary urinary bladder malignancies generally have occurred in patients who had previously developed drug-induced hemorrhagic cystitis. Although no causal relationship to the drug has been established, the possibility of secondary malignancy, based on available data, should be considered in any benefit-to-risk assessment for the use of the drug.

Dosage and Administration: *Orally* and *Parenterally.* Because potentially hazardous and fatal complications can occur, it is recommended that the drug be administered only by physicians who are fully aware of the associated risks. Dosage must always be carefully individualized and should be adjusted on the basis of blood count studies and the patient's tolerance. For patients who have not received prior radiation or chemotherapy, the initial loading dose is 40 to 50 mg/kg of body weight, usually administered *intravenously* at a rate of 10 to 20 mg/kg/day for 2 to 5 days. Patients who have had prior radiation or chemotherapy or those with tumor infiltration of the bone marrow may require reduction of the initial loading dose by 1/3 to 1/2. If given *orally,* a dose of 1 to 5 mg/kg/day can be administered. The white blood cell count should be monitored closely during induction therapy. For maintenance therapy, the suggested *oral* dosage is 1 to 5 mg/kg daily and the suggested *intravenous* dosage is 10 to 15 mg/kg every 7 to 10 days, or 3 to 5 mg/kg twice weekly. The total leukocyte count is a good objective guide for regulating the maintenance dose. For the preparation and handling of solutions, the physician should consult the package literature.

Availability:
CYTOXAN®: **(Mead Johnson)**
Injection, 100, 200 and 500 mg vials in cartons of 12.
Tablets, 25 and 50 mg in bottles of 100 and 1000; the 50 mg tablets are also available in unit-dose packages of 100.

CYCLOSERINE

Chemical Name: D-4-Amino-3-isoxazolidinone.

Description: Cycloserine is a broad-spectrum antibiotic which is produced by a strain of *Streptomyces orchidaceous* and has also been synthesized. It occurs as a hygroscopic, amphoteric, white, crystalline powder that is freely soluble in water, soluble in alcohol, and is stable in alkaline solutions. It is rapidly destroyed at neutral or acid pH.

Cycloserine inhibits cell-wall synthesis in susceptible strains of gram-positive and gram-negative bacteria and in *Mycobacterium tuberculosis.* It is rapidly absorbed following an oral dose, reaching peak plasma levels within 3 to 4 hours, diminishing to barely detectable quantities after 12 hours. The value of the drug is enhanced by the fact that it diffuses throughout the body fluids and tissues and readily crosses the blood-brain barrier reaching approximately the same cerebrospinal fluid concentrations as those found in the plasma.

Indications: Treatment of active pulmonary and extrapulmonary tuberculosis (including renal disease) when the organisms are susceptible to this drug and after failure of adequate treatment with the primary medications (streptomycin, isoniazid, and aminosalicylic acid). Like all antituberculosis drugs, cycloserine should be administered in conjunction with other effective chemotherapy and not as the sole therapeutic agent. It may be effective in the treatment of acute urinary tract infections caused by susceptible strains of gram-positive and gram-negative bacteria, especially *Enterobacter* and *Escherichia coli.* It is generally no more and is usually less effective than other antimicrobial agents in the treatment of urinary tract infections caused by bacteria other than mycobacteria. Use of cycloserine in these infections should be considered only when the more conventional therapy has failed and when the organism has been demonstrated to be sensitive to the drug.

Contraindications: Administration is contraindicated in patients with hypersensitivity to cycloserine, epilepsy, depression, severe anxiety, or psychosis, severe renal insufficiency, and excessive concurrent use of alcoholic beverages.

Warnings: Administration of cycloserine should be discontinued or the dosage reduced if the patient develops allergic dermatitis or symptoms of central nervous system toxicity, such as convulsions, psychosis, somnolence, depression, confusion, hyperreflexia, headache, tremor, vertigo, paresis, or dysarthria. The toxicity of cycloserine is closely related to excessive blood levels (above 30 mcg/ml), which are due to high dosage or inadequate renal clearance. The ratio of toxic dose to effective dose in tuberculosis is small. The risk of convulsions is increased in chronic alcoholics. Patients should be monitored by hematologic, renal excretion, blood level, and liver function studies. Safe use during pregnancy has not been established nor has safe use and dosage for the pediatric age group been established.

Precautions: Before treatment with cycloserine is initiated, cultures should be taken and the organism's susceptibility to the drug should be established. In tuberculous infections, its sensitivity to the other antituberculosis agents in the regimen should also be demonstrated. Blood levels should be determined at least weekly for patients having reduced renal function, for individuals receiving a daily dosage of more than 500 mg, and for those showing signs and symptoms suggestive of toxicity. The dosage should be adjusted to keep the blood level below 30 mcg/ml. Anticonvulsant drugs or sedatives may be effective in controlling symptoms of CNS toxicity, such as convulsions, anxiety, and tremor. Patients receiving more than 500 mg of cycloserine daily should be closely observed for such symptoms. The value of pyridoxine in preventing CNS toxicity from cycloserine has not been proved. Administration of this drug and other antituberculosis drugs has been associated in a few instances with vitamin B-12 and/or folic acid deficiency, megaloblastic anemia, and sideroblastic anemia. If evidence of anemia develops during treatment, appropriate studies and therapy should be instituted.

Adverse Reactions: Most adverse reactions occurring during therapy with cycloserine involve the nervous system or are manifestations of drug hypersensitivity. The following side effects have been observed: Nervous system symptoms (which appear to be related to higher dosages of the drug, i.e., more than 500 mg daily) include convulsions, drowsiness and somnolence, headache, tremor, dysarthria, vertigo, confusion and disorientation with loss of memory, psychoses (possibly with suicidal tendencies), character changes, hyperirritability, aggression, paresis, hyperreflexia, paresthesias, major and minor (localized) clonic seizures, coma, and allergic skin rash (apparently not related to dosage). Miscellaneous reactions include elevated serum transaminase, especially in patients with preexisting liver disease. Symptoms of overdosage include CNS depression with accompanying drowsiness, somnolence, dizziness, hyperreflexia, mental confusion, convulsions, and allergic dermatitis. Pyridoxine, 300 mg or more daily, and anticonvulsants may be given to relieve convulsions. General management may include symptomatic and supportive therapy, such as gastric lavage, oxygen, artificial respiration, intravenous fluids, standard measures for management of circulatory shock, and maintenance of body temperature.

Dosage and Administration: *Orally.* Cycloserine is currently administered only by this route. If used alone, adults should receive as initial dosage 250 mg twice daily at intervals of 12 hours for 2 weeks. Blood concentrations below 25 to 30 mcg/ml without clinical signs of toxicity may be an indication for increase in dosage to 250 mg every 8 hours. If optimal blood levels of 25 to 30 mcg/ml are not obtained in 2 weeks, 1 gm daily (not to be exceeded) in 4 divided doses may be considered, especially if there is inadequate therapeutic response with minimum evidence of clinical toxicity. Blood level determinations should be made 3 to 4 hours after a dose of the drug is given. When the drug is combined with isoniazid, a dosage of 500 mg/day is believed adequate and at present should not be exceeded. For combined therapy, the dosage schedule of 250 mg of cycloserine with 150 mg of isoniazid, administered every 12 hours, should be followed, since this reduces the incidence of side effects. In patients with normal renal function, urinary tract infections due to susceptible organisms may be treated with 250 mg of cycloserine every 12 hours. The drug in combination with other antituberculosis agents is more effective than when used alone.

Availability:
SEROMYCIN® Pulvules® (Capsules), 250 mg in bottles of 40 and 500. **(Lilly)**

CYCLOTHIAZIDE: see The Thiazide Diuretics

CYCRIMINE HYDROCHLORIDE

Chemical Name: α-Cyclopentyl-α-phenyl-1-piperidinepropanol hydrochloride.

Description: An antispasmodic agent occurring as a white, odorless, solid with a bitter taste, slightly soluble in water and sparingly soluble in alcohol. An analogue of trihexyphenidyl, its anticholinergic activity may be characterized by blocking the uptake of catecholamines into the corpus striatum.

Indications: As an adjunctive measure in the syndrome known as parkinsonism, whether arteriosclerotic, idiopathic or postencephalitic in origin.

Contraindications: Should not be administered to patients in whom parasympathetic inhibition is undesirable or to those showing hypersensitivity to this drug.

Warnings: Caution should be observed in treating patients with glaucoma because the possible consequent dilation of the pupil might be harmful. Safe use of cycrimine during pregnancy has not been established.

Precautions: Use cautiously in the aged particularly those with arteriosclerotic changes; in patients with tachycardia, or a tendency toward urinary retention.

Adverse Reactions: Transient nausea and anorexia, blurred vision, dry mouth, or sore mouth and tongue are minor and often disappear upon withdrawal of the drug. Epigastric distress can often be ameliorated if the medication is administered with meals or with a glass of milk. Lightheadedness, weakness, tachycardia, elevated temperature, flushing, rash, transitory confusional states, have also been reported. Symptoms of overdosage include dryness of mucous membranes, dilatation of pupils, hot, dry and flushed skin, hyperpyrexia, tachycardia, nausea and vomiting, restlessness and confusion with coma, circulatory collapse, and respiratory depression. Treatment is symptomatic and consists of gastric lavage, maintaining respiratory support, and oxygen therapy. Urinary retention may require catheterization. Instillation of 0.5% pilocarpine nitrate into the eyes to counteract mydriasis may be required.

Dosage and Administration: *Orally* with meals. The recommended initial dosage administered 3 times daily is: postencephalitic, 5 mg; idiopathic and arteriosclerotic, 1.25 mg. Individualization of dosage and administration schedules are essential for successful usage. The maximal recommended dosage is usually 20 mg daily; however, some postencephalitic patients may require more.

Availability:
PAGITANE® Tablets, 1.25 and 2.5 mg in bottles of 100 and 1000. **(Lilly)**

CYPROHEPTADINE HYDROCHLORIDE

Chemical Name: 4-(5*H*-Dibenzo[a,d]cyclohepten-5-ylidene)-1-methylpiperidine hydrochloride monohydrate.

Description: A serotonin and histamine antagonist with anticholinergic and sedative effects, it occurs as a white to slightly yellowish, crystalline solid that is slightly soluble in water. Unlike the phenothiazines it does not contain sulfur or nitrogen in the tricyclic ring system.

Indications: Symptomatic relief of perennial and seasonal allergic rhinitis; vasomotor rhinitis; allergic conjunctivitis due to inhalant allergens and foods; mild, uncomplicated allergic skin manifestations of urticaria and angioedema; amelioriation of allergic reactions to blood or plasma in patients with a known history of such reactions; dermographism; as therapy for anaphylactic reactions adjunctive to epinephrine and other standard measures after the acute manifestations have been controlled. It may be useful in mild, local allergic reactions to insect bites; physical allergy; minor drug and serum reactions characterized by pruritus. It may also be useful in itching caused by allergic dermatoses including contact dermatitis or that due to chicken pox.

Contraindications: Not to be used in patients with angle-closure glaucoma and in those predisposed to urinary retention, stenosing peptic ulcer, symptomatic prostatic hypertrophy, bladder-neck obstruction, or pyloroduodenal obstruction, current use of MAO inhibitors, hypersensitivity to the drug, in elderly, debilitated patients, in newborn and premature infants, nursing mothers, and during an asthmatic attack, or with other lower respiratory symptoms.

Warnings: Since drowsiness, dizziness and hypotension particularly in elderly patients frequently occurs with the use of cyproheptadine, patients should be cautioned against engaging in activities requiring alertness or skill such as driving a car. Cyproheptadine may diminish alertness, or conversely, may cause excitement in children. Use of the drug during pregnancy, or lactation, or in women of childbearing potential requires that the intended benefit be weighed against the possible hazards to the mother and child. Also an inhibition of lactation may be experienced. Overdosage of antihistamines, particularly in infants and children, may produce hallucinations, CNS depression, convulsions and death.

Precautions: Patients using this drug should be cautioned against the ingestion of alcohol and other CNS depressants. Use with caution in patients with bronchial asthma because of a possible drying effect on bronchial secretion, in the presence of increased intraocular pressure, hyperthyroidism, cardiovascular disorders, or hypertension. The occurrence of blood dyscrasias has not, as yet, been reported. The physician should consider carefully the concomitant use of MAO inhibitors with cyproheptadine, since they prolong and intensify the anticholinergic effects of antihistamines.

Adverse Reactions: The most frequently occurring side effects are sedation and sleepiness (often transient); dryness of mouth, nose, and throat; thickening of bronchial secretions, dizziness, epigastric distress, and disturbed coordination. Other adverse reactions that may accompany antihistamine therapy in susceptible patients include fatigue, confusion, restlessness, excitation, nervousness, tremor, irritability, paresthesias, acute labyrinthitis, hysteria, neuritis, convulsions, excessive perspiration, chills, hallucinations, insomnia, euphoria, anorexia, nausea, vomiting, diarrhea, constipation, faintness, hypotension, extrasystoles, tightness of chest and wheezing, urticaria, allergic manifestations of rash and edema, anaphylactic shock, blurred vision, diplopia, vertigo, tinnitus, headache, tachycardia, nasal stuffiness, urinary frequency, difficult urination, urinary retention, early menses, photosensitivity, hemolytic anemia, leukopenia, agranulocytosis, and thrombocytopenia. Overdosage may vary from

CNS depression to stimulation especially in children; also an atropine-like reaction (dry mouth; fixed, dilated pupils; flushing; etc.) as well as gastrointestinal symptoms may occur.

Dosage and Administration: *Orally.* Adults, 4 to 20 mg daily in divided doses. Dosage must be individualized and should not exceed 0.5 mg/kg/day. Children, 0.25 mg/kg daily divided into 3 or 4 doses. The total daily dose should not exceed 16 mg for children 7 to 14 years of age, and 12 mg for children 2 to 6 years of age.

Availability:
PERIACTIN® HYDROCHLORIDE: **(Merck Sharp & Dohme)**
Syrup, 2 mg/5 ml in bottles of 1 pint.
Tablets, 4 mg (white, scored) in bottles of 100.

CYTARABINE

Chemical Name: 1-β-D-arabinofuranosyl cytosine.

Description: Cytarabine, a chemotherapeutic agent markedly cytotoxic to a variety of mammalian cell lines in culture, is a synthetic nucleoside which differs from the normal nucleosides, cytidine and deoxycytidine, in that the sugar moiety is arabinose rather than ribose or deoxyribose.

Detailed in vitro studies indicate that the primary action of cytarabine is inhibition of the synthesis or utilization of deoxycytidine, although inhibition of cytidylic acid kinases and incorporation of the compounds into nucleic acids may also play a role in its cytostatic and cytocidal actions. The drug has also been reported to cause chromosome breakage in human leukocytes, and additional studies using mammalian cell cultures showed that the drug promptly inhibits DNA synthesis. Cytarabine has also been found to be immunosuppressive as demonstrated by inhibition of hemagglutinin synthesis in mice.

The human liver and kidney contain an enzyme which deaminates cytarabine to arabinofuranosyl uracil, an inactive metabolite. Within 12 to 24 hours following intravenous administration, only 5 to 8% of the dose is excreted in the urine unchanged; 90% of the dose is excreted as the deamination product, arabinofuranosyl uracil. Cytarabine appears to be metabolized rapidly, primarily by the liver and, perhaps, by the kidney, and to be excreted chiefly as the deamination product. After the intravenous administration of a single, high dose, blood levels fall to unmeasurable levels within 15 minutes in most patients; some patients have no demonstratable circulating drug as early as 5 minutes after injection.

In animal toxicological studies, the primary toxic effect observed in all species was bone marrow depression with leukopenia. The drug also causes abnormal cerebellar development in the neonatal hamster and is teratogenic to the rat fetus. This latter finding is interesting in view of the low order of toxicity of cytarabine in the rat and the lack of significant systemic antitumor activity in this species.

Indications: Primarily for the induction of remission in acute granulocytic leukemia (adults) and, secondarily, for other acute leukemias (adults and children). It has been noted that the response rates in other forms of acute leukemias (adults and children) have been roughly comparable to those seen in granulocytic leukemia. The drug has been used experimentally in patients with a variety of neoplastic diseases. In general, few with solid tumors have benefited from the drug; occasional tumor responses have been reported in patients with lymphomas and Hodgkin's disease.

Contraindications: As initial therapy in patients with preexisting, drug-induced bone-marrow depression unless, in the opinion of the clinician, such management offers the most optimistic alternative for the patient.

Warnings: Cytarabine is a potent bone-marrow suppressant. Patients taking the drug must be under close medical supervision and, during induction therapy, should have leukocyte and platelet counts performed daily. Facilities should be available for the management of complications of bone-marrow suppression, e.g., infection resulting from granulocytopenia and other impaired body defenses, and hemorrhage secondary to thrombocytopenia. This drug is known to be teratogenic in some animal species. It may be used in women who are or may become pregnant only after due consideration of the potential benefit and potential hazard to mother and child.

Only physicians experienced in cancer chemotherapy should use this drug. For induction therapy, patients should be confined in a hospital with adequate laboratory and supportive resources in order to monitor drug tolerance and protect and maintain a patient compromised by drug toxicity.

Precautions: Therapy should be suspended or modified when drug-induced bone-marrow depression has resulted in a platelet count under 50,000 or a polymorphonuclear granulocyte count under 1000/cu mm. Counts of formed elements in the peripheral blood may continue to fall after the drug is withdrawn and reach lowest values after drug-free intervals of 5 to 7 days. If indicated, therapy may be reinstituted when definite signs of marrow recovery appear (on successive bone-marrow studies). Patients from whom the drug is withheld until "normal" peripheral blood values are attained may escape from drug (cytarabine) control. The problem of nausea and vomiting following the rapid intravenous injection of large doses may be averted by infusing the drug. Because of possible detoxification by the liver, the drug should be used cautiously in those patients with poor liver function. Bone marrow, liver and kidney function should be evaluated periodically in patients receiving this drug. Safe use in infants has not been established. As with other cytotoxic drugs, cytarabine may induce hyperuricemia secondary to rapid lysis of neoplastic cells. The clinician should monitor the blood uric acid level and be prepared to use such supportive and pharmacologic measures as might be necessary to control this problem.

Adverse Reactions: The incidence of reactions in *adults* with leukemia has been reported in the following descending order of frequency: leukopenia, thrombocytopenia, bone-marrow suppression, nausea, megaloblastosis, vomiting, anemia, diarrhea, oral inflammation or ulceration, thrombophlebitis, hepatic dysfunction, fever. The following occurred in less than 2% of patients: renal dysfunction, abdominal pain, anorexia, gastrointestinal hemorrhage, sepsis, cellulitis at injection site, pneumonia, neuritis or neurotoxicity, rash, freckling, esophagitis, cutaneous and mucosal bleeding, chest pain, joint pain, sore throat and reduced reticulocytes. In *children,* reactions occurred in the following descending order of frequency: leukopenia, thrombocytopenia, vomiting, nausea, bone-marrow suppression, oral inflammation or ulceration, anemia, megaloblastosis, bleeding (all sites), diarrhea, hepatic dysfunction, rash and anorexia. The following occurred in less than 2.5% of children: sepsis, esophagitis or esophageal ulceration, cutaneous and mucosal ulceration, pain at injection site, thrombophlebitis, urinary retention, fever, jaundice, dizziness, sore throat, purpura, reduced reticulocytes and alopecia. Although megaloblastosis probably occurs in all patients receiving cytarabine, it is not considered a serious complication.

Dosage and Administration: *Intravenously or subcutaneously; the drug is not active when given orally.* Using the *rapid injection-continuous treatment method,* therapy may be initiated with 2 mg/kg/day for 10 days, then increased to 4 mg/kg/day in the absence of a therapeutic or toxic response. With the *infusion-continuous treatment method,* therapy may be started with 0.5 to 1 mg/kg/day over a period of 1 to 24 hours for 10 days. Results with 1-hour infusions have been satisfactory and these will be most convenient for most patients. In the absence of a therapeutic or toxic response, dosage may be increased to 2 mg/kg/day. With both methods, the blood count should be monitored daily. *Maintenance therapy:* All remissions must be maintained with periodic injections. Weekly or semi-weekly subcutaneous injections of 1 mg/kg have been satisfactory for this purpose. For additional dosage information, consult package literature.

Availability:
CYTOSAR® for Injection (freeze-dried) in multiple-dose vials of 100 mg with a 5-ml ampul of diluent and 500 mg with a 10-ml ampul of diluent. When reconstituted, the resulting solution contains 20 and 50 mg/ml of cytarabine respectively. Reconstituted solutions may be stored at room temperature for 7 days. Discard any solution in which a slight haze develops. **(Upjohn)**

DACARBAZINE

Chemical Name: 5-(3, 3-Dimethyl-1-triazeno)-imidazole-4-carboxamide.

Description: An antineoplastic agent dacarbazine is used primarily for the treatment of metastatic malignant melanoma. It occurs as a colorless to an ivory-colored solid that is extremely sensitive to light.

The precise mechanism (or mechanisms) of cytotoxic action has not been defined; however, it has been reported that the pharmacologic effect may be due to: (1) inhibition of DNA synthesis by functioning as a purine analog; (2) by acting as an alkylating agent; or (3) by interacting with SH groups. It has been noted that the volume of distribution of the drug exceeds total body water content, suggesting localization in some body tissue, probably the liver. When administered intravenously, the plasma half-life of dacarbazine has been found to be about 35 minutes, and only 5% of the drug is protein bound. Animal studies have shown that approximately 46% of a radio-labeled dose can be recovered from the urine after 6 hours with about ½ of this amount as unchanged drug and an equal amount as the metabolite (amino imidazole carboxamide). Also, animal studies have shown that the drug can cause carcinogenic and teratogenic effects. Dacarbazine is subject to renal tubular secretion rather than glomerular filtration.

Indications: Treatment of metastatic malignant melanoma. The drug may be used concurrently with other standard modalities of therapy.

Contraindications: Patients with known hypersensitivity to the drug.

Warnings: Dacarbazine is a highly toxic drug and should be used only under constant supervision of a physician experienced in cancer chemotherapy. Since facilities for necessary studies must be available, hospitalization of the patient is necessary. Hemopoietic depression is the most serious toxic effect and involves primarily the leukocytes and platelets, although mild anemia may sometimes occur. Leukopenia and thrombocytopenia may be severe enough to cause death. The possible bone marrow depression requires careful monitoring of white blood cells, red blood cells and platelet levels. Hemopoietic toxicity may warrant temporary suspension or cessation of therapy. This drug should not be administered to pregnant women or to women of childbearing age who might become pregnant, except when the intended benefits to the patient outweigh the possible risk to the fetus.

Precautions: Because of the highly toxic nature of dacarbazine, the physician must weigh carefully the possibility of achieving therapeutic benefit against the risk of developing severe complications. The drug should be administered preferably to patients who are hospitalized and who can be observed carefully and frequently before and after treatment.

Adverse Reactions: Anorexia, nausea, and vomiting occur frequently, and over 90% of the patients are affected with the first few doses. Vomiting lasts from 1 to 12 hours and may be completely, but unpredictably, relieved with phenobarbital and/or prochlorperazine. Uncontrolled nausea and vomiting have rarely required discontinuation of treatment. Infrequently, the drug has caused diarrhea. This may be avoided by restricting the patient's oral intake of food and fluids from 4 to 6 hours prior to drug administration. In some patients, these symptoms usually subside within a day or two. Patients have experienced an influenza-like syndrome, manifested by fever up to 39°C (102.2°F), myalgia, and malaise. These occur usually after the administration of large single doses approximately 7 days after the start of treatment and last from 7 to 21 days, and they may recur with successive treatment. Alopecia, facial flushing, facial paresthesias, and a few cases of significant abnormalities in liver or renal function have also been reported. Extravasation of the drug subcutaneously during the intravenous administration may result in tissue damage and severe pain.

Dosage and Administration: *Intravenously.* The recommended dosage is 2 to 4.5 mg/kg of body weight/day for 10 days; may be repeated every 4 weeks. It has been observed that in some cases the lower dosage was just as effective as the higher dosage. An alternate recommended dosage is 250 mg/square meter of body surface/day for 5 days; may be repeated every 3 weeks. The injection should be prepared by adding Sterile Water for Injection, USP; 9.9 ml to the 100 mg vial and 19.7 ml to the 200 mg vial. The resulting solution contains 10 mg/ml of dacarbazine, and has a pH of about 3 to 4. Injection may be completed in approximately 1 minute. Any solution remaining in the vial may be stored at 4°C for up to 72 hours; if stored at 20°C, the solution is not stable for more than 8 hours.

Availability:

DTIC Injection in vials of 100 and 200 mg in cartons of 12. **(Dome)**

DACTINOMYCIN

Chemical Name: Actinomycin D.

Description: Dactinomycin is an antibiotic obtained as the principal component of the mixture of actinomycins produced by *Streptomyces parvullus.* This organism, unlike other species, yields an essentially pure substance that contains only traces of similar compounds differing in the amino acid content of the peptide side chains. It is available for clinical use as a yellow, lyophilized powder which, in aqueous solution, produces a clear gold color.

Although the actinomycins have demonstrated some antibiotic activity, their toxicity in relation to antibacterial properties is such as to preclude their use in the treatment of gram-positive and gram-negative infections and in some fungi infections. However, because the actinomycins are cytotoxic, they have an antineoplastic effect. This cytotoxic action is the basis for using actinomycins in the palliative treatment of certain types of cancer. Although the precise mechanism of action is not fully understood, available evidence implies that the drug acts primarily by interfering with the normal transcription during DNA and RNA synthesis.

Indications: Recommended only in the treatment of *hospitalized patients* with Wilm's tumor (a malignant tumor of the kidney region with metastases often to the lungs and regional lymph nodes), rhabdomyosarcoma, and carcinoma of the testes and uterus (embryonal, teratocarcinoma, choriocarcinoma). Currently available information is inadequate to justify its use in other types of cancer.

Contraindications: If dactinomycin is given at or about the time of infection with chicken pox, a severe generalized disease, which may result in death, may occur.

Warnings: Dactinomycin is recommended for use in treating only hospitalized patients with Wilm's tumor, rhabdomyosarcoma, and carcinoma of the testes and uterus (embryonal, teratocarcinoma, and choriocarcinoma). All other indications for dactinomycin, such as Ewing's sarcoma, osteogenic sarcoma, lymphomas, malignant melanoma, sarcoma botryoides, neuroblastoma, cancer of the stomach or intestines, breast carcinoma, and cancer of the lung, are as yet experimental.

Precautions: Dactinomycin is a toxic drug and very careful and frequent observation of the patient is essential. Adverse reactions may involve any tissue of the body. The possibility of an anaphylactoid reaction should be considered. A variety of abnormalities of renal, hepatic, and bone marrow function have been reported. It is advisable to determine frequently the function of these organs. Increased incidence of gastrointestinal toxicity and bone marrow suppression has been reported when dactinomycin was administered with radiation therapy. Since teratogenic effects have been observed in the offspring of animals, considerable precautions in its use during pregnancy is advised. The use of this drug in infants under 6 months of age is not recommended.

Adverse Reactions: Toxic effects, except for nausea and vomiting, usually do not become apparent until 2 to 4 days after a course of therapy is discontinued, and may not be maximal before 1 to 2 weeks have elapsed. Deaths have been reported with the use of dactinomycin. However, adverse reactions are usually reversible on discontinuance of therapy. Those reported include: *Miscellaneous*—malaise, fatigue, lethargy, fever, myalgia, proctitis, and hypocalcemia. *Oral*—cheilitis, dysphagia, esophagitis, ulcerative stomatitis, and pharyngitis. *Gastrointestinal*—anorexia, nausea, vomiting, abdominal pain, diarrhea, and gastrointestinal ulceration. Nausea and vomiting, which occur during the first few hours after initiation of therapy, may be alleviated by giving antiemetics. *Hematologic*—anemia, even to the point of aplastic anemia, agranulocytosis, leukopenia, thrombocytopenia, pancytopenia, and reticulopenia. White cell counts should be performed *daily* and platelet counts every 3 days to detect severe hemopoietic depression. If either count markedly decreases, the drug should be withheld until recovery occurs. *Dermatologic*—alopecia, skin eruptions, acne, flare-up of erythema or increased pigmentation of previously irradiated skin. *Soft tissues*—dactinomycin is extremely corrosive. If extravasation occurs during intravenous use, severe damage to soft tissues will occur. In at least one instance this has led to contracture of the arms.

Dosage and Administration: *Intravenously.* Adults, usually 0.5 mg daily for a maximum of 5 days. Children, a dose of 15 mcg/kg may be given daily for 5 days. An alternative dosage schedule is a total of 2.4 mg/sq meter of body surface given over a period of 1 week. In both adults and in children, a second course may be given after at least 2 weeks have elapsed, provided all evidence of toxicity has disappeared. The dosage necessarily will vary depending upon the tolerance of the patient, the size and location of the neoplasm, and the use of other forms of therapy. It may be necessary to reduce the usual dosage when other chemotherapy or x-ray therapy is used concomitantly or has been employed previously. To avoid extravasation, the drug should be injected into the tubing of a running intravenous infusion; any unused portion must be discarded. If the drug is given directly into the vein without the use of an infusion, the two-needle technique should be employed. This involves using one sterile needle to withdraw [after reconstitution] the calculated dose from the vial, and a second sterile needle for direct injection into the vein. **Note:** The powder is reconstituted by adding 1.1 ml of Sterile Water for Injection only. Other diluents may cause precipitation.

Availability:
COSMEGEN® Injection Lyovac® (Lyophilized) in vials containing dactinomycin, 0.5 mg and mannitol, 20 mg. **(Merck Sharp & Dohme)**

DAINITE

Description: Both formulations have been designed specifically to provide extensive therapeutic action in the asthmatic patient without the high frequency of gastric intolerance usually associated with aminophylline. Each tablet contains:

	Dainite	*Dainite-KI*
Aminophylline	200 mg	200 mg
Pentobarbital sodium	16 mg	——
Ephedrine hydrochloride	16 mg	16 mg
Aluminum hydroxide gel, dried	160 mg	160 mg
Benzocaine	16 mg	16 mg
Phenobarbital	——	16 mg
Potassium iodide	——	325 mg

Indications: Symptomatic relief of mild and severe bronchial asthma, for the bronchospastic type of pulmonary emphysema, and prophylactically to prevent or lessen asthmatic attacks. The Dainite-KI formulation is recommended, in addition, in chronic asthma and in those patients who consistently develop a thick, viscous, tenacious sputum and thus have difficulty in expectorating accumulated secretions in the bronchial tree during or following an asthmatic attack.

Contraindications: Neither preparation should be given to patients sensitive to aminophylline or sympathomimetic drugs. Dainite-KI is specifically contraindicated in those patients who have had a severe reaction or are sensitive to or have an idiosyncrasy to potassium iodide.

Warnings: Pentobarbital and phenobarbital may be habit-forming.

Precautions: Both formulations should be used with caution in patients with cardiovascular disease and hypertension.

Adverse Reactions: Nausea, vomiting and gastric irritation occur occasionally. Potassium iodide may cause acne, rhinorrhea, a metallic taste and parotitis.

Dosage and Administration: *Orally. Dainite*—1 tablet upon arising and 1 at 4 PM. Dosage may be increased, as indicated, to 1 or 2 tablets before meals. *Dainite-KI*—1 tablet upon arising, 1 at 4 PM and 1 or 2 tablets at bedtime.

Availability:
DAINITE® Tablets (pink) in bottles of 100. **(Mallinckrodt)**
DAINITE-KI Tablets (mottled, tri-colored) in bottles of 100 and 500. **(Mallinckrodt)**

DANAZOL

Chemical Name: 17α-pregna-2, 4-dien 20-yno[2,3-*d*]-isoxazol-17-ol.

Description: The antigonadotropic properties of danazol, an isoxazol derivative of 17alpha-ethinyl testosterone, are effective in managing most cases of endometriosis. It has been established that the drug is neither estrogenic nor progestational, but that it inhibits the release of gonadotropins (FSH and LH) from the pituitary gland. This action suppresses ovarian function resulting in anovulation with associated amenorrhea. In addition, the normal and ectopic endometrial tissue is altered so that it becomes inactive and atrophic. Complete resolution of endometrial lesions has been reported to occur in the majority of patients. Generally, the pituitary-suppressive action of the drug is reversible, since ovulation and cyclic bleeding usually return within 2 to 3 months after therapy has been discontinued. Mild, dose-related androgenic activity has also been reported with danazol.

Indications: Treatment of endometriosis. It is indicated for use only in those patients who cannot tolerate other drug therapy, in whom other effective drugs are contraindicated, or who fail to respond to other effective drug therapy when given in adequate doses. It is not indicated for use in patients in whom surgery alone is considered the treatment of choice.

Contraindications: Undiagnosed abnormal genital bleeding, markedly impaired hepatic, renal, or cardiac function, and in mothers who are breast feeding their babies.

Warnings: While no embryotoxic or teratogenic effects attributable to danazol have been observed during reproduction studies in animals, safe use in pregnant patients has not been established. If a patient becomes pregnant during treatment, the drug should be withdrawn. Since some androgenic effects may not be reversible, even after discontinuation of therapy, patients should be observed carefully for signs of virilization or other unfavorable response.

Precautions: Because the drug may cause some degree of fluid retention, conditions that might be influenced by this factor, such as epilepsy, migraine, cardiac or renal dysfunction, require careful observation. Although there have been no embryotoxic or teratogenic effects attributable to danazol thus far, safe use during pregnancy has not been confirmed.

Adverse Reactions: The androgenic effects reported include acne, edema, mild hirsutism, decrease in breast size, deepening of the voice, oiliness of the skin or hair, weight gain, and rarely clitoral hypertrophy. The hypoestrogenic effects reported include flushing, sweating, vaginitis including itching, dryness, and burning, and vaginal bleeding, nervousness, and emotional instability. Although the following adverse reactions have also been reported, a causal relationship to danazol has been neither confirmed nor disproved. These include *allergic*—skin rashes, and rarely, nasal congestion; *CNS*—dizziness, headache, sleep disorders, fatigue, tremor, and rarely, paresthesia in the extremities, visual disturbances, changes in appetite, and chills; *gastrointestinal*—gastroenteritis, and rarely, nausea, vomiting, and constipation; *musculoskeletal*—muscle cramps or spasms, and pain in the back, neck, or legs; *genitourinary*—rarely, hematuria; *other*—loss of hair, changes in libido, elevation in blood pressure, and rarely, pelvic pain.

Dosage and Administration: *Orally.* The recommended dosage is 400 mg twice daily (without interruption) for 3 to 6 months; however, some patients may require 9 months of therapy. It is advised to initiate therapy during menstruation to rule out any possibility of pregnancy thus avoiding the institution of appropriate tests. If, after termination of therapy, symptoms recur, treatment can be reinstituted.

Availability:
DANOCRINE® Capsules (orange), 200 mg in bottles of 100. **(Winthrop)**

DANTROLENE SODIUM

Chemical Name: 1-{[5-(*p*-nitrophenyl) furfurylidene] amino} hydantoin sodium hydrate.

Description: Dantrolene is a skeletal muscle relaxant agent that produces an effect directly on the muscle itself. It occurs as an orange powder that is slightly soluble in water, and only slightly more soluble in alkaline solutions. The anhydrous salt has a molecular weight of 336, and the hydrated salt, which contains about 15% water, has a molecular weight of 399.

In isolated nerve-muscle preparations, the drug has been shown to produce relaxation of the contractile state of skeletal muscle, probably due to its effect on the sarcoplasmic reticulum.

There is no demonstrable effect on peripheral nerve conduction or neuromuscular transmission. Clinical studies have found that absorption of the drug following oral administration is incomplete and slow but consistent, and that the duration and intensity of skeletal muscle relaxation is related to dosage and blood levels. The mean biologic half-life in adults is 8.7 hours following a 100-mg dose. Since dantrolene is probably metabolized in the liver, enhancement of its metabolism by other drugs is therefore possible, although it has been reported that neither phenobarbital nor diazepam appears to affect its metabolism.

Long-term studies with animals receiving large doses of the drug demonstrated a depression of growth or weight, and signs of liver and kidney toxicity. These effects were reversible upon cessation of treatment. Other studies with Sprague-Dawley female rats given 15, 30 and 60 mg/kg/day showed an increased incidence of benign and malignant tumors of the liver, and at the highest dosage an increase of lymphangiomas and angiocarcinomas of the liver. Therefore, dantrolene's possible carcinogenic potential cannot be fully discounted.

Indications: Symptomatic treatment of skeletal muscle spasm resulting from spinal cord injury, stroke, cerebral palsy, or multiple sclerosis. It is not indicated in the treatment of those resulting from rheumatic disorders. It is usually of help in patients with reversible spasticity where relief will aid in restoring residual function. Treatment for prolonged periods may be justified if the drug produces a significant reduction in painful and/or disabling spasticity, markedly reduces the intensity and/or degree of nursing care required, or relieves the patient of the annoying manifestations of muscle spasm.

Contraindications: In patients in whom the spastic state is utilized to sustain an upright posture and balance in locomotion, or to obtain or maintain increased function, and in the presence of acute hepatitis or active cirrhosis.

Warnings: Because of the drug's potential hepatotoxic effect, it should not be used in conditions other than those recommended. When administered for 60 days or longer, fatal hepatitis has been reported in 0.1 to 0.2% of patients and symptomatic hepatitis has been observed in approximately 0.35 to 0.5% of patients. In addition, liver dysfunction, as evidenced by abnormalities in the blood chemistry, has been observed in about 0.7 to 1% of all patients who have taken the drug for varying periods of time. The risk of hepatic injury appears to be greater in female patients, and in all patients over 35 years of age. No serious hepatic injury has been reported in patients receiving the drug for less than 60 days, although elevations of liver enzymes have occurred. Dantrolene should be used only in conjunction with appropriate monitoring of hepatic function including frequent determinations of SGOT and SGPT. If no observable benefit is derived from the administration of the drug after a total of 45 days, therapy should be discontinued. Safe use during pregnancy has not been proven; therefore, it should not be given to women who are or who may become pregnant unless the expected benefits have been weighed against the possible hazards to the mother and child. It is not recommended for use in nursing mothers or in children under 5 years of age. Because possible adverse effects may not become apparent until after many years, a benefit-risk consideration is particularly important in pediatric patients. The concomitant use of tranquilizers, or estrogens (especially in women over 35 years of age) requires special care.

Precautions: Care should be exercised when administering this drug to patients with impaired pulmonary function, particularly those with obstructive pulmonary disease, and in those with severely impaired cardiac function due to myocardial disease. Patients with preexisting liver disease require special care since a few cases of hepatitis (including fatalities) have been reported. Because CNS depression may occur, patients should be advised against engaging in activities requiring alertness or skill. Also, they should be told to refrain from exposing themselves to sunlight as a drug-induced photosensitivity reaction may occur.

Adverse Reactions: The most frequently encountered unfavorable effects of dantrolene have been drowsiness, dizziness, weakness, general malaise, fatigue, and diarrhea. The CNS reactions usually occur early in treatment and can often be prevented by initiating therapy with a low dose, then proceeding with gradual increments until an optimal regimen is established. Diarrhea may be severe and may necessitate withdrawal of the drug. If diarrhea recurs upon readministration of therapy, the drug should be withdrawn permanently. Alterations of liver function studies attributable to dantrolene have been noted in a few patients. Other complications reported include constipation, gastrointestinal bleeding, anorexia, difficulty in swallowing, gastric irritation, abdominal cramps; speech disturbance, seizure, headache, lightheadedness, visual disturbance, diplopia, alteration of taste, insomnia; tachycardia, erratic blood pressure, phlebitis; mental depression, mental confusion, increased nervousness; increased urinary frequency, crystalluria, difficult erection, urinary incontinence and/or nocturia, difficult urination and/or urinary retention; abnormal hair growth, acne-like rash, pruritus, urticaria, eczematoid eruption, sweating; myalgia, backache; feeling of suffocation; excessive tearing; and chills and fever.

Dosage and Administration: *Orally.* It is important that the dosage be titrated and individualized for maximal effect. The lowest dose compatible with optimal therapeutic response is recommended. *For adults:* Initially, 25 mg once daily, then 2, 3 or 4 times daily, followed by increments of 25 mg up to as high as 100 mg 2, 3 or 4 times daily if necessary. Only occasionally will doses greater than 100 mg 4 times daily be required, and in such cases, the dosage should gradually be increased to 200 mg 4 times daily. *For children:* Initially, 1 mg/kg of body weight once daily, then 2, 3 or 4 times daily, followed by increments of 0.5 mg/kg up to as high as 3 mg/kg 2, 3 or 4 times daily if required. Dosages greater than 100 mg 4 times daily should not be given to children. *Oral Suspension:* For children weighing 9 to 13 kg, the suggested daily dosage is 2.5 ml initially followed by increments up to a maximum of 30 ml; 14 to 20 kg, 5 ml initially followed by increments up to a maximum of 40 ml; 21 to 27 kg, 7.5 ml initially followed by increments up to a maximum of 60 ml. The total daily dose should be given in 2, 3, or 4 evenly divided doses.

Availability:
DANTRIUM®: **(Norwich-Eaton)**
Capsules, 25 mg in bottles of 50 and 500 and in unit-dose cartons of 100; 50 and 75 mg in bottles of 100; 100 mg in bottles of 50 and in unit-dose cartons of 100.
Oral Suspension, 5 mg/ml in bottles of 118 and 470 ml.

DAPSONE

Chemical Name: Diaminodiphenylsulfone.

Description: The sulfone, dapsone, occurs as a white, odorless, crystalline powder very slightly soluble in water and soluble in alcohol, methanol, acetone, and dilute hydrochloric acid. The sulfones are bacteriostatic, and although the nature of their action has not been confirmed, they probably work in a manner similar to that of the sulfonamides, since both exhibit about the same range of antibacterial activity and both are antagonized by paraaminobenzoic acid.

Following oral administration, the drug is rapidly and almost completely absorbed from the gastrointestinal tract and reaches peak concentrations in 4 to 8 hours. Daily administration for at least 8 days is necessary to achieve a plateau level, ranging from 0.5 to 0.7 mg% with doses of 50 mg daily to 0.7 to 0.9 mg% with doses of 100 mg daily. About 85% of the daily dosage is recoverable from the urine, mainly in the form of a water-soluble metabolite. Since excretion of the drug is rather slow, a constant blood level can be maintained with relatively low doses.

Indications: The treatment of all forms of leprosy.

Contraindications: Hypersensitivity to dapsone or its derivatives; advanced renal amyloidosis.

Warnings: Severe anemia should be treated prior to initiation of therapy. In the occasional case of severe anemia developing, it may be necessary to temporarily discontinue administration of the drug, with resumption at a lower dosage level when the anemia is under control. The drug should be withdrawn immediately at the very first sign of a hypersensitive reaction, and appropriate measures instituted. Since safe use during pregnancy has not been established, all due considerations should be observed when given to pregnant patients.

Precautions: As with any sulfone preparation, periodic hemograms are advised during the course of treatment with this drug. The hemolytic effect may be exaggerated in patients deficient in the enzyme glucose-6-phosphate dehydrogenase. When complications such as a lepra reaction (e.g., erythema nodosum leprosum) develop, treatment should be suspended, and may be resumed at smaller doses 1 or 2 weeks after all signs of the reaction have subsided. It may not be prudent to increase the dosage beyond the level at which the reaction appeared. Patients with lepromatous leprosy may be extremely sensitive to dapsone; therefore, attempts should be made to build up tolerance by starting therapy with minute doses before employing the full therapeutic regimen. Liver function tests such as the determination of urine bilirubin and serum transaminase (SGOT) are advisable in patients complaining of loss of appetite, nausea and vomiting.

Adverse Reactions: Shortly after initiation of therapy, transient cyanosis and pallor may occur. Anorexia, nausea, vomiting, headache, giddiness and tachycardia are uncommon provided dosage is induced gradually. Psychosis has been reported, but is not likely with the lower dosage schedules recommended. Anemia, methemoglobinemia, rarely agranulocytosis and leukopenia; drug fever with general dermatitis; hepatitis; inflammation (with or without allergic manifestations); lymphadenitis; peripheral motor neuropathy (rare) etc., and febrile reactions usually are manifestations of excessive dosage and can be reversed by reducing the dosage or withdrawing the drug temporarily. See monograph on Sulfoxone Sodium for a full spectrum of possible adverse reactions.

Dosage and Administration: *Orally.* Treatment should be initiated at a low dosage level with gradual increments, depending upon the response of the patient, until an optimal level is reached. *For lepromatous leprosy, a spaced regimen* (twice-weekly dosage schedule) is recommended. The initial dose is 25 mg and is increased every 4th week in increments of 25 mg (1st to 4th, 25 mg; 5th to 8th, 50 mg; 9th to 12th, 75 mg; 13th to 16th, 100 mg), followed by 100 mg 3 times weekly for the next 4 weeks (17th to 20th), then 100 mg 4 times weekly from the 21st to 24th week. *For uncomplicated tuberculoid and dimorphous leprosy,* a similar dosage regimen as recommended for lepromatous leprosy, however, the maximal dosage should not exceed 200 mg weekly in tuberculoid leprosy, and 300 mg weekly in dimorphous leprosy. Children's dosage should be reduced from 1/4 to 1/2 the adult dosage. *Daily regimen,* a dose of 10 to 15 mg for 6 days a week may be given. The increase in dose should be gradual, and the maximum should be reached in about 4 to 6 months. The total weekly dosage for each regimen should be the same.

Availability:
AVLOSULFON® Tablets, 25 and 100 mg (scored) in bottles of 100. **(Ayerst)**

DEANOL ACETAMIDOBENZOATE

Chemical Name: *p*-Acetamidobenzoic acid compound with 2-(dimethylamino)ethanol.

Description: Deanol acetamidobenzoate, the *p*-acetamidobenzoic acid salt of 2-(dimethylamino)ethanol, is a tertiary amine which differs structurally from the quaternary amine, choline, only in that a methyl group is absent. It occurs as a white to off-white, crystalline powder very soluble in water and sparingly soluble in alcohol.

The concept that deanol is a precursor of acetylcholine which affects the CNS is supported by evidence derived from biochemical and pharmacologic studies. Studies with carbon 14-labelled deanol indicate that it crosses the blood-brain barrier and probably is converted intracellularly to acetylcholine. The drug does not depress the appetite or cause jitteriness, as does amphetamine, and also does not affect the BMR (basal metabolic rate), blood pressure or pulse rate. Deanol is not an MAO (monoamine oxidase) inhibitor. Toxicity is relatively low.

Indications: (1) Learning problems: learning less than that usually associated with apparent level of intelligence, reading difficulties and shortened attention span; (2) behavior problems: hyperkinetic behavior problem syndrome characterized by distractibility, motor disinhibition, dissociation and perserveration; and (3) or, as more frequently encountered, hyperkinetic behavior and learning disorders incorporating varying combinations of both of the above: underachievers, reading and speech difficulties, impaired motor coordination and hyperactive, impulsive, compulsive behavior, often described as asocial, antisocial, delinquent, stimulus-governed. Clinical studies have not been adequate to confirm beneficial effects in these conditions.

Contraindications: Grand mal epilepsy and mixed epilepsy with a grand mal component are relative contraindications; absolute contraindications are not known.

Adverse Reactions: Mild overstimulation; dull occipital headache early in therapy; constipation; tenseness in neck, masseter and quadriceps muscles; insomnia; pruritus; transient rash; and rarely, postural hypotension. These usually disappear with continued treatment or reduced dosage.

Dosage and Administration: *Orally.* Initially, 500 mg daily. If satisfactory improvement is perceptible after 3 weeks, most children may be maintained on 250 to 500 mg daily. The maintenance dosage should be adjusted to the patient's needs.

Availability:
DEANER® Tablets, 25 mg in bottles of 100; 100 and 250 mg in bottles of 50. **(Riker)**

DECAMETHONIUM BROMIDE

Chemical Name: Decamethylenebis[trimethylammonium bromide].

Description: Decamethonium bromide is a potent, synthetic, relatively short-acting skeletal muscle relaxant. It occurs as a white, crystalline powder freely soluble in water and in alcohol. It is miscible in any proportion and compatible with solutions of thiopental sodium. It exerts the same mode of action as does succinylcholine; however, it is not hydrolyzed by plasma cholinesterase, is free from histamine-like effects, exerts no significant effect on the myocardium, and is completely compatible with procaine and pentothal sodium in customary dilutions.

The mechanism by which it acts is similar to that of acetylcholine; it depolarizes nerve impulses of the motor end plate at the myoneural junction resulting in neuromuscular blockade. On a weight basis, 3 mg of the drug relaxes skeletal muscle to about the same extent as that produced by 15 mg of tubocurarine chloride. However, muscle relaxation is more prompt and of shorter duration than that produced by tubocurarine but of longer duration than that produced by succinylcholine. Following intravenous administration of 3 mg, the drug produces acceptable relaxation for 4 to 8 minutes, muscular activity begins to return in 8 to 10 minutes and reverts to normal in about 20 minutes. The drug is excreted in the urine, unchanged, and in almost the same amount as that administered.

Indications: As an adjunct to general anesthesia to produce skeletal muscle relaxation and minimize the amount of anesthetic required. Also as an adjunct in electroconvulsive therapy thus reducing the severity of convulsions and minimizing the danger of trauma. It has also been used in conjunction with thiopental sodium to facilitate endotracheal intubation.

Contraindications: In patients with hypersensitivity to the drug or to bromides.

Warnings: Decamethonium bromide is a potent drug which may cause respiratory depression. For this reason, the drug should be used only by those experienced in the technique of artificial respiration and the administration of oxygen under positive pressure. Facilities for these procedures should be immediately available at all times. Some authorities recommend endotracheal intubation routinely when administering drugs of this type. Anticholinesterases such as neostigmine are not effective antidotes or inhibitors, and artificial respiration must be relied on in all cases of respiratory depression. As with any drug its use in pregnant patients, particularly during the first trimester, relies on the expected results versus the potential hazards to the fetus. If other skeletal muscle relaxants are to be used during the same procedure, the possibility of a synergistic or antagonistic effect should be considered. The action of this drug may be enhanced by certain antibiotics. It should be used only after becoming thoroughly familiar with the precautions, indications and dosage. The physician is urged to read carefully the package literature.

Precautions: Special care must be exercised when using the drug in very young or very old patients, and in patients undergoing operation in the Trendelenburg or lithotomy position, in those with impaired renal function (delayed excretion may markedly sustain muscular paralysis), severe burns, and in recently digitalized patients, or patients who may be overdigitalized as serious cardiac arrhythmias or cardiac arrest may occur. Utmost caution is advised in patients with fractures or neuromuscular disorders as the muscle fasciculations may invoke additional trauma.

Adverse Reactions: Bradycardia, tachycardia, hypertension, hypotension, arrhythmias, cardiac arrest, respiratory depression, apnea, hyperthermia, postoperative muscle pain, and excessive salivation have been reported. Intense and continued muscle relaxation may occur, and may cause prolonged respiratory depression or apnea. These are usually the result of the drug's extended pharmacological actions. Should apnea occur, artificial respiration and the administration of oxygen are essential in order to prevent hypoxia and hypercapnia. If the primary depolarizing block has become a nondepolarizing block, edrophonium or neostigmine, preceded by atropine, may be used as adjunctive treatment aids.

Dosage and Administration: *Intravenously.* The usual initial dose is 2 to 2.5 mg administered at a rate of 1 mg/min, but may vary from 0.5 to 3 mg depending on the response and the degree of muscle relaxation desired. Additional doses of 0.5 to 1 mg may be given at intervals of 10 to 30 minutes, as required. Full relaxing doses of 2 to 2.5 mg may be given 30 to 40 minutes later without danger of cumulative effect.

Availability:
SYNCURINE® Injection, 1 mg/ml in multiple-dose vials of 10 ml. **(Burroughs Wellcome)**

DEFEROXAMINE MESYLATE

Chemical Name: *N*-{5-[3-[(5-Aminopentyl)hydroxycarbamoyl]propionamido]pentyl}-3-[[5-(*N*-hydroxyacetamido)pentyl]carbamoyl]propionohydroxamic acid.

Description: Deferoxamine is a chelating agent with a particular affinity for iron. It chelates iron by binding ferric ions to the 3 hydroxamic groups of the molecule to form ferrioxamine, a stable chelate which prevents the iron from entering into further chemical reactions. This chelate is readily soluble in water and passes easily through the kidney, giving the urine a characteristic reddish color. Theoretically, 100 parts by weight of deferoxamine mesylate are capable of binding about 8.5 parts by weight of ferric iron. It also promotes iron excretion in patients who have secondary iron overload from multiple transfusions, such as occur in the treatment of Cooley's anemia and other chronic anemias. One controlled study has found that long-term therapy with deferoxamine slows accumulation of hepatic iron and retards or eliminates progression of hepatic fibrosis. Clinical and animal studies thus far have shown that the drug does not cause any demonstrable increase in the excretion of electrolytes and trace metals.

Indications: To facilitate the removal of iron in the treatment of acute iron intoxication, and for the management of chronic iron overload. It is not indicated for the treatment of primary hemochromatosis (phlebotomy is the method of choice). The drug is an adjunct to, not a substitute for, standard measures generally used in treating acute iron intoxication which may include induction of emesis with syrup of ipecac; gastric lavage; suction and maintenance of a clear airway; control of shock with intravenous fluids, blood, oxygen and vasopressors; correction of acidosis.

Contraindications: Since the drug and the chelate which it forms with iron are excreted primarily by the kidney, the drug is contraindicated in patients with severe renal disease or anuria.

Warnings: Studies with dogs have revealed that long-term administration of deferoxamine mesylate produces cataracts. Rarely have cataracts been reported in 3 patients who were on prolonged therapy. However, slit lamp examinations performed in some patients treated with this agent for acute iron intoxication did not reveal any cataracts. Since skeletal anomalies were noted in the fetuses of 2 animal species at doses just above those recommended for clinical use, the drug should not be administered to women of childbearing potential, particularly during early pregnancy, except when in the judgment of the physician the potential benefits outweigh the possible hazards to the mother and fetus.

Precautions: The drug should be given intramuscularly or by *slow* intravenous infusion to avoid such reactions as flushed skin, urticaria, hypotension and shock. Since iron mobilization by this drug is relatively poor in patients under 3 years of age, it should therefore be withheld in such patients unless significant iron mobilization (e.g., 1 mg of iron/day or more) can be demonstrated.

Adverse Reactions: Occasionally, pain and induration at the injection site. Side effects reported in patients treated for acute iron intoxication include generalized erythema, urticaria and hypotension, which occurred with rapid IV injection. Adverse effects reported in patients receiving long-term therapy for chronic iron storage diseases include allergic-type reactions (cutaneous wheal formation, generalized pruritus, rash, anaphylactic reaction), blurred vision, dysuria, abdominal discomfort, diarrhea, leg cramps, fever and tachycardia. These reactions may also occur in an occasional patient treated for acute iron intoxication.

Dosage and Administration: Preferably *intramuscularly,* especially in patients in shock. Initially, 1 gm followed by 0.5 gm every 4 hours for 2 doses. Subsequent doses of 0.5 gm may be given every 4 to 12 hours, depending upon clinical response. Dosage should not exceed 6 gm in 24 hours. *Intravenous* administration should be reserved for those patients who are in a state of cardiovascular collapse and given *only by slow infusion* at a rate not exceeding 15 mg/kg/hour. As soon as the clinical condition permits, IV administration should be discontinued and the drug given intramuscularly. Simultaneous IM and IV should be avoided. *For chronic iron overload,* 0.5 to 1 gm daily administered intramuscularly. In addition, 2 gm should be administered intravenously (not to exceed 15 mg/kg/hour) with, but separate from, each unit of blood transfused.

Availability:
DESFERAL® Parenteral (lyophilized) in ampuls of 500 mg in cartons of 4. **(Ciba)**

DEHYDROCHOLIC ACID

Chemical Name: 3,7,12-Trioxo-5β-cholanic acid.

Description: Unlike the naturally occurring salts of cholic acid present in ox bile extract, dehydrocholic acid is an unconjugated, oxidized acid made synthetically by oxidizing the cholanic acids (chiefly cholic acid) found in natural bile. It occurs as a white, fluffy, odorless powder, having a bitter taste, and is practically insoluble in water and slightly soluble in ether and in alcohol.

Dehydrocholic acid and its sodium salt are capable of increasing the volume of bile of relatively high water content and low viscosity. However, it probably is much less effective than natural bile salts (glycocholates and taurocholates) in lowering surface tension to promote the absorption of fat and fat-soluble vitamins. Following administration, unconjugated ketocholanic preparations, such as dehydrocholic acid, leave the absolute amount of solid bile constituents unchanged or actually somewhat decreased without evidence of suppressing hepatic function.

Indications: For temporary relief of constipation. Also, as an adjunct, primarily for its "flushing" action, in the management of the following conditions involving the biliary tract: recent surgery of the biliary tract, recurring biliary calculi or strictures, recurring noncalculous cholangitis, biliary dyskinesia, chronic partial obstruction of the common bile duct, and sclerosing choledochitis. Prophylactically, the drug has been used in patients following surgery on the biliary tract to prevent accumulation of debris and possibly bacteria in the common duct and/or drainage tube, and with chronic partial obstruction of the common bile duct. The addition of digestants are recommended for the symptomatic relief of digestive disorders associated with enzyme deficiency. The sodium salt is used intravenously as a diagnostic agent to determine arm-to-tongue circulation time [of blood].

Contraindications: In cholelithiasis, jaundice, hepatic insufficiency (viral hepatitis, suppurative cholangitis and advanced cirrhosis), or in complete obstruction of hepatic or common bile ducts, gastrointestinal or genitourinary tract due to any cause. It should not be used as a diuretic or as an adjunct to diuretics.

Precautions: Dehydrocholic acid increases the flow and volume of bile by hydrocholeretic action. If promotion of true bile flow is desired, a cholagogue should be used. Since evidence is lacking that bile acids improve liver function or accelerate the clearance rate in jaundice, the drug should not be used for these purposes. Cautious use is recommended in patients with prostatic hypertrophy, acute hepatitis or acute yellow atrophy of the liver, partial obstruction of the gastrointestinal or genitourinary tract, in children under 6 years of age, and in elderly patients. Intravenously, the drug may produce allergic reactions in sensitive individuals and, therefore, should not be used in asthmatics or those with a history of allergy without preliminary skin testing.

Adverse Reactions: Dehydrocholic acid reportedly has not caused any toxic effects when used as recommended.

Dosage and Administration: *Orally,* 1 or 2 tablets 2 to 4 times daily with or after meals. Dosage should be adjusted to suit the needs of the patient, since no predetermined schedule will be equally effective for all patients. In the presence of biliary fistula or in any condition in which the bile is draining away from the intestinal tract, and during prolonged administration, the concomitant administration of bile salts may be indicated in order to assure adequate digestion and absorption of nutrients. *Intravenously for hydrocholeresis,* a 20% solution is used: 5 to 10 ml the first day, and 10 ml on the second and third days. Intravenous therapy should be replaced by oral therapy as soon as possible. For the determination of *arm-to-tongue circulation time,* 3 to 5 ml of a 20% solution is injected rapidly [*intravenously*] into the cubital vein with the patient in the supine position. The end point is reached when the patient senses a bitter taste passing quickly from the base to the tip of the tongue. The normal range, from the beginning of the injection to the first perception of a bitter taste, is 8 to 16 seconds.

Availability:

Dehydrocholic Acid

CHOLAN-DH® Tablets, 250 mg (white, uncoated) in bottles of 100. **(Pennwalt)**

CHOLAN-HMB® Tablets (pink, scored), 250 mg with phenobarbital, 8 mg (**Warning:** may be habit-forming) and homatropine methylbromide, 2.5 mg in bottles of 100 and 1000. **(Pennwalt)**

CHOLAN® V Tablets, 250 mg with homatropine methylbromide, 5 mg in bottles of 100. **(Pennwalt)**

GASTROENTERASE® Tablets, 50 mg with pepsin (in outer layer), 150 mg; standardized pancreatic enzyme, 100 mg and standardized cellulose (in enteric core), 25 mg in bottles of 100. **(Wallace)**

KETOCHOL® Tablets, 250 mg of ketocholanic acids equivalent to 250 mg of dehydrocholic acid in bottles of 100 and 500. **(Searle)**

NEOCHOLAN® Tablets, 250 mg in bottles of 100. **(Dow)**

Sodium Dehydrocholate

DECHOLIN® SODIUM Injection, 20% in ampuls of 5 ml. **(Dome)**

DEMECARIUM BROMIDE

Chemical Name: (*m*-Hydroxyphenyl)trimethylammonium bromide, decamethylenebis [methylcarbamate].

Description: A quaternary ammonium anticholinesterase drug, it occurs as a slightly hygroscopic, white, crystalline powder freely soluble in water and in alcohol.

Demecarium bromide is a cholinesterase inhibitor with sustained activity, and acts mainly on true (erythrocyte) cholinesterase. Its efficacy and toxicity are comparable to those of similar drugs such as physostigmine, isoflurophate and echothiophate. When applied to the eye demecarium produces an intense miosis and ciliary muscle contraction. These effects are accompanied by increased capillary permeability of the ciliary body and iris, increased permeability of the blood-aqueous barrier, and vasodilation. Myopia may be induced, or if present, may be augmented by the increased refractive power of the lens that results from the accommodative effect of the drug. Because of its potency, prolonged action, and ease of absorption through the conjunctival sac as well as the intact skin, demecarium is capable of producing systemic effects.

Following instillation of the drug in the eye, miosis appears within 1 hour and attains its maximum in about 2 to 4 hours. Reduction of intraocular pressure occurs within a few hours and is often preceded by a slight rise in pressure. In some instances, the concomitant administration of a carbonic anhydrase inhibitor may enhance the effectiveness of demecarium in controlling intraocular pressure. Residual pupillary constriction and decreased intraocular pressure may persist for 1 week or more following a single application.

Indications: Treatment of open-angle glaucoma; conditions obstructing aqueous outflow, such as synechial formation, that are amenable to miotic therapy; following iridectomy, and in the management of accommodative convergent strabismus (accommodative esotropia).

Contraindications: Hypersensitivity to demecarium bromide, active uveal inflammation, and narrow-angle glaucoma.

Warnings: Demecarium should be administered with extreme caution to patients with myasthenia gravis who are receiving systemic anticholinesterase therapy; conversely, the cautious use of systemic anticholinesterase drugs in patients with myasthenia gravis who are receiving demecarium bromide is also advised. The safe use of an anticholinesterase drug during pregnancy has not been established, nor has the absence of adverse effects on the fetus or respiration of the neonate. Therefore, the use of demecarium during pregnancy requires that the potential benefits be weighed against its possible hazards.

Precautions: It is recommended that gonioscopy be performed before initiating therapy with this drug. The intensity and persistence of miosis during treatment with demecarium bromide necessitate that it be used with caution, if at all, in ocular hypertension accompanied by intraocular inflammatory processes. Systemic effects are infrequent when the ophthalmic solution is applied topically by the proper technique and in recommended doses. The use of demecarium should be discontinued if salivation, urinary incontinence, diarrhea, profuse sweating, muscle weakness, respiratory difficulties, shock, or cardiac irregularities occur. Individuals receiving cholinesterase inhibitors who are exposed to organophosphate-type insecticides and pesticides, such as gardeners, organophosphate-manufacturing plant or warehouse workers, farmers, residents of communities which are undergoing insecticide or pesticide spraying or dusting, should be warned of the added systemic effects possible from absorption through the respiratory tract or skin. Wearing of respiratory masks, frequent washing, and clothing changes may be advisable. Anticholinesterase drugs should be used with extreme caution, if at all, in patients with marked vagotonia, bronchial asthma, spastic gastrointestinal disturbances, peptic ulcer, pronounced bradycardia and hypotension, recent myocardial infarction, epilepsy, parkinsonism, and other disorders that may respond adversely to vagotonic effects. Extreme caution should be exercised before intraocular surgery because of the possibility of hyphema. However, despite observance of all precautions and the use of only the recommended dose, there is some evidence that repeated administration may cause depression of the concentration of cholinesterase in the serum and erythrocytes, with resultant systemic effects.

Adverse Reactions: Stinging, burning, lacrimation of the eyes, twitching of eye lid, conjuctival and ciliary redness, browache, headache, induced myopia with visual blurring, and activation of latent iritis or uveitis may occur. Retinal detachment has been reported occasionally. Iris cysts may form, enlarge, and obscure vision (particularly in children), and frequent examination for this condition is advisable. Prolonged use may result in conjunctival thickening and obstruction of nasolacrimal canals. Should systemic effects occur such as salivation, urinary incontinence, nausea, abdominal cramps, vomiting, diarrhea, dyspnea, bradycardia, cardiac irregularities, atropine sulfate in a dose (for adults) of 0.4 to 0.6 mg or more should be given parenterally. A proportionately smaller amount should be given to children. Artificial respiration may be required. A paradoxical increase in intraocular pressure may follow anticholinesterase therapy which may be alleviated by a mydriatic agent.

Dosage and Administration: *By instillation.* Chronic simple glaucoma: Treatment may range from 1 drop of an 0.125% solution twice weekly to 2 drops of an 0.25% solution twice daily depending on response. The drug should be used at the lowest effective concentration and no more frequently than is necessary to control intraocular pressure. Reduction in intraocular pressure occurs in about 12 hours and is usually preceded by a slight rise in pressure. Pupillary constriction and decreased intraocular pressure may persist for a week or more following a single instillation. For glaucoma or strabismus in children, the initial dose is 1 drop. Subsequent dosage is regulated, preferably with the aid of periodic tonometric measurements. Strabismus: In the management of esotropia uncomplicated by amblyopia or anisometropia, the solution may be used in both eyes, but no more than 1 drop at a time every day for 2 to 3 weeks, then 1 drop every other day for 3 to 4 weeks. Further dosage is dependent upon clinical response.

Availability:
HUMORSOL® Ophthalmic Solution, 0.125 and 0.25% in Ocumeter® (plastic-dispenser bottles) of 5 ml. **(Merck Sharp & Dohme)**

DEMECLOCYCLINE HYDROCHLORIDE

Chemical Name: 7-Chloro-4-dimethylamino-1,4,4α,5,5α,6,11,12α-octahydro-3,6,10,12,12α-pentahydroxy-1,11-dioxo-2-naphthacenecarboxamide hydrochloride.

Description: A broad-spectrum antibiotic produced by *Streptomyces aureofaciens,* it differs chemically from chlortetracycline by the absence of a methyl group in the sixth position. It occurs as an odorless, bitter-tasting, yellow, crystalline powder. In vitro the compound has a similar spectrum of activity as the tetracyclines. Tetracyclines are primarily bacteriostatic and are thought to exert their antimicrobial effect by the inhibition of protein synthesis. They are active against a wide range of gram-negative and gram-positive organisms. The drugs of this class have closely similar antimicrobial spectra, and cross-resistance among them is common. They are readily absorbed and are bound to plasma proteins in varying degrees, are concentrated by the liver in the bile and excreted in the urine and feces at high concentrations and in a biologically active form.

Indications: *Demeclocycline hydrochloride* is indicated in infections caused by the following microorganisms: Rickettsiae: (Rocky Mountain spotted fever, typhus fever and the typhus group, Q fever, rickettsialpox, tick fevers.) *Mycoplasma pneumoniae* (PPLO, Eaton agent). Agents of psittacosis and ornithosis. Agents of lymphogranuloma venereum and granuloma inguinale. The spirochetal agent of relapsing fever (*Borrelia recurrentis*). The following gram-negative microorganisms: *Haemophilus ducreyi* (chancroid), *Pasteurella pestis* and *Pasteurella tularensis, Bartonella bacilliformis, Bacteroides* species, *Vibrio comma* and *Vibrio fetus. Brucella* species (in conjunction with streptomycin). Because many strains of microorganisms have been shown to be resistant to tetracyclines, culture and susceptibility testing are recommended.

Demeclocycline is also indicated for treatment of infections caused by the following gram-negative microorganisms, when bacteriologic testing indicates appropriate susceptibility to the drug: *Escherichia coli, Enterobacter aerogenes* (formerly *Aerobacter aerogenes*), *Shigella* species, *Mima* species and *Herellea* species, *Haemophilus influenzae* (respiratory infections), *Klebsiella* species (respiratory and urinary infections).

Demeclocycline is indicated for treatment of infections caused by the following gram-positive microorganisms when bacteriologic testing indicates appropriate susceptibility to the drug: *Streptococcus pyogenes* (For upper respiratory infections due to Group A beta-hemolytic streptococci, penicillin is the usual drug of choice, including prophylaxis of rheumatic fever.) Alpha-hemolytic streptococci (viridans group), Enterococcus group (*Streptococcus faecalis*), *Staphylococcus (Diplococcus) pneumoniae, Staphylococcus aureus,* skin and soft tissue infections. Tetracyclines are not the drugs of choice in the treatment of any type of staphylococcal infection. When penicillin is contraindicated, tetracyclines are alternative drugs in the treatment of infections due to: *Neisseria gonorrhoeae, Treponema pallidum* and *Treponema pertenue* (syphilis and yaws), *Listeria monocytogenes, Clostridium* species, *Bacillus anthracis, Fusobacterium fusiforme* (Vincent's infection), *Actinomyces* species. In acute intestinal amebiasis, the tetracyclines may be a useful adjunct to amebicides.

Demeclocycline hydrochloride is indicated in the treatment of trachoma, although the infectious agent is not always eliminated, as judged by immunofluorescence. Inclusion conjunctivitis may be treated with oral tetracyclines or with a combination of oral and topical agents. Combined with the antifungal antibiotic nystatin for added protection against monilial superinfection.

Contraindications: In patients hypersensitive to tetracyclines.

Warnings: The use of drugs of the tetracycline class during tooth development (last half of pregnancy, infancy and childhood to the age of 8 years) may cause permanent discoloration of the teeth (yellow-gray-brown). This adverse reaction is more common during long-term use of the drugs but has been observed following repeated short-term courses. Enamel hypoplasia has also been reported. Tetracycline drugs, therefore, should not be used in this age group unless other drugs are not likely to be effective or are contraindicated. If renal impairment exists, even usual oral or parenteral doses may lead to excessive systemic accumulation of the drug and possible liver toxicity. Under such conditions, lower than usual total doses are indicated and, if therapy is prolonged, serum level determinations of the drug may be advisable. Phototoxic reactions can occur in individuals taking demeclocycline, and are characterized by severe burns of exposed surfaces resulting from direct exposure of patients to sunlight during therapy with moderate or large doses of demeclocycline. Patients apt to be exposed to direct sunlight or ultraviolet light should be advised that this reaction can occur, and treatment should be discontinued at the first evidence of skin erythema. The antianabolic action of the tetracyclines may cause an increase in BUN. While this is not a problem in those with normal renal function, in patients with significantly impaired function higher serum levels of demeclocycline may lead to azotemia, hyperphosphatemia, and acidosis. Results of animal studies indicate that tetracyclines cross the placenta, are found in fetal tissues and can have toxic effects on the developing fetus (often related to retardation of skeletal development). Evidence of embryotoxicity has also been noted in animals treated early in pregnancy; therefore, due consideration should be given when administering this antibiotic to pregnant patients with regard to the therapeutic benefits to be obtained as against the risk to the developing fetus. All tetracyclines form a stable calcium complex in any bone forming tissue. A decrease in the fibula growth rate has been observed in prematures given oral tetracycline in doses of 25 mg/kg every 6 hours. This reaction was shown to be reversible when the drug was discontinued. Tetracyclines are present in the milk of lactating women who are taking a drug in this class.

Precautions: As with other antibiotic preparations, use of this drug may result in overgrowth of nonsusceptible organisms, including fungi. If superinfection occurs, the antibiotic should be discontinued and appropriate therapy should be instituted. In venereal diseases when coexistent syphilis is suspected, darkfield examination should be done before treatment is started and the blood serology repeated monthly for at least 4 months. Because demeclocycline has been shown to depress plasma prothrombin activity, patients who are on anticoagulant therapy may require downward adjustment of their anticoagulant dosage. In long-term therapy, periodic laboratory evaluation of organ systems, including hematopoietic, renal and hepatic studies should be performed. All infections due to Group A beta-hemolytic streptococci should be treated for at least 10 days. Since bacteriostatic drugs may interfere with the bactericidal action of penicillin, it is advisable to avoid giving demeclocycline in conjunction with penicillin. Following a course of therapy, persistence for several days in both urine and blood of bacterio-suppressive levels of demeclocycline may interfere with culture studies. These levels should not be considered therapeutic.

See monograph on Nystatin for additional information.

Adverse Reactions: *Gastrointestinal:* Anorexia, nausea, vomiting, diarrhea, glossitis, dysphagia, enterocolitis, and inflammatory lesions (with monilial overgrowth) in the anogenital region. These reactions have been caused by both the oral and parenteral administration of tetracyclines. *Skin:* Maculopapular and erythematous rashes. Exfoliative dermatitis has been reported but is uncommon. Photosensitivity is discussed above. (See "Warnings".) *Renal toxicity:* Rise in BUN has been reported and is apparently dose-related. *Hypersensitivity reactions:* Urticaria, angioneurotic edema, anaphylaxis, anaphylactoid purpura, pericarditis and exacerbation of systemic lupus erythematosus. Bulging fontanels have been reported in young infants following full therapeutic dosage. This sign disappeared rapidly when the drug was discontinued. *Blood:* Hemolytic anemia, thrombocytopenia, neutropenia and eosinophilia have been reported. When given over prolonged periods, tetracyclines have been reported to produce a brown-black microscopic discoloration of thyroid glands. No abnormalities of thyroid function studies are known to occur. Those occasionally associated with large doses of nystatin are nausea, vomiting, gastrointestinal distress and diarrhea.

Dosage and Administration: *Orally* in 2 to 4 divided doses. Adults, 600 mg/day. Infants and children, 6 to 12 mg/kg/day. Should not be given with milk formula or calcium containing food and should be administered 1 hour prior to feeding. Therapy should be continued for 24 to 48 hours after fever or other symptoms have subsided.

Availability:

Demeclocycline Hydrochloride

DECLOMYCIN®: **(Lederle)**

Capsules, 150 mg in bottles of 16 and 100 and in unit-dose packages of 100 (10 x 10).
Syrup, 75 mg/5 ml in bottles of 60 ml and 1 pint.
Tablets, 75 mg in bottles of 25; 150 mg in bottles of 16 and 100 and in unit-dose packages of 100 (10 x 10); 300 mg in bottles of 12 and 48 and in unit-dose packages of 100 (10 x 10).

w/Nystatin

DECLOSTATIN®: **(Lederle)**

Capsules, 150 mg with nystatin, 250,000 units in bottles of 16 and 100.
Tablets, 300 mg with nystatin, 500,000 units in bottles of 12 and 48.

DERMA MEDICONE-HC

Description: Each gm contains:

Hydrocortisone acetate	10 mg
Benzocaine	20 mg
Oxyquinoline sulfate	10.5 mg
Ephedrine hydrochloride	1.1 mg
Menthol	4.8 mg
Ichthammol	10 mg
Zinc oxide	136 mg

Suppresses inflammation, pain, swelling, burning and itching.

Indications: Contact dermatitis, eczematoid dermatitis, atopic dermatitis, neurodermatitis, seborrheic dermatitis, allergic dermatitis, rhus dermatitis, and pruritus ani and/or vulvae.

Contraindications: Tuberculosis of the skin.

Precautions: Observe the usual adrenocorticosteroid precautions. Exercise care if patient is taking other corticosteroid preparations, if infection is present, or if a rash or irritation develops. Not to be used in the eyes.

Dosage and Administration: *Topically.* Apply to affected area 2 to 4 times daily.

Availability:

DERMA MEDICONE®-HC Ointment in tubes of 7 and 20 gm. **(Medicone)**

DESERPIDINE

Chemical Name: 11-Desmethoxyreserpine.

Description: Deserpidine is an alkaloid derived from *Rauwolfia canescens* and differs structurally from reserpine in that a methoxy group is absent at position 11. It occurs as a white to light yellow, crystalline powder insoluble in water and very slightly soluble in alcohol. Pharmacologically, the actions of deserpidine are similar to those of reserpine.

Indications: Management of mild essential hypertension and as a supplement to more potent agents in the treatment of more severe hypertension. It has been combined with benzothiadiazines such as hydrochlorothiazide for use in hypertension that is unresponsive to diuretics or rauwolfia alone. It is also indicated for the relief of symptoms in agitated psychosis such as schizophrenia primarily in those individuals who are unable to tolerate phenothiazine derivatives or those who also require antihypertensive medication.

Contraindications: In patients with known hypersensitivity and in those with severe mental depression, suicidal tendencies, active peptic ulcer or ulcerative colitis or who are receiving electroconvulsive therapy. Thiazide diuretics should not be used in patients known to be sensitive to the drug, nor should they be used in patients with severe renal disease (except nephrosis) or complete renal shutdown, severe liver disease and/or impending hepatic coma.

Warnings: Extreme caution should be exercised in treating patients with a history of mental depression. Therapy should be discontinued at the first sign of despondency, early morning insomnia, loss of appetite, impotence, or self-deprecation. Drug-induced depression may persist for several months after drug withdrawal and may be severe enough to result in suicide. The deserpidine-hydrochlorothiazide combination is not indicated for initial therapy of hypertension since this condition requires that the dosage be titrated to the individual patient. Safe use of deserpidine in pregnant or lactating women has not been established, and should therefore be used in pregnant women or women of childbearing potential only when it is deemed essential to the welfare of the patient. Since it crosses the placental barrier and appears in cord blood, increased respiratory secretion, nasal congestion, cyanosis, and anorexia may occur in infants born to mothers treated with this drug.

Precautions: Deserpidine should be used with caution in patients with a history of peptic ulcer, ulcerative colitis, or gallstones because the drug causes a rise in free and total hydrochloric acid and an increase in volume of gastric secretion. If symptoms suggest a recurrence of peptic ulcer, the drug should be withdrawn. Caution is also required when treating hypertensive patients with renal insufficiency since they adjust poorly to lowered levels of blood pressure. Cardiac arrhythmias have developed when rauwolfia preparations were administered together with digitalis or quinidine. Dosage should be reduced or the drug withdrawn at least 2 weeks before elective surgery. Hypotension and bradycardia have been reported in patients receiving anesthesia while taking rauwolfia alkaloids. Those taking anticonvulsant drugs should have the dosage of these drugs adjusted to avoid interaction with rauwolfia. Electroconvulsive therapy within 7 days following administration of deserpidine is hazardous. Preexisting depression should be differentiated from the transient lethargy, physical fatigue, or change in mood that may occur during initial therapy. Patients should be observed for symptoms of depression, particularly in those whose histories are questionable. The action of deserpidine may be potentiated by alcohol, barbiturates or narcotics. For the precautions associated with the thiazide component, see monograph on Hydrochlorothiazide (The Thiazide Diuretics).

Adverse Reactions: Are similar to those of reserpine, but the incidence, particularly lethargy and depression, is lower. The following reactions are usually reversible and disappear when the drug has been discontinued. They include gastric hypersecretion, anorexia, diarrhea, nausea and vomiting; angina-like symptoms, arrhythmias, and bradycardia; drowsiness, depression, nervousness, paradoxical anxiety, nightmares, extrapyramidal tract symptoms, CNS sensitization manifested by dull sensorium and deafness; pruritus, rash, and asthma in susceptible patients; glaucoma, uveitis, optic atrophy, and conjunctival injection; thrombocytopenic purpura; nasal congestion, weight gain, impotence or decreased libido, dysuria, dyspnea, muscular aches, dryness of mouth, dizziness, and headache; rarely, water retention with edema in patients with hypertensive vascular disease. Hypotension, hypothermia, central respiratory depression and bradycardia may develop in cases of severe overdosage. Treatment consists of the careful evacuation of stomach contents followed by the usual procedures for the symptomatic management of CNS-depressant overdosage. Severe hypotension should be treated with a direct-acting vasopressor such as levarterenol. For adverse reactions associated with the thiazide component, see monograph on Hydrochlorothiazide (The Thiazide Diuretics).

Dosage and Administration: *Orally.* For mild hypertension, the usual initial dosage for adults is 0.25 mg 3 or 4 times daily. For maintenance, a single daily dose of 0.25 mg may be adequate for some patients. For mild anxiety, a starting dose of 0.1 mg daily is suggested, increased gradually if needed. For psychiatric disorders, the usual initial dose is 0.5 mg daily. Dosage may then be adjusted from 0.1 to 1 mg according to the patient's response. The usual adult dosage of deserpidine-hydrochlorothiazide ranges from 1 to 2 tablets 3 times daily. The choice of a particular potency ratio depends upon the severity of the hypertension. When indicated, the higher strength may be given initially and the dosage then reduced gradually as the condition becomes stabilized. When other antihypertensive agents are added to the regimen, this should be done gradually. Ganglionic blocking agents should be given at only half the usual dose, since their effect is potentiated by hydrochlorothiazide.

Availability:

Deserpidine **(Abbott)**

HARMONYL® Tablets, 0.1 mg (yellow) in bottles of 100; 0.25 mg (pink, grooved) in bottles of 100 and 1000.

ORETICYL® 25 Tablets, 0.125 mg with hydrochlorothiazide, 25 mg in bottles of 100 and 1000. **(Abbott)**

ORETICYL 50 Tablets, 0.125 mg with hydrochlorothiazide, 50 mg in bottles of 100 and 1000.

ORETICYL FORTE Tablets, 0.25 mg with hydrochlorothiazide, 25 mg in bottles of 100 and 1000.

DESIPRAMINE HYDROCHLORIDE

Chemical Name: 10,11-Dihydro-5-[3-(methylamino)propyl]-5*H*-dibenz[b,f]azepine hydrochloride.

Description: Desipramine hydrochloride is a dibenzazepine derivative representing the desmethyl analog of imipramine hydrochloride and differs from the latter in that it has only 1 methyl group on the side chain nitrogen. It occurs as a white, crystalline powder soluble in water and in alcohol.

An active metabolite of imipramine, desipramine is structurally and pharmacologically similar to the parent compound although it appears to be less potent, it provides a more rapid onset of action. The mechanism by which this drug exerts its antidepressant action is rather vague, but like other tricyclic compounds it does not inhibit MAO activity nor does it act primarily as a CNS stimulant. Since depression is associated with a deficiency or depletion of catecholamines, the mode of action of this drug may be involved in increasing the amount of amine available at the synaptic receptor. It has been shown in experimental animals, however, that the drug exhibits a disruptive action on the electroencephalogram and on operant behavior, an energetic anticonvulsant action, a peripheral atropine-like action, antihistamine and antiserotonin effects, some adrenergic blockade, and a gastric antisecretory effect.

Following oral administration of usual doses, the drug is well absorbed from the gastrointestinal tract, is distributed in lung and brain tissue, and in the liver where it is detoxified and subsequently excreted in the urine as the *N*-demethyl analog and as glucuronides. Full treatment benefit is seldom attained before the end of the second week.

Indications: For relief of depressive symptoms especially those of endogenous origin.

Contraindications: The drug should not be given in conjunction with or within 2 weeks of treatment with a MAO inhibitor. It should not be administered during the acute recovery period following myocardial infarction, or to patients who have shown prior hypersensitivity to the drug. Cross sensitization between this drug and other dibenzazepines is a possibility.

Warnings: Extreme care should be employed when used in patients with cardiovascular disease because of the possibility of conduction defects, arrhythmias, tachycardias, strokes and acute myocardial infarction, in those with a history of urinary retention or glaucoma, or with a history of epilepsy since desipramine has been shown to lower the seizure threshold. Special care is recommended in patients with thyroid disease or those on thyroid medication. This drug should not be given to patients receiving guanethidine or related adrenergic neuron-blocking agents since it has been noted to block their pharmacologic action. Other agents that may potentiate the effects of desipramine include other CNS drugs or alcohol. Patients should be cautioned about the possibility of impaired ability to operate a motor vehicle or other dangerous machinery. Elderly and adolescent patients should receive lower dosages than those usually recommended. Although teratogenic studies in experimental animals have proved negative, the safety of the drug's use in pregnant women or in women of childbearing potential has not been established. Use of the drug in these women, therefore, should be withheld unless the clinical situation justifies the potential risks. Since experience with children is lacking, the drug is not recommended at this time for patients under 12 years of age.

Precautions: Considering the structural similarity, certain precautions associated with its parent compound (imipramine) should be exercised. Therapy with desipramine should not be substituted for hospitalization or restraint if the risk of homicide or suicide is considered grave.

In patients with manic depressive illness, the drug may induce a hypomanic state following the end of the depressive phase, or may exacerbate psychosis in schizophrenic patients. Deliberate ingestion of large doses [suicidal] may prove fatal. Therapy should be discontinued prior to elective surgery since hypertensive episodes have been observed during surgical procedures. Close supervision and careful adjustment of dosage are required when this drug is administered concomitantly with anticholinergic or sympathomimetic drugs. Clinical experience is insufficient to warrant concurrent administration of electroconvulsive therapy and antidepressant drugs. Thus, if such treatment is essential, the possibility of increased risk relative to therapeutic benefit should be carefully considered. Patients should be cautioned that while taking this drug their response to alcoholic beverages may be exaggerated. Desipramine causes both elevation and lowering of blood sugar; therefore diabetic patients may require special consideration. Leukocyte and differential counts should be performed in any patient who develops fever and sore throat during therapy; the drug should be withdrawn if there is evidence of pathological neutrophil depression. In all patients undergoing extended courses of therapy, periodic blood and liver studies for signs of toxicity should supplement careful clinical observations.

Adverse Reactions: Desipramine hydrochloride is well tolerated by most patients and severe complications or adverse reactions are infrequent. Those most often reported following the administration of tricyclic compounds in general cause little discomfort and seldom require discontinuation of the drug. These include the *Nervous system:* Dizziness, weakness, fatigue, drowsiness, insomnia, headache, mydriasis, and disturbed visual accommodation have been reported. In addition, numbness, tingling, ataxia, peripheral neuropathy, seizures, tremor, unsteadiness, tinnitus and paresthesias have been reported. Occasionally, mild extrapyramidal activity, falling and neuromuscular incoordination have been noted. A confusional state (with such symptoms as hallucinations, disorientation, delusions, anxiety, restlessness, agitation, insomnia, nightmares, and hypomania) may be produced, particularly in older patients and at higher dosage and may require discontinuation of the drug. Changes in EEG patterns and exacerbation of psychosis have been observed. Epileptiform seizures may occur. A reduction in dosage may help control some of these adverse reactions. *Gastrointestinal tract:* Anorexia, dryness of the mouth, nausea, epigastric distress, constipation, paralytic ileus, and diarrhea have been reported in patients receiving desipramine. Peculiar taste, abdominal cramps, stomatitis, and black tongue have been reported with the administration of tricyclic compounds. *Skin:* Skin rashes (including photosensitization), perspiration and flushing sensations have been reported during therapy. *Liver:* Transient jaundice, apparently of an obstructive nature, and liver damage have been observed in rare cases. Elevation in transaminase and changes in alkaline phosphatase have occurred and should indicate repeated liver-function profiles. If progressive elevation occurs, the drug should be discontinued. *Blood:* Bone-marrow depression, agranulocytosis, thrombocytopenia and purpura have been reported. If these occur, the drug should be discontinued. Transient eosinophilia has been observed in some instances. *Cardiovascular system:* Hypotension, hypertension, tachycardia, palpitation, arrhythmias, heart block, myocardial infarction and stroke have been observed and may require discontinuation of treatment. Patients who require concomitant vasodilating therapy should be carefully supervised, particularly during the initial phases. *Genitourinary system:* Urinary frequency or retention, nocturia, delayed micturition, dilatation of urinary tract, and impotence have been reported. *Endocrine system:* Occasional hormonal effects, including gynecomastia, galactorrhea and breast enlargement have been reported with desipramine. In addition, decreased libido and estrogenic effects have been noted. The exact relationship of these adverse effects to the administration of the drug has not been established. *Sensitivity:* Urticaria edema (face, tongue, or general), and rare instances of drug fever and cross-sensitivity with imipramine have been observed.

Dosage and Administration: *Orally.* Initially in mild cases, 25 mg 3 times daily. More severe cases may require initial doses of up to 50 mg 3 times daily. When necessary, dosage may later be increased to not more than 200 mg daily in divided doses. Following a satisfactory response, the patient may be maintained on 50 to 100 mg/day. Geriatric and adolescent patients, 25 to 100 mg daily in divided doses.

Availability:

NORPRAMIN® Tablets, 25 mg (lemon-yellow) and 50 mg (light green) in bottles of 100, 500 and 1000 and in (unit-dose) packages of 100; 75 mg (orange), 100 mg (peach) and 150 mg

(white) in bottles of 50 and in unit-dose packages of 100. **(Merrell-National)**
PERTOFRANE® Capsules, 25 mg (pink) and 50 mg (maroon and pink) in bottles of 100 and 1000. **(USV)**

DESMOPRESSIN ACETATE

Chemical Name: 1-(3-Mercaptopropionic acid)-8-D-argininevasopressin monoacetate trihydrate.

Description: Desmopressin is an analog of the *naturally* occurring antidiuretic hormone arginine vasopressin. The drug has been found to have significant therapeutic value in the control or prevention of the symptoms and complications of severe central or cranial diabetes insipidus such as polyuria, polydypsia and dehydration. It is of no value in the treatment of nephrogenic diabetes insipidus. A synthetic substance administered as a nasal spray, the drug is generally free of the allergic reactions usually observed with hormonal antidiuretic replacement therapy. It also has the advantages of a longer duration of action, usually lasting from 10 to 12 hours, and a lower incidence of adverse effects as well as insignificant pressor and oxytocic effects and decreased visceral smooth muscle activity resulting from modifications in the structural formula of arginine vasopressor. Thus 1 ml (0.1 mg) has been found to provide antidiuretic activity of about 400 IU as compared with that of arginine vasopressin. Clinical studies indicate that the twice daily regimen is effective in restoring normal urine volume and osmolality in adults and children afflicted by the disease. The biphasic half-lives for demopressin have been found to be 7.8 and 75.5 minutes compared with 2.5 and 14.5 minutes for lysine vasopressin, another form of the hormone used for this condition, thus assuring a prompt onset of action with a continuing duration of response after each administration.

Studies with pregnant rats and rabbits given doses up to 12.5 times the clinical intranasal dose have revealed no evidence of harmful effects on the fetus. However, there are no documented reports on the drug's effect in pregnant patients.

Indications: Antidiuretic replacement therapy in the management of central diabetes insipidus and its complications.

Contraindications: Undue sensitivity to the drug.

Warnings: *For intranasal use only.* Because water retention with resultant hyponatremia are possible occurrences with antidiuretic therapy, fluid intake should be carefully regulated, particularly in very young and elderly patients.

Precautions: When given in high dosage, the drug has occasionally produced a slight elevation in blood pressure which generally disappeared when the dosage was reduced. Cautious use is recommended in patients with coronary artery insufficiency and/or hypertensive cardiovascular disease. Safe use during pregnancy has not been confirmed.

Adverse Reactions: Excessive use may produce transient headache and nausea. Nasal congestion, rhinitis and flushing have been reported occasionally, as well as mild abdominal cramps and vulval pain. These complications disappeared with a reduction in dosage. There is no specific antidote in the event of overdosage. If considerable fluid retention is causing concern, a saluretic such as furosemide may be given to induce diuresis.

Dosage and Administration: *Intranasally.* The optimal dose is judged by urinary volume and plasma osmolalities. The usual dosage range for adults is 0.1 to 0.4 ml daily, either as a single dose or in 2 or 3 divided doses. Most adults generally respond well to 0.2 ml daily in 2 divided doses. The usual dosage range for children 3 months to 12 years of age is 0.05 to 0.3 ml daily, either as a single dose or in 2 divided doses. The morning and evening doses should be separately adjusted for an adequate diurnal rhythm of water turnover. For proper usage a graduated plastic catheter for instillation is provided. **Note:** The product should be stored under refrigeration at 4°C.

Availability:
DDAVP® Aqueous Solution, 0.1 mg in vials of 2.5 ml in cartons of 1 containing 2 applicator tubes. **(Ferring)**

DESONIDE: see The Adrenal Corticosteroids

DESOXIMETASONE: see The Adrenal Corticosteroids

DESOXYCORTICOSTERONE: see The Adrenal Corticosteroids

DESQUAM-X5/-X10

Description: Contains benzoyl peroxide, 5 or 10%; polyoxyethylene lauryl ether, 6%; disodium edetate, diisopropanolamine and water. The wash contains benzoyl peroxide, 4% triton X-200, water, sodium dioctyl sulfosuccinate, sodium lauryl sulfoacetate, magnesium aluminum silicate, methocel A4M and disodium edetate. The combination provides drying and peeling of the skin of patients with acne. Also provides antibacterial action especially against Propionibacterium acnes.

Indications: Control of acne vulgaris.

Contraindications: Hypersensitivity to any of the components.

Precautions: Avoid contact with the eyes, mucous membranes, highly inflamed or denuded skin, or thin, highly sensitive skin. Discontinue use if painful irritation develops. Recommended for external use only. **Note:** May bleach colored fabrics.

Dosage and Administration: *Topically.* After cleansing the skin, apply to or wash the affected area twice daily. For fair-skinned individuals or when weather conditions are excessively dry, it is suggested that therapy be initiated with 1 application daily.

Availability:
DESQUAM-X5/-X10® Gel in tubes of 42.5 and 90 gm. **(Westwood)**
DESQUAM-X® Wash in plastic bottles of 141.8 gm. **(Westwood)**

DEXBROMPHENIRAMINE MALEATE: see Brompheniramine Maleate

DEXPANTHENOL

Chemical Name: *Dextro* pantothenyl alcohol.

Description: *Dextro* pantothenyl alcohol differs structurally from pantothenic acid only in that the carboxyl group of the latter is reduced to a primary alcohol group. It occurs as a viscous liquid freely soluble in water. Following parenteral administration, it is converted to and excreted as pantothenic acid.

Pantothenic acid apparently is essential to normal epithelial function. It is a precursor to the formation of coenzyme A which is involved with the conversion of succinic acid in the metabolism of fat and carbohydrate, with phosphorylation and with acetylation reactions in tissues. The presence of pantothenic acid is therefore essential to the acetylation of choline to acetylcholine, the transmitter substance required for normal intestinal motility.

Indications: For prophylactic use immediately after major abdominal surgery to minimize the possibility of paralytic ileus. Intestinal atony causing abdominal distention; postoperative or postpartum retention of flatus, or postoperative delay in resumption of intestinal motility; paralytic ileus. Dexpanthenol with choline bitartrate may be helpful in relieving patients with gas retention associated with the splenic flexure syndrome, cholecystitis, gastritis, gastric hyperacidity, irritable colon, regional ileitis, postantibiotic and postoperative gas retention or during laxative withdrawal.

Contraindications: None known.

Warnings: There have been rare instances of allergic reaction of unknown cause during the concomitant use of this drug and other drugs such as antibiotics, narcotics, and barbiturates. Administration of full-strength dexpanthenol directly into the vein is not advised.

Precautions: Patients taking cholinesterase inhibitors such as neostigmine, or other drugs that stimulate peristalsis, should wait at least 12 hours before receiving dexpanthenol. These same patients should wait at least 1 hour after the withdrawal of succinylcholine before taking dexpanthenol. If there is any evidence of an allergic reaction, treatment should be discontinued. If the ileus is mechanical in nature, appropriate measures to eliminate its cause should not be delayed by the use of the drug. The effectiveness of dexpanthenol-choline may be impaired in the presence of potassium deficiency.

Adverse Reactions: Frequency of bowel movements may be increased.

Dosage and Administration: Adults, 1 or 2 ml *intramuscularly,* repeated in 2 hours and then every 4 to 6 hours until all danger of distention has passed. Administration for 48 to 72 hours or longer may be required. For children, 5 mg/lb is recommended in the same frequency as for adults. *Intravenously,* by slow infusion using a 2-ml dose incorporated in either glucose or lactate-Ringer's solution. *Orally,* for adults, 2 tablets 3 times daily, increased in severe cases of gas retention to 3 tablets or more 3 times daily. After relief is obtained, dosage may be reduced to 1 or 2 tablets daily, or discontinued entirely. Resume full dosage if flatulence recurs.

Availability:
ILOPAN® Solution, 250 mg/ml in ampuls of 2 ml, vials of 10 ml and in Stat-Pak® (2-ml disposable syringes). **(Warren-Teed)**
ILOPAN®-CHOLINE Tablets (pink), 50 mg with 25 mg of choline bitartrate in bottles of 100 and 500. **(Warren-Teed)**

DEXTRAN 40

Description: Dextran 40 is a polysaccharide formed by the action of the bacterium, *Leuconostoc mesenteroides,* on sucrose. It is a low molecular weight polymer of glucose, the average molecular weight being 40,000 and ranging from about 15,000 to 75,000. By partial hydrolysis of the crude dextran and by differential fractionation, a molecular size approximately that of serum albumin is obtained. Its degree of branching is relatively low, with more than 90% of the cross linkage being of the straight chain type.

Indications: As a priming fluid, either as sole primer or as an additive, in pump oxygenators during extracorporeal circulation. In clinical comparisons with homologous blood and/or other hemodiluents, it has been shown that dextran 40 reduces the destruction of erythrocytes and platelets, reduces intravascular hemagglutination (blood sludging), maintains an erythrocyte electronegativity charge and reduces such dangers in the use of homologous blood as serum hepatitis and transfusion reactions. It is also used as an adjunct in the treatment of shock. The drug enhances blood flow, particularly the microcirculation by a combination of mechanisms such as increasing blood volume, venous return, and cardiac output. Rheomacrodex is also indicated for use in prophylaxis therapy against venous thrombosis and pulmonary embolism in patients undergoing procedures known to be associated with a high incidence of thromboembolic complications, such as hip surgery.

Contraindications: It should not be used in the presence of marked thrombocytopenia, hypofibrinogenemia, severe cardiac decompensation, in renal disease with severe oliguria or anuria, and known hypersensitivity to dextran.

Warnings: As a colloidal hypertonic solution, the drug attracts water from the extravascular space. This fluid shift should be considered when given to poorly hydrated patients. Renal excretion of dextran 40 causes an elevation of the urinary specific gravity; only minor elevations occur if the urinary flow is adequate. However, if the flow is diminished, its viscosity and specific gravity can increase appreciably. Serum or urinary osmolarity should be determined in order to assess the patient's state of hydration, and if signs of dehydration are apparent, additional fluid should be administered. The concomitant use of an osmotic diuretic, such as mannitol, also can be used to maintain an adequate flow of urine. There have been reports of renal failure and evidence of tubular vacuolization (osmotic nephrosis) following administration of dextran 40. Also reported were abnormalities in renal and hepatic function, but the effect of the drug specifically could not be determined. Dosages exceeding those recommended may prolong prothrombin time possibly resulting in bleeding. Although the incidence is rare, severe and fatal anaphylactic reactions, consisting of marked hypotension, may develop, especially in patients previously exposed to dextran solutions. Therefore, patients so treated should have their blood pressure monitored and should be observed closely for at least the first 30 minutes of infusion. Equipment for emergency measures should be readily available. Discontinuation of the drug will usually relieve less severe reactions, while more serious reactions may necessitate the use of parenteral administration of antihistaminics (ephedrine or epinephrine), steroids, and resuscitative measures while other means of shock therapy are instituted. Safe use of dextran 40 during pregnancy has not been established with respect to adverse effects on fetal development. Therefore, it should not be used in the first trimester of pregnancy or in women of childbearing potential unless the expected benefits outweigh the potential hazards.

Precautions: Individuals with normal hemostasis receiving up to 15 ml/kg of body weight may show changes in blood coagulation and hemostasis characterized by variable decreases in platelet adhesiveness, fibrinogen, factors V and IX and a marked decrease in factor VIII. Since these changes tend to be more pronounced following trauma or major surgery, all patients should be observed for early signs of bleeding complications. Some of these changes may be reversed by infusing the patient with factor VIII concentrate. It is strongly recommended that central venous pressure be monitored frequently during the initial infusion of the drug. The patient should be carefully observed for signs of circulatory overloading. Care should be taken to prevent a depression of the hematocrit below 30% of volume. Blood sugar determinations employing high concentrations of acid, and blood typing and cross-matching procedures employing enzyme techniques may give unreliable readings if the samples are taken after infusion of dextran 40. It is recommended, therefore, that, whenever possible, blood samples for these determinations should be taken prior to initiating infusion of dextran 40.

Adverse Reactions: Mild urticarial reactions, generalized urticaria, tightness in the chest, wheezing, hypotension, nausea and vomiting may occur in some instances.

Dosage and Administration: *Intravenously.* The dosage used in the priming fluid will vary with the volume of the pump oxygenator available. As a sole primer or as an additive, 10 to 20 ml/kg of body weight generally are added to the perfusion circuit. *As adjunctive therapy in shock,* total dosage during the first 24 hours should not exceed 20 ml/kg of body weight. The first 500 ml should be infused rapidly with the remaining dose being administered more slowly. Should therapy continue beyond 24 hours, the total daily dosage should not exceed 10 ml/kg of body weight and therapy should not continue beyond 5 days. *For the prevention of thromboembolic complications during surgery,* 500 to 1000 ml (approx. 10 ml/kg of body weight) should be administered on the day of the operation. Treatment should be continued at a dose of 500 ml daily for an additional 2 to 3 days. Thereafter, in accordance with the risk of complications or the duration of immobilization, 500 ml may be given every second or third day for up to 2 weeks.

Availability:

DEXTRAN 40 Solution, 10% in either normal saline or in 5% dextrose in infusion bottles of 500 ml. **(Cutter)**

LMD Solution, 10% in either normal saline or 5% dextrose in bottles of 500 ml. **(Abbott)**

RHEOMACRODEX® Solutions, 10% in either normal saline or in 5% dextrose in infusion bottles of 500 ml. **(Pharmacia)**

DEXTRAN 70

Description: Dextran is a polymolecular polysaccharide composed of glucose units formed when the bacterium *Leuconostoc mesenteroides* is cultured in sucrose-containing media. The crude dextran is hydrolyzed and fractionated to an average molecular weight of 70,000 although small portions of the dextran present may be as low as 20,000 or as high as 115,000. This figure is comparable to that of serum albumin.

A plasma volume expander, dextran produces a relatively prolonged hemodilution with an accompanying decrease in total serum proteins and hematocrit values. After infusion about 75% of the dextran is excreted in the urine in a 72-hour period; the remainder is enzymatically degraded to glucose at a rate of 70 to 90 mg/kg of body weight daily. The expansion of plasma volume resulting from administration of dextran gradually diminishes as dextran is eliminated. The administration of 500 ml to normal individuals does not appear to alter pulse rate, blood pressure or respiration, or to produce changes in renal or hepatic functions. It has been known to interfere with blood-typing, cross-matching or Rh determinations. The highly viscous solution containing 32% dextran 70 in dextrose (10% w/v) affords direct visualization of the canal of the uterine cervix and the cavity and lining of the uterus. When introduced into the uterine cavity through the cannula of the hysteroscope, it has been found useful in distending the uterine cavity and in irrigating and visualizing its surfaces.

Indications: Treatment of shock or impending shock caused by hemorrhage, burns, surgery, or other trauma. It is intended for emergency treatment when whole blood or blood products are not available, and must not be regarded as a substitute for whole blood or plasma proteins. The 32% solution is indicated for hysteroscopy.

Contraindications: Marked hemostatic defects of all types (thrombocytopenia, hyperfibrinogenemia, etc.), including those induced by drugs; marked cardiac decompensation, renal disease with severe oliguria or anuria; decreased urinary output secondary to shock is not a contraindication unless there is no improvement in urine output after the initial dose, and known hypersensitivity to dextran. Contraindications to hysteroscopic examination are recent uterine perforation, acute and chronic recurrent infections of the upper genital tract, endometrial carcinoma, or pregnant patients who are beyond 4 gestational weeks.

Warnings: Patients should be observed closely for symptoms of anaphylaxis especially during the first 30 minutes of dextran infusion, since severe and fatal reactions have been reported. These are manifested by sudden marked hypotension, vomiting, nausea, dyspnea, tightness of the chest, and generalized urticaria. If symptoms of an anaphylactoid reaction appear, the infusion should be discontinued immediately and suitable therapy instituted. Effective anaphylactic therapy includes epinephrine hydrochloride (0.3 to 0.5 ml of a 1:1000 solution). Transient prolongation of bleeding time may occur when dextran is administered in doses of more than 1 liter. Care should be taken to prevent a depression of hematocrit below 30% volume. Dextran may also interfere with platelet function, and should be used with caution in patients with thrombocytopenia.

Precautions: Individuals with normal hemostasis receiving up to 15 ml/kg of body weight may show changes in blood coagulation and hemostasis characterized by variable decreases in platelet adhesiveness, fibrinogen, factors V and IX and a significant decrease in factor VIII. Since these changes tend to be more pronounced following trauma or major surgery, all patients should be observed for early signs of bleeding complications. Some of these changes may be reversed by infusing the patient with factor VIII concentrate. The possibility of a circulatory overload should be kept in mind. Special care should be taken in administering dextran 70 to patients with increased risk of pulmonary edema or congestive heart failure. It should also be administered cautiously in patients with uremia or other evidence of impaired renal function, and in those with a history of chronic liver disease. Blood sugar determinations employing high concentrations of acid may give falsely elevated glucose results. Although it does not alter a patient's blood group or type, dextran may interfere with blood grouping, typing and cross-matching due to rouleaux formation (a roll of red blood corpuscles arranged like a pile of coins). Therefore, *it is recommended that blood samples be drawn and reserved for these purposes prior to infusion of dextran.* If difficulties develop with blood drawn afterwards, the cells may be washed with isotonic sodium chloride or other suitable salt solution. The possibility of circulatory overload should be kept in mind.

Adverse Reactions: Allergic reactions including urticaria, nasal congestion, wheezing, tightness in chest, mild hypotension, and nausea, vomiting, fever, and joint pains. If a reaction develops, therapy should be discontinued and the patient treated accordingly.

Dosage and Administration: *Intravenously.* Total dosage and rate of infusion depend upon the magnitude of fluid loss and the resultant hemoconcentration. Adults, usually 500 ml infused at a rate of 20 to 40 ml/minute. Total dosage should not exceed 20 ml/kg during the first 24 hours. For children, the best guide to dosage is the body weight or body surface area (BSA) of the patient; total dosage should not exceed 20 ml/kg of body weight. For hysteroscopic examination, dosage depends on the type and length of the procedure, but the usual dose is 50 to 100 ml. The solution should be infused under low pressure (approximately 100 mm Hg) until the uterus is sufficiently distended to permit adequate visualization. Infusion pressures greater than 150 mm Hg are not recommended.

Availability:
DEXTRAN 70 Solution, 6% in normal saline in bottles of 250 and 500 ml. **(Cutter)**
HYSKON® Solution, 32% in dextrose (10% w/v) in ampuls of 100 ml in cartons of 12. **(Pharmacia)**
MACRODEX® Solution, 6% in normal saline or in 5% dextrose in water in bottles of 500 ml. **(Pharmacia)**

DEXTRANOMER

Description: A polymer of dextran formulated as small, dry, hydrophilic beads designed for the purpose of cleansing and debriding various secreting skin lesions. The beads are made of chain-like dextran macromolecules arranged in a tridimensional network. When applied to the surface of discharging wounds, a combination of absorptive forces and capillary action causes the exudates, bacteria and other contaminants to migrate into the dry beads. The ability of the substance to remove exudates rapidly and continuously results in a simultaneous reduction of inflammation, edema, pain and echar formation, while permitting a therapeutic process to take place on the underlying conditions, such as venous or arterial flow, pressure, etc. This overall action tends to hasten formation of granulation tissue and to reduce the time necessary for wound healing or skin grafting. Because of its chemically inert nature, it does not produce hypersensitivity or local allergic reactions, nor is it absorbed systemically.

Indications: Intended as an adjunctive measure in cleansing and debriding secreting wounds such as occurs in venous stasis ulcers, decubitus ulcers, infected traumatic and surgical wounds and infected burns. It is not effective in cleansing nonsecreting wounds.

Precautions: Cross-contamination may be avoided if the contents of the container are used on no more than one patient. When treating cratered decubitus ulcers, the beads should be packed loosely. It has been observed that during the first few days of treatment, wounds generally appear larger due to reduction of edema.

Adverse Reactions: Occasionally, pain of short duration has been noted when the dressings were changed.

Dosage and Administration: *Topically.* First cleanse the wound with sterile water, saline solution or another appropriate cleansing agent, then pour on a sufficient amount of the beads to cover the area being treated to a thickness of 3 mm or approximately 4 gm and lightly bandage. The procedure should be repeated when the beads turn a greyish-yellow color. The dressing should be changed at least once or twice daily, but as many as 4 changes may be necessary if the wound is draining profusely.

Availability:
DEBRISAN Sterile Beads in containers of 60 and 120 gm and in unit-dose packages of 4 gm. **(Pharmacia)**

DEXTROAMPHETAMINE Ⓒ

Chemical Name: d-α-Methylphenethylamine.

Description: Dextroamphetamine is the *dextro* isomer of amphetamine. The sulfate and monobasic phosphate salts occur as white, odorless, crystalline powders and have a bitter taste.

The phosphate is soluble in water and slightly soluble in alcohol; the sulfate is freely soluble in water and slightly soluble in alcohol. Dextroamphetamine *tannate* occurs as a homogeneous protocolloid complex consisting of dextroamphetamine and tannic acid complex mixed with polygalacturonic acid. The complex is insoluble in water, but free dextroamphetamine becomes available for absorption by ion exchange, depending upon the proper pH. Polygalacturonic acid physically retards drug release in the low pH environment of the stomach and then dissolves in the alkaline media of the intestine where dextroamphetamine is ultimately released.

The pharmacologic actions of dextroamphetamine and its racemic parent, amphetamine, are qualitatively similar to those of ephedrine and include CNS and respiratory stimulation and sympathomimetic activity including pressor response, mydriasis, bronchodilation, and contraction of the urinary bladder sphincter. On a weight basis, dextroamphetamine has a greater influence on the CNS and a lesser activity on the peripheral nervous system than does the racemic amphetamine.

Indications: Treatment of narcolepsy and minimal brain dysfunction in children usually characterized by hyperkinetic behavior disorders, and as an occasional adjunct in short-term (a few weeks) management of exogenous obesity in conjunction with a medically supervised regimen of weight reduction based on caloric restriction. It is also used as adjunctive therapy in Parkinson's disease.

Some combination products used in the treatment of obesity contain methylcellulose that swells in the stomach giving the patient a feeling of fullness. Parenterally, it is used as an analeptic to counteract overdoses of depressant drugs such as barbiturates. A combination with amobarbital is recommended for the relief of symptoms of mental and emotional distress associated with lowered caloric intake. Dextroamphetamine may also be combined with a tranquilizer when mild CNS stimulation is desired in addition to the calming effect of the tranquilizer.

For the contraindications, warnings, precautions and adverse reactions attributable to any of the components in combination with dextroamphetamine, their individual monographs should be consulted.

Contraindications: Advanced arteriosclerosis, symptomatic cardiovascular diseases, moderate to severe hypertension, hyperthyroidism, glaucoma, known hypersensitivity or idiosyncrasy to the sympathomimetic amines, agitated states, and patients with a history of drug abuse. Also, dextroamphetamines are contraindicated during or within 14 days following the administration of MAO inhibitors because a hypertensive crisis may occur.

Warnings: Amphetamines have a significant potential for abuse. In view of their limited short-term anorectic effect and rapid development of tolerance, they should be used with extreme caution and only for limited periods of time in weight reduction programs. Since tolerance to the anorectic effect usually develops within a few weeks, the recommended dosage should not be exceeded in an attempt to increase the effect; rather the drug should be discontinued. Abrupt cessation following prolonged high dosage administration results in extreme fatigue and mental depression; changes are also noted on the sleep EEG. Dextroamphetamines may alter the insulin requirements in patients with diabetes and may decrease the hypotensive effect of guanethidine. Safe use during pregnancy has not been established; therefore, those who are or may become pregnant and especially those in the first trimester of pregnancy, require that the potential benefits of the drug be weighed against the possible hazards to the mother and fetus. Amphetamines are not recommended for use as anorectic agents in children under 12 years of age. Patients should be cautioned that amphetamines may impair their ability to engage in potentially hazardous activities such as operating machinery or driving a motor vehicle.

Precautions: To be used with caution in patients hypersensitive to sympathomimetics and in those with coronary or cardiovascular disease. Excessive use by unstable patients may result in a psychological dependence in which case the drug should be discontinued. Manifestations of chronic intoxication with amphetamines include severe dermatoses, marked insomnia, irritability, hyperactivity, and personality changes. The most severe manifestation of chronic intoxication is psychosis, often clinically indistinguishable from schizophrenia. Caution is to be exercised in prescribing amphetamines for patients with even mild hypertension.

The least amount feasible should be prescribed or dispensed at one time in order to minimize the possibility of overdosage.

For information regarding the component drugs see their respective monographs.

Adverse Reactions: *Cardiovascular*—Palpitations, tachycardia, elevation of blood pressure. *CNS*—Overstimulation, restlessness, dizziness, insomnia, euphoria, dysphoria, tremor, headache; rarely, psychotic episodes at recommended doses. *Gastrointestinal*—Dryness of the mouth, unpleasant taste, diarrhea, other gastrointestinal disturbances. Anorexia and weight loss may occur as undesirable effects when amphetamines are used for other than the anorectic effect. *Allergic*—Urticaria. *Endocrine*—Impotence and changes in libido. Manifestations of acute overdosage include restlessness, tremor, hyperreflexia, rapid respiration, confusion, assaultiveness, hallucinations, and panic states. Fatigue and depression usually follow CNS stimulation. Cardiovascular effects are manifested by arrhythmias, hypertension, hypotension, and circulatory collapse. Complications involving the gastrointestinal tract include nausea, vomiting, diarrhea, and abdominal cramps. Fatal poisoning usually terminates in convulsions and coma. Management of acute intoxication is primarily symptomatic and includes gastric lavage and sedation with a barbiturate. Experience with hemodialysis or peritoneal dialysis has not been sufficient to permit recommendations in this regard. Acidifications of the urine increases amphetamine excretion. Intravenous phentolamine has been suggested for possible acute, severe hypertension, if this complicates the amphetamine overdosage.

Dosage and Administration: *Orally.* Amphetamines should be administered at the lowest effective dosage, and dosage should be individually adjusted. It is advisable to begin treatment with a test dose of 5 mg and to increase the amount progressively until optimal dosage has been determined. *For narcolepsy*—adults 5 to 60 mg daily; children 6 to 12 years of age, initially, 5 mg daily; may be increased in increments of 5 mg at weekly intervals until optimal response is attained; children 12 years of age and older, 10 mg daily; may be raised in increments of 10 mg at weekly intervals until optimal response is obtained. *For minimal brain dysfunction in children*—2.5 to 40 mg or more daily; children 3 to 5 years of age, initially 2.5 mg daily, increased in increments of 2.5 mg weekly if necessary; children 6 years of age and older, initially 5 mg 1 or 2 times daily, then increased in increments of 5 mg at weekly intervals until the desired response is obtained. The first dose should be given upon awakening and additional doses at intervals of 4 to 6 hours. **Not recommended for children under 3 years of age.** *For exogenous obesity*—5 to 10 mg 3 times daily, administered 30 to 60 minutes before each meal, or 1 or 2 extended-release formulations taken in the morning. *Intramuscularly. For the treatment of intoxication by a barbiturate,* 10 to 20 mg initially, repeated at intervals of 30 minutes according to response of the patient. As soon as consciousness returns, parenteral administration should be discontinued and replaced by oral medication. May also be given intravenously.

Availability:

Dextroamphetamine Sulfate

Ⓒ DEXAMPEX™: **(Lemmon)**
Capsules, 15 mg (green and white) in bottles of 100 and 1000.
Tablets, 5 mg (blue) and 10 mg (pink) in bottles of 100 and 1000.

Ⓒ DEXEDRINE®: **(Smith Kline & French)**
Elixir, 5 mg/5 ml in bottles of 1 pint.
Spansule® Capsules, 5 mg in bottles of 50; 10 and 15 mg in bottles of 50 and 500.
Tablets, 5 mg in bottles of 100 and 1000.

w/Amobarbital (Warning: May be habit-forming)

Ⓒ DEXAMYL® (for use in weight control only): **(Smith Kline & French)**
Spansule® Capsules, 10 mg with amobarbital, 65 mg; 15 mg with amobarbital, 97 mg in bottles of 50.
Tablets, 5 mg with amobarbital, 32 mg in bottles of 100.

w/Prochlorperazine

Ⓒ ESKATROL® Spansule® Capsules (sustained release), 15 mg with prochlorperazine (as the maleate), 7.5 mg in bottles of 50. (Only as an adjunct in weight control.) **(Smith Kline & French)**

Dextroamphetamine Tannate

Ⓒ OBOTAN® Tablets, 17.5 mg in bottles of 100. **(Mallinckrodt)**
Ⓒ OBOTAN FORTE Tablets, 26.25 mg in bottles of 100. **(Mallinckrodt)**

DEXTROTHYROXINE SODIUM

Chemical Name: D-3,5,3′,5′,-Tetraiodothyronine sodium.

Description: Sodium dextrothyroxine, the monosodium salt of the *dextro* isomer of thyroxine, which is the major secretion of the thyroid gland. The predominant effect is the reduction of serum cholesterol levels in hyperlipidemic patients; beta lipoprotein and triglyceride fractions may also be reduced from previously elevated levels.

While the exact mechanism of action is still under investigation, most evidence indicates that sodium dextrothyroxine stimulates the liver to increase oxidative catabolism and excretion of cholesterol and its degradation products by way of the biliary route and into the feces. Cholesterol synthesis is not inhibited and abnormal end products do not accumulate in the blood. Dextrothyroxine inhibits iodine uptake by the thyroid but this action does not affect the basal metabolic rate. On a weight basis, it is about one-fifth to one-twenty-fifth as active as the racemic thyroxine and one-tenth to one-fiftieth as potent as the sodium salt.

Following oral administration, dextrothyroxine is not absorbed from the gastrointestinal tract as readily as is the sodium salt, is metabolized in the liver and excreted in the urine and in feces in about equal amounts, unchanged and as metabolites. It is not known whether or not dextrothyroxine crosses the placental barrier or appears in the milk of nursing mothers.

Indications: Antilipidemic agent used as adjunct to diet and other measures for the reduction of elevated serum cholesterol in euthyroid patients with an absence of organic heart disease. Also indicated in the treatment of hypothyroidism in those patients with cardiac disease who cannot tolerate other types of thyroid preparations. Patients taking digitalis require special consideration since both dextrothyroxine sodium and digitalis exert a positive inotropic effect on the heart. The added action may stimulate the myocardium excessively in patients with significant myocardial impairment. When such concomitant therapy is necessary, the dosage of dextrothyroxine should not exceed 4 mg/day, and the total effect of both drugs should be carefully monitored. It has not been established whether the drug-induced lowering of serum cholesterol or lipid levels has a detrimental, beneficial, or no effect on the morbidity or mortality due to atherosclerosis or coronary heart disease.

Contraindications: This is not an innocuous drug. Strict attention should be paid to the indications and contraindications. Sodium dextrothyroxine is contraindicated in euthyroid patients with one or more of the following conditions: known organic heart disease, including angina pectoris; history of myocardial infarction; cardiac arrhythmia or tachycardia, either active or in patients with demonstrated propensity for arrhythmias; rheumatic heart disease; history of congestive heart failure and decompensated or borderline compensated cardiac status; hypertensive states (other than mild, labile systolic hypertension); advanced liver or kidney disease; pregnancy; nursing mothers; history of iodism. If impaired liver or kidney functions are present, the advantages of sodium dextrothyroxine therapy must be weighed against the possibility of deleterious results.

Warnings: Since several studies have shown that sodium dextrothyroxine potentiates the effects of anticoagulants (i.e., warfarin or dicumerol) on prothrombin time, the doses of such anticoagulants should be reduced by 1/3 upon initiation of dextrothyroxine therapy. Subsequent dosage should be based upon laboratory findings which should be instituted at weekly intervals during the first few weeks of therapy. During anticoagulant therapy, attention should also be paid to other clotting factors in some patients (Factors VII, VIII, IX and platelet activity). It is advised that sodium dextrothyroxine be withdrawn 2 weeks prior to surgery if the use of anticoagulants during surgery is being contemplated. When sodium dextrothyroxine is used as thyroid replacement therapy in hypothyroid patients with concomitant coronary artery disease (especially those with a history of angina pectoris or myocardial infarction) or other cardiac disease, treatment should be initiated with care. Special consideration of the dosage schedule of sodium dextrothyroxine is required. This drug may increase the oxygen requirements of the myocardium, especially at high dosage levels. Patients with coronary artery disease who are receiving this drug must be seen at frequent intervals. If aggravation of angina or increased myocardial ischemia, cardiac failure, or clinically significant arrhythmia develops during the treatment of hyperthyroid patients, the dosage should be reduced or the drug discontinued.

Special consideration must be given to the dosage of other thyroid medications used concomitantly with sodium dextrothyroxine. As with all thyroactive drugs, hypothyroid patients are more sensitive to a given dose of sodium dextrothyroxine than euthyroid patients. Epinephrine injection in patients with coronary artery disease may precipitate an episode of coronary insufficiency. This condition may be enhanced in patients receiving thyroid analogues. These possible occurrences should be kept in mind when catecholamine injections are required in sodium dextrothyroxine-treated hypothyroid patients with coronary artery disease. Since the possibility of precipitating cardiac arrhythmias during surgery may be greater in patients treated with thyroid hormones, it may be prudent to discontinue the drug in euthyroid patients at least 2 weeks prior to an elective operation. During emergency surgery in euthyroid patients, and in surgery in hypothyroid patients in whom it may not be advisable to withdraw thyroid therapy, the patients should be carefully observed.

There have been reports that sodium dextrothyroxine in diabetic patients is capable of increasing blood sugar levels with a resultant increase in requirements of insulin or oral hypoglycemic agents. Special attention should be paid to parameters necessary for good control of the diabetic state in dextrothyroxine-treated diabetic subjects and to dosage requirements of insulin or other antidiabetic drugs. If sodium dextrothyroxine is later withdrawn from patients who had required an increase of insulin (or oral hypoglycemic agents) dosage during its administration, the dosage of the antidiabetic drugs should be reduced and adjusted to maintain good control of the diabetic state. Women of childbearing age with familial hypercholesteremia or hyperlipemia should not be deprived of this drug while they are exercising strict birth control procedures. Although teratogenic studies in 2 animal species have revealed no abnormalities in the offspring, risk to fetus must be weighed against possible benefits to the mother.

Precautions: The consideration of dietary regulation must not be precluded in patients with hypercholesterolemia. Increased serum PBI values should not be interpreted as evidence of hypermetabolism. PBI values in the range of 10 to 25 mcg% in treated subjects are common. If signs or symptoms of iodism develop during therapy, the drug should be discontinued. Although no adverse effects on growth has been shown in 1 year treatment of a few children with familial hypercholesteremia, it is recommended for continued use in this age group only if significant cholesterol lowering effect is observed.

Adverse Reactions: Effects are largely due to increased metabolism and may be minimized by adhering to recommended dosages. Adverse effects are least commonly seen in euthyroid patients without evidence of organic heart disease. The incidence of adverse effects is increased in hypothyroid patients, and is highest in those patients with organic heart disease superimposed on the hypothyroid state. In the absence of known organic heart disease, some cardiac changes may be precipitated during therapy. In addition to angina pectoris, arrhythmia consisting of extrasystoles, ectopic beats, or supraventricular tachycardia, ECG evidence of ischemic myocardial changes and increase in heart size have been observed. Myocardial infarctions (both fatal and nonfatal) have occurred but it is not known if any of these infarctions were due to the drug. Changes in clinical status that may be related to the metabolic action of the drug include insomnia, nervousness, palpitations, tremors, weight loss, lid lag, sweating, flushing, fever, hair loss, diuresis, menstrual irregularities; gastrointestinal complaints including dyspepsia, nausea, vomiting, constipation, diarrhea, decreased appetite. Other reactions include headache, increased or decreased libido, hoarseness, tinnitus, dizziness, peripheral edema, malaise, fatigue, visual disturbances, psychic changes, paresthesia, muscle pain, and various bizarre subjective complaints. Skin rashes, itching, gallstones, cholestatic jaundice, worsening of peripheral vascular disease, sensorium, exophthalmos and retinopathy have been reported.

Dosage and Administration: *Orally.* For adults with hypercholesterolemia, the initial daily dosage should be 1 to 2 mg, increased by increments of 1 or 2 mg at intervals of at least 1 month to a maximum of 8 mg daily. Maintenance dosage should be 4 to 8 mg daily. When used as partial or complete substitution therapy for levothyroxine in hypothyroid patients, the more conservative dosage schedule is recommended. Initially, the daily dose is 1 mg for 1 month; the amount may be increased by increments of 1 mg daily at intervals of not less than 1 month to a maximum level of 4 to 8 mg daily. The maximum in patients receiving digitalis therapy is 4 mg. For children with hypercholesterolemia, 0.05 mg/kg initially, increased by increments of 0.05 mg/kg at monthly intervals to a maximum of 4 mg daily. Maintenance dose is about 0.1 mg/kg. If new signs or symptoms of cardiac disease develop during the treatment period, the drug should be discontinued.

Availability:
CHOLOXIN® Tablets, 1 and 6 mg in bottles of 30 and 100; 2, 4 and 6 mg in bottles of 100 and 250. **(Flint)**

DIALOG

Description: Each tablet contains allobarbital, 15 mg and acetaminophen, 300 mg. Combines the sedative action of allobarbital with the analgesic and antipyretic effects of acetaminophen.

Indications: For the relief of pain and discomfort of simple headache; neuralgia, myalgia, musculoskeletal pain; dysmenorrhea; bursitis; sinusitis; fibrositis; to relieve the discomfort and reduce fever caused by respiratory infections, influenza, and other febrile conditions.

Contraindications: In patients sensitive to any of the components, in those with moderate to severe hepatic disease, or with a personal or familial history of acute intermittent porphyria.

Warnings: Allobarbital may be habit-forming. Dosage of coumarin anticoagulants may require adjustment during and on cessation of therapy. Although safe use in pregnant and lactating women has not been established, it may be given only with special attention to the potential benefits versus the risks to the unborn child.

Precautions: Periodic complete blood counts are advised during prolonged therapy.

Adverse Reactions: Nausea, transitory dizziness, anemia, leukopenia, pancytopenia, and rash may occur. Overdosage of allobarbital will produce symptoms typical of acute barbiturate excess. Signs and symptoms of overdosage of acetaminophen consist of gastrointestinal, renal, hepatic, and myocardial damage, severity being directly related to dosage. Gastric emptying, instillation of activated charcoal, diuresis, and intensive supportive care are recommended. Hemodialysis, recommended for removal of allobarbital in severe cases, is apparently not effective for removal of acetaminophen.

Dosage and Administration: *Orally.* Adults, 1 or 2 tablets every 4 hours; not to exceed 8 tablets in 24 hours. Children 6 to 12 years of age, ½ to 1 tablet every 4 hours; not to exceed 4 tablets in 24 hours.

Availability:
DIALOG® Tablets in bottles of 30. **(Ciba)**

DIATRIZOATE MEGLUMINE
DIATRIZOATE SODIUM

Chemical Name: 3,5-Diacetamido-2,4,6-triiodobenzoic acid methylglucamine salts.

Description: Diatrizoate is structurally related to iothalamate. Meglumine and sodium diatrizoate are organic iodide preparations that are radiopaque, water soluble and contain 47% and 59.87% iodine, respectively.

Intravenous administration results in rapid distribution throughout the circulatory system to the renal area where the preparation is excreted in unchanged form by glomerular filtration. X-ray visualization of the kidneys occurs within 3 to 15 minutes but this is influenced by the status of renal function. The gastrointestinal tract can be visualized radiologically following oral or rectal administration. Some absorption of diatrizoate may take place across the gastrointestinal mucosa and the renal area may be visualized to some extent. The drug is also absorbed across the peritoneum and pleura.

Indications: Visualization of the urinary tract by intravenous administration or by retrograde pyelography or cystourethrography and the gastrointestinal tract by oral or rectal administration. Also used for peripheral arteriography and venography; angiocardiography; thoracic aortography; cerebral arteriography, splenoportography, and diskography. The 25% solution is primarily useful for infusion urography and tissue contrast enhancement of endocranial CT scanning procedures.

A combination of *meglumine diatrizoate* and *sodium diatrizoate* is used for combined arteriography and venography of the peripheral vessels and for angiocardiography with accompanying pyelogram; for excretion urography (by direct intravenous or drip infusion); cerebral angiography; operative, T-tube or percutaneous transhepatic cholangiography; splenoportography; arthrography; and discography.

The combination of *meglumine diatrizoate* and *iodipamide* is used when combined visualization of the biliary and renal systems is desired and for hysterosalpingography.

Contraindications: Hypersensitivity to the preparation. Acute thrombophlebitis is usually a contraindication for venography. Cerebral angiography should be used with caution, if at all, if recent cerebral embolism or thrombosis is suspected. Arthrography is inadvisable when there is infection in or near the joint; urography in the presence of anuria; discography in the presence of an infection or open wound near the region to be examined. Specific contraindications to percutaneous transhepatic cholangiography include prothrombin time below 50%, significant thrombocytopenia and evidence of coagulation defects. Splenoportography should not be performed on any patient for whom splenectomy is contraindicated, since complications of the procedure at times make splenectomy necessary, and any condition which may increase the possibility of rupture of the spleen.

The presence of the menstrual period or genital tract infection precludes hysterosalpingography as does pregnancy or a suspicion of pregnancy. This diagnostic procedure should not be utilized for 6 months after pregnancy is terminated or for 1 month following curettage of the uterus or conization of the cervix.

Diatrizoate 60% should not be used for myelography or for examination of dorsal cysts or sinuses which might communicate with the subarachnoid space, since even a small amount of the medium in the subarachnoid space may produce convulsions and result in fatality. Epidural injection is also contraindicated.

Warnings: Since serious and sometimes fatal reactions have occurred with the administration of radiopaque media, it is therefore of the utmost importance that a course of action be carefully planned in advance for the immediate treatment of serious reactions, and that adequate and appropriate facilities be readily available in case a severe reaction occurs. Safe use during pregnancy has not been established; therefore, the anticipated therapeutic benefits must be weighed against the possible hazards to the mother and fetus. In addition, most clinicians consider elective contrast radiography of the abdomen contraindicated during pregnancy. Intravascular administration of contrast media may promote sickling in patients who are homozygous for sickle cell disease. The results of PBI and RAI uptake studies, which depend on iodine estimations, will not reflect thyroid function for up to 16 days following administration of iodinated urographic media. However, function tests that do not depend on iodine estimations, such as T_3 resin uptake or direct thyroxine assays, are not affected.

Administration of angiographic media to patients known or suspected to have pheochromocytoma can cause dangerous changes in blood pressure. A minimum dose should be injected. The blood pressure should be carefully monitored and measures for controlling major fluctuations should be available.

During aortography by the translumbar technique, extreme care is advised to avoid inadvertent intrathecal injection since the injection of even small amounts (5 to 7 ml) of the contrast medium may cause convulsions, permanent sequelae or fatality. Should the accident occur, the patient should be placed upright to confine the hyperbaric solution to a low level, anesthesia may be required to control convulsions, and if there is evidence of a large dose having been administered, a careful cerebrospinal fluid exchange-washout should be considered. Selective spinal arteriography, or arteriography of trunks providing spinal branches, can cause mild to severe muscle spasm. However, serious neurologic consequences, including permanent paralysis, have occasionally been reported. Selective visceral arteriography should be performed with extreme caution in patients with severe generalized artherosclerosis, specifically with plagues or aneurysms at the level of the iliac or femoral arteries.

Precautions: The clinician should have a thorough understanding of the particular procedure, including the indications for specific contrast media and the associated hazards and possible complications. Caution is advised with the use of radiopaque media in severely debilitated patients and in those with marked hypertension. The possibility of thrombosis should be considered when percutaneous techniques are employed. Serious and fatal anaphylactic reactions may result from administration of these preparations including even a test dose of 0.5 to 1 ml intravenously; therefore, it is essential that the patient be observed for at least 15 minutes following parenteral administration. Prophylactic premedication of allergic patients with antihistamines may be desirable and emergency medication (such as oxygen, vasopressors, barbiturates, antihistamines and adrenocortical steroids) should be immediately available should a reaction occur. These preparations should be utilized cautiously in patients with severe liver or kidney disease, asthmatic patients and in those with a history of iodide sensitivity. In severely ill patients the value of the information to be gained from the diagnostic procedure must be weighed against the possible complications of the procedure. Evaluation of thyroid function, if indicated, should be performed prior to administration of these preparations because the iodine in the preparation may interfere with thyroid function tests. Also, contrast agents may interfere with some chemical determinations made on urine specimens; therefore, urine should be collected before administration of the medium or 2 or more days afterwards. Preparatory dehydration may be hazardous in infants, young children, the elderly, and azotemic patients, especially those with polyuria, oliguria, anuria, diabetes, advanced vascular disease, or preexisting dehydration. The undesirable dehydration in these patients may be accentuated by the osmotic diuretic action of the medium.

Adverse Reactions: Reactions accompanying the use of contrast media may vary directly with the concentration of the substance, the amount used, the technique employed, and the underlying pathology. Adverse reactions, usually of a minor nature, have occurred in 10 to 14% of patients who have received these solutions intravenously. Rarely, atheromatous or other embolic phenomena can occur in angiography. *Hemodynamic reactions* include vasodilatation with flushing, hypotension and, rarely, vein cramp or thrombophlebitis. Serious *cardiovascular reactions* include cardiac arrhythmias (such as ventricular fibrillation), shock, and cardiac arrest. Transient proteinuria may occur occasionally following the injection of radiopaque material and oliguria and anuria (renal shutdown) have been reported as a secondary effect of hypotensive reaction. *Allergic reactions* include asthmatic attacks, nasal and conjunctival symptoms, dermal reactions such as urticaria and, rarely, anaphylactoid shock. Rare fatalities have been reported due to the medium employed or from unknown causes. Severe reactions may also be characterized by signs and symptoms relating to the *respiratory* system (dyspnea, cyanosis, pulmonary or laryngeal edema), or to the *nervous system* (restlessness, confusion, or convulsions). Infrequently, immediate or delayed chills can occur, sometimes accompanied by hyperpyrexia. Other reactions include nausea, vomiting, excessive salivation, and sweating. Discomfort and colic because of ureteropelvic spasm occasionally may follow the examination. In some instances anxiety, headache, and dizziness may be noted. Infrequently, iodism (salivary gland swelling) from organic compounds appears 2 days after exposure and usually subsides by the 6th day. Subcutaneous extravasation, chiefly because of hypertonicity of the medium, causes transient stinging. If the volume is small, ill effects are very unlikely. However, if subcutaneous extravasation is extensive, especially in the foot, the physician should consider infiltration with Sterile Water for Injection, or injection of spreading agents.

In percutaneous transhepatic cholangiography, some discomfort is common, but pain is unusual. Complications of the procedure are often serious and have been reported in 4 to 6% of patients. These reactions have included bile leakage and peritonitis, which are more likely to occur in patients with obstructions that cause unrelieved high biliary pressure. Bleeding (sometimes massive with exsanguination) may occur, especially in patients with clotting abnormalities. Hypotension, fever, or chills can occur, suggesting the presence of a blood-bile fistula. Tension pneumothorax, cholangitis, and bacteremia or septicemia have also been noted. Selective renal arteriography can cause nausea, vomiting, hypotension and hypertension. Post-arteriographic changes in laboratory studies include transient elevations in BUN, serum creatinine and glucose. Complications due to this procedure during selective visual arteriography include hematomas, thrombosis, pseudoaneurysms at injection site, and dislodgement of arteriosclerotic plaques. Other reactions that may develop include urticaria, hypotension, hypertension, and insignificant changes in renal function and liver evaluation tests.

Neurological complications may ensue when the contrast media is introduced into the cerebral vasculature and may be manifested by neuromuscular disorders, seizures, loss of consciousness, hemiplegia, unilateral dysesthesias, visual field defects, aphasia, amnesia, and respiratory difficulties. Such untoward reactions are generally temporary, although permanent visual field defects have occurred.

Dosage and Administration: Diatrizoate solutions are available for *oral, intravenous, intra-arterial* and *rectal* administration. It is also available for *instillation* into the genitourinary tract. In infants and children and in certain adults, the medium may be injected intramuscularly. Prior to injection the solution should be warmed. A test dose must be given prior to parenteral administration. The sensitivity test most often performed is the slow injection of 0.5 to 1 ml of the radiopaque medium, administered intravenously, prior to injection of the full diagnostic dose. It should be noted that the absence of a reaction to the test dose does not preclude the possibility of a reaction to the full diagnostic dose.

The details of administration and the dose and type of preparation to be used will depend on the status and size of the patient and the information desired. The physician is referred to the medical literature and the manufacturer's package circular for specific details.

Availability:

Diatrizoate Meglumine

CARDIOGRAFIN® Injection, 85% in vials of 50 ml. **(Squibb)**

CYSTOGRAFIN® Injection, 30% in bottles of 100 and 300 ml with sufficient capacity for dilution up to 500 ml. **(Squibb)**

DIATRIZOATE MEGLUMINE Injection, 76% in vials of 20 and 50 ml. **(Squibb)**

GASTROGRAFIN® Oral Solution, 76% in bottles of 120 ml. **(Squibb)**

HYPAQUE-CYSTO® Injection, 30% in bottles of 300 ml containing 100 ml of solution and in bottles of 500 ml containing 250 ml of solution. **(Winthrop)**

HYPAQUE-DIU® Injection, 30% in bottles of 300 ml with or without infusion set. **(Winthrop)**

HYPAQUE® MEGLUMINE Injection, 60% in vials of 20, 30, 50 and 100 ml. **(Winthrop)**

RENO-M-30® Injection, 30% in vials of 50 and 100 ml. **(Squibb)**

RENO-M-60® Injection, 60% in vials of 10, 30 and 50 ml with sufficient excess for sensitivity testing and in single-dose bottles of 100 ml. **(Squibb)**

RENO-M-DIP Solution, 30% in bottles of 300 ml with administration set. The solution also contains the sequestering agent disodium edetate, 0.04%, and is used for drip infusion pyelography. **(Squibb)**

w/Iodipamide Meglumine

SINOGRAFIN® Injection, 40% with meglumine iodipamide, 20% in vials of 10 ml. **(Squibb)**

w/Diatrizoate Sodium

HYPAQUE®-M 75% Injection, 50% with sodium diatrizoate, 25% in vials of 20 and 50 ml containing 15 and 37.5 gm respectively of the radiopaque medium. **(Winthrop)**

HYPAQUE-M 90% Injection, 60% with sodium diatrizoate, 30% in vials of 50 ml containing 45 gm of the radiopaque medium. **(Winthrop)**

RENOGRAFIN®-60 Injection, 52% with sodium diatrizoate, 8% in vials of 10, 30 and 50 ml and in single-dose bottles of 100 ml. **(Squibb)**

RENOGRAFIN-76 Injection, 66% with sodium diatrizoate, 10% in vials of 20 and 50 ml with sufficient excess for sensitivity testing and in single-dose bottles of 100 and 200 ml. **(Squibb)**

RENOVIST® Injection, 34.3% with sodium diatrizoate, 35% in vials of 50 ml. **(Squibb)**

RENOVIST® II Injection, 28.5% with sodium diatrizoate, 29.1% in vials of 30 and 60 ml. **(Squibb)**

Diatrizoate Sodium

HYPAQUE® SODIUM Injection, 20% in bottles of 100 ml (for retrograde pyelography only). **(Winthrop)**

HYPAQUE SODIUM Injection, 25% in bottles of 300 ml with or without infusion set. **(Winthrop)**

HYPAQUE SODIUM Injection, 50% in vials of 20, 30 and 50 ml. **(Winthrop)**

HYPAQUE SODIUM ORAL: **(Winthrop)**

Liquid, 249 mg/ml of iodine in bottles of 120 ml containing 50 gm.

Powder for Solution, 600 mg/gm iodine in cans of 250 gm with measuring spoon (approx. 10 gm capacity).

DIAZEPAM Ⓒ IV

Chemical Name: 7-Chloro-1,3-dihydro-1-methyl-5-phenyl-2*H*-1,4-benzodiazepin-2-one.

Description: Diazepam, a benzodiazepine derivative, is a psychotherapeutic agent structurally and pharmacologically related to chlordiazepoxide and to oxazepam. It occurs as a colorless, crystalline powder insoluble in water and sparingly soluble in alcohol and in propylene glycol. Its molecular weight is 284.74.

The drug presumably acts on parts of the limbic system, the thalamus and hypothalamus, producing calming effects. Unlike chlorpromazine and reserpine, diazepam has no demonstrable blocking action on the peripheral autonomic system, nor does it produce extrapyramidal adverse reactions; however, animals treated with high doses of diazepam did have transient ataxia. In clinical studies, pregnant patients were found to have measurable blood levels of the drug in both maternal and cord blood, indicating placental transfer of the drug.

Following oral administration, the drug appears to be well absorbed from the gastrointestinal tract and exerts its effects within ½ to 1 hour. Following intramuscular injection, effects of the drug appear in 15 to 30 minutes. The onset of action is much more rapid after IV administration and the effects may persist for as long as 3 hours. The drug is detoxified in the liver to a metabolite which may be further metabolized to an amino acid derivative. The metabolites of diazepam are excreted primarily as glucuronides in the urine and feces.

Indications: Symptomatic relief of tension and anxiety states brought about by stress or environment; aids in the treatment of somatic complaints of emotional origin; in psychoneurotic states where tension, anxiety, apprehension or agitation exists alone or associated with depressive symptoms; in the relief of symptoms of acute alcohol withdrawal, including acute agitation, tremor, impending or acute delirium tremens, and hallucinosis; adjunctively for relief of apprehension, anxiety and acute stress reaction prior to surgical procedures; in convulsive disorders; and in the alleviation of skeletal muscle spasm associated with local pathology, cerebral palsy, paraplegia, athetosis, stiff-man syndrome, and tetanus. Parenteral diazepam is a useful adjunct in status epilepticus, severe recurrent convulsive seizures, prior to cardioversion or endoscopic procedures. The physician is advised to reevaluate the status of drug treatment when given for periods extending beyond 4 months.

Contraindications: In infants, in patients with known hypersensitivity to diazepam, acute narrow-angle glaucoma, and in open-angle glaucoma unless patients are receiving appropriate therapy.

Warnings: When administered intravenously the solution should be injected slowly, directly into the vein, taking at least 1 minute for each 1 ml (5 mg) given. The solution should not be mixed or diluted with other solutions or drugs, and should not be added to other intravenous fluids. Although rare, apnea and cardiac arrest have been noted, usually following intravenous administration, especially in elderly or very ill patients and in those with limited pulmonary reserve. Resuscitative equipment including that necessary to support respiration should be readily available. Parenteral diazepam is not recommended as the sole treatment for psychotic or severely depressed patients. Also, it should not be administered to patients in shock, coma, or in acute alcoholic intoxication with depression of vital signs. Because of its CNS-depressive effects, patients should be cautioned not to engage in activities requiring alertness or skill. When oral diazepam is used as an adjunct in treating convulsive disorders, the possibility of an increase in the frequency and/or severity of grand mal seizures may require an increase in the dosage of the anticonvulsant. Additionally, abrupt withdrawal of diazepam in such cases may temporarily increase the frequency and/or severity of seizures. Patients should also be advised against the simultaneous ingestion of alcohol and similar acting drugs. Withdrawal symptoms (similar to those noted with barbiturates and alcohol) have occurred following abrupt discontinuance of diazepam (convulsions, tremor, abdominal and muscle cramps, vomiting and sweating). These were usually limited to those patients who had received excessive doses over an extended period of time. Addiction-prone individuals should be under careful supervision when receiving diazepam because of the predisposition of such patients to habituation and dependence. Concomitant use with a narcotic agent requires that the dosage of the narcotic be reduced by at least ⅓ and administered in small increments. There have been reports of an increased risk of congenital malformations and the use of diazepam during the first trimester of pregnancy. Therefore, unless the need is urgent, use of the drug during the gestation period should be avoided. Also, measureable amounts of diazepam have been found in maternal and cord blood indicating placental transfer. Until additional information regarding safe use is available, it is not recommended for obstetrical use.

Precautions: Caution is advisable when combined with other drugs which may potentiate the action of diazepam: phenothiazines, narcotics, barbiturates, MAO inhibitors and other depressants; in severely depressed patients, especially those with suicidal tendencies; in patients with impaired renal or hepatic function. In elderly and debilitated patients, dosage should be limited to the smallest effective amount to preclude the development of ataxia or oversedation. Injectable diazepam is not recommended for obstetric use. Since an increase in the cough reflex and laryngospasm may occur with peroral endoscopic procedures, the use of a topical anesthetic and the availability of specific countermeasures are recommended. The safety and efficacy of injectable diazepam in children under 12 years of age have not been established.

Adverse Reactions: Most commonly reported were drowsiness, fatigue and ataxia. Infrequently encountered were confusion, constipation, depression, diplopia, dysarthria, headache, hiccups, hypoactivity, hypotension, incontinence, jaundice, changes in libido, nausea, phlebitis at injection site, changes in salivation, skin rash, slurred speech, syncope, tremor, urinary retention, urticaria, vertigo and blurred vision. Paradoxical reactions such as acute hyperexcited states, anxiety, hallucinations, increased muscle spasticity, insomnia, rage, sleep disturbances and stimulation have been reported; should these occur, use of the drug should be discontinued. Because of isolated reports of neutropenia and jaundice, periodic blood counts and liver function tests are advisable during long-term therapy. Minor changes in EEG patterns, usually low-voltage fast activity, have been observed in patients during and after diazepam therapy and are of no known significance. Slow intravenous administration, 5 mg (1 ml)/minute is advised in order to minimize the possibility of venous thrombosis, phlebitis, local irritation, swelling and, rarely, vascular impairment. It is essential not to use small veins such as those on the dorsum of the hand or wrist; also extreme care should be taken to avoid intraarterial administration or extravasation.

Dosage and Administration: *Orally, intramuscularly* (deep into the muscle) or *intravenously* (slow administration). Must be individualized according to diagnosis, severity of symptoms and degree of response. While the usual daily dosages will meet the needs of most patients, there will be some who may require higher doses. In the first few days of administration a cumulative effect of the drug may occur, and therefore the dosage should be increased only after stabilization is apparent. *Orally.* Adults—symptomatic relief of anxiety and tension in psychoneurosis and anxiety reactions: 2 to 10 mg, 2 to 4 times daily depending upon severity of symptoms. Symptomatic relief in acute alcohol withdrawal: 10 mg 3 or 4 times during the first 24 hours, reducing to 5 mg 3 or 4 times daily as needed. Adjunctively for relief of skeletal muscle spasms: 2 to 10 mg 3 or 4 times daily and for convulsive disorders, 2 to 10 mg 2 to 4 times daily. Elderly and debilitated patients, or in the presence of debilitating disease: 2 to 2.5 mg 1 or 2 times daily initially, increase gradually as needed and tolerated. Children because of varied responses, therapy should be initiated—with lowest dose and increase as required—1 to 2.5 mg 3 or 4 times daily initially; increase gradually as needed and tolerated. *Parenterally.* Treatment of moderate to severe psychoneurotic reactions: 2 to 10 mg, may be repeated in 3 to 4 hours, if required. Symptomatic relief of acute alcohol withdrawal syndrome: 10 mg initially, then 5 to 10 mg in 3 or 4 hours depending upon the clinical response. Adjunctively for the relief of acute stress prior to endoscopic procedures: up to 20 mg *intravenously* or 5 to 10 mg *intramuscularly* approximately 30 minutes prior to the procedure. Adjunctively for the relief of muscle spasm: 5 to 10 mg initially, may be repeated in 3 or 4 hours, if necessary. Tetanus may require large doses. Adjunctively in status epilepticus and in severe recurrent convulsive seizures, 5 to 10 mg initially, may be repeated in 2 to 4 hours, if required. For relief of preoperative anxiety and tension: 10 mg *intramuscularly* (preferred route) prior to surgical procedure. If atropine, scopolamine or other premedications are desired, they must be administered in separate syringes. For management of acute stress reactions prior to cardioversion, 5 to 15 mg *intravenously* within 5 to 10 minutes prior to the procedure. Lower doses (usually 2 to 5 mg) and slow increase in dosage should be used for elderly or debilitated patients and when other sedative drugs are administered. Not for use in children under 6 months. The physician is urged to read carefully the package literature for the management of overdosage.

Availability:

Ⓒ IV VALIUM®: **(Roche)**

Injectable, 5 mg/ml in ampuls of 2 ml, in Tel-E-Ject® (disposable syringes) of 2 ml and in vials of 10 ml.

Tablets, 2, 5 and 10 mg in bottles of 100 and 500, in Prescription Paks of 50 and in Tel-E-Dose packages of 100.

DIAZOXIDE

Chemical Name: 7-Chloro-3-methyl-2*H*-1, 2, 4-benzothiadiazine 1,1-dioxide.

Description: Diazoxide, a nondiuretic thiazide derivative, is a rapid-acting antihypertensive agent. It shares with the diuretic benzothiadiazines the capacity to reduce blood pressure in hypertensive patients. The injection is a clear, colorless, aqueous solution in which the pH has been adjusted to approximately 11.6 with sodium hydroxide.

Following intravenous administration, a decrease in peripheral resistance occurs due to selective smooth-muscle relaxation of the arterioles. A prompt reduction in blood pressure generally appears within 5 minutes (usually within 1 or 2 minutes) followed by a relatively rapid increase in blood pressure in the next 10 to 30 minutes, which continues more slowly over the following 2 to 12 hours, almost reaching, but rarely exceeding, pretreatment levels. This blood-pressure reduction increases cardiac output. A second administration may be required for a satisfactory reduction of blood pressure if the first injection fails to produce an adequate response within 30 minutes. Renal blood flow is increased after an initial decrease while coronary and cerebral blood flow are maintained. Following oral administration, an increase in blood glucose concentration occurs without appreciably affecting hypertension. Patients with normal kidney function respond to the drug within 1 hour and may experience hyperglycemia for up to 8 hours.

While it has been demonstrated that an antihypertensive response has been obtained with slow injection of diazoxide, a greater antihypertensive effect is induced with rapid intravenous administration, usually within 30 seconds.

Over 90% of diazoxide is bound to serum protein. This binding may displace other substances or drugs also bound to protein, such as bilirubin or coumarin anticoagulants. These potential interactions must be considered when administering the drug intravenously. When thiazides or other commonly used potent diuretics are added to the treatment regimen, the hyperglycemic, hyperuricemic, and antihypertensive effects of diazoxide may be potentiated. The plasma half-life of the drug ranges from 19.7 to 36.3 hours; however, the duration of the antihypertensive effect is variable, generally lasting less than 12 hours.

Animal studies in several species have shown that the drug exerts its action through its direct effect on peripheral arterioles. This effect does not impair cardiac function or seriously diminish perfusion of the kidneys. In addition, in each species tested, diazoxide was reported to elicit hyperglycemia, increased serum-free fatty acids and decreased plasma-insulin levels by a mechanism thought to involve both suppression of insulin release and enhanced catecholamine action. Cataracts have also been observed in a few animals receiving repeated daily doses of intravenous or oral diazoxide.

Although the data are not conclusive, reproduction and teratology studies in several species of animals indicate that the drug, when administered during the critical period of embryo formation, may interfere with normal fetal development, possibly through altered glucose metabolism. Parturition was occasionally prolonged in animals treated at term.

Indications: For the emergency reduction of blood pressure in malignant hypertension in hospitalized patients, when prompt and urgent decrease of diastolic pressure is required. Treatment with orally effective antihypertensive agents should be instituted as soon as the hypertensive emergency is controlled. **Note:** Diazoxide is not effective against hypertension due to pheochromocytoma. Diazoxide has also been found useful in the management of hypoglycemia due to hyperinsulism associated with the following conditions: *Adults:* Inoperable islet cell adenoma or carcinoma, or extrapancreatic malignancy. *Infants and children:* Leucine sensitivity, islet cell hyperplasia or adenoma, or adenomatosis, nesidioblastosis, extrapancreatic malignancy. Its use is limited to hypoglycemia resulting from these conditions, and should be employed only after the diagnosis has been firmly established. The drug may be used preoperatively as a temporary measure, and postoperatively if the hypoglycemia persists.

Contraindications: *Parenterally,* in patients with compensatory hypertension, such as that associated with aortic coarctation or arteriovenous shunt, and in those hypersensitive to diazoxide or to other thiazides, unless the potential benefits outweigh the possible risks. *Orally,* in patients with functional hypoglycemia.

Warnings: Safe use of the drug in pregnant women or in children has not been established.

Clinical observation suggests that the drug crosses the placental barrier and appears in cord blood. The drug may produce fetal or neonatal hyperbilirubinemia, thrombocytopenia, altered carbohydrate metabolism, and possibly other adverse reactions reported to have occurred in adults. Hyperglycemia and hyperosmolar coma associated with transient cataracts developed in one infant receiving repeated daily doses of oral diazoxide. The disturbed carbohydrate metabolism was successfully treated with insulin. Since thiazides can appear in breast milk, this possibility should be considered with diazoxide. Hyperglycemia occurs in the majority of patients, but usually requires treatment only in patients with diabetes mellitus; this reaction responds to the usual management including insulin. Therefore, blood glucose levels should be monitored especially in patients with diabetes or in those requiring multiple injections of this drug. Since diazoxide causes sodium retention, repeated injections may precipitate edema and congestive heart failure—the extracellular fluid may be a cause of treatment failure in nonresponsive patients. This retention responds characteristically to diuretic agents if adequate renal function is present. Although no evidence of excessive anticoagulant effects has been reported, patients, especially those who are hypoalbuminemic and who are receiving diazoxide and coumarin or its derivatives, may require a reduction in dosage of the anticoagulant. Parenteral administration requires special care when used concurrently with other drugs which act by direct peripheral vasodilation, especially hydralazine, the nitrites and papaverine-like compounds.

Precautions: Frequent monitoring of the patient's blood pressure is required until it has stabilized. Hypotension may occur; therefore, adequate facilities to treat such untoward reactions including sympathomimetic drugs should be readily available. The injection should be administered *only* into a peripheral vein. Because the alkalinity of the solution is irritating to tissue, extravascular injection or leakage should be avoided. Subcutaneous administration has produced inflammation and pain but without necrosis. If leakage into subcutaneous tissues occurs, the area should be treated conservatively. Special care is required in patients who have impaired cerebral or cardiac circulation, i.e., patients in whom abrupt and brief reduction in blood pressure might be detrimental. Patients undergoing peritoneal dialysis or hemodialysis may require more than one injection of diazoxide.

Adverse Reactions: Frequently noted following parenteral administration was sodium and water retention after repeated injections. Less frequently noted were hypotension which may progress to shock levels; myocardial ischemia, usually transient, but possibly leading to thrombosis and manifested by anginal pain, atrial and ventricular arrhythmias, and marked electrocardiographic changes; cerebral ischemia, also usually transient may lead to thrombosis which may be manifested by unconsciousness, convulsions, paralysis or confusion, or by focal neurological deficit such as numbness of the hands; persistent retention of nitrogenous wastes after repeated injections; and sensitivity reactions, such as rash, leukopenia, fever and, rarely, acute pancreatitis. One patient experienced papilledema which was induced by plasma volume expansion secondary to the administration of diazoxide. Other adverse reactions noted were orthostatic hypotension, sweating, flushing, and generalized or localized sensation of warmth, supraventricular tachycardia and palpitation; bradycardia; various transient neurological findings secondary to alterations in regional blood flow to the brain, such as headache (sometimes throbbing), dizziness, lightheadedness, sleepiness (also reported as lethargy, somnolence or drowsiness), euphoria, tinnitus and momentary hearing loss, and weakness of short duration; chest discomfort or nonanginal "tightness in the chest"; transient hyperglycemia in nondiabetic patients; dyspnea, cough and choking sensation; nausea and vomiting and/or abdominal discomfort, anorexia, alteration in taste, parotid swelling, salivation, dry mouth, lacrimation, ileus, constipation, and diarrhea; warmth or pain along the injected vein; cellulitis without sloughing and/or phlebitis at the site of extravasation; back pain; and increased nocturia. Rarely noted were apprehension or anxiety, malaise and blurred vision.

Patients receiving oral diazoxide may experience, in addition to some of the foregoing, diabetic ketoacidosis and hyperosmolar nonketotic coma which may develop quite rapidly and may be counteracted with insulin and restoration of fluid and electrolyte balance. Prolonged surveillance is essential in view of the long half-life of the drug. Other frequently noted complications include hirsutism of the lanugo type, appearing mainly on the forehead, back and limbs, and is most commonly seen in women and children. This phenomenon usually subsides on discontinuation of therapy. Hyperglycemia or glycosuria may require reduction in dosage in order to avoid progression to ketoacidosis or hyperosmolar coma. Thrombocytopenia, with or without purpura, may require discontinuation of the drug. Neutropenia, skin rash, headache, weakness, and malaise may also occur. Other adverse reactions which have been observed include transient hypertension, chest pains (rare); decreased hemoglobin/hematocrit; excessive bleeding; decreased immunogammaglobulinemia; increased SGOT, alkaline phosphatase, azotemia, decreased creatinine clearance, reversible nephrotic syndrome, decreased urinary output, hematuria, albuminuria; insomnia, polyneuritis, paresthesia, pruritus, extrapyramidal signs; transient cataracts, subconjunctival hemorrhage, ring scotoma, blurred vision, diplopia, lacrimation; monilial dermatitis, herpes, advance in bone age, alopecia; fever, lymphadenopathy, gout, acute pancreatitis/pancreatic necrosis, galactorrhea, and enlargement of lump in breast. Overdosage is characterized by an undesirable hypotension and excessive hyperglycemia. The hypotension can usually be controlled by sympathomimetic agents, such as norepinephrine, and the hyperglycemia will usually respond to the conventional agents for treating this condition. Diazoxide may be removed from the blood by peritoneal dialysis or hemodialysis.

Dosage and Administration: *Intravenously only.* With the patient recumbent, the contents of 1 ampul are administered in 30 seconds or less. The dosage for children may be calculated on the basis of 5 mg/kg of body weight (0.3 ml/kg). Slow intravenous injection may fail to reduce the blood pressure or may produce an exceedingly short response. Successive injections frequently produce a better response. When the blood pressure is stabilized, oral therapy with other antihypertensive agents should be substituted. *Orally.* Patients should be under close medical supervision, and blood glucose level should be carefully monitored until the patient's condition has stabilized satisfactorily; in most instances, this may be accomplished in several days. *For adults and children,* the usual daily dosage is 3 to 8 mg/kg of body weight, divided into 2 or 3 equal doses every 8 or 12 hours. In certain instances, patients with refractory hypoglycemia may require higher dosages. Ordinarily, an appropriate starting dosage is 3 mg/kg/day, divided into 3 equal doses every 8 hours. Thus, an average adult patient would receive a starting dosage of approximately 200 mg daily. *For infants and newborns,* the usual daily dosage is 8 to 15 mg/kg of body weight, divided into 2 or 3 equal doses every 8 or 12 hours. An appropriate starting dosage is 10 mg/kg/day, divided into 3 equal doses every 8 hours.

Availability:
HYPERSTAT® I.V. Injection, 300 mg in ampuls of 20 ml. **(Schering)**
PROGLYCEM®: **(Schering)**
Capsules, 50 and 100 mg in bottles of 100.
Oral Suspension, 50 mg/ml in bottles of 30 ml with calibrated dropper.

DIBUCAINE HYDROCHLORIDE

Chemical Name: 2-*n*-Butoxy-*N*-(2-diethylaminoethyl)-cinchoninamide hydrochloride.

Description: Specially prepared solutions containing dibucaine hydrochloride in concentrations of 1:200 (5 mg/ml), 1:400 (2.5 mg/ml) and 1:1500 (0.667 mg/ml). A long-acting local anesthetic when applied to mucous membranes and in infiltration and spinal anesthesia, occurring as colorless or white crystals or white, crystalline powder freely soluble in water and in alcohol.

Dibucaine, a quinoline derivative, is approximately 20 times as potent and as toxic as procaine when injected and is thus used in smaller concentrations. Duration of spinal anesthesia ranges from 3 to 4 hours, but can be prolonged up to 6 hours by the addition of epinephrine. As with procaine, its toxicity is manifested by CNS stimulation followed by depression.

Indications: In spinal anesthesia, particularly the saddle-block method for relief of obstetric pain.

Contraindications: It is absolutely contraindicated in the presence of meningitis, cranial hemorrhage, tumors, poliomyelitis, moribund patients, blood infections, pernicious anemia with cord symptoms, arthritis, spondylitis, tuberculosis or metastatic lesions in the spinal column; also in those conditions rendering spinal puncture impossible. It is relatively contraindicated in hysteria or excessive nervous tension, chronic backache, preoperative headache or history of migraine, hypersensitivity to drugs, possibility of severe hemorrhage during surgery, shock, hypotension, hemorrhagic spinal fluid, cardiac decompensation, massive pleural effusions, and markedly increased intraabdominal pressure. In obstetrics, pelvic disproportion, abruptio placentae praevia with significant bleeding, unengaged head, need for intrauterine manipulation, and during the early stages of labor are additional contraindications to its use.

Warnings: Ephedrine, oxygen and a quick-acting barbiturate should be in readiness in case toxic symptoms of overdosages such as sudden fall in blood pressure, respiratory difficulties or CNS stimulation occur. Patients with known drug sensitivities should be pretested before a local anesthetic agent is administered.

Precautions: Anesthetist should be equipped to provide a rigidly aseptic technique; be prepared to remain in constant attendance; be equipped to deal with complications or side effects that may arise; be familiar with the contraindications to spinal anesthesia.

Adverse Reactions: Cessation of respiration, hypotension, postanesthetic headache, nausea and vomiting, palsies, meningitis, myelitis, and drug idiosyncrasy.

Dosage and Administration: For dosage schedule see package insert. Careful adherence to prescribed technique is necessary if satisfactory results are to be achieved. Attention must be given to proper type of needle, correct site for injection, positioning of patient, speed of injection, extent of analgesia and availability of measures for control of possible complications of hypotension. Complete information on technique of saddle block anesthesia may be obtained from the manufacturer.

Availability:
NUPERCAINE®: **(Ciba)**
Heavy Solution, 1:400 in 5% dextrose in ampuls of 2 ml.
Spinal Anesthesia, 1:200 in ampuls of 2 ml; 1:1500 in ampuls of 20 ml.

DICHLORPHENAMIDE

Chemical Name: 4,5-Dichloro-m-benzenedisulfonamide.

Description: Dichlorphenamide, a potent carbonic anhydrase inhibitor, occurs as a white or nearly white, crystalline compound with a molecular weight of 305.16. It is very slightly soluble in water but soluble in dilute solutions of sodium carbonate and sodium hydroxide. Dilute alkaline solutions of the drug are stable at room temperature.

Dichlorphenamide interferes with the catalytic activity of carbonic anhydrase, which is concerned with the formation of $H+$ and HCO_3- ions and the conservation of base as sodium bicarbonate. Under the influence of dichlorphenamide, the renal excretion of sodium, potassium, chloride, and bicarbonate is increased and an alkaline urine is produced. The activity of this agent is not impaired in the presence of an acid urine such as that accompanying the use of ammonium chloride.

As with all carbonic anhydrase inhibitors, it can cause a metabolic (renal) acidosis by depressing tubular reabsorption of bicarbonate and increasing the renal excretion of sodium and potassium ions in excess of chloride ions. However, the drug has been shown to cause a relatively greater chloruresis than similar compounds, and thus the potential for significant metabolic acidosis is lessened.

Dichlorphenamide does not appear to be concentrated in gastric mucosa in sufficient amounts to influence materially the activity of carbonic anhydrase in this tissue. Thus, in dogs gastric motility or secretion is not affected to any significant degree by this compound.

Considerable evidence indicates that carbonic anhydrase inhibitors reduce intraocular pressure by partially suppressing the secretion of fluid (inflow), although the mechanism of this function is not fully understood. Evidence suggests that bicarbonate ions are produced in the ciliary body by hydration of carbon dioxide under the influence of carbonic anhydrase and diffuse into the posterior chamber with sodium ions. The aqueous fluid contains more sodium and bicarbonate ions than does plasma and is consequently hypertonic. Water is attracted to the posterior chamber by osmosis. Systemic administration of a carbonic anhydrase inhibitor has been shown to inactivate carbonic anhydrase in the ciliary body of the rabbit's eye and to reduce the high concentration of bicarbonate ions in ocular fluids.

Dichlorphenamide has been given to dogs for 6 months with essentially no sign of toxicity. Instillation of a 1% solution into the conjunctival sac of the rabbit's eye produced no evidence of local anesthetic activity or irritation. Clinical studies show that dichlorphenamide in high doses causes some decrease in renal blood flow and glomerular filtration rate.

Intraocular pressure begins to fall within 1 hour after oral administration, reaches a maximal level within 2 to 4 hours, and is maintained at a reduced level for approximately 6 to 12 hours.

Indications: Adjunctive treatment of chronic simple (wide-angle) glaucoma, secondary glaucoma (acute phase), and for preoperative control of intraocular tension of glaucoma.

Contraindications: In order to avoid the likelihood of blood pH decreases below 7.2, dichlorphenamide should not be used if the arterial pCO_2 is greater than 63 mm Hg. It is also contraindicated in the presence of hepatic insufficiency, renal failure, adrenocortical insufficiency, hyperchloremic acidosis, or in conditions in which sodium and/or potassium serum levels are depressed. The drug should not be used in patients with severe pulmonary obstruction who are unable to increase their alveolar ventilation since increased acidosis may occur.

Warnings: Laboratory studies with rats have demonstrated teratogenic effects (skeletal anomalies) with high doses. There has been no evidence of these effects in patients treated with dichlorphenamide; however, the drug should not be used in women of childbearing potential or during pregnancy, especially during the first trimester, unless the expected benefits outweigh the potential hazards to the mother and fetus.

Precautions: Potassium excretion is increased by dichlorphenamide and hypokalemia may develop with brisk diuresis, when severe cirrhosis is present, or during concomitant use of steroids or ACTH. Interference with adequate oral electrolyte intake will also contribute to hypokalemia. Digitalis therapy may exaggerate the metabolic effects of hypokalemia especially with reference to myocardial activity. Therefore, close monitoring of the electrolyte balance, blood pH and blood gases of the patient should be performed during therapy. Dichlorphenamide should be used with caution in patients with severe degrees of respiratory acidosis. Therapy with this drug should be discontinued if the pH of the blood falls below 7.2. The possible occurrence of agranulocytosis, thrombocytopenia, or the formation of renal calculi should be considered.

Adverse Reactions: Gastrointestinal disturbances such as anorexia, nausea, and vomiting; loss of weight; constipation; urinary frequency; renal colic; renal calculi; mild skin eruptions; pruritus; leukopenia, agranulocytosis, thrombocytopenia; headache; weakness; nervousness; globus hystericus; sedation; lassitude; depression; confusion, disorientation; dizziness; ataxia; tremor; tinnitus; and paresthesias of the hands, feet, and tongue. The occurrence of one or more of these reactions requires a reduction in dosage or temporary discontinuance of the drug.

Dosage and Administration: *Orally.* For glaucoma, the usual dose is 100 to 200 mg initially, followed by 100 mg every 12 hours until the desired response has been obtained. Maintenance therapy, 25 to 50 mg 1 to 3 times daily. Therapy is more successful when administered in conjunction with miotics such as pilocarpine, physostigmine, isoflurophate, demecarium bromide, or carbachol.

Availability:
DARANIDE® Tablets, 50 mg in bottles of 100. **(Merck Sharp & Dohme)**
ORATROL® Tablets, 50 mg in bottles of 250. **(Alcon)**

DICLOXACILLIN: see The Penicillins

DICYCLOMINE HYDROCHLORIDE

Chemical Name: (Bicyclohexyl)-1-carboxylic acid 2-(diethylamino)ethyl ester hydrochloride.

Description: Dicyclomine hydrochloride, an anticholinergic, is an amino ester of a substituted alicylic carboxylic acid. It occurs as a white, odorless, crystalline powder freely soluble in water.

The compound has a direct relaxant effect on smooth muscle as well as a depressant effect on parasympathetic function. These dual actions produce relief of spasm with minimum atropine-like side effects; nevertheless, there is no conclusive evidence as to whether or not anticholinergic-antispasmodic agents will facilitate healing of the peptic ulcer, or prevent complications or recurrences. Phenobarbital is added for its sedative action.

Indications: Adjunctive therapy in the treatment of peptic ulcer. May also be of use in the management of the irritable bowel syndrome (irritable colon, spastic colon, mucous colitis, acute enterocolitis, and functional gastrointestinal disorders), and in neurogenic bowel disturbances including the splenic flexure syndrome and neurogenic colon. The *syrup* is also indicated for infant colic.

Contraindications: Anticholinergic-antispasmodics are contraindicated in obstructive uropathy (bladder neck obstruction due to prostatic hypertrophy), obstructive disease of the gastrointestinal tract such as achalasia, and pyloroduodenal stenosis, paralytic ileus, intestinal atony of the elderly or debilitated patient, unstable cardiovascular status in acute hemorrhage, severe ulcerative colitis, toxic megacolon complicating ulcerative colitis, and myasthenia gravis.

Warnings: Intolerance to high environmental temperature may occur with the use of this drug and may lead to heat prostration (fever and heat stroke) due to reduced perspiration. Since diarrhea may be an early symptom of incomplete intestinal obstruction, especially in patients with ileostomy or colostomy, the use of this drug in this instance would be inappropriate and possibly harmful. Patients should be forewarned that in the event of drowsiness and/or dizziness, they should not undertake activities requiring alertness or physical coordination.

Precautions: Should be used with caution in patients known to have or are suspected of having glaucoma or prostatic hypertrophy. Use with caution in patients with autonomic neuropathy, hepatic or renal disease, ulcerative colitis (since large doses may suppress intestinal motility to the point of producing a paralytic ileus and the use of this drug may precipitate or aggravate the serious complication of toxic megacolon), hyperthyroidism, coronary heart disease, congestive heart failure, cardiac arrhythmias, hypertension, and hiatal hernia associated with reflux esophagitis since drugs of this type may aggravate this condition. In the treatment of gastric ulcer, the drug may cause a delay in gastric emptying time and may complicate such therapy (antral stasis). Dicyclomine may not be effective in the presence of complications due to billiary tract disease. Tachycardia should be ruled out prior to therapy since an increase in heart rate may occur. Overdosage may produce a curare-like action.

Adverse Reactions: Most of the unwanted effects associated with the use of anticholinergic agents are manifestations of their pharmacologic actions. Those that may occur include xerostomia, urinary hesitancy and retention, blurred vision, tachycardia, palpitations, mydriasis, cycloplegia, increased ocular tension, loss of taste, headache, nervousness, drowsiness, weakness, dizziness, insomnia, nausea, vomiting, impotence, suppression of lactation, constipation, bloated feeling, severe allergic reaction or drug idiosyncrasies including anaphylaxis, urticaria and other dermal manifestations, some degree of mental confusion and/or excitement, especially in elderly patients, and decreased perspiration. With the injectable form patients may experience a temporary sensation of lightheadedness, and occasionally local irritation.

Dosage and Administration: *Orally,* 3 or 4 times daily. Adults, 1 tablet or 1 or 2 capsules or teaspoonsful of syrup. Children, 1 capsule or 1 teaspoonful of syrup. Infants, 1/2 teaspoonful of syrup. *Intramuscularly* only. Adults, 10 to 20 mg every 4 to 6 hours.

Availability:

Dicyclomine Hydrochloride

Tablets, 10 and 20 mg in bottles of 1000. **(Lederle)**

BENTYL®: **(Merrell-National)**

Capsules, 10 mg in bottles of 100, 500 and 1000 and in unit-dose dispensers of 100.

Injection, 10 mg/ml in ampuls and prefilled syringes of 2 ml and in multiple-dose vials of 10 ml.

Syrup, 10mg/5 ml in bottles of 1 pint.

Tablets, 20 mg in bottles of 100, 500 and 1000 and in unit-dose dispensers of 100.

w/Phenobarbital (**Warning:** May be habit forming)
Capsules, 10 mg with phenobarbital, 15 mg in bottles of 100, 500 and 1000.
Syrup, 10 mg with phenobarbital, 15 mg/5 ml in bottles of 1 pint.
Tablets, 20 mg with phenobarbital, 15 mg in bottles of 100 and 500.

DIENESTROL: see The Estrogens

DIETHYLCARBAMAZINE CITRATE

Chemical Name: *N,N*-Diethyl-4-methy-l-piperazinecarboxamide dihydrogen citrate.

Description: An antihelminthic agent, composed of a synthetic organic compound that is free of toxic metallic elements; exhibits specific action against several species of filaria. The piperazine ring may be of fundamental importance in the activity of this compound, although piperazine itself has no activity against filaria.

Indications: Treatment of Bancroft's filariasis resulting from *Wuchereria bancrofti;* onchocerciasis resulting from *Onchocerca volvulus,* creeping eruptions (larva migrans) caused by *Ancylostoma braziliense* or *Ancylostoma canium* worms, loiasis, ascariasis, particularly those types due to *Ascaris lumbricoides* infestations; and tropical eosinophilia—of which symptoms were relieved and normal eosinophil counts were established.

Precautions: Should be administered carefully to avoid or control allergic and other unpleasant reactions.

Adverse Reactions: Mild side reactions following treatment of Wuchereria bancrofti infestations are transient but fairly frequent. Headache, lassitude, weakness, or general malaise are most commonly observed. Nausea and vomiting occur in some patients and skin rash is occasionally seen. These effects are not considered serious and do not usually require discontinuation of therapy, unless severe allergic phenomena appear in conjunction with skin rash. Facial edema and pruritus, especially of the eyes, are frequently encountered when given to patients with onchocerciasis. Severe reactions may develop after a single dose when intense infestations are treated, and in such instances patients should be given 1 dose on the first day, 2 doses on the second day, and 3 doses on the third day. If very severe reactions occur, the drug should be withdrawn and antihistamine therapy initiated. After 1 or 2 days, therapy may be resumed, but if severe allergic phenomena again supervene, the drug should be used thereafter only with extreme caution. Giddiness, nausea, vomiting, and malaise may occur more frequently following treatment of ascariasis in children who are malnourished or who suffer from various debilitating diseases. Reactions are specific to the type of infestation being treated, and a proportion of them may be due to disintegration of the worms.

Dosage and Administration: *Orally.* Usual dosage is 2 mg/kg of body weight 3 times daily immediately following meals. A man weighing between 150 and 160 lb would require 150 mg 3 times daily. Acute cases should be treated for 3 to 4 weeks. For ascariasis, 13 mg/kg given once daily for 7 days should reduce the number of worms by 85 to 100%. No pretreatment fasting or post-treatment purging is required. Expulsion of the ascaride generally begins 1 or 2 days after initiation of therapy. The recommended children's dose is 6 to 10 mg/kg 3 times daily for 7 to 10 days. In obstinate cases an additional course of treatment consisting of 10 mg/kg 3 times daily is indicated. The usual dose for tropical eosinophilia is 13 mg/kg once daily for 4 to 7 days.

Availability:
HETRAZAN® Tablets, 50 mg in bottles of 100. **(Lederle)**

DIETHYLPROPION HYDROCHLORIDE Ⓒ IV

Chemical Name: 1-Phenyl-2-diethylamino-1-propanone hydrochloride.

Description: Diethylpropion hydrochloride, a congener of amphetamine, is used clinically solely for the purpose of curbing the appetite. It occurs as a white, crystalline powder soluble in water and in alcohol.

Indications: As a short-term adjunct (a few weeks) in a regimen of weight reduction based on caloric restriction.

Contraindications: Advanced arteriosclerosis, severe hypertension, hyperthyroidism, known hypersensitivity, or idiosyncrasy to sympathomimetic amines, glaucoma, agitated states, patients with a history of drug abuse, during or within 14 days following administration of monoamine oxidase inhibitors (may precipitate a hypertensive crisis).

Warnings: If tolerance to the effect of the drug develops, it is emphasized that the recommended dose not be exceeded but that the drug be withdrawn. Patients should be advised that their ability to engage in hazardous occupations requiring alertness or skill such as driving a motor vehicle or operating machinery may be impaired. The physician should be aware that some patients may develop psychic dependence from the use of amphetamine-like agents, and the possibility of abuse should be kept in mind. The least amount feasible should be prescribed in order to minimize the possibility of overdosage. Extreme fatigue, mental depression, and changes on the EEG usually occur following abrupt withdrawal in patients on prolonged use with high doses. It is generally recognized that when treating pregnant patients all medications should be used with the greatest consideration of the potential harmful effects on the fetus, especially during the first trimester. Diethylpropion is not recommended for use in children under 12 years of age.

Precautions: The physician is urged to use caution in prescribing this drug for patients with hypertension or with symptomatic cardiovascular disease including arrhythmias. Dosage should be well titrated in diabetic patients since their insulin requirements may be altered, in epileptic patients who may experience an increase in convulsive episodes, and in patients taking guanethidine since the hypotensive effect of this drug may be decreased.

Adverse Reactions: Rarely severe enough to require discontinuation of therapy, unpleasant symptoms with diethylpropion hydrochloride have been reported to occur in relatively low incidence. As is characteristic of sympathomimetic agents, it may occasionally cause *CNS effects* such as overstimulation, nervousness, restlessness, dizziness, jitteriness, insomnia, anxiety, euphoria, dysphoria, tremor and, rarely, psychotic episodes at recommended doses. In contrast, CNS depression has been reported. In a few epileptics an increase in convulsive episodes has also been noted. Sympathomimetic *cardiovascular effects* reported include tachycardia, precordial pain, arrhythmia, palpitation, and increased blood pressure. One published report described T-wave changes in the ECG of a healthy young male after ingestion of diethylpropion hydrochloride. *Allergic phenomena* reported include such conditions as rash, urticaria, ecchymosis and erythema. *Gastrointestinal effects* such as unpleasant taste, diarrhea, constipation, nausea, vomiting, and abdominal discomfort have occurred. Specific reports on the hematopoietic system include two instances each of bone marrow depression, agranulocytosis, and leukopenia. A variety of miscellaneous adverse reactions have been noted by physicians. These include dry mouth, increased sweating, dyspnea, menstrual upset, gynecomastia, hair loss, muscle pain, decreased libido, impotence, dysuria, and polyuria. Acute overdosage results in accentuation of the usual pharmacological effects of this class of drugs. They include excitement, agitation, tachycardia, hypertension, mydriasis, slurred speech, ataxia, tremor, chills, hyperreflexia, tachypnea, fever, and toxic psychoses characterized by auditory and visual hallucinations and paranoid delusions. Circulatory failure and death may result from severe overdosage. Management is largely symptomatic and includes gastric lavage and sedation with barbiturates. Intravenous phentolamine is recommended to counteract acute, severe hypertension should this occur.

Dosage and Administration: *Orally.* For adults and children over 12 years of age, one 25-mg tablet 3 times daily 1 hour before meals, and in midevening if desired to overcome night hunger or 1 continuous-release 75-mg tablet daily, swallowed whole, in midmorning.

Availability:
Ⓒ TENUATE®: **(Merrell-National)**
Dospan® Tablets, 75 mg (continuous release) in bottles of 100 and 250.
Tablets, 25 mg in bottles of 100 and 1000.

Ⓒ TEPANIL®: **(Riker)**
Tablets, 25 mg in bottles of 100.
Ten-Tab® Tablets, 75 mg (continuous release) in bottles of 30, 100 and 250.

DIETHYLSTILBESTROL: see The Estrogens

DIFLORASONE DIACETATE: see The Adrenal Corticosteroids

DIGITALIS

Description: Digitalis is the dried leaf of *Digitalis purpurea* and occurs as a dark green powder insoluble in water and in alcohol. The potency is such that 100 mg is equivalent to 1 Digitalis unit, U.S.P. When Digitalis is prescribed, Powdered Digitalis is to be dispensed. The chemical nature of the digitalis glycosides is due to the composition of a steroid nucleus, a lactone ring and a sugar molecule in its molecular structure.

The principal action of digitalis appears to be its ability to enhance the force of myocardial contraction. In patients with clinically latent or overt congestive heart failure, this increased contractile force produces increased cardiac output and decreased heart size, venous pressure and blood volume, with diuresis and relief of existing edema. In patients with atrial fibrillation or atrial flutter, the drug exerts additional effects by way of vagal stimulation and depression of atrio-ventricular conduction to reduce ventricular rate and enhance ventricular efficiency.

Following oral administration, digitalis is adequately, though partially, absorbed from the intestinal tract. The onset of action after oral administration occurs in 1 to 2 hours. Peak of action follows in 6 to 8 hours and the duration of therapeutic action is approximately 24 to 48 hours. A given dose of digitalis is totally eliminated in about 14 days. Existing toxic effects may last for nearly the same period.

Since digitalis glycosides are metabolized in the liver and the unchanged and metabolized components of the drug are excreted chiefly by the kidneys, the elimination of digitalis may be delayed by hepatic or renal dysfunction.

Indications: Congestive heart failure, regardless of etiology. Also useful in controlling cardiac arrhythmias such as atrial fibrillation and flutter, even in the absence of left ventricular failure. Its effectiveness in other types of arrhythmias is less certain, although good results have been obtained in paroxysmal atrial tachycardia. Its value has not been established in cardiogenic shock.

Contraindications: Hypersensitivity to digitalis, evidence of digitalis intoxication, in shock or when there is a mechanical impediment to myocardial contraction such as cardiac tamponade, constrictive pericarditis, and may be ineffective in severe mitral stenosis. Ventricular tachycardia and ventricular fibrillation are contraindications. However, if congestive failure supervenes after a protracted episode of tachycardia and the patient has not received digitalis treatment, the drug may be used.

Warnings: Many of the arrhythmias for which digitalis is advised are identical with those reflecting digitalis intoxication. When the possibility of digitalis intoxication cannot be excluded, cardiac glucosides should be withheld temporarily if the clinical situation permits. Patients with idiopathic hypertrophic subaortic stenosis must be managed with extreme care. Unless cardiac failure is severe, it is doubtful whether digitalis should be employed.

Precautions: Before initiating therapy, it is essential to take a careful history regarding any previous or recent use of digitalis glycosides and an electrocardiogram to aid in later evaluation of digitalis effects. Careful consideration must be given to dosage requirements whenever digitalis is to be used, and patients must be observed closely during the period of digitalization. Attention to digitalis dosage is required in the aged and in the infant. Situations requiring unusual care include acute myocardial infarction, severe pulmonary disease, or far-advanced heart failure, incomplete atrioventricular block, Adams-Stokes syndrome, chronic constrictive pericarditis, acute glomerulonephritis accompanied by congestive failure, rheumatic carditis (especially when severe), electrolyte disturbances particularly hypercalcemia and hypokalemia, renal or hepatic dysfunction, and the use of drugs that may enhance digitalis toxic effects, e.g., rauwolfia and veratrum alkaloids and sympathomimetics of the ephedrine group.

Adverse Reactions: Digitalis intoxication is most common and is dose-related; electrocardiographic monitoring may be necessary to avoid this condition. In patients on thiazide diuresis, the therapeutic and the toxic doses may become identical, because of potassium loss and increased cardiac susceptibility. Digitalis intoxication may be recognized by the following signs and symptoms: *Gastrointestinal*—Anorexia, nausea, vomiting, salivation, diarrhea, abdominal discomfort. *Eyes*—Blurring of vision, scotomata, colored vision usually for yellow or green and occasionally for red, brown or blue. Retrobulbar neuritis has been reported. *Neurological*—Headache, fatigue, malaise, drowsiness, disorientation, confusion, aphasia, hallucinations, and rarely, convulsions. Neuralgic pain, sometimes simulating trigeminal neuralgia, may rarely occur. *Cardiac effects*—Almost every known type of arrhythmia such as extrasystoles, pulsus bigeminus, atrioventricular block, dropped beats, atrioventricular dissociation, sinus arrhythmia, paroxysmal atrial tachycardia, atrioventricular nodal tachycardia, atrial standstill. Ventricular fibrillation is the most common cause of death from digitalis intoxication. Manifestations of toxicity call for prompt cessation or adjustment of therapy. Serum potassium levels should be determined, and supplemental potassium considered in the event of hypokalemia. Allergic reactions to digitalis are rare, but have been reported as follows: Skin reactions, pruritus or urticaria, eosinophilia, thrombopenia, joint tenderness, fever. Gynecomastia, especially in males, has been reported after prolonged administration. There is no evidence that digitalis is transferred across the placental barrier. Many pregnant women have received digitalis and no reports are known of harmful effects on the fetus or the newborn.

Dosage and Administration: A narrow margin of safety exists between the therapeutic and toxic doses. Each patient should be digitalized on an individual basis. Body weight is used only as a rough guide for dosage calculation. *Orally* for adults: for full digitalization, the average dosage is 1.2 to 1.8 gm. Initial dosage is 0.7 gm followed by 0.4 gm every 6 hours for 2 doses in the following 24 hours. Maintenance dosage is 100 mg daily after full digitalization is obtained.

Availability:
DIGIFORTIS®: **(Parke-Davis)**
Capsules (Kapseals®), 100 mg in bottles of 100 and 500.
Tablets, 100 mg in bottles of 1000 and in unit-dose packages of 100.
DIGIGLUSIN® Tablets, 1 N.F. unit of digitalis glycosides in bottles of 100. **(Lilly)**
DIGITALIS Capsules, 100 mg in bottles of 100. **(Lilly)**
PIL-DIGIS Tablets, 100 mg in bottles of 100 and 1000. **(Key Pharm.)**

DIGITOXIN

Description: Digitoxin is a crystalline-pure single cardiac glycoside obtained from *Digitalis purpurea* and is identical, pharmacologically, with whole-leaf digitalis. It is noted for its uniform potency, complete absorption and lack of gastrointestinal irritation. It occurs as a white or pale buff, crystalline powder insoluble in water and slightly soluble in alcohol. Acetyldigitoxin is an intermediate pure cardiac glycoside obtained by enzymatic degradation of lanatoside-A with a loss of one molecule of glucose.

The digitalis glycosides have qualitatively the same therapeutic effect on the heart. They increase the force of myocardial contraction, increase the refractory period of the atrioventricular (AV) node and, to a lesser degree, affect the sinoatrial (SA) node and conduction system by way of the parasympathetic and sympathetic nervous systems.

Following intravenous injection, the therapeutic action starts in 25 minutes to 2 hours, is maximal in 4 to 12 hours, regresses in 2 to 3 days and disappears in 2 to 3 weeks. Following oral administration, the therapeutic action starts in 2 to 3 hours, is maximal in 12 to 24 hours, regresses in 2 to 3 days and disappears in 2 to 3 weeks. Onset of action for orally administered acetyldigitoxin occurs in 4 to 10 hours with therapeutic action persisting for 5 to 10 days.

Indications: All degrees of congestive heart failure, atrial flutter, atrial fibrillation and paroxysmal atrial tachycardia. May be employed in cardiogenic shock, especially when the condition is accompanied by pulmonary edema. Digitoxin is not indicated in sinus tachycardia or premature systoles in the absence of heart failure. May be given parenterally when the patient cannot take medication orally. Parenteral digitoxin is not the drug of choice for very rapid digitalization in emergencies, because of its slow onset of action.

Contraindications: Ventricular tachycardia or fibrillation, digitalis intoxication and known hypersensitivity to the cardiac glycosides.

Warnings: Many of the arrhythmias for which digitalis is advised are identical with those reflecting digitalis intoxication. When the possibility of digitalis intoxication cannot be excluded, cardiac glycosides should be withheld temporarily if the clinical situation permits. Patients with congestive heart failure may complain of nausea and vomiting. Since these symptoms may also be associated with digitalis intoxication, a clinical determination of their cause must be attempted before further administration of the drug. Considerable care is necessary in the presence of idiopathic hypertrophic subaortic stenosis, and unless cardiac failure is severe, it is doubtful whether digitalis should be employed. Very young infants (1st month) have a sharply defined tolerance to digitalis, and impaired renal function must be considered. Premature and immature infants are particularly sensitive, and reduction of dosage may be necessary. The presence of acute glomerulonephritis accompanied by congestive failure requires extreme care. A relatively low total dose, administered in divided doses, and concomitant use of reserpine or other antihypertensive agents have been recommended. Constant ECG monitoring is essential, and it is recommended that the drug be discontinued as soon as possible. Patients with rheumatic carditis, especially when severe, are unusually sensitive to digitalis and are prone to disturbances of rhythm. If heart failure develops, the drug may be tried with relatively low doses, and then cautiously increased until a beneficial effect is obtained. If a therapeutic trial does not result in improvement, the drug should be withdrawn. **Note:** Digitalis glycosides are an important cause of accidental poisoning in children.

Precautions: Parenteral digitoxin should be given with utmost caution to patients still under the influence of digitalis from previous medication; to patients with hypercalcemia; and in the presence of multiple ventricular extrasystoles, ventricular tachycardia, hypersensitivity of the carotid sinus, Adams-Stokes syndrome, or heart block. Patients under the influence of digitalis should not receive calcium intravenously, because elevation of the serum calcium concentration increases the effect of digitalis, and deaths have been reported from intoxication induced in this manner. Potassium depletion, usually caused by concomitant use of diuretics, corticosteroids, hemodialysis, or which may accompany such conditions as malnutrition, old age and longstanding congestive failure, sensitizes the heart to digitalis intoxication and may produce arrhythmias even with recommended doses. Hypokalemia also tends to reduce the positive inotropic effect of digitalis. Acute myocardial infarction, severe pulmonary disease, or far advanced heart failure are apt to be more sensitive to digitalis and more prone to disturbances of rhythm. Special care and reduced doses are required in the presence of myxedema and renal insufficiency. Electrical conversion of arrhythmias may also require adjustment of digitalis dosage.

Adverse Reactions: Reactions are due chiefly to overdosage and include mental depression, anorexia, nausea, vomiting, diarrhea, premature heart beats, complete heart block, AV (atrioventricular) dissociation, ventricular tachycardia and fibrillation, restlessness, headache, weakness, apathy, visual disturbances, mental confusion, disorientation and delirium. Although rare, gynecomastia may occur.

Dosage and Administration: *Orally. Slow digitalization:* 0.2 mg twice daily for a period of 4 days, followed by maintenance dosage. *Rapid digitalization:* preferably 0.6 mg initially, followed by 0.4 mg and then 0.2 mg at intervals of 4 to 6 hours. Maintenance dosage ranges from 0.05 to 0.3 mg daily; the most common dose is 0.15 mg daily. *Intravenously.* The average digitalizing dose is about the same as that used when digitoxin is given orally. The dose must be reduced proportionately for partially digitalized patients. A single injection of an average digitalizing dose is not recommended. Patients who have extensive myocardial damage or conduction defects may require a much smaller dose than those with less abnormal hearts. Digitoxin may be given intramuscularly when IV administration is not practical. If the IM route is used, the glycoside should be injected deeply into the gluteal muscle. For infants, the digitalizing dose may approximate 0.3 mg, maintenance, 0.02 to 0.05 mg daily.

Availability:

Digitoxin

Tablets, 0.1 mg in bottles of 500. **(Abbott)**

Tablets, 0.2 mg in bottles of 1000. **(Lederle)**

Tablets, 0.1 and 0.2 mg in bottles of 1000. **(Parke-Davis)**

ACYLANID® (acetyldigitoxin) Tablets, 0.1 mg in bottles of 100. **(Sandoz)**

CRYSTODIGIN®: **(Lilly)**

Injection, 0.2 mg/ml in ampuls of 1 ml.

Tablets, 0.05, 0.15 and 0.2 mg in bottles of 100 and 500; 0.1 mg in bottles of 100, 500 and 5000 and in unit-dose packages of 100.

PURODIGIN® Tablets, 0.1, 0.15 and 0.2 mg in bottles of 100 and 500. **(Wyeth)**

DIGOXIN

Description: Digoxin is a pure, stable, cardiotonic glycoside isolated from the leaves of *Digitalis lanata.* It differs structurally from digitoxin in that a hydroxyl group is present on carbon 12 of the nucleus. It occurs as clear to white crystals or as a white, crystalline powder insoluble in water and soluble in dilute alcohol.

The oral administration of digoxin usually produces an initial effect within 1 hour, the action becoming maximal in about 6 hours. The intravenous administration of digoxin usually produces an initial effect within 5 to 10 minutes, the action becoming maximal in 1 or 2 hours. With intramuscular injection the onset of effect occurs within 30 minutes, the action becoming maximal in 4 to 6 hours.

In cases of atrial fibrillation, dramatic slowing of the ventricular rate may occur. When the rhythm is normal, there may be no substantial change in the cardiac rate; however, it has been observed that in either case a rapid fall in venous pressure may take place, followed by diuresis (and consequent loss of body weight) and symptomatic relief. The rapid development of the maximal action of digoxin permits the physician to assess the full effect of the previous dose before administering subsequent doses. The moderately rapid dissipation of the drug permits vigorous therapy without danger of prolonged toxicity.

Indications: Treatment of all degrees of congestive heart failure, atrial fibrillation, atrial flutter, supraventricular tachycardia and premature extrasystoles. Its indications are the same as those for digitalis leaf or other digitalis drugs.

Contraindications: Evidence of digitalis intoxication; ventricular paroxysmal tachycardia or ventricular fibrillation *only* in refractory cases not induced by digitalis intoxication and if heart failure has developed.

Warnings: Many of the arrhythmias for which digitalis is advised are identical with those reflecting digitalis intoxication. If the possibilty of digitalis intoxication cannot be excluded, cardiac glycosides should be temporarily withheld if permitted by the clinical situation. Nausea and vomiting may be indicative of congestive heart failure or of digitalis intoxication; therefore, clinical determination of the cause of these symptoms must be attempted before further drug administration.

Precautions: If the patient has taken digoxin or any other less rapidly excreted drug of the digitalis group during the preceding week or two, the dose of digoxin must be reduced accordingly. Patients who have impaired renal function and excretion frequently require doses lower than those recommended. Because of possible diminished tolerance to digitalis due to immaturity of hepatic and renal functions, the total digitalizing dose for newborn and premature infants should be reduced accordingly. Potassium loss, usually due to diuretics or electrolyte manipulations, sensitizes the heart to digitalis intoxication, in which case it may be necessary to reduce the usual dosages during digitalization and maintenance. Digoxin usually is ineffective in cases of cardiac failure due to mechanical causes which are independent of myocardial disease (e.g., cardiac tamponade), or to disorders not primarily of cardiac origin (e.g., severe anemia). Despite a variable or poor response to digoxin in the presence of active rheumatic carditis, the development of cardiac failure is an indication for its use.

Adverse Reactions: Reactions are due chiefly to overdosage and are quite similar to those occurring with other digitalis preparations. The most common toxic manifestations are anorexia, nausea, vomiting, diarrhea, and various cardiac arrhythmias, including ventricular extrasystoles and paroxysmal supraventricular tachycardia or fibrillation with atrioventricular block which may proceed to complete heart block. In general, the gastrointestinal manifestations of toxicity [digoxin] precede the arrhythmias. Headache, weakness, apathy, and visual disturbances are indications of CNS toxicity. Because of the rapid dissipation of the drug, manifestations of toxicity are of short duration, usually lasting from a few hours to 1 or 2 days.

Dosage and Administration: In all cases, both the digitalizing and maintenance dosages should be individually adjusted. *Orally.* The average amount of digoxin that patients must accumulate to be digitalized with digoxin tablets is 1 to 1.5 mg. Digitalization may be accomplished by any of several approaches that vary in dosage and frequency of administration, but reach the same endpoint in terms of total amount accumulated. In previously undigitalized patients, a single loading dose of 0.5 to 0.75 mg usually produces a detectable effect in 1 to 2 hours that becomes maximal within 6 to 8 hours. Additional doses of 0.25 to 0.5 mg may be given cautiously at intervals of 6 to 8 hours until full digitalization is achieved. The average daily maintenance dose is 0.125 to 0.5 mg (usually 0.25 mg), and if the loading dose is not given, serum concentrations reach a steady state plateau in about 7 days in patients with normal renal function. In the elderly patient, 0.125 to 0.25 mg should be considered the average maintenance dose. *Intravenously.* The usual dosage initially is 1 mg and ranges from 0.5 to 2 mg; maintenance dosage is 0.5 mg and ranges from 0.25 to 0.75 mg. Since potassium depletion usually occurs with digitalis intoxication, oral and intravenous administration of potassium chloride may correct the arrhythmias. In the absence of renal failure, potassium chloride may be given *orally* in divided doses totalling 4 to 6 gm daily for adults and 1 to 2 gm daily for children. For critical cases, 40 mEq of potassium chloride in 500 ml of a 5% dextrose solution may be given by slow intravenous infusion over a 1-hour period and repeated, if required, until a total of 120 mEq have been given. For children, the intravenous infusion dosage is 5 to 10 mEq in 100 ml of a 5% dextrose solution over a 1-hour period repeated, if required, to a total of 15 to 30 mEq. Electrocardiographic monitoring should be conducted and the infusion halted immediately upon the appearance of peaking of the T-waves. For detailed dosage regimens used to achieve various degrees of digitalization, see package literature.

Availability:

Digoxin

Injection, 0.25 mg/ml in Tubex® (sterile cartridge-needle unit) of 1 and 2 ml. **(Wyeth)**

Tablets, 0.25 mg in bottles of 1000. **(Lederle)**

Tablets, 0.125 mg in bottles of 1000 and in unit-dose cartons of 100. **(Philips Roxane)**

LANOXIN®: **(Burroughs Wellcome)**

Injection, 0.1 mg/ml (Pediatric) in ampuls of 1 ml; 0.25 mg/ml in ampuls of 2 ml.

Pediatric Elixir, 0.05 mg/ml in bottles of 60 ml with calibrated dropper.

Tablets, 0.125 mg (yellow, scored) in bottles of 100 and 1000 and in unit-dose packages of 30, 100 and 1000; 0.25 mg (white, scored) in bottles of 100, 500, 1000 and 5000 and in unit-dose strip packages of 30, 100 and 1000; 0.5 mg (green, scored) in bottles of 100 and 1000.

SK-DIGOXIN Tablets, 0.25 mg in bottles of 1000. **(Smith Kline & French)**

DIHYDROERGOTAMINE MESYLATE

Description: A hydrogenated ergotamine compound used in the symptomatic treatment of migraine. It directly stimulates the smooth muscles of peripheral and cranial blood vessels while central vasomotor centers are depressed. Compared with ergotamine, dihydroergotamine exhibits more marked adrenergic blocking properties, but less pronounced vasoconstrictive action. It is capable of exerting a marked oxytocic effect on the gravid uterus at term. Following intramuscular injection, onset of action occurs in 15 to 30 minutes and relief is sustained for 3 to 4 hours.

Indications: Vascular headache, e.g., migraine, histaminic cephalalgia (cluster headache).

Contraindications: Peripheral vascular disease, coronary heart disease, hypertension, impaired hepatic or renal function, sepsis, infectious states, and pregnancy; also hypersensitivity to the drug.

Warnings: Failure to observe the upper limits of repeated parenteral dosage may result in eventual onset of the peripheral toxic signs and symptoms of ergotism. Lactating women should be cautioned not to nurse their babies while taking this drug.

Adverse Reactions: Numbness and tingling of fingers and toes, muscle pains in the extremities, weakness in the legs, precordial distress and pain, transient tachycardia or bradycardia, nausea, vomiting, localized edema and itching. Large doses have been found to raise arterial pressure, induce coronary vasoconstriction and slow the heart rate both by a direct action and its effect on the vagus nerve. Under this condition, ergotamine also displays oxytocic and spasmolytic properties.

Dosage and Administration: *Intramuscularly* or *intravenously*. For vascular headache, 1 ml at the first warning sign of headache, repeated at 1-hour intervals to a total of 3 ml intramuscularly or 2 ml intravenously.

Availability:
D.H.E. 45® Solution, 1 mg/ml in ampuls of 1 ml. **(Sandoz)**

DIHYDROTACHYSTEROL

Chemical Name: 9, 10-Secoergosta-5,7,22-trien-3β-ol.

Description: A stable, oil-soluble steroid, obtained by reducing tachysterol, an irradiated product of ergosterol, which exerts a specific influence on the calcium level of the blood—prevents tetany in patients with hypoparathyrodism by elevating serum calcium. In contrast to parathyroid extract, dihydrotachysterol is active when taken orally; it exerts a slow but persistent effect, and tolerance does not develop with prolonged use.

Indications: For patients with acute, chronic, and latent forms of postoperative tetany, idiopathic tetany, and hypoparathyroidism.

Contraindications: In patients with hypercalcemia, abnormal sensitivity to vitamin D, and hypervitaminosis D.

Warnings: Since animal reproduction studies have shown fetal abnormalities in several species associated with hypervitaminosis D, its use during pregnancy should be carefully considered by the physician in view of the potential hazards to the fetus.

Precautions: Because of its effect on serum calcium, dihydrotachysterol should be administered to pregnant patients or to patients with renal stones only when it is deemed essential to the welfare of the patient. In patients with renal osteodystrophy accompanied by hyperphosphatemia, maintenance of a normal serum phosphorus level by dietary phosphate restriction and/or administration of aluminum gels as intestinal phosphate binders is essential to prevent metastatic calcification. Adequate dietary calcium is essential for satisfactory clinical response to the drug. To prevent hypercalcemia, treatment should alway be controlled by routine determinations of the blood calcium level. Administration of thiazide diuretics to hypoparathyroid patients who are concurrently being treated with dihydrotachysterol may cause hypercalcemia. Polyuria, polydipsia, and albuminuria are manifestations of impaired renal function. Wide-spread calcification of soft tissues, including heart, blood vessels, kidneys, and lungs, can occur, with death resulting from cardiovascular or renal failure. The effects of the drug may persist for up to one month after cessation of therapy.

Adverse Reactions: Usually due to overdosage are manifested by languor, anorexia, nausea and vomiting, diarrhea, osteoporosis, weight loss, metastatic calcifications, renal damage, anemia, band keratitis, convulsions; in extreme overdosage by vertigo, tinnitus, headache, abdominal cramps, polyuria, thirst, stupor, ataxia of lower extremities, albuminuria, and exanthema.

Dosage and Administration: *Orally.* Individualized to maintain blood calcium levels between 9 and 10 mg/100 ml. Initial dose in parathyroid insufficiency, 3 to 10 ml or 6 to 20 capsules daily for several days, weekly maintenance dosage is 1 to 7 ml or 2 to 14 capsules as required for normal blood and urine calcium levels. May be supplemented with 10 to 15 gm of calcium lactate or gluconate daily. Following thyroid operation, 1 ml or 2 capsules daily with 6 gm of calcium lactate until danger of tetany has passed.

Availability:
DIHYDROTACHYSTEROL Tablets, 0.125 and 0.4 mg in bottles of 50; 0.2 mg in bottles of 100 and in unit-dose blister packs of 100. **(Philips Roxane)**
HYTAKEROL®: **(Winthrop)**
Capsules, 0.125 mg in bottles of 50.
Solution in oil, 0.25 mg/ml in bottles of 15 ml.

DIIODOHYDROXYQUIN

Chemical Name: 5,7-Diiodo-8-quinolinol.

Description: An antiinfective agent closely related chemically and pharmacologically to iodochlorhydroxyquin; it occurs as a light yellowish-tan, microcrystalline powder relatively insoluble in water and sparingly soluble in alcohol. It contains 63.9% iodine.

Possesses amebacidal, antitrichomonal and slight antibacterial and antifungal activity. It has been suggested that the 8-hydroxyquinolines function as antibacterial agents by chelating, at bacterial surfaces, trace metals essential for bacterial growth. Antieczematous and antiseborrheic properties have also been attributed to the hydroxyquinoline drugs. Diiodohydroxyquin is especially destructive to amebae, is relatively nontoxic and does not cause gastrointestinal irritation.

Indications: Treatment of asymptomatic intestinal amebiasis (ameba and cysts carrier states) and mild symptomatic amebic dysentery. It is not recommended for the treatment of nonspecific diarrhea.

Contraindications: Hypersensitivity to the drug or to iodine, hepatic damage, and preexisting optic neuropathy.

Warnings: Optic atrophy, optic neuritis and peripheral neuritis have been reported in patients, primarily in children, following prolonged therapy with high dosages. It is therefore essential that the recommended dosage or duration of administration not be exceeded. Safe use during pregnancy and lactation has not been established.

Precautions: Routine caution is advised in patients with thyroid disease. Protein-bound iodine levels may be increased during treatment with this drug and may therefore interfere with the results of certain thyroid function tests. These effects may persist for as long as 6 months after discontinuation of therapy.

Adverse Reactions: Rarely iodism. Optic neuritis, optic atrophy, and peripheral neuropathy have been reported following prolonged therapy with high dosage. Although rare, an occasional sensitive patient may develop severe generalized furunculosis (iodine toxicoderma), mild or severe dermatitis, chills, fever, anal irritation, itching, transitory abdominal discomfort, diarrhea, or headache. Other side effects reported were hair loss, elevated serum PBI levels, agranulocytosis, and thyroid hypertrophy. Long-term use of these drugs should be avoided.

Dosage and Administration: *Orally.* Intestinal amebiasis in adults, 650 mg 3 times daily for 20 days. If required, this course of treatment may be repeated after a drug-free interval of 2 to 3 weeks. Intestinal amebiasis in children, 30 to 40 mg/kg of body weight daily, divided into 2 or 3 doses for 20 days. Total daily dose should not exceed 650 mg 3 times daily. The powder may be *insufflated* into the vagina in an amount sufficient for a thin coating of the vaginal walls.

Availability:
Diiodohydroxyquin
Tablets, 650 mg in bottles of 1000. **(Panray)**

YODOXIN: **(Glenwood)**
Powder in bottles of 25 gm.
Tablets, 210 mg in bottles of 100 and 1000.

DIMACOL

Description: A combination of a vasoconstrictor, antihistamine, non-narcotic cough suppressant and a stimulating expectorant which has been chosen and formulated to help reduce nasal and bronchial congestion, suppress cough and ameliorate allergic manifestations associated with the common cold and other upper respiratory disorders. Each capsule or teaspoonful (5 ml) contains:

Pseudoephedrine hydrochloride	30 mg
Dextromethorphan hydrobromide	15 mg
Guaifenesin	100 mg

Liquid contains 4.75% alcohol.

Indications: The management of cough, mucosal congestion, edema, and nasal hypersecretion associated with the common cold, upper respiratory infection and sinusitis.

Contraindications: Hypersensitivity to any of the components, and in patients receiving MAO inhibitors.

Precautions: Should be used cautiously in the presence of hypertension, heart disease, peripheral vascular disease, diabetes mellitus, hyperthyroidism, prostatic hypertrophy or glaucoma.

Adverse Reactions: Those that may occur include nausea, vomiting, dry mouth, nervousness, insomnia.

Dosage and Administration: *Orally* 3 times daily. Adults and children 12 years of age and older, 1 capsule or teaspoonful of liquid; children 6 to 12 years, ½ teaspoonful; children under 6 years, as directed by the physician.

Availability:
DIMACOL® (OTC): **(Robins)**
Capsules (orange and green) in bottles of 100 and 500 and in Pre-Pak® cartons of 12 and 24.
Liquid (orange-colored, chocolate-flavored) in bottles of 1 pint and 1 gallon.

DIMENHYDRINATE

Chemical Name: 2(Diphenylmethoxy)-*N,N*-dimethylethylamine-8-chlorotheophyllinate.

Description: A centrally acting antiemetic of the nonphenothiazine group. It occurs as a white, crystalline, odorless powder slightly soluble in water and freely soluble in alcohol. Exhibits some antihistaminic properties, but is employed chiefly in the treatment and prevention of motion sickness. Dimenhydrinate acts primarily by reducing excitability of the labyrinth and depressing conduction in vestibular-cerebellar pathways, thereby relieving those symptoms caused by excessive vestibular stimulation.

Indications: Prevention and treatment of nausea, vomiting and vertigo due to motion sickness.

Warnings: Caution should be used when dimenhydrinate is administered in conjunction with those antibiotics which cause ototoxic symptoms, as these symptoms may be masked by the drug and an irreversible state may ensue. Patients should be cautioned against engaging in activities requiring alertness or skill.

Adverse Reactions: Drowsiness, especially with high doses.

Dosage and Administration: *Orally.* Adults, initial dose 50 to 100 mg, repeated every 4 hours if needed. Children 8 to 12 years of age, 25 to 50 mg 3 times daily, *orally* or *rectally;* younger children may use the oral liquid, but only on the advice of the physician. *Intramuscularly.* In adults, 50 to 100 mg at intervals determined by the physician. *Intravenously.* Each 1 ml (50 mg) of solution should be diluted in 10 ml of Sodium Chloride Injection U.S.P. and injected over a period of 2 minutes. Children's parenteral doses should be smaller than those given by other routes. *Rectally.* Adults, 1 moistened suppository 1 or 2 times daily inserted past the sphincter. Children's doses depend on weight and age.

Availability:
Dimenhydrinate
Injection, 50 mg/ml in Tubex® (sterile cartridge-needle unit) of 1 ml in cartons of 10. **(Wyeth)**
Tablets, 50 mg in bottles of 1000. **(Lederle)**
DRAMAMINE®: **(Searle)**
Injection, 50 mg/ml in ampuls of 1 ml and in vials of 5 ml.
Oral Liquid (OTC), 12.5 mg/4 ml in bottles of 1 pint.
Rectal Suppositories (Supposicones®), 100 mg in cartons of 12.
Tablets (OTC), 50 mg in bottles of 100, 1000 and 2500, packets of 12 tablets in cartons containing 20 packets and in unit-dose cartons of 1000 (10 x 100).

DIMERCAPROL

Chemical Name: 2,3-Dimercapto-1-propanol.

Description: A chelating agent used as an antidote in metal poisoning. It occurs as a colorless liquid, with a disagreeable, mercaptan-like odor, freely soluble in water and soluble in alcohol. Combines with metals to form relatively stable, nonionized ring complexes. It promotes the excretion of arsenic, gold and mercury by removing them from the tissues with the formation of stable, relatively nontoxic mercaptides. Dimercaprol prevents inhibition of sulfhydryl enzymes by metals and to a lesser degree may reactivate affected enzymes; however, it is most effective when administered prior to significant enzyme damage. Following intramuscular injection, maximal blood levels are achieved within 30 to 60 minutes, and degradation and excretion are essentially complete within 4 hours.

Indications: Treatment of arsenic, gold and mercury poisonings; also acute lead poisoning in combination with calcium disodium edetate. Results in the treatment of other heavy metal poisonings have been inconclusive. Dimercaprol has proved to be an effective drug for acute poisoning by mercury salts if therapy is begun within 1 or 2 hours following ingestion. It has not been found to be very effective for chronic mercury poisoning.

Contraindications: In most instances of hepatic insufficiency with the exception of postarsenical jaundice. The drug should be discontinued or used only with extreme caution if acute renal insufficiency develops during therapy.

Warnings: There may be local pain at the site of the injection. A reaction apparently peculiar to children is fever which may persist during therapy. It occurs in approximately 30% of children. A transient reduction of the percentage of polymorphonuclear leukocytes may also be observed.

Precautions: Because the dimercaprol-metal complex breaks down easily in an acid medium, production of an alkaline urine affords protection to the kidney during therapy. Iron should not be administered to patients undergoing therapy with this drug. Since no adequate clinical reports are available regarding the use of dimercaprol during pregnancy, it should therefore not be used unless judged by the physician to be necessary in the treatment of life-threatening acute poisoning.

Adverse Reactions: One of the most consistent responses to dimercaprol is a rise in blood pressure accompanied by tachycardia. This rise is roughly proportional to the dose administered. Doses larger than those recommended may cause other transitory signs and symptoms such as nausea and, in some instances, vomiting; headache; a burning sensation in the lips, mouth and throat; a feeling of constriction, even pain, in the throat, chest, or hands; conjunctivitis, lacrimation, blepharospasm, rhinorrhea, and salivation; tingling of the hands; a burning sensation in the penis; sweating of the forehead, hands and other areas; abdominal pain, and an occasional appearance of painful sterile abscesses. Many of the above symptoms are accompanied by a feeling of anxiety, weakness, and unrest and often are relieved by administration of an antihistamine.

Dosage and Administration: *Intramuscularly only. For mild arsenic or gold poisoning,* 2.5 mg/kg of body weight 4 times daily for 2 days, 2 times on the 3rd day, then once daily thereafter for 10 days; for *severe arsenic or gold poisoning,* 3 mg/kg every 4 hours for 2 days, 4 times on the 3rd day, then twice daily thereafter for 10 days. *For mercury poisoning,* 5 mg/kg initially, followed by 2.5 mg/kg 1 or 2 times daily for 10 days. *For acute lead encephalopathy,* Initially, 4 mg/kg of dimercaprol alone; thereafter in combination with calcium disodium edetate at 4-hour intervals. The EDTA should be administered at a separate site. For less severe poisoning the dose can be reduced to 3 mg/kg after the initial dose. Treatment should continue for 2 to 7 days depending on the clinical response. Successful treatment depends on beginning injections at the earliest possible moment and on the use of adequate amounts at frequent intervals. Other supportive measures should always be used in conjunction with dimercaprol therapy.

Availability:
BAL In OIL Solution, 100 mg/ml in ampuls of 3 ml in cartons of 10.
(Hynson, Westcott & Dunning)

DIMETANE EXPECTORANT

Description: Each 5 ml contains brompheniramine maleate, 2 mg; phenylephrine hydrochloride, 5 mg; phenylpropanolamine hydrochloride, 5 mg; guaifenesin, 100 mg and alcohol, 3.5%; in addition the DC expectorant also contains codeine phosphate, 10 mg.

Indications: Relief of coughing, and of the allergic response of nasal tissue and for the symptomatic relief of many manifestations of allergic states in which expectorant action is desired. Codeine has been added to the formulation to enhance its antitussive properties.

Contraindications: Hypersensitivity to any of the components, pregnant patients, nursing mothers, newborn or premature infants, lower respiratory tract symptoms, including asthma, and concurrent use with MAO inhibitors.

Warnings: Codeine phosphate may be habit-forming. Special care should be exercised in patients with narrow-angle glaucoma, stenosing peptic ulcer, pyloroduodenal obstruction, symptomatic prostatic hypertrophy, and bladder neck obstruction. Hallucinations, convulsions, and possibly death may occur particularly in infants and children who are more susceptible to toxic dosages of antihistamines, and dizziness, sedation, and hypotension are more likely to occur in elderly patients. Because of the atropine-like action of brompheniramine, special precautions are necessary in patients with a history of bronchial asthma, increased intraocular pressure, hyperthyroidism, cardiovascular disorders, and hypertension.

Precautions: Administer with care to patients with cardiac or peripheral vascular disease or hypertension. Until the response has been determined, patients should be cautioned against engaging in activities requiring alertness or skill. Those receiving antihistamines should be warned against the possible additive effects with CNS depressants such as alcohol, hypnotics, sedative, tranquilizers, and drugs of similar action.

Adverse Reactions: Those affecting the *cardiovascular system* are manifested by hypotension, hypertension, headache, palpitation, tachycardia, and extrasystoles; the *hematologic system* by hemolytic anemia, thrombocytopenia, and agranulocytosis; the *nervous system* by sedation, sleepiness, dizziness, disturbed coordination, fatigue, confusion, restlessness, excitation, nervousness, tremor, irritability, insomnia, euphoria, paresthesias, blurred vision, diplopia, vertigo, tinnitus, acute labyrinthitis, hysteria, neuritis, and convulsions; the *gastrointestinal system* by epigastric distress, anorexia, nausea, vomiting, diarrhea, and constipation; the *genitourinary system* by urinary frequency, difficult urination, urinary retention, and early menses; the *respiratory system* by thickening of bronchial secretions, tightness of chest and wheezing, and nasal stuffiness. Miscellaneous reactions that may be encountered include urticaria, drug rash, anaphylactic shock, photosensitivity, excessive perspiration, chills, dryness of mouth, nose and throat. Appropriate measures and practices to counteract the signs and symptoms of overdosage which may range from CNS depression to excitement should be initiated.

Dosage and Administration: *Orally.* Adults, 1 to 2 teaspoonsful 4 times daily, or more if required. Children, 1/2 to 1 teaspoonful 3 or 4 times daily.

Availability:
DIMETANE® EXPECTORANT in bottles of pints and gallons. **(Robins)**
Ⓒ DIMETANE EXPECTORANT-DC in bottles of pints and gallons. **(Robins)**

DIMETAPP

Description: Each 5 ml of elixir and each Extentab contain respectively: brompheniramine maleate, 4 mg and 12 mg; phenylephrine hydrochloride, 5 mg and 15 mg; phenylpropanolamine hydrochloride, 5 mg and 15 mg. The elixir contains 2.3% alcohol.

A combination of ingredients producing potent antihistaminic, decongestant and bronchodilator action, which reduces or abolishes the allergic response of nasal tissue.

Indications: For the prevention and symptomatic relief of allergic manifestations of upper respiratory illnesses, as in seasonal and perennial allergies, acute sinusitis, rhinitis, pharyngitis, bronchitis, otitis, and the common cold in which the drug reduces inflammatory edema, nasal congestion and/or secretions, thereby affording relief from nasal stuffiness and postnasal drip.

Contraindications: Hypersensitivity to antihistamines. Not recommended for use during pregnancy. Dimetapp should be used with caution, if at all, in patients taking MAO inhibitors. Because of its drying and thickening effect on the lower respiratory secretions, this drug is not recommended in the treatment of bronchial asthma. The Extentabs are contraindicated in children under 12 years of age.

Warnings: Overdosage in infants and children may produce convulsions and death.

Precautions: Administer with care to patients with cardiac or peripheral vascular disease or hypertension. Until the response has been determined, patients should be cautioned against engaging in operations requiring alertness or skill. Those receiving antihistamines should be warned against the possible additive effects with CNS depressants such as alcohol, hypnotics, sedatives, tranquilizers, and drugs of similar action.

Adverse Reactions: May include hypersensitivity reactions such as rash, urticaria, leukopenia, agranulocytosis and thrombocytopenia, drowsiness, lassitude, giddiness, dryness of the mucous membranes, tightness of the chest, thickening of bronchial secretions, urinary frequency and dysuria, palpitation, hypotension or hypertension, headache, faintness, dizziness, tinnitus, incoordination, visual disturbances, mydriasis, CNS-depressant and (less often) stimulant effect, anorexia, nausea, vomiting, diarrhea, constipation, and epigastric distress.

Dosage and Administration: *Orally.* Adults, 1 Extentab morning and evening or 1 or 2 teaspoonsful of the elixir 3 or 4 times daily. Children, 1 to 6 months of age, 1/4 teaspoonful; 7 months to 2 years, 1/2 teaspoonful; 2 to 4 years, 3/4 teaspoonful; 4 to 12 years, 1 teaspoonful. Dosages to be taken 3 or 4 times daily.

Availability:
DIMETAPP®: **(Robins)**
Elixir in bottles of 120 ml, pints and gallons.
Extentabs® (extended-action tablets) in bottles of 100 and 500.

DIMETHINDENE MALEATE

Chemical Name: 2-[1-[2-(2-Dimethylaminoethyl)inden-3-yl]ethyl]pyridine maleate.

Description: An antihistaminic and antipruritic drug related to the group of antihistamines including pheniramine, brompheniramine, chlorpheniramine, and pyrrobutamine, which contain a diarylpropylamine structure. Occurs as white, crystalline powder sparingly soluble in water, freely soluble in alcohol, sensitive to light.

Antihistamines are competitive antagonists of histamine. In varying degree they antagonize most, but not all, of the pharmacological effects of histamine. They also have effects on the CNS which are both stimulant and depressant, and exhibit peripheral anticholinergic (atropine-like) action.

Following oral administration, the effects of dimethindene appear within 30 minutes and persist for 6 to 8 hours.

Indications: Symptomatic treatment of seasonal and perennial allergic rhinitis, vasomotor rhinitis, allergic conjunctivitis due to inhalant allergens and foods, mild, uncomplicated allergic skin manifestations of urticaria, angioedema; dermographism; as therapy for anaphylactic reactions adjunctive to epinephrine and other standard measures after the acute manifestations have been controlled. For the amelioration and prevention of allergic reactions to blood or plasma in patients with a known history of such reactions.

Contraindications: Premature infants, neonates, or nursing mothers; in patients receiving MAO inhibitors or in those with narrow angle glaucoma, stenosing peptic ulcer, symptomatic prostatic hypertrophy, bladder neck obstruction, pyloroduodenal obstruction, lower respiratory tract symptoms (including asthma), or hypersensitivity to dimethindene or related compounds.

Warnings: Antihistamines often produce drowsiness. Therefore, patients should be cautioned about activities requiring alertness such as driving a car or operating dangerous machinery. The depressant effects of this drug may be additive to those of other CNS depressants such as hypnotics, sedatives, tranquilizers, etc. A paradoxical excitation may occur, particularly in children. Safe use of this drug in pregnant women or during lactation has not been established; therefore, the expected benefits must be weighed against the potential hazards. Overdosage may result in convulsions which may have a fatal outcome in susceptible patients, particularly infants and children.

Precautions: Because of its atropine-like, anticholinergic activity, it should be used with care in patients with increased intraocular pressure, hyperthyroidism, cardiovascular disease, hypertension, or in those with a history of bronchial asthma.

Adverse Reactions: Those frequently noted were sedation or drowsiness; dryness of mouth, nose, and throat; thickening of bronchial secretions; dizziness; disturbed coordination, and epigastric distress. Other complications which may be noted include fatigue; chills; confusion; restlessness; excitation; nervousness; irritability; insomnia; euphoria; anorexia; nausea; vomiting; diarrhea; constipation; hypotension; tightness in the chest; wheezing; blurred vision; diplopia; vertigo; tinnitus; headache; convulsions; palpitation; tachycardia; extrasystoles; nasal stuffiness; urinary frequency; difficult urination; urinary retention; hemolytic anemia; leukopenia; thrombocytopenia; agranulocytosis; aplastic anemia; allergic or hypersensitivity reactions, including drug rash, urticaria, anaphylactic shock, and photosensitivity. The following reactions associated with some antihistaminics and may or may not occur with dimethindene should nevertheless be anticipated. These include excessive perspiration, tremor, paresthesias of the extremities, acute labyrinthitis, neuritis, and early menses. The greatest problem from acute overdosage with antihistaminics is their CNS effects which produce depression and/or stimulation. In children particularly, stimulation predominates initially in a syndrome which may include excitement, hallucinations, ataxia, incoordination, athetosis, and convulsions followed by postictal depression. Dry mouth, fixed dilated pupils, flushing of the face and fever are common and resemble the syndrome of atropine poisoning. Death may occur following deep coma and cardiovascular collapse. Since there is no specific therapy to counteract acute overdosage, general symptomatic and supportive measures should be instituted promptly and maintained for as long as required.

Dosage and Administration: *Orally.* Adults and children over 6 years of age, 1 tablet once or twice daily.

Availability:
FORHISTAL® Lontab® (long-acting tablets), 2.5 mg in bottles of 100. **(Ciba)**
TRITEN® Tab-In™ (delayed-release tablets), 2.5 mg in bottles of 100. **(Marion)**

DIOXYLINE PHOSPHATE

Chemical Name: 1-(4-Ethoxy-3-methoxybenzyl)-6,7-dimethoxy-3-methylisoquinoline phosphate.

Description: Dioxyline phosphate is a synthetic, crystalline, non-narcotic compound which possesses the ability to relax smooth-muscle spasm. It occurs as a white, crystalline powder soluble in water and in alcohol. Dioxyline is structurally and pharmacologically similar to papaverine; it differs structurally in the presence of a methyl group at the 3 position on the isoquinoline ring and in the replacement of a methoxy with an ethoxy group on the benzyl ring.

Its primary action is on cardiac and smooth muscle, especially those of the larger arteries. This spasmolytic effect is a direct one and is unrelated to muscle innervation. The direct action on the heart tends to slow the rate and increase the fibrillation threshold of the ventricle, and to depress conduction and prolong the refractory period of the myocardium. Dioxyline acts as a relaxant on various smooth muscles and if spasm exists, the relaxation may be prominent. The drug causes practically no effect on the CNS.

Indications: Treatment of angina pectoris and conditions in which there is reflex spasm of blood vessels in arms, legs, or lungs. May also be useful in those conditions involving spasm of the smooth muscle.

Contraindications: There are no known contraindications to the oral administration of dioxyline phosphate.

Adverse Reactions: Although rarely noted, complications when they do occur are generally mild and may include nausea, dizziness, sweating, flushing, sedation, and abdominal cramps. These symptoms may be exacerbated when doses in excess of those recommended are ingested. Gastric lavage should be instituted as soon as feasible followed by general procedures for symptomatic therapy.

Dosage and Administration: *Orally,* administered 3 or 4 times daily. Adults, 100 to 400 mg.

Availability:
PAVERIL® Phosphate Tablets, 100 and 200 mg in bottles of 100 and 500. **(Lilly)**

DIPHEMANIL METHYLSULFATE

Chemical Name: 4-Diphenylmethylene-1,1-dimethylpiperidinium methylsulfate.

Description: A quaternary ammonium anticholinergic agent, diphemanil occurs as a bitter, white, crystalline powder sparingly soluble in water and in alcohol. Structurally, it resembles mepenzolate, piponzolate, and piperidolate in that the molecule contains 2 benzene rings and a piperidine ring.

As with other related compounds, diphemanil produces effects quantitatively similar to those of atropine. It inhibits motility of the gastrointestinal tract and diminishes the volume of perspiration, saliva, gastric and pancreatic secretions. Diphemanil has little or no direct spasmolytic (papaverine-like) action on smooth muscle and high doses may block ganglionic and skeletal neuromuscular transmission. Following oral administration, effects appear in 1 to 2 hours and persist for about 4 hours. It is excreted in the urine mainly unaltered.

Indications: Adjunctive treatment of gastric hyperacidity associated with duodenal ulcer. The drug neither heals peptic ulcer, decreases the rate of recurrences nor prevents complications.

Contraindications: Hypersensitivity to diphemanil methylsulfate, in the presence of glaucoma, and in myasthenia gravis. It is also contraindicated in obstructive uropathy (bladder neck obstruction due to prostatic hypertrophy), obstructive disease of the gastrointestinal tract (pyloroduodenal stenosis), paralytic ileus, intestinal atony of the elderly or debilitated patient, unstable cardiovascular status in acute hemorrhage, severe ulcerative colitis, and toxic megacolon complicating ulcerative colitis.

Warnings: The use of this drug during pregnancy and lactation or in women of childbearing potential requires that the anticipated benefits be weighed against the possible hazards to the fetus or infant. Safe and effective use in children has not been established. In the presence of high environmental temperature, heat prostration (fever and heat stroke due to decreased sweating) can occur with use of this drug. Treatment with diphemanil in patients with diarrhea due to incomplete intestinal obstruction, especially those with ileostomy or colostomy would be inappropriate and possibly harmful. The drug is capable of inducing drowsiness and dizziness, in which case the patient should refrain from performing any hazardous operation requiring alertness and physical coordination. Overdosage may invoke a curare-like action.

Precautions: Cautious use is recommended when treating elderly patients, and patients with autonomic neuropathy, hepatic or renal disease, hyperthyroidism, coronary heart disease, congestive heart failure, cardiac tachyarrhythmias, tachycardia, hypertension, prostatic hypertrophy, or with hiatal hernia associated with reflux esophagitis, since anticholinergic drugs tend to aggravate this condition. Large doses in patients with ulcerative colitis may suppress intestinal motility to the degree of precipitating a paralytic ileus which can lead to toxic megacolon.

Adverse Reactions: Most untoward effects associated with the use of anticholinergic agents are manifestations of their pharmacologic action and may be expected to appear following administration of full therapeutic doses. Generally, patients may experience one or more of the following: xerostomia, decreased sweating, urinary hesitance and retention, blurred vision, tachycardia, palpitations, mydriasis, cycloplegia, increased ocular tension, loss of taste, headaches, nervousness, mental confusion, drowsiness, weakness, dizziness, insomnia, nausea, vomiting, constipation, bloated feeling, impotence, suppression of lactation, severe allergic reactions or drug idiosyncrasies including anaphylaxis, urticaria and other dermal manifestations. Symptoms of overdosage generally progress from an intensification of the usual side effects of CNS disturbances which range from restlessness and excitement to psychotic behavior, in addition to circulatory changes (flushing, fall in blood pressure, circulatory failure), respiratory failure, paralysis and coma. Measures taken are generally those commensurate with other anticholinergic-induced toxic symptoms.

Dosage and Administration: *Orally.* One to 1½ or 2 tablets every 4 to 6 hours. Once a satisfactory result has been achieved, the dose may be reduced to ½ to 1 tablet every 4 to 6 hours.

Availability:
PRANTAL® Tablets 100 mg in bottles of 100. **(Schering)**

DIPHENADIONE

Chemical Name: 2-Diphenylacetyl-1,3-indandione.

Description: An anticoagulant agent, diphenadione occurs as pale yellow, odorless crystals practically insoluble in water and slightly soluble in alcohol. It is chemically related to phenindione and is a potent and long-acting depressant of prothrombin complex activity. It inhibits hepatic synthesis of factors II, VII, IX and X, thereby lowering the prothrombin concentration in the blood; its relatively long period of action favors a steadily controlled prothrombin level.

Following oral administration, peak anticoagulant effect occurs within 48 to 72 hours, and prothrombin depression may persist for approximately 20 days.

Indications: Prophylaxis and treatment of venous thrombosis and its extension, treatment of atrial fibrillation with embolization, prophylaxis and treatment of pulmonary embolism, and as adjunct in the treatment of coronary occlusion. It is suitable for ambulant, long-term, maintenance anticoagulant therapy.

Contraindications: Patients who are bleeding or who have hemorrhagic tendencies, those with open wounds, ulcerating or granulomatous lesions or extensive denudation of skin, visceral carcinoma, ulcerations of the gastrointestinal tract, subacute bacterial endocarditis, severe liver or kidney disease, severe uncontrolled hypertension, recent or contemplated surgery of the eye, brain, or spinal cord, continuous tube drainage of the stomach or small intestine, and initial elevated prothrombin time, or deficiency of vitamin K or ascorbic acid.

Warnings: The effects of the drug tend to be cumulative and prolonged; therefore, caution should be exercised when administered in any condition where added risk of hemorrhage is present. At the earliest sign of bleeding the drug should be withdrawn. Dosage should be controlled by periodic determination of prothrombin time, since determinations of clotting and bleeding times are not effective measures for control of therapy. Agranulocytosis and hepatitis have been associated with the use of oral anticoagulants; patients should be instructed to report promptly any prodromal symptoms such as marked fatigue, chills, fever, or sore throat. Periodic blood studies and liver function tests are required, and therapy should be terminated if leukopenia or symptoms of hypersensitivity (dermatitis or fever) occur. Rash, persistent albuminuria, or fever of undetermined origin are signs of impending toxicity. Because of the possibility of renal damage, urine should be tested periodically. Oral anticoagulants pass through the placental barrier, and have been reported to cause fetal hemorrhage and intrauterine death. Also, it has been strongly suggested that they may be responsible for the congenital malformations (nasal hypoplasia and other abnormalities consistent with a diagnosis of chondrodysplasia punctata) appearing in children born to mothers who received oral anticoagulants during pregnancy. Consequently, if these drugs must be used in pregnant patients, such patients should then be made well aware of the potential risk.

Precautions: Use with caution in patients with active tuberculosis, moderate hypertension, mild liver or kidney disease, severe diabetes, in patients with indwelling catheters, during menstruation, and the postpartum period, or in patients with a past history of ulcerative disease of the gastrointestinal tract, or any occupation which carries a hazard of significant physical injury, or exposure to DDT and chlordane. Special care is needed in the presence of hepatic disorders, vitamin K deficiency, congestive heart failure, diarrhea, poor nutritional state, collagen disease, disorders of the pancreas, fever, cachexia, renal insufficiency, x-ray therapy, scurvy, and alcoholism since these conditions increase the response to these agents. Conversely, edema, hyperlipidemia, diabetes mellitus, hypercholesterolemia, visceral carcinoma, myxedema, and hereditary resistance to the oral anticoagulants decrease the reponse.

It is of utmost importance that no other drug be administered with diphenadione without full appreciation of its potential for interacting with it, thereby increasing or decreasing its anticoagulant effect. Fatalities have been reported from interactions affecting the metabolism of oral anticoagulants or their binding to plasma proteins. Drugs which may stimulate metabolic degradation of this anticoagulant include phenobarbital as well as other barbiturates, glutethimide, meprobamate, rifampin, ethchlorvynol, and griseofulvin. In addition, oral contraceptives, ACTH, and adrenocorticosteroids have been reported to reduce the response to oral anticoagulants. Patients receiving these drugs may require larger doses of diphenadione to achieve an optimal anticoagulant effect. When these drugs are discontinued, it may be necessary to reduce the dose of diphenadione. Such drugs as phenylbutazone, oxyphenbutazone, diazoxide, chloral hydrate, and mefenamic, ethacrynic, and nalidixic acids may increase the quantity of free drug available by displacing diphenadione from protein binding sites. Quinine, quinidine, and salicylates in large doses depress prothrombin formation in the liver, and thus may increase the patient's sensitivity to diphenadione and cause hemorrhage. Broad spectrum antibiotics, which suppress the organisms comprising the normal bacterial flora of the intestine and reduce production of vitamin K, may increase anticoagulant activity, but this is not usually observed unless there is a dietary deficiency of vitamin K. Other drugs which have been reported to cause an exaggerated response and a prolonged prothrombin time include methylthiouracil, prophylthiouracil, phenyramidol, disulfiram, dextrothyroxine, clofibrate, glucagon, chloramphenicol, nortriptyline, and various anabolic steroids. Oral anticoagulants have been reported to inhibit the enzymatic degradation of phenytoin in the liver thus leading to increased serum levels and prolonged half-life of phenytoin which could result in drug intoxication. Conversely, phenytoin stimulates the metabolism of oral anticoagulants, thereby decreasing their serum levels and thus increasing the plasma prothrombin-proconvertin concentrations. Oral anticoagulants also are known to potentiate the hypoglycemic effect of tolbutamide by inhibiting its degradation in the liver. They have also been known to elevate the serum levels of chlorpropamide and phenobarbital. Therefore, with the addition or withdrawal of any of these drugs, there is the danger of either inadequate anticoagulant response to diphenadione or bleeding. In such cases, the dosage of this drug should be carefully regulated, or its use discontinued.

Adverse Reactions: Occasionally, nausea and hemorrhagic complications at toxic dosage levels. Because of its close chemical similarity to phenindione which has caused agranulocytosis, diphenadione possesses the potential to cause similar blood dyscrasias, as well as other severe reactions.

Dosage and Administration: *Orally,* 20 to 30 mg the first day followed by 10 to 15 mg the second day. The average maintenance dose is 3 to 5 mg daily. The initial dose should not be taken until the prothrombin time has been determined. Subsequent dosage should be dictated by periodic changes in prothrombin level.

Availability:
DIPAXIN® Tablets, 5 mg in bottles of 100. **(Upjohn)**

DIPHENHYDRAMINE HYDROCHLORIDE

Chemical Name: 2-Diphenylmethoxy-*N,N*-dimethylethylamine hydrochloride.

Description: Diphenhydramine hydrochloride is an antihistamine of the ethanolamine type and occurs as a white, crystalline powder freely soluble in water and in alcohol. Readily absorbed following oral administration, it reaches peak tissue concentrations in approximately 1 hour, and the effects persist for about 4 to 6 hours. It is excreted in the urine within 24 hours primarily as degraded products, although a small portion of unchanged drug may also be excreted. This drug shares the actions and uses of other antihistamines. It also exerts antitussive, antiemetic, antispasmodic and sedative action.

Indications: Has been found useful in allergic diseases such as hay fever, allergic rhinitis, vasomotor rhinitis, allergic conjunctivitis, urticaria, angioedema, serum sickness, atopic dermatitis, contact dermatitis, gastrointestinal allergy, pruritus, physical allergies, reactions to injection of contrast media, reactions to therapeutic preparations and allergic transfusion reactions; for the relief of cough due to colds or allergy and for the symptomatic relief of other cold symptoms; as therapy for anaphylactic reactions adjunctive to epinephrine and other standard measures after the acute manifestations have been controlled; also postoperative nausea and vomiting, nausea of pregnancy, motion sickness, parkinsonism and drug-induced extrapyramidal reactions and quieting hyperactive, emotionally disturbed children, and for intractable insomnia and insomnia predominant to certain medical disorders. Parenteral administration is indicated where, in the judgment of the physician, prompt action is necessary and oral therapy would be inadequate.

Contraindications: This drug should not be used in premature or newborn infants, in nursing mothers, or in patients with hypersensitivity to diphenhydramine, in those with lower respiratory tract symptoms including asthma. Preparations containing diphenhydramine should not be given to patients receiving MAO inhibitors and should be used with considerable care, if at all, in patients with narrow-angle glaucoma, prostatic hypertrophy, stenosing peptic ulcer, pyloroduodenal obstruction and bladder-neck obstruction.

Warnings: Overdosage of antihistamines may produce hallucinations, convulsions or death, especially in infants and children. As in the case of other preparations containing CNS depressant drugs, patients receiving diphenhydramine should be cautioned about the additive effects with alcohol and other CNS depressants (hypnotics, sedatives, and tranquilizers). Patients who become drowsy when taking diphenhydramine should be cautioned against engaging in activities requiring alertness or skill, such as driving a car or operating heavy machinery or appliances. Dizziness, sedation, and hypotension are more likely to occur in elderly patients; and a paradoxical excitation may occur in the young child. Although there is no evidence that the use of this drug is detrimental to the mother or fetus, use during pregnancy should be carefully assessed. As with all anticholinergic drugs, an inhibitory effect on lactation may occur. Hypersensitivity reactions to diphenhydramine including anaphylactic shock, are more likely to occur following parenteral administration than oral administration.

Precautions: Avoid subcutaneous or perivascular injection. Diphenhydramine has an atropine-like action which should be considered when prescribing this agent. Use with caution in patients with a history of bronchial asthma, increased intraocular pressure, hyperthyroidism, cardiovascular disease, or hypertension.

Adverse Reactions: Those commonly occurring consist of sedation, sleepiness, dizziness, disturbed coordination, epigastric distress, and thickening of bronchial secretions. Other reactions that may be noted are urticaria; drug rash; anaphylactic shock; photosensitivity; excessive perspiration; chills; dryness of mouth, nose, and throat; hypotension; headache; palpitation; tachycardia; extrasystoles; hemolytic anemia; thrombocytopenia; agranulocytosis; fatigue; confusion; restlessness; excitation; nervousness; tremor; irritability; insomnia; euphoria; paresthesias; blurred vision; diplopia; vertigo; tinnitus; acute labyrinthitis; hysteria; neuritis; convulsions; anorexia; nausea; vomiting; diarrhea; constipation; urinary frequency; difficult urination; urinary retention; early menses; tightness of chest and wheezing, and nasal stuffiness.

Dosage and Administration: *Orally.* Adults, 25 to 50 mg 3 or 4 times daily. Children under 12 years of age, 10 to 20 mg 3 or 4 times daily. As much as 300 to 400 mg daily may be required by adults in acute, generalized or chronic urticaria and allergic-eczema. Maintenance dosage for adults, 25 mg 1 to 4 times daily. *Intravenously* or *intramuscularly, Adults,* 10 to 50 mg not to exceed 400 mg daily. Children, 5 mg/kg of body weight divided into 3 or 4 doses not to exceed 300 mg daily. To control motion sickness: 1 tablet ½ hour before departure and 1 or 2 tablets every 4 hours thereafter. As an antitussive: adults, 1 or 2 teaspoonsful 4 times daily. Children 2 years of age and over, ½ to 1 teaspoonful 3 or 4 times daily.

Availability:

Diphenhydramine Hydrochloride

Injection, 50 mg/ml in ampuls of 1 ml. **(Knoll)**
Capsules, 25 and 50 mg in bottles of 1000. **(Lederle)**
Elixir, 10 mg/5 ml in bottles of 1 pint and 1 gallon; 12.5 mg/5 ml in bottles of 5 ml. **(Lederle)**
Injection, 50 mg/ml in Tubex® (disposable syringes) of 1 ml with needle. **(Wyeth)**
BENADRYL®: **(Parke-Davis)**
Capsules (Kapseals®), 25 and 50 mg in bottles of 100 and 1000 and in unit-dose packages of 100.
Cream, 2% in tubes of 30 and 60 gm.
Elixir, 12.5 mg/5 ml in bottles of 120 ml, 1 pint and 1 gallon and in unit-dose bottles of 5 ml.
Injection, 10 mg/ml in Steri-Vials® of 10 and 30 ml; 50 mg/ml in Steri-Vials® of 10 ml and in ampuls and Steri-Dose® (disposable syringes) of 1 ml.
BENYLIN® Cough Syrup, 12.5 mg/5 ml; alcohol, 5% in bottles of 120 ml, pints and gallons and in unit-dose bottles of 5 and 10 ml. **(Parke-Davis)**
SK-DIPHENHYDRAMINE™ HYDROCHLORIDE: **(Smith Kline & French)**
Capsules, 25 and 50 mg in bottles of 100 and 1000.
Elixir, 12.5 mg/5 ml in bottles of 1 pint.

Combinations

BENADRYL® with EPHEDRINE SULFATE Capsules (Kapseals®), 50 mg with ephedrine sulfate, 25 mg in bottles of 100. **(Parke-Davis)**
DIPHENHYDRAMINE HYDROCHLORIDE Expectorant, 13.3 mg/5 ml with ammonium chloride, 130 mg; sodium citrate, 54 mg and alcohol, 5% in bottles of pints and gallons. **(Lederle)**

DIPHENIDOL

Chemical Name: α,α,Diphenyl-1-piperidinebutanol.

Description: An antiemetic compound, structurally related to chlophedianol and trihexyphenidyl, it occurs as a white, crystalline powder insoluble in water and sparingly soluble in alcohol. Diphenidol apparently exerts a specific antivertigo effect on the vestibular apparatus to control vertigo, and inhibits the chemoreceptor-trigger zone to control nausea and vomiting.

When given orally, peak blood concentration of the drug generally occurs in 1½ to 3 hours and is excreted in the urine and feces within 3 to 4 days. In clinical studies with 936 pregnant patients, 8% (72) of the patients experienced some fetal abnormality. Of the 72 patients, 6 had premature but otherwise normal infants, 40 aborted, 10 had stillbirths, and 16 had infants with miscellaneous defects such as hernias, congenital heart defects, hydrocephalus, internal strabismus, anencephalus, enlarged thyroid, and hypospadia; whether or not these were drug-induced has not been fully substantiated.

Indications: Peripheral (labyrinthine) vertigo and associated nausea and vomiting as seen in Meniere's disease, and in middle- and inner-ear surgery. Also for the prevention and control of nausea and vomiting as seen in postoperative states, malignant neoplasms and labyrinthine disturbances including motion sickness.

Contraindications: Known hypersensitivity to the drug, and in anuria.

Warnings: Auditory and visual hallucinations, disorientation and confusion have been reported in patients treated with diphenidol. Use of the drug is therefore limited to hospitalized patients or to patients under comparable close medical supervision. When prescribing diphenidol, the physician should carefully weigh the benefits against the possible risks and give due consideration to alternate therapeutic measures. The frequency of these reactions appears to be less than 0.5%. Thus far, they have occurred within 3 days of initiating the drug in recommended dosage and have subsided spontaneously usually within 3 days after discontinuation of the drug. Therefore, patients on diphenidol should be observed closely, and if these reactions occur the drug should be discontinued. Use during pregnancy, lactation or in women of childbearing potential requires that the expected benefits be weighed against its possible hazards to the mother and child. Diphenidol is not indicated for use in nausea and vomiting of pregnancy, since therapeutic value and safety have not been determined.

Precautions: Because drowsiness may occur, patients should be cautioned not to engage in any activity requiring alertness or skill. The antiemetic action of the drug may mask signs of overdosage of drugs (e.g., digitalis) or may obscure diagnosis of conditions such as intestinal obstruction and brain tumor. Patients should be observed regularly for signs of idiosyncratic reactions. Should be used with care in patients with glaucoma, obstructive lesions of the gastrointestinal and genitourinary tracts such as stenosing peptic ulcer, prostatic hypertrophy, pyloric and duodenal obstruction and organic cardiospasm. Intravenous administration to patients with a history of sinus tachycardia may be undesirable because this procedure may initiate an attack in such patients. Several patients were reported to have experienced a transient decrease in systolic and diastolic blood pressure up to 20 mm Hg, following parenteral use of this drug.

Adverse Reactions: Auditory and visual hallucinations, disorientation, confusion, drowsiness, overstimulation, depression, sleep disturbances, dry mouth, gastrointestinal irritation (nausea and indigestion), blurred vision, rarely dizziness, skin rash, malaise, headache, heartburn, and transient lowering of blood pressure. Mild jaundice of questionable relationship to the drug has been reported. Treatment of overdosage is essentially supportive, with maintenance of blood pressure plus careful observation of the patient. Large doses orally may require immediate gastric lavage.

Dosage and Administration: *Orally,* usual adult dose, 1 or 2 tablets every 4 hours. For rapid control of acute symptoms inject 1 to 2 ml *intramuscularly* (deep into the muscle) or *intravenously* directly or through venoclysis. Another 1 ml may be injected after 1 hour if symptoms persist. Thereafter, if intravenous method is used switch to intramuscular or oral route. In children, the unit doses are best calculated by body weight and should not be administered more often than every 4 hours. The total daily dose should not exceed 2.5 mg/lb *orally,* or 1.5 mg/lb *intramuscularly.* **Note:** The drug is not recommended for use in infants under 6 months of age or 25 lb of body weight. *Intravenous* or *subcutaneous* administration is not recommended in children of any age.

Availability:

Diphenidol (as hydrochloride)

VONTROL®: **(Smith Kline & French)**

Injection, 20 mg/ml in ampuls of 2 ml.

Tablets, 25 mg in bottles of 100.

DIPHENOXYLATE HYDROCHLORIDE ©

Chemical Name: 1-(3-Cyano-3,3-diphenylpropyl)-4-phenylisonipecotic acid ethyl ester.

Description: A synthetic constipating drug, structurally related to alphaprodine, anileridine and meperidine, it occurs as a white, crystalline powder slightly soluble in water. Diphenoxylate acts on the smooth muscle of the intestinal tract to inhibit gastrointestinal motility.

In experimental studies, large doses (40 to 60 mg) of diphenoxylate have been shown to produce a morphine-like euphoria, and toxic doses may cause respiratory depression and coma. Narcotic antagonists are the usual effective antidotes. A subtherapeutic dose of atropine sulfate has been added to discourage deliberate overdosage.

Indications: Adjunctive therapy in the management of diarrhea.

Contraindications: In patients with known hypersensitivity to diphenoxylate, or atropine, or in those with jaundice, and in children less than 2 years of age. Also contraindicated in diarrhea associated with pseudomembranous enterocolitis.

Warnings: Should be used with caution, if not contraindicated, in patients with cirrhosis or advanced liver disease and in those receiving addicting drugs and barbiturates because of the potentiating effects of these drugs. Diphenoxylate may be habit forming. **This product is not an innocuous drug and dosage recommendations should be strictly adhered to, especially in children.** It should be used with special care in children since signs of atropinism may occur even with recommended doses. Special care is also advised in young children because of the variable response to the drug in this age group. The concurrent use of diphenoxylate with MAO inhibitors may precipitate a hypertensive crisis. Diphenoxylate may potentiate the action of barbiturates, tranquilizers, and alcohol; therefore, patients should be closely observed when these medications are used concomitantly. Drug-induced inhibition of peristalsis may result in fluid retention in the colon which may lead to dehydration and electrolyte imbalance. If severe dehydration or electrolyte imbalance develops, the drug should be withheld until appropriate corrective therapy has been initiated. The drug must be used with caution in patients acutely ill with ulcerative colitis since it can precipitate adynamic ileus of the colon and possibly toxic dilatation (megacolon). Consequently, such patients should be carefully observed and therapy should be discontinued promptly if abdominal distension occurs or if other untoward symptoms develop. The use of diphenoxylate during pregnancy, lactation or in women of childbearing age requires that the potential benefits be weighed against any possible hazard to the mother and child. The effects of diphenoxylate or atropine sulfate may be evident in the infants of nursing mothers, since these compounds are excreted in breast milk.

Precautions: Patients should be cautioned to adhere strictly to recommended dosage schedules. Diphenoxylate should be administered with considerable caution to patients who are receiving addicting drugs or to individuals known to be addiction prone or to those who may increase their dosage on their own initiative. The medication should be kept out of reach of children since accidental overdosage may cause severe, even fatal, respiratory depression.

Adverse Reactions: Nausea, sedation or drowsiness, dizziness, vomiting, pruritus, restlessness, abdominal bloating, or cramps, numbness of the extremities, angioneurotic edema, giant urticaria, coma, lethargy, anorexia, atropine effects, paralytic ileus, headache, swelling of the gums, euphoria, depression, and general malaise. Dryness of the skin and mucous membranes, flushing, hyperthermia and tachycardia followed by lethargy or coma, hypotonic reflexes, nystagmus, pinpoint pupils, and respiratory depression may occur with overdosage. Patients should be carefully observed for a period of at least 48 hours since respiratory depression may not be evident until 12 to 30 hours afterwards. Gastric lavage, establishment of a patent airway and, if necessary, mechanically assisted respiration are advised. Administration of nalorphine or levallorphan is effective in reversing respiratory depression.

Dosage and Administration: *Orally.* Adults, 2 teaspoonsful or 2 tablets 4 times daily. Children, 2 to 5 years of age, 6 mg; 5 to 8 years, 8 mg; 8 to 12 years, 10 mg administered in divided doses.

Availability:
Ⓒ COLONIL™: **(Mallinckrodt)**
Liquid, each 5 ml contains 2.5 mg with atropine sulfate, 0.025 mg in bottles of 60 ml with calibrated plastic dropper.
Tablets, 2.5 mg with atropine sulfate, 0.025 mg in bottles of 100, 500, 1000 and 2500.
Ⓒ LOMOTIL®: **(Searle)**
Liquid, each 5 ml contains 2.5 mg with atropine sulfate, 0.025 mg in bottles of 60 ml with calibrated plastic dropper.
Tablets, 2.5 mg with atropine sulfate, 0.025 mg in bottles of 100, 500, 1000 and 2500, in individually blister-sealed, unit-dose cartons of 100 (2 × 50) and in tablet-dispenser packs of 30.
SK-DIPHENOXYLATE™ Tablets, 2.5 mg with atropine sulfate, 0.025 mg in bottles of 100 and 1000. **(Smith Kline & French)**

DIPHENYLHYDANTOIN: see Phenytoin

DIPHENYLPYRALINE HYDROCHLORIDE

Chemical Name: 4-Diphenylmethoxy-l-methylpiperidine hydrochloride.

Description: A potent antihistaminic agent with anticholinergic and sedative effects, related to diphenhydramine in chemical structure and pharmacologic action. The action of antihistamines appears to be due to competition with histamine for cell receptor sites on effector cells. It occurs as a white, odorless, crystalline powder freely soluble in water and in alcohol. Diphenylpyraline provides prompt and prolonged relief for a variety of allergic conditions.

Indications: Symptomatic treatment of seasonal hay fever and perennial allergic rhinitis, vasomotor rhinitis, allergic conjunctivitis due to inhalant allergans and foods, mild, uncomplicated allergic skin manifestations of urticaria and angioedema.

Contraindications: Known hypersensitivity to the drug, newborn or premature infants, nursing mothers, in lower respiratory symptoms including asthma, and concomitant use with monoamine oxidase inhibitors.

Warnings: Considerable caution is required in patients with narrow-angle glaucoma, stenosing peptic ulcer, symptomatic prostatic hypertrophy, bladder neck obstruction, and pyloroduodenal obstruction. Overdosage of this drug in infants and children may result in hallucinations, convulsions, and possibly death. The drug may diminish alertness in children, and in the young child particularly, it may produce excitement. Until more data is available, diphenylpyraline should be used in pregnant patients only when the anticipated benefits outweigh the possible risks. Because of an additive effect, patients should be cautioned not to take alcohol or other CNS depressants such as hypnotics, sedatives, tranquilizers, antianxiety agents, etc. while on this drug. Elderly patients are more likely to experience drug-induced dizziness, sedation and hypotension.

Precautions: Should drowsiness occur, patients should be cautioned not to engage in activities requiring alertness or skill such as driving a car or operating machinery. Due to its atropine-like action, this drug requires special care when given to patients with a history of bronchial asthma, increased intraocular pressure, hyperthyroidism, cardiovascular disease, and hypertension. Monoamine oxidase inhibitors (MAOI) can prolong and intensify the anticholinergic effects of antihistamines.

Adverse Reactions: The most frequently reported are sedation, sleepiness; dry mouth, nose, throat; thickening of bronchial secretions, dizziness, epigastric distress, and disturbed coordination. Other side effects which may occur are fatigue, confusion, restlessness, excitation, nervousness, insomnia, euphoria, anorexia, nausea, vomiting, diarrhea, constipation, hypotension, tightness of chest and wheezing, chills, urticaria, drug rash, anaphylactic shock, blurred vision, diplopia, vertigo, tinnitus, headache, palpitation, tachycardia, extrasystoles, paresthesias, acute labyrinthitis, hysteria, neuritis, convulsions, nasal stuffiness, urinary frequency, difficult urination, urinary retention, early menses, photosensitivity, excessive perspiration, hemolytic anemia, thrombocytopenia, and agranulocytosis. Manifestations of overdosage include arrhythmias, hypertension or hypotension and circulatory collapse. Gastrointestinal symptoms are characterized by nausea, vomiting, diarrhea, and abdominal cramps. Acute intoxication may vary from CNS depression to stimulation especially in children. Also, atropine-like reactions such as dry mouth; fixed, dilated pupils; flushing, etc., as well as gastrointestinal symptoms and marked cerebral irritation may occur. Treatment involves induced vomiting or gastric lavage. Saline cathartics are valuable for their action in rapid dilution of bowel content. **Stimulants should not be employed.** Hypotension may be counteracted by administering levarterenol bitartrate by means of intravenous drip.

Dosage and Administration: *Orally.* Adults, 1 capsule every 12 hours or 1 tablet every 4 hours. Children 6 to 12 years of age, 1 capsule daily or 1 tablet every 6 hours; 2 to 6 years of age, ½ to 1 tablet every 8 hours. May be given to children under 2 years of age at the direction of the physician.

Availability:
DIAFEN® Tablets, 2 mg in bottles of 100. **(Riker)**
HISPRIL® Spansule® (sustained-release capsules), 5 mg in bottles of 50. **(Smith Kline & French)**

DIPHTHERIA AND TETANUS TOXOIDS, ALUM PRECIPITATED

Description: A combination of purified alum-precipitated tetanus and diphtheria toxoids, 1 ml representing one human (antigenic) dose of each toxoid. The quantity of tetanus toxoid in a single dose (0.5 ml) of this preparation is about 7.5 Lf units, the same as that contained in an individual dose of regular tetanus toxoid. The quantity of diphtheria toxoid is about 1.5 Lf units, or one-sixteenth that in regular diphtheria toxoid for adults and 25 Lf units (equal to that of regular toxoid) for children.

Indications: For primary immunization against diphtheria and tetanus toxins. Stimulates formation of specific antibodies producing an immunization response at least equal to that of each antigen injected separately. To maintain immunity against these diseases, a booster dose may be given every 3 to 4 years.

Contraindications: Acute respiratory disease or other active infections; a history of CNS damage or convulsions.

Precautions: The parenteral administration of any biological product should be attended by every known precaution for the prevention and arrest of allergic and other untoward reactions. A careful history should review possible sensitivity of the patient to the type of protein to be injected. Any acute respiratory disease or other active infection if present, should indicate postponement of the injection. A separate heat-sterilized syringe and needle or new disposable equivalent should be used for each individual patient to prevent transmission of homologous serum hepatitis or other infectious agents from one individual to another. Care should be taken to avoid injecting into a blood vessel. Patients with a history of serious allergic reactions to tetanus toxoid, should be given a small test dose before the full booster dose is administered. Adrenocorticotropin, adrenal corticosteroids or other immunosuppressive agents reduce host resistance to disease; therefore, they should not be administered following exposure to infectious agents (mumps, rabies, tetanus) as the host-parasite relationship may be altered sufficiently to cause severe or fatal illness in spite of prophylactic administration of a vaccine. Since almost all biological products have the capability of producing serious neurological disorders, the possibility of their occurrence must be appreciated by those who have the responsibility to immunize individuals against infectious disease. However, neurologic disorders in infants and children do not constitute a valid reason for deferring or withholding routine immunization, since there is no conclusive evidence that children with brain damage or convulsive disorders have a higher incidence of serious reaction from routine immunizations procedures than do normal children. Should a CNS reaction occur shortly after any dose of antigen, immunization should be postponed until the child reaches at least 1 year of age and evidence of active cerebral involvement has subsided.

Adverse Reactions: Reactions are usually mild and may be *local,* characterized by edema, erythema and/or pain or *systemic* with chills, fever, and general malaise occurring.

Dosage and Administration: *Intramuscularly.* Immunizing dosage consists of 2 injections of 0.5 ml each, 4 to 6 weeks apart. An 0.5 ml booster dose is recommended 6 to 12 months later and then, to maintain immunity, every 3 to 4 years. *For pediatric use:* Immunizing dosage consists of 3 injections of 0.5 ml doses given at intervals of 3 to 4 weeks. The injections are given *subcutaneously* at sites away from previous immunizations. The booster dose is 0.5 ml for children under 6 years of age. The toxoids are best administered at body temperature.

Availability:
DIPHTHERIA AND TETANUS TOXOIDS, COMBINED (ALUMINUM PHOSPHATE ADSORBED) and Purogenated® *for pediatric use* in vials of 5 ml and in disposable syringes (Lederject®) of 0.5 ml. **(Lederle)**
DIPHTHERIA AND TETANUS TOXOIDS (ALUMINUM PHOSPHATE ADSORBED) and Purogenated® *for adult use* in vials of 5 ml and in disposable syringes (Lederject®) of 0.5 ml. **(Lederle)**
DIPHTHERIA AND TETANUS TOXOIDS (FLUID) and purified *for pediatric use* in vials of 7.5 ml. **(Lilly)**
DIPHTHERIA AND TETANUS TOXOIDS (ALUMINUM PHOSPHATE ADSORBED) *for adult use* in vials of 5 ml. **(Lilly)**
DIPHTHERIA AND TETANUS TOXOIDS (ALUMINUM PHOSPHATE ADSORBED) and purified (biologic) *for pediatric use* in vials of 5 ml. **(Lilly)**
DIPHTHERIA AND TETANUS TOXOIDS (ALUMINUM PHOSPHATE ADSORBED) and purified *for pediatric use* in vials of 5 ml. **(Parke-Davis)**
DIPHTHERIA AND TETANUS TOXOIDS (ALUMINUM PHOSPHATE ADSORBED) and ultrafined *for adult use* in vials of 5 ml and in Tubex® (sterile cartridge-needle unit) of 0.5 ml. **(Wyeth)**
DIPHTHERIA AND TETANUS TOXOIDS (ALUMINUM PHOSPHATE ADSORBED) and ultrafined *for pediatric use* in vials of 5 ml and in Tubex® (sterile cartridge-needle unit) of 0.5 ml. **(Wyeth)**

DIPHTHERIA-TETANUS TOXOIDS AND PERTUSSIS VACCINE COMBINED

Description: A suspension of purified alum precipitated or plain diphtheria and tetanus toxoids and of extracted pertussis antigen in 0.3 M glycine solution. The concentration of the antigen is such that the total dose for primary immunization (1.5 ml) contains 12 protective units of pertussis antigen, about 15 Lf units of tetanus toxoid and about 50 Lf units of diphtheria toxoid. The extracted pertussis antigen is as effective as whole-cell vaccine in the stimulation of pertussis antibodies; the incidence and severity of local and systemic reactions are less and it contains considerably less protein nitrogen than does the whole-cell vaccine.

Indications: For active immunization against diphtheria, tetanus and whooping cough in infants and children from 2 months to 6 years of age.

Contraindications: In the presence of acute respiratory disease or other active infection.

Precautions: This combination of antigens should be employed *only* as a prophylactic agent and *only* in patients 6 years of age and under. Not to be used as a therapeutic agent at any time. Postvaccinal neurological disorders, such as convulsions or encephalophy, have been reported following use of this agent. Although these reactions are uncommon, they may be serious, and the possibility of their occurrence must be considered. It has been suggested that individuals with a history of serious allergic reactions to tetanus toxoid be given a small test dose of Tetanus Toxoid, Fluid, intradermally before the full booster dose is administered. A history of CNS damage or convulsions is generally regarded as an indication to use fractional doses of the individual antigens or to start with $^1/_{10}$ the recommended dosage and then follow with standard doses if no untoward reactions occur. Adrenocorticotropin, adrenal corticosteroids and other immunodepressants suppress the antibody response following immunization, and reduce host resistance to the disease. Therefore, they should not be administered following exposure to infectious agents (mumps, rabies, tetanus) as the host-parasite relationship may be altered sufficiently to cause severe or fatal illness in spite of prophylactic administration of a vaccine. Inoculations should be postponed in the presence of acute infection. In older individuals, reactions due to sensitivity to the proteins of the diphtheria and pertussis organisms are more frequent and more severe. This effect is more evident with combined than with single antigens. Care should be exercised against injecting this vaccine into a blood vessel.

Adverse Reactions: Local and systemic reactions have been less frequent with this product than with vaccines containing whole pertussis cells. When local reactions have occurred, they have consisted primarily of erythema, induration and tenderness. Pain at the injection site has been minimal. Following injection, a small nodule may develop at the site of injection and may remain for a few weeks before being completely absorbed. Occasionally, liquefaction develops about the nodule, which, in rare exceptions, may increase sufficiently to require incision and drainage. Postvaccinal reactions, such as chills, fever, malaise, and restlessness, have been reported infrequently. Rarely noted were reactions involving the CNS. A small but significant number of cases of encephalopathy, with mental and physical symptoms which may be irreversible, or even fatal, have been reported. These were presumed to be due to the pertussis vaccine component. Epinephrine, 1:1000 and other emergency drugs and equipment should be readily available to combat severe systemic reactions should they develop.

Dosage and Administration: *Intramuscularly,* at sites away from previous immunizations and in areas with abundant subcutaneous tissue. Skin should be sponged with a suitable antiseptic before injection. Primary immunization consists of 3 doses of 0.5 ml each, administered 4 to 6 weeks apart. Booster injections of 0.5 ml are recommended 1 year after primary immunization and again before entry into school.

Availability:
DIPHTHERIA-TETANUS TOXOIDS AND PERTUSSIS VACCINE COMBINED (aluminum phosphate adsorbed) *for adult use* in vials of 7.5 ml. **(Merrell-National)**
TRI-IMMUNOL® (aluminum phosphate adsorbed) in vials of 7.5 ml. **(Lederle)**
TRIOGEN® (aluminum phosphate adsorbed) in vials of 7.5 ml. **(Parke-Davis)**
TRIPLE ANTIGEN (aluminum phosphate adsorbed) in vials of 7.5 ml and in Tubex® (sterile cartridge-needle unit) of 0.5 ml. **(Wyeth)**

DIPYRIDAMOLE

Chemical Name: 2,6-bis-(Diethanolamino)-4,8-dipiperidinopyrimido-(5,4-d)pyrimidine.

Description: A coronary vasodilatory compound unrelated chemically to the nitrates or to digitalis. It occurs as a bitter, odorless, yellow, crystalline powder very slightly soluble in water and freely soluble in alcohol. Its mode of action is unknown but the drug apparently acts directly on the coronary vessels and the myocardial cell. It increases coronary blood flow without significantly altering blood pressure, heart rate or myocardial oxygen consumption.

Indications: Chronic angina pectoris. Prolonged therapy may reduce the frequency or eliminate anginal episodes, improve exercise tolerance and reduce nitroglycerin requirements. The drug is not intended to abort the acute anginal attack.

Contraindications: No specific contraindication is known.

Precautions: Use cautiously in patients with hypotension.

Adverse Reactions: Headache, dizziness, nausea, flushing, weakness or syncope, mild gastrointestinal distress and skin rash. A possible aggravation of angina pectoris has been noted.

Dosage and Administration: *Orally,* 50 mg 3 times daily taken at least 1 hour before meals. Clinical response may not be noted before the 2nd or 3rd month of continuous therapy. Prompt cessation of undesirable symptoms usually follows withdrawal of the drug.

Availability:
PERSANTINE® Tablets, 25 mg in bottles of 100 and 1000. **(Boehringer Ingelheim)**

DISODIUM EDETATE

Chemical Name: (Ethylenedinitrilo) tetraacetic acid disodium salt. (EDTA).

Description: Disodium edetate is a chelating agent which differs structurally from calcium disodium edetate in that the calcium chelate is absent in the molecule. It occurs as a white powder freely soluble in water.

The drug forms chelates with the cations of calcium and many divalent and trivalent metals. Because of its affinity for calcium, disodium edetate will produce a lowering of the serum calcium level during intravenous infusion. Slow infusion over a protracted period may cause mobilization of extracirculatory calcium stores. The chelate thus formed is excreted in the urine. Disodium edetate exerts a negative inotropic effect upon the heart. It also forms chelates with other polyvalent metals and produces increases in urinary excretion of magnesium, zinc and other trace elements. The drug does not form a chelate with potassium but may reduce the serum level and increase urinary loss of potassium.

Indications: In selected patients for the emergency treatment of hypercalcemia and for the control of ventricular arrhythmias associated with digitalis toxicity.

Contraindications: In anuric patients. It is not indicated for the treatment of generalized arteriosclerosis associated with advancing age.

Warnings: The use of this drug in any particular patient is recommended only when the severity of the clinical condition justifies the aggressive measures associated with this type of therapy. Rapid intravenous infusion or attainment of high serum concentration of disodium edetate may cause a precipitous drop in the serum calcium level and may result in fatality. Toxicity appears to be dependent upon both total dosage and speed of administration. The rate of administration and dosage should not exceed those recommended. Because of its irritant effect on the tissues and because of the danger of serious side effects if administered in the undiluted form, disodium edetate injection should be diluted before infusion. Renal excretory function should be assessed prior to treatment. Periodic BUN and creatinine determinations and daily urinalysis should be performed on patients receiving this drug. Because of the possibility of inducing an electrolyte imbalance during treatment with disodium edetate, appropriate laboratory determinations and studies to evaluate the status of cardiac function should be performed. Repetition of these tests is recommended as often as clinically indicated, particularly in patients with ventricular arrhythmia and those with a history of seizure disorders or intracranial lesions. If clinical evidence suggests any disturbance of liver function during treatment, appropriate laboratory determinations should be performed and withdrawal of the drug may be required. The oxalate method of determining serum calcium tends to give low readings in the presence of disodium edetate; modification of this method, as by acidifying the sample, or use of a different method may be required for accuracy. The least interference will be noted immediately before a subsequent dose is administered. Safe use of disodium edetate has not been established with respect to adverse effects on fetal development. Therefore, it should be used in women of childbearing potential and particularly during early pregnancy only when, in the judgment of the physician, the potential benefits outweigh the possible hazards.

Precautions: After the infusion of disodium edetate the patient should remain in bed for a short time because of the possibility of postural hypotension. The possibility of an adverse effect on myocardial contractility should be considered when administering the drug to patients with heart disease. Caution is dictated in the use of this drug in patients with limited cardiac reserve or incipient congestive failure. Disodium edetate therapy should be used with caution in patients with clinical or subclinical potassium deficiency states. In such cases it is advisable to perform serum potassium blood levels for possible hypokalemia and to monitor ECG changes. The possibility of hypomagnesemia should be kept in mind during prolonged therapy. Treatment with disodium edetate has been shown to cause a lowering of blood sugar and insulin requirements in patients with diabetes who are being treated with insulin.

Adverse Reactions: Gastrointestinal symptoms such as nausea, vomiting, and diarrhea are fairly common following administration of this drug. Transient symptoms such as circumoral paresthesia, numbness and headache and a transient drop in systolic and diastolic blood pressure may occur. Thrombophlebitis, febrile reactions, hyperuricemia, anemia, exfoliative dermatitis and other toxic skin and mucous membrane reactions have been reported. Nephrotoxicity and damage to the reticuloendothelial system with hemorrhagic tendencies have been reported with excessive dosages. Overdosage may cause a precipitous fall in serum calcium level; therefore the means for intravenous calcium replacement should be readily available. Extreme caution must be exercised in the use of intravenous calcium in the treatment of tetany, especially in patients receiving digitalis because the action of the drug and the replacement of calcium ions may reverse the desired digitalis effect.

Dosage and Administration: *Intravenous infusion only.* The solution must be diluted before injection. The recommended daily dosage is 50 mg/kg of body weight for adults and 40 mg/kg for children; the adult dosage should not exceed 3 gm and the children's should not exceed 70 mg/kg in 24 hours. After dilution with 500 ml of 5% dextrose injection, or sodium chloride injection, the resultant volume should be administered over a period of 3 to 4 hours. Toxicity depends upon both *total dosage* and *rate of flow;* administration, therefore, must not be hurried. The usual regimen consists of daily infusions for 5 days, followed by a rest period of 2 days. This cycle is repeated 3 times until the drug has been given for a total of 15 days. Therapy should then be discontinued for several weeks while the results are being assessed. Subsequent courses of treatment may be indicated.

Availability:
ENDRATE® Injection, 150 mg/ml in ampuls of 20 ml (adjusted with sodium hydroxide).

(Abbott)

DISOPYRAMIDE PHOSPHATE

Chemical Name: α-[2-(diisopropylamino)ethyl]-α-phenyl-2-pyridineacetamide phosphate.

Description: Disopyramide is an antiarrhythmic agent that suppresses cardiac ventricular arrythmias, and is specifically designed to reduce or prevent those types of arrhythmias that can lead to ventricular fibrillation. Although chemically unique among the antiarrhythmic agents, its pharmacologic actions are similar to those of quinidine and procainamide. The chief characteristics of the drug are that it suppresses or prevents the recurrence of unifocal, multifocal and paired premature ventricular contractions, in addition to episodes of ventricular tachycardia. Disopyramide is appropriate whether these arrythmias occur singly or in combination, or if they are primary or occur in association with coronary artery disease; and it is effective in both digitalized and nondigitalized patients. Animal studies have shown that the drug has no effect on alpha- or beta-adrenergic receptors. Electrophysiologic studies demonstrated that the drug produces quinidine-like effects on atrial and AV node refractory periods, but the effects differed on AV node or His-Purkinje conduction times in that there were little or no significant results; also the sinus node recovery time was decreased. Disopyramide's usefulness in patients with acute myocardial infarction, persistent ventricular tachycardia, atrial arrhythmias or arrhythmias due to digitalis intoxication, as well as its value in preventing sudden death in patients with serious ventricular ectopic activity awaits further clinical studies.

Following oral administration, the drug is rapidly and almost completely absorbed from the gastrointestinal tract, reaching peak plasma levels within 2 hours, and a mean plasma half-life of 6.7 hours. The usual therapeutic plasma levels are 2 to 4 mcg/ml, and approximately 50% of the plasma concentration is bound to protein. In healthy individuals the urinary excretion of disopyramide and its metabolites accounts for about 80% of the dose with close to 50% as unchanged drug, 20% as the mono-N-dealkylated metabolite, and 10% as other metabolites. Altering the urinary pH does not affect the plasma half-life or the amount of drug excreted in the urine. About 10% of disopyramide is excreted in the feces.

Results of studies in pregnant rats and rabbits have revealed only minimal evidence of impaired fertility and no evidence of fetal anomalies.

Indications: Treatment of patients with unifocal or multifocal premature ventricular contractions, paired premature ventricular contractions, and episodes of ventricular tachycardia (persistent ventricular tachycardia is generally treated with DC cardioversion).

Contraindications: Cardiogenic shock, preexisting second- or third-degree AV block (if no pacemaker is present), or known hypersensitivity to the drug.

Warnings: The drug should be discontinued promptly if severe hypotension, not associated with cardiac arrhythmia, develops in patients with primary cardiomyopathy or inadequately compensated congestive heart failure. Patients with a poorly compensated or uncompensated congestive heart failure should not receive this drug unless the condition is exacerbated by or caused by an arrhythmia, and until proper treatment including optimal digitalization has been accomplished. The drug may then be useful in suppressing the ectopy. Careful monitoring of the patient is essential under these circumstances. In some patients with marginally compensated heart failure, the drug may cause cardiac decompensation. In these patients, progressive congestive heart failure should generally be treated with cardiac glycosides and diuretics and the course of treatment closely followed. If adequate control of congestive heart failure is not attained, the disopyramide dosage should be reduced or the drug discontinued. A reduced dosage should be administered if first-degree heart block develops, and if the block persists, continuation of treatment must depend upon an assessment of the benefits versus the risk of higher degrees of heart block. Development of second- or third-degree AV block or uni-, bi-, or trifascicular block requires cessation of treatment unless the ventricular rate is adequately controlled by a pacemaker. Because of its anticholinergic properties, disopyramide should be used with caution in patients with glaucoma or with urinary retention.

Precautions: The occurrence of significant widening (greater than 25%) of the QRS complex on the electrocardiogram warrants withdrawal of the drug. Patients with atrial flutter or fibrillation should be digitalized prior to disopyramide administration to ensure that drug-induced enhancement of AV conduction does not allow a ventricular rate beyond physiologically acceptable limits. The effects of the drug are presently uncertain in patients with sick sinus (bradycardia/tachycardia) syndrome, Wolff-Parkinson-White syndrome, or bundle branch block. The drug should be administered cautiously to patients who are receiving or who have recently received other antiarrhythmic drugs, since excessive widening of the QRS complex may occur in such instances. Dosage should be reduced in patients with impaired renal or hepatic function and the ECG carefully monitored for signs of overdosage. Antiarrhythmic drugs may be ineffective in patients with hypokalemia; therefore, any potassium deficit should be corrected before instituting therapy with this drug. Safe use during pregnancy has not been established; consequently, it should be used in pregnant women only when it is clearly indicated and the benefits/risks ratio has been carefully evaluated. It is not known whether or not disopyramide is excreted in human milk. However, studies in rats have shown that the concentration of the drug and its metabolites in milk is up to 3 times greater than in plasma. If use of the drug is deemed essential, an alternate method of infant feeding should be instituted. Safe and effective use in pediatric patients has not been confirmed.

Adverse Reactions: *Anticholinergic reactions* include dry mouth; urinary hesitancy; constipation; blurred vision; dryness of the nose, eyes and throat; and urinary retention. *Genitourinary effects* include urinary frequency and urgency, and dysuria. *Gastrointestinal reactions* are manifested by nausea; abdominal pain; bloating and gas; anorexia, diarrhea, and vomiting. *CNS reactions* include nervousness, depression, insomnia, impotence, dizziness, generalized fatigue, muscle weakness, headache, and malaise. A single case of acute psychosis has been reported following therapy, with prompt return to normal mental status when therapy was discontinued. *Cardiovascular effects* observed were edema, and weight gain, disturbances of cardiac conduction, shortness of breath, syncope, chest pain, and hypotension. *Dermatologic reactions* include a generalized rash and dermatoses.

Dosage and Administration: *Orally.* The recommended initial dosage for adults is a 300-mg loading dose, followed by 150 mg every 6 hours. For patients of small stature or those with renal or hepatic insufficiency, cardiomyopathy, or possible cardiac decompensation, a 200-mg loading dose is recommended, followed by a maintenance dosage of 100 mg every 6 hours. Dosage must be individualized based on each patient's response and tolerance.

Availability:
NORPACE® Capsules, 100 mg (white and orange) and 150 mg (brown and orange) in bottles of 100. **(Searle)**

DISULFIRAM

Chemical Name: Bis(diethylthiocarbamoyl) disulfide.

Description: An antioxidant compound used as an adjunct in the treatment of chronic alcoholism. It occurs as a white to off-white, odorless and almost tasteless powder very slightly soluble in water and soluble in alcohol.

Indications: For the alcoholic patient who wants to remain in a state of enforced sobriety so that supportive and psychotherapeutic treatment may be applied.

Contraindications: Patients who are receiving or have recently received metronidazole, paraldehyde, alcohol, or alcohol-containing preparations, such as cough syrups, tonics, and the like, should not be given disulfiram. Disulfiram is contraindicated in the presence of severe myocardial disease or coronary occlusion, psychoses or hypersensitivity.

Warnings: Disulfiram should never be administered to a patient when he is in a state of alcohol intoxication or without his full knowledge. The physician should instruct relatives accordingly. The patient must be fully informed of the disulfiram-alcohol reaction. He must be strongly cautioned against surreptitious drinking while taking the drug, and he must be fully aware of possible consequences. He should be warned to avoid alcohol in disguised forms, *i.e.* in sauces, vinegars, cough mixtures, and even aftershave lotions and back rubs. He should also be warned that reactions may occur with alcohol up to 14 days after ingesting disulfiram. Disulfiram plus alcohol, even small amounts, produces flushing, throbbing in head and neck, throbbing headache, respiratory difficulty, nausea, copious vomiting, sweating, thirst, chest pain, palpitation, dyspnea, hyperventilation, tachycardia, hypotension, syncope, marked uneasiness, weakness, vertigo, blurred vision, and confusion. In severe reactions there may be respiratory depression, cardiovascular collapse, arrhythmias, myocardial infarction, acute congestive heart failure, unconsciousness, convulsions, and death. The intensity of the reaction varies with each individual, but is generally proportional to the amounts of disulfiram and alcohol ingested. Mild reactions may occur in the sensitive individual when the blood alcohol concentration is increased to as little as 5 to 10 mg/100 ml. Symptoms are fully developed at 50 mg/100 ml, and unconsciousness usually results when the blood alcohol level reaches 125 to 150 mg. The duration of the reaction varies from 30 to 60 minutes to several hours in the more severe cases, or as long as there is alcohol in the blood.

Disulfiram appears to decrease the rate at which certain drugs are metabolized and so may increase the blood levels and the possibility of clinical toxicity of drugs given concomitantly. The drug should be used with caution in those patients receiving phenytoin and its congeners, since toxic levels of these antiepileptic agents have been reported during concomitant disulfiram therapy. It may be necessary to adjust the dosage of oral anticoagulants upon beginning or stopping disulfiram, since disulfiram may prolong prothrombin time. Patients taking isoniazid when disulfiram is given should be observed for the appearance of unsteady gait or marked changes in mental status and the disulfiram discontinued if such signs appear. Because of the possibility of an accidental disulfiram-alcohol reaction, disulfiram should be used with extreme caution in patients with any of the following conditions: diabetes mellitus, hypothyroidism, epilepsy, cerebral damage, chronic and acute nephritis, hepatic cirrhosis or insufficiency. The safe use of this drug in pregnant women has not been established. Therefore, it should be used during pregnancy only when, in the judgment of the physician, the probable benefits outweigh the possible risks.

Precautions: It is suggested that every patient under treatment carry an *Identification Card,* stating that he is receiving disulfiram, describing the disulfiram-alcohol reaction, and showing name of physician or institution to be contacted in case of emergency. Alcoholism may accompany or be followed by dependence on narcotics or sedatives. Barbiturates have been administered concurrently with disulfiram without untoward effects, but the possibility of initiating a new abuse should be considered. Base line and follow-up transaminase tests (10 to 14 days) are suggested to detect any hepatic dysfunction that may result with disulfiram therapy. In addition, a complete blood count and a sequential multiple analysis (SMA-12) test should be performed every 6 months.

Adverse Reactions: Occasional skin eruptions are, as a rule, readily controlled by concomitant administration of an antihistaminic drug. In a small number of patients, a transient mild drowsiness, fatigability, impotence, headache, acneform eruptions, allergic dermatitis, or a metallic or garlic-like aftertaste may be experienced during the first 2 weeks of therapy. These complaints usually disappear spontaneously with the continuation of therapy or with reduced dosage. Psychotic reactions have been noted, attributable in most cases to high dosage, combined toxicity (with metronidazole or isoniazid), or to the unmasking of underlying psychoses in patients stressed by the withdrawal of alcohol. There have been reports of polyneuritis and peripheral neuritis, and rare instances of optic neuritis. One case of cholestatic hepatitis has been reported, but its relationship to the drug has not been verified.

Dosage and Administration: *Orally.* Before initiating therapy, abstinence from alcohol for at least 12 hours is necessary. Should be administered for at least 4 days before adequate blood levels can be expected. *Initial dosage,* up to 500 mg for 1 or 2 weeks. *Maintenance dosage,* 125 mg up to 500 mg (average 250 mg) daily. Due to a transitory sedative effect, a decrease in alertness, and fatigue may occur; it has therefore been suggested that the drug be administered at bedtime. Consult package literature for further details.

Availability:
ANTABUSE® Tablets, 250 mg in bottles of 100; 500 mg in bottles of 50 and 1000. **(Ayerst)**

DOBUTAMINE HYDROCHLORIDE

Chemical Name: (±)-4-[2-[[3-(*p*-Hydroxyphenyl)-1-methylpropyl]amine]ethyl]-pyrocatechol hydrochloride.

Description: Dobutamine, a synthetic catecholamine, is a potent cardiac stimulant with minimal effects on heart rate and blood pressure. A direct-acting inotropic agent, its primary activity results from stimulation of the beta receptors of the heart while producing comparatively mild chronotropic, hypertensive, arrhythmogenic, and vasodilative effects. Its biochemical nature is such that it does not cause the release of endogenous norepinephrine as does dopamine. In preclinical, comparative studies with isoproterenol, dobutamine was found to be less inclined to increase heart rate and to decrease peripheral vascular resistance. In patients with depressed cardiac function, both drugs augment cardiac output to a similar degree, but whereas improvement in cardiac output with isoproterenol is more a reflection of increased heart rate while the stroke volume changes little or declines, the reverse is true of dobutamine which does not appreciably increase heart rate (although tachycardia has occasionally been observed) but stroke volume is generally increased. With dobutamine, facilitation of atrioventricular conduction has been observed in clinical electrophysiologic studies and in patients with atrial fibrillation. Also, systemic vascular resistance is usually decreased, and minimal vasoconstriction has rarely been observed. While most clinical experience with the drug has been of short duration (up to several hours), a limited number of patients underwent studies for 24, 48 and 72 hours, and some of these showed a persistent increase in cardiac output whereas in others output returned toward base-line values.

The onset of action occurs within 1 to 2 minutes; however, as much as 10 minutes may be required to obtain the peak effect of a particular infusion rate. An ultra-short plasma half-life of 2 minutes has been reported. The major excretion products in the urine are conjugates of dobutamine and 3-0-methyl dobutamine, the latter being an inactive metabolite. Studies in animals have provided evidence that the actions of dobutamine are not dependent on presynaptic mechanisms, since alteration of synaptic concentrations of catecholamines with either reserpine or tricyclic antidepressants does not apparently modify its effects.

Reproduction studies performed in rats and rabbits have revealed no evidence of impaired fertility, harm to the fetus, or teratogenic effects.

Concurrent administration with drugs including digitalis preparations, furosemide, spironolactone, lidocaine, glyceryl trinitrate, isosorbide dinitrate, morphine, atropine, heparin, protamine, potassium chloride, folic acid, and acetaminophen produced no evidence of drug interactions. Preliminary studies indicate that the concomitant use of dobutamine and nitroprusside results in a higher cardiac output and, usually, a lower pulmonary wedge pressure than when either drug is used alone.

Indications: *Short-term* treatment of adults with cardiac decompensation due to depressed contractility resulting either from organic heart disease or from cardiac surgical procedures. Patients who have atrial fibrillation with rapid ventricular response should be digitalized prior to instituting therapy with dobutamine.

Contraindications: Idiopathic hypertrophic subaortic stenosis.

Warnings: A dose-related increase in heart rate or blood pressure, especially systolic pressure may occur. Approximately 10% of patients in clinical trials have had rate increases of 30 beats/minute or more, and about 7.5% have had a 50-mmHg or greater increase in systolic pressure. These effects are promptly reversed by a reduction in dosage. Because the drug facilitates atrioventricular conduction, patients with atrial fibrillation are at risk of developing rapid ventricular response, and those with preexisting hypertension appear to face an increased risk of developing an exaggerated pressor response. The drug may precipitate or exacerbate ventricular ectopic activity, but it rarely has caused ventricular tachycardia.

Precautions: ECG and blood pressure should be continuously monitored, and pulmonary wedge pressure and cardiac output should be checked whenever possible to aid in the safe and effective use of the drug. If hypovolemia exists, it should be corrected with suitable volume expanders before treatment is initiated. Patients who have recently received a beta-blocking agent may not respond to the drug, and the peripheral vascular resistance may be increased. No improvement may be observed in the presence of marked mechanical obstruction, such as severe vascular aortic stenosis. The drug should be used in pregnant patients only when the expected benefits clearly outweigh the potential risks to the fetus. Currently, no clinical data are available on the safe and effective use in children.

Adverse Reactions: Most patients generally experienced a 10- to 20-mmHg increase in systolic blood pressure and an increase in heart rate of 5 to 15 beats/minute. Moreover, 5% of patients have had increases in premature ventricular beats during infusions. The incidence of nausea, headache, anginal pain, nonspecific chest pain, palpitations, and shortness of breath was noted in 1 to 3% of patients. No abnormal laboratory values attributable to dobutamine have been observed. Infusions of up to 72 hours have produced no additional adverse effects. In case of overdosage, as evidenced by excessive alteration of blood pressure or by tachycardia, a reduction in the rate of administration or a temporary suspension of treatment is required until the patient's condition stabilizes. Because the duration of action is short, usually no additional remedial measures are necessary.

Dosage and Administration: *Intravenously.* For reconstitution, Sterile Water for Injection or 5% Dextrose Injection may be used. Since the drug is incompatible with alkaline solutions, it should *not* be mixed with products such as 5% Sodium Bicarbonate Injection. To reconstitute, add 10 ml of diluent to the vial, and if not completely dissolved, another 10 ml may be added. The reconstituted solution may be stored under refrigeration for 48 hours or at room temperature for 6 hours. Before administration, the solution must be further diluted to at least 50 ml in 5% dextrose, isotonic sodium chloride solution or sodium lactate injection. The rate of infusion needed to increase cardiac output usually ranges from 2.5 to 10 mcg/kg/minute, but up to 40 mcg/kg/minute may be required to obtain the desired effect. The final volume administered should be determined by the fluid requirements of the patient.

Availability:
DOBUTREX® Powder for Injection (lyophilized) in 20-ml vials of 250 mg. **(Lilly)**

DOLONIL

Description: Each dark maroon, coated square tablet contains:

Phenazopyridine hydrochloride	150 mg
Hyoscyamine hydrobromide	0.3 mg
Butabarbital	15 mg

A combination of antiinflammatory, parasympatholytic and sedative agents for the symptomatic relief of urinary tract complications that may arise from infection, trauma, surgery, endoscopic procedures, or from the passage of sounds or catheters.

Indications: Symptomatic relief of pain, frequency, urgency, burning and dysuria arising from inflammation of the urothelium, the mucosal lining of the lower urinary tract, particularly when accompanied by detrusor muscle spasm and apprehension.

Contraindications: Renal or hepatic insufficiency, glaucoma, porphyria, sensitivity to any component; also in patients with bladder neck obstruction.

Warnings: Butabarbital may be habit-forming.

Precautions: The development of a yellowish tinge of the skin or sclerae may indicate accumulation due to impaired renal excretion and may warrant withdrawal of the drug.

Adverse Reactions: Dry mouth, drowsiness or dizziness is noted in more than one third of patients (and may occur in half of the patients of older age groups). These symptoms seldom require discontinuation of medication. Other atropine-like effects such as blurred vision may also occur. There may be occasional gastrointestinal disturbances.

Dosage and Administration: *Orally.* Average adult dose, 1 tablet 4 times daily taken after each meal and at bedtime. Urine becomes reddish-orange in color.

Availability:
DOLONIL® Tablets in bottles of 100. **(Warner/Chilcott)**

DONNAZYME

Description: Each green, coated tablet contains in the acid-soluble outer layer:

Hyoscyamine sulfate	0.0518 mg
Atropine sulfate	0.0097 mg
Hyoscine hydrobromide	0.0033 mg
Phenobarbital	8.1 mg
Pepsin N.F. equivalent	150 mg
In the enteric-coated core:	
Pancreatin N.F. equivalent	300 mg
Bile salts	150 mg

The antispasmodic action decreases spasm and hypermotility; the phenobarbital calms the patient and the digestive enzymes supplement the patient's own enzymes.

Indications: Symptomatic relief of gastrointestinal disorders, chronic pancreatitis and/or gastritis, postcholecystectomy syndrome and chronic biliary disorders.

Contraindications: Acute glaucoma, advanced renal or hepatic disease, biliary tract obstruction, or a hypersensitivity to any of the ingredients.

Warnings: Phenobarbital may be habit-forming.

Precautions: Administer with caution to patients with incipient glaucoma or with prostatic hypertrophy.

Adverse Reactions: Rarely, blurred vision, dry mouth, difficult urination with recommended dosage.

Dosage and Administration: *Orally.* Two tablets after each meal. To preserve the integrity of the enteric coating, do not crush or chew tablets.

Availability:
DONNAZYME® Tablets in bottles of 100 and 500. **(Robins)**

DOPAMINE HYDROCHLORIDE

Chemical Name: 3, 4-Dihydroxyphenethylamine hydrochloride.

Description: Dopamine hydrochloride is a naturally occurring biochemical catecholamine that undergoes β-hydroxylation to form norepinephrine. It is an α-adrenergic drug that is currently being used for the treatment of shock. The compound occurs as a white, odorless, crystalline powder that is freely soluble in water and soluble in alcohol. It is sensitive to light, alkali, iron salts and oxidizing agents.

Dopamine increases cardiac output by exerting a direct inotropic effect on the heart muscle. The myocardial demand for oxygen is increased less with this drug than it is with isoproterenol, and it usually does not produce tachycardia. Also, increase in cardiac output produced by dopamine does not result in substantial decreases in systemic vascular resistance as may occur with isoproterenol. Clinical studies reveal that dopamine increases the pulse and systolic pressure with little or no increase in diastolic pressure. Total peripheral resistance is usually unchanged when the drug is administered at low or moderate doses. Blood flow to the peripheral vasculature usually decreases while mesenteric flow increases. Dopamine has also been reported to dilate the renal vessels presumably by activating a specific receptor thus resulting in increases in glomerular filtration rate, renal blood flow, and sodium excretion. Although the urinary output is increased, the osmolarity of the urine usually remains the same and is not decreased. Prognosis is better in patients whose renal flow and blood pressure have not undergone profound deterioration. Nevertheless, in a number of oliguric or anuric patients, administration of dopamine resulted in an increase in urine flow which in some cases reached normal limits. It should be considered that concurrent administration with diuretic agents may produce an additive or potentiating effect.

Studies in pregnant animals have not produced any evidence of teratogenic effects in the offspring, but they did reveal that the number of offsprings that did survive was less, and those that did survive carried the potential for cataract formation.

Indications: To correct hemodynamic imbalances present in the shock syndrome due to myocardial infarction, trauma, endotoxic septicemia, open heart surgery, renal failure, and chronic cardiac decompensation as in congestive heart failure. Hypovolemia should be fully corrected with either a suitable plasma expander or whole blood prior to the administration of dopamine.

Contraindications: In patients with pheochromocytoma.

Warnings: Because of the danger of excessive cardiac irritability, dopamine should not be administered in the presence of uncorrected tachyarrhythmias or ventricular fibrillation. Prior treatment of patients with MAO inhibitors requires that the initial dose of dopamine be reduced to at least 1/10 the usual dose in order to avoid a prolonged and potentiated effect. The drug may be used in pregnant patients when, in the judgment of the physician, the expected benefits outweigh the potential risk to the fetus. Since studies have not been adequate to define proper dosage and limitation of use in pediatric patients, the safe and effective use of dopamine in these patients has not been established. **Note:** This drug should not be added to alkaline diluent solutions.

Precautions: If a disproportionate rise in diastolic pressure (i.e., a marked decrease in the pulse pressure) is observed in patients receiving this drug, the infusion rate should be decreased and the patient observed carefully for further evidence of predominant vasoconstrictor activity unless such an effect is desired. Although in clinical trials the inadvertent subcutaneous infiltration did not produce any evidence of tissue necrosis, the usual precautions should nevertheless be taken. Patients with a history of occlusive vascular disease such as atherosclerosis, arterial embolism, Raynaud's disease, cold injury, diabetic endarteritis, and Buerger's disease should be closely monitored for any changes in color or temperature of the skin in the extremeties. If a change occurs and it is thought to be the result of compromised circulation, the benefits of continuing the infusion should be weighed against the risk of possible necrosis. The condition may be reversed by either decreasing or discontinuing the rate of infusion. Extreme caution is particularly indicated in patients inhaling cyclopropane or halogenated hydrocarbon anesthetics since these agents may increase cardiac autonomic irritability and, consequently, may sensitize the myocardium to the action of this drug. Close monitoring of urine flow, cardiac output and blood pressure is necessary when infusing dopamine.

Adverse Reactions: Those frequently observed included ectopic beats, nausea, vomiting, tachycardia, anginal pain, palpitation, dyspnea, headache, hypotension, and vasoconstriction. Those infrequently observed included aberrant conduction, bradycardia, piloerection, widened QRS complex, azotemia, and elevated blood pressure.

Dosage and Administration: Slow *intravenous* infusion is the usual route. Dopamine is a potent drug and must be diluted before administration. Transfer the contents of 1 ampul to a 250 or 500 ml bottle of physiological saline, 5% dextrose or lactated Ringer's solution. Consult package literature for complete details. Initially, 2 to 5 mcg/kg/minute is given by continuous infusion to patients who are likely to respond to modest increments of heart force and renal perfusion. In more seriously ill patients, the initial dose is 5 mcg/kg/minute, and increase gradually using increments of 5 to 10 mcg/kg/minute up to 20 to 50 mcg/kg/minute as needed. If doses in excess of 50 mcg/kg/minute are required, it is suggested that the urine output be checked frequently. Administration at rates greater than 50 mcg/kg/minute have safely been used in advance circulatory decompensation states. If unnecessary fluid expansion is of concern, adjustment of drug concentration may be preferred over increasing the flow rate of a less concentrated dilution.

Availability:
INTROPIN® Injection, 40 mg/ml in ampuls of 5 ml. **(Arnar-Stone)**

DOXAPRAM HYDROCHLORIDE

Chemical Name: 1-Ethyl-4-(2-morpholinoethyl)-3,3-diphenyl-2-pyrrolidinone hydrochloride hydrate.

Description: A centrally acting respiratory stimulant, it occurs as a white, crystalline powder sparingly soluble in water and in alcohol. Doxapram increases the depth, and may to some extent increase the rate of respiration by stimulation of the medullary respiratory centers.

The onset of respiratory stimulation usually occurs within 20 to 40 seconds with peak effect attained in 1 to 2 minutes. The duration of effect is variable usually 5 to 12 minutes. Doxapram is used primarily for the purpose of stimulating respiration or hastening arousal and return to protective reflexes. The respiratory stimulant action results principally in an increase in tidal volume and a moderate increase in respiratory rate. Blood pressure and pulse rate may also be increased. The drug may cause a decrease in arterial carbon dioxide tension, an increase in blood pH and an increase in arterial oxygen tension by increasing alveolar ventilation. In anesthetized patients who are apneic subsequent to the use of controlled ventilation, doxapram may be effective in restoring adequate spontaneous breathing provided the apnea is not due to the residual effects of muscle relaxant drugs. The pressor response appears to be due primarily to stimulation of brain-stem vasomotor areas and is mediated through the sympatho-adrenal system.

Indications: To stimulate respiration in patients with postanesthetic respiratory depression or apnea other than that due to muscle relaxant drugs; to increase depth of respiration in postoperative cases; to hasten arousal and return of protective pharyngeal and laryngeal reflexes, and to aid in the differential diagnosis of postanesthetic respiratory depression, and as a temporary measure in hospitalized patients with acute respiratory insufficiency superimposed on chronic obstructive pulmonary disease.

Contraindications: Epilepsy and other convulsive states, incompetence of the ventilatory mechanism due to muscle paresis, flail chest, pneumothorax, airway obstruction, extreme dyspnea, severe hypertension, cerebrovascular accidents, evidence of head injury, strongly suspected or confirmed pulmonary embolism, acute bronchial asthma, respiratory failure due to neuromuscular disorders, in restrictive respiratory diseases such as pulmonary fibrosis, coronary artery disease, frank uncompensated heart failure, and hypersensitivity to the drug. Doxapram is not recommended in children under 12 years of age.

Warnings: Doxapram is an analeptic agent; it is neither an antagonist to muscle relaxant drugs nor a specific narcotic antagonist. Since it has an acid pH, it should not be mixed with alkaline solutions such as thiopental sodium. Narcosis may recur after stimulation with doxapram; therefore, care should be taken to maintain close observation until the patient has been fully alert for ½ to 1 hour. Doxapram is an adjunct to well-accepted supportive measures and resuscitative techniques. It may not stimulate adequate spontaneous breathing or provide sufficient arousal in patients who are severely depressed with CNS-depressant drugs. When administered to postoperative patients or to patients in a state of narcosis with chronic pulmonary insufficiency, oxygen should be administered concomitantly. Failure to do so may result in further oxygen debt and more severe dyspnea. Doxapram should be administered with considerable care and only under close supervision to patients with cerebral edema, bronchial asthma, severe tachycardia, cardiac arrhythmia, cardiac disease, hyperthyroidism and pheochromocytoma. No adequate clinical studies have been performed to determine safe use during pregnancy. Until further clinical experience has been obtained, the physician must weigh the need against possible risks in using the drug in pregnant patients or in women of child-bearing potential.

Precautions: Doxapram should be administered with caution to patients receiving sympathomimetics or monoamine oxidase inhibitors since a synergistic pressor effect may occur; in postoperative patients with marked dyspnea due to obstructive pulmonary emphysema, acute or chronic asthma, profound metabolic disorders, severe to moderately severe hypertension, increased cerebrospinal fluid pressure, convulsive disorders, acute agitation and in patients who had received muscle relaxant drugs. Since the drug stimulates basal gastric secretion in dogs, it should be used cautiously in patients with peptic ulcer and in those undergoing gastric surgery. Excessive pressor response, tachycardia, skeletal muscle hyperactivity and enhanced deep tendon reflexes may constitute early manifestations of overdosage; therefore, it is important that blood pressure, pulse and deep tendon reflexes be evaluated periodically during and following administration. Sudden development of hypotension or dyspnea demands immediate withdrawal of the drug.

Adverse Reactions: The following have been reported: *Central and autonomic nervous systems reactions* include hyperactivity, feeling of warmth, sweating, muscle tremor, clonus, increased deep tendon reflexes, dizziness, muscle spasticity, pyrexia, confusion, paresthesia, pupillary dilatation, pilomotor erection, headache, bilateral babinski, fasciculation, and carpopedal spasm. A grand mal seizure occurred 95 minutes after drug administration in a known epileptic patient who was taking anticonvulsant medication. *Respiratory reactions* include cough, dyspnea, laryngospasm, bronchospasm, and hiccough. *Cardiovascular reactions* are characterized by hypertension, sinus tachycardia, bradycardia, extrasystoles, lowered T-waves, premature ventricular contractions, irregular heart rhythm, and tightness in chest. Although a mild to moderate increase in blood pressure is not frequent, such an increase may occasionally be of concern in hypertensive patients. *Gastrointestinal complications* include nausea and/or vomiting, salivation, stimulation of lower bowel, and sour taste. *Genitourinary side effects* are characterized by urinary retention, and stimulation of urinary bladder with spontaneous voiding. Other reactions that may occur include pruritus, and thrombophlebitis. A decrease in hemoglobin, hematocrit, or red blood cell count has been observed in postoperative patients. In the presence of preexisting leukopenia, a further decrease in white blood cell was observed following anesthesia and treatment with doxapram hydrochloride. Elevation of BUN and albuminuria have also been observed.

Dosage and Administration: *Intravenously. In the management of postanesthetic respiratory depression:* as a single injection, the usual dose is 0.5 to 1 mg/kg of body weight with a maximum recommended dose of 1.5 mg/kg. When a single injection is used as a priming dose, therapy may be continued with multiple intravenous injections of 0.5 to 1 mg/kg at intervals of 5 minutes up to a maximum of 2 mg/kg. If preferred, it can be given by intravenous infusion at a rate of approximately 5 mg/minute until a satisfactory response is obtained. Then a maintenance infusion rate of 1 to 3 mg/minute is suggested. The recommended maximum dosage by infusion is 4 mg/kg. *To hasten arousal during recovery period:* a total dose of 1 to 1.5 mg/kg *intravenously* is recommended; administered as a single injection or divided into 2 equal doses and given 5 minutes apart. *In the management of chronic obstructive pulmonary disease associated with acute hypercapnia,* the initial rate of infusion is 1 to 2 mg/minute, increased to a maximum of 3 mg/minute if required. Arterial blood gases should be determined prior to and at least every 30 minutes during the 2 hours of infusion. Additional infusions beyond the single maximum 2-hour administration are not recommended. *Not to be used in children under 12 years of age.*

Availability:
DOPRAM® Solution, 20 mg/ml in vials of 20 ml. **(Robins)**

DOXEPIN HYDROCHLORIDE

Chemical Name: *N,N*-Dimethyldibenz[b,e]oxepin-$\Delta^{11(6H)}$, γ-propylamine hydrochloride, *cis*- and *trans*-isomers.

Description: Doxepin hydrochloride is a dibenzoxepin psychotherapeutic agent with antianxiety and antidepressant activity; it possesses the characteristics of other tricyclic compounds, and has been reported to be as effective as imipramine in the treatment of depression. No instances of withdrawal symptoms were reported in patients who were observed systematically for these reactions. This is consistent with the virtual absence of euphoria as a side effect and the lack of potential to addiction that is characteristic of this type of chemical compound. While its mechanism of action is not known, studies have demonstrated that the drug is neither a monoamine oxidase inhibitor nor a primary stimulant of the CNS. The current hypothesis is that the drug may potentiate the central and peripheral action of adrenergic agents by blocking the reuptake of norepinephrine at the adrenergic neurons. Doxepin is well absorbed and rapidly metabolized following oral administration.

In animal reproduction studies, gross and microscopic examination of the offspring showed no evidence of drug-related teratogenic effects. Doses of up to 25 mg/kg/day for 8 to 9 months revealed no observable changes in the number of live births, litter size, or in lactation. A decreased rate of conception was noticed when male rats were given 25 mg/kg/day for prolonged periods—an effect which has occurred with other psychotropic drugs. This phenomenon has been attributed to the drug's effect on the central and/or autonomic nervous system.

Indications: Psychoneurotic anxiety or depressive reactions, or both; psychotic depressive disorders, including involutional depression and manic-depressive reactions, anxiety and/or depression associated with alcoholism or organic disease. The target symptoms of psychoneurosis vulnerable to the drug include anxiety, tension, depression, somatic symptoms and concerns, insomnia, guilt, lack of energy, fear, apprehension and worry.

Contraindications: Hypersensitivity to the drug or to other dibenzoxepines, glaucoma, tendency to urinary retention.

Warnings: Although teratogenic effects have not been seen in animals, doxepin, nonetheless, should not be used during pregnancy unless its use is considered essential for the welfare of the patient. Because safety for its use has not been established, the drug should not be used in children under 12 years of age. Doxepin should not be used concomitantly with MAO inhibitors; at least 2 weeks should elapse between discontinuance of an MAO inhibitor and initiation of therapy with this drug.

Precautions: Patients should be cautioned that their response to alcohol may be potentiated, and that in the event of drowsiness, they should not drive a motor vehicle or engage in any hazardous occupation requiring alertness or skill. Since suicide is an inherent risk, depressed patients should be observed closely during the early phase of therapy and until significant improvement is noted. That latent psychotic symptoms may be activated should be kept in mind. At the usual clinical dosage, 75 to 150 mg/day, doxepin can be given concomitantly with guanethidine and other sympathetic inhibitors without blocking their antihypertensive effect. However, at a daily dosage of 300 mg or more, doxepin does exert a significant blocking effect.

Adverse Reactions: The following undesirable effects are those usually associated with tricyclic compounds in general and may or may not be observed with doxepin. *Anticholinergic effects:* mild and reversible dry mouth, blurred vision, constipation, and urinary retention. *CNS effects:* transient drowsiness is most commonly noted, infrequently noted are confusion, disorientation, hallucinations, paresthesias, ataxia, extrapyramidal symptoms and seizures. *Cardiovascular effects:* infrequent instances of tachycardia and hypotension. *Hematologic effects:* eosinophilia occurred in a few patients, and bone marrow depression manifesting as agranulocytosis, leukopenia, thrombocytopenia and purpura was occasionally noted. *Gastrointestinal effects:* nausea, vomiting, indigestion, taste disturbances, diarrhea, anorexia and aphthous stomatitis. *Endocrine effects:* occasional instances of altered libido, testicular swelling, gynecomastia in males, enlargement of breasts and galactorrhea in females, and hypoglycemia or hyperglycemia. Other infrequently reported effects include skin rash, facial edema, photosensitization, pruritus, dizziness, tinnitus, weight gain, sweating, chills, fatigue, weakness, flushing, jaundice, alopecia, and headache. Overdosage is usually manifested primarily by excessive sedation and anticholinergic effects such as blurred vision and dry mouth, although an increase of any of the reported adverse reactions may occur. Other complications may be a pronounced tachycardia, hypotension and extrapyramidal symptoms. Treatment is essentially symptomatic. The occurrence of hypotension and excessive sedation usually requires supportive therapy.

Dosage and Administration: *Orally.* Mild to moderately severe conditions, initially 25 mg 3 times daily for 4 days. Usual optimal dosage is 75 to 150 mg daily. Dosage adjustment depends upon individual response. More severely ill patients may require 50 mg 3 times daily initially, increased gradually to 300 mg/day if necessary. Nothing is to be gained by exceeding a daily dosage of 300 mg. In patients with very mild symptomatology or emotional symptoms accompanying organic disease, lower doses (e.g., 25 to 50 mg/day) may be adequate. Although optimal antidepressant response may not be manifested for 2 to 3 weeks, antianxiety activity is apparent much more quickly.

Availability:
ADAPIN Capsules, 10, 25, 50 and 100 mg in bottles of 100 and 1000. **(Pennwalt)**
SINEQUAN®: **(Pfizer)**
Capsules, 10, 75 and 100 mg in bottles of 100 and 1000 and in unit-dose packages of 100 (10 strips × 10); 25 and 50 mg in bottles of 100, 1000 and 5000 and in unit-dose packages of 100 (10 strips × 10); 150 mg in bottles of 50 and 500 and in unit-dose packages of 100.
Oral Concentrate, 50 mg/5 ml (equiv.) in bottles of 120 ml with calibrated dropper.

DOXORUBICIN HYDROCHLORIDE

Description: Doxorubicin, a derivative of anthracycline, is an antineoplastic antibiotic isolated from cultures of *Streptomyces peucetius var caesius.* It has been used successfully to produce regression in a number of neoplastic diseases. Its chemical structure resembles that of daunorubicin, differing only in the substitution of a hydroxyl group for a hydrogen atom in the acetyl radical of the aglycone portion of the compound. Clinical experience has shown the drug to possess broad-spectrum activity against a variety of tumors, especially solid tumors, including lung tumors and sarcomas. It has no antiinfective activity.

The cytocidal action of the drug is postulated to be due to interference with DNA and RNA synthesis. It has been reported to be most active in the growth phase of cells and is thus more effective in inducing tumor regression than in maintaining regression. Cell culture studies have demonstrated rapid cell penetration and perinucleolar binding, rapid inhibition of mitotic activity and nucleic acid synthesis, mutagenesis and chromosomal abberations. Pharmacokinetic studies with radiolabeled drug indicate that, when given intravenously, a significant portion of the drug is readily absorbed from the plasma. Slow excretion in urine and bile suggests significant tissue binding, especially in liver, spleen, kidney, heart, and lung tissues. Of particular interest is the finding that doxorubicin binds very tightly to myocardial DNA which is consistent with the unusual cardiomyopathy caused by this drug. Plasma levels of the radioactive drug were about ½ the initial levels in 30 minutes and remained fairly constant for at least 7 to 10 days. Urinary excretion ranges from 4 to 5% and fecal excretion from 40 to 50% in 7 days. The drug does not cross the blood brain barrier. The toxicity of doxorubicin appears to be dose-related with a striking increase in symptoms when the total dosage approaches 550 mg/square meter of body surface. There is no adequate information on whether or not this drug may affect fertility in human males and females or have a teratogenic potential or other adverse effect on the fetus. It has been shown to have carcinogenic properties and immunosuppressive activity when tested in experimental animals.

Indications: Treatment of acute lymphoblastic and myeloblastic leukemias, Wilms' tumor, soft-tissue and osteogenic sarcomas, neuroblastoma, breast carcinoma, ovarian carcinoma, transitional cell bladder tumor, bronchogenic lung carcinoma, thyroid carcinoma, and lymphomas of both Hodgkin's and non-Hodgkin's types. A number of other solid tumors in the pediatric age group have also shown some responsiveness but in numbers too limited to justify specific recommendation. **Important Note:** Doxorubicin should be administered only under the supervision of a qualified physician experienced in the use of cancer chemotherapeutic agents.

Contraindications: Patients with myelosuppression induced by previous treatment with other antiblastic agents and those with impaired cardiac function. Also contraindicated in patients previously treated with maximal doses of doxorubicin and daunorubicin.

Warnings: Initial treatment with this drug requires close observation of the patient and extensive laboratory monitoring. It is recommended that patients be hospitalized, especially during the first phase of treatment, so that the major acute toxic effects can be observed. The total dose administered should also take into consideration any previous therapy with other anthracyclines such as daunorubicin. **Extravasation into subcutaneous tissue may cause severe local tissue necrosis. The most serious complications that may occur involve the cardiovascular and hematopoietic systems. Serious, irreversible myocardial toxicity with delayed congestive failure unresponsive to any cardiac supportive therapy may be encountered as the total dosage approaches 550 mg/m^2**. Bone marrow depression occurs in 60 to 85% of patients and primarily involves the leukocytes. It is recommended that white blood cells, red blood cells and platelets be carefully monitored. Hematopoietic toxicity may require suspension or cessation of drug therapy. Dosage should be reduced in patients with impaired renal or hepatic function. Prior to and during therapy, evaluation of hepatic function is advised using conventional clinical laboratory tests such as SGOT, SGPT, alkaline phosphatase, bilirubin, and BSP. Safe use of doxorubicin during pregnancy has not been established; therefore, the benefits of therapy should be weighed against the potential hazards to the mother and fetus. Patients should be told that the urine will be colored red for 1 or 2 days after drug administration.

Precautions: Doxorubicin may cause cardiac toxicity, particularly in patients who have received a total dosage in excess of 550 mg/square meter of body surface. Acute left ventricular failure has been reported, generally occurring several weeks after administration. The situation is complicated because the cardiac failure usually does not respond to available medical or physical therapy for cardiac support. It is recommended that baseline EKG and a monthly follow-up EKG be taken during and immediately following active drug therapy. EKG changes such as T-wave flattening, S-T depression, voltage reduction, and arrhythmias may serve as indications for suspension of therapy; it must be recognized that fatal cardiotoxicity can occur precipitously without prior EKG alterations.

Adverse Reactions: Myelosuppression and cardiotoxicity are major dose-limiting complications. Patients should be advised that complete alopecia almost uniformly accompanies therapy. Stomatitis and esophagitis, which can be quite severe, are commonly associated with this drug and could result in ulceration. Gastrointestinal symptoms that are less commonly noted include nausea, vomiting, anorexia, and diarrhea. Hyperpigmentation of nail beds and dermal creases may occur in pediatric patients. Severe cellulitis, vesication, and tissue necrosis result if the drug is extravasated during administration. Erythematous streaking along the vein proximal to the site of injection has been reported as well as phlebosclerosis which may develop when small veins or a single vein is used for repeated administration. Occasionally, fever, chills, urticaria, and rarely, conjunctivitis and lacrimation have been noted. Anaphylaxis may be an additional complication. A case of an apparent cross sensitivity to lincomycin has been observed.

Dosage and Administration: *Intravenously* only. The recommended dosage schedule for adults is 60 to 75 mg/square meter of body surface in a single dose administered at intervals of 21 days. The lower dose is preferred in patients with inadequate bone marrow reserve, prior therapy or neoplastic marrow infiltration. An alternate dosage schedule, which is preferred in pediatric patients, is 30 mg/m^2 in a single dose on 3 successive days, repeated every 4 weeks. The total dose should not exceed 550 mg/m^2 otherwise irreversible myocardial toxicity may occur. A dose level of 40 to 55 mg/m^2 at each administration is recommended if hepatic function is impaired. Toxicity in patients with renal impairment is inconsistent so that dosage must be carefully monitored. It is advised that the drug be added to a freely running intravenous infusion of normal saline or 5% dextrose in order to minimize the possibility of extravasation and consequent tissue damage. Following reconstitution with 5 ml of sodium chloride for injection, the product may be stored for 24 hours at room temperature or for 48 hours if refrigerated (4 to 10°C).

Availability:
ADRIAMYCIN™ Powder for Injection (lyophylized) in vials of 10 and 50 mg with 50 and 250 mg of lactose respectively in cartons of 10. **(Adria)**

DOXYCYCLINE

Chemical Name: alpha-6-Deoxy-5-oxytetracycline.

Description: Doxycycline hyclate is a salt of a yellow, crystalline antibiotic powder prepared by the catalytic hydrogenation of methacycline or by the Raney nickel reduction of a benzyl mercaptan methacycline derivative; it is sparingly soluble in water. Doxycycline monohydrate, an amphoteric base prepared from the hyclate, is insoluble in water. The drug is closely related chemically and in action and uses to other antibiotics of the tetracycline group.

Doxycycline is a broad-spectrum antibiotic and has been shown to be active against a wide range of gram-positive and gram-negative organisms. It is primarily bacteriostatic and is thought to exert its antimicrobial effect by the inhibition of protein synthesis. The drugs in the tetracycline class have closely similar antimicrobial spectra. Microorganisms may be considered highly sensitive if the M.I.C. (minimum inhibitory concentration) is less than 4 mcg/ml, and slightly sensitive if the M.I.C. is 4 to 12.5 mcg/ml. It is readily absorbed and is bound to plasma proteins in varying degrees. It is concentrated by the liver in the bile, and excreted in the urine and feces at high concentrations and in a biologically active form. The biological activity and concentration of doxycycline in the feces has not yet been accurately determined.

The drug is virtually completely absorbed after oral administration. Following a 200-mg dose, normal adult volunteers averaged peak serum levels of 2.6 mcg/ml of doxycycline at 2 hours decreasing to 1.45 mcg/ml at 24 hours. Excretion of doxycycline by the kidney is about 40%/72 hours in individuals with normal function (creatinine clearance about 75 ml/min). This percentage excretion may fall as low as 1 to 5%/72 hours in individuals with severe renal insufficiency (creatinine clearance below 10 ml/min). Studies have shown no significant difference in serum half-life of doxycycline (range 18 to 22 hours) in individuals with normal and severely impaired renal function. Hemodialysis does not alter serum half-life.

If the Kirby-Bauer method of disc susceptibility testing is used, a 30 mcg doxycycline disc should give a zone of at least 16 mm when tested against a doxycycline-susceptible bacterial strain.

Indications: Has been found clinically effective in the treatment of a variety of infections caused by susceptible strains of gram-positive and gram-negative organisms, such as pneumonia, other respiratory tract infections, genitourinary tract infections, soft tissue infections, ophthalmic infections, gastrointestinal infections, other infections due to susceptible strains of Bacteroides, Pasteurella, Brucella (in combination with streptomycin), Psittacosis, Listeria, Rickettsia, *Mycoplasma pneumoniae* (Eaton agent, PPLO), *H. pertussis, B. anthracis, C. welchii, N. meningitidis,* spirochetes (Treponema), *Donovania granulomatis,* prostatitis and trigonitis due to Proteus and Pseudomonas; also may be useful in the treatment of acne vulgaris and/or conglobata.

Contraindications: In patients known to be or suspected of being hypersensitive to tetracyclines.

Warnings: The use of doxycycline during tooth development (last half of pregnancy, infancy and childhood to the age of 8 years) may cause permanent discoloration of the teeth (yellow-gray-brown). This adverse reaction is more common during long term use of the drug but has been observed following repeated short-term courses. Enamel hypoplasia has also been reported with this antibiotic. *Therefore, doxycycline should not be used in this age group unless other drugs are not likely to be effective or are contraindicated.* Photosensitivity manifested by an exaggerated sunburn reaction has been observed in some individuals taking doxycycline. Patients apt to be exposed to direct sunlight or ultraviolet light should be advised that this reaction can occur with this drug and treatment should be discontinued at the first evidence of skin erythema. Doxycycline forms a stable calcium complex in any bone-forming tissue. In vitro, this antibiotic binds calcium less strongly than other tetracyclines. A decrease in the fibula growth rate has been observed in prematures given oral tetracycline in doses of 25 mg/kg every 6 hours. This reaction was shown to be reversible when the drug was discontinued. The antianabolic action of doxycycline may cause an increase in BUN. Studies to date indicate that this does not occur with the use of this drug in patients with impaired renal function.

Precautions: As with other antibiotics, use of doxycycline may result in overgrowth of nonsusceptible organisms, including fungi. If superinfection occurs, appropriate therapy should be instituted. In venereal disease when coexistent syphilis is suspected, a dark-field examination should be done before treatment is started and the blood serology repeated monthly for at least 4 months. Because doxycycline has been shown to depress plasma prothrombin activity, patients who are on anticoagulant therapy may require downward adjustment of their anticoagulant dosage. In long-term therapy, periodic laboratory evaluation of organ systems, including hematopoietic, renal and hepatic studies should be performed. Since bacteriostatic drugs may interfere with the bactericidal action of penicillin, it is advisable to avoid giving doxycycline in conjunction with penicillin.

Adverse Reactions: In clinical efficacy studies, doxycycline was generally well tolerated. Due to its virtually complete absorption, side effects of the lower bowel, particularly diarrhea, have been infrequent. The following adverse reactions may occur in those receiving doxycycline: *Gastrointestinal:* anorexia, nausea, vomiting, diarrhea, glossitis, dysphagia, enterocolitis, and inflammatory lesions (with monilial overgrowth) in the anogenital region. These reactions have been caused by both the oral and parenteral administration of tetracyclines. *Skin:* maculopapular and erythematous rashes. Exfoliative dermatitis has been reported but is uncommon. *Renal:* rise in BUN has been reported and is apparently dose-related. *Hypersensitivity reactions:* urticaria, angioneurotic edema, anaphylaxis, anaphylactoid purpura, pericarditis, and exacerbations of systemic lupus erythematosus. When given over prolonged periods, tetracyclines have been reported to produce brown-black microscopic discoloration of thyroid glands. No abnormalities of thyroid function studies are known to occur. Bulging fontanels have been reported in young infants following full therapeutic dosage of doxycycline. This sign disappeared rapidly when the drug was discontinued. *Blood:* hemolytic anemia, thrombocytopenia, neutropenia, and eosinophilia may occur with this drug.

Dosage and Administration: *Orally* or *intravenously.* **The usual dose and frequency of administration of doxycycline differ from those of the other tetracyclines. Exceeding the recommended dosage may result in an increased incidence of side effects.** Adults and children over 100 lbs of body weight, 100 mg every 12 hours followed by a maintenance dose of 100 mg/day, administered as a single dose or 50 mg every 12 hours. *In severe infections,* 100 mg every 12 hours. Children weighing 100 lbs or less, 2 mg/lb of body weight divided into 2 doses on the first day, followed by 1 mg/lb of body weight given as a single daily dose or divided into 2 doses, on subsequent days. *For severe infections,* up to 2 mg/lb of body weight may be used. *In streptococcal infections,* therapy should be continued for 10 days to prevent the development of rheumatic fever or glomerulonephritis. If gastric irritation occurs, the drug should be given with food or milk. Simultaneous administration with aluminum hydroxide gel has been shown to decrease absorption of doxycycline.

Availability:
DOXY-II® Capsules (as hyclate), 50 mg in bottles of 50; 100 mg in bottles of 50 and 500. **(USV)**

VIBRAMYCIN®: **(Pfizer)**
Capsules (as hyclate), 50 mg in bottles of 50, in X-Pak® of 5 capsules in cartons of 10 packs and in unit-dose cartons of 100; 100 mg in bottles of 50 and 500, in V-Paks® of 5 capsules in cartons of 5 packs and in unit-dose cartons of 100.
Intravenous Sterile Powder (as hyclate) in vials of 100 and 200 mg.
Powder for Oral Suspension (as monohydrate), 25 mg/5 ml in bottles of 60 ml.
Syrup (as calcium salt), 50 mg/5 ml in bottles of 30 ml and 1 pint.

DROMOSTANOLONE PROPIONATE

Chemical Name: 17β-Hydroxy-2α-methyl-5α-androstan-3-one propionate.

Description: A synthetic steroid hormone, related to testosterone in chemical structure and physiologic action, it differs structurally from testosterone by the presence of a methyl group at the alpha-2 position and in saturation at the 4-5 position. It occurs as a white, crystalline powder insoluble in water and soluble in alcohol. The compound produces retention of nitrogen, potassium and phosphorus, increase in protein anabolism and decrease in amino acid catabolism.

Indications: Palliative treatment of advanced or metastatic carcinoma of the breast in women who are inoperable and are 1 to 5 years postmenopausal at the time of diagnosis or who have been proved to have hormone-dependent cancer by previous beneficial response to castration.

Contraindications: In carcinoma of the male breast and premenopausal women.

Precautions: The usual precautions for testosterone should be observed for dromostanolone propionate. Patients with edema may require diuretics before and during treatment with this steroid; also in the presence of bone metastases, serum calcium levels should be determined before and at intervals during the course of treatment. Hypercalcemia may require corticosteroid therapy or other management. If an increase in libido occurs, the use of sedation may be helpful. Although not reported with dromostanolone thus far, drug-induced jaundice or masculinization of the fetus has been known to occur with the use of other anabolic agents. At the present time, there are no reports of the use of this drug in carcinoma of the breast during pregnancy or in carcinoma of the breast in male patients with or without associated carcinoma of the prostate. Objective evidence of tumor progression should be evaluated periodically by physical examination, x-rays and determinations of serum calcium and alkaline phosphatase levels. The drug should be used with caution in liver disease, cardiac decompensation, nephritis, nephrosis, during pregnancy or in carcinoma of the prostate.

Adverse Reactions: The most likely to be seen are mild virilism, such as deepening of the voice, acne, facial hair growth, and enlargement of the clitoris. Rarely noted were edema, hypercalcemia, severe CNS effects, and local reaction at the site of injection.

Dosage and Administration: *Intramuscularly.* Recommended dosage, 100 mg 3 times weekly for as long as satisfactory results are obtained. Treatment should continue for at least 8 to 12 weeks before any conclusions are drawn as to the efficacy of this steroid. If a significant progression of the disease occurs during the first 6 to 8 weeks of therapy another form of treatment should be considered.

Availability:
DROLBAN® Solution, 50 mg/ml in ampuls of 10 ml. **(Lilly)**

DROPERIDOL

Chemical Name: 1- {1-[3-(*p*-Fluorobenzoyl)propyl]-1,2,3,6-tetrahydro-4-pyridyl}-2-benzimidazolinone.

Description: Droperidol is a sedative-tranquilizer of the butyrophenone class. It occurs as a white to light-tan amorphous to microcrystalline powder very slightly soluble in water, slightly soluble in alcohol, and freely soluble in chloroform. The pH (3.0 to 3.8) of the aqueous solution is adjusted with lactic acid.

Following intramuscular or intravenous administration of a single dose, autonomic and brain stem activity is reduced within 3 to 10 minutes but the full effect may not be apparent for 30 minutes. Although the duration of activity usually diminishes within 2 to 4 hours, some effects may persist for up to 12 hours. Premedication with this drug significantly reduced the incidence of postoperative nausea and vomiting in patients who have been given strong anesthetics. It has no effect on motion sickness. Results of controlled studies with droperidol have shown that there is little or no effect on respiration or myocardial contractile force, heart rate, and cardiac output. Blood pressure is lowered due in part to a direct vasodilator effect and in part to adrenergic blockade. Clinical evidence suggests that droperidol is an epinephrine antagonist and that it potentiates the action of pentobarbital and the analgesic effect of fentanyl and other narcotic analgesics. Metabolic studies in laboratory animals indicate that most of the ingested drug is excreted in the urine and feces.

Indications: Preoperatively to allay anxiety in and calm the surgical patient; during induction and during maintenance for smooth emergence and to help minimize the incidence of postoperative nausea and vomiting; as a supplement to general or regional anesthesia in such procedures as neurosurgical, ophthalmologic, otolaryngologic, thoracic, cardiovascular, abdominal, gynecologic and genitourinary, orthopedic, plastic and reconstructive, diagnostic and radiotherapeutic. Droperidol may be given concurrently with a narcotic analgesic to help prolong anesthesia into the postoperative period, thus minimizing the dosage of any necessary narcotics postoperatively.

Contraindications: Hypersensitivity to the drug.

Warnings: Since safe use of droperidol during the gestation period has not been established, the potential risks to mother and fetus should be weighed against the anticipated benefits. Whether the drug is safe to use in children up to 2 years of age has not been determined. Since hypotension may occur, drugs to treat this complication should be readily available.

Precautions: When the patient has been given another CNS depressant (e.g., barbiturates, narcotics, major tranquilizers, and general anesthetics), the effects of which may parallel those of droperidol, the dose of the latter should be reduced to at least 1/4 to 1/3 that usually recommended to avoid excessive CNS depression. Because of their vital role in the metabolism and excretion of many drugs, impaired function of liver or kidneys should serve as a reminder to use droperidol with caution. The physician should be aware of the additional problems that may be encountered in elderly, debilitate or other poor-risk patients, and it is advised that the initial dose be appropriately reduced until their response to the drug can be evaluated. Droperidol is capable of blocking the pressor response to pressor amines and possibly precipitating severe hypotension in the immediate postoperative period. In the absence of a hypertensive response to fluid therapy, consideration should be given to the use of pressor agents other than epinephrine. Care should be exercised in positioning the patient because of the possibility of orthostatic hypotension. When used for postoperative monitoring of the patient, it has been found that the EEG pattern generally returns to normal *slowly*.

Adverse Reactions: Dizziness, chills or shivering, laryngospasm, bronchospasm, restlessness, hyperactivity, anxiety, or transitory moderate hypotension and tachycardia may occur. A low incidence of extrapyramidal symptoms (dystonia, akathisia and oculogyric crisis) has been observed, controllable or reversible with antiparkinsonian agents. Rarely, hallucinatory episodes (possibly emergence delirium) have been seen. When used with a narcotic analgesic, respiratory depression, apnea and muscular rigidity may result in respiratory arrest unless treated promptly. Elevated blood pressure, with or without preexisting hypertension, has been reported following administration of droperidol combined with fentanyl or other parenteral analgesics. The manifestations of overdosage are an extension of the drug's pharmacologic actions, and are treated with the usual standard measures and procedures that are applied to similarly acting drugs.

Dosage and Administration: Before determining the individual dose the following factors should be taken into account: age, body weight, physical status, underlying pathological condition, use of other drugs, type of anesthesia to be used, and the surgical procedure involved. Adults: *as premedication,* 2.5 to 10 mg intramuscularly or intravenously 1/2 to 1 hour before induction. *For induction,* 2.5 mg/20 to 25 lbs, usually intravenously. *As maintenance,* 1.25 to 2.5 mg, usually intravenously. Children 2 to 12 years of age, as little as 1 to 1.5 mg/20 to 25 lbs is recommended.

Availability:
INAPSINE® Injection, 2.5 mg/ml in ampuls of 2 and 5 ml and in multiple-dose vials of 10 ml.

(McNeil)

DYCLONINE HYDROCHLORIDE

Chemical Name: 3-Piperidino-4′-butoxypropiophenone hydrochloride.

Description: Dyclonine hydrochloride, an organic ketone, is a synthetic local anesthetic agent. It occurs as white crystals or as a white, crystalline powder that is soluble in water. It exhibits a local anesthetic effect when placed on the tongue.

Dyclonine suppresses sensory perception by reversibly blocking the conduction of impulses in peripheral nerve fibers. Following topical application, the onset of action is rapid (within 2 to 10 minutes) and the intensity and duration of anesthesia are similar to those of other local anesthetic agents.

Indications: Whenever topical anesthesia of the skin or mucous membranes is desired. May be useful in dentistry, dermatology, urology, gynecology, proctology, otolaryngology, ophthalmology and in various instrumentation (endoscopy) procedures.

Contraindications: In cystoscopic procedures following intravenous pyelography, and in individuals hypersensitive to dyclonine.

Warnings: The solution is not to be used for injection, nor should it be used in the eyes. Resuscitative equipment and drugs, especially vasopressors, should be immediately available whenever this drug is employed. Extreme caution should be exercised in the administration of dyclonine where traumatized mucosa and/or sepsis in the region of proposed application exists, due to the possibility of rapid systemic absorption. Since its effect on fetal development has not been established, safe use during pregnancy, particularly during the first trimester, requires that the anticipated benefits outweigh the unknown hazards to the mother and fetus.

Precautions: Topical application of any local anesthetic may produce the same untoward effects as those following parenteral administration. Therefore, this anesthetic should be administered only under adequate medical supervision. Dyclonine should be used with utmost care in patients sensitive to various allergens or to those with a strong family history of allergy.

Adverse Reactions: Reactions usually result from high plasma levels due to excessive dosage or rapid absorption, or from hypersensitivity, idiosyncrasy, or diminished tolerance. Those involving the CNS are characterized by excitation and/or depression; nervousness, dizziness, blurred vision, or tremors may occur followed by convulsions, unconsciousness, drowsiness, and possibly respiratory arrest. Excitement may be transient or absent and the first manifestations may be drowsiness merging into unconsciousness and respiratory arrest. Reactions involving the cardiovascular system include depression of the myocardium, hypotension, bradycardia, and possibly cardiac arrest. Local manifestations include irritation, stinging, urethritis with or without bleeding. Allergic reactions are characterized by cutaneous lesions of delayed onset, or urticaria, swelling and edema. Skin testing to detect sensitivity is of doubtful value. Whenever local anesthetics are being used, the means for giving oxygen, artificial respiration, and cardiac massage should always be readily available. CNS effects, including convulsions, are best counteracted by the intravenous administration of an ultra-short-acting barbiturate, or a short-acting muscle relaxant together with oxygen.

Dosage and Administration: *Topically.* The amount of anesthetic used and the exact technique of administration vary with the training and experience of physicians in the administration of topical anesthetics. Barring rare instances of idiosyncrasy or sensitivity, it should be safe to use as much as 40 ml of 0.5% solution or 200 mg of dyclonine hydrochloride or 30 ml of 1% solution or 300 mg of dyclonine hydrochloride. Although higher doses have been used, the recommended maximal dose is about 40 ml of the 0.5% solution and 30 ml of the 1% solution. For the exact dosages used in the indications listed previously, see package literature.

Availability:
DYCLONE® Solution, 0.5 and 1% in bottles of 30 ml. **(Dow)**

DYDROGESTERONE

Chemical Name: 10α-Pregna-4,6-diene-3,20-dione.

Description: Dydrogesterone is the 6-dehydro derivative of the stereoisomer of progesterone, retroprogesterone. It occurs as a white or pale yellow, crystalline powder slightly soluble in water and freely soluble in alcohol.

Clinical studies have shown that the drug produces a progestational reaction in the estrogen-primed endometrium and withdrawal bleeding (in the absence of pregnancy). Dydrogesterone differs from other progesterones in that it does not consistently inhibit ovulation, and is nonthermogenic. It appears to be nontoxic, without androgenic or estrogenic activity. In animals, a myometrial relaxing action has been produced which may be a factor in the alleviation of dysmenorrhea. It is metabolized to retropregnenalone which can be demonstrated in the urine within 20 minutes reaching a maximum at 2½ hours after oral administration.

Indications: Treatment of primary and secondary amenorrhea and abnormal uterine bleeding due to hormonal imbalance in the absence of organic pathology, such as submucous fibroids or uterine cancer.

Contraindications: In patients with undiagnosed vaginal bleeding, carcinoma of the breast, missed abortion, markedly impaired liver function, thrombophlebitis, thromboembolic disorders, cerebral apoplexy, pulmonary embolism or those with a history of these conditions.

Warnings: The medication should be discontinued, pending examination, if there is a sudden partial or complete loss of vision or if there is a sudden onset of proptosis, diplopia or migraine. If examination reveals papilledema or retinal vascular lesions, the drug should be withdrawn. Because of the increased risk of thrombotic disorders observed in patients taking estrogen-progestogen combinations, the physician should be alert to the earliest manifestations of these disorders (thrombophlebitis, cerebrovascular disorders, pulmonary embolism, and retinal thrombosis); should any of these occur or be suspected, the drug should be discontinued immediately. Detectable amounts of progestogens have been found in the milk of mothers receiving them. The effect on the nursing infant has not been determined. Use of the drug during the first 4 months of gestation is not recommended.

Precautions: Before hormonal therapy is considered in patients with excessive or abnormal uterine bleeding, the cause should be determined. Appropriate procedures should be used to determine whether an organic lesion or systemic disease is the cause of the bleeding. Pretreatment examination should include breasts and pelvic organs, as well as a Papanicolau smear. Endocrine and liver function studies, if they become abnormal, should be repeated 2 months after the drug has been withdrawn. Patients should be observed for signs of fluid retention and conditions which might be influenced by this factor. Adequate diagnostic measures are indicated in cases of undiagnosed vaginal bleeding. Patients with a history of psychic depression should be observed and the drug discontinued if the depression recurs to a serious degree. Because of a decrease in glucose tolerance in some patients on estrogen-progestogen combinations, diabetics should be carefully observed during therapy. The pathologist should be advised of progestogen therapy when relevant specimens are submitted.

Adverse Reactions: A significant association has been demonstrated between the use of estrogen-progestogen combination drugs and the occurrence of thrombophlebitis, pulmonary embolism, and cerebral thrombosis. Also the following serious occurrences have been observed in patients taking this combination: Neuro-ocular lesions, such as retinal thrombosis and optic neuritis; a rise in blood pressure in susceptible patients; premenstrual-like syndrome; changes in libido; changes in appetite; cystitis-like syndrome; headache; nervousness; dizziness; fatigue; backache; hirsutism; loss of scalp hair; erythema multiforme; erythema nodosum; hemorrhagic eruption; and itching. The following laboratory tests may be altered: *Hepatic function:* Increased sulfobromophthalein retention and other tests. *Coagulation tests:* Increase in prothrombin, Factors VII, VIII, IX, and X. *Thyroid function:* Increase in PBI, and butanol extractable protein bound iodine, and a decrease in T_3 uptake values. Also affected are the metyrapone test and the pregnanediol determination test.

Dosage and Administration: *Orally. For primary and secondary amenorrhea,* 10 to 20 mg daily in divided doses, from day 15 to day 25 of the cycle, continued for several cycles. In oligomenorrhea (functional amenorrhea), 10 mg daily in divided doses for 5 days will induce withdrawal bleeding in most patients. *For abnormal uterine bleeding due to hormonal imbalance in the absence of organic pathology,* initially, 10 to 20 mg in divided doses for 5 to 10 days. Thereafter, successive courses of treatment will usually consist of 10 mg in divided doses daily for 5 days on the 21st through the 25th day of the cycle.

Availability:
DUPHASTON® Tablets, 5 mg in bottles of 40; 10 mg in bottles of 40 and 100. **(Philips Roxane)**
GYNOREST® Tablets, 5 mg in bottles of 50; 10 mg in bottles of 100. **(Mead Johnson)**

DYPHYLLINE

Chemical Name: 7-(2,3-Dihydroxypropyl) theophylline.

Description: Dyphylline occurs as extremely bitter crystals freely soluble in water and slightly soluble in alcohol and in chloroform. It is completely soluble over the physiological pH range, is stable in gastric juice and appears to produce less gastric irritation than most theophylline compounds.

Dyphylline exhibits all the pharmacologic effects of theophylline including bronchodilation, vasodilation, myocardial stimulation and mild diuresis. It also improves pulmonary function as determined by spirometric measurement.

Indications: Relief of acute bronchial asthma and for reversible bronchospasm associated with chronic bronchitis and emphysema. It is combined with guaifenesin in order to relieve bronchospasm and its associated dyspnea, nonproductive cough and tracheobronchial irritation. When combined with ephedrine, phenobarbital, and guaifenesin, it provides bronchodilating, expectorant and sedative action.

Contraindications: Unusual sensitivity to the drug, concomitant use with other xanthine containing formulations.

Warnings: Phenobarbital may be habit-forming. Since status asthmaticus is a medical emergency, high doses of this drug can be expected to be toxic.

Precautions: Use cautiously in the presence of severe cardiac disease, hypertension, acute myocardial injury, renal or hepatic malfunction, glaucoma, hyporthyroidism, and peptic ulcer. Cautious use is also indicated when dyphylline is administered concomitantly with other CNS stimulating drugs; and when administered to children. Postprandial administration may help to avoid gastric discomfort.

Adverse Reactions: The most consistent unfavorable reactions include *gastrointestinal* symptoms manifested by irritation, nausea, vomiting, and epigastric pain, generally preceded by headache, hematemesis, and diarrhea; *CNS* by stimulation, irritability, restlessness, insomnia, reflex hyperexcitability, muscle twitching, clonic and tonic generalized convulsions, and agitation; *respiratory* by tachypnea, and respiratory arrest; *renal* by albuminuria, increased excretion of renal tubule and red blood cells; *miscellaneous* by fever, and dehydration.

Dosage and Administration: *Orally* or *intramuscularly.* Usual adult dosage is 200 mg 3 or 4 times daily. In acute asthmatic attacks, 5 tablespoonsful of the elixir may be given. The usual parenteral administration is 250 to 500 mg injected slowly. Children, 2 to 3 mg/lb of body weight in divided doses, but should not exceed 6 mg/lb/day. Combined with guaifenesin or with ephedrine, phenobarbital and guaifenesin, the usual dosage is 1 tablet or 2 tablespoonsful of elixir 3 or 4 times daily. Dosage for children has not been established; therefore, these agents are not recommended for children under 6 years of age. Older children should be started on low doses which are then gradually increased to the lowest effective dosage, but should not exceed 5 mg/lb/day.

Availability:

LUFYLLIN®: **(Mallinckrodt)**

Elixir, 100 mg/15 ml (20% alcohol) in bottles of pints and gallons.

Injection, 500 mg in ampuls of 2 ml in cartons of 25.

Tablets, 200 mg in bottles of 100 and 1000; 400 mg in bottles of 100.

LUFYLLIN-EPG: **(Mallinckrodt)**

Elixir, 100 mg/10 ml with guaifenesin, 200 mg; ephedrine hydrochloride, 16 mg, and phenobarbital, 16 mg (5.5% alcohol) in bottles of 1 pint.

Tablets, 100 mg with guaifenesin, 200 mg; ephedrine hydrochloride, 16 mg and phenobarbital, 16 mg in bottles of 100.

LUFYLLIN-GG: **(Mallinckrodt)**

Elixir, 200 mg/30 ml with guaifenesin, 200 mg (17% alcohol) in bottles of pints and gallons.

Tablets, 200 mg with guaifenesin, 200 mg in bottles of 100, 500 and 1000 and in unit-dose packages of 100 and 1000.

NEOTHYLLINE®: **(Lemmon)**
Elixir, 160 mg/15 ml (18% alcohol) in bottles of pints and gallons.
Injection, 500 mg in ampuls of 2 ml in cartons of 10.
Tablets, 200 mg in bottles of 100 and 1000; 400 mg in bottles of 100 and 500.
NEOTHYLLINE®-G: **(Lemmon)**
Elixir, 100 mg/5 ml with guaifenesin 50 mg (20% alcohol) in bottles of pints and gallons.
Tablets, 100 mg with guaifenesin, 50 mg in bottles of 100 and 1000.
PHYLDROX Tablets, 100 mg with ephedrine sulfate, 25 mg and phenobarbital, 15 mg in bottles of 1000. **(Lemmon)**
NEOSPECT® Tablets, 100 mg with guaifenesin, 100 mg; ephedrine sulfate, 25 mg and phenobarbital, 15 mg in bottles of 100 and 1000. **(Lemmon)**

ECHOTHIOPHATE IODIDE

Chemical Name: (2-Mercaptoethyl) trimethylammonium iodide *O,O*-diethyl phosphorothioate.

Description: A quaternary thiophosphinyl cholinesterase inhibitor, it occurs as a hygroscopic, white, crystalline powder freely soluble in water and soluble in alcohol.

In common with isoflurophate, demecarium and physostigmine, echothiophate inhibits cholinesterase. The resulting accumulation of acetylcholine produces miosis and stimulates contraction of the iris and of the ciliary muscle, thus reducing intraocular pressure by increasing the facility of aqueous outflow. This effect is accompanied by vasodilatation of conjunctival vessels and increased permeability of the blood-aqueous barrier. An indirect decrease in activity of extraocular muscles of convergence also occurs.

Indications: Treatment of chronic open-angle glaucoma; subacute or chronic angle-closure glaucoma after iridectomy or in cases in which surgery is not advisable; certain nonuveitic secondary types of glaucoma, especially glaucoma following cataract surgery; and in the diagnosis and treatment of concomitant esotropias.

Contraindications: Active uveal inflammation; most cases of angle-closure glaucoma due to the possibility of increasing angle block; hypersensitivity to any of the components in the preparation.

Warnings: Succinylcholine should be administered only with extreme care, if at all, prior to or during general anesthesia to patients receiving anticholinesterase medication because of possible respiratory or cardiovascular collapse. In those patients under treatment of myasthenia gravis where other anticholinesterase medication is employed, echothiophate should only be used with full awareness of the likelihood of pharmacologic interactions. Safe use during pregnancy has not been established with regard to adverse effects on the fetus or on the respiration of the neonate.

Precautions: Gonioscopy is recommended prior to initiation of therapy with this drug. The drug should be used cautiously, if at all, in the presence of a quiescent uveitis or a history of this condition since an intense and persistent miosis and ciliary muscle contraction may occur. Caution is also advised in patients with a history of retinal detachment. Digital compression of the nasolacrimal ducts will minimize drainage into the nasal chamber, and may reduce the likelihood of systemic effects. Temporary discontinuance of medication is necessary if salivation, urinary incontinence, diarrhea, profuse sweating, muscle weakness, respiratory difficulties, or cardiac irregularities develop. Because of the synergistic effect of echothiophate with carbamate or organo-phosphate pesticides such as parathion, TEPP, malathion, etc., patients regularly exposed to them should be warned to use all the protective measures recommended. The physician should be aware of potential problems in the presence of marked vagotonia, bronchial asthma, gastrointestinal spasm, peptic ulcer, pronounced bradycardia and hypotension, epilepsy, urinary tract obstruction, vascular hypertension, recent myocardial infarction, or Parkinson's disease and other disorders that may respond adversely to vagotonic effects. The risk of the possible occurrence of hyphema should be considered when used prior to eye surgery.

Adverse Reactions: Stinging, burning, lacrimation, twitching of the eye, conjunctival and ciliary redness, browache, induced myopia with visual blurring, retinal detachment (occasional), and activation of latent iritis or uveitis may occur. Cysts of the iris may develop with prolonged use of the drug, and if treatment is continued, they may enlarge and obscure vision. These cysts which occur more frequently in children than in adults usually disappear when echothiophate therapy is discontinued, or when the strength of the drops or the frequency of instillation is reduced. Regular examinations are advisable when the drug is being prescribed for the treatment of accommodative esotropia. Prolonged use may cause conjunctival thickening, obstruction of the nasolacrimal canals, and lens opacities. A paradoxical rise in intraocular pressure may follow instillation of this drug. This may be alleviated by the use of a sympathomimetic mydriatic such as phenylephrine.

Dosage and Administration: *Topically.* In chronic simple glaucoma, initially, 1 drop of a 0.03 to 0.06% solution is instilled in each eye twice daily, just before retiring and in the morning. The dosage regimen prescribed should specify the lowest effective concentration and frequency of application that is necessary to maintain a reduction in intraocular pressure. In accommodative esotropia, initially, 1 drop of a 0.125% solution is instilled in each eye once daily, on retiring, for a period of 2 to 3 weeks. Further administration depends upon the clinical response.

Availability:
ECHODIDE Powder for Ophthalmic Solution, 1.5, 3, 6.25 and 12.5 mg with 5 ml diluent to make 0.03%, 0.06%, 0.125% and 0.25%, respectively. **(Alcon)**
PHOSPHOLINE IODIDE® Powder for Ophthalmic Solution, 1.5, 3, 6.25 and 12.5 mg with 5 ml diluent to make 0.03%, 0.06%, 0.125%, and 0.25% solutions, respectively. **(Ayerst)**

EDROPHONIUM CHLORIDE

Chemical Name: Ethyl(*m*-hydroxyphenyl)dimethylammonium chloride.

Description: A short and rapid-acting cholinergic compound used as a differential diagnostic agent in suspected cases of myasthenia gravis; it produces increased muscle strength without fasciculations in myasthenic patients in contrast to possible fasciculations but no increase in muscle strength in nonmyasthenic patients. Its pharmacologic action is due to the inhibition or inactivation of acetylcholinesterase at sites of cholinergic transmission. When used in myasthenia gravis, the drug results in a pronounced increase in strength; its onset of action is rapid (within 30 to 60) seconds and persists for an average of 10 minutes. In addition edrophonium reverses the neuromuscular block produced by curare.

Indications: In differential diagnosis and as adjunct to the evaluation of treatment requirements in myasthenia gravis. Also may be employed for evaluating emergency treatment in myasthenic crises; or whenever a curare antagonist is needed to terminate the action of curare, *d*-tubocurarine, gallamine triethiodide, or dimethyltubocurarine. It may be used adjunctively with assisted respiration and oxygen in the treatment of respiratory depression caused by curare overdosage. Because of its brief duration of action, it is not recommended for maintenance therapy in myasthenia gravis.

Contraindications: In patients with known hypersensitivity to anticholinesterase agents, and in mechanical intestinal and/or urinary obstruction.

Warnings: In the event of a severe cholinergic reaction which may occur in hypersensitive individuals, whether normal or myasthenic, 1 mg of atropine sulfate should be immediately available to be administered in aliquots intravenously. Edrophonium should be used with caution in patients with bronchial asthma or cardiac dysrhythmias. The transient bradycardia which may develop can be relieved with atropine sulfate. Although rarely occurring, patients should nevertheless be closely observed for any development of cardiac and respiratory arrest in which specialized assistance may be required. Care should be given when administering this drug to patients with symptoms of myasthenic weakness who are also on anticholinesterase drugs. Since symptoms of anticholinesterase overdose (cholinergic crisis) may mimic underdosage (myasthenic weakness), the patient's condition may be worsened by the use of this drug. Safe use during pregnancy or lactation has not been established. Therefore, use of this drug in women of childbearing potential requires that the expected benefits outweigh the possible hazards to the mother and child.

Precautions: An insensitivity reaction to the drug may develop; therefore, patients should be carefully watched for any development of respiratory difficulties in which assistance may be required. Dosages of anticholinesterase drugs should be reduced or withheld until patients regain their sensitivity to them. The drug may be used adjunctively in the treatment of respiratory depression caused by curare and curarimimetic drugs; it is not effective as an antidote for decamethonium bromide and succinylcholine chloride.

Adverse Reactions: Careful observation should be made for severe cholinergic reactions in the hyperreactive individual. The myasthenic patient in crisis who is being tested with this drug should be observed for bradycardia or cardiac standstill and cholinergic reactions if an overdose is given. The following reactions, common to anticholinesterase agents, may occur although not all of these reactions have been reported with the use of this drug. These include increased lacrimation, pupillary constriction, spasm of accommodation, diplopia, conjunctival hyperemia; convulsions, dysarthria, dysphonia, dysphagia; increased tracheobronchial secretions, laryngospasm, bronchiolar constriction, paralysis of the respiratory muscles, central respiratory paralysis; cardiac arrhythmias (especially bradycardia), fall in cardiac output leading to hypotension; increased salivary, gastric and intestinal secretion, nausea and vomiting, increased gastrointestinal peristalsis, diarrhea, abdominal cramps; weakness of skeletal muscles, fasciculations; increased urinary frequency and incontinence, diaphoresis. A cholinergic crisis usually occurs with overdosage and is manifested by nausea, vomiting, diarrhea, sweating, increased bronchial and salivary secretions and bradycardia. Obstruction of the airway by bronchial secretions is a hazardous complication that may be managed with suction and by the use of atropine. In the event of respiratory depression, artificial respiration with adequate respiratory exchange should be maintained.

Dosage and Administration: *Intravenously* or *intramuscularly.* For diagnosis, adults, 2 mg is injected *intravenously* within 15 to 30 seconds. Leaving the needle in situ, if no response occurs within 45 seconds the remaining 8 mg should be given. A dose of 10 mg may be given *intramuscularly.* For children weighing up to 75 lbs., 1 mg and those above this weight, 2 mg injected intravenously; if no response occurs within 45 seconds, the dose may be titrated up to 5 mg for children weighing up to 75 lbs. and 10 mg for those above this weight. The dose should be given in increments of 1 mg every 30 to 45 seconds. For infants, the recommended dose is 0.5 mg preferably by the intramuscular route. Patients who demonstrate a cholinergic reaction should be retested after ½ hour with a 2 mg dose to rule out a false-negative reaction. Patients over 50 years of age should be given 0.4 mg of atropine sulfate *subcutaneously* 10 minutes prior to the institution of this drug to prevent bradycardia and hypotension. As a curare antagonist, 10 mg *intravenously* administered slowly over a period of 30 to 45 minutes; may be repeated whenever necessary. For additional dosage information, consult package literature.

Availability:
TENSILON® Solution, 10 mg/ml in ampuls of 1 ml and in vials of 10 ml. (pH is adjusted to approx. 5.4.) **(Roche)**

ELDEC

Description: Each dark blue capsule with light blue band contains:

Vitamin A (acetate)	(1667 units)	0.5 mg
Thiamine mononitrate		10 mg
Riboflavin		0.87 mg
Pyridoxine hydrochloride		0.67 mg
Niacinamide		16.7 mg
Ascorbic acid		66.7 mg
dl-Panthenol		10 mg
Ferrous sulfate, dried		16.7 mg
Iodine (as potassium iodide)		0.05 mg
Calcium carbonate		66.7 mg
Vitamin E (*dl*-alpha tocopheryl acetate)		10 IU

Cyanocobalamin (vitamin B-12)	2 μg
Folic acid	0.33 mg

Indications: To correct vitamin, mineral and folic acid deficiencies.

Contraindications: Hypersensitivity to any of the components.

Precautions: Folic acid may obscure pernicious anemia in that the peripheral blood picture may revert to normal while the neurological manifestations remain progressive.

Dosage and Administration: *Orally.* One Kapseal 3 times daily before meals.

Availability:
ELDEC® Kapseals® (Capsules) in bottles of 100. **(Parke-Davis)**

EMESERT Ⓒ III

Description: Each insert contains:

	Pink #1	*Green #2*	*Blue #3*
Pyrilamine maleate	25 mg	50 mg	50 mg
Pentobarbital	30 mg	45 mg	100 mg

In a colored base of polyethylene glycol.

A synergistic combination of an antinauseant with a fast-acting sedative.

Indications: Recommended as follows: No. 1 for nausea and vomiting in children from 6 months to 12 years of age. No. 2 for older children (above 12 years) and adults. No. 3 for severe nausea and vomiting in adults.

Contraindications: Hypersensitivity to any of the components; acute intermittent porphyria; in patients with anorectal disease or severe hepatic impairment; in the presence of uncontrolled pain; in acute head injury associated with vomiting or other signs of CNS trauma; and in patients previously addicted to barbiturates. *Emesert is not recommended in infants under 6 months of age.*

Warnings: Safe use of this drug during pregnancy has not been established. Therefore, it should not be given to women who are or may become pregnant unless, in the judgment of the physician, the potential benefits outweigh the possible risks. Administration of these inserts to patients with severe psychologic disturbances may result in confusion, delirium and accentuation of the condition. Pentobarbital may be habit-forming, and may have an additive effect with alcohol or other CNS depressants. Prolonged administration, even at doses contained in this product, may produce psychic dependence, thus, withdrawal symptoms can occur following large doses which may result in delirium, convulsions, and death. Since barbiturates are respiratory depressants, caution is essential when the drug is administered in the presence of any respiratory difficulty.

Precautions: Special care is needed when administering this drug to patients with a history of drug dependence or suicidal tendencies, or to those who are concurrently receiving other sedative, hypnotic or narcotic agents. Patients should be cautioned that pentobarbital may impair their ability to engage in potentially hazardous activities such as operating machinery or driving a motor vehicle. Cautious use is indicated in patients with hyperthyroidism, diabetes mellitus, severe anemia, or congestive heart failure.

Adverse Reactions: Complications occurring with pyrilamine maleate usually include tremor; dryness of mouth, nose and throat; tinnitus; pupillary dilation; urinary retention; excitement; hypotension; palpitation; tachycardia; fatigue; vertigo; incoordination and muscle weakness. Those due to pentobarbital include respiratory depression, allergic reactions; severe depression of the CNS; drowsiness; lethargy; hangover; paradoxical excitement; apnea and circulatory collapse. Symptoms of overdosage are coma; diminished or absent reflexes; respiratory depression; hypothermia followed by fever and gradual appearance of circulatory collapse and pulmonary edema. Treatment consists of maintaining and assisting respiration; supporting circulation with vasopressors and intravenous fluids; dialysis, if indicated; aspiration of the stomach if the inserts are ingested; and administration of osmotic diuretic and antibiotics as needed.

Dosage and Administration: *Rectally.* Insert 1 Emesert of appropriate form into the rectum; may be repeated according to the following schedule; children 6 months to 2 years of age, #1 insert every 6 to 8 hours, not to exceed 3 doses within a 24-hour period; 2 to 12 years of age, every 6 to 8 hours, not to exceed 4 doses within a 24-hour period; older children and adults less severely affected, #2 insert every 4 to 6 hours, not to exceed 4 doses within a 24-hour period; adults severely affected, #3 insert every 6 to 8 hours, not to exceed 4 doses within a 24-hour period. Use is not recommended in infants under 6 months of age.

Availability:
Ⓒ EMESERT® Rectal inserts, #1, #2 and #3 strip-packed in cartons of 12 and 50.
(Arnar-Stone)

EMETINE HYDROCHLORIDE

Description: The hydrated hydrochloride of an alkaloid obtained from ipecac or prepared synthetically, emetine is used primarily in the treatment of amebiasis; it exerts a direct lethal action on *Entamoeba histolytica.*

Indications: Intestinal amebiasis, extraintestinal amebiasis, other parasitic infections such as balantidiasis, fascioliasis, and paragonimiasis.

Contraindications: Organic disease of the heart or kidney, except those with amebic abscess or hepatitis not controlled by chloroquin; pregnancy; in children, except those with uncontrolled severe dysentery; in patients who have received a course of emetine less than 6 weeks to 2 months previously.

Precautions: Utmost caution should be exercised in administering emetine to aged or debilitated patients. **Since emetine is a potentially dangerous drug, strict medical supervision of the patient, with daily examination, is mandatory. All patients must be confined to bed during treatment and for several days afterward.** Pulse rate and blood pressure should be checked 2 or 3 times daily and an electrocardiogram should be taken before the drug is administered, and after the fifth dose, upon completion of therapy, and 1 week later. Discontinue medication if tachycardia, precipitous fall in blood pressure, neuromuscular symptoms, marked gastrointestinal effects, and considerable weakness occur.

Adverse Reactions: Emetine produces a variety of toxic manifestations which, depending on individual susceptibility, may occur at any dose level. Local reactions, consisting of aching, tenderness and muscle weakness in the area of the injection site, are common. Eczematous, urticarial or purpuric lesions may also appear. Systemic reactions involve the gastrointestinal, neuromuscular and cardiovascular systems. Severe gastrointestinal side effects are unusual; nausea and vomiting, in association with dizziness and headache, are more common. Neuromuscular symptoms consist of weakness, aching, tenderness and skeletal-muscle stiffness. The weakness and muscle pain tend to persist until emetine is discontinued; they usually appear before more serious symptoms develop and thus serve as a guide for avoiding overdosage. The most important toxic effects are related to the cardiovascular system. Hypotension, tachycardia, precordial pain, dyspnea, electrocardiographic abnormalities, gallop rhythm, cardiac dilatation, congestive failure, and death have been reported.

Dosage and Administration: *Subcutaneously* (preferable) or *intramuscularly.* **The intravenous route is considered dangerous and is contraindicated.** In acute fulminating amebic dysentery, emetine should be administered only long enough to control the diarrheal or dysenteric symptoms. In adults, 65 mg daily or 32 mg morning and evening, administered for 3 to 5 days, will usually suffice. In amebic hepatitis or abscess, emetine may be administered for 10 days in a daily dose of 65 mg or 32 mg morning and evening, subcutaneously or intramuscularly. The dose of emetine should not exceed 65 mg/day; this may be given in a single injection or in 32-mg portions morning and evening. Some clinicians recommend 1 mg/kg/day not to exceed 65 mg/day. For children under 8 years of age, give no more than 10 mg of emetine daily; for those over 8 years of age, no more than 20 mg. A course should not be repeated in less than 6 weeks.

Availability:
EMETINE HYDROCHLORIDE Solution, 65 mg/ml in ampuls of 1 ml. **(Lilly)**

EMPRAZIL
EMPRAZIL-C (C III)

Description: Each Emprazil tablet contains pseudoephedrine hydrochloride, 20 mg; phenacetin, 150 mg; aspirin, 200 mg; caffeine, 30 mg. Emprazil-C contains in addition codeine phosphate, 15 mg. Formulated to provide analgesic, antipyretic and decongestant action; the codeine component provides in addition antitussive action.

Indications: Relief of distressing symptoms of upper respiratory tract infections such as coughs, aches, pain, malaise, fever, swollen respiratory mucosa associated with colds and flu, and as prophylaxis against secondary otitis media or sinusitis.

Warnings: Codeine phosphate may be habit-forming.

Precautions: Use with caution in hypertensive patients.

Adverse Reactions: Mild stimulation may occur in sensitive patients.

Dosage and Administration: *Orally.* Adults and children over 12 years of age, 1 or 2 tablets 3 times daily. Children 6 to 12 years of age, 1 tablet 3 times daily.

Availability:
EMPRAZIL® Tablets in bottles of 100 and 1000. **(Burroughs Wellcome)**
(C III) EMPRAZIL-C® Tablets in bottles of 100. **(Burroughs Wellcome)**

EN-CEBRIN F

Description: Each capsule contains:

Vitamin A (synthetic)	(4000 units)	1.2 mg
Ergocalciferol	(400 units)	10 μg
Thiamine monohydrate		3 mg
Riboflavin		2 mg
Niacinamide		10 mg
Pyridoxine hydrochloride		2 mg
Folic acid		1 mg
Cyanocobalamin (vitamin B-12 equiv.)		5 μg
Pantothenic acid (as calcium pantothenate, racemic)		5 mg
Ascorbic acid		50 mg
Calcium carbonate		250 mg
Iron (as ferrous fumarate)		30 mg
Iodine (as potassium iodide)		0.15 mg
Copper sulfate		1 mg
Magnesium hydroxide		5 mg
Manganese glycerophosphate		1 mg
Zinc chloride		1.5 mg

Indications: For the prophylaxis and treatment of vitamin-mineral and folate deficiencies associated with pregnancy and lactation, and for the prevention of megaloblastic anemia especially during the third trimester of pregnancy.

Contraindications: None known.

Precautions: Folic acid may obscure the hematologic symptoms of pernicious anemia while neurological manifestations remain progressive. Parenteral vitamin B-12 is therefore essential in patients with this disease. In susceptible patients, hypersensitivity or idiosyncrasy to any of the components may occur.

Adverse Reactions: Infrequently noted were nausea and vomiting.

Dosage and Administration: *Orally.* The usual dosage is 1 capsule daily.

Availability:
EN-CEBRIN® F Pulvules (capsules) in bottles of 100. **(Lilly)**

ENGRAN-HP

Description: Each tablet contains:

Vitamin A (as acetate)	(8000 units)	2.4 mg
Ergocalciferol (vitamin D)	(400 units)	10 μg
Vitamin E	(30 units)	30 mg
Thiamine mononitrate		1.7 mg
Riboflavin		2 mg
Pyridoxine hydrochloride		2.5 mg
Cyanocobalamin		0.8 μg
Folic acid		0.8 mg
Niacinamide		20 mg
Sodium ascorbate		60 mg
Calcium, elemental (as carbonate)		650 mg
Iodine, elemental (as potassium iodide)		0.15 mg
Iron, elemental (as stabilized ferrous carbonate)		18 mg
Magnesium oxide		100 mg

Indications: Vitamin-mineral supplement during pregnancy and lactation.

Precautions: Pernicious anemia should be ruled out before starting treatment. While folic acid corrects the blood picture of pernicious anemia, it does not ameliorate the attendant neurologic involvement. Parenteral use of vitamin B-12 is recommended to assure essential medical supervision of the patient.

Adverse Reactions: Allergic sensitization has been reported following both oral and parenteral administration of folic acid.

Dosage and Administration: *Orally.* Two tablets daily, or as required.

Availability:
ENGRAN®-HP High Potency tablets in bottles of 100. **(Squibb)**

ENTOZYME

Description: Each white-coated tablet contains:

In the acid-soluble outer layer	
Pepsin N.F. (equivalent)	250 mg
In the enteric-coated core	
Pancreatin N.F. (equivalent)	300 mg
Bile salts	150 mg

Entozyme enhances proteolysis by its peptic and tryptic activity, carbohydrate digestion by amylolytic activity, and fat emulsification and transport by lipolytic activity and the action of the bile salts. The components of 6 tablets will digest in vitro 60 gm of fat, 48 gm of protein, and 48 gm of carbohydrate.

Indications: Management of gastrointestinal disturbances associated with diminished secretion of pancreatic enzymes, such as pancreatitis, pancreatic fibrosis, and postpancreatectomy states; for relief of steatorrhea, pyrosis, flatulence, belching associated with cholecystitis, postcholecystectomy syndrome, subtotal gastrectomy and miscellaneous vague digestive complaints. Also useful in maintaining adequate nutrition for geriatric patients.

Contraindications: Biliary tract obstruction; hypersensitivity to any of the components.

Adverse Reactions: A rash may develop in highly sensitive patients.

Dosage and Administration: *Orally*, 2 tablets after each meal, adjusted to the needs of the patient. *Do not crush or chew tablets.*

Availability:
ENTOZYME® Tablets in bottles of 100 and 500. **(Robins)**

EPHEDRINE SULFATE

Chemical Name: *l*-α-[1-(methylamino)ethyl]benzyl alcohol sulfate.

Description: Ephedrine sulfate is the sulfate salt of a *levo*rotatory alkaloid obtained from *Ephedra equisetina* or prepared synthetically. It is an adrenergic drug which exerts peripheral effects resembling those of epinephrine and central effects resembling those of the amphetamines. Ephedrine produces a more sustained action but is less potent than epinephrine. It stimulates both α and β receptors and its peripheral actions are due partly to norepinephrine release and partly to direct effects on receptors. The drug stimulates the heart, elevating the systolic and usually the diastolic blood pressure. Its vasopressor effect results largely from increased cardiac output and to a lesser extent from peripheral vasoconstriction. Ephedrine produces relaxation of bronchial muscle which is more sustained but less pronounced than that produced by epinephrine. It also stimulates the CNS to a greater extent than does epinephrine but its central action is less potent than that of the amphetamines. The central effects of ephedrine are overshadowed to a large extent by its peripheral actions. It produces sympathomimetic effects when administered orally, parenterally or topically.

Indications: For oral or parenteral treatment of allergic disorders, such as bronchial asthma, and for local treatment of nasal congestion in acute coryza, vasomotor rhinitis, acute sinusitis and hay fever. The drug has long been used as a pressor agent, particularly during spinal anesthesia when hypotension occurs frequently. In Stokes-Adams syndrome with complete heart block, the drug has a value similar to that of epinephrine. It is given as a CNS stimulant in narcolepsy, depressive states and poisoning due to central depressant drugs. It has also been used in enuresis and myasthenia gravis. A barbiturate is added to the formulation for its calming effect on the tense, anxious, asthmatic patients and for decreasing the incidence of undesirable effects associated with sympathomimetic agents; atropine for its parasympatholytic activity, and iodide for its liquefying action on viscid secretions from mucous membranes.

Contraindications: In patients with known hypersensitivity to the drug, and in those with angle-closure glaucoma. Parenteral administration should not be given to those patients anesthetized with agents such as cyclopropane or halothane.

Warnings: The solution containing ephedrine and procaine is not intended for intraspinal or intravascular administration.

Precautions: Special care should be used when administering the drug to patients with heart disease including coronary insufficiency, angina pectoris, diabetes, hyperthyroidism, prostatic hypertrophy or hypertension, as well as to patients receiving digitalis. Caution is required in patients taking MAO inhibitors or tricyclic antidepressant or to those undergoing general anesthesia, particularly with cyclopropane or the halogenated hydrocarbon agents. If vasopressor drugs are intended for use in correcting hypotension during parturition, the obstetrician should be mindful that some oxytocic drugs may cause severe hypertension which may result in cerebral hemorrhage during the postpartum period. Prolonged use may produce a syndrome resembling an anxiety state. Tolerance to ephedrine may develop, but temporary withdrawal of the drug restores its original effectiveness. Parenteral administration should not be used to overcome hypotension due to acute hemorrhage or noncardiogenic shock.

Adverse Reactions: Acute toxic reactions are usually extensions of the therapeutic actions of the drug and are most often due to overdosage. Administration of ephedrine may be followed by throbbing headache, restlessness, insomnia, anxiety, tension, tremor, weakness, dizziness, confusion, delirium, hallucinations, pallor, respiratory difficulty, palpitation, precordial pain (occasional), sweating, nausea or vomiting. These effects are usually transient and can be minimized by rest and recumbency. Repeated injections of ephedrine may cause contraction of the bladder sphincter and interfere with voluntary urination. The possibility of urinary retention, especially in the elderly male, should be considered.

Dosage and Administration: The usual dose for adults is 25 to 50 mg, given *subcutaneously, intramuscularly,* or *intravenously* (slowly), or 25 to 50 mg *orally,* repeated every 3 to 4 hours if necessary. In enuresis, standard texts recommend 25 to 50 mg orally at bedtime. In myasthenia gravis, standard texts recommend 25 mg orally 3 or 4 times daily. Combined with barbiturates, 1 capsule every 4 to 6 hours or 1 teaspoonful of elixir every 2 to 4 hours.

Availability:

Ephedrine Sulfate

Capsules, 25 mg (OTC) in bottles of 100 and 1000; 50 mg in bottles of 100. **(Lilly)**
Injection, 25 mg/ml in ampuls of 1 ml. **(Lilly)**
Injection, 50 mg/ml in ampuls of 1 ml. **(Abbott, Lilly and Parke-Davis)**
Syrup, 4 mg/ml in bottles of 1 pint. **(Lilly)**

Combinations

ENURETROL® Chewable Tablets, 7.5 mg with atropine sulfate, 0.15 mg in bottles of 50. **(Cooper)**

EPHED-ORGANIDIN: **(Wallace)**
Elixir, 16 mg with iodinated glycerol, 30 mg and phenobarbital, 8 mg/5 ml (**Warning:** may be habit-forming) in bottles of 1 pint.
Tablets, 24 mg with methapyrilene fumarate, 70 mg and iodinated glycerol, 60 mg in bottles of 100.

CIII EPHEDRINE and AMYTAL® Capsules, 25 mg with amobarbital, 50 mg (**Warning:** may be habit-forming) in bottles of 100 and 500. **(Lilly)**

EPHEDRINE and NEMBUTAL®-25 Capsules, 25 mg (as hydrochloride) with sodium pentobarbital, 25 mg (**Warning:** may be habit-forming) in bottles of 100. **(Abbott)**

EPHEDRINE and PROCAINE Injection, 50 mg (as hydrochloride) with procaine hydrochloride, 10 mg/ml in ampuls of 1 ml. **(Lilly)**

CIII EPHEDRINE and SECONAL® Sodium Capsules, 25 mg with sodium secobarbital, 50 mg (**Warning:** may be habit-forming) in bottles of 100. **(Lilly)**

EPINEPHRINE

Chemical Name: *l*-3,4-Dihydroxy-α-[(methylamino)methyl]benzyl alcohol.

Description: Epinephrine is an active principal of the adrenal medulla. The *lev*orotatory form available commercially occurs as a white to nearly white, microcrystalline, odorless powder very slightly soluble in water and in alcohol. With acids, it forms salts that are readily soluble in water, e.g., hydrochloride and bitartrate. Epinephrine bitartrate occurs as a white, grayish-white or brownish-gray, crystalline powder freely soluble in water.

Because of poor absorption from the gastrointestinal tract, epinephrine is ineffective orally, but it is effective when administered parenterally or topically. A potent sympathomimetic drug, it activates an adrenergic receptive mechanism on effector cells and imitates all actions of the sympathetic nervous system, except those on the arteries of the face and sweat glands. Epinephrine acts on both alpha and beta receptors and is the most potent alpha receptor activator. It stimulates the heart to increased output; raises the systolic blood pressure; relaxes bronchial spasm; decreases intestinal peristalsis; mobilizes liver glycogen, resulting in hyperglycemia and glycosuria.

Its actions on the beta receptors of the heart, vascular and other smooth muscles are quite prominent. When given by rapid intravenous injection, the drug evokes a rapid rise in blood pressure, mainly systolic, by (1) direct stimulation of cardiac muscle which increases the strength of ventricular contraction, (2) increasing the heart rate, and (3) constriction of the arterioles in the skin, mucosa and splanchnic areas of the circulation.

When administered by slow intravenous injection, epinephrine usually produces only a moderate rise in systolic and a fall in diastolic pressures. Although some increase in pulse pressure occurs, there is usually no significant elevation in mean blood pressure. Accordingly, the compensatory reflex mechanisms that come into play with a pronounced increase in blood pressure do not antagonize the direct cardiac actions of epinephrine as much as with catecholamines that have a predominant action on alpha receptors. Total peripheral resistance decreases by action of epinephrine on beta receptors of the skeletal muscle vasculature and blood flow is thereby enhanced. Usually this vasodilator effect of the drug on the circulation predominates so that the modest rise in systolic pressure which follows slow injection or absorption is mainly the result of direct cardiac stimulation and increase in cardiac output. In some instances peripheral resistance is not altered or may even rise owing to a greater ratio of alpha to beta activity in different vascular areas.

Epinephrine is rapidly inactivated in the body and is degraded by enzymes in the liver and other tissues. The major portion of injected doses is excreted in the urine as inactivated compounds and the remainder either partly unchanged or conjugated.

Indications: The most common uses of epinephrine are to relieve respiratory distress due to bronchospasm, to provide rapid relief of hypersensitivity reactions to drugs or other allergens, and to prolong the action of infiltration anesthetics. Its cardiac effects may be of use in restoring cardiac rhythm in cardiac arrest due to various causes, but it is not intended for use in cardiac failure or in hemorrhagic, traumatic, or cardiogenic shock. As a topical hemostatic agent; the treatment of mucosal congestion in hay fever, rhinitis, acute sinusitis; to bring about vasoconstriction conjunctively with local anesthetics; the relief of bronchial asthmatic paroxysms, the suspension is recommended for the symptomatic treatment of bronchial asthma, and reversible bronchospasm of chronic bronchitis and emphysema; in syncope due to com plete heart block or carotid sinus hypersensitivity; the symptomatic relief of serum sickness, urticaria, angioneurotic edema; for resuscitation in cardiac arrest following anesthetic accidents. May also be used in chronic, simple (open-angle) glaucoma, for relaxation of uterine musculature and inhibition of uterine contraction, as adjunctive therapy with miotics, and in selected cases with carbonic anhydrase inhibitors.

Contraindications: In anesthesia with cyclopropane, or halogenated hydrocarbons or with local anesthetics in areas supplied by end-arteries (digits, nose, ear, penis), cardiac resuscitation in the presence of ventricular fibrillation; in patients in shock or with organic brain damage; in women in labor; in the presence of cardiac dilatation and coronary insufficiency. Since epinephrine may occasionally increase intraocular pressure significantly, it is contraindicated in narrow-angle glaucoma.

Warnings: When used in the eyes, eye pain or ache, browache, headache, conjunctival hyperemia and allergic lid reactions may occur. Adrenachrome deposits in the conjunctiva and cornea after prolonged use have been reported. Since macular edema may occur in some aphakic patients, it should be used with caution in these patients. Caution is advised when administering epinephrine to elderly patients; to those with cardiovascular disease, hypertension, diabetes or hyperthyroidism; in psychoneurotic individuals; and during pregnancy. Extreme caution is required in patients with long-standing bronchial asthma and emphysema who have developed degenerative heart disease. Overdosage or inadvertant intravenous injection of epinephrine may induce cerebrovascular hemorrhage resulting from the sharp rise in blood pressure. Fatalities may result from pulmonary edema because of the peripheral constriction and cardiac stimulation produced. Rapidly acting vasodilators such as nitrites, or alpha blocking agents may counteract the marked pressor effects of epinephrine. It is not recommended to use epinephrine with excessive doses of digitalis, mercurial diuretics, or other drugs that sensitize the heart to arrhythmias. Additionally, simultaneous use with isoproterenol may induce serious cardiac arrhythmias due to their combined effects. Anginal pain may be induced when coronary insufficiency is present.

Precautions: Tricyclic antidepressants, certain antihistamines such as diphenhydramine, tripelennamine, *d*-chlorpheniramine; MAO inhibitors, and sodium *1*-thyroxine may potentiate the effects of epinephrine. If vasopressor drugs are intended for use during parturition, the obstetrician should bear in mind that some oxytocic drugs may cause severe hypertension which may result in cerebral hemorrhage during the postpartum period. Caution should be exercised when used for cardiac resuscitation in cases of asystole. **Note:** Epinephrine is readily destroyed by alkalies and oxidizing agents.

Adverse Reactions: May cause anxiety, palpitation, vertigo, headache (especially in hyperthyroid patients), cardiac arrhythmias when given to patients with heart disease, ventricular fibrillation when given during inhalation anesthesia with various drugs, and cerebral hemorrhage in patients with hypertension or cerebral arteriosclerosis, necrosis at the injection site, and "Epinephrine Fastness" due to prolonged use. Prolonged topical use in the eye may produce extracellular pigmentation in the palpebral conjunctiva. On rare occasions systemic side effects characterized by occipital headaches, browache, palpitation, pallor, tachycardia, extrasystoles, hypertension, trembling, and sweating have been observed. Stinging with rebound redness may occur following instillation of ophthalmic solution.

Dosage and Administration: *Subcutaneously* or *intramuscularly*. 1:1000 solution: Adults: 0.06 to 1 ml. Children: 0.01 to 0.3 ml. *Topically*. As hemostatic: in solutions from 1:15,000 to 1:1000. In glaucoma: 1 drop of a 1 to 2% solution instilled into conjunctival sac once or twice daily. Conjunctively with local anesthetics: 1:100,000 to not greater than 1:50,000. For resuscitation: (1:1000 solution) 0.5 ml *intracardially* and 0.05 to 0.2 ml diluted 200 times *intravenously (slowly)*. For *intraspinal* use, add 0.2 to 0.4 ml of a 1:100,000 to 1:20,000 concentration to the anesthetic spinal fluid mixture.

Availability:

Epinephrine

SUS-PHRINE® Suspension, 5 mg/ml in ampuls of 0.5 ml and multiple-dose vials of 5 ml. **(Cooper)**

Epinephrine Hydrochloride

Injection, 0.1 mg/ml (1:10,000) in Abboject® syringes of 10 ml with or without intracardiac needle. **(Abbott)**

Injection, 0.1 mg/ml (1:10,000) in Bristoject® (prefilled disposable syringes) of 10 ml. **(Bristol)**

Injection, 1 mg/ml (1:1000) in disposable syringes of 1 ml with needle (Tubex®). **(Wyeth)**

Ophthalmic Solution, 1 mg/ml in Dropperettes Applicators of 1 ml. **(Smith Miller & Patch)**

ADRENALIN®: **(Parke-Davis)**

Injection, 1 mg/ml (1:1000) in ampuls of 1 ml and Steri-Vials of 30 ml.

Solution for Inhalation, 10 mg/ml in bottles of 7.5 ml.

Topical Solution (OTC), 1 mg/ml (1:1000) in screw-cap bottles of 30 ml.

EPIFRIN® Ophthalmic Solution, 0.25% in dropper bottles of 15 ml; 0.5, 1 and 2% in dropper bottles of 5 and 15 ml. **(Allergan)**

GLAUCON® Ophthalmic Solution, 0.5, 1 and 2% in dropper bottles of 10 ml. **(Alcon)**

Epinephrine Bitartrate

E-PILO Ophthalmic Solution, 1% with pilocarpine hydrochloride, 1, 2, 3, 4 or 6% in plastic squeeze bottles of 10 ml with dropper-tip and in Dropperettes® applicators of 1 ml. **(Smith, Miller & Patch)**

EPITRATE® Ophthalmic Solution, 2% in dropper bottles of 7.5 ml. **(Ayerst)**

LYOPHRIN® Ophthalmic Solution, 2% in vials of 5 ml with 5-ml vial of diluent. **(Alcon)**

MEDIHALER-EPI® Suspension, 7 mg/ml in vials of 15 ml with or without oral adapter. Each measured dose contains 0.3 mg epinephrine bitartrate, equivalent to 0.16 mg epinephrine base. **(Riker)**

Epinephryl Borate

EPINAL® Ophthalmic Solution, 0.25, 0.5 and 1% in plastic dropper bottles of 7.5 ml. **(Alcon)**

EPPY® Ophthalmic Solution, 0.5 and 1% in dropper bottles of 7.5 ml. **(Barnes-Hind)**

EPPY N Ophthalmic Solution, 0.5 and 1% with erythorbic acid, boric acid, polyvinyl pyrrolidone, polyoxyl 40 stearate and benzalkoniun chloride in bottles of 7.5 ml. **(Barnes-Hind)**

EPRAGEN (CIII)

Description: Each capsule contains ephedrine hydrochloride, 22 mg; aspirin, 130 mg; phenacetin, 227 mg and amobarbital, 50 mg.

Indications: Allergic conditions.

Contraindications: Hypersensitivity to any of the components.

Warnings: Amobarbital may be habit-forming.

Precautions: Use with caution in the presence of peptic ulcer, serious cardiovascular-renal disease, hyperthyroidism or diabetes mellitus. Phenacetin may aggravate renal disease. The CNS-depressant effect of amobarbital may be additive with that of other centrally depressant drugs such as alcohol.

Adverse Reactions: Patients hypersensitive to sympathomimetics may develop nervousness, insomnia, palpitation and other symptoms of stimulation.

Dosage and Administration: *Orally.* Adults, 1 capsule in the morning and 1 or 2 at night. Children, dosage varies with age; part of the contents of a capsule may be removed in order to adjust the dose.

Availability:
Ⓒ III EPRAGEN® Pulvules in bottles of 100 and 500. **(Lilly)**

ERGOCALCIFEROL

Chemical Name: Irradiated Ergosta-5,7,22-trien-3β-Ol.

Description: Ergocalciferol, or vitamin D, occurs as white, odorless crystals insoluble in water and soluble in alcohol, chloroform, ether, and fatty oils. One hundred IU of vitamin D are equivalent to 2.5 mcg. **Note:** 1.25 mg is equal to 50,000 units; 12.5 mg is equal to 500,000 units.

Ergocalciferol regulates calcium-phosphorus metabolism and is essential for normal bone development. In hypoparathyroidism, the administration of large doses of this vitamin increases serum calcium levels and decreases serum phosphorus levels. It is active when taken orally, exerting a prolonged antitetanic effect. The biologically active metabolites of ergocalciferol are synthesized in the liver and kidneys. About 1/2 of an oral dose is excreted via the bile into the feces with only very small amounts appearing in the urine. The vitamin is stored chiefly in the liver but it is also found in the skin, brain, spleen, and bones. In the plasma, vitamin D is bound to alpha globulins and albumin. There is a time lag of 12 to 24 hours between the administration of the vitamin and initiation of its action in the body.

Indications: Treatment of refractory rickets, hypoparathyroidism, and familial hypophosphatemia.

Contraindications: In patients with hypercalcemia, malabsorption syndrome, abnormal sensitivity to the toxic effects of vitamin D, hypervitaminosis D, and impaired renal function.

Warnings: The safe use of ergocalciferol in excess of 400 IU daily during pregnancy has not been established. Studies with several species of pregnant animals have demonstrated fetal abnormalities associated with hypervitaminosis D. For the protection of the fetus, therefore, the use of this vitamin in excess of the recommended dietary allowance during normal pregnancy should be avoided. Hypersensitivity to vitamin D may be one etiologic factor in infants with idiopathic hypercalcemia. In these instances vitamin D must be severely restricted.

Precautions: Very large doses of ergocalciferol should be considered potentially dangerous. Hence, the effect must be carefully controlled by periodic determinations of calcium in the blood and urine. Several fatalities resulting from prolonged use of excessive doses have been reported. Large doses of ergocalciferol should be used only with caution in elderly patients. Ingestion of supplemental vitamin-D containing products should be evaluated. Additionally, when high therapeutic doses are employed, progress should be followed with frequent serum and urinary calcium, potassium, and urea determinations. Intravenous calcium, parathyroid hormone, and/or dihydrotachysterol may be supplementary requirements in the treatment of hypoparathyroidism. Patients should be cautioned not to take mineral oil since it interfers with the absorption of vitamin D. Maintenance of a normal serum phosphorus level by dietary phosphate restriction and/or administration of aluminum gels as intestinal phosphate binders is essential in patients with hyperphosphatemia, as frequently seen in renal osteodystrophy, in order to prevent metastatic calcification. Concurrent administration of thiazide diuretics to hypoparathyroid patients may result in hypercalcemia. The physician should bear in mind that the effects of the drug can persist for 2 or more months after cessation of therapy.

Adverse Reactions: Toxic effects may occur when ergocalciferol is ingested for several months by adults in doses of 100,000 units or more daily or by children in doses of 20,000 units daily. Patients should be kept under observation in order to detect symptoms of toxicity, which may include anorexia; nausea; weakness; weight loss; vague aches and stiffness; constipation; diarrhea; convulsions; mental retardation; anemia; mild acidosis; impairment of renal function with polyuria, nocturia, polydipsia, hypercalciuria, azotemia (reversible), hypertension, nephrocalcinosis, generalized vascular calcification, irreversible renal insufficiency which may be fatal, albuminuria, or urinary casts; widespread calcification of the soft tissues, including the heart, blood vessels, renal tubules, and lungs; osteoporosis in adults; and dwarfism in infants and children due to a decline in the average rate of linear growth and increased mineralization of bones. These reactions gradually disappear if treatment is discontinued at the first sign of symptoms. Toxic effects are usually associated with hypercalcemia. Treatment consists in immediate withdrawal of the vitamin, a low calcium diet, generous intake of fluids, and acidification of the urine along with symptomatic and supportive treatment. Corticosteroids have been used successfully in severe cases. Deaths due to renal or cardiovascular failure have been reported.

Dosage and Administration: *Orally* or *intramuscularly.* The range between therapeutic and toxic doses is narrow; therefore, dosage must be individualized under close medical supervision. Calcium intake must be adequate so that the blood concentration is kept between 9 and 10 mg/100 ml. *For refractory rickets,* generally 50,000 units; however, dosage may range from 12,000 to 500,000 units. *For hypoparathyroidism,* the initial dose is from 100,000 to 200,000 units daily; maintenance dose is from 50,000 to 200,000 units daily. Blood calcium, phosphorus, and urea determinations should be made every 2 weeks or more frequently if necessary. The bones should be x-rayed every month until the condition is corrected and stabilized. **Note:** Intramuscular injections should be given slowly, preferably deeply into the gluteal muscle, taking care to avoid injection into a vein.

Availability:

CALCIFEROL™: **(Kremers-Urban)**
Injection in oil, 12.5 mg/ml in vials of 10 ml.
Tablets, 1.25 mg in bottles of 100.

DRISDOL®: **(Winthrop)**
Capsules, 1.25 mg in bottles of 50.
Liquid for Oral Use, 0.25 mg/gm (in propylene glycol) in bottles of 60 ml.

VITAMIN D Capsules, (GELTABS®), 1.25 mg in bottles of 100. **(Upjohn)**

Synthetic Oleovitamin D

DELTALIN® Capsules (Gelseals®), 1.25 mg in bottles of 100 and 500. **(Lilly)**

ERGONOVINE MALEATE

Description: Ergonovine is the hydroxyisopropylamide of lysergic acid. The maleate is the salt of one of the principal alkaloids of ergot obtained from the dried sclerotium of *Claviceps purpurea.* It occurs as a white to grayish-white or faintly yellow, odorless, microcrystalline powder sparingly soluble in water and slightly soluble in alcohol. Methylergonovine maleate is produced semi-synthetically and shares the actions and uses of ergonovine maleate.

Ergonovine maleate has been shown to possess all of the desirable oxytocic activity of ergot itself. It produces a firm contraction of the uterus, the onset of which ranges from immediately to 15 minutes depending upon route of administration. Upon the initial tetanic contraction is superimposed a succession of minor relaxations and contractions. The extent of relaxation increases gradually over a period of about 1½ hours, but vigorous rhythmic contractions continue for a period of 3 hours or more after an injection. The prolonged initial contraction is the type necessary to control uterine hemorrhage.

Indications: Prevention and treatment of postpartum and postabortal hemorrhage due to uterine atony; subinvolution.

Contraindications: In those patients who have shown allergic or idiosyncratic reactions to the drug. Also contraindicated for the induction of labor and in cases of threatened spontaneous abortion; and in patients with toxemia or hypertension.

Warnings: This drug should **not** be administered intravenously because of the possibility of inducing sudden hypertensive and cerebrovascular accidents. If intravenous administration is essential, it should be given *slowly* over a period of no less than 60 seconds with careful monitoring of blood pressure.

Precautions: Because of the high uterine tone produced, the drug is not recommended for routine use before delivery of the placenta unless the operator is versed in the technique described by Davis and others and has adequate facilities and personnel at his disposal. Prolonged use is to be avoided. Although unreported thus far, it is quite possible that hypersensitive individuals may develop ergotism. Caution should be exercised in the presence of sepsis, obliterative vascular disease, hepatic or renal involvement.

Adverse Reactions: Nausea and vomiting; dizziness; headache; tinnitus; diaphoresis and palpitation; temporary chest pain and dyspnea; allergic phenomena, including shock; in a few individuals elevations of blood pressure (sometimes extreme), most frequently in association with regional anesthesia (caudal or spinal), previous administration of a vasoconstrictor, and the intravenous administration of the oxytocic. The mechanism of such hypertension is obscure since it may occur in the absence of anesthesia, vasoconstrictors and oxytocics. They usually subside promptly following intravenous administration of 15 mg of chlorpromazine. Other complications that may occur include dizziness, headache, tinnitus, diaphoresis and palpitation, temporary chest pain, and dyspnea.

Dosage and Administration: The immediate postpartum dose usually is 0.2 mg, *intramuscularly* or *orally*. In emergencies (see Warnings), the dose may be given *intravenously*. To minimize late postpartum bleeding, 0.2 or 0.4 mg may be given orally 2 to 4 times daily for a maximum of 1 week or until the danger of uterine atony has passed (usually 48 hours). The tablets may also be taken *perlingually*, and by *rectum* (suspended in water as a retention enema). In calcium-deficient patients, the uterus may fail to respond, in which case calcium salts should be given intravenously and with caution; they should not be given intravenously to patients taking digitalis concomitantly.

Availability:
ERGONOVINE MALEATE Injection, 0.2 mg/ml in disposable syringes (Tubex®) of 1 ml with needle. **(Wyeth)**
ERGOTRATE® MALEATE: **(Lilly)**
Injection, 0.2 mg/ml in ampuls of 1 ml.
Tablets, 0.2 mg in bottles of 100 and 1000 and in 10 strips of 10 individually labeled blisters each containing 1 tablet.
METHERGINE® (Methylergonovine Maleate): **(Sandoz)**
Injection, 0.2 mg/ml in ampuls of 1 ml.
Tablets, 0.2 mg in bottles of 100 and 1000 and in SandoPaks® (unit-dose) packages of 100 (10 × 10).

ERGOT ALKALOIDS, DIHYDROGENATED

Description: Intended for the treatment of idiopathic cerebral dysfunction which is generally expressed by such symptoms as mood depression, confusion, unsociability, dizziness, and lack of self care. Each tablet contains 0.167 or 0.33 mg each of dihydroergocornine, dihydroergocristine and dihydroergokryptine. There is no specific evidence which clearly establishes the mechanism by which the drug produces its mental effects nor is there conclusive evidence that it particularly affects cerebral arteriosclerosis or cerebrovascular insufficiency. However, experimental evidence from animal studies involving isolated brain tissue from cats suggests that these alkaloids may enhance neuronal uptake and utilization of oxygen and other nutrients. Clinical studies revealed that patients taking dihydrogenated ergot alkaloids showed greater symptomatic improvement than those taking papaverine. The drug also lacks the vasoconstrictor properties of the natural ergot alkaloids.

Indications: Treatment of selected symptoms in elderly patients. Short-term clinical studies have shown moderate improvement in self care and in such symptoms as depression, confusion, unsociability, and dizziness.

Contraindications: Known hypersensitivity to the drug.

Precautions: Because the target symptoms are of unknown etiology, the clinician is urged to make a careful diagnosis before prescribing this medication.

Adverse Reactions: Sublingual irritation, transient nausea, and gastric disturbance may occur.

Dosage and Administration: *Orally* or *sublingually,* 1 or 2 tablets 3 times daily. Since alleviation of symptoms is usually gradual, results may not be observed for 3 to 4 months.

Availability:
CIRCANOL® Sublingual Tablets, 0.5 and 1 mg in bottles of 100 and 1000. **(Riker)**
DEAPRIL®-ST Sublingual Tablets, 1 mg in bottles of 100. **(Mead Johnson)**
HYDERGINE®: **(Sandoz)**
Oral Tablets, 1 mg in packages of 100 and 500.
Sublingual Tablets, 0.5 mg in packages of 100 and 1000; 1 mg in packages of 100, 500 and 1000.

ERGOTAMINE TARTRATE

Description: Ergotamine is a complex alkaloid; it is a derivative of lysergic acid obtained from ergot. Ergotamine tartrate occurs as colorless crystals or as a white to yellowish-white, crystalline powder slightly soluble in alcohol and in water; it is slightly more soluble in the presence of a slight excess of tartaric acid.

Ergotamine is an alpha adrenergic blocking agent with a direct stimulating effect on the smooth muscle of peripheral and cranial blood vessels, and also induces depression of central vasomotor centers. It is effective in relieving the pain of migraine, apparently because of its direct action on the cranial vessels in which the amplitude of contraction is reduced. Ergotamine is frequently combined with caffeine on the theory that caffeine acts synergistically with ergotamine and thus lowers the effective dose of ergotamine in the treatment of migraine. The combination is said to be effective by constricting the cerebral arteries during the vasodilation phase of the migraine syndrome. When migraine headaches are further complicated by excessive nausea and vomiting, a formulation containing belladonna alkaloids for their anticholinergic and antiemetic effects and pentobarbital for its CNS-depressant effects has been provided.

Indications: Treatment of vascular headache and recurrent, throbbing vascular headaches: typical or atypical migraine, migraine variants, histaminic cephalalgia (cluster headache) and related conditions in which distention of the cranial vessels appears to be the precipitating factor.

Contraindications: In patients with occlusive vascular disease (thromboangiitis obliterans, luetic arteritis, marked arteriosclerosis, coronary artery disease, thrombophlebitis, Raynaud's disease), sepsis, impaired liver or kidney function, severe pruritus, and during pregnancy. It should be used with caution in elderly and undernourished patients, and in those hypersensitive to any of the components.

Warnings: Avoidance of excessive dosage and careful supervision of the patient is advised. **Because of the possible cumulative effects of ergotamine tartrate, it is essential that the dosage be limited to no more than 6 tablets during 1 attack and no more than 10 tablets in 1 week.** Patients should be counseled to use the minimal effective dose to control their symptoms. Symptoms of chronic ergotism include cold, pale and numb extremities, muscle pains both with and without activity, decreased or even obliterated peripheral pulses and gangrene of the fingers and toes. Other symptoms of ergotism may occur including anginal pain, tachycardia, bradycardia, changes in blood pressure (increase or decrease), headache, nausea, vomiting, diarrhea, itching, formication, anal burning, weakness, miosis, confusion, depression, drowsiness, increase in muscle tone with pain and trismus and rarely convulsions and hemiplegia.

Precautions: In rare instances, patients, particularly those who have used the medication indiscriminately over long periods of time, will display withdrawal symptoms consisting primarily of headache upon discontinuation of the drug.

Adverse Reactions: When ergotamine is administered in the recommended dosages in the absence of contraindications, it is regarded as a safe and useful drug; few serious side effects have been reported from its use in the migraine syndrome. Unpleasant complications which may occur include nausea and vomiting, weakness in the legs, muscle pains in the extremities, numbness and tingling of fingers and toes, percordial distress and pain, and transient tachycardia or bradycardia. Localized edema and itching may occur in an occasional hypersensitive patient. Most of these effects are generally not serious enough to necessitate interruption of therapy. Pentobarbital may cause drowsiness. Overdosage is manifested by vomiting; numbness, tingling, pain and cyanosis of the extremities associated with diminished or absent peripheral pulses; hypertension or hypotension; drowsiness, stupor, coma, convulsions and shock. One patient who had received 5 times the recommended daily adult dose over a period of 14 days experienced reversible bilateral papillitis with ring scotomata. Treatment is supportive and consists of the induction of emesis, gastric lavage, and catharsis; maintenance of adequate pulmonary ventilation, correction of hypotension, and the control of convulsions. Treatment of peripheral vasospasm should consist of warmth, *but not heat,* and protection of the ischemic limbs. Vasodilators may be beneficial but caution is advised in order to avoid aggravating an already existent hypotension.

Dosage and Administration: *Injection test:* relief of throbbing, recurrent headache following intramuscular injection of 1 ml (0.5 mg) is almost conclusive evidence that the headache is of vascular origin and may serve to confirm the diagnosis. *Relief of acute attack:* 0.5 to 1 ml *intramuscularly* or *subcutaneously,* or 2 to 6 tablets *orally* (no more than 10 tablets in 1 week), or 1 to 2 suppositories *rectally* (no more than twice weekly). The minimal effective dose should be established for each patient by titrating the amount required to control headaches in that patient. This is best done by starting with 0.5 ml or 1 tablet at onset of attack, repeated at ½- to 1-hour intervals if required. The total amount required to control headache should then be used at the first warning sign of subsequent attacks as the optimal dose for that patient. Maximal dose/week is 2 ml or 10 tablets; amount and duration of treatment should be established by the physician. May also be used by *oral inhalation.* A single inhalation at the first sign of an attack, repeated at intervals of 5 minutes if relief is not obtained. No more than 6 inhalations should be administered in any 24-hour period.

Availability:
ERGOMAR® Sublingual Tablets, 2 mg (foil-wrapped) in dispenser containers of 20. **(Fisons)**
ERGOSTAT™ Sublingual Tablets, 2 mg (individually sealed in foil pouch) in vials of 24. **(Parke-Davis)**
GYNERGEN®: **(Sandoz)**
Injection, 0.5 mg/ml in ampuls of 0.5 ml and 1 ml.
Tablets, 1 mg in bottles of 100.
MEDIHALER ERGOTAMINE® for Oral Inhalation in metal vials of 2.5 ml with adapter. Each depression on the vial delivers 0.36 mg of ergotamine tartrate. **(Riker)**

Combinations
CAFERGOT®: **(Sandoz)**
Suppositories, 2 mg with caffeine, 100 mg in cartons of 12.
Tablets, 1 mg with caffeine, 100 mg in packages of 100 and 1000 and in SandoPak® (unit-dose) packages of 100.
CAFERGOT® P-B (**Warning:** pentobarbital may be habit-forming). **(Sandoz)**
Suppositories, 2 mg with caffeine, 100 mg; Bellafoline®, 0.25 mg and 60 mg of pentobarbital, in cartons of 12.
Tablets, 1 mg with caffeine, 100 mg; Bellafoline®, 0.125 mg and sodium pentobarbital, 30 mg in packages of 100 and in SandoPak® (unit dose) packages of 100.
MIGRAL® Tablets, 1 mg with caffeine, 50 mg and cyclizine hydrochloride, 25 mg in bottles of 100. **(Burroughs Wellcome)**
WIGRAINE®: **(Organon)**
Suppositories, 1 mg with caffeine, 100 mg; belladonna alkaloids (*levorotatory*), 0.1 mg (hyoscyamine, 87.5% and atropine sulfate, 12.5%) and phenacetin, 130 mg in cartons of 12.
Tablets in cartons of 20 and 100. Composition is the same as that of the suppositories.

ERYTHRITYL TETRANITRATE

Description: Erythrityl tetranitrate is the nitric acid ester of erythritol, and occurs as a white, crystalline powder insoluble in water and soluble in alcohol.

Taken orally, sublingually or chewed, it provides prolonged prophylaxis of anginal attacks. The basic action of the nitrites is to relax smooth muscles, especially those of the finer blood vessels; this is independent of innervation. The postarteriolar vessels (capillaries and venules) are most susceptible although the larger veins and arteries also are relaxed to some extent. Appreciable effects are noted within 5 minutes following sublingual administration, are fully developed within 30 to 45 minutes and generally persist for 2 hours. Noticeable effects appear within 30 minutes after oral use, reaching maximal in about 60 to 90 minutes followed by a variable duration of action.

Indications: The prophylaxis and long-term treatment of patients with frequent or recurrent anginal pain and reduced exercise tolerance, rather than for the treatment of the acute attack of angina pectoris since the onset of action, while evident in 5 minutes, is somewhat slower than that of nitroglycerin. Formulated with phenobarbital to alleviate anxiety and tension which may be precipitating factors.

Precautions: Some fall in blood pressure may occur with large doses. Caution should be exercised in patients with recent cerebral hemorrhage. Patients should be cautioned that freedom from anginal attacks is not to be interpreted as a signal to drop all restrictions.

Adverse Reactions: In common with nitroglycerin, temporary vascular headache may occur during the first few days of therapy, but usually can be controlled by reducing the dosage temporarily. Oral administration is less likely to cause headache. Mild gastrointestinal disturbances occur occasionally with larger doses and may be controlled by temporary reduction of dosage. Sublingual administration may produce a tingling sensation at the point of contact with the mucous membrane.

Dosage and Administration: Initially, 5 mg *sublingually* or 10 mg *orally* or *chewed*, 3 times daily; an additional dose at bedtime is recommended for those patients subject to nocturnal attacks. This dosage may be increased in 2 or 3 days if necessary. Up to 100 mg are generally well tolerated, although some individuals are more likely to develop temporary headache at the higher level. Combined sublingual-oral administration may be obtained by allowing a tablet to dissolve partially under the tongue for 2 or 3 minutes and swallowing the remaining portion, or by using a chewable tablet. Chewable tablets produce an effect within 5 minutes; sublingual tablets in about 5 minutes. Maximal action develops in 30 to 45 minutes. Administered orally, an effect appears in about 30 minutes and reaches a peak in 60 to 90 minutes. Total duration of effect is up to 4 hours. Dosage for erythrityl tetranitrate with phenobarbital is 1 tablet, *orally only,* 3 or 4 times daily.

Availability:
CARDILATE®: **(Burroughs Wellcome)**
Chewable Tablets, 10 mg in bottles of 100.
Tablets, (oral or sublingual use), 5 and 15 mg in bottles of 100; 10 mg in bottles of 100 and 1000.
CARDILATE-P® Tablets (oral use only), 10 mg with phenobarbital, 15 mg (**Warning:** may be habit-forming) in bottles of 100. **(Burroughs Wellcome)**

THE ERYTHROMYCINS

Description: Erythromycin, a macrolide antibiotic, is isolated from cultures of *Streptomyces erythraeus.* It is a basic compound which contains an amino sugar, desosamine, and a nitrogen-free sugar, cladinose, attached to erythronolide, the aglycone portion of the molecule. The spectrum of activity of erythromycin is similar to that of penicillin. Erythromycin base and its salts and esters, with the exception of erythromycin estolate, are reduced in activity in acid solutions. Therefore, they should be administered in the fasting state and never with or prior to the ingestion of fruit juices or acid beverages.

The precise mechanism of erythromycin is unknown; however, it appears to inhibit protein synthesis without affecting nucleic acid synthesis. It may act as a bacteriostatic or bactericidal agent depending upon the nature of the organism and the concentration of the drug. Nevertheless, some strains of *Haemophilus influenzae* and *staphylococci* have demonstrated resistance to erythromycin. Culture and susceptibility testing should be performed. If the Kirby-Bauer method of disc susceptibility is used, a 15 mcg erythromycin disc should give a zone diameter of at least 18 mm when tested against an erythromycin susceptible organism.

It is readily absorbed from the upper small intestinal tract, producing peak concentration within 2 hours and with adequate concentrations continuing for 6 hours. The estolate produces higher, more predictable and more prolonged levels than the base or stearate.

Following absorption, erythromycin diffuses readily into most body fluids. In the absence of meningeal inflammation, low concentrations are normally found present in the spinal fluid, but passage of the drug across the blood-brain barrier increases in meningitis. In the presence of normal hepatic function, erythromycin is concentrated in the liver and excreted in the bile; the effect of hepatic dysfunction on excretion of erythromycin by the liver into the bile is not known. Approximately 2 to 5% of an orally administered dose and 12 to 15% of an intravenously administered dose can be recovered as the active form in the urine. When large doses of erythromycin are given orally, the feces may contain as much as 0.5 mg/gm. Erythromycin crosses the placental barrier, but fetal plasma levels appear to be low.

Indications: Treatment of *Streptococcus pyogenes* (Group A beta hemolytic streptococcus): Upper and lower respiratory tract, skin, and soft tissue infections of mild to moderate severity. Injectable benzathine penicillin G is considered to be the drug of choice in the treatment and prevention of streptococcal pharyngitis and in long-term prophylaxis of rheumatic fever. When oral medication is preferred for treatment of the above conditions, penicillin, G or V, or erythromycin are alternate drugs of choice. Also, the importance of strict adherence by the patient to the prescribed dosage regimen must be stressed. A therapeutic dose should be administered for at least 10 days. *Alpha-hemolytic streptococci* (viridans group): Short-term prophylaxis of bacterial endocarditis prior to dental or other operative procedures in patients with a history of rheumatic fever or congenital heart disease who are hypersensitive to penicillin. (Erythromycin is not suitable prior to genitourinary surgery where the organisms likely to lead to bacteremia are gram-negative bacilli or the enterococcus group of streptococci.) *Staphylococcus aureus:* Acute infections of skin and soft tissue of mild to moderate severity. Resistant organisms may emerge during treatment. *Diplococcus pneumoniae:* Upper respiratory tract infections (e.g., otitis media, pharyngitis) and lower respiratory tract infections (e.g. pneumonia) of mild to moderate degree. *Mycoplasma pneumoniae* (Eaton agent, PPLO): In the treatment of respiratory tract infections when due to this organism. *Neisseria gonorrhoeae* and *Treponema pallidum:* Erythromycin has been reported to produce good results in the treatment of gonorrhea and primary syphilis in patients allergic to the penicillins. Before treatment of gonorrhea, patients who are suspected of also having syphilis should have a microscopic examination for *T. pallidum* (by immunofluorescence or darkfield) before receiving erythromycin, and monthly serologic tests for a minimum of 4 months. In treatment of primary syphilis, spinal fluid examinations should be performed before treatment and as part of follow up after therapy. *Corynebacterium diphtheriae* and *C. minutissimum:* As an adjunct to antitoxin, to prevent establishment of carriers, and to eradicate the organism in carriers. Erthromycin has been found to be effective in the treatment of erythrasma. *Entamoeba histolytica:* In the treatment of intestinal amebiasis only. Extraenteric amebiasis requires treatment with other agents. *Listeria monocytogenes:* Infections due to this organism. *Haemophilus influenzae:* For upper and lower respiratory tract infections of mild to moderate severity when used concomitantly with adequate doses of sulfonamides. Not all strains of this organism are susceptible at the concentrations ordinarily achieved. The ointment may be effective in the treatment of superficial topical infections due to erythromycin-sensitive organisms.

Contraindications: Erythromycin is contraindicated in patients with known hypersensitivity to this antibiotic.

Warnings: Safe use during pregnancy has not been established. Since intramuscular administration may be irritating and painful, it is not advised in patients with severe infections in whom high doses and/or frequent or prolonged use of the drug is required, and in those patients with insufficient muscle mass such as small children. It may also cause sterile abscess formation and necrosis.

Precautions: Because erythromycin is excreted principally by the liver, utmost caution is advised since variations in liver function have been observed following prolonged therapy with high dosage levels. This is especially important when erythromycin estolate is to be prescribed, and the physician should be aware that hepatic dysfunction, with or without jaundice, may occur and may be accompanied by malaise, nausea, vomiting, abdominal colic and fever. The development of any of these symptoms suggest immediate withdrawal of the drug. Other erythromycin preparations should be considered in preference to the estolate salt in patients with liver disease or those suspected of having impaired liver function. Also, surgical procedures should be performed when indicated.

Adverse Reactions: The most frequent side effects of oral erythromycin preparations are gastrointestinal, such as abdominal cramping and discomfort, and are dose-related. Nausea, vomiting, and diarrhea occur infrequently with usual oral doses. During prolonged or repeated therapy, there is a possibility of overgrowth of nonsusceptible bacteria or fungi. If such infections occur, the drug should be discontinued and appropriate therapy instituted. Mild allergic reactions such as urticaria and other skin rashes have occurred. Serious allergic reactions, including anaphylaxis, have been reported. Jaundice has been reported with erythromycin estolate. An occasional venous irritation has been encountered when erythromycin was administered intravenously, but if the infusion is given slowly, in dilute solution, preferably by continuous intravenous infusion or intermittent rapid infusion in no less than 20 to 60 minutes, pain and vessel trauma are minimized. Intramuscular injection may cause severe pain, with possible sterile abscess formation and necrosis; therefore, it is not indicated in serious to severe infections where high dosage and/or frequent or prolonged administration is required.

The preceding discussed briefly the physiologic, clinical and therapeutic similarities of the erythromycins as a group. In the sections that follow, the individual monographs discuss specifically each of the following erythromycins: Erythromycin (base), Erythromycin Estolate, Erythromycin Ethylsuccinate, Erythromycin Gluceptate, Erythromycin Lactobionate, and Erythromycin Stearate.

ERYTHROMYCIN

Description: Erythromycin occurs as a white, crystalline compound that is soluble in water to the extent of 2 mg/ml and is freely soluble in alcohol.

For indications, contraindications, warnings, precautions and adverse reactions, see general statement.

Dosage and Administration: *Orally.* The usual adult dosage is 250 mg every 6 hours or 500 mg every 12 hours. This may be increased up to 4 gm or more daily according to the severity of the infection. The usual dosage for children is 30 to 50 mg/kg daily in divided doses. Dosage may be doubled for more serious infections. Optimal blood levels are obtained when doses are given on an empty stomach. *For the treatment of streptococcal infections,* a therapeutic dosage should be administered for at least 10 days. In continuous prophylaxis of streptococcal infections in patients with a history of rheumatic heart disease, the dosage is 250 mg twice daily. When erythromycin is administered prior to surgery to prevent endocarditis caused by alpha-hemolytic streptococcus, the recommended dosage for adults is 500 mg before the procedure and 250 mg every 6 hours for 4 doses following the procedure. The recommended dosage for children is 30 mg/kg of body weight daily divided into 3 or 4 evenly spaced doses. *For the treatment of primary syphilis,* 30 to 40 gm given in divided doses over a period of from 10 to 15 days. *For the treatment of dysenteric amebiasis,* 250 mg 4 times daily for 10 to 14 days for adults, and 30 to 50 mg/kg of body weight daily in divided doses for 10 to 14 days for children. *For the treatment of gonorrhea-induced acute inflammatory disease,* see erythromycin lactobionate. *Topically.* Apply the ointment to the infected area 3 to 4 times daily; for ocular infections, 1 or more times daily. The infected area should be cleansed before application and covered if necessary by a light dressing.

Availability:
E-MYCIN® Tablets, 250 mg in bottles of 100 and 500 and in unit-dose blister packages of 20 and 100. **(Upjohn)**
ERYTHROMYCIN Filmtab Tablets, 250 and 500 mg in bottles of 100; 250 mg are also available in Abbo-Pac® (unit-dose) packages of 100 in strips of 10. **(Abbott)**
ILOTYCIN®: **(Dista)**
Ointment, 10 mg/gm in tubes of 15 and 30 gm and in jars of 1 lb.
Ophthalmic Ointment, 5 mg/gm in tubes of 3.5 gm.
Tablets, 250 mg in bottles of 24 and 100 and in blister packs of 100 (10 × 10) and in dispenser rolls of 500 (5 × 100).
ROBIMYCIN™ Tablets (pale green), 250 mg in bottles of 100 and 500. **(Robins)**

ERYTHROMYCIN ESTOLATE

Description: Erythromycin estolate is the lauryl sulfate salt of the propionic acid ester of erythromycin. It occurs as long needles that are poorly soluble in water but are soluble in alcohol, acetone, and chloroform. Since it is stable in gastric acid, it can thus be taken with meals.

When administered orally, it is readily absorbed from the gastrointestinal tract, especially when given on an empty stomach. Following a 250-mg dose, peak serum levels ranging from 0.4 to 1.3 mcg/ml are detected in 2 hours.

For indications, contraindications, other warnings, precautions and adverse reactions, see general statement.

Warnings: Erythromycin estolate appears to be the only erythromycin ester that is associated with an allergic type of cholestatic hepatitis. Patients receiving this drug for 10 days or more or in repeated regimens have shown an incidence of jaundice in the range of 2 to 4%, accompanied by right upper quadrant pain, fever, nausea, vomiting, eosinophilia, and leukocytosis. Liver function tests should be monitored in patients on such dosage schedules, and the drug should be discontinued if abnormalities develop. The use of other erythromycin preparations is suggested in patients with preexisting liver disease or in those suspected of having impaired liver function. In some individuals, associated gastrointestinal symptoms have simulated the colic of biliary tract disease or an acute abdominal surgical problem. In others, clinical symptoms and results of liver function tests have resembled findings in extrahepatic obstruction jaundice. Safe use during pregnancy has not been established.

Dosage and Administration: *Orally.* Adults—250 mg to 1 gm every 6 hours. Children—30 to 50 mg/kg of body weight daily, in divided doses. *For the treatment of streptococcal infections*—dosage should be administered for at least 10 days. *For prophylaxis of rheumatic fever*—the recommended dosage is 250 mg daily. When administered prior to surgery *to prevent endocarditis*—a dosage of 250 mg 4 times daily is recommended for adults and older children, 40 mg/kg of body weight daily for younger children. *For primary syphilis*—500 mg 4 times daily for 15 days. *For gonorrhea*—500 mg 4 times daily for 5 days. *For erythrasma*—1 gm daily for 5 days. *For dysenteric amebiasis*—adults, 500 mg 4 times daily for 4 to 5 days; children, 20 to 40 mg/kg of body weight in divided doses for 4 to 5 days.

Availability:
ILOSONE®: **(Dista)**
Capsules (Pulvules®), 125 mg in bottles of 24 and 100; 250 mg in bottles of 24 and 100 and in Blister Pak (unit dose) cartons of 100 (10 × 10).
Chewable Tablets, 125 and 250 mg in bottles of 50.
Liquid (Oral Suspension), 125 and 250 mg/5 ml in bottles of 60 ml and 1 pint and in unit-dose packages of 100.
Powder for Oral Suspension, 125 mg/5 ml in bottles of 60 and 150 ml.
Ready-Mixed Drops, 100 mg/ml in bottles of 10 ml with calibrated dropper.
Tablets, 500 mg in bottles of 50 and in Blister Pak cartons of 100 (10 × 10).

ERYTHROMYCIN ETHYLSUCCINATE

Description: The ethylsuccinate ester of erythromycin is stable as an aqueous suspension for 7 days when stored at 2 to 15° C.

Readily and adequately absorbed following oral administration, particularly when the stomach is empty; however, the suspension and chewable tablet have been claimed to produce consistent, predictable serum levels when administered in either the fasting or nonfasting state. Adequate therapeutic concentrations are generally maintained by giving the drug at 6-hour intervals.

For indications, contraindications, warnings, precautions and adverse reactions, see general statement.

Dosage and Administration: Dosage of erythromycin ethylsuccinate is expressed in terms of erythromycin base. *Orally.* The usual dosage for adults and older children is 400 mg every 6 hours. Dosage may be increased up to 4 or more gm/day according to the severity of the infection. Pediatric dosage is based on 30 to 50 mg/kg (14 to 23 mg/lb) of body weight daily in 4 or 5 divided doses for moderate infections. For more severe infections this dosage may be doubled. If twice-a-day dosage is desired in either adults or children, ½ the total daily dose may be given every 12 hours, 1 hour before meals. When used prior to surgery to prevent endocarditis, a recommended dosage schedule for adults and older children is 800 mg before the procedure and 400 mg every 6 hours for 4 doses after the procedure. For small children, 30 to 50 mg/kg/day divided into 3 or 4 evenly spaced doses. For treatment of primary syphilis, the recommended dose is 48 to 64 gm given in divided dosage over a period of 10 to 15 days. For the treatment of intestinal amebiasis, the recommended dosage is 400 mg 4 times daily for adults and 30 to 50 mg/kg daily in divided doses for children; treatment should continue for a period of 10 to 14 days. **Note:** Chewable tablets may be either chewed or swallowed whole.

Availability:

E.E.S.™-200 (ERYTHROCIN® ETHYLSUCCINATE): **(Abbott)**

Chewable Wafers, 200 mg in packages of 50.

Drops (for oral suspension), 100 mg/2.5 ml in bottles of 50 ml; 200 mg/5 ml (dropperful) in bottles of 30 ml.

Granules (for oral suspension), 200 mg/5 ml in bottles of 60, 100 and 200 ml and in Abbo-Pac® (unit-dose) bottles of 5 ml in packages of 100.

Liquid, 200 and 400 mg/5 ml in bottles of 100 ml in packages of 6 and in 1 pint.

E.E.S.™-400 Filmtabs® (pink), 400 mg in bottles of 100. **(Abbott)**

PEDIAMYCIN®: **(Ross)**

Chewable Tablets, 200 mg in bottles of 50.

Drops (for oral suspension), 100 mg/2.5 ml (dropperful) in bottles of 30 and 50 ml.

Liquid, 200 and 400 mg/5 ml in bottles of 100 ml and 1 pint.

Suspension (for oral use), 200 mg/5 ml in bottles of 60, 90 and 150 ml.

WYAMYCIN® Liquid (for oral use), 200 and 400 mg/5 ml in bottles of 1 pint. **(Wyeth)**

ERYTHROMYCIN GLUCEPTATE

Description: The glucoheptonate salt of erythromycin, for intravenous administration, is stable as an aqueous solution for 7 days when stored at 2 to 15° C. Following intravenous administration of a 200-mg dose, peak serum levels of 3 to 4 mcg/ml are reached in 1 hour diminishing to 0.5 mcg/ml in 6 hours. From 12 to 15% of intravenously administered erythromycin is excreted in the active form in the urine.

For indications, contraindications, warnings, precautions and adverse reactions, see general statement.

Dosage and Administration: *Intravenously.* The initial solution is prepared by adding at least 10 ml of sterile water for injection to the 250 or 500 mg ampul or at least 20 ml of sterile water for injection to the 1 gm ampul, and shaking the vial until the antibiotic is completely dissolved. This solution should then be added to normal sodium chloride or to a 5% dextrose solution to give 1 gm/liter for slow, continuous infusion. If the medication is to be given by intermittent injection, 1/4 of the total daily dose can be given in 20 to 60 minutes by slow intravenous injection of 250 to 500 mg in 100 to 250 ml of normal sodium chloride or 5% dextrose solution. Injection should be sufficiently slow to avoid pain along the vein. The recommended intravenous dosage for severe infections in adults and children is 15 to 20 mg/kg of body weight daily. Higher doses may be given in very severe infections. Although continuous infusion is preferable, administration in divided doses no more frequently than every 6 hours is also effective. Patients receiving intravenous erythromycin should be changed to the oral dosage form as soon as possible. For additional information on dilution procedures, consult package literature.

Availability:
ILOTYCIN® GLUCEPTATE Injection (IV), 250 mg in vials of 20 ml; 500 mg in vials of 30 ml; 1 gm in vials of 50 ml. **(Dista)**

ERYTHROMYCIN LACTOBIONATE

Description: The lactobionate salt of erythromycin, for intravenous use, is stable as a 5% solution for 2 weeks when stored at 4 to 15° C; however, when it is further diluted prior to intravenous administration, the solution should be used within 8 hours since it is not suitable for storage; pH is approximately neutral.

Intravenous injection of 200 mg of erythromycin lactobionate produces peak serum levels of 3 to 4 mcg/ml almost immediately, 2 mcg/ml at 1 hour, and 0.5 mcg/ml at 6 hours; approximately 12 to 15% of the active form is excreted in the urine.

For indications, contraindications, warnings, precautions and adverse reactions, see general statement.

Dosage and Administration: *Intravenously.* If the medication is to be given by intermittent injection, 1/4 of the total daily dose can be given in 20 to 60 minutes by slow intravenous injection of 250 to 500 mg in 100 to 250 ml of normal sodium chloride or 5% dextrose solution. Injection should be sufficiently slow (60 drops/minute) to avoid pain along the vein. The recommended intravenous dosage for severe infections in adults and children is 15 to 20 mg/kg of body weight daily; up to 4 gm may be administered. Although continuous infusion is preferable, administration in divided doses at intervals not greater than every 6 hours is effective. For the treatment of gonorrhea-induced acute pelvic inflammatory disease, the recommended regimen is 500 mg every 6 hours for 3 days, followed by 250 mg of erythromycin stearate or base every 6 hours for 7 days. Occasionally, venous irritation has been encountered, but this can be kept at a minimum if the injection is given slowly, in dilute solution, and by continuous infusion over 20 to 60 minutes. Patients receiving intravenous administration should be changed to the oral dosage form as soon as possible.

Availability:
ERYTHROCIN® LACTOBIONATE (IV) in vials of 500 mg and 1 gm. **(Abbott)**

ERYTHROMYCIN STEARATE

Description: The stearic acid salt of erythromycin for oral administration only. Optimal levels are reached when the drug is taken in the fasting state or immediately before meals. Less than 5% of the active form is present in the urine.

For indications, contraindications, warnings, precautions and adverse reactions, see general statement.

Dosage and Administration: *Orally.* Adults: The usual dosage is 250 mg every 6 hours or 500 mg every 12 hours; severe infections may require 4 gm or more daily. Children: The usual dosage is 30 to 50 mg/kg/day in 3 or 4 divided doses; severe infections may require 60 to 100 mg/kg/day. If dosage is desired on a twice-a-day schedule for either adults or children, 1/2 of the total daily dose may be given every 12 hours, 1 hour before meals. *For the treatment of streptococcal infections,* a therapeutic dosage should be administered for at least 10 days. In continuous prophylaxis of streptococcal infections in patients with a history of rheumatic heart disease, the dosage is 250 mg twice daily. When used prior to surgery to prevent endocarditis, a recommended schedule for adults is 500 mg before the procedure and 250 mg every 6 hours for 4 doses after the procedure. For small children, 30 to 50 mg/kg/day divided into 3 or 4 evenly spaced doses. *For treatment of primary syphilis,* 30 to 40 gm given in divided doses over a period of from 10 to 15 days. *For treatment of gonorrhea,* 500 mg 4 times daily for 3 days followed by 250 mg every 6 hours for 7 days. *For dysenteric amebiasis,* adults—250 mg 4 times daily for 10 to 14 days; children—30 to 50 mg/kg/day in divided doses for 10 to 14 days.

Availability:

Erythromycin Stearate

Tablets (Film-coated), 250 mg in bottles of 100. **(ICN)**

Tablets, 250 mg in bottles of 100 and 500; 500 mg in bottles of 100 and in unit-dose packages of 100. **(Lederle)**

Tablets, 250 mg in bottles of 100 and 250. **(Philips Roxane)**

BRISTAMYCIN® Tablets, 250 mg in bottles of 100 and 500 and in Dosa-Trol® (unit-dose) packages of 100. **(Bristol)**

ERYPAR® FILMSEAL® (Film-coated tablets, yellow), 250 mg in bottles of 100 and 500 and in unit-dose packages of 100; 500 mg in bottles of 100. **(Parke-Davis)**

ERYTHROCIN® STEARATE FILMTAB® (Tablets, pink), 125 mg in bottles of 50; 250 mg in bottles of 20, 100 and 500; 500 mg in bottles of 100. **(Abbott)**

ETHRIL® Tablets, 250 mg in bottles of 100; 500 mg in bottles of 50. **(Squibb)**

PFIZER-E® Tablets, 250 mg in bottles of 100 and 500 and in unit-dose cartons of 100; 500 mg in bottles of 100 and in unit-dose cartons of 100. **(Pfipharmecs)**

SK-ERYTHROMYCIN™ Tablets, 250 mg in bottles of 100 and 500; 500 mg in bottles of 100. **(Smith Kline & French)**

WYAMYCIN® Tablets (Film-coated), 250 mg in bottles of 100 and 500; 500 mg in bottles of 100. **(Wyeth)**

ESTRADIOL: see The Estrogens

THE ESTROGENS

Description: The naturally occurring estrogenic substances are steroidal compounds—they have in common an unsaturated steroid ring A and a hydroxyl group in position 3. When derived from the urine of pregnant mares, the mixture is composed principally of sodium estrone sulfate with variable amounts of equilin sodium sulfate. Of the various natural estrogenic substances available, estradiol, estrone, and estriol are considered to be the most important, and the most potent of these is esthinyl estradiol. Its 3-methyl ether (Mestranol) is frequently used in combination with progesterone-like compounds for the regulation of the menstrual cycle and for the control of fertility. The natural (free) estrogens are oil soluble and are effective when administered subcutaneously or intramuscularly, but have little potency when given orally. Esterification increases both the effect and duration of action, and conjugation makes them more resistant to enzymatic destruction in both the gastrointestinal tract and liver, thus rendering them more effective orally. These chemical alterations of the natural (free) estrogens render them effective by mouth, largely through protection from inactivation by the liver. The natural (free) estrogens are insoluble in water, but when conjugated with either sulfate or glucuronic acid, these hormones become water soluble. Conjugation, in addition to increasing oral effectiveness, also facilitates excretion in the urine.

Estrogens are believed to be removed rapidly from the plasma by excretion in the bile. They are then reabsorbed from the intestine and transported to the liver by way of the enterohepatic circulation. The liver is the principal site of conjugation of the estrogens with glucuronic acid. Estrogens also appear to circulate as conjugated steroids bound to protein.

In addition to the naturally occurring estrogens, a number of highly potent nonsteroidal estrogens are available which are capable of producing all the pharmacologic and therapeutic responses attributed to natural estrogens. Although there appears to be little or no structural relationship between the two groups of compounds, the synthetic nonsteroidal compounds are converted to steroids in the body, and exert the same biological effects as do the naturally occurring hormones. All are effective when administered orally. These estrogens are slowly degraded in the body but little is known of their mode of action or of their excretion products.

Estrogens promote growth of the endometrium; promote thickening, stratification, and cornification of the vagina, and cause enlargement of mammary gland ducts. It is possible that they inhibit secretion of hypothalmic releasing factor to the pituitary gland. The ability of estrogens to promote the development of both primary and secondary sex characteristics is of benefit in female hypogonadism. In the menopausal syndrome, whether natural or induced, the estrogens aid in relieving nervous symptoms as well as the hot flushes, perspiration, and other vasomotor disorders. Senile vaginitis and other vulvar and vaginal conditions associated with estrogen deficiency respond promptly to estrogen therapy. Indirectly, they contribute to the shaping of the skeleton, maintenance of tone and elasticity of urogenital structures and changes in the epiphyses of the long bone that allow for pubertal-growth spurt and termination. Estrogens are also involved in the psychologic and emotional aspects of feminine behavior. As estrogen levels increase during the menstrual cycle, there is a sense of vigor and well-being. Decline of estrogen activity at the end of the menstrual cycle can bring on menstruation, although the cessation of progesterone secretion is the most important factor in the mature ovulatory cycle. However, in the pre- or non-ovulatory cycle, estrogen is the primary determinant in the onset of menstruation; however, estrogens do not induce ovulation. They affect calcium and phosphorus metabolism and are involved in the maintenance of normal bone structure. In prolonged estrogen deficiency states, administration of estrogen acts to prevent associated bone degenerative changes. These agents appear to be responsible for the relatively greater amount of alpha-lipoprotein and correspondingly lower amount of beta-lipoprotein found in premenopausal women as compared with men. The palliative effects of estrogens on the local discomfort of prostatic carcinoma and its metastases are achieved through suppression of androgenic activity, with resultant desexualization that serves as an adjunct to, or a substitute for castration. In mammary cancer in women who have undergone castration or who are 5 years or more postmenopausal, the drug has an analgesic, euphoric effect and produces temporary objective improvement in some patients.

Indications: As replacement therapy in the control of the menopausal syndrome, both natural and artificial; in the treatment of senile vaginitis, kraurosis vulvae, with and without pruritus vulvae; hypogenitalism and sexual infantilism; amenorrhea and other symptoms of female hypogonadism; certain types of dysfunctional uterine bleeding; relief of breast engorgement in suppressed lactation; to retard the progress of osteoporosis; relief of prostatic carcinoma, and palliation of mammary cancer in women who have undergone castration or who are more than 5 years postmenopausal and whose disease is not amenable to surgery or irradiation. May also be used for estrogen deficiency-induced osteoporosis, only when used in conjunction with other therapeutic measures such as diet, calcium, physiotherapy, and other general health-promoting measures.

Contraindications: In patients with markedly impaired liver function; known or suspected carcinoma of the breast, except those cases of progressing disease not amenable to surgery or irradiation occurring in women who are at least 5 years postmenopausal; known or suspected estrogen-dependent neoplasia such as carcinoma of the endometrium; thromboembolic disorders including thrombophlebitis, cerebrovascular disorders, retinal thrombosis, or pulmonary embolism, or in patients with a past history of these disorders; in undiagnosed abnormal genital bleeding; in markedly impaired liver function, and in known hypersensitivity to estrogens.

Warnings: A significant association has been reported between maternal ingestion of estrogens particularly **diethylstilbestrol** during pregnancy, especially within the first 12 weeks, and the appearance of vaginal adenosis developing years later (postpubertal stage) in the offspring. The significance of this finding with respect to the possible development of vaginal adenocarcinoma is not known; nonetheless, such patients should be examined periodically. It is not known at present whether such an association is applicable to all estrogens; however, pregnancy is a definite contraindication to the use of diethylstilbestrol and its closely related congeners (dienestrol, hexestrol, benzestrol, and promethestrol). There is also some evidence of abnormalities in male offspring. The other estrogens are not recommended for use during pregnancy.

A complete pretreatment examination should be performed with special attention to pelvic and breast organs, and should include a Papanicolaou smear. Estrogen therapy should not be administered to women with recurrent chronic mastitis or abnormal mammograms unless therapeutic benefit is anticipated despite the possibility of aggravation of the mastitis or stimulation of undiagnosed estrogen-dependent neoplasia. Failure to control abnormal uterine bleeding or its unexpected recurrence is an indication for curettage. Constant observation of the patient is necessary so that the earliest manifestations of thrombotic disorders (thrombophlebitis, cerebrovascular disorders, pulmonary embolism, and retinal thrombosis) may be evaluated. If these occur or are suspected, the drug should be discontinued immediately. A sudden onset of proptosis, diplopia or migraine may occur, especially when estrogens are given conjunctively with progesterones, and if examination reveals papilledema or retinal vascular lesions, therapy should be terminated. Safe use of estrogens in pregnant women has not been established, and when used in association with progesterones, it is recommended that pregnancy be ruled out in any patient who has missed two consecutive periods, before continuing the regimen. Therapy also should be discontinued if hypercalcemia occurs in patients with metastatic breast cancer, since this indicates progression of bone metastasis. In view of individual variation in endogenous estrogen production, relative overdosage may occur which could result in abnormal or excessive uterine bleeding, mastodynia, edema, and enlargement of fibromyomas of the uterus. Large doses may produce urinary stress incontinence in nonpregnant females. Postmenopausal women appear to be at greater risk of developing estrogen-induced endometrial carcinoma, gallbladder complications, and increases in blood pressure, particularly when high doses and prolonged therapy are employed. Since these substances are excreted in the mother's milk, the estrogenic effect on the nursing infant should be considered when estrogens are administered to lactating women.

Precautions: Close medical supervision is mandatory when estrogens are used for the treatment of mammary or prostatic carcinoma, and careful use is advised in patients with a history of cerebrovascular accident. If irregular bleeding persists, nonfunctional causes should be suspected and adequate diagnostic measures instituted. Patients with a history of psychic depression should be carefully observed and the drug discontinued if the depression recurs to a serious degree. Because of the effects of estrogens on epiphyseal closure, these substances should be used judiciously in young patients in whom bone growth is incomplete. It has been found that high doses of estrogens will inhibit anterior pituitary function, and this should be considered when treating patients in whom fertility is desired. Caution also is advised when used in the female in order to avoid continuous stimulation of the breast and uterus, and cyclic therapy is recommended (3 week regimen with 1 week rest period—withdrawal bleeding may occur during the 1 week rest period). In the male, prolonged continuous therapy may produce gynecomastia, loss of libido, and testicular atrophy. Because of salt and water retention associated with estrogenic-anabolic activity, estrogens should be used with caution when epilepsy, migraine, asthma, cardiac or renal disease are present; also in diabetes because of decrease in glucose tolerance. Estrogens may elevate PBI levels by increasing the level of serum binding proteins, and determinations of serum PBI should not be considered definitive unless estrogens have been discontinued for at least 60 days. Certain liver and endocrine function tests may be affected by exogenous estrogen administration. If test results are abnormal in a patient taking estrogen, they should be repeated after the estrogen has been withdrawn for one cycle. Although the age of the patient constitutes no absolute limiting factor, treatment with estrogens may mask the onset of the climacteric. Estrogens induce changes in menopausal vaginal epithelium, uterine endothelium and breast tissue and these changes should be considered when specimens are sent for pathology examination.

Adverse Reactions: The following effects may occur with estrogens alone but they usually occur when administered concomitantly with progesterones. These include thrombophlebitis, pulmonary embolism and cerebrovascular accidents; neuro-ocular lesions such as retinal thrombosis and optic neuritis; nausea, vomiting, anorexia, gastrointestinal symptoms (abdominal cramps, bloating or mild diarrhea); edema; spotting or withdrawal bleeding; breast tenderness and enlargement; changes in body weight (increase or decrease); headache; increase in cervical mucus; allergic rash; loss of libido, and tenderness of breast; sterile abscess; reactivation of endometriosis; aggravation of migraine headaches; hepatic cutaneous porphyria becoming manifest; areolar pigmentation. The following adverse effects are known to occur in patients receiving both estrogens and progesterones: thrombophlebitis, pulmonary embolism, cerebral thrombosis, coronary thrombosis, and neuro-ocular lesions; chloasma or melasma; cholestatic jaundice; rise in blood pressure in susceptible individuals; mental depression; amenorrhea during and after treatment; post-treatment anovulation; cystitis-like syndrome; hirsutism; loss of scalp hair; erythema nodosum, and erythema multiforme; hemorrhagic eruption; premenstrual-like syndrome; changes in libido; changes in appetite; nervousness; dizziness; fatigue, irritability, and malaise; backache; itching, and changes in menstrual flow. The following laboratory tests may give altered results by concomitant use of estrogens and progesterones: hepatic function (increased BSP retention); coagulation tests (increase in prothrombin and Factors VII, VIII, IX, X); metyrapone test; pregnanediol determination and thyroid function tests (Increase in PBI and butanol extractable iodine, decrease in T_3 uptake value). A possible diminution in lactation may occur when given immediately postpartum; also hypercalcemia may develop.

NATURAL
Estradiol
Estrogenic Substances, Conjugated
Estrogenic Substances, Esterified
Estrogenic Substances, Mixed
Estrone
Hormonin

SYNTHETIC
Chlorotrianisene
Dienestrol
Diethylstilbestrol

THE NATURAL ESTROGENS

ESTRADIOL

Chemical Name: Estra-1,3,5(10)-triene-3,17-*B*-diol.

Description: Estradiol, the most biologically active estrogen, is the primary ovarian follicular hormone, and is readily oxidized in the body to estrone, which is subsequently hydrated to estriol. It can be obtained from both natural and synthetic sources. Estradiol occurs as an odorless, hygroscopic, white or creamy white, crystalline substance that is almost insoluble in water and freely soluble in alcohol. Conversion of estradiol to its esters (benzoate, cypionate and valerate) produces compounds that exert a slow release of the hormone from the site of intramuscular administration. Of these preparations estradiol benzoate exerts its effect for only a short period (2 to 3 days), the cypionate for about 3 weeks, while the valerate is intermediate in its duration of action. There is no depot effect at the site of injection—90% of the injected dose of estradiol leaves the bloodstream within 24 hours. Passive storage occurs in the reticuloendothelial system. As circulating levels of estradiol drop, more returns to the bloodstream from the storage site for an even, continuous therapeutic effect. Increasing the dose acts to prolong the duration of pharmacologic action rather than to increase blood levels. These compounds are not considered suitable for use in menstrual disturbances where a limited duration of action is desirable, or for replacement purposes when cyclic therapy is indicated.

For indications, contraindications, warnings, precautions and adverse reactions, see general statement.

Dosage and Administration: *Orally, intramuscularly or subcutaneous implantation.*

Menopausal symptoms, atrophic vaginitis, pruritus vulvae: Initially, 1 to 1.5 mg of estradiol intramuscularly 2 or 3 times weekly; maintenance dosage is 0.5 to 1 mg twice weekly. May also be treated by subcutaneous implantation of 25 mg repeated every 3 months, or orally with 0.3 to 0.6 mg of estradiol with estrone and estriol, daily. Estradiol benzoate, 1 to 1.66 mg 2 or 3 times weekly, maintenance dosage of 2 to 5 mg every 3 to 4 weeks. Ethinyl estradiol, 0.01 to 0.05 mg (up to 0.15 mg for severe cases) daily by oral administration.

Hypogenitalism and sexual infantilism: Estradiol, 1.5 mg intramuscularly 2 or 3 times weekly or 25 mg by subcutaneous implantation. Estradiol benzoate, 1.66 mg 2 or 3 times weekly.

Amenorrhea, oligomenorrhea associated with hypogonadism: Estradiol, 1.5 mg intramuscularly 2 or 3 times weekly during the first 2 weeks of a 28-day menstrual cycle followed by progesterone during the last 2 weeks; regimen should be continued for 3 to 6 months followed by a 2-month rest period. Ethinyl estradiol, treatment schedule the same as for estradiol using a dose of 0.02 to 0.15 mg.

To achieve hemostasis in functional uterine bleeding: Ethinyl estradiol, 0.5 mg 1 or 2 times daily after bleeding is controlled, then 0.05 mg 1 to 3 times daily during the first 2 weeks of menstrual period and progesterone the last 2 weeks.

Postpartum breast engorgement: Estradiol, 1.5 mg intramuscularly. Estradiol benzoate, 1.66 mg daily. Estradiol valerate, a single dose of 10 to 25 mg administered at the end of the first stage of labor. Ethinyl estradiol, 0.02 to 1 mg daily.

Prostatic carcinoma: Estradiol, 1.5 mg intramuscularly 3 times weekly or by subcutaneous implantation, 25 mg. Estradiol benzoate, 1.66 mg 3 or more times weekly. Estradiol valerate, 30 mg or more every 1 to 2 weeks. Ethinyl estradiol, 0.05 to 3 mg daily. Polyestradiol phosphate, deep intramuscular injection only, 40 or up to 80 mg every 2 to 4 weeks. Response is usually noted within 3 months from start of therapy.

Mammary carcinoma: Estradiol, 1.5 mg 3 or more times weekly. Estradiol benzoate, 1.66 mg 3 or more times weekly. Estradiol valerate, 20 to 40 mg every 2 to 3 weeks. Ethinyl estradiol, 0.15 to 3 mg daily.

Availability:

Estradiol

ESTRACE® Tablets, 1 and 2 mg (micropulverized) in bottles of 100. **(Mead Johnson)**

PROGYNON® Pellets (for subcutaneous implantation), 25 mg in vials of 1 pellet in cartons of 3. **(Schering)**

Estradiol Benzoate

ESTRADIOL BENZOATE Injection (in sesame oil), 0.5 and 1 mg/ml in multiple dose vials of 10 and 30 ml. **(Various Mfrs.)**

Estradiol Cypionate

DEPO®-ESTRADIOL Injection (in cottonseed oil), 1 mg/ml in vials of 10 ml; 5 mg/ml in vials of 5 ml. **(Upjohn)**

w/Testosterone Cypionate (DEPO-TESTADIOL®) Injection, 2 mg/ml with testosterone cypionate, 50 mg/ml in vials of 1 and 10 ml. **(Upjohn)**

Estradiol Valerate

DELESTROGEN® Injection, 10 mg/ml (in sesame oil) in vials of 5 ml; 20 and 40 mg/ml (in castor oil) in vials of 5 ml. **(Squibb)**

Ethinyl Estradiol

ESTINYL® Tablets, 0.02 and 0.05 mg in bottles of 100 and 250; 0.5 mg in bottles of 100. **(Schering)**

FEMINONE® Tablets, 0.05 mg in bottles of 100 and 1000. **(Upjohn)**

GYNETONE® Tablets, 0.02 and 0.04 mg with methyltestosterone, 5 and 10 mg respectively in bottles of 100. **(Schering)**

Polyestradiol Phosphate

ESTRADURIN® Secules, 40 mg with 2-ml ampul of sterile diluent. **(Ayerst)**

ESTROGENIC SUBSTANCES, CONJUGATED

Description: Naturally occurring, orally active, water-soluble estrogens, usually obtained from pregnant mares' urine, and containing not less than 90% and not more than 115% of the labeled amount of conjugated estrogens. They contain not less than 50% and not more than 65% of sodium estrone sulfate, and not less than 20% and not more than 35% of sodium equilin sulfate, calculated on the basis of the total conjugated estrogens content.

Indications: Menopausal syndrome, postmenopause, osteoporosis, senile vaginitis, kraurosis vulvae with and without pruritus, abnormal uterine bleeding, hypogenitalism, amenorrhea, mammary and prostatic carcinoma, and prevention of postpartum breast engorgement. Combined with *meprobamate*, to provide added relief of anxiety and tension and to promote muscular relaxation and normal sleeping habit. Combined with *phenobarbital* for control of vasomotor symptoms of the climacteric, prompt amelioration of its nervous manifestations, particularly when symptoms of tension, irritability and insomnia are superimposed on those of declining ovarian function. Combined with *testosterone* for relief of postpartum breast engorgement (when lactation is to be suppressed); osteoporosis, Paget's disease, in nonunion and delayed union of fractures in the elderly, as adjunct to prolonged corticoid therapy, dysmenorrhea, climacteric (male and female), malnutrition (in the female). The Vaginal Cream is indicated in postmenopausal and senile vulvovaginitis, pruritus vulvae caused by atrophic changes in the vulval epithelium, dyspareunia associated with atrophic vaginal epithelium and for use prior to plastic pelvic surgery in menopausal cases. Topical Cream, adjunctively in the treatment of acne vulgaris. Intravenously for abnormal uterine bleeding. Intravenous administration (Premarin®) has been used in patients to control spontaneous capillary bleeding, to reduce excessive capillary oozing during surgery, to decrease postoperative bleeding and to control dysfunctional uterine bleeding.

Contraindications: Known hypersensitivity to any of the components; markedly impaired liver function; known or suspected carcinoma of the breast, except those cases of progressing disease not amenable to surgery or irradiation occurring in women who are at least 5 years postmenopausal; known or suspected estrogen-dependent neoplasia, such as carcinoma of the endometrium; undiagnosed abnormal vaginal bleeding; in patients with a history of thromboembolic disorders, thrombophlebitis, cerebral embolism. Contraindications to meprobamate, methyltestosterone, and phenobarbital should be observed.

For warnings, precautions and adverse reactions, see general statement.

Dosage and Administration: *Orally. Severe menopausal symptoms,* cyclic therapy is recommended. The dose is 1.25 mg daily, increased to 2.5 to 3.75 mg daily if a satisfactory response is not obtained in 3 or 4 days, and gradually decreased to maintenance levels of from 0.625 mg daily or less as symptoms are controlled. *Mild to moderately severe menopausal symptoms,* 0.3 to 1.25 mg daily depending upon the individual condition. *Female hypogonadism,* dosage is adjusted according to the development of secondary sex characteristics. *Dysfunctional uterine bleeding,* 3.75 to 7.5 mg daily in divided doses for 2 to 5 days or until bleeding stops. *Relief of breast engorgement,* 5 mg daily for 2 or more days. *Senile vaginitis and related disorders* in which tissue changes are desirable, 1.25 to 3.75 mg or more daily. *Prostatic carcinoma,* not less than 3.75 mg daily for several weeks followed by ½ the dosage for maintenance therapy. *Inoperable and terminal mammary cancer,* 30 mg daily for at least 2 months for subjective response and 5 months for objective response. *Intravaginally or topically:* Apply 2 to 4 gm of cream daily (provides 1.25 to 2.5 mg of naturally occurring conjugated estrogens). *Intravenously or intramuscularly* (Premarin®). *To control spontaneous hemorrhage and dysfunctional uterine bleeding and to reduce blood loss during surgery,* adults—25 mg, may be repeated; children—5 to 10 mg. Injection should be made slowly to obviate the occurrence of flushes. *Tablets with meprobamate,* 1 tablet 3 times daily in 21-day courses with a rest period of 7 days is recommended. *Tablets with methyltestosterone,* in amounts according to the condition being treated. *Tablets with phenobarbital,* 1 tablet or more daily, or as directed by the physician.

Availability:

Estrogenic Substances, Conjugated

Tablets, 0.625, 1.25 and 2.5 mg in bottles of 100 and 1000. **(ICN)**

GENISIS® Tablets, 0.625 and 1.25 mg in bottles of 100 and 500; 2.5 mg in bottles of 100. **(Organon)**

PREMARIN®: **(Ayerst)**
Intravenous, 25 mg (dry powder) with a 5-ml vial of sterile diluent.
Tablets, 0.3 and 2.5 mg in bottles of 100 and 1000; 0.625 and 1.25 mg in bottles of 100 and 1000 and in unit-dose packages of 100.
Vaginal Cream, 0.625 mg/gm in tubes of 45 gm with applicator.

w/Meprobamate

MILPREM® Tablets, 0.45 mg with meprobamate, 200 or 400 mg in bottles of 100. **(Wallace)**
PMB® Tablets, 0.45 mg with meprobamate, 200 or 400 mg in bottles of 60 and 500. **(Ayerst)**

Other Combinations

PREMARIN with METHYLTESTOSTERONE Tablets, 0.625 mg with methyltestosterone, 5 mg and 1.25 mg with methyltestosterone, 10 mg in bottles of 100 and 1000. **(Ayerst)**

ESTROGENIC SUBSTANCES, ESTERIFIED

Description: Esterified estrogens are a mixture of purified, esterified, orally active, water-soluble estrogens expressed as sodium estrone sulfate. Since the ratio of estrone to equilin in the urine of pregnant mares varies with the period of gestation, the mixture is standardized by adjustment with sodium estrone sulfate. Esterified estrogens contain not less than 75% and not more than 85% of sodium estrone sulfate, and not less than 6.5% and not more than 15% of equilin sodium sulfate, in such proportions that the total of these two components is not less than 90% and not more than 110%.

Indications: *In the female* as replacement therapy in the management of symptoms generally associated with the menopausal syndrome, (natural or surgical), female hypogonadism (hypogenitalism), amenorrhea, or primary ovarian failure. Also indicated in patients with abnormal uterine bleeding due to hormonal imbalance in the absence of organic pathology, senile vaginitis, kraurosis vulvae with or without pruritus, and in the treatment of inoperable carcinoma in patients who are at least 5 years past the menopause. *In the male* as palliative therapy for inoperable or advanced prostatic carcinoma. The addition of chlordiazepoxide is for the relief of anxiety, tension and/or apprehension which may be significant components of the clinical profile. Combined with testosterone for the treatment of postpartum breast engorgement and moderate to severe menopausal vasomotor symptoms not controlled by estrogens alone.

For contraindications, warnings, precautions and adverse reactions, see general statement.

Dosage and Administration: *Orally. For relief of menopausal symptoms,* cyclic therapy is recommended. The average daily dose is 1.25 mg; may be increased to 2.5 or 3.75 mg. *For senile vaginitis and related disorders,* the recommended dosage is 0.3 to 1.25 mg daily. *For female hypogonadism,* cyclic therapy is recommended, and dosage should be regulated according to the development of secondary sex characteristics. *For dysfunctional uterine bleeding,* a dose of 7.5 mg daily for 3 to 5 days or until bleeding stops. *For relief of breast engorgement,* the recommended dosage is 5 mg daily for 2 or more days, starting as soon as possible following delivery. *For relief of prostatic carcinoma,* a dose of 3.75 mg or more daily for several weeks; for maintenance, ½ the initial dose is usually satisfactory. *For inoperable and terminal mammary cancer,* a dose of 30 mg daily for at least 2 months for a subjective response, and a total of 5 months for an objective response is recommended. When administering Menrium tablets, the usual dosage is 1 tablet 3 times daily. Combined with *chlordiazepoxide,* 1 tablet 3 times daily, and with *methyltestosterone,* 1 or 2 tablets daily.

Availability:

Estrogenic Substances, Esterified

AMNESTROGEN® Tablets, 0.625, 1.25 and 2.5 mg in bottles of 100. **(Squibb)**
EVEX® Tablets, 0.625 mg (orange), 1.25 mg (pink) and 2.5 mg (yellow) in bottles of 100. **(Syntex)**
MENEST® Tablets, 0.3 mg (yellow) in bottles of 100; 0.625 mg (orange) and 1.25 mg (green) in bottles of 100 and 1000; 2.5 mg (pink) in bottles of 50 and 1000. **(Beecham)**
SK-ESTROGENS™ Tablets, 0.3, 0.625, 1.25 and 2.5 mg in bottles of 100. **(Smith Kline & French)**

ZESTĒ™ Tablets, 0.625 and 1.25 mg in bottles of 100. **(Ascher)**

w/Chlordiazepoxide

MENRIUM® 5-2 tablets (light green), 0.2 mg with chlordiazepoxide, 5 mg; 5-4 tablets (dark green), 0.4 mg with chlordiazepoxide, 5 mg; 10-4 tablets (purple), 0.4 mg with chlordiazepoxide, 10 mg in bottles of 100 and 500. **(Roche)**

w/Methyltestosterone

ZESTĒ M.T. Tablets, 1.25 mg with methyltestosterone, 2.5 mg in bottles of 100. **(Ascher)**

ESTROGENIC SUBSTANCES, MIXED

Description: A suspension of crystalline estrogenic steroids, principally estrone derived from pregnant mares' urine (equine); also small amounts of equilen and equilenin with traces of estrogenic diols are present. When combined with other steroids, each modifies the specific action of the other and lessens the side effects which may occur when used alone. The potency is expressed in milligrams of crystalline estrone or International Units; 1 mg equals 10,000 I.U. of estrone.

Indications: Menopausal syndrome (natural or surgical); kraurosis vulvae, pruritus vulvae, senile vaginitis and vulvitis; hypomonorrhea, oligomenorrhea, primary and secondary amenorrhea; dysfunctional uterine bleeding (menorrhagia, metrorrhagia); painful breast engorgement during lactation (prevention and treatment) and prostatic cancer. Combined with progesterone in the treatment of functional uterine bleeding, in threatened or repeated abortion, amenorrhea, dysmenorrhea and monopausal syndrome.

Contraindications: When genital or mammary carcinoma is suspected or when there is a family history of cancer incidence; in existing amenorrhea of nonendocrine origin. Should not be used when rhythmic ovarian function with fertility is desirable. See general statement.

Warnings: See general statement.

Precautions: Periodic pelvic examinations should be performed before and after therapy to rule out genital malignancy. See general statement.

Adverse Reactions: Local erythema, inflammation, local pain and lump at site of injection; withdrawal bleeding; nausea. In the male: gynecomastia, loss of libido, and testicular atrophy. See general statement.

Dosage and Administration: *Intramuscularly.* Average dosage is 1 to 3 mg 1 or more times weekly. *In breast engorgement,* 5 mg 1 or 2 times daily for 2 or more days. *Prostatic cancer,* 3 mg daily for 2 or 3 weeks. With *progesterone,* 1 ml daily for 3 to 5 days.

Availability:

Estrogenic Substances, Mixed

ESTROGENIC SUBSTANCES Aqueous Suspension, 2 mg/ml in vials of 10 ml; 5 mg/ml in vials of 5 ml. **(Various Mfrs.)**

MENAGEN® Capsules, 1 mg in bottles of 100. **(Parke-Davis)**

NEO-AMNIOTIN® Aqueous Suspension, 2 and 5 mg/ml in vials of 10 ml. **(Squibb)**

URESTRIN® Injection in Oil, 2 mg/ml in vials of 10 ml. **(Upjohn)**

w/Progesterone

CYCLOGESTERIN®: **(Upjohn)**

Solution, 1 mg/ml with progesterone, 10 mg/ml; 2.5 mg/ml with progesterone, 25 mg/ml in vials of 5 ml.

Tablets, 1 mg with progesterone, 30 mg in bottles of 15.

ESTRONE

Chemical Name: 3-Hydroxyestra-1,3,5(10)-trien-17-one.

Description: A steroidal estrogen obtained from natural or synthetic sources, it occurs as small, white crystals or as a white to creamy white, crystalline powder practically insoluble in water and soluble in alcohol. Structurally, it differs from estradiol in that it has a keto group rather than a secondary alcohol group at the 17 position on ring D of the steroid nucleus.

Laboratory studies show that the estrogenic activity of 1 mg of crystalline estrone is equal to 10,000 International Units (IU) or about 1/3 the amount of crystalline estrone required to induce estrus with complete cornification of the vaginal epithelium.

Estrone piperazine sulfate is an oral preparation of pure crystalline estrone conjugated as the sulfate and stabilized with piperazine. It is soluble in water and has almost no odor or taste. Although the amount of piperazine in the compound is not sufficient to exert pharmacologic action, its addition ensures solubility, stability and uniform potency of the estrogen. Absorption from the gastrointestinal tract is usually prompt and complete.

Estrone is ordinarily administered intramuscularly, since enzymatic degradation in the gastrointestinal tract and liver greatly reduces its oral activity.

Indications: Replacement therapy of estrogen deficiency associated with the menopausal syndrome, moderate to severe vasomotor symptoms, female hypogonadism (hypogenitalism), amenorrhea, female castration, or primary ovarian failure, in the management of senile vaginitis, kraurosis vulvae with or without pruritus, abnormal uterine bleeding due to hormonal imbalance in the absence of organic pathology, for the prevention of postpartum breast engorgement, and in inoperable progressing prostatic cancer (for palliation only when castration is not feasible).

Contraindications: Cancerous or precancerous lesions of the breasts or genital tract, prolonged high dosage in premenopausal patients when rhythmic ovarian function with fertility is desired, uterine bleeding due to blood dyscrasias, estrogen-producing or dependent tumors. See general statement.

Warnings: Thromboembolic phenomena especially in the postpartum patient has been reported. See general statement.

Precautions: Bleeding or spotting should be thoroughly investigated in both premenopausal and postmenopausal women. Preexisting fibroid tumors may become enlarged during treatment. Since a number of thyroid tests may be altered, it is advisable that therapy be discontinued for at least 3 to 6 weeks before undertaking these tests. See general statement.

Adverse Reactions: The most frequently encountered side effect was nausea. Less commonly noted were sodium and water retention, breast swelling and tenderness, anorexia, vomiting, headaches, changes in liver function and breakthrough bleeding. Rare reactions to estrogens usually include allergies, jaundice, increased blood sugar levels and decreased glucose tolerance and loss or increase of libido. Estrogens may also precipitate or aggravate porphyria cutanea tarda in predisposed individuals. Increased amounts of estrogens used with progestational agents have been associated with thromboembolic phenomena, although a direct causal relationship has not been clearly established. **Note:** In male patients receiving high doses of estrogens for prostatic carcinoma, testicular atrophy and certain signs of feminization can be expected to occur in a significant number of patients.

Dosage and Administration: *Orally* or *intramuscularly. Estrogen deficiency states,* 1.5 to 4.5 mg daily depending on the needs of the patient. The most effective dosage in the majority of patients is 3 mg. Maintenance dosage is given for 3 to 4 weeks alternating with rest period of 5 to 7 days. Withdrawal bleeding may occur toward the end of the rest period. It may be preferable in some patients to give piperazine estrone sulfate continuously and to add a progestational agent every 4 to 6 weeks to evoke a menstrual period. *For senile vaginitis, kraurosis vulvae and pruritus vulvae,* 1.25 mg 1 to 3 times daily. *For treatment of female hypogonadism,* the dosage should be regulated according to the development of secondary sex characteristics. Usually a dosage of 1.25 mg 1 to 3 times daily is administered for the first half of a theoretical cycle followed by progesterone administration for the last half. After 3 to 6 months on this regimen, the patient receives no medication to determine if the cycle can be maintained without hormonal therapy; if not, therapy is continued. *Postpartum breast engorgement,* 4.5 mg every 4 hours for 5 doses following delivery. *Dysfunctional uterine bleeding,* a daily dosage of 4.5 to 9 mg in divided doses will usually be sufficient. *Carcinoma of the prostate,* 3 to 6 mg 3 times daily. For complete details on dosage schedule, see package literature.

Availability:

Estrone

Aqueous Suspension, 2 and 5 mg/ml in vials of 10 ml. **(Various Mfrs.)**
Aqueous Suspension, 2 mg/ml in vials of 10 ml; 5 mg/ml in vials of 5 ml. **(Lilly)**
Injection in Oil, 1 mg/ml in vials of 10 ml. **(Lilly)**
THEELIN®: **(Parke-Davis)**
Aqueous Suspension, 1, 2 and 5 mg/ml in ampuls of 1 ml; 2 mg/ml in Steri-Vials® of 10 ml; 5 mg/ml in Steri-Vials of 5 ml.
Injection in Oil, 1 mg/ml in ampuls of 1 ml and in Steri-Vials® of 10 ml.
Vaginal Suppositories, 0.2 mg in cartons of 6.

Combinations

THEELIN R-P® Aqueous Suspension, 2 mg/ml with potassium estrone sulfate, 1 mg/ml in Steri-Vials® of 10 ml. **(Parke-Davis)**

Estrone Piperazine Sulfate

OGEN®: **(Abbott)**
Tablets, 0.75, 1.5, 3 and 6 mg in bottles of 100; 1.5 mg tablets in Pak-Dispensers of 21 tablets in cartons of 6.
Vaginal Cream, 1.5 mg/gm in tubes of 42.5 gm with applicator.

HORMONIN

Description: Each tablet contains:

	Hormonin No. 1	*Hormonin No. 2*
Estriol	0.135 mg	0.27mg
Estrone	0.7 mg	1.4 mg
Estradiol	0.3 mg	0.6 mg

Indications: As replacement therapy in the treatment of the menopausal and postmenopausal syndromes. The estrogens employed are those normally present in premenopausal women. Thus, by replacing these physiologically normal hormones which are in low endogenous production during the climacteric, a smoother and more predictable response may be expected.

Contraindications: In women with a familial or personal history of mammary or genital cancer. See general statement.

Warnings: Estrogens should not be administered to women with recurrent mastitis or abnormal mammograms except in instances in which treatment is warranted despite the possibility of aggravation of this condition or of stimulation of undiagnosed estrogen-dependent neoplasia. Constant observation of the patient is essential so that the earliest manifestations of thrombotic disorders (thrombophlebitis, cerebrovascular disorders, pulmonary embolism, and retinal thrombosis) may be noted. If these occur or are suspected, the drug should be discontinued immediately. Since these substances are excreted in the mother's milk, the estrogenic effect on the nursing infant should be regarded when estrogens are administered to lactating women. Therapy should be discontinued if hypercalcemia occurs in patients with metastatic breast cancer, since this indicates progression of bone metastases. A significant relationship between the maternal ingestion of diethylstilbestrol during pregnancy and the occurrence of vaginal adenocarcinoma in the offspring has been demonstrated. In view of this finding the use of any estrogen preparation during pregnancy is not recommended. See general statement.

Precautions: A complete pretreatment physical examination should be performed with special attention to the pelvic and breast areas of the body. Patients may experience abnormal or excessive vaginal bleeding while on medication; the incidence of any pathological change should necessarily be ruled out. Estrogens may cause preexisting fibromyomata to increase in size, may mask the onset of the climacteric, and may also alter liver and endocrine function tests. To avoid continuous stimulation of the breast and uterus, cyclic therapy is recommended (3 weeks on medication with 1 week rest period—withdrawal bleeding may occur during this 1 week rest period). Estrogens have been found to induce changes in menopausal vaginal epithelium, uterine endothelium and breast tissue; these changes should be considered when specimens are sent for pathology examination. See general statement.

Adverse Reactions: Those generally encountered with the use of this drug include breakthrough bleeding, spotting, change in menstrual flow, dysmenorrhea, premenstrual-like syndrome, amenorrhea during and after treatment, increase in size of uterine fibromyomata, vaginal candidiasis, change in cervical eversion and in degree of cervical secretion, cystitis-like syndrome, breast tenderness, enlargement or secretion, nausea, vomiting, abdominal cramps, bloating, cholestatic jaundice, chloasma or melasma which may persist when the drug is discontinued, erythema multiforme, erythema nodosum, hemorrhagic eruption, loss of scalp hair, hirsutism, steepening of corneal curvature, intolerance to contact lenses, headache, dizziness, mental depression, chorea, increase or decrease in weight, reduced carbohydrate tolerance, aggravation of porphyria, edema, and changes in libido. Overdosage may cause withdrawal bleeding in women.

Dosage and Administration: *Orally.* For relief of menopausal symptoms, 1 or 2 tablets of No. 1 or 1 tablet of No. 2 daily depending upon the severity of symptoms. The initial dosage subsequently may be reduced for maintenance therapy. To avoid possible continuous stimulation of the breast and uterus, cyclic therapy may be employed. In severe cases the initial therapy may be supplemented with parenteral estrogens.

Availability:
HORMONIN® No. 1 Tablets (pink and white) in bottles of 100 and 500. **(Carnrick)**
HORMONIN® No. 2 Tablets (aqua and white) in bottles of 100 and 500. **(Carnrick)**

THE SYNTHETIC ESTROGENS

CHLOROTRIANISENE

Chemical Name: Chlorotris(*p*-methoxyphenyl)ethylene.

Description: Chlorotrianisene, a synthetic estrogenic substance derived from diethylstilbestrol, occurs as white crystals or as a white, crystalline powder very slightly soluble in water, slightly soluble in alcohol and soluble in vegetable oils.

Because chlorotrianisene is stored in fatty tissue, its onset of action may be delayed and because of its slow release from these tissues, the drug's effect persists for some time after its administration has been discontinued.

Indications: Prevention and treatment of painful engorgement of the breast when suppression of lactation is desired; palliative control of prostatic carcinoma; and estrogen deficiency states such as the menopausal syndrome; senile vaginitis, kraurosis vulvae, pruritus vulvae—conditions in which prolonged or severe estrogen deficiency is a conditioning factor; also in female hypogonadism.

Contraindications: Estrogen therapy may aggravate breast carcinoma, particularly in patients who are less than 5 years past the menopause. See general statement.

For warnings and precautions, see general statement.

Adverse Reactions: Prolonged continuous administration can lead to endometrial hyperplasia and breakthrough bleeding. Gynecomastia and reduced potency may occur in the male. Nausea, vomiting, urticarial and other cutaneous reactions have been reported. Although edema is rare, caution should be exercised when estrogen must be given to patients whose renal functional reserve is low, such as those with borderline cardiac decompensation. See general statement.

Dosage and Administration: *Orally. Postpartum breast engorgement:* one 12-mg capsule 4 times daily for 7 days, or two 25-mg capsules every 6 hours for 6 doses. For immediate postpartum use, the first dose should be given within 8 hours after delivery. *Prostatic carci-*

noma: 12 to 25 mg daily. *Menopausal syndrome:* 12 to 25 mg daily for 30 days; 1 or more courses may be given. *Senile vaginitis, kraurosis vulvae, pruritus vulvae:* 12 to 25 mg daily for 30 to 60 days. *Female hypogonadism:* 12 to 25 mg daily for 21 days, followed if desired by an immediate intramuscular injection of 100 mg of progesterone; alternatively, an oral progesterone may be given during the last 5 days of therapy with chlorotrianisene. The next course may begin on the 5th day of the induced uterine bleeding.

Availability:
TACE® Capsules, 12 mg (green, soft gelatin) in bottles of 28, 100 and 500; 25 mg (two-tone green, hard gelatin) in bottles of 60; 72 mg in cartons of 48 (12 x 4). **(Merrell-National)**

DIENESTROL

Chemical Name: 4,4′-(Diethylideneethylene)diphenol.

Description: Dienestrol is a synthetic estrogen that differs structurally from diethylstilbestrol in that the 2 diethyl groups of the latter are replaced by 2 unsaturated ethylidene groups. Dienestrol occurs as colorless, white, or practically white, needle-like crystals or as a white or practically white, crystalline powder practically insoluble in water and soluble in alcohol.

Indications: Recommended for the treatment of postmenopausal and senile vulvovaginitis, atrophic vaginitis, pruritus vulvae caused by atrophic changes in the vulval epithelium, dyspareunia associated with an atrophic vaginal epithelium, and for use prior to plastic pelvic surgery in menopausal cases.

Contraindications: Malignancy of the vulva or vagina. A significant association has been reported between maternal ingestion of **diethylstilbestrol** during pregnancy and the appearance of vaginal carcinoma developing years later in the offspring. It is not known at present whether such an association is applicable to all estrogens. However, pregnancy is a definite contraindication to the use of diethylstilbestrol or any of its closely related congeners (dienestrol, hexestrol, benzestrol and promethestrol). The other estrogens are not indicated for use during pregnancy. See general statement.

For warnings, precautions and adverse reactions, see general statement.

Dosage and Administration: *Intravaginally,* 1 applicatorful of cream or 1 suppository once or twice daily for 7 to 14 days, then reduced gradually to once every 48 hours for a similar period. For maintenance, 1 applicatorful or 1 suppository 1 to 3 times weekly after the vaginal mucosa has been restored.

Availability:
DIENESTROL Cream, 0.1 mg/gm in tubes of 78 gm with or without applicator. **(Ortho)**
DV®: **(Merrell-National)**
Cream, 0.01% in tubes of 90 gm with applicator.
Suppositories, 0.7 mg in cartons of 16 with applicator.

DIETHYLSTILBESTROL

Chemical Name: α,α'-Diethyl-4,4′-stilbenediol.

Description: Diethylstilbestrol is a nonsteroidal, synthetic stilbene derivative possessing estrogenic activity. It occurs as a white, crystalline powder practically insoluble in water and soluble in vegetable oils. The *diphosphate* occurs as a white, crystalline powder soluble in water. On a molecular basis, diethylstilbestrol is equivalent to about 1.6 mg of diethylstilbestrol diphosphate. Apparently, it is capable of producing all the pharmacologic and therapeutic responses attributed to natural estrogens.

Indications: Whenever an estrogenic effect is desired. It has proved useful as replacement therapy in states of estrogen deficiency, and it is also used for specific effects in the absence of deficiency. It has been found of value in moderate to severe vasomotor symptoms, menopausal symptoms or female castration; postmenopausal and senile vulvovaginitis; kraurosis vulvae with or without pruritus; dyspareunia; painful engorgement of the breast postpartum; as a palliative for inoperable progressing carcinoma of the prostate only when castration is not feasible, and for breast cancer in women who are more than 5 years postmenopausal. Also, in the male in whom bilateral orchiectomy cannot be performed. Under restricted conditions for postcoital (contraceptive use). With *methyltestosterone,* it is indicated in the treatment of osteoporosis due wholly or partly to gonadal deficiency (postmenopausal osteoporosis).

Contraindications: A significant association has been reported between maternal ingestion of **diethylstilbestrol** during pregnancy, especially within the first 12 weeks, and the appearance of vaginal adenosis developing years later (postpubertal stage), in the offspring. The significance of this finding with regard to the possible development of vaginal adenocarcinoma is not known; nonetheless, such patients should be examined periodically. It is not known at present whether such an association is applicable to all estrogens. However, pregnancy is a definite contraindication to the use of diethylstilbestrol and its closely related congeners (dienestrol, hexestrol, benzestrol, and promethestrol). There is suggestive evidence that male offspring may develop abnormalities. The other estrogens are not indicated for use during pregnancy. See general statement.

For warnings, precautions, and adverse reactions, see general statement. See monograph on Testosterone for additional reactions.

Dosage and Administration: *Orally. Menopausal symptoms:* 0.2 to 0.5 mg daily, increased as needed. *Senile vaginitis:* 0.5 mg daily. *Painful breast engorgement postpartum:* 5 mg 1 to 3 times daily for a total of 30 mg. *Functional uterine bleeding:* usually 5 mg 3 to 5 times daily until bleeding stops. *Prostatic carcinoma:* 1 to 3 mg daily, increased in advanced cases, then reduced to an average of 1 mg daily, or 50 mg (initially) of the diphosphate salt 3 times daily with subsequent increases to 200 mg or more 3 times daily, then reduced to an average of 1 mg daily. *Mammary carcinoma:* 15 mg daily. *Intravaginally.* Up to 1 mg may be administered daily in suppository form for 10 to 14 days in addition to 0.5 to 2 mg/day orally. For maintenance, as much as 5 mg can be given weekly in suppository form when treatment is not supplemented by oral administration. *Intramuscularly. Menopause and senile vaginitis:* 0.25 to 1 mg 2 or 3 times a week. *Postpartum breast engorgement:* 5 mg once or twice daily for a total of 2 to 4 days. *Functional uterine bleeding:* 5 mg 2 or 3 times daily until checked. *Prostatic carcinoma: Intravenously.* On the first day, inject 0.5 gm of the diphosphate salt dissolved in 300 ml of saline or 5% dextrose solution. On subsequent days inject 1 gm dissolved in the same volume of solution. The infusion should be administered slowly (20 to 30 drops/minute) during the first 10 to 15 minutes and then the rate of flow adjusted so that the entire amount is given in a period of 1 hour. This procedure should be followed for 5 days or more depending upon the response of the patient. For maintenance, the recommended dosage is 0.25 to 0.5 gm administered in a similar manner once or twice weekly or the oral form may be substituted. *For postcoital (contraceptive) use in emergency situations:* the recommended dosage is 25 mg twice daily for 5 consecutive days beginning, preferably, within 24 hours and no later than 72 hours after exposure. To be effective, the patient must be warned to take the full course of the drug regardless of the nausea which commonly occurs. Dosage for combination products should coincide with dosage for diethylstilbestrol alone.

Availability:

Diethylstilbestrol

DIETHYLSTILBESTROL: **(Lilly)**

Enseals® (enteric-coated tablets), 0.1, 0.25, 0.5, 1 and 5 mg in bottles of 100 and 1000. *Not for postcoital (contraceptive) use.*

Suppositories, 0.1 and 0.5 mg in cartons of 6 and 50.

Tablets, 0.25 mg in bottles of 100; 0.1, 0.5, 1 and 5 mg in bottles of 100 and 1000; the 5 mg tablets are also available in 10 strips of 10 individually labeled blisters each containing 1 tablet. *Not for postcoital (contraceptive) use.*

TYLOSTERONE®: Tablets, 0.25 mg with methyltestosterone, 5 mg in bottles of 100 and 1000. **(Lilly)**

Diethylstilbestrol Diphosphate *(for prostatic carcinoma only)*

STILPHOSTROL® (as sodium salt): **(Dome)**

Injection, 50 mg/ml in ampuls of 5 ml.

Tablets, 50 mg in bottles of 50.

ETHACRYNIC ACID

Chemical Name: [2,3-Dichloro-4-(2-methylenebutyryl)phenoxy] acetic acid.

Description: An alpha-beta unsaturated ketone derivative of an aryloxyacetic acid, it occurs as a white or nearly white, crystalline powder very slightly soluble in water and soluble in alcohol; the sodium salt of ethacrynic acid is soluble in water.

The pharmacologic action of ethacrynic acid is similar to that of furosemide but its direct mode of action has not been clearly defined. It appears to react with critical renal sulfhydryl groups in a manner similar to that of organomercurials, but whether or not this biochemical interplay contributes to its diuretic action has not been determined. It apparently inhibits the reabsorption of sodium in the ascending limb of Henle's loop and also exerts a direct effect on electrolyte transport at the proximal tubule. It appears to decrease distal tubular reabsorption of sodium and chloride.

It has been used in the management of all types of edema. Patients with congestive heart failure involving acute pulmonary edema, renal edema, hepatic cirrhosis with ascites have responded well. Water and electrolyte excretion may be increased several times over that observed with thiazide diuretics, and it appears effective whether or not there is clinical acidosis or alkalosis. The onset of action occurs within 30 minutes after an oral dose, and within 5 minutes after an intravenous dose. Following oral administration, peak diuretic-saluretic activity occurs in about 2 hours with a duration of action lasting from 6 to 8 hours.

Indications: Treatment of edema associated with congestive heart failure, renal disease, including the nephrotic syndrome, hepatic cirrhosis with ascites and ascites due to malignancy; idiopathic edema and lymphedema; also in pediatric patients with the nephrotic syndrome or congenital heart disease. Intravenous use is indicated when rapid diuresis is desired as in acute pulmonary edema, or when gastrointestinal absorption is impaired or oral medication is not practical.

Contraindications: In anuria; if an increase in electrolyte imbalance, azotemia and/or oliguria occurs during treatment of severe progressive renal disease; if severe watery diarrhea occurs; also in infants, and in nursing mothers.

Warnings: Excessive diuresis with water and electrolyte depletion may occur if given in excessive dosage or to patients with massive fluid accumulation. It is not recommended for use in pregnant patients; however, use in women of childbearing age requires that its potential benefits be weighed against possible hazards to the fetus. The safety and efficacy of this drug in toxemia of pregnancy has not been established. **Careful attention must be given to the directions for use and to the individual patient's response to the drug.** Frequent serum electrolyte, CO_2 and BUN determinations should be performed when therapy is initiated and periodically thereafter during diuresis. Any electrolyte abnormalities should be corrected or the drug temporarily withdrawn. Patients with advanced cirrhosis of the liver, particularly those with a history of previous episodes of electrolyte imbalances or hepatic encephalopathy, should be carefully observed for signs of impending hepatic coma and death. Too vigorous a diuresis, as evidenced by a rapid and excessive weight loss, may induce an acute hypotensive episode. In elderly cardiac patients, rapid contraction of plasma volume with homoconcentration may result in thromboembolic episodes such as cerebrovascular thrombosis and pulmonary emboli which may be fatal. In digitalized patients acute hypokalemia may precipitate fatal cardiac arrhythmias. To avoid or minimize possible excessive water or electrolyte losses, the physician is advised to weigh the patient throughout treatment, adjust the dosage carefully, administer small initial doses, employ intermittent dosage schedule when possible, and monitor the electrolytes initially and frequently during active diuresis. When excessive diuresis or electrolyte loss occurs, the drug should be withdrawn until homeostasis is restored. Supplementary potassium chloride may be required. Enteric-coated potassium chloride tablets, either alone or with nonenteric coated thiazides have been implicated in stenosis and ulceration of the small bowel. These small bowel lesions have caused obstruction, hemorrhage, and perforation. Surgery was frequently required and deaths have occurred. Such preparations should be withdrawn immediately if gastrointestinal symptoms (abdominal pain, distention, nausea, vomiting, bleeding) occur. Lithium generally should not be given with diuretics because they reduce its renal clearance and add to the high risk of lithium toxicity.

Precautions: Weakness, muscle cramps, paresthesias, thirst, anorexia, and signs of hyponatremia, hypokalemia, and/or hypochloremic alkalosis; rarely tetany may occur following vigorous or excessive diuresis and these may be accentuated by rigid salt restriction; therefore, additional salt and potassium intake is advised. Safety and efficacy of ethacrynic acid in hypertension have not been established and the dosage of coadministered antihypertensive agents may require adjustment to avoid a severe hypotensive effect. A transient increase in serum urea nitrogen may occur, which is reversible when the drug is discontinued. It should be kept in mind that the drug may displace warfarin from plasma proteins and may therefore necessitate a reduction in the anticoagulant dosage. Ototoxic effects have been reported with the use of ethacrynic acid, and these effects may be enhanced when used concurrently with aminoglycoside antibiotics. Also, patients being treated for renal edema may develop hypoproteinemia which may require the addition of a salt-poor albumin solution to the regimen.

Adverse Reactions: Hyperuricemia, decreased urinary urate excretion, acute gout, acute symptomatic hypoglycemia with convulsions may occur. Anorexia, malaise, abdominal discomfort or pain, dysphagia, nausea, vomiting, diarrhea, melena; acute nonhemorrhagic pancreatitis, hyperglycemia, jaundice, liver dysfunction; agranulocytosis or severe neutropenia, thrombocytopenia have been noted. Deaths have occurred in patients with severe myocardial disease and in patients with severe hepatic cirrhosis with ascites with or without accompanying encephalopathy. Reported rarely were acute vertigo, deafness, tinnitus with a sense of fullness in the ears, skin rash, headache, fever, chills, blurred vision, fatigue, apprehension confusion, and Henoch-Schonlein purpura in rheumatic heart patients. Ethacrynate sodium has caused local irritation, pain and local thrombophlebitis.

Dosage and Administration: *Orally or intravenously.* Dosage must be regulated carefully to prevent a more rapid or substantial loss of fluid or electrolyte than is required or necessary. To initiate diuresis in adults 50 to 100 mg; maintenance 50 to 200 mg daily. In children 25 mg with careful increments of 25 mg to achieve effective maintenance. Small alterations in dose may effectively prevent a massive diuretic response. The usual intravenous dose is 50 mg for adults. Occasionally a second dose at a new injection site to avoid thrombophlebitis may be required. Insufficient pediatric experience precludes recommendation for this age group.

Availability:
EDECRIN® Tablets 25 mg (white) and 50 mg (green) in bottles of 100.
(Merck Sharp & Dohme)
EDECRIN SODIUM Intravenous in vials of 50 ml containing ethacrynate sodium equivalent to 50 mg of ethacrynic acid. **(Merck Sharp & Dohme)**

ETHAMBUTOL HYDROCHLORIDE

Chemical Name: *d*-2,2′-(Ethylenediimino)di-1-butanol dihydrochloride.

Description: Ethambutol is an oral chemotherapeutic agent which is effective specifically against actively growing microorganisms of the genus *Mycobacterium*, including *M. tuberculosis*. It occurs as a white, odorless, crystalline powder freely soluble in water and slightly soluble in alcohol.

Following a single oral dose of 25 mg/kg of body weight, peak serum levels of 2 to 5 mcg/ml are attained in 2 to 4 hours. In patients with normal renal function, the serum level falls to undetectable amounts in 24 hours. The intracellular concentrations of erythrocytes reach peak values approximately twice those of plasma and maintain this ratio throughout the 24 hours. During the 24-hour period following oral administration of ethambutol, approximately 50% of the initial dose is excreted unchanged in the urine, while an additional 8 to 15% appears in the form of 2 metabolites. The main path of metabolism appears to be an initial oxidation of the alcohol to an aldehydic intermediate, followed by conversion to a dicarboxylic acid derivative. From 20 to 22% of the initial dose is excreted in the feces unchanged. No drug accumulation has been observed with consecutive single daily doses of 25 mg/kg of body weight in patients with normal kidney function, although marked accumulation has been found in patients with renal insufficiency.

Ethambutol diffuses into actively growing mycobacterium cells such as tubercle bacilli. It appears to inhibit the synthesis of one or more metabolites, thus causing impairment of cell metabolism, arrest of multiplication, and cell death. No cross resistance with other available antimycobacterial agents has been demonstrated. It has been shown to be effective against strains of *Mycobacterium tuberculosis* but does not seem to be active against fungi, viruses, or other bacteria. Ethambutal appears to reduce the incidence of mycobacterial resistance to isoniazid when both drugs are used concurrently.

An agar diffusion microbiologic assay, based upon inhibition of *Mycobacterium smegmatis* (ATCC 607) may be used to determine concentrations of ethambutol in serum and urine.

Toxicological studies in animals on prolonged high doses of ethambutol produced evidence of myocardial damage and cardiac failure, degenerative changes in the CNS (not dose related), and depigmentation of the tapetum lucidum of the eyes. In few instances of fetuses born of mice treated with prolonged high doses, a low incidence of cleft palate, exencephaly and abnormality of the vertebral column was observed.

Indications: Pulmonary tuberculosis. It should not be used as the sole agent, but rather in conjunction with at least one other antituberculous drug, depending upon its comparative safety and appropriate susceptibility studies.

Contraindications: Known hypersensitivity to the drug, and in patients known to have optic neuritis unless clinical judgment determines that it may be used.

Precautions: While no detectable adverse effects on fetal development have been noted during clinical trials, it should nonetheless be used with considerable caution in pregnant patients and in women of childbearing potential, and then only when the therapeutic benefits outweigh the possible risks to the fetus. Since the drug is excreted in the urine, dosage should be reduced for those patients with impaired renal function; reduction will depend upon serum levels of the drug. Careful consideration should be given to the possibility of adverse effects on vision and to patients with existing visual defects; physical examination should include ophthalmoscopy, finger perimetry and testing of color discrimination. In some cases, evaluation of visual changes may be difficult. Renal, hepatic and hematopoietic functions should be assessed periodically during long-term therapy. Ethambutol is not recommended for use in children under 13 years of age because safe use has not been established.

Adverse Reactions: The most notable problem is the development of optic neuritis, resulting in diminished visual acuity and loss of color discrimination. The intensity of the visual difficulty, which may be unilateral or bilateral, is related to dosage and duration of treatment. Patients should be advised to report any visual aberration, and if symptoms persist or if a progressive decrease in visual acuity is apparent, the drug should be withdrawn promptly. Recovery generally occurs when treatment is discontinued; the time required usually corresponds to the degree of visual impairment; however, the effect may possibly be irreversible. Other adverse reactions reported include: anaphylactoid reactions, dermatitis, pruritus and joint pain; anorexia, nausea, vomiting, gastrointestinal upset, abdominal pain; fever, malaise, headache, and dizziness; mental confusion, disorientation and possible hallucinations. Numbness and tingling of the extremities due to peripheral neuritis have been reported infrequently. Elevated serum uric acid levels occur and precipitation of acute gout has been reported. Transient impairment of liver function as indicated by abnormal liver function tests is not an unusual finding. Since ethambutol is recommended for therapy in conjunction with one or more other antituberculous drugs, these changes may be related to the concurrent therapy.

Dosage and Administration: *Orally.* Ethambutol should not be used alone either in the initial phase or in treating reactivated cases. Nor should it be used in children under 13 years of age. *Initial treatment:* 15 mg/kg (7 mg/lb) as a single dose once every 24 hours. In the more recent studies, isoniazid has been given concurrently in a single daily dose. *Retreatment:* A single dose of 25 mg/kg (11 mg/lb) is given once every 24 hours, concurrently with at least one other antituberculous drug shown to be sensitive to the second drug. After 60 days of therapy with ethambutol, dosage should be reduced to 15 mg/kg (7 mg/lb) and given as a single dose once every 24 hours.

Availability:

MYAMBUTOL® Tablets, 100 mg in bottles of 100 and 1000; 400 mg in bottles of 100. **(Lederle)**

ETHAVERINE HYDROCHLORIDE

Chemical Name: 6,7-Diethoxy-1-(3,4-diethoxybenzyl)isoquinoline hydrochloride.

Description: Ethaverine, a synthetic non-narcotic derivative of isoquinoline, is closely related to papaverine in both chemical structure and clinical action. In ethaverine, the 4 ethoxy groups replace the 4 methoxy groups of papaverine. The isoquinoline group of compounds have been reported to be of value as peripheral vasodilators in vasoconstrictive conditions in which there is no significant organic occlusion. The spasmolytic effect of ethaverine is claimed to be from 2 to 4 times as potent as that of papaverine, and to be less toxic. It appears to effect a direct smooth muscle relaxation that is independent of innervation, and also to have almost no effect on the CNS. It is particularly effective in cases where spasm exists, especially conditions affecting the larger blood vessels such as the systemic, cardiac, peripheral and pulmonary vessels, the smooth muscle of the intestine, the biliary tract and ureters.

Indications: Treatment of coronary, peripheral and cerebral vascular insufficiency associated with arterial spasm. It is also indicated to improve coronary circulation following occlusion and infarction, thus reducing frequency and severity of attacks of angina pectoris.

Contraindications: In the presence of complete atrioventricular dissociation.

Warnings: Phenobarbital may be habit-forming.

Precautions: Cautious use of ethaverine is required in patients with glaucoma. All xanthine preparations should be used with extreme care in patients with tachycardia or palpitations. Since safe use of this drug in pregnant or lactating women has not been established, it should therefore not be prescribed for these patients unless its use is deemed essential to the welfare of the patient.

Adverse Reactions: Those that may occur in susceptible individuals include nausea, anorexia, abdominal distress and ischemia, CNS stimulation, dryness of throat, hypotension, malaise, lassitude, drowsiness, flushing, sweating, vertigo, respiratory depression, cardiac depression, cardiac arrhythmia, and headache. If these occur, the dosage should be reduced or the drug withdrawn.

Dosage and Administration: *Orally.* The usual dosage is 1 or 2 tablets every 3 or 4 hours, with or directly after meals. Because of the chronic nature of the disease, long-term therapy may be necessary.

Availability:
ETHAQUIN® Tablets, 100 mg in bottles of 100, 500, 1000, 2500 and 5000. **(Ascher)**
ETHATAB® Tablets, 100 mg in bottles of 100 and 1000. **(Meyer)**
LAVERIN® Tablets, 100 mg in bottles of 100 and 1000. **(Lemmon)**

ETHCHLORVYNOL C-IV

Chemical Name: Ethyl B-chlorovinyl ethynyl carbinol.

Description: Ethchlorvynol is a *tertiary* carbinol which contains neither nitrogen nor a benzene ring. It is chemically unrelated to the barbiturates and to nonbarbiturate hypnotics such as chloral hydrate, bromides, paraldehyde or glutethimide. Ethchlorvynol occurs as a colorless or yellowish liquid which darkens when exposed to air and light, has a pungent, aromatic odor, is not miscible with water, but is miscible with most organic solvents.

Ethchlorvynol is rapidly absorbed from the gastrointestinal tract. Following administration of the usual hypnotic dose (500 mg), sleep occurs within 15 minutes to 1 hour, and lasts for approximately 5 hours. If necessary, patients may be aroused in much the same way as from normal sleep.

In normal individuals less than 0.1% of the usual dose is excreted either unchanged or conjugated to glucuronic acid or sulfate in the urine within 24 hours after ingestion. In vitro studies show that the drug is dialyzable and is bound to plasma proteins only to a very small extent.

Although animal studies have not clearly established an adverse effect on reproduction, studies in rodents have shown a somewhat higher percentage of stillbirths and a lower survival rate of progeny.

Indications: As a short-term hypnotic in the management of insomnia.

Contraindications: In patients known to be hypersensitive to the drug, and in those with porphyria.

Warnings: Should not be used during the first and second trimesters of pregnancy, and only with considerable caution during the third trimester as the drug may cause CNS depression and transient withdrawal symptoms in the newborn. Safe use during lactation has not been established. Patients should be cautioned about the possible combined exaggerated effects with alcohol, barbiturates, tranquilizers or other CNS depressants. Such exaggerated effects may result in blurring of vision, paralysis of accommodation and profound hypnosis. Also, patients should be cautioned that shortly after taking a dose, they should refrain from performing hazardous occupations requiring alertness or skill. **The drug is capable of developing psychological and physical dependence. Severe withdrawal symptoms, including convulsions and toxic psychoses clinically similar to those seen with barbiturates, have been reported in patients taking regular doses as low as 1 gm daily for prolonged periods followed by sudden withdrawal of the drug.** Therefore, prolonged administration of the drug is not recommended. Patients, particularly those known to be suicidal or addiction-prone, or those who are likely to increase the dosage of ethchlorvynol on their own initiative, should be observed for signs of drug abuse. These include unusual anxiety, tremor, ataxia, slurring of speech, memory loss, perceptual distortions, irritability, agitation and delirium. Other less well defined signs and symptoms may include anorexia, nausea or vomiting, weakness, dizziness, sweating, muscle twitching and weight loss. Pulmonary edema of rapid onset has resulted from intravenous abuse. Ethchlorvynol has been reported to decrease the prothrombin time in patients taking coumarin anticoagulants. Until further clinical trials assure its safe and effective use, it is not recommended for use in the pediatric age group.

Precautions: The dosage of this drug should be reduced when given to patients taking MAO inhibitors or tricyclic antidepressants, and should be limited for elderly and debilitated patients to the smallest effective amount. Transient delirium has been reported when ethchlorvynol was combined with antidepressants such as amitriptyline. Although rare, reversible toxic amblyopia has been seen with long-term continuous use, and permanent visual defects have been known to occur. Routine caution is advised in patients with impaired hepatic or renal function. The drug is not recommended for use in patients who are taking alcohol or barbiturates. In some individuals ethchlorvynol appears to be absorbed rapidly and may produce ataxia or transient giddiness. Should this occur, a glass of milk or other food should be taken with subsequent doses of the drug, or therapy should be discontinued.

Adverse Reactions: Those that may develop include hypotension, nausea or vomiting, gastric upset, aftertaste, blurred vision, dizziness, facial numbness, allergic reactions (urticaria), thrombocytopenia (few cases), drowsiness, mild "hangover" and symptoms of mild excitation. There have been rare reports of cholestatic jaundice. A few instances of prolonged hypnosis, profound muscular weakness, excitement, hysteria, or syncope without marked hypotension have been noted. Nystagmus and pancytopenia resulting from acute overdosage have been noted in addition to prolonged deep respiratory depression, hypothermia, hypotension and relative bradycardia. Treatment of acute overdosage is essentially the same as that employed for any CNS depressant. An adequate airway must be maintained for the comatose patient and oxygen should be administered. Emphasis should be placed on pulmonary care and monitoring of blood gases. Peritoneal or hemodialysis have been reported to be of value in the treatment of massive overdosage. The usefulness of analeptic agents in such cases is controversial, and may aggravate the condition of patients in deep coma. Successful management of overdosage depends on continuous support of vital functions until consciousness is fully regained. The possibility of pulmonary edema occurring should be kept in mind. General supportive measures should be employed supplemental to immediate gastric lavage. In the unconscious patient, gastric lavage should be preceded by tracheal intubation with a cuffed tube.

Dosage and Administration: *Orally for adults only.* Usually from 500 mg to 1 gm at bedtime as a hypnotic. Patients who awaken during the early morning hours, or those who awaken prematurely following the 500-mg bedtime dose, may take 100 to 200 mg upon awakening.

Availability:
Ⓒ PLACIDYL® Capsules, 100 and 200 mg in bottles of 100; 500 mg in bottles of 100 and 500, and in Abbo-Pac®s (unit-dose packages) of 100; 750 mg in bottles of 100 and in Abbo-Pacs (unit-dose packages) of 100. **(Abbott)**

ETHINAMATE Ⓒ

Chemical Name: 1-Ethynylcyclohexyl carbamate.

Description: Ethinamate is a nonbarbiturate sedative and hypnotic drug that is chemically similar to ethchlorvynol. It occurs as a white, odorless, crystalline powder slightly soluble in water and freely soluble in alcohol. The drug has a more rapid onset of action and a shorter duration of sedation than any oral barbiturate. It is inactivated at least partly by the liver due to hydroxylation of the cyclohexyl ring; the product is then conjugated and excreted as the glucuronide.

Indications: As a hypnotic in those patients in whom sleep will continue once it has been induced.

Contraindications: Known hypersensitivity to the drug.

Warnings: Not recommended for use during pregnancy or lactation, or in pediatric patients. The concurrent ingestion of ethinamate with alcohol or other CNS depressants, especially in overdosage, will increase the potential hazards of these agents. Patients should be cautioned not to perform any hazardous occupation requiring alertness for at least 4 or 5 hours after taking the drug. Psychically predisposed patients have developed a dependency on the drug after prolonged overdosage. In such cases, gradual withdrawal should be accomplished in a controlled hospital setting. The addictive daily dose should be reduced 1 or 2 capsules every 2 or 3 days until the drug has been withdrawn. Psychiatric follow-up care is also indicated. An abrupt withdrawal can precipitate dangerous reactions.

Precautions: Elderly or debilitated patients should start with lower doses (e.g., ½ capsule). Patients with unrelieved pain should not be heavily sedated.

Adverse Reactions: There have been reports of thrombocytopenic purpura, drug idiosyncrasy with fever, paradoxical excitement in children, mild gastrointestinal symptoms and skin rashes. CNS and respiratory depression may occur with overdosage and treatment requires the same procedures attendant with barbiturate intoxication.

Dosage and Administration: *Orally for adults only.* For insomnia, 1 or 2 capsules 20 minutes before retiring. Treatment should be limited to 14 days.

Availability:
Ⓒ VALMID® Pulvules® (capsules), 500 mg in bottles of 100. **(Dista)**

ETHIONAMIDE

Chemical Name: 2-Ethylthioisonicotinamide.

Description: Ethionamide is an antibacterial agent which is bacteriostatic against *Mycobacterium tuberculosis.* It occurs as a yellow, crystalline substance that is practically insoluble in water and soluble in alcohol. It has a faint-to-moderate sulfide odor and is stable at all ordinary temperatures and levels of humidity.

Administration of 1 gm orally yields maximal plasma concentrations of approximately 20 mcg/ml in 3 hours, diminishing to 3 mcg/ml in 9 hours. Its half-life is shorter than that of isoniazid. Pharmacokinetic studies show that the drug is rapidly and widely distributed throughout the body with approximate concentration in the blood and various organs, but with significant concentration in the cerebrospinal fluid. Less than 1% is excreted in the urine in the active form, the rest as metabolites.

Indications: Treatment of all forms of pulmonary tuberculosis, particularly when primary therapy with streptomycin, isoniazid and aminosalicylic acid has failed because of patient intolerance or bacterial resistance. Ethionamide should not be used as the sole agent, but rather in conjunction with other effective antituberculous drugs.

Contraindications: Severe hypersensitivity and severe hepatic damage.

Warnings: Since teratogenic effects have been observed in rabbits and rats receiving doses in excess of those recommended in clinical use, use of the drug should be avoided during pregnancy or in women of childbearing potential, unless the benefits outweigh the possible hazards. Optimal dosage for children has not been established. However, this does not preclude use of the drug when its use is crucial to therapy.

Precautions: Pretreatment examinations should include in vitro susceptibility tests of recent cultures of *M. tuberculosis* from the patient as measured against ethionamide and the usual primary antituberculous drugs. Serum transaminase (SGOT, SGPT) levels should be determined prior to and every 2 to 4 weeks during therapy. Patients with diabetes mellitus may be more difficult to manage and they develop hepatitis more frequently. Ethionamide may intensify the adverse effects of other antituberculous drugs given concomitantly. Convulsions have occurred, requiring special care, particularly when ethionamide is given with cycloserine.

Adverse Reactions: Gastrointestinal intolerance (most common), peripheral neuritis, optic neuritis, psychic disturbances (including mental depression), postural hypotension, skin rashes, thrombocytopenia, pellagra-like syndrome, jaundice and/or hepatitis, increased difficulty in management of diabetes, stomatitis, gynecomastia and impotence.

Dosage and Administration: *Orally.* Should be given with at least one other effective antituberculous drug. Average adult dosage is 0.5 to 1 gm daily in divided doses, concomitantly with pyridoxine.

Availability:
TRECATOR®-SC Tablets, 250 mg (orange, sugar-coated) in bottles of 100 and 500. **(Ives)**

ETHOBRAL (C-II)

Description: One member from each of 3 classes of barbiturates has been combined in quantities less than those usually used for each to promote sleep. The capsule exerts a prompt hypnotic effect and sustains sound sleep for 7 to 8 hours with minimal aftereffects. Each capsule contains secobarbital sodium, 50 mg; butabarbital sodium, 30 mg and phenobarbital, 50 mg.

Indications: In insomnia when a prompt and sustained hypnotic effect is desired. Not recommended for daytime sedation.

Contraindications: In patients hypersensitive or previously addicted to barbiturates, or in those with chronic intermittent porphyria, uncontrolled pain because of the possibility of producing excitement, and severe respiratory conditions.

Warnings: Barbiturates may be habit-forming. May also impair the mental and/or physical abilities required for the performance of potentially hazardous tasks, such as driving a vehicle or operating machinery. Psychic dependence may occur with prolonged use, even with therapeutic dosages; therefore, gradual withdrawal of the medication is advised in order to avoid the potential occurrence of delirium, convulsions, or death. When prescribed for pregnant patients, the physician should carefully consider the benefits versus the risks to the fetus. Barbiturates readily cross the placental barrier and if administered during labor may have a depressant effect on the infant. These drugs are also found in the milk of nursing mothers, and their use is not recommended during lactation. Barbiturates, by inducing liver microsomal enzyme activity, increase the rate of hepatic metabolism of many drugs; thus, adjustment in dosages of these other agents may be necessary. The potency of coumarin anticoagulants may be decreased so that patients receiving such concomitant therapy should have frequent prothrombin determinations. The dose of barbiturates should be reduced when given simultaneously with other CNS-depressant agents. They must be used with caution in patients receiving MAO inhibitors, since these drugs may potentiate the depressant effects of barbiturates.

Also, barbiturates should be administered with special care to patients with borderline hypoadrenal function, whether of pituitary or primary adrenal origin, since the systemic effects of hydrocortisone (exogenous or endogenous) may be diminished.

Precautions: Use with caution in severe anemia, congestive heart failure, chronic pulmonary emphysema, or other conditions in which respiratory depression may be undesirable, and in elderly or debilitated patients or in those with renal or hepatic impairment or psychoneuroses, or in those suffering from shock.

Adverse Reactions: Respiratory depression, apnea, circulatory collapse, skin rash, allergic reactions, severe CNS depression, vertigo, drowsiness, lethargy, residual sedation (hangover effect), nausea, vomiting, diarrhea, paradoxical excitement (especially in elderly patients) are commonly observed in sensitive individuals or in those taking excessive doses. Jaundice is occasionally seen in patients who have become hypersensitive to barbiturates or who are suffering from barbiturate poisoning. Hypersensitivity reactions may occur, especially in those individuals with asthma, urticaria, angioneurotic edema or similar conditions. In addition, megaloblastic anemia has been reported in a few patients receiving prolonged antiepileptic therapy with phenobarbital. Although the anemia responds rapidly to folic acid or vitamin B-12, such therapy may precipitate epileptic seizures.

Dosage and Administration: *Orally,* 1 capsule at bedtime.

Availability:
Ⓒ ETHOBRAL® Capsules, 130 mg (green) in bottles of 100. **(Wyeth)**

ETHOHEPTAZINE CITRATE

Chemical Name: Hexahydro-1-methyl-4-phenylazepine-4-carboxylate citrate.

Description: A non-narcotic analgesic, ethoheptazine differs structurally from meperidine in that the six-membered piperidine ring is replaced by a seven-numbered hexamethylenimine ring. It occurs as a white, crystalline powder sparingly soluble in water and very slightly soluble in alcohol.

Following oral administration, ethoheptazine is readily absorbed from the gastrointestinal tract, is partially detoxified by the liver, and is excreted in the urine within 48 hours, intact and as the hydroxy and de-esterified metabolites. Its site and mode of action in the CNS have not been clearly defined.

Indications: Treatment of mild to moderate pain, particularly in those patients who cannot tolerate aspirin. In combination with aspirin, the drug may be used for the pain of arthritis and other musculoskeletal disorders; it is not to be used in those severe types of pain which require the use of the potent narcotic analgesics for relief. The addition of a tranquilizer such as meprobamate may be useful in relieving pain accompanied by either skeletal muscle spasm or tension and anxiety or both.

Contraindications: Hypersensitivity or intolerance to any of the components.

Warnings: Aspirin should be used cautiously in patients with peptic ulceration or gastritis. Prolonged use of phenacetin may produce anemia, methemoglobinemia, hypersensitivity and renal disease; nephrotoxicity may result.

Precautions: Salicylates may prolong the prothrombin time induced by anticoagulants. Ethoheptazine alone or in combination with other drugs should be used with caution during pregnancy or lactation and in women of childbearing potential. The potential benefits must outweigh the possible hazards. Precautions pertaining to the use of meprobamate and other components must be observed. Patients should be cautioned, in the event of dizziness, not to perform hazardous operations requiring alertness or skill.

Adverse Reactions: Nausea, with or without vomiting, epigastric distress and dizziness. Overdosage with ethoheptazine and aspirin resulted in symptoms of CNS depression including drowsiness and lightheadedness. On the basis of pharmacologic data, CNS stimulation, nausea and vomiting may occur. Adverse reactions associated with meprobamate must be kept in mind.

Dosage and Administration: *Orally.* The usual adult dosage is 75 to 150 mg of ethoheptazine alone or in combination with aspirin or with APC 3 to 4 times daily. Ethoheptazine in combination with meprobamate is not recommended for children 12 years of age or younger.

Availability:

Ethoheptazine Citrate

ZACTANE® Tablets, 75 mg (equiv. to 44 mg of base) in bottles of 100. **(Wyeth)**

Combinations

ZACTIRIN® Tablets, 75 mg with aspirin, 325 mg in bottles of 48 and 1000. **(Wyeth)**

ZACTIRIN COMPOUND-100 Tablets, 100 mg with aspirin, 227 mg; phenacetin, 162 mg and caffeine, 32.4 mg in bottles of 100 and 1000 and in Redipak® (strip-pack) cartons of 100. **(Wyeth)**

Ⓒ EQUAGESIC® Tablets, 75 mg with meprobamate, 150 mg and aspirin, 250 mg in bottles of 50 and in Redipak (strip-pack) cartons of 25 and 100. **(Wyeth)**

ETHOPROPAZINE HYDROCHLORIDE: see The Phenothiazines

ETHOSUXIMIDE

Chemical Name: 2-Ethyl-2-methylsuccinimide.

Description: Ethosuximide is an anticonvulsant succinimide structurally and pharmacologically related to phensuximide and to methsuximide. It occurs as a white, waxy solid practically insoluble in water.

The site and mode of action remain vague; the frequency of epileptiform attacks is reduced apparently by depressing the motor cortex and raising the threshold of the CNS to convulsive stimuli.

Readily and completely absorbed from the gastrointestinal tract, the drug reaches maximum plasma concentration in 1 to 7 hours after ingestion. The average biological half-life is approximately 30 hours in children and 60 hours in adults. Ethosuximide is not significantly bound to plasma proteins, and about 10 to 20% is excreted unchanged in the urine; the remainder is metabolized by hepatic microsomal enzymes to various metabolites of which the inactive hydroxyethyl derivative accounts for almost 40% of the administered drug.

Animal reproduction studies have shown an increase in the number of stillbirths and ossification defects in neonatal rodents.

Indications: For the control of petit mal epilepsy. When petit mal coexists with grand mal and other forms of epilepsy, ethosuximide may be given in combination with other anticonvulsants in an effort to control the seizures.

Contraindications: In patients with a history of hypersensitivity to succinimides.

Warnings: Blood dyscrasias, including some with fatal outcome, have been reported to be associated with ethosuximide; therefore, periodic blood studies should be performed. The drug should be used with extreme caution in patients with known hepatic or renal disease or dysfunction; routine urinalyses and frequent liver function studies are advisable. Clinical reports suggest that the use of anticonvulsant drugs in pregnant women may have a teratogenic effect on the unborn child. While a definite cause and effect relationship has not been firmly established, it is recommended that the medication be discontinued prior to and during pregnancy, primarily in patients in whom withdrawal would not pose a serious threat. However, treatment with these drugs should not be interrupted in patients inclined to major seizures because of the strong possibility of precipitating status epilepticus with its attendant hypoxia and risk to both mother and fetus. At present, it is not known whether or not even minor seizures incur some hazard to the developing embryo or fetus. Patients should be cautioned that in the event of drowsiness, they should not perform any hazardous operation requiring alertness or skill. Instances of systemic lupus erythematosus have been reported.

Precautions: When used alone in mixed types of epilepsy, ethosuximide may increase the frequency of grand mal attacks. Dosage must be individualized according to the patient's response and tolerance, and plasma drug levels should be monitored regularly in order to obtain maximal seizure control with minimal side effects. Abrupt withdrawal may precipitate petit mal status.

Adverse Reactions: *Gastrointestinal System:* Gastrointestinal symptoms occur frequently and include anorexia, vague gastric upset, nausea and vomiting, cramps, epigastric and abdominal pain, weight loss, and diarrhea. *Hemopoietic System:* Hemopoietic complications include leukopenia, agranulocytosis, pancytopenia, aplastic anemia, and eosinophilia. *Nervous System:* Neurologic and sensory reactions are manifested by drowsiness, headache, dizziness, euphoria, hiccups, irritability, hyperactivity, lethargy, fatigue, and ataxia. Psychiatric or psychological aberrations such as disturbances of sleep, night terrors, inability to concentrate, and aggressiveness have been reported. These effects may be noted particularly in patients who have previously exhibited psychological abnormalities. There have been rare reports of paranoid psychosis, increased libido, and increased state of depression with overt suicidal intentions. *Integumentary System:* Dermatologic manifestations include urticaria, Stevens-Johnson syndrome, systemic lupus erythematosus, and pruritic erythematous rashes. *Miscellaneous:* Other reactions noted were myopia, vaginal bleeding, swelling of the tongue, gum hypertrophy, and hirsutism.

Dosage and Administration: *Orally.* Initially for children 3 to 6 years of age, 250 mg daily. For adults and children over 6 years of age, 500 mg daily. The daily dose may then be increased by increments of 250 mg every 4 to 7 days until control is achieved with minimal side effects. If it becomes necessary to increase the daily dosage beyond 1 to 1.5 gm, it should be done slowly, and the patient's response carefully evaluated.

Availability:
ZARONTIN®: **(Parke-Davis)**
Capsules, 250 mg in bottles of 100.
Syrup, 250 mg/5 ml in bottles of 1 pint.

ETHOTOIN

Chemical Name: 3-Ethyl-5-phenylhydantoin.

Description: A synthetic drug, it is a useful anticonvulsant in the treatment of grand mal epilepsy. It exerts an anticonvulsant effect without causing CNS depression. Duration of activity was found to be 3 to 4 hours, and the principal site of metabolism is the liver. On a weight to weight basis with many common anticonvulsants, it is less effective but considerably less toxic. Since ethotoin may not always provide complete control of seizures, it is often administered concomitantly with other anticonvulsant drugs.

Indications: For the control of grand mal epilepsy and in psychomotor seizures.

Contraindications: In patients with hepatic abnormalities or hematologic disorders.

Warnings: Recent reports strongly suggest an association between the use of anticonvulsant drugs and an increased incidence of birth defects in the offspring. Therefore, use during pregnancy, lactation or in women of childbearing age requires that the potential benefits be weighed against possible hazards to the patient and fetus. It is strongly advised that anticonvulsant therapy not be discontinued in patients in whom the drug is administered to prevent major seizures because of the potential of precipitating status epilepticus with attendant hypoxia, and risk to both the mother and the unborn child. Consideration should, nevertheless, be given to discontinuation of anticonvulsants prior to and during gestation when the nature, frequency and severity of the seizures do not constitute a serious threat to the patient. At present, it is not known whether even minor seizures pose some risk to the developing embryo or fetus.

Precautions: Blood counts and urinalyses should be performed when therapy is initiated and at monthly intervals for several months thereafter; also liver function studies should be done. Its use in combination with other drugs known to adversely affect the hematopoietic system should be avoided, and physicians should be alert for general malaise, sore throat, and other symptoms indicative of early blood dyscrasias. Medication should be discontinued, if signs of liver damage or a marked depression of the blood count occurs. Folic acid metabolism may be affected, precipitating a megaloblastic anemia; if this occurs during gestation, supplemental folic acid should be considered. Considerable caution should be exercised if ethotoin is administered concurrently with phenacemide, since paranoid symptoms have occurred with use of this combination. For other potential drug interactions, see monograph on Phenytoin. Neonatal hemorrhage has occurred in infants born to mothers treated with anticonvulsant drugs. It has been suggested that vitamin K be given prophylactically to such infants at birth.

Adverse Reactions: Occasionally, nausea, vomiting, fatigue, insomnia, dizziness, headache, diplopia, nystagmus, skin rash, numbness, fever, diarrhea and chest pain have occurred. Rarely noted were ataxia and gum hypertrophy. Some cases of systemic lupus erythematosus, and lymphadenopathy have occurred. Therefore, if a lymphoma-like syndrome develops, the drug should be withdrawn and the patient closely observed for regression of symptoms before treatment is resumed. Overdosage is manifested by drowsiness, visual disturbances, nausea, and ataxia, and excessive doses by coma. Treatment is initiated by inducing emesis, although gastric lavage may be considered as an alternative. General supportive measures will be necessary. A careful evaluation of blood-forming organs should be made following recovery.

Dosage and Administration: *Orally,* in 4 to 6 divided doses daily. The drug should be taken after meals and doses should be spaced as evenly as possible. Initial dosage should not be more than 1 gm daily for adults, 0.75 gm for children. The usual adult maintenance dosage is 2 to 3 gm daily; less than 2 gm has been found ineffective. Daily dosages of 0.5 to 1 gm have been found effective in children, but 2 to 3 gm have also been necessary. When used after another anticonvulsant drug, the other drug should not be discontinued but should be reduced gradually, as ethotoin is increased.

Availability:
PEGANONE® Tablets, 250 and 500 mg in bottles of 100. **(Abbott)**

ETHOXAZENE HYDROCHLORIDE

Chemical Name: 4-[(*p*-Ethoxyphenyl)azo]-*m*-phenylenediamine hydrochloride.

Description: An azo dye structurally similar to phenazopyridine hydrochloride, it occurs as a reddish powder insoluble in water.

In common with phenazopyridine, ethoxazene may exhibit some bacteriostatic effect in vitro but imparts little or no antibacterial activity to the urine after oral administration. Its chief value lies in its local anesthetic action on urinary tract mucosa; it provides rapid relief of pain while sulfonamides, streptomycin or other antibiotics are being employed.

Indications: Relief of pain associated with acute or chronic urinary tract infections, particularly cystitis, urethritis and pyelitis.

Contraindications: Severe liver disease, chronic glomerulonephritis, uremia, and in pyelonephritis of pregnancy with gastrointestinal disturbances.

Precautions: Should be used with caution in all gastrointestinal conditions. Patients should be forewarned that ethoxazene colors the urine orange or red.

Dosage and Administration: *Orally,* before meals. Adults and children 8 years of age or over, 1 tablet 3 times daily. Children under 8 years of age, 1 tablet twice daily.

Availability:
SERENIUM® Tablets, 100 mg in bottles of 50. **(Squibb)**

ETHOXZOLAMIDE

Chemical Name: 6-Ethoxybenzothiazole-2-sulfonamide.

Description: Ethoxzolamide is an orally effective carbonic anhydrase inhibitor structurally and pharmacologically related to acetazolamide and occurs as a white, odorless, tasteless powder insoluble in water and soluble in alcohol. Weight for weight, ethoxzolamide is about twice as potent as acetazolamide.

In addition to suppressing the enzyme, carbonic anhydrase, in the renal tubules, ethoxzolamide also suppresses carbonic anhydrase in the ciliary body of the eye, thus decreasing the aqueous inflow and reducing intraocular pressure. By its action it increases the excretion of sodium, potassium and bicarbonate ions with diuresis. Its effectiveness in reducing intraocular pressure is also believed to be associated with decreased formation of bicarbonate in the secretory process in the ciliary body with resultant lowered osmotic pressure in the posterior chamber of the eye. Also, carbonic anhydrase inhibitors reduce the incidence of convulsive attacks in epileptic patients. Following oral administration, maximal plasma levels are reached in about 2 hours; its activity persists for 8 to 12 hours. Its metabolic rate has not been determined.

Indications: Treatment of chronic simple (open-angle) glaucoma, preoperative acute congestive (narrow-angle) glaucoma, preoperative chronic congestive glaucoma, acute secondary glaucoma, and in preoperative control of intraocular pressure. Because it increases the excretion of sodium, potassium and bicarbonate ions, it has been used as a diuretic in the prevention and treatment of edema associated with congestive heart failure. It has also been used in the treatment of epilepsy.

Contraindications: Idiopathic renal hyperchloremic acidosis, renal failure, hyponatremia, hypokalemia, Addison's disease.

Warnings: Studies with ethoxzolamide in rats and mice have demonstrated teratogenic and embryocidal effects at exceedingly large doses. Although evidence of these effects in clinical use is lacking, the drug should not be used during gestation, especially during the first 3 months, unless the clinical situation justifies the risk, and then only with extreme caution.

Precautions: It is advised that caution be used in patients with hepatic cirrhosis, and with advanced pulmonary disease with impaired respiratory capacities and elevated pCO_2 values. Electrolyte balance should be assessed frequently.

Adverse Reactions: Adverse effects most frequently encountered include polyuria, nausea, occasional dizziness, paresthesia of the fingers, toes or mucocutaneous junctions of the lips and anus, and diarrhea. Other less frequent adverse responses include drowsiness, fatigue, headache, anorexia, dry mouth, tinnitus, dysuria, disorientation, confusion, globus hystericus, ataxia, lassitude, depression, tremor, and mild skin eruptions. As with other carbonic anhydrase inhibitors, the possibility of agranulocytosis, thrombocytopenia, and the formation of renal calculi should be kept in mind.

Dosage and Administration: *Orally. Glaucoma*: 62.5 to 250 mg concomitantly with miotics 2 to 4 times daily. If the response is unsatisfactory, the drug should be discontinued or supplemented as indicated. In *congestive heart failure* and *edema,* 62.5 to 250 mg after breakfast for 3 days, wait 4 days, and repeat cycle, or alternatively, administer every other day.

Availability:
CARDRASE® Tablets, 125 mg in bottles of 100. **(Upjohn)**
ETHAMIDE® Tablets, 125 mg in bottles of 100. **(Allergan)**

ETHYLESTRENOL

Chemical Name: 17 α-Ethylestr-4-en17β-ol.

Description: Ethylestrenol is a member of a series of synthetic 3-deoxo nortestosterone steroids characterized by the absence of an oxygen atom at carbon 3. The removal of the oxygen atom from this position has resulted in a reduction of androgenic activity with the retention and enhancement of anabolic properties. Because of this structural alteration, it is claimed that ethylestrenol is about 19 times more effective than methyltestosterone and about 6 times more effective than norethandrolone. Ethylestrenol occurs as a white, crystalline powder practically insoluble in water and soluble in alcohol.

Indications: Management of a broad range of conditions amenable to therapy with anabolic agents. Therapy is most effective when combined with a good dietary regimen, adequate amounts of nutrients including vitamins, minerals and proteins. The drug exhibits all the classic properties of anabolic agents including the promotion of tissue building and weight gain, stimulation of appetite and euphoria, renewed vigor, as an aid in bone matrix reconstitution and in combating the depression and weakness of chronic illness or prolonged convalescence. It can also prevent or reverse certain catabolic effects associated with corticosteroid therapy.

Contraindications: In male patients with known or suspected prostatic carcinoma, in those with benign prostatic hypertrophy with obstructive symptoms, in carcinoma of the male breast, in patients with nephroses or the nephrotic phase of nephritis, in those with a history of hypersensitivity or toxic reaction to the drug, in patients with cardiac, hepatic or renal decompensation, hypercalcemia, impairment of liver function, in prepubertal males, and in patients easily stimulated. It should not be given to pregnant or lactating women, because masculinization of the female fetus or the breast-fed infant may occur.

Warnings: Anabolic agents will not enhance athletic ability. Female patients, particularly those who may be overly sensitive to the drug, should be carefully observed for signs of virilization (hoarseness or deepening of the voice, oily skin, acne, hirsutism, enlarged clitoris, stimulation of libido, and menstrual irregularities). Some of these changes, such as voice changes, may be irreversible even after withdrawal of the drug. Therapy should be discontinued if hypercalcemia occurs in patients who are immobilized or in those with breast cancer.

Precautions: In common with other anabolic steroids, this drug may produce reversible biochemical signs of hepatic dysfunction, usually manifested by increased BSP retention, elevated transaminase levels or bilirubin values. These changes, in the absence of clinical evidence of liver disease, suggest that these agents exert a peculiar effect on the excretory system of the liver and are not essentially hepatotoxic. If jaundice or other signs of hepatic dysfunction are noted, the drug should be discontinued. Any drug-induced menstrual irregularities which may occur should disappear upon cessation of therapy and resumption of normal cycling. Androgenic-anabolic steroids have been reported to increase prothrombin time response in patients receiving anticoagulants and may thus precipitate hemorrhagic complications. They have also been shown to alter glucose tolerance tests; consequently, diabetic patients should be followed carefully and the dosage of insulin or oral hypoglycemic agent should be adjusted accordingly. Because of its hypercholesterolemic effects, caution is required when administering this drug to patients with a history of myocardial infarction or coronary artery disease. Additionally, serial determinations of serum cholesterol should be performed at regular intervals and therapy adjusted in accordance with the clinical response. Edema may occur due to the retention of sodium and water; this complication may be further provoked by the concomitant administration of adrenal corticosteroids or ACTH. Careful observation of patients receiving this combination of drugs is essential. Cautious use of this drug in young boys is advised in order to avoid possible premature epiphyseal closure or precocious sexual development. If priapism occurs, the drug should be withdrawn.

Adverse Reactions: The following have been observed with anabolic-androgen preparations in general and may or may not occur with ethylestrenol. They include oligospermia, decreased ejaculatory volume, inhibition of testicular function, testicular atrophy, impotence, epididymitis, bladder irritability, hypercalcemia (particularly in patients with metastatic breast carcinoma, usually indicative of progression of bone metastases), sodium and water retention, priapism, gynecomastia, virilization in the female, menstrual irregularities, hypersensitivity reactions including rash and dermatitis, rarely, anaphylactoid reaction. Alterations may occur in the following clinical laboratory tests: metyrapone test, fasting blood sugar and glucose tolerance test, thyroid function test (decrease in PBI, thyroxine-binding capacity and radioactive iodine uptake, and an increase in T^3 uptake by the red blood cells or resin; free thyroxine levels remain normal and the altered tests usually persist for 2 to 3 weeks after discontinuing anabolic therapy), electrolyte imbalance (retention of sodium, chloride, water, potassium, calcium, and inorganic phosphates), blood coagulation tests (increase in clotting factors II, V, VII and X), and miscellaneous laboratory tests (decreased creatinine and creatinine excretion lasting up to 2 weeks after discontinuing therapy and increased 17-ketosteroid excretion). The following have been reported to occur in both male and female patients: increased or decreased libido, flushing of the skin, acne (especially in females and prepubertal males), habituation, excitation and insomnia, chills, leukopenia, bleeding in patients on concomitant anticoagulant therapy, and premature closure of epiphyses in children. Oral preparations have been associated with nausea, vomiting, diarrhea, as well as with symptoms resembling those of peptic ulcer.

Dosage and Administration: *Orally.* Adults: The average patient will respond, in terms of weight gain and subjective response, to a daily dosage of 4 mg. As a guide to correct dosage, it should be emphasized that the drug will produce an anabolic effect in daily dosage which need not exceed 0.1 mg/kg of body weight. Some patients may require 6 or 8 mg daily, at least initially. The higher dosage should be reduced following a satisfactory response. For children, the average dosage is 2 mg daily; however, this will vary depending upon the age and size of the child and the nature of the underlying disease. In general, satisfactory responses will be noted in most children within a range of 1 to 3 mg daily.

Availability:
MAXIBOLIN®: **(Organon)**
Elixir, 2 mg/5 ml in bottles of 120 ml.
Tablets, 2 mg in bottles of 100.

ETHYNODIOL DIACETATE + ETHINYL ESTRADIOL

Description: Each tablet contains 1 mg of the progestogen, ethynodiol diacetate, and 0.05 mg of the estrogen, ethinyl estradiol. Together they prevent ovulation by inhibiting the output of gonadotropins from the pituitary gland. They depress the output of both the follicle stimulating hormome (FSH) and the luteinizing hormone (LH).

The lower than usual estrogen content provides added assurance in today's climate of increased concern that the incidence and severity of adverse reactions can be minimized.

Important Note: Clinical studies have revealed an increased risk of thromboembolic disease associated with the use of hormonal contraceptives. Patients over 40 years of age, or those who smoke, or who have a history of preeclampsia toxemia, hypercholesterolemia, diabetes, hypertension, or obesity have a greater risk of developing fatal or nonfatal myocardial infarction. Although the potential carcinogenic effect of estrogens has not been substantiated, close clinical surveillance of all women taking oral contraceptives must be undertaken.

Indications: Prevention of pregnancy.

Contraindications: Past history or presence of thrombophlebitis, thromboembolic disorders or cerebrovascular accident; known or suspected carcinoma of the breast; impaired liver function; undiagnosed abnormal vaginal bleeding and in known or suspected estrogen-dependent neoplasia.

Warnings: Medications should be discontinued immediately if any of the following conditions exist or are suspect: thrombotic and thromboembolic disorders such as thrombophlebitis, cerebrovascular disorders including hemorrhage, and pulmonary embolism; sudden partial or complete loss of vision; sudden onset of proptosis, diplopia or migraine; papilledema or retinal vascular lesions. It is generally recognized that cigarette smoking increases the risk of serious cardiovascular complications, particularly in women over 35 years of age; therefore, women should be strongly advised not to smoke while taking this drug. Since fetal abnormalities have been reported to occur in the offspring of women who have taken progesterone and/or estrogens during pregnancy, the safe use of oral contraceptives in pregnant patients has not been confirmed; therefore, pregnancy should be ruled out before continuing the contraceptive program in any patient who has missed 2 consecutive periods. If the patient has not adhered to the prescribed schedule, the possibility of pregnancy should be considered when the first period is missed. A small fraction of the hormones has been found in the milk of mothers taking oral contraceptives. The long-range effect on the nursing infant has not been determined to date. Also reported during short-term as well as long-term use of oral contraceptives were hepatic lesions (adenomas, hepatomas, hamartomas, regenerating nodules, etc.), occasionally fatal, which may present as an abdominal mass or with the signs and symptoms of an acute abdominal condition. These lesions should be suspected if the patient complains of abdominal pain or shows signs of intraabdominal bleeding.

Precautions: The drug should not be given to nursing mothers because of the possible estrogenic responses in the infant. Before initiating therapy, physical examination of the breast and pelvic organs and a Papanicolaou smear should be performed. Treatment should be discontinued for 2 months before endocrine and liver function tests are undertaken. Use with caution in patients with a history of psychic depression, and in those with a history of metabolic disease or conditions that might be aggravated by possible estrogen-induced fluid retention, such as epilepsy, migraine, asthma, and cardiac and renal dysfunctions. Preexisting uterine fibromyomas may increase in size during therapy and patients with these tumors should be examined periodically. If breakthrough bleeding persists, nonfunctional causes should be considered. Because ethynodiol may cause a decrease in glucose tolerance, the status of patients with overt diabetes should be evaluated frequently. Women should be advised of the possibility of an increase in the amount of estrogen-induced cervical mucus. It should be used judiciously in young patients in whom bone growth is not complete.

Adverse Reactions: The following were reported with varying degrees of incidence: thrombophlebitis, pulmonary embolism, cerebrovascular accidents with hemorrhage, retinal thrombosis and optic neuritis, hepatic lesions with or without intraabdominal bleeding, gallbladder disease, nausea, vomiting, gastrointestinal symptoms such as abdominal cramps and bloating, breakthrough bleeding, spotting, change in menstrual flow, amenorrhea during and after treatment, edema, chloasma or melasma, breast changes (tenderness, enlargement, and secretion), decrease or increase in weight, vaginitis, changes in cervical erosion and cervical secretions, suppression of lactation when given immediately postpartum, cholestatic jaundice, migraine, rash (allergic), rise in blood pressure, mental depression, anovulation (posttreatment), premenstrual-like syndrome, changes in libido, changes in appetite, cystitis-like syndrome, headache, nervousness, dizziness, fatigue, backache, hirsutism, loss of scalp hair, erythema multiforme, erythema nodosum, hemorrhagic eruption, itching; the following laboratory tests may be altered by the use of this drug: liver function (increased BSP and other values); increased prothrombin, Factors VII, VIII, IX and X; increased PBI and butanol-extractable PBI and decreased T^3 values; metyrapone test and the pregnanediol determination.

Dosage and Administration: *Orally.* Starting on any given day, 1 tablet daily for 21 consecutive days, then 7 days off. This schedule is repeated cycle after cycle. For specific details, consult package literature.

Availability:
DEMULEN®-21 Tablets, 1 mg in Compack® Dispensers of 21 in cartons of 126 (6 × 21); refills (12 × 21) in cartons of 252 (12 × 21) and (48 × 21) in cartons of 1008 (48 × 21). **(Searle)**
Triopak™ Containers (10). Each Triopak contains 1 Compack and 2 refills.
DEMULEN-28® Tablets, 1 mg (21 white and 7 pink placebos) in Compack Dispensers of 28 in cartons of 168 (6 × 28); refills (12 × 28) in cartons of 336. **(Searle)**
Triopak™ Containers (10). Each Triopak contains 1 Compack and 2 refills.

ETIDOCAINE HYDROCHLORIDE

Chemical Name: (±)-2-(*N*-Ethylpropylamino)-2′,-6′-butyroxylidide hydrochloride.

Description: A synthetic local anesthetic of the amide type, etidocaine is similar in chemical structure and pharmacological action to lidocaine. Additionally, it possesses a greater degree of lipid solubility and protein binding capacity, and also provides a longer duration of analgesic action. In common with other local anesthetics, the drug blocks transmission of nerve impulses by stabilizing the neuronal membrane potential, thus preventing the initiation and conduction of nerve impulses.

Following administration, onset of action occurs within 3 to 5 minutes and usually lasts for 5 to 10 hours. In peridural nerve block, the drug has been found to produce a profound degree of motor blockade and abdominal muscle relaxation with a duration of analgesic action 1.5 to 2 times longer than that produced by lidocaine. In addition, the difference in analgesic duration between etidocaine and lidocaine may be even greater following peripheral nerve blockade than following central nerve block. Also, the duration of analgesia is prolonged, often extending beyond 9 hours, when used for peripheral nerve blocks such as brachial plexus blockade.

Due to its high tissue solubility, the drug is rapidly distributed following absorption from the injection site. Its volume of tissue distribution has been reported to be larger than that seen with comparable local anesthetic agents. It is metabolized in the liver at a rate similar to that of lidocaine, and is excreted by the kidney with little unchanged drug appearing in the urine. Animal studies apparently indicate that no single metabolite will account for more than 10% of the administered dose. Clinical studies to date demonstrate that etidocaine does not produce either methemoglobinemia or tissue irritation.

Indications: Recommended for percutaneous infiltration anesthesia, peripheral nerve blocks, and central neural blocks such as caudal or epidural blocks.

Contraindications: History of hypersensitivity to local anesthetic agents of the amide type.

Since the warnings, precautions and adverse reactions are generally those associated with other amide type of local anesthetics, see monographs on Lidocaine Hydrochloride, Mepivacaine Hydrochloride and Prilocaine Hydrochloride.

Dosage and Administration: The dosage varies considerably and depends upon the area to be anesthetized, the vascularity of the tissues, the number of neuronal segments to be blocked, the type of regional anesthetic technique and the status and tolerance of the individual patient. Although single injections of 450 mg have been employed for regional anesthesia without observable adverse effects, at present, it is strongly recommended that the maximal dose of a single injection should not exceed 400 mg (approx. 5.5 mg/kg or 2.7 mg/lb) when used in combination with epinephrine 1:200,000 or 300 mg (approx. 4 mg/kg or 2 mg/lb) when used without epinephrine. Incremental doses may be repeated at intervals of 2 to 3 hours. The following dosages of etidocaine with epinephrine 1:200,000 generally have proved satisfactory and are therefore suggested as a guide. *For percutaneous infiltration,* from 1 to 80 ml of an 0.5% solution. *For peripheral nerve block,* from 5 to 80 ml of an 0.5% solution or 5 to 40 ml of a 1% solution. *For central neural block,* from 10 to 30 ml of a 1% solution or 10 to 20 ml of a 1.5% solution. *For vaginal obstetrical and gynecologic procedures,* from 10 to 30 ml of an 0.5% solution or 5 to 20 ml of a 1% solution. *For caudal block,* from 10 to 30 ml of an 0.5 or 1% solution. Dosage should be reduced for elderly or debilitated patients and for those with severe renal disease. **Important Note:** Since toxicity is influenced by the rate of administration, it is recommended that injection into vascular areas be made *slowly.*

Availability:
DURANEST® Injection, 0.5% with or without epinephrine 1:200,000 in vials of 30 ml and with epinephrine in vials of 50 ml; 1% with or without epinephrine in vials and ampuls of 30 ml; 1.5% with epinephrine in ampuls of 20 ml. **(Astra)**

ETIDRONATE DISODIUM

Chemical Name: 1-Hydroxyethylidene diphosphonic acid disodium.

Description: Etidronate disodium is a unique, oral osteochemotherapeutic agent designated for the treatment of symptomatic Paget's disease. The drug inhibits bone resorption and abnormal new bone formation, by modifying the crystal growth of calcium hydroxyapatite, resulting in a fall in elevated urinary hydroxyproline excretion and elevated serum alkaline phosphatase levels. These biochemical changes appear to correspond to changes toward more normal bone formation as shown by a reduction in bone turnover as well as a reduction in the uptake of radionuclide bone-imaging agents at active pagetic bone sites. Besides relieving bone pain and improving mobility, the drug also reduces the hypervascularity of affected bone, thereby diminishing the abnormally elevated cardiac output associated with active pagetic conditions. This leads to a reduction in temperature over superficially located bone lesions. However, hyperphosphatemia (reversible), which appears to be drug-induced, has been observed, but apparently this phenomenon does not require discontinuation of the medication. This occurrence appears to be the result of increased tubular reabsorption of phosphate by the kidney, and serum values in excess of 7 mg% have been observed with high doses. No adverse effects have been noted and the serum phosphate levels generally return to normal about 2 to 4 weeks after discontinuing treatment. Depending on concentration, the drug may also either inhibit crystal resorption or crystal growth. Accumulation of unmineralized osteoid has been frequently observed in patients taking the recommended clinical regimen. Therapy with etidronate disodium does not appear to be accompanied by clinically significant changes in serum parathyroid hormone or serum calcium levels. It occurs as a white powder, has a molecular weight of 250, and is highly soluble in water. Since no metabolic process takes place, it is excreted intact by the kidneys. Absorption from the gastrointestinal tract is dose-dependent and averages about 1% at 5 mg/kg of body weight, 2.5% at 10 mg/kg, and 6% at 20 mg/kg administered daily. Most of the absorbed drug is cleared from the blood within 6 hours, and within 24 hours approximately ½ is excreted in the urine with the remainder chemically absorbed on the bone which is then slowly eliminated.

Indications: Treatment of symptomatic Paget's disease of bone (osteitis deformans). Clinical effectiveness has been demonstrated primarily in patients with polyostotic pagetic lesions.

Contraindications: None known.

Warnings: Adherence to the recommended dose regimen is advised in order to avoid overtreatment. Although the initial response may be very slow, it may then continue for months after the drug has been discontinued. Consequently, dosage should not be increased prematurely nor should treatment be resumed before there is convincing evidence of reactivation of the disease process, and then retreatment should not be instituted until the patient has had at least a 3-month drug-free interval. Because the incidence of osteogenic sarcoma is known to be increased in Paget's disease, pagetic lesions, with or without therapy, may appear on x-ray to progress markedly, possibly with some loss of definition of periosteal margins. Therefore, such lesions should be evaluated carefully to differentiate them from osteogenic sarcoma.

Precautions: Etidronate disodium retards mineralization of osteoid formed during the accretion process. This effect is dose and time dependent. Extended periods of medication should be approached cautiously, since some patients receiving higher doses may show an overlap of beneficial and mineralization inhibition effects. When administered at a dose of 20 mg/kg/day, the drug suppresses bone turnover and essentially halts mineralization of new bone in pagetic lesions, and, to a lesser extent, in the uninvolved skeleton, although mineralization generally proceeds normally after discontinuation of treatment. The patient's nutritional intake, particularly calcium and vitamin D intake should be adequate, since they may be particularly sensitive to drugs that affect calcium homeostasis; also patients with impaired renal function should be approached very carefully, if at all, as well as those with enterocolitis because of increased frequency of bowel movements and diarrhea which can occur at doses of 20 mg/kg/day and sometimes at a lower dose regimen. The drug should be used only when clearly needed in women who are or who may become pregnant. There are no data available to support the use of the drug in children; also, nursing should not be undertaken while the patient is taking this medication.

Adverse Reactions: Increased or recurrent bone pain at existing pagetic sites and/or the appearance of pain at sites previously asymptomatic occurred in 1 out of 10 patients receiving 5 mg/kg/day, and in 2 out of 10 patients receiving higher doses; however, the pain resolved while therapy was continued in some patients but persisted for several months in others. The risk of fractures, a common feature in Paget's disease, may be increased when 20 mg/kg/day of the drug is given in a time-span exceeding 3 months. This risk may be greater in patients with extensive and severe disease, a history of multiple fractures, and/or rapidly advancing osteolytic lesions. It is recommended that the drug be discontinued when fractures occur and that therapy not be reinstated until healing of the fracture has been completed. Gastrointestinal problems such as diarrhea, loose bowel movement, and nausea are increased in some patients when given doses greater than 5 mg/kg/day. The incidence is about 1 out of 15 and rises to about 2 out of 10 patients when given doses of 20 mg/kg/day. Hypocalcemia may occur with overdosage.

Dosage and Administration: *Orally.* The recommended initial dose is 5 mg/kg/day for no more than 6 months. Doses greater than 10 mg/kg/day should be reserved for use when there is an overriding requirement for suppression of increased bone turnover in Paget's disease or when the patient requires more prompt reduction of elevated cardiac output. In any event, doses above 10 mg/kg/day should not be given for longer than 3 months, and doses in excess of 20 mg/kg/day are not recommended. The dose should be administered as a single dose 2 hours before meals with fruit juice or water. As a guide to therapy and patient's response, urinary hydroxyproline excretion and/or serum alkaline phosphatase levels should be monitored periodically during the course of treatment.

Availability:
DIDRONEL® Tablets, 200 mg in bottles of 250. **(Proctor & Gamble)**

EXTRALIN

Description: *Extralin* is a liver-stomach concentrate resulting from the interaction of a liver extract and stomach tissue. Each capsule contains 50 mg of the concentrate.

Each capsule of *Extralin B* contains: liver-stomach concentrate, 67 mg; vitamin B-12 activity equivalent, 3 mcg; thiamine hydrochloride, 1 mg and riboflavin, 0.25 mg. Other vitamin B complex factors also are present in the liver-stomach concentrate.

Each capsule of *Extralin F* contains: special liver-stomach concentrate (containing intrinsic factor), 390 mg; cobalamin concentrate equivalent to cobalamin, 15 mcg and folic acid, 1 mg. The total vitamin B-12 activity in the special liver-stomach concentrate, and the cobalamin concentrate, is 30 mcg.

Indications: Both *Extralin* and *Extralin B* are effective in the treatment of pernicious anemia. *Extralin F* is effective in the treatment of pernicious anemia and other megaloblastic anemias.

Contraindications: Hypersensitivity to any of the components.

Precautions: In cases of vitamin B-12 deficiency anemia associated with malabsorption syndrome, or in those cases of pernicious anemia in which resistance is encountered to the potentiation of absorption of physiologic doses of vitamin B-12, parenteral therapy, or oral therapy with massive doses of vitamin B-12, may be necessary for adequate treatment. The status of the patient is the final criterion for judging adequacy of treatment. Periodic clinical and laboratory studies are considered essential. The use of folic acid without adequate vitamin B-12 therapy in patients with pernicious anemia may result in hematologic remission but neurologic progression.

Dosage and Administration: *Orally.* The usual dosage of *Extralin* is 4 capsules 3 times daily with meals; of *Extralin B,* 3 capsules 3 times daily with meals. One capsule of *Extralin F* produces a standard response in the average uncomplicated case of pernicious anemia and other megaloblastic anemias.

Availability:
EXTRALIN® Capsules (Pulvules®) in bottles of 84. **(Lilly)**
EXTRALIN® B Capsules in bottles of 84. **(Lilly)**
EXTRALIN® F Capsules in bottles of 30. **(Lilly)**

FENFLURAMINE HYDROCHLORIDE Ⓒ IV

Chemical Name: N-ethyl-α-methyl-m-(trifluoromethyl) phenethylamine hydrochloride.

Description: Fenfluramine, an anorectic agent, is a phenethylamine compound (with some sympathomimetic properties) that is related chemically to the amphetamines; it differs pharmacologically in that it appears to display little or no stimulatory effects on the CNS. The drug has been reported to possess sedative or tranquilizing properties. At clinically effective doses, the drug exhibits the desired anorexiant properties of the prototype compound. This anorectic effect usually diminishes after a few weeks.

Fenfluramine has shown potential embryoteratogenic effects in rats. However, additional reproduction studies in rabbits, mice and monkeys yielded negative results.

Indications: A short-term (a few weeks) adjunctive agent in the management of exogenous obesity in conjunction with a medically supervised regimen of weight reduction based on caloric restriction.

Contraindications: Glaucoma; hypersensitivity to fenfluramine or other sympathomimetic amines; during or within 14 days following the administration of monoamine oxidase inhibitors (MAOI) since a hypertensive crisis may result; and patients with a history of drug abuse or alcoholism.

Warnings: Tolerance to the anorectic effect usually develops within a few weeks. When this occurs, the maximum recommended dose should not be exceeded in an attempt to increase the effect, rather the drug should be discontinued. Because of the drug's effect on the CNS, patients should be cautioned, that in the event of drowsiness, they should not engage in activities requiring alertness or skill. The possibility that fenfluramine may produce physical and psychological dependence should be considered when evaluating the desirability of including the drug in the weight reduction programs of individual patients. Alcoholic patients may respond with paranoia, depression, and psychosis. Safe use in pregnant women and in children under 12 years of age has not been established.

Precautions: Physicians should be aware that the effects of concomitant administration of fenfluramine with other CNS-acting drugs may be potentiated; also, patients with a history of mental depression may experience an exacerbation of the depression. The effect of antihypertensive drugs such as guanethidine, methyldopa, and reserpine may be slightly increased. Although the drug may be used in mild hypertension with monitoring of blood pressure, it is not recommended for use in severe hypertension or in the presence of symptomatic heart disease including arrhythmias.

Adverse Reactions: Those not associated with other anorectic drugs, but have been reported to occur with fenfluramine are diarrhea, sedation, and depression. The most common reactions reported were drowsiness, diarrhea, and dryness of mouth; less frequently reported were: *CNS:* Dizziness; confusion; incoordination; headache; euphoria; depression; anxiety, nervousness or tension; insomnia; weakness or fatigue; increased or decreased libido; agitation; dysarthria. *Gastrointestinal:* Constipation; abdominal pain; nausea. *Autonomic:* Sweating; chills; blurred vision. *Genitourinary:* Dysuria; urinary frequency. *Cardiovascular:* Palpitation; hypotension; hypertension; fainting. *Dermatologic:* Skin rash; urticaria; burning sensation. *Miscellaneous:* Eye irritation; myalgia; fever; chest pain; bad taste. The monograph on Amphetamine should be consulted for overdosage and treatment.

Dosage and Administration: *Orally.* The initial dosage regimen is 1 tablet 3 times daily, taken before meals. The dosage thereafter should be adjusted to the needs and response of the patient. If a satisfactory anorexiant effect is not obtained and toleration has been good, the dosage may be increased at weekly intervals by 1 tablet daily until a maximum dosage of 2 tablets 3 times daily is attained. In patients in whom the initial dosage is not well tolerated, dosage may be reduced to 2 tablets daily and thereafter gradually increased in order to minimize adverse reactions.

Availability:
Ⓒ-IV PONDIMIN® Tablets, 20 mg (orange, scored) in bottles of 100 and 500. **(Robins)**

FENOPROFEN CALCIUM

Chemical Name: α-Methyl-3-phenoxybenzeneacetic acid dihydrate calcium.

Description: Fenoprofen calcium is a nonsteroidal antiinflammatory, antiarthritic compound with analgesic and antipyretic activity. A propionic acid derivative, the drug is a unique chemical entity in that it differs from aspirin, indomethacin, phenylbutazone and adrenal corticosteroids. It occurs as a white, crystalline powder that is slightly soluble in water, soluble in alcohol (95%) to the extent of about 15 mg/ml at 25°C, and insoluble in benzene.

The exact mode of action is not fully understood; however, antiinflammatory response has been found not to be due to adrenal stimulation. In studies with rats the drug was found to inhibit the development of redness and edema in acute inflammatory conditions and to reduce soft-tissue swelling and bone damage associated with chronic inflammation. Improvement in patients treated with fenoprofen for rheumatoid arthritis has been shown by a reduction in joint swelling, pain, morning stiffness and in disease activity as demonstrated by a reduction in the number of joints with limited motion, thus helping to restore function and mobility. There is no evidence that it alters the progressive course of the underlying disease.

Under fasting conditions, fenoprofen is rapidly absorbed, achieving peak plasma levels of 50 mcg/ml within 2 hours of oral administration of a 600-mg dose. It is significantly bound to serum albumin and the plasma half-life has been reported to be about 3 hours. Approximately

90% of a single oral dose is eliminated within 24 hours, primarily as fenoprofen glucuronide and 4'-hydroxyfenoprofen glucuronide. The coadministration of aspirin decreases the biologic half-life due to an increase in metabolic clearance which results in a greater amount of hydroxylated drug in the urine. Although the mechanism of the interaction of these two drugs is not known, enzyme induction or displacement of fenoprofen from plasma albumin binding sites are possibilities. Chronic administration of phenobarbital, a known enzyme inducer, may also be associated with a decrease in the drug's plasma half-life. Fenoprofen-treated patients show less suppression of collagen-induced platelet aggregation than do aspirin-treated patients. In the symptomatic treatment of arthritis, it was reported that the drug hasn't clearly shown itself to be more efficacious than aspirin, but that it is generally better tolerated with less frequent gastrointestinal upset (nausea, dyspepsia), tinnitus or impaired hearing when administered in the recommended dosage range. Whether or not it causes less peptic ulceration than does aspirin has not been established.

In-vitro studies have shown that fenoprofen, because of its affinity for albumin, may displace from their binding sites other drugs which are also albumin bound and may lead to drug interactions. Fenoprofen, as well as other nonsteroidal antiinflammatory agents, could likewise be displaced, thus making increased quantities of the free drug available which could lead to toxic results. Patients receiving hydantoin, sulfonamides, or sulfonylureas should be observed for signs of toxicity to these drugs. Since the drug is capable of displacing coumarin-type anticoagulants from their binding sites, this could lead to prolonged prothrombin time, and hemorrhage may result. Patients receiving both drugs should be under careful observation.

Indications: For relief of the signs and symptoms of rheumatoid arthritis and osteoarthritis. It is indicated in the treatment of acute flare-ups and exacerbations and in the long-term management of these diseases. May be used as the sole therapeutic agent or in combination with gold or corticosteroids. In the treatment of rheumatoid arthritis it is not recommended for patients who are in the acute stages of the disease (e.g., severely incapacited, bedridden or confined to a wheelchair) until safe and effective use has been confirmed.

Contraindications: Patients with known hypersensitivity to the drug. Fenoprofen should not be given to patients in whom aspirin and other nonsteroidal antiinflammatory drugs induce the symptoms of asthma, rhinitis, or urticaria.

Warnings: Since gastrointestinal bleeding, sometimes severe, has been reported with the use of this drug, patients with active peptic ulcer or those with a history of upper gastrointestinal tract disorders should be under close medical supervision. In such cases, attempts should be made to treat the arthritis with nonulcerogenic drugs, such as gold salts. However, if fenoprofen must be given, the patient should be carefully observed for signs of ulcer perforation or severe gastrointestinal bleeding. In subacute and chronic studies in rats, fenoprofen caused interstitial nephritis, glomerulonephritis and renal papillary necrosis. These abnormalities were found to be dose-related, and usually appeared when the dose approximated the clinical dose. In chronic studies in monkeys, interstitial nephritis also occurred, although this was seen at doses considerably above the clinical dose. Lower doses were not studied in this species. During the course of the clinical trials, one patient developed renal failure and died. Death was attributed to septicemia, bilateral suppurative pyelonephritis and renal papillary necrosis; however, it was not determined if these were drug-induced. A few patients developed mild elevations of BUN. Since the drug is eliminated primarily by the kidney, it should not be administered to patients with significantly impaired renal function. Periodic renal function tests should be performed in all patients under treatment with this drug.

Precautions: Hepatic effects ranging from alterations in liver function tests (increased serum levels of transaminase, LDH, and alkaline phosphatase) to hepatocellular hypertrophy have been reported. It is therefore recommended that periodic liver function tests be performed, and the drug withdrawn if abnormalities occur. Reproduction studies in rats have shown the drug to be associated with prolonged labor and difficult parturition when given during late pregnancy. Evidence suggests that this may be due to decreased uterine contractility probably resulting from the inhibition of prostaglandin synthesis. The safety of this drug during pregnancy and lactation has not been established, and its use during these events is not recommended. In patients receiving concomitant fenoprofen-steroid therapy, any reduction of steroid dose should be gradual to avoid the possible complications of sudden steroid withdrawal. Patients with initial low hemoglobin values who are receiving long-term treatment should have a hemoglobin determination at reasonable intervals. The drug should be used cautiously in patients with compromised cardiac function, or with impaired hearing, and in those who may be adversely affected by prolongation of the bleeding time, since fenoprofen decreases platelet aggregation. Although there have been no reports of drug-induced eye changes, it is recommended that eye examinations be performed during the initial phase of therapy and at periodic intervals thereafter. Caution should be exercised by patients whose activities require alertness or skill if they experience drowsiness, dizziness, or other manifestation of CNS-depressant effects. Until further clinical trials establish safe and effective use in children, it is not recommended for use in patients in this age group.

Adverse Reactions: The most common side effects are gastrointestinal. Dyspepsia, the most frequent, has been seen in 1 out of 7 patients. Other adverse reactions in descending order of frequency were constipation, nausea, vomiting, abdominal pain, anorexia, occult blood in the stool, diarrhea, flatulence, dry mouth. Rarely reported were peptic ulceration and/or gastrointestinal hemorrhage. Another common adverse reaction was pruritus (1 of 10) followed by rash, increased sweating, urticaria; somnolence (1 of 7) followed by dizziness, tremor, confusion, insomnia; tinnitus (1 of 10) followed by blurred vision, decreased hearing; palpitations (1 of 25) followed by tachycardia; anemia (1 of 500)—1 patient required discontinuation of therapy due to anemia—followed by increase in alkaline phosphatase, LDH, SGOT; headache (1 of 7) followed by nervousness, asthenia, dyspnea, peripheral edema, fatigue, malaise, dysuria.

Dosage and Administration: *Orally.* The recommended initial dosage for rheumatoid arthritis is 600 mg and for osteoarthritis is 300 to 600 mg 4 times daily. Many patients show improvement within a few days, but some may require an additional 2 to 3 weeks before symptoms start to diminish. Dosage should be adjusted according to the patient's condition, but more than 3200 mg/day is not advised. To receive maximal benefit, the drug should be administered 30 minutes before or at least 2 hours after meals. If gastrointestinal symptoms occur, the drug should then be taken with meals or with milk.

Availability:
NALFON®: **(Dista)**
Pulvules (capsules), 300 mg in bottles of 60 and 500.
Tablets, 600 mg in bottles of 500 and in Rx paks of 100.

FENTANYL CITRATE Ⓒ II

Chemical Name: *N*-(1-Phenethyl-4-piperidyl)propionanilide citrate.

Description: A synthetic, narcotic analgesic derived from the piperidine group of preparations. It occurs as a white, crystalline powder with a bitter taste, and is sparingly soluble in water and soluble in alcohol.

It is similar to morphine and meperidine in its pharmacologic effects, but differs in that it produces the same degree of analgesia at approximately 1/100 and 1/750 the dose respectively. It causes virtually no emesis or histamine release in dogs. However, clinical signs and symptoms typical of narcotic analgesics such as miosis, euphoria, and respiratory depression have been observed. Respiratory depression may be of sufficient degree to cause apnea. Bradycardia, muscular rigidity, and bronchial and laryngeal constriction may also be experienced. As with morphine, drug-induced bradycardia is blocked or reversed by atropine and most of its effects, including analgesia, are reversed by nalorphine hydrochloride.

The mechanism of action of fentanyl in producing analgesia has not been completely defined. It has been suggested that it suppresses pain by elevating the threshold to pain sensitivity through its thalamic and reticular activity and that it produces a feeling of indifference to pain through its cortical activity. When used preoperatively, during, and in the immediate postoperative period (recovery room) with general or regional anesthesia, fentanyl prevents or relieves pain of any type or degree.

When administered intravenously, fentanyl produces analgesia almost immediately. Peak effect occurs within 3 to 5 minutes. The duration of analgesia is 30 to 60 minutes which is considerably shorter than that of morphine and meperidine. Following intramuscular administration, the onset of action is somewhat slower, usually 7 to 8 minutes and duration of anesthesia lasts for 1 to 2 hours. Increasing the dose does not prolong the duration of anesthesia. Combined with droperidol, the onset of action occurs in 3 to 10 minutes following intravenous or intramuscular administration; the duration of action usually diminishes within 2 to 4 hours. Up to 10% of the drug is excreted unchanged in the urine; the remainder is believed to be metabolized in the liver.

Indications: For analgesic action in the preoperative and in the immediate postoperative period (recovery room). May also be used to prevent or relieve tachypnea and postoperative emergence delirium. Fentanyl citrate may be used as a supplement in the anesthetic technique called neuroleptanalgesia. A muscle relaxant is usually administered to complete this technique. It has been used effectively as an analgesic supplement to anesthesia in plastic and reconstructive, otolaryngologic, ophthalmologic, neurosurgical, cardiovascular, gynecologic and genitourologic, orthopedic, thoracic, abdominal, diagnostic, dental, and radiotherapeutic procedures. Combined with droperidol it is employed to produce tranquilization and analgesia during surgical and diagnostic procedures, and as premedication, induction and maintenance as an adjunct to general or regional anesthesia.

Contraindications: In patients in whom muscle relaxants should not be used, because of the possibility of skeletal muscle rigidity, and in those hypersensitive to either component. It should be used with extreme caution, if at all, in patients who may be particularly susceptible to respiratory depression, such as comatose patients who may have head injury or brain tumor. In addition, the drug may obscure the clinical course of patients with head injury.

Warnings: Fentanyl may be habit-forming and its use should be attended with the same cautionary measures as those used for morphine. The patient should be observed closely for signs of apnea, hypotension or both. Appropriate drugs and facilities for assisted or controlled respiration should be readily available, and vital signs should be monitored routinely. Judicious use is recommended in patients receiving other drugs known to cause alterations in blood pressure. Severe and unpredictable potentiation by MAO inhibitors has been reported with narcotic analgesics. Since safe use of fentanyl in this regard has not been established, the use of this analgesic in patients who have received MAO inhibitors within 14 days is not recommended. Also safe use in pregnant patients and in children under 2 years of age has not been substantiated.

Precautions: Cautious use is necessary in patients with severe impairment of pulmonary function, and should respiratory depression be compromised by muscle rigidity, muscle relaxants and assisted respiration may be required. The respiratory and sedative effects of fentanyl are enhanced by other CNS depressants (e.g., barbiturates, major tranquilizers, narcotics, and general anesthetics). Therefore, the dose of these agents should be reduced by $^1/_4$ to $^1/_3$ when they are administered concomitantly with this drug. Caution should be exercised when administering to patients with known Parkinson's disease, in those with liver and kidney dysfunction, or with cardiac arrhythmias, especially cardiac bradyarrhythmias, and in elderly or poor-risk patients. Care should also be exercised in the moving and positioning of patients because of the possibility of orthostatic hypotension.

Adverse Reactions: The most common adverse reactions reported to occur are respiratory depression, apnea, muscular rigidity, bradycardia, and hypotension. If these remain untreated, respiratory arrest, circulatory depression, or cardiac arrest may occur. Those less frequently reported are nausea and emesis. Rarely reported are dizziness, visual difficulty, itching, euphoria, bronchoconstriction, and episodes suggestive of Oddi spasm.

The monograph on Droperidol should be consulted for additional contraindications, warnings, precautions and adverse reactions.

Dosage and Administration: *Intramuscularly* or *intravenously.* Fentanyl: *For premedication,* 1 to 2 ml intramuscularly 30 to 60 minutes prior to the procedure. *For induction,* initially 1 to 2 ml intravenously; may be repeated at 2- to 3-minute intervals until desired effect is achieved. *For maintenance,* 0.5 to 1 ml intravenously or intramuscularly. *For postoperative* (recovery room), 1 to 2 ml intramuscularly. *For adjunctive use to regional anesthesia,* 1 or 2 ml intramuscularly or by slow intravenous administration. Fentanyl with droperidol: *For premedication,* 0.5 to 2 ml intramuscularly 45 to 60 minutes prior to surgery with or without atropine. *For induction,* 1 ml/20 to 25 lbs of body weight intravenously or by intravenous drip (10 ml are added to 250 ml of 5% dextrose in water and the drip administered rapidly until the onset of somnolence). *For maintenance,* 0.5 to 1 ml intravenously or intramuscularly.

Availability:
Ⓒ SUBLIMAZE® Injection, 0.05 mg/ml in ampuls of 2 and 5 ml. **(McNeil)**
Ⓒ INNOVAR® Injection, 0.05 mg/ml with droperidol, 2.5 mg/ml in ampuls of 2 and 5 ml. **(McNeil)**

FEOSOL PLUS

Description: Each capsule contains:

Ferrous sulfate, dried (equivalent to 325 mg ferrous sulfate; 65 mg of iron)	200 mg
Folic acid	0.4 mg
Ascorbic acid	50 mg
Thiamine hydrochloride	2 mg
Riboflavin	2 mg
Pyridoxine hydrochloride	2 mg
Vitamin B-12 (activity equivalent)	5 μg
Niacin	20 mg

Indications: In iron-deficiency anemias where additional nutritional support is needed, i.e., convalescence, adolescence, pregnancy and malnutrition.

Warnings: Use of folic acid in patients who have or may develop pernicious anemia involves the serious hazard of permitting progressive degeneration of the spinal cord while treating the anemia characteristic of the disease. Parenterally administered cyanocobalamin is the therapy of choice in pernicious anemia and should be employed in patients receiving folic acid unless pernicious anemia has been ruled out.

Precautions: Since iron salts significantly impair absorption of oral tetracyclines, these agents should not be given within 2 hours of each other.

Adverse Reactions: Nausea, constipation or diarrhea. Gastrointestinal effects may be minimized by administration with meals. Lethargy, vomiting, diarrhea, weak and rapid pulse, and low blood pressure are distinctive signs of overdosage.

Dosage and Administration: *Orally,* 2 capsules daily after meals. Children 4 years of age and over, 1 or 2 capsules daily.

Availability:
FEOSOL PLUS® Capsules in bottles of 30 and 100. **(Smith Kline & French)**

FERO-FOLIC-500

Description: Each red Filmtab contains:

Ferrous sulfate (equivalent to 105 mg iron)*	525 mg
Folic acid	0.8 mg
Ascorbic acid (as sodium ascorbate)	500 mg

*In controlled-release form.

Indications: Prophylaxis and treatment of iron and folate deficiency anemias. Especially indicated during pregnancy.

Contraindications: Patients with pernicious anemia.

Warnings: Folic acid alone is improper therapy in the treatment of pernicious anemia and other megaloblastic anemias where vitamin B-12 is deficient.

Precautions: Folic acid does not control the neurological symptoms of pernicious anemia; however, the dose of folic acid in this preparation is designed to meet the increased folate demands of pregnancy while mitigating the danger of obscuring a deficiency of vitamin B-12. Accordingly, in older patients and those with conditions tending to lead to vitamin B-12 depletion, serum B-12 levels should be regularly assessed during treatment with this product. Concomitant parenteral therapy with vitamin B-12 may be necessary in patients with a deficiency of this vitamin.

Adverse Reactions: Allergic sensitization has been reported following both oral and parenteral administration of folic acid. Acute overdosage may be manifested by increased capillary permeability, reduced plasma volume, increased cardiac output, and sudden cardiovascular collapse. An emetic should be administered as soon as possible, followed by gastric lavage if indicated.

Dosage and Administration: *Orally,* 1 tablet daily may be taken on an empty stomach. Best taken after meals if gastric intolerance prevails.

Availability:
FERO-FOLIC-500® Filmtab® Tablets in bottles of 100 and 500. **(Abbott)**

FERRITRINSIC

Description: Each tablet contains Intrinase® (vitamin B-12 with intrinsic factor concentrate), 1/3 N.F. XI oral unit; iron (from 187.7 mg dried ferrous sulfate), 60 mg; desiccated liver, 100 mg; folic acid, 0.133 mg; ascorbic acid (as sodium ascorbate and ascorbic acid), 50 mg; thiamine mononitrate, 2 mg; riboflavin, 2 mg; niacinamide, 10 mg.

Indications: Treatment of patients with iron deficiency anemia, which may be associated with mild blood loss, restricted dietary regimens, certain metabolic diseases, convalescence and old age; also in the treatment of nutritional macrocytic anemias.

Precautions: Not all patients with pernicious anemia show satisfactory therapeutic responses to oral vitamin B-12-intrinsic factor preparations. In addition, some patients with an initial good response appear to become refractory to intrinsic factor after varying periods of oral therapy. Periodic examinations and laboratory studies of pernicious anemia patients are essential and recommended. Failure of response, or inadequate response, is an indication for parenteral vitamin B-12 (cobalamin), generally recognized as the preferred treatment of this condition. Although toxic effects of Intrinase have not been reported, the possibility of gastrointestinal allergy should be kept in mind.

Adverse Reactions: Occasional gastrointestinal intolerance to ferrous sulfate may be noted. This may be minimized by taking the medication immediately after meals.

Dosage and Administration: *Orally.* Adults, 1 tablet 3 times daily. Children, 1 to 3 tablets daily according to age.

Availability:
FERRITRINSIC® Tablets in bottles of 50 and 500. **(Upjohn)**

FESTALAN

Description: Each tablet contains:

In the outer layer:
Atropine methyl nitrate .... 1 mg
In the enteric-coated core:
Lipase .... 10 WU*
Amylase .... 10 WU*
Protease .... 17 WU*

Hemicellulase	50 mg
Bile constituents	25 mg

*Willstaetter Units of digestive activity.

A combination of enzymes and bile salts to promote digestion with an antispasmodic agent to reduce spasm and hypermotility of the gastrointestinal tract.

Indications: Treatment of gastrointestinal disorders involving insufficient digestive enzymes, hypermotility and nonspecific spasms. It may be helpful in the relief of discomfort due to excess gas, pancreatic insufficiency, enteritis, chronic pancreatitis, chronic hepatitis, and gallbladder disease. It may also be helpful in patients who have undergone pancreatectomy, cholecystectomy, subtotal gastrectomy, or other surgery of the upper gastrointestinal tract, and in those with functional bowel distress, nervous indigestion, irritable bowel syndrome, mucous colitis or spastic colon.

Contraindications: In the presence of glaucoma, prostatic hypertrophy, and a sensitivity to atropine.

Precautions: Urinary retention may result from prostatic hypertrophy and may necessitate reducing the dosage or discontinuing medication. It should be used with caution in patients with cardiac disease. Overdosage may result in the usual symptoms of atropine toxicity.

Adverse Reactions: Mild dryness of mouth, blurring of vision, dysuria, and constipation have been noted, but did not necessitate a reduction in dosage. Skin rash and flushing may occur in patients sensitive to atropine. The dosage or frequency of administration should be decreased if severe dryness of the mouth, mydriasis, or rapid or irregular pulse occurs.

Dosage and Administration: *Orally.* Usual adult dosage is 1 or 2 tablets 3 times daily, taken with each meal.

Availability:
FESTALAN® Tablets (orange, enteric-coated) in bottles of 100 and 1000. **(Hoechst)**

FIBRINOLYSIN

Description: Fibrinolysin (human) is a purified, lyophilized preparation of the naturally occurring proteolytic enzyme contained in the Cohn Fraction III of normal human blood plasma. It is prepared by fractional extraction from the plasma and subsequent activation with purified, pyrogen-free streptokinase. It occurs as a white powder very soluble in water. Potency is expressed in terms of units; 1 unit is defined as that amount that will lyse a standard fibrin clot in 10 minutes under standard conditions of pH, temperature and concentration.

Fibrinolysin (bovine) is a nondialyzable proteolytic enzyme that is extracted from bovine plasma as profibrinolysin and activated with chloroform; it is insoluble in water and soluble in sodium chloride solution. Potency is expressed in units based on the amount of enzyme that will lyse a standard fibrin clot in the same interval as does a reference standard preparation. Desoxyribonuclease, a proteolytic enzyme, is obtained by fractional precipitation of an acidic extract of beef pancreas and occurs as a white powder very soluble in water. Potency is expressed in units based on the rate and extent to which the enzyme reduces the viscosity of highly polymerized desoxyribonucleic acid. Fibrinolysin and desoxyribonuclease, combined, is compatible with penicillin, chloramphenicol, streptomycin and tetracycline. A topical preparation is available in which the 2 proteolytic enzymes are combined with chloramphenicol.

Indications: *Fibrinolysin (human):* The treatment of thrombophlebitis, phlebothrombosis, pulmonary embolism and thrombosis of arteries, except cerebral and coronary arteries. Treatment is more likely to be of benefit when it is started within 5 days of a thrombotic incident. Used in adequate doses, the drug may be given adjunctively to conventional anticoagulant therapy. *Bovine:* Combined with desoxyribonuclease, it produces lysis of fibrin and liquefication of pus. The enzymatic debridement produced by the drug makes it useful in the removal of necrotic debris, fibrin and purulent exudates. The combination is used to reduce the viscosity and tenacity of purulent exudates and to promote debridement of necrotic debris in the treatment of vaginitis and cervicitis; to promote healing of wounds, burns and ulcers; and to irrigate abscess cavities, superficial hematomas, sinus tracts and fistulas. Chloramphenicol may be added to combat infection by sensitive organisms.

Contraindications: Hemorrhagic diathesis, major liver dysfunction or hypofibrinogenemia.

Precautions: Because of the possibility of increasing clotting time, and affecting the amount of heparin required to achieve the desired prolongation of clotting time, determination of the clotting time should be made whenever more than 200,000 units of human fibrinolysin are used in any one day. It should be used with caution immediately after anesthesia or surgery. Bleeding from open wounds during therapy can be controlled by plasma or whole blood. Antibodies are known to develop against streptokinase; the possibility of an allergic reaction should therefore be kept in mind. Usual precautions should be observed regarding allergic reactions, particularly in patients highly sensitive to materials of bovine origin.

Adverse Reactions: Febrile reactions, chills, nausea, vomiting, dizziness, headache, muscle pain, backache, tachycardia, hypotension, symptomatic hypertension, facial flushing, chest pain, pain in abdomen and local hyperemia.

Dosage and Administration: *Intravenous infusion.* The contents of 1 vial are dissolved, without shaking, in 25 ml of sterile water for injection or 5% dextrose injection **(sodium chloride injection is not to be used)** and then added to 250 ml of 5% dextrose injection and administered at the rate of 50,000 to 100,000 units/hour for 1 to 6 hours each day. Dosage may be repeated for 3 or 4 consecutive days, depending upon patient response. A single dose of 100,000 units may be adequate in uncomplicated thrombophlebitis, but extensive or organized venous thrombi may require a total of 250,000 to 400,000 units. For arterial thrombosis, 250,000 to 500,000 units have been given daily for 1 to 3 days. Doses of 50,000 to 200,000 units (2000 units/ml) have been infused directly into thrombosed arteries. *Fibrinolysin with desoxyribonuclease:* When used to irrigate abscesses, empyema cavities, fistulae, sinus tracts, or subcutaneous hematomas, the solution should be drained and replaced at intervals of 6 to 10 hours. Traces of blood in the discharge usually indicate active filling in of the cavity. *Intravaginally.* In mild to moderate vaginitis and cervicitis, 5 ml of ointment should be deposited deep into the vagina each night for 5 nights, or until the contents of 1 tube have been used. In severe conditions, it may be advisable to apply a solution initially, wait 1 or 2 minutes for dispersal, then insert a vaginal tampon and remove the next day, followed by as many applications of ointment as appear necessary. *Topically.* For skin surface lesions, amount of ointment to be applied is best left to the discretion of the physician. For best effect, the ointment must remain in contact with substrate and be reapplied at least once daily; necrotic debris to be removed periodically. Enzymatic activity is rapidly and progressively diminished after application, especially the solution, and probably exhausted for practical purposes after 24 hours. The manufacturer's package circular should be consulted for specific details.

Availability:

Fibrinolysin (Human)

THROMBOLYSIN® LYOVAC® (lyophilized) in vials of 50,000 units. **(Merck Sharp & Dohme)**

Fibrinolysin (Bovine) and Desoxyribonuclease

ELASE® in vials containing 25 units of fibrinolysin (bovine) and 15,000 units of desoxyribonuclease. **(Parke-Davis)**

ELASE® Ointment containing in each gram 1 unit of fibrinolysin and 666.6 units of desoxyribonuclease in tubes of 10 and 30 gm with or without vaginal applicator. **(Parke-Davis)**

ELASE®-CHLOROMYCETIN® Ointment containing in each gram the same amounts of fibrinolysin and desoxyribonuclease as above and, in addition, 10 mg of chloramphenicol in tubes of 10 and 30 gm. **(Parke-Davis)**

FILIBON F.A.

Description: Each capsule-shaped tablet contains:

Folic acid		1 mg
Vitamin A (as acetate)	(8000 units)	2.4 mg
Vitamin D (as yeast)	(400 units)	10 μg
Thiamine (as mononitrate)		1.7 mg

Riboflavin	2 mg
Pyridoxine hydrochloride	4 mg
Vitamin C (as calcium ascorbate)	60 mg
Vitamin E	30 IU
Niacinamide	20 mg
Cyanocobalamin (vitamin B-12)	8 μg
Calcium (as carbonate)	250 mg
Iron (as ferrous fumarate)	45 mg

Trace elements supplied as magnesium oxide, and potassium iodide.

Indications: As a vitamin-mineral supplement during pregnancy and lactation.

Precautions: Pernicious anemia should be ruled out before starting treatment. While folic acid corrects the blood picture of pernicious anemia, it does not ameliorate the attendant neurologic involvement.

Dosage and Administration: *Orally.* One tablet daily. Additional calcium may be needed.

Availability:
FILIBON® F.A. Tablets (pink) in jars of 100. **(Lederle)**

FILIBON FORTE

Description: Each tablet contains:

Vitamin A (as acetate)	(8000 units)	2.4 mg
Vitamin D	(400 units)	10 μg
Vitamin E (as *d*-α-tocopheryl acid succinate)		45 IU
Ascorbic acid		90 mg
Niacinamide		30 mg
Pyridoxine hydrochloride		3 mg
Thiamine mononitrate		2 mg
Riboflavin		2.5 mg
Folic acid		0.8 mg
Vitamin B-12		12 μg
Calcium (as carbonate)		300 mg
Iron (as ferrous fumarate)		45 mg

Trace elements supplied as magnesium oxide and potassium iodide.

Indications: As a dietary supplement in pregnant and lactating women.

Precautions: Folic acid may obscure pernicious anemia in that the peripheral blood picture may revert to normal while the neurological manifestations remain progressive.

Dosage and Administration: *Orally.* One tablet daily. Additional calcium may be required.

Availability:
FILIBON® FORTE Tablets in jars of 100. **(Lederle)**

FIORINAL Ⓒ III

FIORINAL w/CODEINE Ⓒ III

Description: Each Fiorinal capsule or tablet contains butalbital, 50 mg; caffeine, 40 mg, aspirin, 200 mg; phenacetin, 130 mg. Each Fiorinal with Codeine capsule contains, in addition to the above formula, codeine phosphate, 7.5 mg, 15 mg or 30 mg.

Possessing analgesic, sedative, antipyretic and, in the case of Fiorinal w/Codeine, antitussive action, Fiorinal compliments and increases the time-tested action of codeine, thus enhancing the analgesic-sedative effect, which is particularly well-suited for acute, short-range periods of pain and discomfort.

Indications: Nervous tension and sleeplessness associated with pain, headache or general malaise; nervous and muscular pain accompanied by hyperexcitability and nervousness; and all conditions requiring relief of pain or reduction of fever. The codeine component raises the pain threshold and the combined drug is indicated for all types of pain associated with medical and surgical aftercare, postpartum pain, dysmenorrhea, neuritis, pleurisy, sciatica, neuralgia, sinusitis, pharyngitis, tonsillitis, otitis, febrile diseases, dental pain following extractions, tension headache, bursitis, arthritis, rheumatism, low back pain, dislocations, strains, sprains, fractures; also indicated in upper respiratory tract infections such as acute colds, bronchitis, influenza, and pneumonia.

Contraindications: Hypersensitivity to any of the components, and in patients with porphyria.

Warnings: Butalbital and codeine may be habit-forming. Excessive and prolonged use of butalbital can produce drug dependence, characterized by psychic dependence, and less frequently, physical dependence and tolerance; therefore, caution should be exercised when prescribing for patients accustomed to taking large quantities of drugs, which is not uncommon in patients with chronic tension headache. Patients should be cautioned that their mental and/or physical abilities for the performance of potentially hazardous tasks may be impaired. Concurrent use with other CNS-depressant drugs should be avoided; however, if such combined therapy is essential, the dose of each may need to be reduced. The drug should be used in pregnant and lactating women only when the clinical manifestations show a definite need. Safe and effective use in children under 12 years of age has not been established.

Precautions: Patients with peptic ulcer, coagulation disorders, or renal disease require special consideration because of the salicylate and phenacetin components.

Adverse Reactions: Drowsiness and dizziness are the most frequent occurring reactions, while lightheadedness, nausea, vomiting, flatulence occur less frequently. Overdosage is primarily manifested by drowsiness. For possible adverse effects attributable to codeine, see specific monograph.

Dosage and Administration: *Orally.* Adults, 1 or 2 capsules or tablets, repeated if necessary up to 6 per day, or as directed.

Availability:
(C-III) FIORINAL®: **(Sandoz)**
Capsules (bright kelly green and lime green) in bottles of 100 and 500.
Tablets (white, compressed) in bottles of 100 and 1000 and in SandoPaks® of 100.
w/Codeine
Capsules, No. 1 (7.5 mg) [red and yellow] in bottles of 100, No. 2 (15 mg) [gray and yellow] and No. 3 (30 mg) [blue and yellow] in bottles of 100.

FLAVOXATE HYDROCHLORIDE

Chemical Name: Beta-piperidinoethyl 3-methyl-4-oxo-2-phenyl-4*H*-1-benzopyran-8-carboxylate hydrochloride.

Description: Flavoxate is a urinary tract spasmolytic agent employed specifically for the relief of symptoms associated with various urologic disorders. Because its antispasmodic action is exerted directly on the muscle, it counteracts smooth muscle spasm of the urinary tract.

Indications: Symptomatic relief of dysuria, urgency, nocturia, suprapubic pain; frequency and incontinence as may occur in cystitis, prostatitis, urethritis, urethrocystitis and/or urethrotrigonitis. It is not indicated for definitive treatment, but is compatible with drugs used for the treatment of urinary tract infections.

Contraindications: Patients with pyloric or duodenal obstruction, obstructive intestinal lesions or ileus, achalasia, gastrointestinal hemorrhage, and obstructive uropathies of the lower urinary tract.

Warnings: To be given cautiously to patients with suspected glaucoma.

Precautions: In the event of drowsiness and blurred vision, patients should be cautioned not to engage in activities requiring alertness or physical coordination. Safe use in women who are or may become pregnant has not been established; therefore, the drug should not be given except when the expected benefits outweigh the possible hazards to the mother and fetus.

Adverse Reactions: Although relatively uncommon, the following have been reported: nausea and vomiting, dry mouth, nervousness, vertigo, headache, drowsiness, blurred vision, increased ocular tension, disturbance in eye accommodation, urticaria and other dermatoses, mental confusion especially in the elderly patient, dysuria, tachycardia and palpitation, hyperpyrexia, eosinophilia and leukopenia (one case which was reversible upon discontinuation of the drug).

Dosage and Administration: *Orally.* Adults and children over 12 years of age—1 or 2 tablets 3 or 4 times daily. Dosage should be individualized according to the degree of relief of symptoms of the patient. **Note:** This drug is not recommended for infants and children under 12 years of age because safe and effective use have not been established.

Availability:
URISPAS® Tablets, 100 mg in bottles of 100 and in single-unit packages of 100.
(Smith Kline & French)

FLEET THEOPHYLLINE RECTAL UNIT

Description: Aqueous solutions containing in each 37 ml either 312 mg or 625 mg of theophylline monoethanolamine. However, each unit delivers an average volume of 30 ml containing either 250 mg or 500 mg of the drug. The solutions are preserved with methyl- and propylparabens.

Following rectal installation, clinically effective plasma levels are usually obtained within 1/2 hour. It relaxes the bronchial smooth muscle, stimulates both cardiac muscle and the CNS, and produces diuresis.

Indications: Symptomatic relief of acute bronchial asthma, and for reversible bronchospasm associated with chronic bronchitis and emphysema.

Contraindications: Hypersensitivity to any component; in patients with coronary artery disease or angina pectoris where, in the physician's judgment, myocardial stimulation may prove harmful; in those with severe renal or liver impairment, and in pediatric patients—deaths have resulted from the rectal administration of adult doses in children.

Precautions: Cautious use is required in patients with a history of peptic ulcer. Rectal administration of theophylline may be irritating.

Adverse Reactions: Administration of theophylline by any route may cause nausea and vomiting. Harmful results may be manifested by gastric irritation and pain, reactivation of peptic ulcer, intestinal bleeding, kidney irritation, albuminuria, palpitation, nervousness, and insomnia. In acute toxicity, symptoms may include fever, delirium, agitation, convulsions, hematemesis, bloody diarrhea, shock, dehydration, and even death.

Dosage and Administration: *Rectally for adults only.* The rectal unit is ready to use. Remove cover, gently insert prelubricated rectal tube, squeeze out contents of plastic bottle. The dose should not be repeated in intervals of less than 8 hours, nor should more than 2 doses be administered within 24 hours.

Availability:
FLEET® THEOPHYLLINE Rectal Unit, 250 and 500 mg in ready-to-use, single-dose squeeze bottles in packages of 6. **(Fleet)**

FLOXURIDINE

Chemical Name: 2′-Deoxy-5-fluorouridine.

Description: Floxuridine is a fluorinated pyrimidine compound that contains a furanose ring in its molecular structure. It occurs as a white, crystalline powder freely soluble in water.

When administered intraarterially, floxuridine appears to be rapidly catabolized to 5-fluorouracil, and thus produces the same toxic and antimetabolic effects in the body as does 5-fluorouracil. It is believed to exert its antimetabolic action primarily by interfering with the synthesis of desoxyribonucleic acid (DNA) and to a lesser degree ribonucleic acid (RNA) during cell reproduction. This effect is seen in all rapidly proliferating normal and malignant cells. When floxuridine is given by continuous intraarterial infusion, its direct anabolism to floxuridine monophosphate is enhanced, thus increasing the inhibition of DNA.

Laboratory studies have revealed the drug to be teratogenic and mutagenic in animals; such possible effects occurring in patients should be considered.

Indications: Palliative management of carcinoma in carefully selected patients who are considered incurable by surgery or by other means. However, patients with known disease that has extended beyond an area capable of infusion by way of a single artery should, except in unusual circumstances, be considered for systemic therapy with other chemotherapeutic agents. This drug is not intended as an adjuvant to surgery.

Contraindications: Patients in a poor nutritional state, those with bone marrow depression, or with potentially serious infections.

Warnings: *Floxuridine should be administered only by or under the supervision of a qualified physician who is experienced in cancer chemotherapy and intraarterial drug therapy. Because of the possibility of severe toxic reactions, it is imperative that all patients be hospitalized during the first course of treatment.* Extreme caution is advised in poor risk patients with impaired hepatic or renal function, in those who have had high-dose pelvic irradiation, or who had previous therapy with alkylating agents. Safe use during pregnancy has not been established; therefore, floxuridine should not be used during pregnancy, particularly in the first trimester, unless in the judgment of the physician, the potential benefits to the patient outweigh the possible adverse effects on fetal development. Floxuridine should be discontinued *immediately* whenever one of the following signs of toxicity appears: stomatitis or esophagopharyngitis; a leukocyte count of less than 3500 or a rapidly decreasing leukocyte count; intractable vomiting; diarrhea, frequent bowel movements or watery stools; gastrointestinal ulceration and bleeding; thrombocytopenia (a platelet count under 100,000) and hemorrhage from any site.

Precautions: Patients should be carefully supervised since floxuridine is a highly toxic drug with a narrow margin of safety, and also since therapeutic response is unlikely to occur without some evidence of toxicity. Patients should be well informed of expected toxic manifestations, particularly the oral manifestations, of the drug before therapy is begun. Careful monitoring of the leukocyte and platelet count is recommended. Severe hematological toxicity, gastrointestinal hemorrhage and even death may result despite meticulous selection of patients and careful adjustment of dosage. Although severe toxicity is more likely to occur in poor-risk patients, fatalities may be encountered even in patients in relatively good condition.

Adverse Reactions: The most common are: nausea, vomiting, diarrhea, enteritis, stomatitis, localized erythema; anemia, leukopenia, elevations of alkaline phosphatase, serum transaminase, serum bilirubin, and lactic dehydrogenase. Others include: *functional gastrointestinal reactions*—anorexia, cramps and pain; *mucosal gastrointestinal reactions*—duodenal ulcer, duodenitis, gastritis, gastroenteritis, glossitis and pharyngitis; *dermatological reactions*—alopecia, dermatitis, edema, excoriation, maceration, nonspecific skin reactions, pruritus, rash and ulceration; *other clinical reactions*—abscess, ataxia, blurred vision, convulsions, depression, dysuria, fever, hemiplegia, hiccups, hypoadrenalism, lethargy, malaise, nystagmus, pain, vertigo and weakness; *laboratory abnormalities*—alterations in BSP, prothrombin, total proteins, sedimentation rate, and thrombopenia; *procedural complications of regional arterial infusion*—arterial aneurysm, arterial ischemia, arterial thrombosis, bleeding at catheter site, blocked catheter, displaced or leaking embolism, fibromyositis, infection at catheter site and thrombophlebitis. Any form of therapy which adds to the stress of the patient, interferes with nutrition, or depresses bone marrow function will increase the toxicity of floxuridine.

Dosage and Administration: *Intraarterially* only. The recommended therapeutic dose regimen by continuous arterial infusion is 0.1 to 0.6 mg/kg of body weight daily. For hepatic artery infusion, a dose of from 0.4 to 0.6 mg/kg daily is usually employed because the liver metabolizes the drug, thus reducing the potential for systemic toxicity. Therapy should be continued for as long as the patient responds or until adverse reactions appear. Administration of the infusion is best achieved with the use of an appropriate pump in order to overcome pressure in the large arteries and to ensure a uniform rate of infusion. For reconstitution, add 5 ml of water for injection to the vial which, if not used promptly, should be stored under refrigeration for no more than 2 weeks.

Availability:
FUDR Soluble Powder, 500 mg in vials of 5 ml. **(Roche)**

FLUCYTOSINE

Chemical Name: 5-Fluorocytosine.

Description: Flucytosine, an antifungal agent, is a fluorinated pyrimidine chemically related to fluorouracil and floxuridine. It occurs as a white to off-white, crystalline powder with a molecular weight of 129.1.

Flucytosine is not metabolized significantly when administered orally. Although its exact mode of action is not known, results from in vitro and in vivo studies indicate that it is active against *Candida* and *Cryptococcus* organisms. Nevertheless, about 40 to 50% of the pretreatment clinical isolates of *Candida* have been reported to be resistant to flucytosine. Most strains of *Cryptococcus* initially isolated from clinical material have shown that the drug's minimal inhibitory concentrations ranged from 0.46 to 7.8 mcg/ml. It has been determined that any isolate with a minimal inhibitory concentration greater than 100 mcg/ml for *Candida* and 12.5 mcg/ml for *Cryptococcus* be considered resistant. It is advised that susceptibility studies be performed as early as possible and be repeated during therapy. For in vitro studies, the broth medium and procedure described by Shadomy is recommended for interpretations of susceptibility. It should be noted that teratogenic effects have occurred in rats which metabolize flucytosine to fluorouracil.

Indications: Treatment of systemic candidal and cryptococcal infections such as septicemia, endocarditis, meningitis, and in those of the pulmonary and genitourinary systems.

Contraindications: Hypersensitivity to the drug.

Warnings: Since flucytosine is excreted primarily by the kidneys, extreme caution is advised in patients with impaired renal function, and careful monitoring of renal excretion is recommended. Extreme caution is also advised in patients with bone marrow depression, especially those patients who have a hematologic disease, who are being treated or who have a history of treatment with radiation or drugs which depress the bone marrow. The hematopoietic system and hepatic function should be carefully assessed during treatment. Safe use during pregnancy has not been established; therefore, flucytosine should not be given to pregnant or lactating women or to women of childbearing potential unless, in the judgment of the physician, the potential benefits to the patient outweigh the possible adverse effects on fetal development.

Precautions: Close monitoring of the patients is essential, and before initiating therapy, their hematologic and renal status should be determined. Blood levels of alkaline phosphatase, SGOT and SGPT should be checked at frequent intervals throughout the course of treatment.

Adverse Reactions: Frequently reported were nausea, vomiting, diarrhea, rash, anemia, leukopenia, thrombocytopenia, and elevation of hepatic enzymes, BUN, and creatinine levels. Less frequently reported were confusion, hallucinations, headache, sedation, and vertigo.

Dosage and Administration: *Orally.* The usual dosage is 50 to 150 mg/kg of body weight daily administered at 6-hour intervals. Nausea and vomiting may be reduced or avoided if the capsules are given a few at a time over a 15-minute period. If the BUN or the serum creatinine level is elevated, or if there are other signs of renal impairment, the initial dose should be at the lower level.

Availability:
ANCOBON® Capsules, 250 and 500 mg in bottles of 100. **(Roche)**

FLUDROCORTISONE ACETATE: see The Adrenal Corticosteroids

FLUMETHASONE PIVALATE: see The Adrenal Corticosteroids

FLUOCINOLONE ACETONIDE: see The Adrenal Corticosteroids

FLUOCINONIDE: see The Adrenal Corticosteroids

FLUORAC: see The Fluoride-Vitamins

FLUORESCEIN SODIUM

Description: Fluorescein sodium is a dye closely related chemically to phenolphthalein. It is available as a solution and as lint-free paper strips chemically treated and impregnated with fluorescein sodium. It is used for the diagnosis of corneal lesions and for the detection of minute foreign bodies embedded in the cornea. The normal cornea will not accept the stain, whereas abraded corneas will stain green and remain green for quite some time; affected conjunctival areas will stain orange-yellow.

Indications: *Topical:* As an aid in the diagnosis of abrasions and foreign bodies of the cornea, in fitting conventional contact lenses and in applanation tonometry. *Injection:* For retinal angiography; to distinguish viable from nonviable, malignant from nonmalignant tissue, and to determine vascular circulatory relationship. Benoxinate is added for its anesthetic effect.

Contraindications: Known hypersensitivity to any of the components.

Warnings: Prolonged use of a topical ocular anesthetic is not recommended, since it may produce permanent corneal opacification with accompanying visual loss.

Precautions: Not to be used in an eye with a known penetrating injury. For the dry eye or for special tests, the solution should be used. Use with caution in patients with known allergies, asthma, and related conditions; if signs of sensitivity develop, use of the drug should be discontinued.

Adverse Reactions: Occurring occasionally were temporary stinging, burning and conjunctival redness. Rarely noted were severe, immediate-type, apparently hyperallergic corneal reaction, with acute, intense and diffuse epithelial keratitis, a gray, ground-glass appearance, sloughing of large areas of necrotic epithelium, corneal filaments and at times, iritis with descemetitis. Injection of the solution may cause moderate to marked nausea and headache; gastrointestinal distress, urticaria and other symptoms and signs of hypersensitivity; cardiac arrest, basilar artery ischemia, thrombophlebitis at the injection site, severe shock and temporary yellowish skin discoloration. Urine attains a bright yellow color. Discoloration of the skin fades in 6 to 12 hours, urine fluorescence in 24 to 36 hours.

Dosage and Administration: *Topically.* To test for corneal lesions, instill a few drops of a 2% solution into the conjunctival sac, washing out the dye before observation. Anesthetize the eye or moisten end of applicator with a drop of sterile water, and place the applicator strip at the fornix in the lower cul-de-sac close to the punctum. For best results, the patient should close lids tightly over the applicator. *Injection.* For ophthalmology, inject contents of syringe rapidly into the antecubital vein. To avoid possible serious allergic reaction, it is advised that a very small test dose be injected prior to the diagnostic procedure. Within 9 to 14 seconds, luminescence appear in the retinal vessels which can be observed with standard viewing equipment. The children's dose is calculated on the basis of 35 mg/10 lbs of body weight. To combat any grave consequences, 0.1% epinephrine for intravenous or intramuscular use, an antihistamine and oxygen should be readily available.

Availability:
FLUORESCEIN SODIUM:
Ophthalmic Solution, 2% in Drop-Tainer®s of 15 ml. **(Alcon)**
Ophthalmic Solution, 2% in Dropperettes® applicators of 1 ml. **(Smith, Miller & Patch)**
FLUORESCITE® Injection, 5% in ampuls of 10 ml; 10% in ampuls of 5 ml and in disposable syringes of 10 ml prefilled with 5 ml of fluorescein sodium. (IV use only as diagnostic aid and for angiography of retinal vessels); 25% in ampuls of 2 ml. **(Alcon)**

FLUOR-I-STRIP® Sterile Applicators in cartons of 200. **(Ayerst)**
FLUOR-I-STRIP®-A.T. Sterile Applicators (for applanation tonometry) in envelopes of 2 applicators in cartons of 200. **(Ayerst)**
FUL-GLO® Strips, 0.6 mg in cartons of 300. **(Barnes-Hind)**
FUNDUSCEIN® Injection, 10% in ampuls of 5 ml; 25% in ampuls of 3 ml. **(Smith, Miller & Patch)**

Combinations

FLURESS® Ophthalmic Solution, containing sodium fluorescein, 0.25% and benoxinate hydrochloride, 0.4% in bottles of 5 ml with dropper. **(Barnes-Hind)**

THE FLUORIDE-VITAMINS

Introduction: A 1959 report of the Joint Committee of the American Academy of Pediatrics and the American Society of Dentistry for Children pointed out that the foundation for dental health is established early in life, and that dental caries, the greatest single cause of dental disease, is largely a problem of the first 2 decades. The deciduous teeth are no less susceptible than the permanent, and disease in them is not without serious consequence for permanent dentition. Caries susceptibility during tooth development may be influenced by nutritional alterations. The best recognized of these is the ingestion of appropriate amounts of the fluoride ion during calcification of the teeth. A well-defined increase in caries resistance occurs due to the incorporation of the fluoride ion in the crystal lattice of the enamel and dentin.

Nutritional Influences on Tooth Development: Vitamin deficiencies cause characteristic malformations in tooth structure. It has been shown that a deficiency of vitamin A in the diet results in a disturbance of the keratin matrix of enamel, while a deficiency of vitamin C causes a similar disturbance of the "collagen" matrix of dentin. Lack of vitamin D results in poor calcification, the signs of which are histologically indistinguishable from those produced by a lack of calcium or phosphorus in the diet, or an improper balance of these elements. Pyridoxine supplementation has been reported to decrease the incidence of dental caries in pregnant women, children, and various experimental animals.

The Role of Fluoride in Prophylaxis of Caries: The most important known dietary component that influences the chemical composition of the developing tooth and its susceptibility to caries is the fluoride ion. In communities where drinking water naturally contains no detectable amounts or very small amounts and where the diet also is low in fluorides, the incidence of tooth decay among the children raised in these areas is high. In communities where the drinking water supplies 1 ppm (parts per million) or more of fluoride and the diet remains low in fluoride, the children's teeth will have 50 to 60% less tooth decay. Wherever surveys have been made, the individuals in communities with high-fluoride waters uniformly have a low caries-index in comparison with individuals in neighboring communities with low-fluoride waters.

The optimal level of fluoride intake has been established at 1 ppm (1 mg/liter) above which the incidence of mottled enamel increased and below which there was an increased susceptibility to caries, malocclusion and tooth mortality.

Safety of Fluorides: Studies of children who have drunk artificially fluoridated waters (1 ppm) for periods up to 10 years have failed to disclose any adverse effects on growth, or general health and well being, or any changes in skeletal density or rate of skeletal maturation. The incidence of dental fluorosis increases as the concentration of fluoride exceeds 1 ppm. Bone changes have been reported associated with long-term intake (15 to 25 years) of 5 to 24 mg of fluoride/day, which is far in excess of the recommended dosage.

Indications: Fluoride with vitamins is indicated as a nutritional measure in the prevention of caries, and as a dietary supplement for the prevention of vitamin deficiencies.

Contraindications: Fluoride-vitamins should be used only in areas where the fluoride content of the drinking water is 1 ppm or less, and the total daily intake from this source does not exceed 0.3 mg for children under age 3, and 0.5 mg for those age 3 and over.

Precautions: Like all medications, these preparations should be kept out of the reach of children. To avoid dental fluorosis, which may be a consequence of excessive fluoride intake, it is well to limit these preparations to the recommended dosage. The oral dose of sodium fluoride that may be lethal for an adult is not known with certainty but it is estimated to be between 5 and 10 gm. Calculated for a 2-year-old child, the lowest lethal dose would be about 700 mg. As a safety measure, the Council on Dental Therapeutics has suggested that no more than 264 mg of sodium fluoride be dispensed at one time.

Adverse Reactions: Reports include skin rashes, gastrointestinal upset and headache. These disappeared when administration was discontinued.

Dosage and Administration: *Orally.* For infants and children, 0.6 ml daily or 1 tablet daily. Chewable tablets may be chewed, dissolved in the mouth, swallowed, or crushed and sprinkled on food. Drops may be placed directly on the tongue or mixed with milk, formula, water, fruit juice or food.

The preceding discussion applies equally to virtually all the preparations in the pages that follow. It will not be necessary, therefore, to repeat the indications, contraindications, precautions and adverse reactions, unless, of course, there is a significant deviation from the previous description.

Therefore, only the formulas and how they are packaged will be mentioned; included are the following:

Sodium Fluoride
ABDEC Drops w/Fluoride
Ad-Cebrin w/Fluoride
The Adeflors
Cari-Tab
Fluorac
Initia Drops w/Fluoride
Mulvidren-F
Natabec w/Fluoride
Novacebrin w/Fluoride
Palaflor
Vi-Daylin/F
Vi-Daylin/F ADC
Vi-Daylin/F w/Iron
The Vi-Flors
Vi-Penta F

SODIUM FLUORIDE

Description: Sodium fluoride is used for the effect of the fluoride ion in increasing resistance to dental caries. It occurs as an odorless, white, crystalline powder soluble in water and insoluble in alcohol.

It is prepared from a naturally occurring fluoride such as fluorospar or cryolite. It contains approximately 45% fluoride ion; its solutions have a pH of 7 and are stable, but should be stored and dispensed in plastic, or in paraffin-lined glass, or U.S.P. type I borosilicate glass containers.

Dosage and Administration: *Orally,* for infants, 0.5 to 1 mg.

Availability:
LURIDE®: **(Hoyt)**
Oral Liquid, 5.5 mg/ml (1 mg/0.4 ml) in bottles of 30 and 40 ml with calibrated dropper.
Tablets (LOZI-TABS®), 0.25 and 0.5 mg in bottles of 120 and 1200; 1 mg in bottles of 120, 1000 and 5000.
PEDIAFLOR® Drops, 0.5 mg/ml in dropper bottles of 50 ml. **(Ross)**

ABDEC DROPS WITH FLUORIDE

Description: Each 0.6 ml represents:

Sodium fluoride*		1.1 mg
Vitamin A palmitate	(5000 units)	1.5 mg
Ergocalciferol	(400 units)	10 μg
Ascorbic acid		50 mg
Thiamine hydrochloride		1 mg
Pyridoxine hydrochloride		1 mg
Riboflavin phosphate sodium*		1.65 mg
Niacinamide		10 mg
Sodium *d*-pantothenate*		5.5 mg

*Equivalent to 1.2 mg riboflavin, 5 mg pantothenic acid and 0.5 mg fluoride.

Availability:
ABDEC® DROPS with FLUORIDE in bottles of 50 ml with dropper. **(Parke-Davis)**

AD-CEBRIN WITH FLUORIDE DROPS

Description: Each 0.6 ml contains:

Fluoride (as sodium fluoride)		0.5 mg
Vitamin A synthetic	(2500 units)	0.75 mg
Vitamin D synthetic	(400 units)	10 μg
Vitamin C (as sodium ascorbate and ascorbic acid)		60 mg

Availability:
AD-CEBRIN® with FLUORIDE DROPS in bottles of 30 ml with calibrated dropper. **(Lilly)**

ADEFLOR(S)

Description: Each 0.6 ml of Adeflor Drops contains:

Fluoride (as sodium fluoride)		0.5 mg
Vitamin A	(2000 units)	0.6 mg
Vitamin D	(400 units)	10 μg
Ascorbic acid		50 mg
Pyridoxine hydrochloride		1 mg

Each Adeflor Chewable Tablet contains:

Fluoride (as sodium fluoride)		0.5 mg or 1 mg
Vitamin A	(4000 units)	1.2 mg
Vitamin D	(400 units)	10 μg
Ascorbic acid (as sodium ascorbate)		75 mg
Thiamine mononitrate		2 mg
Riboflavin		2 mg
Niacinamide		18 mg
Pyridoxine hydrochloride		1 mg
Calcium pantothenate		5 mg
Cyanocobalamin		2 μg

Each Adeflor M Tablet contains:

Fluoride (as sodium fluoride)	1 mg
Vitamin A	1.8 mg
Vitamin D	10 μg
Thiamine mononitrate	1.5 mg
Riboflavin	2.5 mg
Ascorbic acid (as sodium ascorbate)	100 mg
Niacinamide	20 mg
Pyridoxine hydrochloride	10 mg

Calcium pantothenate		10 mg
Cyanocobalamin		2 μg
Folic acid		0.1 mg
Calcium (as calcium carbonate)		250 mg
Iron (from ferrous fumarate, 91.27 mg)		30 mg

Availability:
ADEFLOR®: **(Upjohn)**
Drops in bottles of 30 and 50 ml with calibrated dropper.
Chewable Tablets, 0.5 and 1 mg in bottles of 100 and 500.
M Tablets in bottles of 100 and 500.

CARI-TAB

Description: Each tablet contains:

Fluoride (as sodium fluoride)		0.5 mg
Vitamin A	(2000 units)	0.6 mg
Ergocalciferol	(200 units)	5 μg
Ascorbic acid		75 mg

Availability:
CARI-TAB® SOFTAB® Tablets in bottles of 100. **(Stuart)**

FLUORAC

Description: Each chewable tablet provides:

Fluoride (as sodium fluoride)		0.5 mg
Vitamin A palmitate	(5000 units)	1.5 mg
Ergocalciferol	(400 units)	10 μg
Vitamin C (as ascorbic acid, 31 mg and sodium ascorbate, 50 mg)		75 mg
Pyridoxine hydrochloride		2 mg

Availability:
FLUORAC® Chewable Tablets in bottles of 100. **(USV)**

INITIA DROPS WITH FLUORIDE

Description: Each 0.6 ml contains:

Fluoride (as sodium fluoride)		0.5 mg
Vitamin A palmitate	(1500 units)	0.45 mg
Ergocalciferol	(200 units)	5 μg
Ascorbic acid		50 mg
Pyridoxine hydrochloride		1 mg

Availability:
INITIA® DROPS with FLUORIDE in bottles of 50 ml with calibrated dropper. **(Parke-Davis)**

MULVIDREN-F

Description: Each tablet contains:

Fluoride (as sodium fluoride)		1 mg
Vitamin A	(4000 units)	1.2 mg
Ergocalciferol	(400 units)	10 μg
Ascorbic acid		75 mg
Thiamine mononitrate		2 mg

Riboflavin	2 mg
Pyridoxine hydrochloride	1.2 mg
Cyanocobalamin	3 µg
Niacinamide	10 mg
Calcium pantothenate	3 mg

Dosage and Administration: *Orally.* Infants and children under 3 years of age, ½ tablet daily; children 3 years of age and older, 1 tablet daily.

Availability:
MULVIDREN®-F Softab® Tablets in bottles of 100. **(Stuart)**

NATABEC WITH FLUORIDE

Description: Each capsule (Kapseal®) contains:

Fluoride (as sodium fluoride)		1 mg
Vitamin A acetate	(4000 units)	1.2 mg
Ergocalciferol	(400 units)	10 µg
Ascorbic acid		50 mg
Thiamine mononitrate		3 mg
Riboflavin		2 mg
Pyridoxine hydrochloride		3 mg
Cyanocobalamin		5 µg
Niacinamide		10 mg
Ferrous sulfate, exsiccated		150 mg
Calcium carbonate, precipitated		600 mg

Availability:
NATABEC® with FLUORIDE Kapseals® in bottles of 100 and 1000. **(Parke-Davis)**

NOVACEBRIN WITH FLUORIDE

Description: Each 0.6 ml of drops and each chewable tablet contain:

		Drops	*Tablet*
Fluoride (as sodium fluoride)		0.5 mg	1 mg
Vitamin A	(4000 units)	1.2 mg	1.2 mg
Vitamin D	(400 units)	10 µg	10 µg
Ascorbic acid		60 mg	60 mg
Thiamine (as hydrochloride or mononitrate)		1 mg	1.5 mg
Riboflavin		1 mg	2 mg
Pyridoxine hydrochloride		1 mg	1 mg
Niacinamide		10 mg	12 mg
Cyanocobalamin		—	3 µg
Pantothenic acid (as panthenol)		—	2.5 mg

Availability:
NOVACEBRIN® with FLUORIDE: **(Lilly)**
Chewable Tablets in bottles of 100.
Drops in bottles of 30 ml with calibrated dropper.

PALAFLOR

Description: Each tablet represents:

Fluoride (as sodium fluoride)		2.2 mg
Vitamin A acetate	(4000 units)	1.2 mg
Ergocalciferol	(400 units)	10 µg
Ascorbic acid		50 mg

Thiamine mononitrate	3 mg
Riboflavin	3 mg
Pyridoxine hydrochloride	1 mg
Cyanocobalamin	5 μg
Niacinamide	20 mg
Calcium pantothenate	5.4 mg
dl-Tocopheryl acetate	10 IU
Calcium phosphate, dibasic	78 mg
Potassium sulfate	5.5 mg
Ferric phosphate	13.5 mg
Magnesium oxide	1.65 mg

Availability:
PALAFLOR® Chewable Tablets in bottles of 120. **(Parke-Davis)**

VI-DAYLIN/F

Description: Each 1 ml of drops and each chewable tablet contain:

		Drops	*Tablet*
Fluoride (as sodium fluoride)		0.5 mg	1 mg
Vitamin A		0.45 mg	0.75 mg
Vitamin D	(400 units)	10 μg	10 μg
Thiamine (as hydrochloride or mononitrate)		0.4 mg	1.02 mg
Riboflavin		0.6 mg	1.2 mg
Ascorbic acid		30 mg	60 mg
Pyridoxine hydrochloride		0.4 mg	1.28 mg
Niacinamide		6 mg	13.4 mg
Cobalamin		—	4.5 μg
Folic acid		—	0.2 mg
Vitamin E (*dl*-alpha tocopheryl acetate)		5 IU	15 IU

Each 1 ml of Vi-Daylin/F ADC Drops contains:

Fluoride (as sodium fluoride)		0.5 mg
Vitamin A	(1500 units)	0.45 mg
Vitamin D	(400 units)	10 μg
Ascorbic acid		30 mg

Availability:
VI-DAYLIN®/F: **(Ross)**
Chewable Tablets in bottles of 100.
Drops in bottles of 50 ml with calibrated dropper.
VI-DAYLIN®/F ADC Drops in bottles of 50 ml with calibrated dropper.

VI-DAYLIN/F with IRON

Description: Each 1 ml of drops contains:

		Drops	*ADC w/Iron Drops*
Fluoride (as sodium fluoride)		0.5 mg	0.5 mg
Vitamin A	(1500 units)	0.45 mg	0.45 mg
Vitamin D	(400 units)	10 μg	10 μg
Thiamine		0.5 mg	—
Riboflavin		0.6 mg	—
Niacin		8 mg	—
Pyridoxine hydrochloride		0.4 mg	—
Iron (as ferrous sulfate)		10 mg	10 mg
Ascorbic acid		35 mg	35 mg
Vitamin E		5 IU	—

Availability:
VI-DAYLIN®/F with IRON Drops in bottles of 50 ml with calibrated dropper. **(Ross)**
VI-DAYLIN/F ADC with IRON Drops in bottles of 50 ml with calibrated dropper. **(Ross)**

VI-FLOR(S)

Description: Each 1 ml of drops and each chewable tablet of **Poly-Vi-Flor** contain:

	Drops	*Tablets*
Fluoride (as sodium fluoride)	0.5 mg	1 mg
Vitamin A	0.45 mg	0.75 mg
Vitamin D (400 units)	10 μg	10 μg
Vitamin E (*dl*-alpha tocopheryl acetate)	5 IU	15 IU
Ascorbic acid	35 mg	60 mg
Folic acid	—	0.3 mg
Thiamine	0.5 mg	1.05 mg
Riboflavin	0.6 mg	1.2 mg
Niacin	8 mg	13.5 mg
Pyridoxine	0.4 mg	1.05 mg
Cyanocobalamin (vitamin B-12)	2 μg	4.5 μg

Each 1 ml of drops and each chewable tablet of **Poly-Vi-Flor with Iron** contain, in addition, iron, 10 and 12 mg respectively. *The drops do not contain cyanocobalamin.*

Each 1 ml and each chewable tablet of **Tri-Vi-Flor** contains:

	Drops	*Tablets*
Fluoride	0.25 or 0.5 mg	1 mg
Vitamin A	0.45 mg	0.75 mg
Calciferol (400 units)	10 μg	10 μg
Ascorbic acid	35 mg	60 mg

Dosage and Administration: *Orally.* For infants and children under 3 years of age—1 ml of drops daily. For children 3 years of age and over—1 tablet daily. **Note:** As with all products containing iron, parents should be cautioned against excessive dosage.

Availability:
Vi-Flor® **(Mead Johnson)**
POLY-VI-FLOR®:
Drops in bottles of 30 and 50 ml with calibrated dropper.
Chewable Tablets in bottles of 100 and 1000.
w/Iron Drops in bottles of 50 ml with Safti-Dropper®.
w/Iron Tablets in bottles of 100 and 1000.
TRI-VI-FLOR®:
Drops in bottles of 30 and 50 ml with calibrated dropper.
Chewable Tablets in bottles of 100 and 1000.

VI-PENTA F

Description: Each **Zestabs** Chewable Tablet contains:

Fluoride (as sodium fluoride)	1 mg
Vitamin A acetate (5000 units)	1.5 mg
Ergocalciferol	10 μg
Ascorbic acid	60 mg
Thiamine mononitrate	1.2 mg
Riboflavin	1.5 mg
Pyridoxine hydrochloride	1.2 mg
Cyanocobalamin	3 μg
d-Biotin	40 μg

Niacinamide		10 mg
dl-α-Tocopheryl acetate		2 IU
Calcium pantothenate		10 mg

Each 0.6 ml of **Multivitamin Drops** contains:

Fluoride (as sodium fluoride)		0.5 mg
Vitamin A palmitate	(5000 units)	1.5 mg
Ergocalciferol	(400 units)	10 μg
Ascorbic acid		50 mg
Thiamine hydrochloride		1 mg
Riboflavin (as 5' phosphate sodium)		1 mg
Pyridoxine hydrochloride		1 mg
dl-α-Tocopheryl acetate		2 IU
d-Biotin		30 μg
Niacinamide		10 mg
d-Panthenol		10 mg

Each 0.6 ml of **Infant Drops** contains:

Fluoride (as sodium fluoride)		0.5 mg
Vitamin A palmitate	(5000 units)	1.5 mg
Ergocalciferol	(400 units)	10 μg
Ascorbic acid		50 mg
dl-α-Tocopheryl acetate		2 IU

Availability:

VI-PENTA® F: **(Roche)**

Chewable Tablets (Zestabs®) in bottles of 100.

Infant Drops in bottles of 30 ml with calibrated dropper.

Multivitamin Drops in bottles of 30 ml with calibrated dropper.

FLUOROMETHOLONE: see The Adrenal Corticosteroids

FLUOROURACIL

Chemical Name: 5-Fluorouracil.

Description: A fluorinated pyrimidine antagonist belonging to the category of antimetabolites, it occurs as a white, crystalline powder sparingly soluble in water and very slightly soluble in alcohol.

The rationale for its therapeutic usefulness is based on the suggestion that uracil may be utilized preferentially for nucleic acid biosynthesis in some tumors. Fluorouracil resembles the natural uracil molecule in structure, except that a fluoride atom has replaced a hydrogen atom in the 5th position of the pyrimidine ring. However, fluorouracil appears to function as an antimetabolite in at least 3 different ways: it interferes with the synthesis of deoxyribonucleic acid (DNA); it incorporates itself, to a small extent, into ribonucleic acid (RNA), thus producing a fraudulent RNA, and it inhibits utilization of preformed uracil in RNA synthesis by blocking uracil phosphatase. Since DNA and RNA are essential for cell division and growth, the effect of this compound may be to create a thymine deficiency, which provokes unbalanced growth and death of the cell. This action is most marked on those cells which grow more rapidly and which take up fluorouracil at a more rapid pace.

It has been shown that this drug inhibits the growth of human neoplasms and that its toxic effects are greatest on cells of the bone marrow, the intestinal mucosa and certain tumors of the breast, rectum and colon. While there is no evidence to indicate that the drug prolongs survival time, it has been a useful agent in relieving pain and other symptoms in certain types of human malignancies. There has also been an occasional regression in tumor size.

Following intravenous administration, fluorouracil is distributed into tumors, intestinal mucosa, bone marrow, liver, and other tissues; however, studies have shown a higher concentration of the drug or its metabolites in the tumor than in surrounding tissue or in corresponding normal tissue. A significant percentage of the drug is excreted intact in the urine within a few hours following intravenous administration, but the major portion of fluorouracil is metabolized primarily in the liver, and is excreted as respiratory carbon dioxide and as urea.

Clinical studies using radioactive fluorouracil topically showed that absorption, as measured by C^{14} content of plasma, urine and respiratory carbon dioxide, was considered insignificant. The activity in normal skin adjacent to a lesion is less frequent and intense because of the drug's cytotoxic selectivity.

Indications: Palliative management of carcinoma of the breast, stomach, pancreas, colon or rectum in carefully selected patients who are considered incurable by surgery or other means. The drug is not intended as an adjuvant to surgery, or for prophylactic use in any other manner. Also for the topical treatment of multiple actinic or solar keratoses.

Contraindications: In patients in a poor nutritional state, those with bone marrow previously depressed by other therapy or those with potentially serious infections. Also contraindicated in patients known to be hypersensitive to any component of the topical preparations.

Warnings: The daily dose of fluorouracil should not exceed 0.8 gm. It should be used with utmost care in patients who have undergone recent major surgery or who have a history of high-dose pelvic irradiation or who have had previous use of alkylating agents. Also it should be administered with considerable care in those who have a widespread involvement of bone marrow by metastatic tumors or who have extensive liver impairment or jaundice. When applied topically, the use of an occlusive dressing may result in inflammatory reactions in the adjacent normal skin. Because of possible potentiation, excessive exposure to ultraviolet rays should be avoided while under topical treatment. Safe use during pregnancy has not been established, and since the risk of mutagenesis has not been evaluated, such possible effects occurring in male and female patients must be considered.

Precautions: It is imperative that all patients be hospitalized during their first course of intravenous treatment. Severe hematological toxicity, gastrointestinal hemorrhage and even death may result despite meticulous selection of patients and careful adjustment of dosage. Although severe toxicity is more likely in poor risk patients, fatalities may be encountered even in patients in relatively good condition. Therapy should be discontinued promptly whenever signs of toxicity appear such as leukopenia, thrombocytopenia, stomatitis, esophagopharyngitis, intractable vomiting, diarrhea, gastrointestinal ulceration and bleeding, hemorrhage from any site.

Although topical application with bare fingers is not recommended, the hands should be washed immediately following each such application. Medication should be applied very carefully near eyes, nose and mouth. Biopsy of those areas unresponsive to or recurring after topical treatment should be performed to rule out frank neoplasm.

Adverse Reactions: Stomatitis and esophagopharyngitis which may lead to sloughing and ulceration; diarrhea, anorexia, nausea and emesis are commonly seen during therapy. Leukopenia usually follows every course of adequate therapy, and the lowest white blood cell counts are commonly observed between the 9th and 14th days after the first course of therapy, but may be delayed for as long as 20 days. By the 30th day the count has usually returned to the normal range. Alopecia and dermatitis may be seen in a substantial number of patients, and they should be informed that it is a transient effect. The dermatitis most often seen is a pruritic maculopapular rash generally appearing on the extremities and less frequently on the trunk. Dry skin and fissuring have also been observed. Photosensitivity, as manifested by erythema or increased pigmentation of the skin, occurs occasionally. Other toxic manifestations are photophobia, lacrimation, epistaxis, euphoria, acute cerebellar syndrome which may persist following discontinuation of therapy, and nail changes, including loss of nails.

Local pain, pruritus and hyperpigmentation and burning at application [topical] site occurred most frequently. Other reactions [topical] included dermatitis, scarring, soreness, tenderness, insomnia, stomatitis, suppuration, scaling, swelling, irritability, medicinal taste, photosensitivity, lacrimation, leukocytosis, thrombocytopenia, toxic granulation and eosinophilia.

Dosage and Administration: *Intravenously*, 12 mg/kg of body weight once daily for 4 successive days, not to exceed 800 mg/day. If no toxicity is observed, 6 mg/kg are given on the 6th, 8th, 10th and 12th days unless toxicity occurs before then. No therapy is given on the 5th, 7th, 9th and 11th days. Therapy is to be discontinued at the end of the 12th day, even if no toxicity has become apparent. In poor risk or undernourished patients, 6 mg/kg daily for 3 days, not to exceed 400 mg/day. If no toxicity is observed, 3 mg/kg may be given on the 5th, 7th, and 9th days unless toxicity occurs in the interim. No therapy is given on the 4th, 6th and 8th days. In cases where toxicity has *not* been a problem, it is recommended that courses be repeated at intervals of 1 month following the last injection of the previous course. In cases where toxicity has occurred, a single weekly dose of 10 to 15 mg/kg, not to exceed 1 gm/week may be given after the toxic signs have subsided.

Topically, twice daily for 2 to 4 weeks. Medication should be applied with a nonmetallic applicator or suitable glove in a quantity sufficient to cover the lesion. Response to treatment is manifested by erythema, usually followed in sequence by vesiculation, erosion, ulceration, necrosis and epithelization. Medication should be continued until the inflammatory reaction reaches the stage of erosion, necrosis and ulceration, at which time the drug should be withdrawn. Complete healing of the lesion may not be evident for 1 to 2 months following termination of therapy.

Availability:
ADRUCIL Injection, 50 mg/ml in ampuls of 10 ml. **(Adria)**
EFUDEX®: **(Roche)**
Cream, 5% in a vanishing cream base in tubes of 25 gm.
Solution, 2 and 5% (w/w) in dropper bottles of 10 ml.
FLUOROPLEX®: **(Herbert)**
Topical Cream, 1% in tubes of 30 gm.
Topical Solution, 1% in dropper bottles of 30 ml.
FLUOROURACIL® Aqueous Solution containing 500 mg in ampuls of 10 ml. **(Roche)**

FLUOXYMESTERONE

Chemical Name: 9α-Fluoro-11β, 17β-dihydroxy-17α-methyl-4-androsten-3-one.

Description: A halogenated derivative of testosterone, it is an orally effective anabolic and androgenic agent. It has up to 5 times the androgenic and anabolic activity of methyltestosterone. Weight for weight, it has an even greater therapeutic potency than parenterally administered testosterone derivatives. It occurs as a white, odorless, crystalline powder that is practically insoluble in water, sparingly soluble in alcohol and slightly soluble in chloroform.

Fluoxymesterone causes minimal retention of sodium, and edema and hypertension do not generally complicate therapy. Nitrogen and potassium excretion is reduced with therapeutic doses; it also decreases the urinary level of calcium and causes recalcification of osseous metastases and regression of soft-tissue lesions. It produces positive nitrogen balance, increases protein anabolism, and decreases amino acid catabolism in both sexes.

In the male, fluoxymesterone stimulates the growth and development of the genital organs and secondary sexual structures, and induces a gain in muscle mass and strength. In the female, the drug induces atrophy of the vaginal epithelium and uterine endometrium and antagonizes the effects of estrogens. When combined with ethinyl estradiol, it minimizes the undesirable side effects of long-term therapy.

Indications: In males, the primary indication is replacement therapy in conditions associated with a deficiency or absence of endogenous testicular hormone; primary eunuchoidism and eunuchism; male climacteric symptoms when these are secondary to androgen deficiency; impotence due to androgen deficiency; delayed puberty, provided that it has been definitely established as such and is not just a familial trait; and those symptoms of panhypopituitarism related to hypogonadism. In the latter case, appropriate adrenal cortical and thyroid hormone replacement therapy are still necessary and are actually of primary importance.

In females, therapy is indicated in the palliation of androgen-responsive, advanced, inoperable female breast cancer in women who are more than 1, but less than 5 years postmenopausal or who have been proven to have a hormone-dependent tumor as shown by previous beneficial response to castration, and in postmenopausal osteoporosis as adjunctive therapy to diet, calcium balance, physiotherapy, and general health promoting measures. Combined with ethinyl estradiol for the relief of symptoms of the menopause, male climacteric and osteoporosis of various etiologies.

Contraindications: Androgens are contraindicated in male patients with prostatic or breast cancer, in those cases of benign prostatic hypertrophy with obstructive symptoms, and in prepubertal males. Fluoxymesterone is contraindicated in women with advanced, inoperable mammary carcinoma when they are less than 1 or more than 5 years postmenopausal, or if they have a tumor that is not hormone-dependent as shown by a lack of beneficial response following castration, and during pregnancy and lactation. Fluoxymesterone is also contraindicated in patients with severe cardio-renal disease, nephrosis or the nephrotic phase of nephritis, in cases of severe liver damage, in hypercalcemic states, in patients easily stimulated, and, because of its hypercholesterolemic effects, in patients with a history of myocardial infarction; also in patients hypersensitive to the drug or to the component.

Warnings: If jaundice occurs, therapy should be discontinued immediately unless, in the opinion of the physician, the benefits of continued therapy outweigh the potential danger. Rarely, continued therapy may cause hepatic coma and death due to intrahepatic cholestasis. The jaundice is usually reversible if therapy is discontinued at once. The use of fluoxymesterone in infants is not recommended since evidence of beneficial effects in prematures and newborns is lacking and the consequences of such therapy in these patients are unknown. Also, it is not recommended for use in athletes since it has been shown to be of no value as an ergogenic aid. Female patients should be carefully observed for symptoms or signs of virilization. Hypercalcemia may develop both spontaneously and as a result of hormonal therapy in women with disseminated breast carcinoma. These patients should be watched carefully for the development of this complication. If hypercalcemia occurs, discontinue therapy and institute appropriate measures. If abnormal vaginal bleeding develops, the drug should be discontinued until the etiology is determined.

Precautions: Caution is required in administering this drug to patients with cardiac, renal, or hepatic disease. Edema may occur occasionally. Concomitant administration with adrenal steroids or ACTH may add to the edema. Fluoxymesterone may increase sensitivity to anticoagulants. Dosage of the anticoagulant may have to be decreased in order to maintain the prothrombin time at the desired therapeutic level. Anabolic steroids have been shown to alter glucose tolerance tests. Patients with diabetes should be followed carefully and their insulin or oral hypoglycemic dosage adjusted accordingly. Liver function should be checked at regular intervals in patients receiving 17-alpha alkyl preparations, including fluoxymesterone. Hepatocellular carcinoma and peliosis hepatis (blood-filled cysts in the liver) have been observed in patients with congenital or acquired aplastic anemia who were treated with androgens for prolonged periods. In some cases, regression of the lesions occurred when therapy was discontinued. Serum cholesterol may increase or decrease during therapy. Serial determinations of serum cholesterol should be made and therapy adjusted accordingly. The adverse consequences of therapy with this drug in young children are not fully understood, but the possibilities of serious disturbance of growth (e.g., premature closure of the epiphyses) and precocious sexual development do exist; therefore, before instituting therapy the possible beneficial effect must be weighed carefully. Since skeletal stimulation may continue for 6 months after therapy has been terminated, fluoxymesterone should be discontinued at the first sign of accelerated bone maturation. If prolonged use in children is anticipated, x-rays of the wrists prior to initial administration followed by roentgenographic observation every 3 to 6 months is recommended. Adequate amounts of calories and protein must be given if an optimal anabolic effect is to be observed.

Adverse Reactions: In males, the following postpubertal adverse reactions have occurred: inhibition of testicular function, testicular atrophy, and diminished ejaculatory volume; oligospermia; impotence; chronic priapism; gynecomastia; epididymitis; and bladder irritability. Prepubertal adverse reactions consist of phallic enlargement and increased frequency of erection. **In females,** hirsutism, male-pattern baldness, deepening of the voice, and clitoral enlargement may occur. These changes are usually irreversible even after prompt discontinuance of therapy and are not prevented by concomitant use of estrogens. Menstrual irregularities may also develop; hypercalcemia may occur, particularly in patients with metastatic breast carcinoma. **In both male and female,** the following reactions are known to occur with the use of anabolic steroids: increased or decreased libido, flushing of the skin, acne (especially in females and prepubertal males), habituation, excitation and sleeplessness, chills, leukopenia, bleeding in patients on concomitant anticoagulant therapy, and premature closure of epiphyses in children. Oral preparations have been associated with nausea, vomiting, diarrhea, as well as with symptoms resembling those of peptic ulcer. Jaundice may occur, but is usually reversible with prompt discontinuance of therapy. Occasionally, hepatic necrosis and death have been noted. Hypersensitivity reactions including rash and dermatitis have been reported. Also, anaphylactic reactions, while rare, can occur. Alterations may occur in the following clinical laboratory tests: metyrapone test, fasting blood sugar (FBS) and glucose tolerance test, thyroid function tests [decrease in protein bound iodine (PBI), thyroxine-binding capacity, and radioactive iodine uptake, and an increase in T^3 uptake by the red blood cells or resin; free thyroxine levels remain normal and the altered tests usually persist for 2 to 3 weeks after discontinuing therapy], electrolytes (retention of sodium, chloride, water, potassium, calcium, and inorganic phosphates), hepatic function tests [increased bromsulphalein (BSP), increased or decreased serum cholesterol, increased serum glutamic oxaloacetic transaminase (SGOT), increased serum bilirubin, and increased alkaline phosphatase], blood coagulation tests (increase in clotting factors II, V, VII, and X), and miscellaneous laboratory tests (increased creatine and creatinine excretion lasting up to 2 weeks after therapy has been terminated).

Dosage and Administration: *Orally.* Dosage must be strictly individualized. *In the male*, a dosage of 2 to 5 mg daily is usually adequate. Doses as high as 10 mg daily may be necessary, but should be used cautiously. *In the female* for the prevention of postpartum breast pain and engorgement in the non-nursing mother, a dosage of 5 mg 2 or 3 times daily for 4 to 6 days, beginning as soon after delivery as possible. For inoperable breast cancer, 20 to 30 mg daily as palliative therapy. Subjective improvement may be noted within 1 month and objective improvement should be noted within 3 months in responsive patients. *Combined with ethinyl estradiol,* the recommended starting dosage in the menopause and for the male climacteric is 1 tablet 2 or 3 times daily. In osteoporosis, 1 or 2 tablets 3 or 4 times daily—this dosage should be approached carefully and increased gradually with necessary caution to the development of side effects.

Availability:

Fluoxymesterone

HALOTESTIN® Tablets, 2 mg in bottles of 100; 5 and 10 mg in bottles of 50 and 100; the 10 mg are also available in unit-dose bottles of 30. **(Upjohn)**

ORA-TESTRYL® Tablets, 5 mg in bottles of 50. **(Squibb)**

w/Ethinyl Estradiol

HALODRIN® Tablets, 1 mg with ethinyl estradiol, 0.02 mg in bottles of 100. **(Upjohn)**

FLUPHENAZINE: see The Phenothiazines

FLUPREDNISOLONE: see The Adrenal Corticosteroids

FLURANDRENOLIDE: see The Adrenal Corticosteroids

FLURAZEPAM HYDROCHLORIDE (C-IV)

Chemical Name: 7-Chloro-1-[2-(diethylamino)ethyl]-5-(o-fluorophenyl)-1,3-dihydro-2*H*-1,4-benzodiazepin-2-one dihydrochloride.

Description: Flurazepam hydrochloride, a nonbarbiturate hypnotic agent, has a molecular weight of 460.826 and occurs as a pale yellow, crystalline compound very soluble in water and freely soluble in USP alcohol.

Animal studies reveal that the drug reduces the pressor response to electrical stimulation of the hypothalamus, and increases the arousal threshold to stimulation of the amygdala and hypothalamus; however, the exact site and mode of action are unknown.

Clinical studies have demonstrated that flurazepam reduces sleep induction time and increases duration of sleep. The drug usually induces sleep within 17 minutes and provides 7 to 8 hours of sleep, decreases sleep latency and number of awakenings while increasing total sleep time.

Indications: All types of insomnia characterized by difficulty in falling asleep, frequent nocturnal awakenings and/or early morning awakening. Since insomnia frequently is transient and intermittent, prolonged use of the drug generally is not necessary or recommended.

Contraindications: Hypersensitivity to the drug.

Warnings: Patients should be cautioned about possible combined effects with alcohol and other CNS depressants, and against engaging in any hazardous occupation requiring complete alertness or skill. Whether or not the drug is safe to use during pregnancy has not been established. Therefore, it should be given to women of childbearing potential only after due consideration of the potential benefits and possible hazards to mother and child. The drug currently is not recommended for patients under 15 years of age. As with any hypnotic, the customary precautions must be exercised when giving the drug to addiction-prone individuals.

Precautions: The usual precautions are indicated for severely depressed patients or those in whom there is any evidence of latent depression or of suicidal tendencies. In the latter instance, appropriate protective measures may be necessary. When flurazepam is used for prolonged periods, blood counts and liver and kidney function should be determined periodically. Patients with impaired renal or hepatic function should be carefully observed and the usual precautions undertaken.

Adverse Reactions: Dizziness, drowsiness, lightheadedness, staggering, ataxia and falling (particularly in the elderly or debilitated), severe sedation, lethargy, disorientation and coma (probably indicative of drug intolerance or overdosage), headache, heartburn, upset stomach, nausea, vomiting, diarrhea, constipation, gastrointestinal pain, nervousness, talkativeness, apprehension, irritability, weakness, palpitations, chest pains, body and joint pains and genitourinary complaints. There have also been rare occurrences of leukopenia and granulocytopenia, sweating, flushes, difficulty in focusing, blurred vision, burning eyes, faintness, hypotension, dyspnea, pruritus, skin rash, dry mouth, bitter taste, excessive salivation, anorexia, euphoria, depression, slurred speech, confusion, restlessness, hallucinations, and elevated SGOT, SGPT, total and direct bilirubins, and alkaline phosphatase. Paradoxical reactions, e.g., excitement, stimulation and hyperactivity also have been reported in rare instances. Manifestations of overdosage include somnolence, confusion and coma. Respiration, pulse rate and blood pressure should be monitored as in all cases of overdosage. General supportive measures should be employed, including immediate gastric lavage. Intravenous fluids should be administered and an adequate airway maintained. Hypotension and CNS depression may be combated by the judicious use of appropriate therapeutic agents. The value of dialysis has not been determined. If excitation occurs following overdosage, barbiturates should not be used. As with the management of intentional overdosage with any drug, it should be borne in mind that several agents may have been ingested.

Dosage and Administration: *Orally.* Dosage should be individualized for maximal beneficial effects. The usual adult dosage is 30 mg at bedtime. In the elderly or debilitated patient it is recommended that therapy be initiated with 15 mg until individual responses are determined. Limiting the dosage to 15 mg in these patients should serve to preclude the development of oversedation, dizziness and/or ataxia.

Availability:
Ⓒ IV DALMANE® Capsules, 15 mg (orange and ivory) and 30 mg (red and ivory) in bottles of 100 and 500, in Tel-E-Dose® cartons of 100 and 120 and in Prescription Paks of 30 and 300.

(Roche)

FOLBESYN

Description: Each tablet contains:

Thiamine mononitrate	10 mg
Riboflavin	5 mg

Niacinamide	50 mg
Pyridoxine	3 mg
Cyanocobalamin (vitamin B-12)	9 μg
Folic acid	0.4 mg
Ascorbic acid	180 mg

Indications: Preoperative or postoperative treatment of debilitated patients, and whenever there is a threatened depletion of water-soluble vitamin reserves.

Contraindications: Not indicated for the treatment of pernicious anemia and other megaloblastic anemias where vitamin B-12 is deficient.

Precautions: Folic acid may obscure pernicious anemia, in that the hematological remission may occur while the neurological manifestations remain progressive.

Adverse Reactions: Reported was allergic sensitization.

Dosage and Administration: *Orally.* One tablet daily.

Availability:
FOLBESYN® (OTC) Tablets in bottles of 50. **(Lederle)**

FOLIC ACID

Synonym: Pteroylglutamic acid.

Chemical Name: *N*-{*p*-{[(2-Amino-4-hydroxy-6-pteridinyl)methyl]amino}benzoyl}glutamic acid.

Description: A complex organic compound present in liver, yeast, fresh green vegetables and other substances, and which may be prepared synthetically. It occurs as a yellow or yellowish-orange, odorless, crystalline powder very slightly soluble in water and insoluble in alcohol.

An antianemic principle inducing reticulocytosis and erythrocytic maturation in macrocytic anemias. In addisonian pernicious anemia, folic acid alone does not prevent the development or cause improvement of spinal cord lesions.

Indications: Treatment of megaloblastic anemias, including sprue, gestational macrocytic anemia, macrocytic anemia of gastrointestinal origin, and the macrocytic anemias associated with pellagra and similar deficiency states. Whether given by mouth or parenterally, folic acid stimulates specifically the production of red blood cells, white blood cells and platelets in patients suffering from megaloblastic anemias. It is the preferred treatment of all megaloblastic anemias except pernicious anemia, where vitamin B-12 is essential. Combined with iron, it alleviates secondary or iron-deficiency anemia, as may develop in nutritional anemia, primary microcytic anemia and certain anemias of pregnancy.

Warnings: Administration of folic acid alone is not the proper therapy for pernicious anemia and other megaloblastic anemias in which vitamin B-12 is deficient.

Precautions: Folic acid may obscure pernicious anemia in that the peripheral blood picture may revert to normal while neurological manifestations progress.

Adverse Reactions: Although rare, the incidence of allergic sensitization has been reported following both oral and parenteral administration of folic acid.

Dosage and Administration: *Orally, intramuscularly, intravenously,* or *subcutaneously.* The recommended therapeutic dose of folic acid in adults and children (regardless of age) is 0.25 to 1 mg daily. Resistant cases may require larger doses. When clinical symptoms have subsided and the blood picture has become normal, the recommended maintenance daily dose is as follows: For infants, 0.1 mg; for children up to 4 years of age, 0.1 to 0.3 mg; for adults and children 4 years of age and older, 0.4 mg, and for pregnant and lactating women, 0.8 mg. Combined with iron: One or 2 capsules before each meal daily and this therapy should be continued until there is adequate hematopoiesis.

Availability:

Folic Acid

Tablets, 0.1, 0.25, 0.4 and 1 mg in bottles of 100 and 1000. **(Various Mfrs.)**

Tablets, 1 mg in bottles of 100 and 1000. **(ICN)**

Tablets, 1 mg in bottles of 100. **(Lilly)**

FOLVITE®: **(Lederle)**

Injection (as sodium folate), 5 mg/ml in vials of 10 ml.

Tablets, 0.25 mg (yellow) in bottles of 100; 1 mg (orange), in bottles of 100 and 1000 and in unit-dose packages of 100 (10 × 10).

FOLVRON® Capsules, 0.33 mg with ferrous sulfate, 182 mg (equiv. to 57 mg elemental iron) in bottles of 100. **(Lederle)**

FORMATRIX

Description: Each tablet contains:

Conjugated estrogens-equine (Premarin®)	1.25 mg
Methyltestosterone	10 mg
Ascorbic acid (as sodium ascorbate)	400 mg

Combined estrogen and androgen therapy helps arrest the catabolic process in osteoporosis, thus aiding to prevent further fractures and loss of height. It is specially formulated to relieve low back pain and to promote healing of fractures in osteoporosis (bone matrix atrophy). It improves the general well being, sleep pattern, appetite, and muscle tone of the patient.

Indications: Postmenopausal osteoporosis (after natural or surgical menopause); osteoporosis due to immobilization, osteoporosis following corticosteroid hormone therapy and osteoporosis due to malnutrition (notably protein depletion and ascorbic acid deficiency).

Contraindications: Carcinoma of the prostate because of the methyltestosterone component.

Adverse Reactions: Withdrawal bleeding, breast tenderness, and hirsutism.

For complete data on contraindications, warnings, precautions and adverse reactions, refer to the monograph on the individual components, estrogen and methyltosterone.

Dosage and Administration: *Orally,* 1 tablet daily. In the female, a rest period of 1 week is recommended after each 21-day course. In the male, check carefully the status of the prostate gland when protracted therapy is given. Adjunctive measures: a high protein diet is recommended; immobilization should be minimized in order to restore the necessary stress and strain as natural aids to bone repair.

Availability:

FORMĀTRIX® Tablets in bottles of 60 and 500. **(Ayerst)**

FURAZOLIDONE

Chemical Name: 3-(5-Nitrofurfurylideneamino)-2-oxazolidinone.

Description: Furazolidone is a nitrofuran with antibacterial and antiprotozoal properties. Its precise mode of action is not known, but it is thought to inhibit the cycle of carbohydrate metabolism in the bacterial cell. In vitro, it is bactericidal against species of Salmonella, Shigella, Staphylococcus, Aerobacter, and Escherichia and enterococci. The drug is incompletely absorbed with only minute amounts appearing in the urine. Metabolic degradation products may tint the urine brown.

Indications: The specific and symptomatic treatment of bacterial or protozoal diarrhea and enteritis caused by susceptible organisms.

Contraindications: Patients with prior hypersensitivity to the drug. The concurrent ingestion of alcohol, MAO inhibitors, tyramine-containing foods, and indirectly acting sympathomimetic amines are contraindicated or should be used with caution. Also contraindicated in infants under 1 month of age.

Warnings: The drug should be used with caution, if at all, during pregnancy, lactation, and in women of childbearing potential, until safety for its use has been established.

Precautions: To avoid a hypertensive crisis, the dosage of concomitantly administered MAO inhibitors, tyramine-containing foods, sympathomimetic amines, sedatives, antihistamines, tranquilizers and narcotics, should be reduced or the drug used with extreme caution. Orthostatic hypotension and hypoglycemia may occur.

Adverse Reactions: Hypersensitivity reactions including hypotension, urticaria, fever, arthralgia, and a vesicular or morbiliform pruritic rash; nausea; vomiting; headache; malaise; disulfiram-like reaction to alcohol characterized by flushing, mild fever, dyspnea, and constriction in the chest; mild reversible intravascular hemolysis in certain ethnic groups of Mediterranean and Near-Eastern origin and Negroes. Colitis, proctitis, anal pruritus, staphylococci enteritis, or renal or hepatic toxicity have not been significant problems with furazolidone.

Dosage and Administration: *Orally.* Average adult dosage, 100 mg 4 times daily. Average dosage for children 5 years of age or older, 25 to 50 mg 4 times daily. The dosage for the liquid is based on an average dose of 5 mg/kg of body weight in 4 equally divided doses daily. The maximal dosage of 8.8 mg/kg/day should probably not be exceeded because of the possibility of producing nausea or vomiting. If a satisfactory clinical response is not obtained within 7 days, it indicates that the pathogen is refractory to furazolidone, thus necessitating withdrawal of the medication. Not recommended for infants under 1 month of age.

Availability:
FUROXONE®: **(Norwich-Eaton)**
Liquid Suspension, 17 mg with kaolin, 1 gm and pectin, 75 mg/5 ml in bottles of 60 ml and 1 pint.
Tablets, 100 mg in bottles of 20 and 100.

FUROSEMIDE

Chemical Name: 4-Chloro-*N*-furfuryl-5-sulfamoylanthranilic acid.

Description: A non-mercurial diuretic of the sulfonamide group that is chemically distinct not only from the organomercurials, but also from the thiazides and other heterocyclic compounds. It occurs as a white, crystalline powder sparingly soluble in water.

The drug appears to act on the distal portion of the renal tubule but its diuretic effect cannot be attributed to aldosterone antagonism or carbonic anhydrase inhibition. It apparently exerts a direct effect on electrolyte transport at the level of the distal tubule and also inhibits the reabsorption of sodium in the ascending loop of Henle. It also has been found to decrease proximal tubular reabsorption of sodium and chloride, resulting in enhanced excretion of these ions especially sodium. The sodium and potassium excretion ratio during therapy with furosemide is in a higher range than during therapy with thiazides; and diuresis, and total electrolyte and fluid loss is greater than with the thiazides.

Following oral administration, the diuretic effect is apparent within 1 hour, maximal effect occurs in the 1st or 2nd hour, and the duration of action is from 6 to 8 hours. Following intravenous administration, the diuretic effect is apparent within 5 minutes, maximal effect occurs within 30 minutes and the duration of action is about 2 hours. Furosemide is excreted in the urine by glomerular filtration and by secretion from the proximal tubule. Reproduction studies in mice, rats and rabbits receiving 2 to 4 times the recommended clinical dose resulted in embroyonic toxicity and maternal deaths.

Indications: Treatment of edema associated with congestive heart failure, cirrhosis of the liver, and renal disease, including the nephrotic syndrome. Furosemide is recommended for use in hypertension either alone or in combination with other antihypertensive agents.

Contraindications: In anuria; in patients hypersensitive to the compound; in the presence of hepatic coma; and in states of electrolyte depletion. **Because animal reproduction studies have shown that furosemide may cause fetal abnormalities, the drug should not be**

administered to women of childbearing potential, unless the condition is life-threatening, and the use of this diuretic is considered of paramount importance over the use of alternative drugs.

Warnings: Patients should be under careful medical supervision and dosage schedules should be adjusted to the needs of the individual patient. The physician should be aware that excessive diuresis may result in electrolyte depletion, dehydration and reduction in blood volume with circulatory collapse and with the possibility of vascular thrombosis and embolism occurring particularly in elderly patients. Also excessive loss of potassium in patients receiving digitalis glycosides may precipitate digitalis toxicity. Care, therefore, should be exercised in patients receiving potassium-depleting steroids. Frequent serum electrolyte, CO_2 and BUN determinations should be performed and abnormalities corrected or the drug temporarily withdrawn. Patients with hepatic cirrhosis and ascites should be strictly observed because a sudden alteration of fluid and electrolyte balance may precipitate hepatic coma. Supplemental potassium chloride and, if required, an aldosterone antagonist are helpful in preventing hypokalemia and metabolic alkalosis. Patients should be observed regularly, since blood dyscrasias, liver damage or other idiosyncratic reactions have been known to occur. Because there have been reports concerning nonspecific small-bowel lesions consisting of stenosis, with or without ulceration associated with the administration of coated potassium-containing formulations, these should be given only when indicated and should be discontinued if abdominal pain, distention, nausea, vomiting or gastrointestinal bleeding occurs. These lesions have caused obstruction, hemorrhage, and perforation; surgery was frequently required and deaths have occurred. Patients with known sensitivity to sulfonamides may also show an allergic reaction to furosemide.

Precautions: As with any potent diuretic, electrolyte depletion may occur and may manifest itself by weakness, dizziness, lethargy, leg cramps, anorexia, vomiting and/or mental confusion. In edematous hypertensive patients being treated with antihypertensive agents, care should be taken to reduce the dose of these drugs when furosemide is administered since it potentiates the hypotensive effect of these medications. Dehydration may cause asymptomatic hyperuricemia, gout or BUN elevations, and these reactions should be avoided especially in patients with renal insufficiency. The drug should be discontinued if increasing azotemia and oliguria occur during treatment of severe progressing renal disease. Hearing impairment (which may in some instances be irreversible) and tinnitus have been reported. Usually, ototoxicity may occur when the drug is injected rapidly, in doses exceeding those recommended, in patients with severe impairment of renal function and in those who are also receiving drugs known to be ototoxic. Periodic checks on urine and blood glucose in diabetic patients should be made as elevations in blood glucose have been known to occur in patients taking this drug. Serum calcium levels may be decreased and rare cases of tetany have been reported. Patients taking high doses of salicylates in conjunction with furosemide may experience salicylate toxicity at lower doses because of competitive renal excretory sites. Concomitant administration with cephaloridine should be avoided since furosemide enhances the nephrotoxicity of this drug. Utmost caution should be exercised in administering curare or its derivatives to patients undergoing therapy with furosemide as sulfonamide diuretics have been reported to decrease arterial responsiveness to pressor amines and to enhance the effect of tubocurarine. It is advisable to discontinue oral medication for 1 week, and parenteral medication 2 days prior to any elective surgery.

Adverse Reactions: Various forms of dermatitis, including urticaria and rarely exfoliative dermatitis, erythema multiforme, pruritus, paresthesia, blurring of vision, postural hypotension, nausea vomiting, and diarrhea have been noted. Anemia, leukopenia, aplastic anemia, and thrombocytopenia purpura may occur. Rare instances of agranulocytosis have occurred which responded to treatment. Cases of deafness and tinnitus, some of which were irreversible, have been reported. These complications developed when the drug was injected in doses that were several times greater than the usual therapeutic dose. Rarely reported were sweet taste, oral and gastric burning, paradoxical swelling, headache, jaundice, thrombophlebitis, emboli, and acute pancreatitis. It has not been established whether or not these were drug-related. Furosemide-induced diuresis may be accompanied by weakness, fatigue, lightheadedness or dizziness, muscle cramps, thirst, increased perspiration, urinary bladder spasm, and symptoms of urinary frequency. Transient pain at the injection site following intramuscular administration has been experienced.

Dosage and Administration: *Orally, intravenously* or *intramuscularly. For diuresis,* the usual oral dose for adults is 20 to 80 mg given as a single dose, preferably in the morning. Depending on the patient's response, a second dose can be administered 6 to 8 hours later. The usual parenteral dose is 20 to 40 mg given as a single dose. The intravenous injection should be administered slowly preferably over a period of 1 to 2 minutes. If the response is not satisfactory, increments of 20 mg, no sooner than 2 hours after the previous dose, should be administered until the desired diuretic effect has been obtained. This individually determined single dose should then be given once or twice daily. *For hypertension,* the usual dose is 40 mg for initiating therapy and for maintenance. When furosemide is used with other antihypertensive agents, the dose of these agents must be reduced by 50% in order to prevent an excessive drop in blood pressure. The usual initial oral dose for infants and children is 2 mg/kg of body weight given as a single dose. If the response is not satisfactory, increments of 1 or 2 mg/kg, no sooner than 6 to 8 hours after the previous dose, should be administered until the desired diuretic effect has been obtained. The usual parenteral dose is 1 mg/kg of body weight given as a single dose. If the response is not satisfactory, increments of 1 mg/kg, no sooner than 2 hours after the previous dose, should be administered until the desired clinical effect has been achieved. Doses greater than 6 mg/kg of body weight are not recommended. *For acute pulmonary edema,* the usual intravenous regimen is 40 mg injected slowly, followed in 1 to 1½ hours by an additional 40 mg, if required. **Note:** The solution should not be used if it turns yellow.

Availability:
LASIX®: **(Hoechst)**
Injection, 10 mg/ml in ampuls of 2 and 10 ml and in prefilled syringes of 2 ml.
Oral Solution, 10 mg/ml in bottles of 60 ml with calibrated dropper and 120 ml with plastic spoon.
Tablets, 20 mg in bottles of 100; 40 mg in bottles of 100 and 500 and in unit-dose packages of 100.

GENTAMICIN SULFATE

Description: Gentamicin sulfate is a bactericidal antibiotic of the amino glycoside group, derived from *Micromonospora purpura* and *M. echinospora.* It occurs as a white to off-white, crystalline powder freely soluble in water and very slightly soluble in alcohol.

The exact mechanism of action of gentamicin has not been determined but it appears to interfere with protein synthesis of the bacterial cell. Laboratory studies show that gentamicin is active against a number of species and strains of both gram-positive and gram-negative bacteria. It is inactive against filamentous fungi, yeasts and viruses.

The gram-positive organisms, against which gentamicin is active, include coagulase-positive and coagulase-negative staphylococci, including certain strains that are resistant to penicillin; group A beta-hemolytic and nonhemolytic streptococci; and *Diplococcus pneumoniae.* The gram-negative organisms, against which gentamicin is active, include certain strains of *Pseudomonas aeruginosa,* indole-positive and indole-negative *Proteus* species, *Escherichia coli, Klebsiella pneumoniae* (Friedlander's bacillus), *Haemophilus influenzae* and *Haemophilus aegyptius* (Koch-Weeks bacillus), *Aerobacter aerogenes, Moraxella lacunata* (diplobacillus of Morax-Axenfeld), and *Neisseria* species, including *Neisseria gonorrhoeae.* Although infrequent, bacterial resistance to gentamicin has occurred, particularly with widespread topical use. Using a 10 mcg gentamicin disc, a zone of inhibition of 13 mm or more indicates susceptibility, and a zone of 12 mm or less indicates resistance. Organisms resistant to this drug have shown cross resistance to other aminoglycoside antibiotics. Its average half-life following intramuscular injection is slightly more than 2 hours.

Peak serum concentrations occur between 30 and 90 minutes following intramuscular injection, and effective serum levels may persist for 6 to 8 hours. When gentamicin is administered by intravenous infusion over a 2-hour period, the serum concentrations are similar to those obtained by intramuscular administration. An injection of a 1 mg/kg dose usually results in a peak serum concentration of approximately 4 mcg/ml. When administered every 8 hours, it does not accumulate in the serum. In patients with impaired renal function, the serum concentration is usually higher and measurable for longer periods; therefore, the dosage must be adjusted.

Approximately 25 to 30% of the administered dose is bound to serum protein; it is released as the drug is excreted principally in the urine by glomerular filtration. In patients with normal renal function, from 30 to 100% of gentamicin is recoverable in the urine in 24 hours. Following parenteral administration, low concentrations of the drug are found in the bile and in the cerebrospinal fluid. The drug can also be detected in the sputum, the pleural and peritoneal fluids. It crosses both the peritoneal and placental membranes.

Indications: Bacteremia, infected surgical wounds, puerperal sepsis, bone and severe soft tissue infections including burns complicated by sepsis, respiratory tract infections, meningitis, gastrointestinal infections (including peritonitis), and selected cases of urinary tract infections; also for use in primary skin infections such as impetigo contagiosa, superficial folliculitis, erythema, furunculosis, sycosis barbae and pyoderma gangrenosum, and in secondary skin infections such as infectious eczematoid dermatitis, pustular acne, pustular psoriasis, infected excoriations, and bacterial superinfections of fungal or viral infections. Also for conjunctivitis, keratitis and keratoconjunctivitis, corneal ulcers, blepharitis and blepharoconjunctivitis, acute meibomianitis and dacryocystitis. Injectable gentamicin sulfate should be considered for initial presumptive therapy in suspected gram-negative sepsis, and for staphylococcal infections where susceptibility testing and clinical judgment indicate its use. When the infecting organism is unknown in suspected sepsis, gentamicin may be administered together with a penicillin-type drug. Following identification of the organism and its susceptibility, appropriate antibiotic therapy should then be continued. In the neonate with suspected sepsis or staphylococcal pneumonia, a penicillin-type drug is usually indicated as concomitant antimicrobial therapy. The combination of carbenicillin and gentamicin provides effective treatment in life-threatening *Pseudomonas aeruginosa* infections.

Contraindications: In patients with a history of hypersensitivity or toxic reactions to gentamicin.

Warnings: Patients should be under close clinical observation because nephrotoxicity and ototoxicity (vestibular and auditory) can occur in patients, primarily in those with preexisting renal damage. Serum concentrations should be monitored when feasible and prolonged concentrations above 12 mcg/ml are not advised. Patients with normal renal function may develop nitrogen retention manifested by increasing levels of BUN, NPN, and creatinine, and by oliguria. Evidence of ototoxicity requires adjustment of dosage or withdrawal of the drug. In the event of overdose or toxic reactions, peritoneal dialysis or hemodialysis will aid in the removal of gentamicin from the blood. Gentamicin should not be used conjunctively with other neurotoxic and/or nephrotoxic drugs, particularly streptomycin, neomycin, kanamycin, cephaloridine, viomycin, polymyxin B, and polymyxin E (colistin). The concurrent use of gentamicin with potent diuretics should be avoided since certain diuretics by themselves may cause ototoxicity. In addition, when administered intravenously, diuretics may effect a rise in gentamicin serum level and potentiate neurotoxicity. The ophthalmic solution is not for injection, and should never be injected subconjunctivally. Also, it should not be introduced directly into the anterior chamber of the eye. The ophthalmic ointment may retard corneal healing.

Precautions: If irritation, hypersensitivity or superinfection with a nonsusceptible organism occurs, treatment should be discontinued. In patients with impaired renal function in whom serious infection develops, serum concentrations of the drug may rise, with increased risk of ototoxicity. Because gentamicin is potentially nephrotoxic, kidney function tests should be performed especially when the recommended dosage or duration of therapy is exceeded. The potential for fetal ototoxicity, nephrotoxicity or teratogenicity has not been established; therefore, the drug should not be used in pregnant patients or in women of childbearing age unless its use is deemed advisable by the physician. Prolonged use of topical antibiotics may give rise to overgrowth of nonsusceptible organisms such as fungi. Should this occur, discontinue use of the preparation and institute appropriate therapy.

Adverse Reactions: Complications following topical application of gentamicin include transient skin irritation manifested by erythema and pruritus that did not usually require discontinuance of treatment, photosensitization, and occasionally burning and stinging of the eye(s). Those following parenteral use include azotemia, elevated BUN, NPN, and creatinine levels, and oliguria; ototoxicity accompanied by dizziness, vertigo, tinnitus, roaring in the ears, and loss of hearing (rare); numbness, skin tingling, muscle twitching, and convulsions. Other reported complications possibly related to gentamicin include increased serum transaminase activity (SGOT or SGPT), increased serum bilirubin, transient hepatomegaly, decreased serum calcium; splenomegaly, anemia, increased or decreased reticulocyte counts, agranulocytosis, granulocytopenia, thrombocytopenia, purpura; fever, rash, itching, urticaria, generalized burning, joint pain, laryngeal edema; nausea, vomiting, headache, increased salivation, lethargy and decreased appetite, weight loss; pulmonary fibrosis, hypotension, and hypertension.

Dosage and Administration: *Intramuscularly, intravenously* or *topically.* Urinary tract infections, the recommended dosage *for serious infections* in the presence of normal kidney function is 3 mg/kg/day administered in 3 equally divided doses (every 8 hours) for 7 to 10 days. *For life-threatening infections,* up to 5 mg/kg/day administered in 3 or 4 equally divided doses and reduced as indicated. Children, 6 to 7.5 mg/kg/day, administered in 3 equally divided doses every 8 hours. Infants and neonates. 7.5 mg/kg/day, administered in 3 equally divided doses every 8 hours. Premature or full-term neonates 1 week of age or less, the total daily dose of 5 mg should be administered in 2 equally divided doses every 12 hours. *Patients with renal failure undergoing hemodialysis,* the recommended dosage is 1 mg/kg of body weight for adults and 2 mg/kg of body weight for children administered at the end of each dialysis period. Topical application: A small amount of cream or ointment should be applied gently to the lesion 3 or 4 times daily. The area treated may be covered with a gauze dressing if desired. In impetigo contagiosa, the crusts should be removed before application to permit maximum contact. Ophthalmic solution, 1 or 2 drops into eye(s) every 4 hours. In severe infections, dosage may be increased to 2 drops every hour. Ophthalmic ointment, apply a small amount to the affected eye 2 or 3 times daily.

Availability:
GARAMYCIN®: **(Schering)**
Cream, 1 mg/gm in tubes of 15 gm.
Injection, 40 mg/ml in multiple-dose vials of 2 ml and in disposable syringes of 1.5 and 2 ml.
Ointment, 1 mg/gm in tubes of 15 gm.
Ophthalmic Ointment, 3 mg/gm in tubes of 3.5 gm.
Ophthalmic Solution, 3 mg/ml in dropper bottles of 5 ml.
Pediatric Injectable, 10 mg/ml in multiple-dose vials of 2 ml.

GENTIAN VIOLET

Chemical Name: Hexamethyl*para*rosaniline chloride.

Description: Gentian violet is a hexamethyl*para*rosaniline chloride compound usually admixed with pentamethyl*para*rosaniline chloride and tetramethyl*para*rosaline chloride. It occurs as a dark green powder or as greenish, glistening pieces having a metallic luster with a faint odor; soluble in water and freely soluble in alcohol. A bacteriostatic and bactericidal agent to gram-positive organisms and to many fungi.

Indications: Treatment of monilial vaginitis (Candida infection).

Contraindications: Hypersensitivity to gentian violet; other vaginal infections.

Warnings: This medication should not be used in the presence of extensive excoriation or ulceration.

Precautions: Patients should be cautioned not to insert an applicator too deeply into the vagina during the last trimester of pregnancy. They should also be advised to refrain from coitus during treatment. Therapy should be discontinued if the infection persists following treatment.

Adverse Reactions: Acute chemical vulvovaginitis; staining of the skin.

Dosage and Administration: *Intravaginally.* By means of a specially designed, single-dose applicator, the contents are expelled into the vagina once nightly, at bedtime, for about 12 to 14 consecutive nights; or 1 tampon may be inserted and left in situ for 3 to 4 hours, once or twice daily, for a period of 12 days. In resistant infections, an additional tampon may be used and left in overnight. During pregnancy, treatment may be extended to 21 days. If infection persists, a second course of treatment may be required.

Availability:
GENAPAX® Vaginal Tampons, 5 mg in cartons of 12. **(Key Pharm.)**
HYVA® GENTIAN VIOLET Vaginal Tablets, 1 mg in cartons of 14 and 28. **(Holland-Rantos)**

GERILETS

Description: Each tablet contains:

Vitamin A	(5000 units)	1.5 mg
Ergocalciferol	(400 units)	10 μg
Thiamine mononitrate		2.25 mg
Riboflavin		2.6 mg
Pyridoxine hydrochloride		3 mg
Biotin		0.45 mg
Folic acid		0.4 mg
Niacinamide		30 mg
Ascorbic acid		90 mg
Calcium pantothenate		15 mg
Cyanocobalamin (vitamin B-12)		9 μg
Iron (as ferrous sulfate)		27 mg
Vitamin E (as *d*-alpha tocopheryl acetate)		45 IU

Indications: As a dietary supplement and supportive regimen for adults and children 4 years of age and older.

Contraindications: In patients hypersensitive to any of the components.

Precautions: Folic acid may obscure the presence of pernicious anemia by producing a hematologic remission but not affecting progression of neurologic manifestations.

Adverse Reactions: Folic acid may produce allergic reactions.

Dosage and Administration: *Orally,* 1 tablet daily or as prescribed.

Availability:
GERILETS® Filmtab® (film-sealed tablets) in bottles of 100 and 250. **(Abbott)**

GITALIN

Description: Gitalin is a water-soluble mixture of amorphous glycosides obtained from *Digitalis purpurea.* It occurs as a white or pale buff, amorphous powder slightly soluble in water and freely soluble in alcohol. The pharmacologic actions are similar to those of other digitalis glycosides (enhances force of myocardial contraction, increases the refractory period of the A-V node and to a lesser degree the S-A node conduction systems).

Following oral administration, the drug apparently is well-absorbed from the gastrointestinal tract, and its rate of elimination or dissipation is relatively rapid so that symptoms of toxicity, if they occur, are not likely to persist for unduly long periods.

Indications: Treatment of congestive heart failure in cardiac arrhythmias (atrial fibrillation, atrial flutter, and paroxysmal atrial tachycardia) and cardiogenic shock.

Contraindications: Digitalis toxicity and ventricular tachycardia, unless congestive heart failure supervenes.

Warnings: Digitalis-induced arrhythmias are identical to those for which digitalis therapy is advised. If the possibility of digitalis intoxication cannot be excluded, the drug should be temporarily withheld if permitted by the clinical situation. The patient with congestive heart failure may complain of nausea and vomiting. These symptoms may also be indications of digitalis intoxication. A clinical determination of the cause of these symptoms must be attempted before further drug administration.

Precautions: Potassium depletion sensitizes the myocardium to digitalis and toxicity is likely to develop even with usual dosage. Also, hypokalemia tends to reduce the positive inotropic effect of digitalis. Potassium loss may result from diuretic, corticosteroid, hemodialysis and other therapy, and it is likely to accompany malnutrition, old age and long-standing congestive heart failure. Hypokalemia can be minimized by adequate supplementation of potassium either by orange juice or potassium salts. Acute myocardial infarction, severe pulmonary disease, or well-advanced heart failure tends to be more sensitive to digitalis and more prone to arrhythmias. Since calcium affects contractility and excitability of the heart in a manner similar to that of digitalis, it may produce serious arrhythmias in digitalis-treated patients. Intoxication can be prevented in most instances by evaluating therapy frequently and by decreasing the dosage in the presence of factors that tend to cause excessive accumulation such as impaired renal function, or when there is an existing atrioventricular block, chronic constrictive pericarditis, or idiopathic hypertrophic subaortic stenosis. Electrical conversion of arrhythmias may require adjustment of the digitalis dosage.

Adverse Reactions: Gynecomastia, though uncommon, may occur. Toxic manifestations usually are those resulting from overdosage, and may include anorexia, nausea, vomiting, diarrhea; headache, weakness, apathy, visual disturbances; alterations of cardiac rhythm or conduction; mental depression.

Dosage and Administration: *Orally.* Initial rapid digitalization, usually 2.5 mg followed by 0.75 mg every 6 hours until therapeutic effect or toxicity develops. Most patients respond to a total dosage of about 6 mg. *Slow method:* A single daily dose of 1.5 mg for 4 to 6 days. *Maintenance:* Average dose is 0.5 mg in the morning. Dosage must be adjusted to the patient's needs and may be as low as 0.25 mg or as high as 1.25 mg daily.

Availability:
GITALIGIN® Tablets, 0.5 mg in bottles of 100. **(Schering)**

GLOBIN ZINC INSULIN: see The Insulins

GLUCAGON

Description: Glucagon is a hyperglycemic, glycogenolytic substance elaborated by the *alpha cells* of the pancreas (islands of Langerhan). Chemically unrelated to insulin, glucagon is a straight-chain polypeptide that contains 29 amino acid residues and has a molecular weight of 3,485. It occurs as an odorless, tasteless, fine, white or faintly colored, crystalline powder that is relatively insoluble in water but is soluble at a pH of less than 3 or more than 9.5.

Glucagon is useful in hypoglycemia only if liver glycogen is available. It is of little or no help in states of starvation, adrenal insufficiency, or chronic hypoglycemia. When administered parenterally, glucagon produces a prompt increase in blood glucose concentration by converting hepatic glycogen to glucose. Like epinephrine, it activates liver phosphorylase, and thereby increases glycogenolysis; it differs in that its glycogenolytic action is confined to the liver and is not blocked by adrenergic blocking agents. It also stimulates the release of insulin and catecholamines, decreases the contractibility of the gastrointestinal tract and inhibits gastric secretion.

Glucagon is effective when given parenterally, but upon oral administration, it is presumed to be destroyed by the proteolytic enzymes in the gastrointestinal tract. Following injection, peak response is usually attained within 10 to 30 minutes, and the effect may last for 1 to 2 hours, depending upon the dose. Glucagon is metabolized primarily by the liver.

Indications: To counteract severe hypoglycemic reaction in diabetic patients and to terminate insulin coma induced for treatment of psychiatric disturbances. Patients with juvenile-type diabetes should be given a supplementary carbohydrate as soon as possible.

Contraindications: In patients hypersensitive to glucagon.

Precautions: In the treatment of hypoglycemic shock with glucagon, liver glycogen must be available. In the hypoglycemic patient, glucose by the intravenous route or by gavage should be considered. Although glucagon may be used for the treatment of hypoglycemia by the patient during an emergency, the physician must still be notified when hypoglycemic reactions occur, so that the dose of insulin may be adjusted more accurately. Frequent testing of the urine is advised in order that a change in insulin requirement can be foreseen. Patients with diabetes should be instructed to carry sugar, candy or other readily absorbable carbohydrate, and to ingest these at the first warning of an oncoming reaction. Those in diabetic coma should be aroused as quickly as possible, since a prolonged hypoglycemic reaction may result in cortical damage.

Adverse Reactions: Glucagon is relatively free of adverse reactions except for occasional nausea and vomiting, which may also occur with hypoglycemia.

Dosage and Administration: *Intramuscularly, intravenously* or *subcutaneously. Hypoglycemic reactions in the diabetic patient.* 0.5 to 1 mg, repeated if patient does not respond within 20 minutes. *To terminate the coma of insulin shock therapy,* 0.5 to 1 mg is usually administered 1 hour after coma has been achieved; larger doses may be employed if necessary. In extremely severe situations, intravenous glucose should be given in addition to glucagon for a faster response. Glucagon may be added to dextrose solutions, but not to solutions containing chlorides of sodium, potassium or calcium since it will precipitate. For complete dosage information, see package literature.

Availability:
GLUCAGON For injection (as the hydrochloride) in ampuls of 1 and 10 mg with 1 and 10 ml vials of diluent, respectively. **(Lilly)**

GLUCO-CALCIUM

Description: An injectable solution of the calcium salts of sugar acids containing 18 mg/ml of calcium (0.898 mEq/ml) equivalent in calcium content to 2 ml of a 10% solution of calcium gluconate or to 0.67 ml of a 10% solution of calcium chloride.

Calcium is the fifth most abundant element in the body, and the major fraction is in the bony structure. Calcium plays important physiological roles, many of which are poorly understood. It is essential for the functional integrity of the nervous and muscular systems, is necessary for normal cardiac function, and is one of the factors involved in the coagulation of blood.

Indications: Treatment of hypocalcemia for those conditions requiring a prompt increase in blood plasma calcium levels, such as neonatal tetany and tetany due to parathyroid deficiency, vitamin D deficiency, and alkalosis. It is also indicated for the prevention of hypocalcemia during exchange transfusions.

Precautions: Because of its additive effect, the drug should be given with caution to patients who are digitalized or who are taking digitalis or digitalis-like preparations. Administration in infants and young children should be restricted to the intravenous route, whenever possible.

Adverse Reactions: Mild local reactions following intramuscular injection may occur; also a tingling sensation, a calcium taste, and a sense of oppression or heat may be experienced with rapid intravenous injection.

Dosage and Administration: *Intramuscularly,* 2 to 5 ml. *Intravenously,* 5 to 20 ml. The solution should be warmed to body temperature and administered slowly (2 ml/minute). During exchange transfusions in newborns, the usual dose is 0.5 ml following every 100 ml of blood exchanged.

Availability:
GLUCO-CALCIUM® Injection in ampuls of 30 ml in cartons of 10. **(Lilly)**

GLUCOLA

Description: Glucola is a carbonated, cola-flavored preparation used to test carbohydrate tolerance. It is a mixture of rapidly hydrolyzable saccharides with an average molecular weight of 3 glucose molecules. It contains 30% glucose, 18% maltose, 13% maltotriose and 39% shortchain dextrins and trace amounts of sodium and potassium; is caffeine-free.

It has been noted that mixtures of glucose, maltose, dextrins and other disaccharides tend to give a more rapid rise in blood-sugar levels than glucose itself.

Indications: To provide a standard loading dose for use in glucose tolerance tests and as the glucose challenge in diabetic screening.

Dosage and Administration: *Orally.* For most adults, the entire contents of the 210-ml bottle should be consumed; best served when chilled. The usual dose for children is 1.75 mg/kg of body weight (approx. 2.2 ml/lb) or 40 gm/square meter of body surface.

Availability:
GLUCOLA® Solution in bottles of 210 and 300 ml. **(Ames)**

GLUTETHIMIDE Ⓒ III

Chemical Name: 2-Ethyl-2-phenylglutarimide.

Description: Glutethimide is a nonbarbiturate, piperidinedione-derivative sedative and hypnotic drug, and occurs as a white, crystalline powder practically insoluble in water and soluble in alcohol.

The exact mode of action is not known, but its effects on the CNS resemble those of the barbiturates. Its onset of action is rapid, producing sleep usually within 30 minutes and lasting 4 to 8 hours. In recommended doses, the drug does not cause respiratory depression (an advantage in preanesthetic sedation), and is suitable for use in the elderly and those with chronic illness. It is not contraindicated in impaired renal or respiratory function.

Indications: For all types of insomnia, and for inducing sleep preoperatively and during the first stage of labor.

Contraindications: Hypersensitivity to the drug.

Warnings: The hypnotic action of glutethimide is potentiated by barbiturates, methaqualone, alcohol, and other CNS depressants. Patients should be cautioned that shortly after taking the drug, they should not perform any hazardous operations requiring alertness or skill. Dosage of coumarin anticoagulants may require adjustments during and following withdrawal of therapy with glutethimide. Patients may become physically and psychologically dependent; therefore, caution must be exercised when prescribing medication for patients with a known propensity for taking excessive quantities of drugs. Withdrawal symptoms are usually manifested by nausea, abdominal discomfort, tremors, convulsions, and delirium. These may occur in newborn infants of mothers who have been taking this medication. When drug-induced dependence exists, the dosage should be reduced gradually. The use of any drug during pregnancy or lactation requires that potential benefits be weighed against possible hazards.

Precautions: Total daily dosage above 1 gm is not recommended for continued administration. In the presence of pain, which may counteract the effect of the drug, an analgesic also should be given.

Adverse Reactions: A generalized skin rash may occur, in which case the drug should be withdrawn, This rash usually clears spontaneously within a few days after drug withdrawal. Occasionally, a purpuric or urticarial rash may occur; exfoliative dermatitis has been reported. With recommended doses, there have been rare reports of nausea, hangover, paradoxical excitation, and blurring of vision. Rarely, acute hypersensitivity reactions, porphyria, and blood dyscrasias such as thrombocytopenic purpura, aplastic anemia or leukopenia, have been reported. Overdosage may be manifested by CNS depression, including coma; hypothermia, which may be followed by fever; depressed or absence of deep tendon reflexes, or of corneal and pupillary reflexes; dilatation of the pupils; depressed or absent response to painful stimuli, inadequate ventilation (even with relatively normal respiratory rate), sometimes with cyanosis, sudden apnea, and diminished or absent peristalsis.

Dosage and Administration: *Orally.* To avoid oversedation, it is advisable to individualize dosage. Not recommended for children under 12 years of age. *In insomnia:* 0.25 to 0.5 gm at bedtime; the dose may be repeated if necessary but not less than 4 hours before arising. *Preoperatively:* 0.5 gm the night before surgery; then 0.5 to 1 gm 1 hour before surgery. *First stage of labor:* 0.5 gm at onset of labor; may be repeated if necessary.

Availability:

Ⓒ**III** **Glutethimide**

Tablets, 500 mg in bottles of 1000. **(Lederle)**

ⒸIII DORIDEN®: **(USV)**

Capsules, 500 mg in bottles of 100.

Tablets, 250 mg in bottles of 100 and 1000; 500 mg in bottles of 100, 500 and 1000 and in strip-dispenser packages of 100.

GLYCERIN

Description: Glycerin occurs as a syrupy liquid with a sweet, warm taste and is about 0.6 times as sweet as cane sugar. Following oral administration, reduction in intraocular pressure reaches maximal effect in about 1 hour, then returns to pretreatment levels in approximately 5 hours. Anhydrous glycerin is extremely hygroscopic, containing not more than 0.3% moisture. Because of its exceptionally high affinity for water, it removes moisture from the tympanic mucosa with subsequent decongestion of the edematous tissue. This auralgesic action results in rapid relief from pain. It also decongests edematous layers of the cornea, thus reducing corneal edema and clearing impaired vision.

Indications: *Orally,* to reduce intraocular pressure. May be used with miotics and carbonic anhydrase inhibitors in acute primary angle-closure glaucoma to reduce intraocular pressure prior to iridectomy. Its use in primary open-angle glaucoma is usually limited to preoperative treatment. Glycerin is also effective in some secondary glaucomas such as those secondary to anterior uveitis, and may be used preoperatively in congenital glaucoma, retinal detachment surgery, routine cataract extraction, and keratoplasty. *Topically,* for the relief of pain and reduction of inflammation in the congestive and serous stages of acute otitis media; also for relief of discomfort in acute stages of "swimmer's ear". As an aid in softening and removal of excessive or impacted cerumen, and as adjuvant therapy when antibiotics or sulfonamides are administered systemically for otic infections. In the eye, for reduction of corneal edema (cloudy cornea) due to glaucoma; after keratoplasty (allergic edema or maladie du greffon); primary (on basis of dystrophy, not glaucoma); traumatic; idiopathic; in keratomalacia; in corneal dystrophy (Fuchs'); and in postoperative edema (cataract surgery). Diagnostically, to facilitate ophthalmoscopic examination, biomicroscopy, gonioscopy, and funduscopy; to differentiate superficial from deep corneal edema (ineffective in latter case).

Precautions: Oral glycerin should be administered cautiously to diabetic patients in order to avoid the occurrence of hyperglycemia and glycosuria. Caution is also advised when administering to senile or severely dehydrated patients. Keep bottle dry. Advise patient to keep dropper dry, not to wash it with water.

Adverse Reactions: Headache, nausea, vomiting, and occasionally diarrhea may occur following oral administration. The untoward effects that occur with the intravenous osmotic agents are potential hazards but are less likely to occur with glycerin.

Dosage and Administration: *Orally.* Adults and children, 1 to 1.5 gm/kg of body weight once daily, or more if necessary, usually given as a 50% solution. Lemon juice may be added to increase palatability. *Topically.* Carefully warm otic solution to body temperature; do not overheat. *For otitis media,* fill ear canal allowing solution to run along wall of ear canal slowly. Plug ear with cotton previously saturated with the solution. Repeat treatment every 1 or 2 hours or 3 or 4 times daily. *For removal of cerumen,* instill into the ear canal 3 times daily for 2 days. *For reduction of corneal edema,* instill 1 or 2 drops of the *ophthalmic* solution into the eye(s) every 3 or 4 hours. *In diagnostic examinations,* instill 1 drop to clear the cornea.

Availability:

Glycerin, nondehydrated

GLYROL® Oral Solution, 75% in bottles of 120 ml. **(Smith, Miller & Patch)**

OSMOGLYN® Oral Solution, 50% in bottles of 180 ml. **(Alcon)**

Glycerin, dehydrated

AURALGAN® Otic Solution in bottles of 15 ml with dropper. Each ml contains dehydrated glycerin, 1 ml with antipyrine, 54 mg and benzocaine, 14 mg. **(Ayerst)**

OPHTHALGAN® for Ophthalmic Use (pure dehydrated glycerin with chlorobutanol, 0.5%) in bottles of 7.5 ml with dropper. **(Ayerst)**

GLYCOPYRROLATE

Chemical Name: 3-Hydroxy-1,1-dimethylpyrrolidinium bromide α-cyclopentylmandelate.

Description: Glycopyrrolate is an anticholinergic quaternary ammonium compound closely related structurally and pharmacologically to pipenzolate. It occurs as a white, crystalline powder very soluble in water.

In common with other parasympatholytic drugs, glycopyrrolate's effects are qualitatively similar to those of atropine, but unlike atropine, it is completely ionized at physiological pH values. As with most other quaternary anticholinergic drugs, glycopyrrolate has little or no direct spasmolytic action on smooth muscle and secretory glands; high doses may block ganglionic and skeletal neuromuscular transmission. CNS stimulation, seen with tertiary amine anticholinergics, occurs infrequently, if at all, with quaternary ammonium compounds because of the latter's inability to cross the blood-brain barrier.

The drug exerts its influence more specifically on the gastrointestinal tract than on other visceral systems. Following a single 4-mg dose intraduodenally, the volume of gastric acid decreased from 86 to 23 ml and free acid decreased from 5.01 to 0.02 mEq in 3 hours under basal conditions. Clinical findings also indicated that pepsin secretion was also diminished, and comparable results have been reported on a 2-mg dosage. The suppression of gastric secretion was evident 6 to 8 hours after each dose. Clinically, the antimotility effect was noted 25 to 30 minutes after a 2-mg oral dose. Within 35 to 40 minutes, the frequency of gastric antral contractions decreased to 0.4/minute compared with a control reading of 2 to 2.5/minute. Following subcutaneous or intramuscular administration, peak effect occurs within 30 to 45 minutes with vagal blocking effect lasting for up to 2 to 3 hours and antisecretory effect for up to 7 hours. Following intravenous administration, the onset of action is usually evident within 1 minute. However, in spite of these findings there is no conclusive evidence that the drug facilitates the healing of peptic ulcer or prevents complications or recurrences.

Indications: In conjunction with diet, antacids, sedatives, and attention to emotional problems, glycopyrrolate is recommended for the management of gastrointestinal disorders amenable to anticholinergic therapy, such as peptic ulcer, irritable bowel syndrome (irritable colon, spastic colon, mucous colitis, acute enterocolitis, and functional gastrointestinal disorders), and neurogenic colon. May also be used parenterally in the management of acute pancreatitis, treatment of biliary colic and the prevention of sphincter spasm associated with the administration of morphine. When these conditions are associated with psychic overlay, phenobarbital may be indicated.

Contraindications: Acute glaucoma; obstructive uropathy such as bladder neck obstruction due to prostatic hypertrophy; obstructive disease of the gastrointestinal tract as in achalasia, pyloroduodenal stenosis, etc.; paralytic ileus; intestinal atony of the elderly or debilitated patient; unstable cardiovascular status in acute hemorrhage; severe ulcerative colitis; toxic megacolon complicating ulcerative colitis; myasthenia gravis. Phenobarbital in acute intermittent porphyria. Unusual sensitivity to any of the components also constitutes a contraindication.

Warnings: Phenobarbital may be habit-forming. All the customary precautions attending the use of phenobarbital should be exercised. See specific monograph. Because perspiration is reduced in patients taking this drug, heat prostration (fever and heat stroke) may occur in high environmental temperatures. Diarrhea may be an early symptom of incomplete intestinal obstruction, particularly in patients with ileostomy or colostomy; the use of the drug in this instance would be inappropriate and possibly harmful. Patients may experience drowsiness and dizziness, and should therefore be cautioned against engaging in any hazardous activity requiring alertness and skill. Toxic doses may cause a curare-like effect which can result in muscular weakness and respiratory arrest. Use of any drug during pregnancy, lactation or the childbearing years requires that the therapeutic benefits be evaluated against the possible harm to the fetus. Until further experience with regard to safe and effective use has been gained, it is not recommended for use in the pediatric age group.

Precautions: Cautious use is advised in elderly patients and in all patients with autonomic neuropathy; hepatic or renal disease; ulcerative colitis, since large doses may suppress intestinal motility to the point of producing a paralytic ileus which may lead to or aggravate toxic megacolon; hyperthyroidism; coronary heart disease; congestive heart failure; cardiac tachyarrhythmias; tachycardia; hypertension; prostatic hypertrophy, and hiatal hernia associated with reflux esophagitis, since anticholinergic drugs may aggravate this condition.

Adverse Reactions: Effects are those usually associated with anticholinergic agents. They include urinary hesitancy and retention; blurred vision due to mydriasis; increased ocular tension; tachycardia; palpitation; decreased sweating; loss of taste; headache; nervousness; drowsiness; weakness; dizziness; insomnia; nausea; vomiting; impotence; suppression of lactation; constipation; bloated feeling; severe allergic reaction or drug idiosyncrasies including anaphylaxis; urticaria and other dermal manifestations, and some degree of mental confusion and/or excitement, especially in elderly patients.

Dosage and Administration: *Orally.* Average dosage is 1 or 2 mg 3 times daily, with or without phenobarbital. Some patients may require an additional dose at bedtime to assure overnight control of symptoms. For maintenance, 1 mg twice daily affords adequate control. After the more severe symptoms associated with acute conditions have subsided, dosage may be reduced to the minimum required to maintain symptomatic control. *Parenterally,* usually 0.1 mg *subcutaneously, intramuscularly* or *intravenously* at 4-hour intervals 3 or 4 times daily; however, some patients may require 0.2 mg. For additional information, refer to the package literature.

Availability:
ROBINUL®: **(Robins)**
Injectable, 0.2 mg/ml in ampuls of 1 ml and multiple-dose vials of 5 and 20 ml.
Tablets, 1 mg in bottles of 100 and 500.
Forte Tablets, 2 mg in bottles of 100 and 500.
PH Tablets, 1 mg with phenobarbital, 16.2 mg in bottles of 100 and 500.
PH Forte Tablets, 2 mg with phenobarbital, 16.2 mg in bottles of 100 and 500.

GOLD SODIUM THIOMALATE

Chemical Name: [(1,2-Dicarboxyethyl)thio]gold disodium salt.

Description: Gold sodium thiomalate is formed by interaction between sodium thiomalate and a gold halide. It is equivalent to about 50% gold. It occurs as a white to yellowish-white powder, very soluble in water. The pH of a 1 in 10 solution is about 6.

Although the precise mechanism of action is not understood, the drug exerts an antiinflammatory effect in rheumatoid arthritis. Maximal benefit is obtained in the early active stage of the disease, since in the late stages, when cartilage and bone damage have occurred, it can only check the progression of the disorder, and thus prevent further structural damage to the joints. It cannot repair damage caused by the previously active disease.

Gold is absorbed within 1 hour following intramuscular administration. With increasing doses at weekly intervals, the gold plasma concentration increases in a step-wise fashion. Between injections, the daily plasma value may fluctuate somewhat, but generally remains constant or decreases slightly until the next injection. Plasma gold concentrations are higher with large doses, but these concentrations are not directly proportional to the weekly gold intake.

Gold is eliminated mainly by the kidneys, although a small amount appears in the feces. On weekly doses of 50 mg about 1 mg is excreted daily. Thus, more than 80% of a dose is present in the body after 1 week, the usual interval between injections. As increased amounts of gold are given, the urinary excretion increases, but not proportionately. Thus, the percentage of retained gold increases with increasing dosage. Following completion of a course, gold may appear in the plasma and urine for 6 to 12 months when large doses have been administered, and for a correspondingly shorter period with small doses.

Indications: Treatment of active rheumatoid arthritis in both adults and children.

Contraindications: Known hypersensitivity to gold or other heavy metals, or a history of toxic reactions to gold; severely debilitated patients; in those with systemic lupus erythematosus; or with Sjogren's syndrome in rheumatoid arthritis. Safe use during pregnancy has not been established with regard to the possibility of adverse effects upon fetal development. Therefore, it should be used in pregnant patients or in women of childbearing potential only when in the judgment of the physician the potential benefits outweigh the possible hazards. The concomitant use of antimalarials, immunosuppressants, phenylbutazone, or oxyphenylbutazone is contraindicated because of their potential to cause blood dyscrasias.

Warnings: Physicians planning to use this drug should be thoroughly familiar with its usefulness and disadvantages. The possibility of toxic reactions should always be explained to the patient before initiating therapy, and they should be warned to report promptly any symptoms suggesting toxicity. Before treatment is started, the patient's hemoglobin, erythrocyte, leukocyte, differential and platelet counts should be determined, and urinalysis should be performed to serve as basic reference. Urine should be analyzed for protein and sediment changes prior to each injection. Complete blood counts including platelet estimation should be made before every second injection throughout treatment. The appearance of purpura or ecchymosis at any time always requires a platelet count. Treatment should be interrupted immediately when toxic reactions occur. The patient should be instructed to report at once any itching, rash or soreness of the mouth.

Precautions: All gold compounds are toxic. Adrenal corticosteroids may be given to prevent or reduce sensitivity reactions during therapy. Regular examinations of the skin, mouth, blood (red and white cell counts), and urine (albumin, casts and red cells) will usually permit early recognition of toxic reactions. Proper precautions and early discontinuance of the drug will reduce the incidence of severe reactions. Dimercaprol (BAL) is indicated in the treatment of gold poisoning.

Adverse Reactions: Reactions of the "nitritoid type" have been reported. These responses resemble anaphylactoid effects. Flushing, fainting, dizziness and sweating are most frequently reported. Other symptoms which may occur include nausea, vomiting, malaise and weakness. More severe, but less common effects, include syncope, bradycardia, thickening of the tongue, difficulty in swallowing and breathing. These effects occur almost immediately or as late as 10 minutes following injection. Dermatitis, stomatitis and gastrointestinal disturbances are the most common side effects. Skin reactions may include pruritus, exfoliative dermatitis, herpes zoster, lichen planus, hyperkeratosis, intertrigo, pustular dermatitis, dyskeratosis, urticaria, pityriasis rosea, and actinic rash. Conjunctivitis, iritis, corneal ulcer, and gold deposition in ocular tissues also have been reported. Other reactions include leukopenia, erythropenia, decreased hemoglobin level, "gold bronchitis," transitory blurring of vision, meningitis, and a hypersensitivity type of reaction manifested by paresis and polyneuritis. Mild reactions include gastrointestinal disturbances, pruritus, anesthesia of the tongue, eosinophilia (very common), lymphoadenitis, and an irritating, nonproductive cough. Severe reactions include dermatitis, which may proceed to generalized exfoliation; stomatitis (occasionally with ulceration), glossitis, and gingivitis; gastrointestinal disturbances such as nausea, vomiting, diarrhea, colitis, and abdominal pain, sometimes with chills and fever; hematologic reactions such as purpura, thrombopenia, agranulocytosis, and aplastic anemia; hepatitis with jaundice; persistent albuminuria, with or without hematuria, and nephrosis.

Dosage and Administration: *Intramuscularly only.* The recommended initial schedule consists of 16 or 20 weekly injections—10 mg the 1st week, 25 mg the 2nd week, and 50 mg the 3rd and subsequent weeks. If no improvement is evident after this course of treatment, the drug is considered to be of no value and should be discontinued. Improvement usually is not noted before the 6th or 8th week. If the patient has improved and no toxic symptoms have developed, the dosage can be reduced to 50 mg every 2 weeks for 4 doses, then every 3 weeks for 4 doses, and then monthly for a prolonged, indefinite time, if tolerated. Should the disease relapse after maintenance treatment has been established, injections should again be resumed at weekly intervals. In juvenile cases, the dosage should be reduced in accordance with the weight of the child. Children under 12 years of age should not receive more than 25 mg in a single dose. Intramuscular injections should be given with the patient lying down; they should remain recumbent for approximately 10 minutes after the injection.

Availability:
MYOCHRYSINE® Injection: 10, 25 and 100 mg/ml in ampuls of 1 ml; 50 mg/ml in ampuls of 1 ml and in multiple-dose vials of 10 ml. **(Merck Sharp & Dohme)**

GRISEOFULVIN

Chemical Name: 7-Chloro-2′,4,6-trimethoxy-6′β-methylspiro[benzofuran-2(*3H*),1′[2]cyclohexene]-3,4′-dione.

Description: A fungistatic antibiotic obtained from *Penicillium* including *Penicillium griseofulvum.* Griseofulvin microsize particles are produced by a special process that fractures the particles into minute crystals of irregular shape offering a greater and more effective surface area for increased gastrointestinal absorption. Further processing to achieve ultramicrosize particles has been found to double the biological availability in that 125 mg are equivalent to 250 mg of microsize griseofulvin.

In vitro studies have shown griseofulvin to be active against various species of *Microsporum, Epidermophyton* and *Trichophyton.* It has no value in the treatment of other genera of fungi or bacteria.

The precise mechanism of action of griseofulvin has not been determined, but available data suggest that the drug is believed to act by interfering with the synthesis of nucleic acid at steps prior to or at the polymerization stage.

Absorption of griseofulvin from the gastrointestinal tract varies considerably among individuals mainly because of insolubility of the drug in aqueous media in the upper portion of the gastrointestinal tract. The degree of intestinal absorption is also influenced by the particle size of the drug. Peak serum level found in fasting adults given 0.5 gm occurs at approximately 4 hours and ranges between 0.5 to 2 mcg/ml. Increase in the size of the dose leads to earlier and higher levels. The serum level may also be increased by administering griseofulvin with a meal containing a high fat content. Most of the orally ingested drug is eliminated in unchanged form in the feces; only about 0.6% is excreted in the urine.

Griseofulvin is deposited in the keratin-precursor cells and has a greater affinity for diseased tissue. The drug is tightly bound to the new keratin which becomes highly resistant to fungal invasion.

Indications: Recommended for the treatment of ringworm infections of the skin, hair, and nails, namely: tinea corporis, tinea pedis, tinea cruris, tinea barbae, tinea capitis, and tinea unguium (onychomycosis). Prior to the institution of therapy, the type of fungi responsible for the infection should be identified by culture. Griseofulvin has a potent fungistatic action, particularly against those fungi responsible for dermatomycoses, namely: *Microsporum canis, M. gypseum, M. audouini, Epidermophyton floccosum, Trichophyton tonsurans, T. rubrum, T. mentagrophytes, T. megnini, T. gallinae, T. verrucosum, T. sulfureum, T. interdigitale, T. schoenleini,* and *T. crateriform.* The use of this drug is not justified in minor or trivial infections which will respond to topical agents alone. Griseofulvin is *not* effective in the following: bacterial infections, candidiasis (moniliasis), histoplasmosis, actinomycosis, sporotrichosis, chromoblastomycosis, coccidioidomycosis, North American blastomycosis, cryptococcosis (torulosis), tinea versicolor, nocardiosis.

Contraindications: This drug is contraindicated in patients with porphyria, hepatocellular failure, and in individuals with a history of sensitivity to griseofulvin.

Warnings: Safe and effective use of griseofulvin for prophylaxis of fungal infections and safe use during pregnancy have not been established.

Precautions: Patients on prolonged therapy should be under close observation. Periodic monitoring of organ system functions, including renal, hepatic and hematopoietic, should be performed. Since griseofulvin is derived from species of *Penicillium*, the possibility of cross sensitivity with penicillin exists; however, known penicillin-sensitive patients have been treated without difficulty. Because a photosensitivity reaction is occasionally associated with griseofulvin therapy, patients should be warned to avoid exposure to intense natural or artificial sunlight. Should a photosensitivity reaction occur, lupus erythematosus may be aggravated. Griseofulvin decreases the activity of warfarin-type anticoagulants so that patients receiving these drugs concomitantly may require dosage adjustment of the anticoagulant during and after griseofulvin therapy. Barbiturates usually depress griseofulvin activity and concomitant administration may require a dosage adjustment of the antifungal agent.

Adverse Reactions: When adverse reactions occur, they are most commonly of the hypersensitivity type such as skin rashes, urticaria, and rarely, angioneurotic edema, and may necessitate withdrawal of therapy and appropriate countermeasures. Paresthesias of the hands and feet have been reported rarely after extended therapy. Other side effects reported occasionally are oral thrush, nausea, vomiting, epigastric distress, diarrhea, headache, fatigue, dizziness, insomnia, mental confusion, and impairment of performance of routine activities. Proteinuria and leukopenia have been reported rarely. Administration of the drug should be discontinued if granulocytopenia occurs. When rare, serious reactions occur with griseofulvin, they are usually associated with high dosages, long periods of therapy, or both.

Dosage and Administration: *Orally.* Dosage should be individualized according to the severity and type of infection being treated. The usual adult dosage is 0.5 gm daily in divided doses (125 mg 4 times daily or 250 mg twice daily). Widespread lesions may require 0.75 to 1 gm daily. Children, a dosage of 5 mg/lb of body weight daily is usually adequate. Children 30 to 50 lb, 125 to 250 mg/day; children over 50 lb, 250 to 500 mg/day in divided doses.

Availability:

Griseofulvin, microsize

FULVICIN-U/F® Tablets, 250 and 500 mg in bottles of 60 and 250. **(Schering)**

GRIFULVIN V®: **(McNeil)**

Suspension, 125 mg/5 ml in bottles of 120 ml.

Tablets, 125, 250 and 500 mg in bottles of 50, 100 and 500.

GRISACTIN®: **(Ayerst)**

Capsules, 125 and 250 mg in bottles of 100 and 500.

Tablets, 500 mg in bottles of 60.

Griseofulvin, ultramicrosize

FULVICIN P/G® Tablets, 125 and 250 mg in bottles of 100. **(Schering)**

GRIS-PEG® Tablets, 125 mg in bottles of 100 and 500. **(Dorsey)**

GUANETHIDINE

Chemical Name: [2-(Octahydro-1-azocinyl)ethyl]guanidine.

Description: Guanethidine is a potent hypotensive agent chemically and pharmacologically unrelated to other hypotensive agents. It occurs as colorless or white, deliquescent crystals that are freely soluble in water and in alcohol.

Guanethidine inhibits or interferes with the release and/or distribution of the chemical mediator (presumably the catecholamine norepinephrine) at the sympathetic neuroeffector junction. Unlike ganglionic blocking agents, it blocks only the sympathetic and not the parasympathetic pathways. It lowers blood pressure in the standing position and, in most cases, the supine position as well; both systolic and diastolic pressures are reduced.

Following a single oral dose, the initial effect occurs within 2 to 3 days and usually lasts for 7 to 14 days. Upon withdrawal of the drug, the hypotensive effect may persist for as long as a week to 10 days. Although guanethidine is excreted primarily by the kidneys, it tends to be reabsorbed into the bowel because of its assimilation in the bile.

Indications: Patients with severe or sustained elevation of blood pressure, particularly diastolic pressure. It is *not* recommended for labile or milder forms of hypertension which can be controlled with sedatives, rauwolfia derivatives or thiazide diuretics; nor in frank congestive heart failure not due to hypertension. May also be useful in renal hypertension, including hypertension secondary to pyelonephritis, renal artery stenosis, and renal amyloidosis; may be added to thiazide and/or hydralazine therapy when these agents fail to reduce blood pressure sufficiently; in lieu of other hypotensive drugs when patients are refractory and hypertension persists, or when side effects of other medication prevent effective treatment.

Contraindications: *Guanethidine:* Concomitant use with MAO inhibitors; known or suspected pheochromocytoma, frank congestive heart failure not due to hypertension, and hypersensitivity to guanethidine. *Hydrochlorothiazide:* Anuria; hypersensitivity to this or other sulfonamide-derived drugs. The routine use of diuretics in otherwise healthy pregnant women is inappropriate and exposes the mother and fetus to unnecessary hazards.

Warnings: Because of the drug's potency, the physician should become thoroughly familiar with the details of its use before prescribing, and warn patients not to deviate from instructions. Patients should be forewarned about the possibility of orthostatic hypotension, manifested by dizziness, weakness and syncope, and should be instructed in proper relief measures. Concomitant administration of guanethidine and rauwolfia derivatives should be undertaken with caution to avoid excessive postural hypotension, bradycardia, and mental depression. If feasible, guanethidine should be discontinued 2 weeks prior to surgery in order to avoid a potential vascular collapse and to reduce the hazard of cardiac arrest during anesthesia. Pre-anesthetic and anesthetic agents should be administered with caution should emergency surgery be deemed necessary, and oxygen, atropine, and vasopressor solutions should be on hand for immediate use. Vasopressor agents should be administered with care because of potential augmented response. Smaller dosages of guanethidine may be required in the presence of febrile illness. Special care should be exercised when treating patients with a history of bronchial asthma since their condition may be aggravated. Safe use of guanethidine during pregnancy has not been established; therefore, it should be administered only when it is deemed essential to the welfare of the patient.

Precautions: Treatment should be titrated to the individual patient, and reevaluated periodically according to the clinical response. Initially, dosage should be small and increased gradually. Guanethidine may be useful but should be given with extreme caution to hypertensive patients with renal disease complicated by nitrogen retention; coronary disease with insufficiency or recent myocardial infarction; cerebral vascular disease, especially with encephalopathy; and with rising blood urea nitrogen levels, since decreased blood pressure may further compromise renal function. Extreme caution is advised when administering this drug to patients with severe cardiac failure. Patients with incipient cardiac decompensation should be observed for weight gain or edema. This may be averted by the concomitant use of a thiazide. Also to be considered is that both digitalis and guanethidine slow the heart rate. Use with caution in patients with a history of peptic ulcer or other chronic disorders which may be aggravated by an increase in parasympathetic tone. Anorexiants, mild stimulants, tricyclic antidepressants, other psychopharmacologic agents, or oral contraceptives may diminish the hypotensive effect of guanethidine. At least one week should elapse after discontinuing MAO inhibitors before initiating therapy with this drug. When treatment is prolonged, it is advised that periodic blood counts and liver function tests be performed.

Adverse Reactions: Side effects most frequently seen (due to sympathetic blockade) are dizziness, weakness, lassitude, and syncope; bradycardia; increased intestinal peristalsis and diarrhea. Diarrhea may be severe at times and necessitate discontinuance of the medication. Other common reactions include inhibition of ejaculation and a tendency toward fluid retention and edema with occasional development of congestive heart failure. Other adverse reactions reported less frequently include dyspnea, fatigue, nausea, vomiting, nocturia, urinary incontinence, dermatitis, loss of scalp hair, dry mouth, rise in BUN, ptosis of the lids, blurred vision, parotid tenderness, myalgia, muscle tremor, mental depression, chest pains (angina), chest paresthesias, nasal congestion, weight gain, and asthma in susceptible individuals. A few instances of anemia, thrombocytopenia and leukopenia have been reported; whether or not these were drug-related has not been established. Treatment of overdosage consists essentially of restoring blood pressure and heart rate to normal by keeping the patient in a supine position and by the administration of vasopressors. Severe and persistent diarrhea should be treated symptomatically to reduce intestinal hypermotility, with due attention to maintenance of hydration and electrolyte balance.

Dosage and Administration: *Orally.* Individualization of dosage is essential for optimal results. Treatment should begin with small doses (10 mg) which may be increased depending upon the patient's response. Since guanethidine has a long duration of action, increases in the dose should not be made more often than every 5 to 7 days, unless the patient is hospitalized. At every visit, the blood pressure should be taken in both the supine and standing position, and increases in dosage determined only if there has been no decrease in the standing blood pressure from the previous levels. In hospitalized patients, an initial dose of 25 or 50 mg may be used with increases of 25 or 50 mg daily or every other day as indicated. *Guanethidine with hydrochlorothiazide,* initially, a single daily dose of 1 tablet; the daily dose may be increased by 1 tablet at intervals of not less than 1 week, and maximal dosage should not exceed 4 tablets daily.

Availability:
ISMELIN® SULFATE Tablets, 10 and 25 mg in bottles of 100 and 1000 and in Consumer Packs and Accu-Paks® (blister units) of 100. **(Ciba)**
ESIMIL® Tablets (as monosulfate), 10 mg with hydrochlorothiazide, 25 mg in bottles of 100 and in Accu-Paks® (blister units) of 100. **(Ciba)**

GUANIDINE HYDROCHLORIDE

Description: A naturally occurring amine found in plants and animals, guanidine resembles physostigmine in its effect on the muscle. The drug's beneficial action on muscle function in patients with the myasthenic syndrome of Eaton-Lambert—differentiated from myasthenia gravis by its association with small cell carcinoma of the lung—is due to its ability to increase the amount of acetylcholine released from the nerve endings by a nerve impulse. It occurs as a white powder that is freely soluble in water and in alcohol.

Indications: Treatment of the neuromuscular defect, characterized by muscle weakness and easy fatigability, associated with the myasthenic syndrome of Eaton-Lambert. Not indicated for the treatment of myasthenia gravis. Electromyography may be necessary to make the diagnosis.

Contraindications: History of intolerance or allergy to the drug.

Warnings: Fatal bone marrow suppression, apparently dose-related, can occur with guanidine. Safe use during pregnancy has not been established; therefore, the benefits of therapy must be weighed against the potential hazards. Since the drug is excreted in breast milk, patients should be advised to use other methods of feeding their infants.

Precautions: Baseline blood studies should be followed by frequent red and white blood cell and differential counts. The appearance of bone marrow suppression warrants discontinuation of the drug; concomitant use of drugs causing bone marrow suppression should be avoided. Since renal function may be affected, it is advised that patients undergo routine urine examinations and serum creatinine determinations.

Adverse Reactions: Mild gastrointestinal disorders, such as nausea, anorexia, abdominal cramping, or diarrhea are early warnings that tolerance is being exceeded; therefore, a reduction in dosage is warranted. Slight numbness or tingling of the face, feet, lips and fingertips shortly following administration may occur, but is usually not an indication to discontinue treatment or to reduce the dosage. Severe intoxication is characterized by nervous hyperirritability, jitteriness, lightheadedness, emotional lability, psychosis, fibrillary tremors and convulsive contractions of muscle; salivation; vomiting; diarrhea; hypoglycemia; circulatory disturbances; bone marrow depression with anemia, leukopenia, thrombocytopenia; sore throat, rash, fever, folliculitis, petechiae, purpura, ecchymosis, and elevation of blood creatinine; uremia; abnormal liver function tests; palpitation, tachycardia, atrial fibrillation, and hypotension. Calcium gluconate administered intravenously may control the neuromuscular and convulsive symptoms and may provide some relief of other toxic manifestations. Atropine is more effective in relieving the gastrointestinal symptoms, circulatory disturbances and changes in blood sugar.

Dosage and Administration: *Orally,* in 3 or 4 divided doses. Initially, a daily test dose of between 10 and 15 mg/kg of body weight, which is then carefully increased according to the needs and tolerance of the individual patient. Severe cases may require as much as 45 mg/kg daily.

Availability:
GUANIDINE HYDROCHLORIDE Tablets, 125 mg in bottles of 100 and 500. **(Key Pharm.)**

HALCINONIDE: see The Adrenal Corticosteroids

HALOPERIDOL

Chemical Name: 4-[4-(*p*-Chlorophenyl)-4-hydroxypiperidinol]-4'fluorobutyrophenone.

Description: Haloperidol, a member of the butyrophenones, differs structurally from other tranquilizers, and is pharmacologically related to the piperazine group of phenothiazine tranquilizers. It occurs as a white to faintly yellow, amorphous or crystalline powder practically insoluble in water and sparingly soluble in alcohol.

Its site and mechanism of action have not been completely demonstrated. However, it is believed that the drug exerts its effect by indirectly blocking parts of the reticular formation, possibly by way of the caudate nucleus. This can occur through interference with transmission phenomena or neurohormonal uptake in specific areas of the midbrain.

Studies with animals receiving 2 to 20 times the maximal clinical dose of haloperidol by oral and/or parenteral routes showed an increased incidence of resorption, reduced fertility, delayed delivery, dose-related offspring mortality (presumably due to lack of maternal care reflecting CNS depression).

Indications: For the control of symptoms of acute and chronic psychosis. The drug may also be used in controlling the classic symptomatology (involuntary tics, vocal utterances, etc.) observed in patients with Gilles de la Tourette's syndrome, a rare behavioral disorder. Parenteral administration is indicated only in the emergency control of the acutely agitated psychotic patient with moderately severe to very severe symptoms.

Contraindications: In comatose patients, patients severely depressed by alcohol or other centrally acting agents, in patients with Parkinson's disease and in those hypersensitive to haloperidol.

Warnings: Safe use of this drug during pregnancy and lactation has not been established; therefore, its use in pregnant patients, in nursing mothers, or in women of childbearing potential requires that the expected benefits be weighed against the potential hazards. Phocomelia has been reported to occur in two infants whose mothers received haloperidol together with other medications having suspected teratogenic potential, during the first trimester of pregnancy. Whether or not this incident was drug-related has not been determined. Lowered serum cholesterol levels and/or cutaneous and ocular changes have been reported in patients taking chemically related drugs. Although none of these changes has been reported with haloperidol, the physician should be alert to these possibilities. Some cases of fatal bronchopneumonia have followed the use of neuroleptics. It has been postulated that lethargy and decreased sensation of thirst due to central inhibition may lead to dehydration, hemoconcentration and reduced pulmonary ventilation. Therefore, if these signs and symptoms appear, especially in the elderly, the physician should promptly institute remedial therapy. Since haloperidol may impair the mental and physical abilities required for the performance of hazardous tasks such as operating machinery or driving a motor vehicle, patients should be cautioned not to engage in any activity requiring alertness or skill. Patients should also be cautioned about the possible potentiation of alcohol by concurrent use of haloperidol. Safe and effective use in children have not been established; therefore, this drug is not recommended for use in the pediatric age group. An encephalopathic syndrome characterized by weakness, lethargy, fever, tremulousness and confusion, extrapyramidal symptoms, leukocytosis, elevated serum enzymes, BUN and FBS followed by irreversible brain damage has occurred in a few patients treated with lithium plus haloperidol. A causal relationship between these events and the concomitant administration of lithium and haloperidol has not been established; however, patients receiving such combined therapy should be monitored closely for early evidence of neurological toxicity and treatment discontinued promptly if such manifestations appear.

Precautions: Should be administered with caution to patients with severe myocardial insufficiency and to patients taking anticoagulants or anticonvulsant medication, or to those with known allergies, or with a history of allergic reactions to drugs. Patients with thyrotoxicosis may experience severe neurotoxicity manifested by rigidity, and inability to walk or talk. Haloperidol potentiates the primary effects of anesthetics and analgesics, and the CNS-depressant action of barbiturates, but not the anticonvulsant action of barbiturates or other anticonvulsants. If used concomitantly, antiparkinsonism drugs may have to be continued after haloperidol has been discontinued, because tissue levels of the latter persist for some time whereas the former are excreted more rapidly. If both drugs are withdrawn simultaneously, extrapyramidal symptoms may be precipitated. The physician should be aware of the potential increase in intraocular pressure when anticholinergic drugs, including antiparkinsonism agents, are given together with haloperidol. Also, when this drug is used to control mania in cyclic disorders, a rapid mood swing to depression may occur.

Adverse Reactions: *CNS effects:* Extrapyramidal reactions—Neuromuscular (extrapyramidal) reactions during the administration of haloperidol have been reported frequently, often during the first few days of treatment. In most patients, these reactions involved Parkinson-like symptoms which, when first observed, were usually mild to moderately severe and usually reversible. Other types of neuromuscular reactions (motor restlessness, dystonia, akathisia, hyperreflexia, opisthotonos, oculogyric crises) have been reported far less frequently, but were often more severe. Severe extrapyramidal reactions have been reported to occur at relatively low doses. Generally the occurrence and severity of most extrapyramidal symptoms are dose-related since they occur at relatively high doses and have been shown to disappear or become less severe when the dose is reduced. Administration of anti-Parkinson drugs such as benztropine mesylate or trihexyphenidyl hydrochloride may be required for control of such reactions. It should be noted that persistent extrapyramidal reactions have been reported and that the drug may have to be discontinued in such cases. Transient abnormal movements, which in some cases resembled tardive dyskinesia, have occurred in some patients on maintenance therapy when the medication was abruptly discontinued. It is not known whether gradual withdrawal of antipsychotic drugs will reduce the rate of occurrence of withdrawal emergent neurological signs but until further evidence becomes available, it seems reasonable to gradually withdraw use of haloperidol. In addition, a neurological syndrome, known as tardive dyskinesia, is associated with antipsychotic drug use, and may appear in some patients on long-term therapy or after the drug has been discontinued. The risk appears to be greater in elderly patients on high-dose therapy, particularly female patients. The symptoms are persistent and in some patients irreversible. Fine vermicular movements of the tongue may be an early sign of the syndrome which, when allowed to progress, is characterized by rhythmical involuntary movements of tongue, face, mouth or jaw such as protrusion of tongue, puffing of cheeks, puckering of mouth, chewing movements sometimes accompanied by involuntary movement of the extremities. If the medication is withdrawn at the first sign, the syndrome may not develop. There is no known effective treatment, and antiparkinson agents have not proved useful in alleviating the symptoms. *Other CNS effects*—Insomnia, restlessness, anxiety, euphoria, agitation, drowsiness, depression, lethargy, headache, confusion, vertigo, grand mal seizures, and exacerbation of psychotic symptoms including hallucinations. *Cardiovascular effects:* Tachycardia and hypotension. *Hematologic effects:* Reports have appeared citing the occurrence of mild and usually transient leukopenia and leukocytosis, minimal decreases in red blood cell counts, anemia, or a tendency toward lymphomonocytosis. Agranulocytosis has rarely been reported to have occurred with the use of haloperidol, and then only in association with other medication. *Hepatic effects:* Impaired liver function and/or jaundice have been reported. *Dermatologic reactions:* Maculopapular and acneiform skin reactions and isolated cases of photosensitivity and loss of hair. *Endocrine disorders:* Lactation, breast engorgement, mastalgia, menstrual irregularities, gynecomastia, impotence, increased libido, hyperglycemia and hypoglycemia. *Gastrointestinal reactions:* Anorexia, constipation, diarrhea, hypersalivation, dyspepsia, nausea and vomiting. *Autonomic reactions:* Dry mouth, blurred vision, urinary retention and diaphoresis. *Respiratory effects:* Laryngospasm, bronchospasm and increased depth of respiration.

Dosage and Administration: *Orally* or *intramuscularly.* To achieve optimal results and to avoid unnecessary adverse effects, the dosage should be based on the patient's age and physical condition, the severity of symptoms, and the response to treatment. The usual initial, *oral,* adult dosage *for moderate symptoms* is 0.5 to 2 mg; *for moderate-severe symptoms,* 2 to 3 mg, and *for very severe symptoms,* 3 to 5 mg administered 2 or 3 times daily. *Parenterally,* the usual dose is 2 to 5 mg. Subsequent doses may be required usually administered at intervals of from 4 to 8 hours. Dosages of more than 15 mg daily are seldom required.

Availability:
HALDOL®: **(McNeil)**
Concentrate, 2 mg/ml (approx. 0.1 ml/drop) in bottles of 15 and 120 ml with calibrated dropper.
Injection, (as lactate), 5 mg/ml in ampuls of 1 ml and in multi-dose vials of 10 ml.
Tablets, 0.5, 1 and 2 mg in bottles of 100 and 1000; 5 and 10 mg in bottles of 50, 100 and 1000. All potencies are available in unit-dose packages of 100.

HALOPROGIN

Chemical Name: 3-Iodo-2-propynyl 2,4,5-trichlorophenyl ether.

Description: Haloprogin is a synthetic antifungal agent for the treatment of superficial fungal infections of the skin.

Each gm of cream provides 10 mg of haloprogin solubilized in polyethylene glycol 400 and 4000, diethyl sebacate and polyvinylpyrrolidone. Each ml of solution provides 10 mg of haloprogin in a homogeneous vehicle of diethyl sebacate and alcohol.

Indications: Topical treatment of tinea pedis, tinea cruris, tinea corporis, and tinea manuum due to infection by *T. rubrum, T. tonsurans, T. mentagrophytes, M. canis,* and *E. floccosum;* and also useful in tinea versicolor due to *M. furfur.*

Contraindications: Hypersensitivity to any of the components.

Warnings: Safe use during pregnancy has not been established.

Precautions: In the event of sensitization or irritation, treatment should be discontinued and appropriate therapy instituted. Four weeks of trial treatment should be adequate. In mixed infections where bacteria or nonsusceptible fungi are present, supplementary therapy should be instituted.

Adverse Reactions: Local irritation, burning sensation, vesicle formation; increased maceration, pruritus or exacerbation of preexisting lesions have been reported.

Dosage and Administration: *Topically.* Apply liberally to the affected area twice daily for 2 to 3 weeks. Interdigital lesions may require up to 4 weeks of therapy. **Note:** Keep away from eyes.

Availability:
HALOTEX®: **(Westwood)**
Cream in tubes of 15 and 30 gm.
Solution in bottles of 10 and 30 ml with controlled drop tip.

HALOTHANE

Chemical Name: 2-Bromo-2-chloro-1,1,1-trifluoroethane.

Description: Halothane, an inhalation anesthetic, is a clear, colorless liquid with a pleasant, nonirritating odor. It is nonflammable and its vapors mixed with oxygen in proportions from 0.5 to 50% (v/v) are not explosive. It is stabilized by the addition of 0.01% thymol (w/w) and by storage in amber-colored bottles; it is unaffected by contact with warm soda lime.

Halothane is a noninflammable general anesthetic which acts by initially depressing the higher centers of the brain; with continued administration in high concentrations, the respiratory and vasomotor centers of the medulla are affected. It is reported to have a smooth and rapid induction with concentrations of 2 to 2.5% vapor when given with ultra-short acting barbiturates as premedication. Induction and recovery are rapid with little or no excitement.

Halothane is nonirritating to the respiratory tract hence there is little or no increase in salivary or bronchial secretion. Since progressive depression of respiration occurs, ventilation should be assisted to avoid hypoxia, acidosis, and apnea. Pharyngeal and laryngeal reflexes are depressed, as well as contractility of the heart and vascular smooth muscle. Bradycardia and hypotension may develop usually in proportion to the depth of anesthesia while cardiac output, arterial pressure and pulse rate are reduced. Atropine may reverse the bradycardia. Overdosage may result in severe hypotension and circulatory failure. Halothane augments the action of nondepolarizing relaxant and ganglionic blocking agents. It is incompatible with catecholamines and severe cardiac arrhythmias may occur if it is used with epinephrine, norepinephrine or levarterenol.

Indications: Induction and maintenance of general anesthesia.

Contraindications: The use of halothane should be avoided if a previous exposure has been followed by an unexplained fever or jaundice. It is not recommended for obstetrical anesthesia except when uterine relaxation is required.

Warnings: Halothane should be used only in vaporizers that have been calibrated to permit a reasonable approximation of output. The vaporizer should not be placed in a completely closed circuit-rebreathing system because overdosage is difficult to avoid. The patient should be observed closely for signs of overdosage manifested by depression of blood pressure, pulse rate, and respiration, particularly during assisted or controlled ventilation. Safe use of halothane during pregnancy has not been established with respect to possible adverse effects upon fetal development. Therefore, this anesthetic should not be used in women of childbearing potential, and particularly during the first trimester of pregnancy, unless, in the judgment of the physician, the expected benefits outweigh the possible hazards to the fetus.

Precautions: Cirrhosis of the liver or liver dysfunction, including a history of viral hepatitis may be the basis for selecting an agent other than halothane. Unless administration is carefully controlled, marked uterine relaxation can occur which may fail to respond to ergot derivatives or oxytocin. Since halothane increases cerebrospinal fluid pressure, measures ordinarily used to reduce this pressure should be employed in patients with markedly raised intracranial pressure before administering halothane. Ventilation should be carefully evaluated, and it may be necessary to assist or control ventilation to insure adequate oxygenation and carbon dioxide removal. Epinephrine and norepinephrine should be employed cautiously, if at all, during halothane anesthesia since their simultaneous use may induce ventricular tachycardia or fibrillation. The actions of nondepolarizing muscle relaxants and ganglionic blocking agents are augmented by halothane.

Adverse Reactions: Those reported were hepatic necrosis, cardiac arrest, hypotension, respiratory arrest, cardiac arrhythmias, hyperpyrexia, shivering, nausea, and emesis.

Dosage and Administration: *By inhalation.* Halothane may be administered by the nonrebreathing technique, partial rebreathing or closed technique. The induction dose varies with the individual patient; but usually involves a concentration of 1 to 4% vaporized by a flow of oxygen or nitrous oxide-oxygen mixture. For maintenance, 0.5 to 1.5% concentration is used.

Availability:
FLUOTHANE® Liquid in bottles of 125 and 250 ml. **(Ayerst)**
HALOTHANE Liquid in bottles of 250 ml. **(Abbott)**

HEPARIN SODIUM

Description: Sodium heparin is a mixture of active principles, having the property of prolonging the clotting time of blood. It is usually obtained from the liver, lung, intestinal mucosa, or other suitable tissues of domestic animals used for food by man. It occurs as a white or pale-color, amorphous powder soluble in water and practically insoluble in alcohol. The potency of sodium heparin, calculated on the dried basis, is not less than 120 U.S.P. units in each mg. The U.S.P. injection is a sterile solution of sodium heparin in water for injection. It may contain a substance or substances intended to delay the absorption of sodium heparin, for the purpose of prolonging the period of effectiveness, and a suitable antibacterial agent.

Heparin is a potent antithrombin anticoagulant. As a sulfonated mucopolysaccharide with a strong electric charge, heparin appears to function as a biologic ion exchanger. Its anticoagulant effect is achieved by its ability to inhibit platelet agglutination, to block the formation of thromboplastin, and to prevent the conversion of prothrombin to thrombin, thereby hindering the transformation of fibrinogen to fibrin without altering the normal components of the blood. Although therapeutic doses prolong the clotting time, bleeding time is usually unaffected. Heparin interferes with the complement fixation reaction in the Wassermann test and, in general, influences inflammatory and allergic reactions by its effect upon amines such as histamine or serotonin, or by neutralizing histamine liberators. Heparin depresses the low-density lipoprotein content of the blood and accelerates the removal of serum fat.

The drug is inactive when administered orally or rectally; absorption from the sublingual mucosa is variable but never adequate to influence blood clotting.

Indications: Anticoagulant therapy in the prophylaxis and treatment of pulmonary embolism, and venous thrombosis and its extension; in atrial fibrillation with embolization; for diagnosis and treatment of chronic consumptive coagulopathies (coagulation consumption coagulopathy); for prevention of clotting in arterial and heart surgery; and for prevention of cerebral thrombosis in the evolving stroke. As adjunctive therapy in the treatment of coronary occlusion with acute myocardial infarction, and in the prophylaxis and treatment of peripheral arterial embolism. May also be employed as an anticoagulant in blood transfusions and in blood samples for laboratory purposes.

Contraindications: In patients hypersensitive to heparin, during active bleeding of any kind, in blood dyscrasias or other disorders characterized by bleeding tendencies such as hemophilia, purpura of any type, thrombocytopenia; severe hepatic, renal or biliary disease; conditions where capillary permeability is increased; in diverticulitis, colitis, and subacute bacterial endocarditis. This drug is also contraindicated in the presence of threatened abortion, suspected intracranial hemorrhage, inaccessible ulcers (especially of the gastrointestinal tract), visceral carcinoma, regional or lumbar block anesthesia, severe hypertension, continuous tube drainage of the stomach or small intestine, during surgery and the immediate post-operative period following surgery of the eye, brain and spinal cord. Heparin sodium is also contraindicated for use as an anticoagulant in any case where it cannot be kept under careful observation with periodic blood coagulation tests.

Warnings: Dosage should be regulated by frequent clotting time determinations. If the clotting time is unduly prolonged or hemorrhage occurs, therapy with this drug should be promptly discontinued. Heparin sodium prolongs the one-phase prothrombin time. Accordingly, if heparin is given with bishydroxycoumarin or sodium warfarin, a period of 4 to 5 hours after the last intravenous dose or 12 to 24 hours after the last subcutaneous dose of heparin should elapse before blood is drawn, if a valid prothrombin time is to be obtained. Drugs, such as acetylsalicylic acid, which interfere with the platelet aggregation reaction, the main hemostatic defense system of heparinized patients, may induce bleeding and should not be used in patients on heparin therapy. Heparin blocks the eosinopenic response of ACTH, adrenocorticosteroids and insulin. Heparin also has an inhibitory effect on antibodies and anaphylaxis. Larger doses of heparin may be necessary in the febrile state. Digitalis, tetracycline, antihistamines, nicotine and ascorbic acid may partially counteract the anticoagulant action of heparin. An increased resistance to heparin is frequently encountered in cases of thrombosis, thrombophlebitis, myocardial infarction, cancer and postoperative cases. Heparin should be used with caution during pregnancy, especially during the last trimester or the immediate postpartum period. Also, extreme caution is essential in those disease states in which there is an increased risk of hemorrhaging.

Precautions: Patients on long-term daily administration of heparin should be observed for the possible development of osteoporosis and spontaneous fractures of ribs and/or vertebrae. Because heparin is derived from animal tissue, it should be used with caution in patients with a history of allergy. Before a therapeutic dose is given to such a patient, a trial dose of 1000 units may be advisable. Customary care should be exercised in the presence of mild hepatic or renal disease, hypertension, during menstruation, or in patients with indwelling catheters. A higher incidence of bleeding may be found in women over 60 years of age. Caution should be used when administering ACD-converted blood (blood collected in heparin sodium and later converted to ACD blood), since heparin sodium anticoagulant activity persists without loss for as long as 22 days following the conversion of such blood stored at refrigerated temperatures. The heparin sodium of the administered blood may under some clinical circumstances produce alterations in the coagulation mechanism of the recipient, particularly when multiple transfusions of the ACD-converted blood are given. **Note:** Solutions should be protected from freezing.

Adverse Reactions: Hemorrhage is the chief complication which may develop as a result of heparin therapy. An overly prolonged clotting time with minor bleeding during therapy can usually be controlled by withdrawing the drug and by the intravenous administration of protamine sulfate. In the event of massive blood loss, replacement of whole blood may be indicated. When administered intramuscularly, heparin may produce local irritation, mild pain and hematoma at the injection site. These effects are less frequently seen following deep subcutaneous (intra-fat) administration. Histamine-like reactions have also been observed at the site of injection. Hypersensitivity reactions have been reported with chills, fever and urticaria. Asthma, rhinitis, lacrimation, precordial tightness, and anaphylactoid reactions have also been noted. Acute reversible thrombocytopenia has been reported following intravenously administered heparin. Osteoporosis following long-term administration, aldosterone suppression, delayed transient alopecia and rebound hyperlipemia have been observed. There have been a few reports of priapism occurring in patients receiving anticoagulant therapy.

Dosage and Administration: The usual method of administration is to mix thoroughly 10,000 U.S.P. heparin units with 500 or 1000 ml of sodium chloride injection and administer by *intravenous drip.* The amount of solution necessary to prolong clotting time to a desirable level will vary greatly from patient to patient, and occasionally it will vary from day to day in the same patient. Dosage must be controlled by repeated clotting-time determinations. Most investigators recommend maintaining clotting time at levels of 2 to 3 times the normal value, as measured by the Lee-White method. The total period during which the clotting time is prolonged for therapeutic reasons must be determined according to the specific condition for which heparin is given. Average doses by *intramuscular* or *deep subcutaneous* injection usually have been 10,000 units, but the possibility of local hematomata with tenderness and irritation must be kept in mind. The effect of any single dose is transitory and lasts for only a few hours; approximately 25% of intravenously injected heparin is excreted in the urine in the first hour. For prolonged effect, continuous intravenous drip or repeated intramuscular or deep subcutaneous injections are necessary.

Availability:

HEPARIN SODIUM Injection, 1000 units/ml in vials of 10 ml; 10,000 units/ml in vials of 5 ml; 20,000 units/ml in vials of 1 and 2 ml. **(Lilly)**

HEPARIN SODIUM Injection, 1000, 5000, 7500, 10,000 and 20,000 units in Steri-Dose® (disposable syringes) of 1 ml. **(Parke-Davis)**

HEPARIN SODIUM Injection, 1000 units/ml in vials of 10 and 30 ml; 5000 units/ml in vials of 1 and 10 ml; 10,000 units/ml in vials of 1 and 4 ml. **(Upjohn)**

HEPARIN LOCK FLUSH Injection, 1000, 2500, 5000, 7500, 10,000, 15,000 and 20,000 units/ml in Tubex® (sterile disposable syringes) of 1 ml with needle; the 5000 units in Tubex(s) of 0.5 ml. Also available in normal saline solution, 10 and 100 units/ml in Tubex(s) of 1 ml. **(Wyeth)**

HEPRINAR® Injection, 1000 units/ml in vials of 10 ml; 5000 units/ml in vials of 1 and 10 ml; 10,000 units/ml in vials of 1 and 5 ml. **(Armour)**

LIPO-HEPIN® Injection, 5000, 10,000 and 20,000 units/ml in ampuls and single-dose syringes of 1 ml; 1000 units/ml in vials of 10 and 30 ml; 5000 units/ml in vials of 1 and 10 ml; 10,000 units/ml in vials of 1, 4 and 5 ml; 20,000 units/ml in vials of 2, 5 and 10 ml; 40,000 units/ml in vials of 2 and 5 ml; 1000 units, 5000 units, 7500 units, 10,000 units, 15,000 units and 20,000 units in single-dose syringes of 0.5 ml. **(Riker)**

LIQUAEMIN® SODIUM Injection, 1000 units/ml in vials of 10 and 30 ml; 5000 units/ml in ampuls of 1 ml and in vials of 1 and 10 ml; 10,000 units/ml in ampuls of 1 ml and vials of 1 and 4 ml; 20,000 units/ml in ampuls of 1 ml and in vials 1, 2, 5 and 10 ml; 40,000 units/ml in vials of 1 and 5 ml. **(Organon)**

PANHEPRIN® Injection, 1000 units/ml in ampuls of 1 ml and in vials of 10 and 30 ml; 5000 units/ml in ampuls of 1 ml and in vials of 10 ml; 10,000 units/ml in ampuls of 1 ml and multiple-dose vials of 4 and 5 ml; 20,000 units/ml in ampuls of 1 ml and vials of 5 ml; 40,000 units/ml in multiple-dose vials of 2 ml. **(Abbott)**

HEPATITIS B IMMUNE GLOBULIN, HUMAN

Description: A sterile solution containing from 10 to 18% of the immunoglobulin fraction of the serum from human donors who have been hyperimmunized with hepatitis B surface antigen (anti-HB_s). It is prepared by cold alcohol fractionation from pooled venous plasma of individuals with high titers of antibody to anti-HB_s, is stabilized with 0.3 M glycine and preserved with 1:10,000 sodium ethymercurithiosalicylate. The pH is approximately 6.8 adjusted with hydrochloric acid or sodium hydroxide. Each vial contains anti-HB_s antibody equivalent to or exceeding the potency of anti-HB_s of the U.S. Reference Hepatitis B Immune Globulin (Bureau of Biologics, FDA). The product is prepared from units of human plasma that have been tested and found nonreactive for hepatitis B surface antigen.

Indications: Provides passive immunization for individuals exposed to the hepatitis B virus. It is indicated primarily for post-exposure prophylaxis following either parenteral exposure (e.g., accidental needle puncture), direct mucous membrane contact (e.g., accidental splash), or oral ingestion (e.g., pipetting accident). Its clinical value in other situations requires additional studies.

Contraindications: None known.

Warnings: Should be given with caution to patients with a history of prior systemic allergic reactions following the administration of human immune globulin preparations. Epinephrine injection 1:1000 should be readily available for use in the event of an acute response.

Precautions: *This preparation should never be given intravenously.* Injections should be made intramuscularly, and care should be exercised to avoid introduction of the solution into a blood vessel. Live virus vaccines such as measles vaccine should not be given to patients who have recently been immunized with this agent because antibodies in the globulin preparation may interfere with the immune response. No interactions with other products are known. Although studies have not been undertaken in pregnant patients to assure whether or not the fetus will be adversely affected by this agent, clinical experience with other immunoglobulin preparations administered during pregnancy suggests that there are no known hazards to the fetus.

Adverse Reactions: The most frequent adverse reactions involve local pain and tenderness at the site of injection, urticaria and angioedema; rarely, anaphylactic responses.

Dosage and Administration: *Intramuscularly,* preferably in the gluteal or deltoid region. The recommended adult dosage is 3 to 5 ml or 0.06 ml/kg of body weight, administered as soon after exposure as possible (preferably within 7 days) and then repeated at 28 to 30 days.

Availability:
H-BIG Solution in vials of 3, 4 and 5 ml. **(Abbott)**

HEPTUNA PLUS

Description: Each capsule contains:

Ferrous sulfate dried (provides 100 mg elemental iron)	340 mg
Desiccated liver (undefatted)	50 mg
Vitamin B-12 (cobalamin concentrate N.F.)*	5 μg
Intrinsic factor concentrate (noninhibitory)	25 mg
Thiamine mononitrate	3 mg
Riboflavin	2 mg
Pyridoxine hydrochloride	2 mg
Sodium ascorbate	150 mg

Niacinamide	15 mg
Calcium pantothenate	1 mg
Copper (from copper sulfate)	1 mg
Molybdenum (from sodium molybdate)	0.2 mg
Calcium (from dibasic calcium phosphate)	37.4 mg
Iodine (from potassium iodide)	0.05 mg
Manganese (from manganese sulfate)	0.033 mg
Magnesium (from magnesium sulfate)	2 mg
Phosphorus (from dibasic calcium phosphate)	29 mg
Potassium (from potassium sulfate)	1.7 mg

*as Stablets®

Indications: Treatment of anemias amenable to oral therapy.

Contraindications: Copper is contraindicated in Wilson's disease.

Precautions: Not all patients with pernicious anemia show satisfactory therapeutic response to oral vitamin B-12 (intrinsic factor concentrate). In addition, some patients with an initial good response appear to become refractory to intrinsic factor after varying periods of oral therapy. Periodic examinations and laboratory studies of pernicious anemia patients are essential and recommended. Failure of response, or inadequate response, is an indication for parenteral vitamin B-12, generally recognized as the preferred treatment of this condition. The fundamental cause of the anemia should be determined since it is usually a manifestation of an underlying disorder such as blood loss, impaired production of intrinsic factor or other conditions.

Adverse Reactions: Gastrointestinal irritation.

Dosage and Administration: *Orally,* For many patients 1 capsule daily will provide sufficient amounts of hematopoietic factors for therapeutic results. If the severity and etiology of the anemia indicate then 1 capsule 3 times daily may be prescribed.

Availability:
HEPTUNA® PLUS Capsules in bottles of 100. **(Roerig)**

HETACILLIN: see The Penicillins

HEXACHLOROPHENE

Description: Hexachlorophene is a chlorinated phenol compound. It occurs as a white, crystalline powder that is insoluble in water but soluble in dilute alkali as well as in a number of organic solvents.

Hexachlorophene possesses high antibacterial properties of a bacteriostatic nature and is particularly effective on gram-positive organisms. It also possesses some fungicidal properties; however, it is ineffective against spores. The compound's high toxicity following oral or systemic administration restricts its germicidal use to topical application. Following topical application, hexachlorophene provides significant antibacterial effect in 4 hours which usually persists over a period of 1 to 2 days.

Indications: Bacteriostatic skin cleanser and surgical scrub.

Contraindications: Hypersensitivity to the compound. It is also contraindicated for use on burned or denuded skin, as an occlusive dressing, wet pack, or lotion, for routine use in total body bathing, as a vaginal pack or tampon, or on any mucous membranes, and in those patients who have demonstrated photosensitivity to halogenated phenol derivatives because of the possibility of cross-sensitivity to hexachlorophene.

Warnings: Hexachlorophene is a potent human neurotoxin at high levels of use such as a 3% emulsion or a 6% powder. Consequently, it should not be left, diluted or undiluted, on the skin or mucous membrane, and should always be thoroughly rinsed off after each application.

Infants, especially premature infants or those with dermatoses, are particularly susceptible to hexachlorophene absorption. Since this compound is rapidly absorbed, patients should be closely monitored for signs of systemic toxicity. This untoward reaction may be manifested by CNS stimulation resulting in irritation and convulsions. Should these occur, hexachlorophene should be promptly discontinued. Applications to burns have produced neurotoxicity and death. Infants have developed dermatitis, irritability, generalized clonic muscular contractions, and decerebrate rigidity following application of a 6% powder. Examination of the brainstem of those infants revealed vacuolization. Therefore, this agent should not be used in premature infants unless, in the judgment of the physician, its use is required by the unique circumstances of the individual case.

Precautions: If hexachlorophene gets into the eyes accidentally during washing, they should be rinsed out promptly and thoroughly with water.

Adverse Reactions: These may include dermatitis and photosensitivity. Highly sensitive skin may produce a reaction characterized by redness and/or mild scaling or dryness.

Dosage and Administration: *Topically. For external use only.* Apply the emulsion either undiluted or diluted as indicated. Place on a wet palm or sponge, then work into a lather and cleanse skin. Rinse and repeat if necessary. *Rinse off thoroughly after use.*

Availability:
pHisoHex® Emulsion, 3% in plastic bottles of 150 ml, 1 pint and 1 gallon and in packets of 8 ml in cartons of 50. **(Winthrop)**
SOY-DOME® Emulsion, 3% (in a soya protein complex base) in plastic dispenser bottles of 180 ml. **(Dome)**

HEXAFLUORENIUM BROMIDE

Chemical Name: Hexamethylene*bis*[9-fluorenyldimethylammonium]dibromide.

Description: A curarimimetic agent which occurs as a white, crystalline powder soluble in water.

Hexafluorenium inhibits plasma cholinesterases, thus suppressing the enzymatic hydrolysis and prolonging the duration of action of succinylcholine. It does not appear to affect intracellular cholinesterases. It also produces a mild nondepolarizing blocking action (curare-like effect) at the myoneural junction. Skeletal muscle relaxation after intravenous injection is evident only under deep anesthesia.

Hexafluorenium is used only in conjunction with succinylcholine after anesthetization and prior to surgery. With the use of this drug, it is possible to employ succinylcholine in about 1/5 the usual total dosage, thereby reducing or eliminating side effects of succinylcholine such as muscle fasciculations. In anesthetized adults of average weight, an intravenous dose of hexafluorenium bromide followed in 3 minutes by succinylcholine chloride intravenously will produce apnea sufficient for endotracheal intubation within 4 minutes and skeletal muscle relaxation lasting for about 20 minutes. The general anesthetic agent being used has little or no effect on the intensity or duration of action of the drugs.

Indications: An adjunct to succinylcholine during anesthesia to potentiate and prolong that drug's neuromuscular blocking activity and thus modify the amount of the drug required.

Contraindications: In patients with known hypersensitivity to the drug or to bromides.

Warnings: Hexafluorenium bromide should not be administered unless facilities for intubation, artificial respiration and administration of oxygen therapy are instantaneously available. The clinician must be prepared to assist or control respiration. Safe use during pregnancy has not been established. Therefore, it should not be used in women of childbearing potential and particularly during early pregnancy unless in the judgment of the physician the potential benefits outweigh the unknown hazards.

Precautions: Hexafluorenium bromide should be used with caution in patients with cardiovascular, hepatic, pulmonary (e.g., asthma), metabolic or renal disorder. The drug should be administered with extreme caution to patients with severe burns, those who have recently been digitalized, or patients who may have digitalis toxicity as serious cardiac arrhythmias or cardiac arrest may result. It should also be used with utmost caution during ocular surgery and in patients with glaucoma, fractures or muscle spasms or with any type of neuromyopathy (i.e., amyotrophic lateral sclerosis, muscular dystrophy, myasthenia gravis, and similar conditions). The possibility of synergistic or antagonistic effects should be considered when the drug is used concomitantly with other relaxants.

Adverse Reactions: Profound and prolonged muscle spasm may occur resulting in respiratory depression or apnea. Bradycardia, tachycardia, hypertension, hypotension, cardiac arrest, arrhythmias, apnea, bronchospasm, hyperthermia, increased intraocular pressure and salivation may also occur.

Dosage and Administration: *Intravenously* by intermittent injection. Inject 0.4 mg/kg of body weight of hexafluorenium bromide. Wait 3 minutes then inject 0.2 mg/kg succinylcholine. Within 3 to 4 minutes, this dose will produce apnea and adequate conditions for endotracheal intubation. Muscle relaxation usually lasts from 20 to 30 minutes. When the effect of the first dose of succinylcholine begins to wear off, a repeat dose of 0.15 mg/kg of succinylcholine should be given. For continuous relaxation, this dose should be repeated at 15- to 30-minute intervals, keeping in mind that as the effect of hexafluorenium bromide wears off, the doses of succinylcholine will have a progressively shorter duration of effect. **Note:** It is advisable that the initial dose of neuromuscular blocking agents should not be greater than that used in a 90-kg (200 lb) patient.

Availability:
MYLAXEN® Aqueous Solution, 20 mg/ml in vials of 10 ml. **(Mallinckrodt)**

HEXOBARBITAL Ⓒ III

Chemical Name: 5-(1-Cyclohexen-1-yl)-1,5-dimethylbarbituric acid.

Description: A rapidly acting barbiturate with ultrashort duration of action, it occurs as a tasteless, white, crystalline powder very slightly soluble in water and slightly soluble in alcohol.

Hexobarbital is rapidly absorbed through the gastrointestinal mucosa, and as a result, it generally produces sleep within 15 to 30 minutes. It is completely metabolized and cleared from the blood stream within 4 to 5 hours.

Indications: Treatment of simple insomnia or as a preanesthetic, preoperative, or postoperative sedative, and for short-term sedation for diagnostic and minor surgical procedures.

Contraindications: In the presence of impaired liver or kidney function.

Warnings: Hexobarbital may be habit-forming and should therefore be prescribed and administered with the same degree of prudence appropriate for the use of other oral barbiturates, since it can produce drug dependence and subsequently has the potential for abuse.

Dosage and Administration: *Orally. For sleep,* 1 or 2 tablets at bedtime. When sleep has been interrupted, 1 tablet may be taken. May be used preoperatively with atropine when morphine is contraindicated.

Availability:
Ⓒ III SOMBULEX® Tablets, 250 mg in bottles of 100. **(Riker)**

HEXOCYCLIUM METHYLSULFATE

Chemical Name: *N*-(β-Cyclohexyl-β-hydroxy-β-phenylethyl)-*N'*-methylpiperazine methosulfate.

Description: A synthetic anticholinergic quaternary ammonium salt, it occurs as a white powder that is soluble in water or physiological saline yielding a stable solution. Hexocyclium has an antimuscarinic action similar to that of other quaternary ammonium compounds which produce anticholinergic effects. In experimental animals, the drug has been shown to decrease gastric secretion, prevent gastric ulceration, decrease gastrointestinal motility, dilate the pupils, inhibit salivation, increase the heart rate, and counteract the peripheral muscarinic effect of choline esters. With massive overdosage, it may also produce a peripheral curare-like neuromuscular block and ganglionic blockade.

Following oral administration of a single dose, hexocyclium is readily absorbed from the gastrointestinal tract, and blocks the effector cells innervated by postganglionic cholinergic nerves. Its action is prompt and usually persists for 3 to 4 hours. The metabolic fate and route of excretion of the drug are not known.

Clinical studies and laboratory experiments with animals have produced no teratogenic effects. Although the clinical significance is not clear, animal experiments with hexocyclium have shown that daily oral doses of 2.5 to 40 mg/kg/day administered to pregnant rabbits produced an increased number of resorption sites and abortions. No significant effects were observed on the progeny of rats.

Indications: Adjunctive management in the treatment of peptic ulcer. Its usefulness in healing the ulcer, decreasing the rate of recurrences or preventing complications has not been firmly established. Hexocyclium with phenobarbital is indicated in those conditions in which a sedative action would be an additional benefit.

Contraindications: In patients with glaucoma, obstruction of the bladder neck, obstructive disease of the gastrointestinal tract (as in achalasia, paralytic ileus, pyloroduodenal stenosis, etc.), intestinal atony of the elderly or debilitated patient, unstable cardiovascular status, acute hemorrhage, severe ulcerative colitis, toxic megacolon complicating ulcerative colitis, and myasthenia gravis.

Warnings: Phenobarbital may be habit-forming. Since small doses inhibit the production of sweat, heat prostration can occur in the presence of high environmental temperature. Diarrhea may be an early symptom of incomplete intestinal obstruction, especially in patients with ileostomy or colostomy. In this instance treatment with this drug would be inappropriate and possibly harmful. In the event of drowsiness or blurred vision, patients should be cautioned not to engage in activities requiring alertness or skill. As with any drug, special consideration should be taken when prescribing this drug to pregnant or lactating women or to women of childbearing potential. Until further clinical trials establish safe use and proper dosage, it is not recommended for use in children.

Precautions: Use with utmost care in patients with autonomic neuropathy, hepatic or renal disease, early evidence of ileus (as in peritonitis), ulcerative colitis, hyperthyroidism, coronary heart disease, congestive heart failure, cardiac arrhythmias, hypertension, nonobstructing prostatic hypertrophy, and hiatal hernia associated with reflux esophagitis. It is not recommended for use in biliary tract disorders. Medications of this type should be discontinued prior to gastroscopy or esophagoscopy procedures. As with all anticholinergic drugs, an inhibitory effect on lactation may occur. Precautions associated with phenobarbital should be observed.

Adverse Reactions: The following have been noted: xerostomia, urinary hesitancy and retention, blurred vision, mydriasis, cycloplegia, increased intraocular tension, tachycardia, palpitations, headaches, nervousness, drowsiness, weakness, dizziness, insomnia, nausea, vomiting, impotency, dysphagia, altered taste perception, heartburn, bloated feeling, constipation, flushing, decreased sweating, urticaria and other dermal manifestations, severe allergic reaction or drug idiosyncrasies, and some degree of mental confusion and/or excitement especially in elderly patients. Overdosage may produce a curare-like action, and ganglionic blockade manifested by respiratory paralysis and circulatory collapse. Artificial respiration and other supportive measures should be applied if needed.

Dosage and Administration: *Orally. Filmtabs* (with or without phenobarbital): the usual recommended adult dosage is 1 tablet 4 times daily, taken before meals and at bedtime. For optimal therapeutic effect, dosage should be adjusted to the patient's response. *Gradumets:* the usual recommended dosage is 1 tablet twice daily, taken before lunch and at bedtime, or before breakfast and the evening meal. For daytime control, one 50 mg Gradumet tablet in the morning is generally adequate. At bedtime, the 75 mg Gradumet tablet is usually preferred for controlling nocturnal gastric secretion.

Availability:
TRAL®: **(Abbott)**
Filmtab® (film-sealed tablets), 25 mg in bottles of 100.
Gradumet® (long-release tablet), 50 and 75 mg in bottles of 50.
w/Phenobarbital
Filmtab, 25 mg with 15 mg phenobarbital in bottles of 100 and 1000.

HEXYLCAINE HYDROCHLORIDE

Chemical Name: 1-Cyclohexylamino-2-propylbenzoate hydrochloride.

Description: A local anesthetic agent of the benzoic acid ester group, it occurs as a white, crystalline powder that is soluble in water. Its molecular weight is 297.8. Similar in action to other local anesthetic agents, hexylcaine reversibly blocks the conduction of impulses in all nervous tissue. When used for surface anesthesia, its potency corresponds to that of cocaine. Clinical studies have revealed that hexylcaine acts faster and longer than an equal concentration of procaine when used for infiltration or nerve block procedures; however, it is slightly more toxic.

Following topical application, onset of anesthesia begins within 2 to 3 minutes, reaches peak effect in about 12 to 15 minutes and persists for approximately 30 minutes. It is hydrolyzed by serum esterase into inactive compounds. Hexylcaine compares favorably with the more active local anesthetic compounds in duration of anesthesia and in degree of motor paralysis produced.

Indications: For topical anesthesia of intact mucous membranes such as those of the respiratory, upper gastrointestinal, or urinary tracts (e.g., before laryngoscopy, bronchoscopy, esophagoscopy, and cystoscopy).

Contraindications: In traumatized mucosal tissues (either suspected or likely to occur), and in patients known to be hypersensitive to local anesthetics of the ester-linkage group. **Note:** Not for ophthalmic use.

Warnings: Safe use of hexylcaine during pregnancy or in women of childbearing age has not been established. Therefore, use of the drug in these patients should be limited to those conditions serious enough to justify the risks to the fetus. For topical use only, not for injection.

Precautions: Since toxic reactions may occur, the necessary drugs and proper resuscitative equipment must be readily available. Local anesthetics should not be instilled into infected areas, since this may cause the infection to spread. The acid medium of infected tissue can interfere with the activity of the drug thus resulting in poor anesthesia. Because of the reactive hyperemia in the infected area, greater absorption of the drug may occur which can result in high plasma levels. Cautious use is advised in patients with known drug sensitivities, in debilitated or elderly patients, and in children.

Adverse Reactions: Hypersensitivity has been reported, and the possibility of an anaphylactoid reaction should be considered. Sudden attainment of high plasma levels may lead to disturbances of the CNS system manifested by drowsiness, restlessness, twitchings, and excitement, and in some instances ending in convulsions. Frequently, this is followed by CNS depression. Cardiovascular reactions may be manifested by hypotension, cardiac arrhythmias and cardiovascular collapse; also respiratory arrest may develop. Prolonged burning sensation, residual tenderness, tissue irritation, swelling and in some patients, sloughing and tissue necrosis also have been reported.

Dosage and Administration: *Topically,* usually in concentrations of 0.5 to 5% depending on the procedure. May be applied to the mucous membranes by spray or packs or by swabbing with cotton applicators. For antral puncture, a 1% or greater concentration may be required. For peroral endoscopic procedures, adequate anesthesia can be obtained with a total of 2 to 10 ml of a 5% solution. **The patient should not be allowed to swallow any excess solution.** For gastroscopy, the patient should gargle 4 times with a 1 or 2% solution (should not exceed 2%); the procedure is repeated twice at 5-minute intervals. Should the patient accidentally swallow or aspirate the drug, a subsequent dose should not be given. For genitourinary procedures, 5 to 10 ml of a 5% solution may be instilled into the male urethra and retained for approximately 5 to 10 minutes. Anesthesia of the female urethra may be produced by inserting a sterile cotton-tipped applicator soaked with the 5% solution into the urethra for 10 minutes. Package literature should be consulted for more detailed information.

Availability:
CYCLAINE® Topical Solution, 5% (50 mg/ml) in rubber-capped bottles of 60 ml.

(Merck Sharp & Dohme)

HISTAMINE PHOSPHATE

Chemical Name: 4-(2-Aminoethyl)imidazole *bis*(dihydrogen phosphate).

Description: Histamine phosphate is a potent stimulant which acts mainly on the vascular system, smooth muscle, and exocrine glands. It is a basic substance which may be derived from the amino acid histidine by decarboxylation. It is usually administered as the stable, water-soluble acid phosphate; 2 molecules of phosphoric acid are attached to each molecule of histamine. Since the molecular weight of histamine phosphate is approximately 3 times greater than that of histamine itself, 2.75 mg of the salt are required to obtain 1 mg of the active principle. It occurs as colorless, odorless, long prismatic crystals that are freely soluble in water and slightly soluble in alcohol.

Histamine is readily absorbed following parenteral administration and acts rapidly when given by the subcutaneous or intramuscular route. Although its action is transient since it diffuses into tissues and is quickly metabolized, it produces a copious, highly acidic gastric secretion. Only 1% escapes enzymatic destruction and appears in the urine in the free form. In contrast, it is poorly absorbed when administered orally. Large amounts can be given without producing effects, since absorption is scant, and much of the compound is metabolized (mostly acetylated) by the intestinal flora.

Clinically, histamine is used as a diagnostic agent to assess the ability of the stomach to secrete acid. Since it is a potent gastric stimulant, it is a useful means for distinguishing between true and false achylia.

Indications: Subcutaneously to test the ability of the gastric mucosa to produce hydrochloric acid, and intravenously for the presumptive diagnosis of pheochromocytoma.

Contraindications: The gastric test is contraindicated in patients with a history of hypersensitivity to histamine products, in those with hypotension, severe hypertension, vasomotor instability, bronchial asthma, urticaria, or severe cardiac, pulmonary or renal disease. The test for pheochromocytoma is contraindicated in the elderly or in the presence of severe hypertension.

Warnings: Severe attacks of asthma or other serious allergic conditions may be precipitated. The possible benefit that may be derived from the gastric test should be carefully weighed against the serious untoward reactions that may develop in patients with severe allergic conditions. When injected subcutaneously, accidental introduction into a blood vessel must be avoided. Safe use of this preparation during pregnancy or lactation has not been established; therefore, the benefits to be derived must be weighed against the possible hazards to the mother and child. Careful consideration is essential in the use of the gastric histamine test in patients with pheochromocytoma.

Precautions: Average or large doses of histamine may cause flushing, dizziness, headache, nervousness, local or generalized allergic manifestations, marked hypertension or hypotension, tachycardia, and abdominal cramps. These reactions can be alarming and are potentially dangerous. Local reactions at the site of injection may include erythema and edema. Since histamine increases the acid level of the gastric juice, symptoms of peptic ulcer may be experienced. Utmost caution is advised in patients with a history of bronchial asthma, since even small doses of the drug by any route of administration may precipitate an asthmatic attack. Blood pressure and pulse rate should be checked frequently, and epinephrine must always be available to counteract severe reactions such as a dangerous fall in blood pressure. A large dose of histamine may cause severe occipital headache, blurred vision, anginal pain, a rapid drop in blood pressure, and cyanosis. Overdosage by either route may cause severe symptoms including vasomotor collapse, shock, and even death.

Adverse Reactions: Injections of average or large doses of histamine may produce such local reactions as erythema and edema and/or such systemic reactions as flushing, dizziness, headache, bronchial constriction, dyspnea, visual disturbances, faintness, syncope, urticaria, asthma, marked hypertension or hypotension, palpitation, tachycardia, nervousness, abdominal cramps, diarrhea, nausea, vomiting, metallic taste, local or generalized allergic manifestations or collapse with convulsions.

Dosage and Administration: *Subcutaneously.* Package literature should be consulted for specific details. *Gastric Histamine Test:* The test is performed in the morning after the patient has fasted overnight, and the residual gastric contents have been aspirated. A dose of 0.01 mg/kg of body weight is injected subcutaneously. After the histamine has been administered, 4 fifteen-minute samples are taken. The maximal effect of histamine is usually noted in the second and third samples. *Test for Pheochromocytoma:* The test is used only in patients whose resting blood pressure does not exceed 150/110. Antihypertensive drugs, sympathomimetic agents, sedatives, and narcotics should be withheld from the patient for at least 24 hours, preferably 72 hours, before the histamine test is performed. *Food should not be withheld.* The initial dose is 0.01 mg injected intravenously. If no response is observed within 5 minutes, a dose of 0.05 mg should be administered. The blood pressure and pulse rate are to be recorded every 30 seconds for 15 minutes. Epinephrine should be readily available in the event of a severe hypotensive response, and phentolamine should be on hand should the response reach dangerous levels. The expected response in both positive and negative tests are headache, flushing, and a decrease in blood pressure followed within 2 minutes by an increase.

Availability:
HISTAMINE PHOSPHATE Injection, 0.275 mg/ml (0.1 mg of base) in ampuls of 1 ml; 0.55 mg/ml (0.2 mg of base) in ampuls of 5 ml; 2.75 mg/ml (1 mg of base) in ampuls of 1 ml. **(Lilly)**

HISTOPLASMIN

Description: Histoplasmin is a standardized, sterile filtrate from the cultures of *Histoplasma capsulatum* grown on a liquid synthetic medium. It is available for clinical use in the undiluted form equal in potency to Reference Histoplasmin. When diluted according to directions, each 0.01 ml of histoplasmin provides 1 ml (10 doses) of the test solution equivalent in activity to N.I.H. Reference Histoplasmin. The diluted material may be kept for 30 days at refrigerator temperatures without appreciable loss of potency.

Indications: As an aid in the diagnosis of histoplasmosis and the differentiation of possible histoplasmosis from coccidiodomycosis, sarcoidosis and other mycotic or bacterial infections, and in the interpretation of roentgenographic plates showing pulmonary infiltration and calcification.

Precautions: Doses in excess of those recommended may result in severe reactions. Histoplasmin should be injected intradermally only. It is advised that the tuberculin test be employed in conjunction with histoplasmin in order to exclude the possibility of tuberculosis. It is also recommended that patients with suspected histoplasmosis who are ill or have a fever be tested with this agent repeatedly. However, the patient may react at times during the course of the infection. Epinephrine should be readily available in the event that an acute hypersensitivity reaction or an anaphylactoid response occurs.

Adverse Reactions: Urticaria, shortness of breath, and increased perspiration may occur.

Dosage and Administration: *Intradermally only.* Inject 0.1 ml doses into the skin of the flexor surface of the forearm. If the injection is correctly made, a small bleb will rise over the needle point. Reactions should be read under adequate light 24 to 48 hours after the injection.

Availability:
HISTOPLASMIN Injection, 0.01 ml in vials of 1 ml with a 1-ml vial of buffered diluent.
(Parke-Davis)

HOMATROPINE

Chemical Name: Mandelyltropine; tropine mandelate.

Description: Homatropine is a synthetic alkaloid produced by a combination of tropine and mandelic acid. The *hydrobromide* occurs as white crystals or as a white, crystalline powder freely soluble in water and soluble in alcohol. The *methylbromide,* designated chemically as 8 methyl homatropinium bromide, occurs as a white, odorless powder very soluble in water and freely soluble in alcohol.

Indications: Homatropine *hydrobromide* is an effective mydriatic and cycloplegic. It is used to dilate the pupils prior to retinoscopy; in the treatment of uveitis and keratitis; and to paralyze accommodation temporarily. Homatropine *methylbromide* is employed as adjunctive therapy in peptic ulcer. It generally has the same actions on the gastrointestinal tract as do the belladonna alkaloids; however, it is less active, but also less toxic, than belladonna. It is used as a spasmolytic in the treatment of gastrointestinal spasm and hyperchlorhydria as well as in the management of mild spastic conditions of the bile ducts, gallbladder and ureters. Formulated with barbiturates to decrease the psychogenic component, and to allay anxiety resulting from these somatic symptoms.

Contraindications: Glaucoma, obstructive uropathy (e.g. bladder neck obstruction due to prostatic hypertrophy), obstructive disease of the gastrointestinal tract (as in achalasia, paralytic ileus, pyloroduodenal stenosis), intestinal atony of the elderly or debilitated patient, unstable cardiovascular status in acute hemorrhage, toxic megacolon complicating ulcerative colitis, and myasthenia gravis.

Warnings: The use of homatropine during pregnancy, lactation, or in women of childbearing potential requires that the expected benefit of the drug be weighed against its possible hazard to the mother or child. In the presence of high environmental temperature, therapy with this drug can induce fever and heat stroke due to decreased perspiration. Also hiatal hernia with reflux may be aggravated. Diarrhea may be an early symptom of incomplete intestinal obstruction, especially in patients with ileostomy or colostomy. In this instance, treatment with homatropine would be inappropriate and possibly harmful.

Precautions: Use with extreme caution in patients with autonomic neuropathy, hyperthyroidism, coronary heart disease, congestive heart failure, cardiac arrhythmias, hypertension, nonobstructing prostatic hypertrophy, advanced hepatic or renal disease, and in the presence of biliary tract disease. Homatropine may cause a delay in gastric emptying which may complicate gastric ulcer therapy (antral stasis). Overdosage may produce a curare-like action. Tachycardia should be ruled out before initiating therapy with this drug since anticholinergic drugs may increase the heart rate. In the event of drowsiness or blurred vision, patients should be cautioned not to engage in any activity requiring alertness or skill.

Adverse Reactions: These may include xerostomia; urinary hesitancy and retention; blurred vision; tachycardia; palpitations; mydriasis; dilation of the pupils; cycloplegia; increased ocular tension, loss of taste; headaches; nervousness; drowsiness; weakness; dizziness; insomnia; nausea; vomiting; bloated feeling; constipation; impotence; allergic reactions or drug idiosyncrasies including anaphylaxis; urticaria and other dermal manifestations; some degree of mental confusion and/or excitement, especially in elderly patients, and suppression of lactation. Decreased perspiration is another adverse reaction that may occur. It should be noted that adrenergic innervation of the exocrine or eccrine sweat glands on the palms and soles make complete control of sweating impossible. Complete anhidrosis cannot occur because large doses of the drug would be required and this would produce severe side effects from parasympathetic paralysis.

Dosage and Administration: *Orally.* The adult dosage of the *methylbromide* is 2.5 to 10 mg 4 times daily before meals. Infants, 0.3 mg dissolved in water or fruit juice is given 4 to 6 times daily before feedings. *Topically.* As a mydriatic, about 5 drops of a 1% solution (*hydrobromide*) are instilled into the conjunctiva every 15 minutes for a period of 2 hours. For iritis, the solution is instilled 2 or 3 times daily as indicated.

Availability:

Homatropine Hydrobromide

Ophthalmic Solution, 2 and 5% in dropper bottles of 15 ml. **(Allergan)**

Ophthalmic Solution, 2 and 5% in Dropperettes® applicators of 1 and 5 ml. **(Smith, Miller & Patch)**

Ophthalmic Solutions, 1 to 5% in various size bottles. **(Various Mfrs.)**

Isopto® HOMATROPINE Ophthalmic Solution, 2 and 5% in Drop-Tainer® bottles of 5 and 15 ml. **(Alcon)**

Homatropine Methylbromide

SED-TENS SE Tablets, 10 mg in bottles of 100 and 1000. **(Lemmon)**

HORMONIN: see The Estrogens

HYALURONIDASE

Description: Hyaluronidase is a protein enzyme, the exact chemical structure of which is not known. It is found widely distributed in nature but is obtained chiefly from bovine testes. It is a spreading, or diffusing, substance which modifies the permeability of connective tissue through the hydrolysis of hyaluronic acid. Hyaluronidase, existing as a gel, occurs as one of the principal viscous polysaccharides of connective tissue and skin, and is one of the chief ingredients of the "tissue cement" which offers resistance to the diffusion of liquids through tissue.

Intravenous administration of even 75,000 N.F. units (500 times the maximal therapeutic dose) of hyaluronidase in animals causes no significant change in blood pressure, respiration, body temperature or kidney function, and no histological changes in the tissues. Results from an experimental study on the influence of hyaluronidase in bone repair support the conclusion that this enzyme alone, in the usual clinical dosage, does not deter bone healing. Hyaluronidase has no effect on the spread of localized infection provided it is not injected into the infected area, and seems to have no deleterious effect on bacterial or viral infections. But when *crude* testicular extracts which contained tissue *irritants* as well as "spreading factor" were used, an increase in area and virulence of the infection was observed.

Indications: This drug is indicated as an adjuvant to increase the absorption and dispersion of other injected drugs, for hypodermoclysis and as an adjunct in subcutaneous urography for improving resorption of radiopaque agents.

Contraindications: Should not be injected into cancerous, infected or highly inflamed areas because of the danger of spreading the cancer or infection.

Precautions: Occasional sensitivity reactions have been reported; the drug should not be administered before the patient has been tested for sensitivity. To test for sensitivity, about 0.02 ml of solution ready for clinical use is injected intradermally. Evidence of sensitivity is a wheal with pseudopods appearing within 5 minutes and persisting for about 1/2 hour, as well as localized pruritus and transient vasodilation. The absence of a positive reaction may not necessarily rule out hypersensitivity. If there is a history of other allergies, caution should be observed even in the absence of a positive reaction. When epinephrine is injected along with hyaluronidase the usual precautions for the use of epinephrine in cardiovascular disease, thyroid disease, diabetes, digital nerve block, ischemia of the fingers and toes, etc., should be observed. Conditions that affect absorption into the bloodstream, such as congestive heart failure or depletion of blood plasma protein, must be considered in the selection of patients. When hyaluronidase is added to commonly used doses of local anesthetics, the likelihood of toxic local anesthetic reactions is increased; therefore, facilities for treating respiratory distress, cardiac difficulties and convulsions should be readily available.

Adverse Reactions: When dextrose solutions, with or without hyaluronidase, are administered by hypodermoclysis, fluid is drawn from the surrounding tissues into the site of injection. This effect may persist for several hours, causing unnecessary pain and a severe decrease in plasma volume if large amounts of fluid are given. The ensuing fall in systolic blood pressure may have serious sequelae in the critically ill patient. This danger can be avoided by using suitable dextrose solutions that contain electrolytes, or by carefully controlling the volume of fluid to be administered and the rates of administration.

Dosage and Administration: *Parenterally by interstitial injection.* The diluent is added to the vial containing the dry material and the solution then is injected by syringe at the injection site of other solutions or it can be added to them. The contents of 1 vial (150 N.F. units) is considered sufficient for each liter of hypodermoclysis fluid. For nerve block infiltration requiring large amounts of anesthetic solution, 150 units and 0.5 ml of epinephrine 1:1000 solution are added to each 50 ml of solution. In eye surgery, 150 units are dissolved in 1 ml of the anesthetic solution with 0.4% potassium sulfate; for nerve block, 0.4 ml of this mixture is diluted to 10 ml and 0.12 ml of epinephrine 1:1000 is added prior to injection. For cone injection, twice as much epinephrine may be used. In the treatment of traumatic swelling (transudate or hematoma), 150 to 500 units is injected into the center of the affected area, followed by the application of pressure bandages or massage to facilitate diffusion of the enzyme into the tissues.

For infants and children, hyaluronidase should be administered in the ratio of 15 units/100 ml of parenteral fluid. *For premature or very young infants,* not more than 25 mg/kg of body weight daily; *children under 3 years of age,* maximal daily dose is 200 ml. The rate of drip should not exceed 2 ml/minute. The subcutaneous route of administration of urographic contrast media is indicated when intravenous administration cannot be successfully accomplished, particularly in infants and small children. With the patient lying down, 75 units of hyaluronidase is injected subcutaneously over each scapula followed by injection of the contrast medium at the same sites.

Availability:
ALIDASE® in vials of 150 N.F. units. **(Searle)**
WYDASE® (lyophilized) in vials of 150 and 1500 N.F. units; stabilized solution, 150 units/ml in vials of 1 and 10 ml. **(Wyeth)**

HYBEPHEN

Description: The formulations provide alkaloids of belladonna and hyoscyamus for smoother antispasmodic action than is possible with atropine alone. Phenobarbital is added to allay apprehension and reduce psychomotor tension. Each teaspoonful (5 ml) of elixir and each tablet contain:

	Elixir/Tablet
Phenobarbital	15 mg
Hyoscyamine sulfate	0.1277 mg
Atropine sulfate	0.0233 mg
Hyoscine hydrobromide	0.0094 mg

Indications: As a smooth muscle relaxant in conditions of excessive parasympathetic stimulation or increased psychomotor activity, and for the relief or control of visceral spasm. As adjunctive therapy in the treatment of conditions of the stomach, duodenum and intestine, the genitourinary system and in associated disorders where spasm is involved.

Warnings: Phenobarbital may be habit-forming. Hybephen should not be administered to patients with glaucoma or with excessive pressure within the eye, to elderly patients in whom undiagnosed glaucoma or excessive pressure with the eye(s) occurs most frequently, or to children under 6 years of age, unless directed by a physician.

Precautions: Should blurring of vision, rapid pulse, or dizziness occur, therapy with this drug should be terminated. The recommended dosage must not be exceeded. Also frequent or prolonged use is not advised. If dryness of the mouth occurs, the dosage should be reduced. The occurrence of eye pain may indicate undiagnosed glaucoma; the drug should be discontinued immediately and the physician consulted.

For adverse reactions, see the monograph on each of the components.

Dosage and Administration: *Orally.* Adults, 1 or 2 teaspoonsful or 1 or 2 tablets 3 times daily. Children, in proportion to age.

Availability:
HYBEPHEN®: **(Beecham)**
Elixir in pints and gallons.
Tablets in bottles of 100 and 1000.

HYCOMINE Ⓒ III

Description: Each coral-pink, scored tablet of Hycomine Compound contains:

Hydrocodone bitartrate	5 mg
Chlorpheniramine maleate	2 mg
Phenylephrine hydrochloride	10 mg
Acetaminophen (APAP)	250 mg
Caffeine	30 mg

Each teaspoonful (5 ml) of Hycomine Pediatric Syrup contains:

Hydrocodone bitartrate	2.5 mg
Phenylpropanolamine hydrochloride	12.5 mg

Each teaspoonful (5 ml) of Hycomine Syrup contains the same ingredients as the Pediatric Syrup, but the quantities of each have been doubled.

Indications: Symptomatic relief of colds, upper respiratory infections, and simple minor coughs due to colds and for the relief of cough as may occur in tracheitis, bronchitis, and pharyngitis.

Contraindications: In patients sensitive to the individual components. The syrup is contraindicated in patients taking MAO inhibitors.

Warnings: Hydrocodone bitartrate may be habit-forming. In the event of drowsiness, dizziness or blurred vision, patients should be cautioned not to engage in activities requiring alertness or skill.

Precautions: Routine caution should be undertaken in the presence of diabetes, hyperthyroidism, hypertension, cardiovascular disorders, and in geriatric patients. Treatment directed toward suppressing or modifying the cough is symptomatic and has no direct effect on the underlying pathology. Therefore, it is important to ascertain that the underlying cause of the cough is identified, that modification of the cough does not increase the risk of clinical or physiologic complications, and that appropriate therapy for the primary disease is provided.

Adverse Reactions: These products are generally well-tolerated. Occasionally noted were drowsiness, blurred vision, cardiac palpitation, dizziness, nervousness, dryness of the mouth, and gastrointestinal distress.

Dosage and Administration: *Orally. Compound Tablets:* Adults, 1 tablet 4 times daily. Children 6 to 12 years of age, ½ tablet 4 times daily; 2 to 6 years, ½ tablet twice daily. *Pediatric Syrup:* Children 6 to 12 years of age, the usual dosage is 1 teaspoonful every 4 hours after meals and at bedtime. No more than 6 teaspoonsful should be given in a 24-hour period. *Syrup:* Adults, 1 teaspoonful every 4 hours. All dosage forms should be administered after meals and at bedtime at intervals of not less than 4 hours.

Availability:
Ⓒ III HYCOMINE®: **(Endo)**
Compound Tablets in bottles of 100 and 500.
Pediatric Syrup in pints and gallons.
Syrup in pints and gallons.

HYDRALAZINE HYDROCHLORIDE

Chemical Name: 1-Hydrazinophthalazine hydrochloride.

Description: An antihypertensive agent, it occurs as a white, odorless, crystalline powder soluble in water and slightly soluble in alcohol.

Although the factors contributing to the hypotensive effect of hydralazine are incompletely understood, it is thought to exert a direct musculotropic action resulting in relaxation of vascular smooth muscle and reduced peripheral resistance. The drug has been found to possess the dual capacity of reducing pathologically elevated blood pressure and at the same time increasing cardiac output and blood flow through the kidneys. The therapeutic effect develops gradually over a period of 15 to 20 minutes even after intravenous administration. Readily absorbed from the gastrointestinal tract following oral administration, maximal blood levels are generally achieved within 3 to 4 hours with diminishing amounts detectable for as long as 24 hours.

Indications: Either alone or as an adjunctive agent in the treatment of essential hypertension. It may be effective in hypertensive states associated with toxemia of pregnancy and acute glomerulonephritis. When combined with hydrochlorothiazide and reserpine, the drug is indicated for most cases of moderate to severe forms of hypertension, especially when complicated by anxiety, impaired renal circulation and edema; however, it is not recommended for initial therapy. Parenteral administration is generally reserved for those cases in which the hypertension is severe; when the need to lower blood pressure is critical, or when the drug cannot be given orally.

Contraindications: Hypersensitivity to the drug, coronary artery disease, and mitral valvular rheumatic heart disease. For contraindications attributable to any additional component, the individual monograph should be consulted.

Warnings: MAO inhibitors should be administered with care to patients receiving hydralazine. Lupus erythematosus cell preparations, and antinuclear antibody titer determinations as well as complete blood counts are deemed essential before and periodically during prolonged therapy, even though the patient is asymptomatic. These studies are also indicated if the patient develops arthralgia, fever, chest pain, continued malaise, or other unexplained signs or symptoms. The development of an acute rheumatic state and symptoms of acute systemic lupus erythematosus during therapy is an indication for cessation of treatment. The drug should be used during pregnancy only when it is deemed essential to the welfare of the patient. For warnings attributable to any additional component, the individual monograph should be consulted.

Precautions: Myocardial stimulation produced by hydralazine can cause anginal attacks and ECG changes of myocardial ischemia. The drug has also been implicated in causing myocardial infarction; therefore, it must be used with considerable caution in patients with suspected coronary artery disease. The drug is capable of increasing pulmonary artery pressure in patients with mitral valvular disease. Hydralazine may reduce the pressor responses to epinephrine. Special attention is advised in patients with advanced renal damage and cerebral vascular accidents. If peripheral neuritis, evidenced by paresthesias, numbness and tingling develops, the addition of pyridoxine to the regimen may provide some relief. Because blood dyscrasias, consisting of reduction in hemoglobin and red blood cell count, leukopenia, agranulocytosis, and purpura have been reported; periodic blood counts and liver function tests are advised. For precautions attributable to any additional component, the individual monograph should be consulted.

Adverse Reactions: Those commonly noted were headache, palpitations, anorexia, nausea, vomiting, diarrhea, tachycardia, angina pectoris. Less frequently noted were nasal congestion, flushing, lacrimation, conjunctivitis, peripheral neuritis characterized by paresthesias, numbness and tinging; edema, dizziness, tremors, muscle cramps; psychotic reactions characterized by depression, disorientation, or anxiety; hypersensitivity reactions including skin rash, urticaria, pruritus, fever, chills, arthralgia, eosinophilia, and, rarely, hepatitis, constipation, difficulty in micturition, dyspnea, paralytic ileus, lymphadenopathy, splenomegaly; blood dyscrasias consisting of reduction in hemoglobin and red cell count, leukopenia, agranulocytosis, and purpura, hypotension, especially postural hypotension; and paradoxical pressor response. For adverse reactions attributable to any additional component, the individual monograph should be consulted.

Dosage and Administration: *Orally, intramuscularly* or *intravenously.* The usual initial oral dosage is 1 tablet 3 times daily. Maintenance dosage is 1 to 2 tablets 3 times daily. The intramuscular or intravenous dosage is 20 mg up to 6 times a day.

Availability:

Hydralazine Hydrochloride

Tablets, 25 and 50 mg in bottles of 100 and 1000. **(Lederle)**

APRESOLINE®: **(Ciba)**

Injection, 20 mg/ml in ampuls of 1 ml.

Tablets, 10 mg in bottles of 100 and 1000; 25 and 50 mg in bottles of 100, 500 and 1000; 100 mg in bottles of 100. The 25 and 50 mg tablets are also available in Accu-Paks® (blister units) of 100.

DRALZINE™ Tablets, 25 mg in bottles of 1000. **(Lemmon)**

Combinations

APRESAZIDE™ Capsules, 25 mg with hydrochlorothiazide, 25 mg; 50 and 100 mg with hydrochlorothiazide, 50 mg in bottles of 100. **(Ciba)**

APRESOLINE®-ESIDRIX® Tablets, 25 mg with hydrochlorothiazide, 15 mg in bottles of 100. **(Ciba)**

DRALSERP® Tablets, 25 mg with reserpine, 0.1 mg in bottles of 100 and 1000. **(Lemmon)**

SERPASIL®-APRESOLINE® Tablets, 25 mg with reserpine, 0.1 mg; 50 mg with reserpine, 0.2 mg in bottles of 100, 500 and 1000. **(Ciba)**

SER-AP-ES® Tablets, 25 mg with reserpine, 0.1 mg and hydrochlorothiazide, 15 mg in bottles of 100 and 1000 and in Accu-Paks® (blister units) of 100. **(Ciba)**

HYDROCHLOROTHIAZIDE: see The Thiazide Diuretics

HYDROCODONE BITARTRATE Ⓒ II

Chemical Name: 7,8-Dihydrocodeinone bitartrate.

Description: Hydrocodone is a hydrogenated ketone of codeine which bears the same chemical relationship to codeine as hydromorphone does to morphine. It occurs as fine, white crystals or as a fine, white, crystalline powder soluble in water and slightly soluble in alcohol.

Its antitussive properties are similar to those of codeine, but it is effective in smaller doses and its action persists for about 4 to 6 hours. It can be used to relieve pain whenever an opiate analgesic is indicated; analgesia is obtained promptly and with less narcosis than with morphine. Hydrocodone has been combined with homatropine methylbromide, a smooth muscle relaxant, to counteract gastrointestinal upsets which sometimes may occur with codeine and its derivatives.

Indications: Exhausting, unproductive cough associated with acute respiratory tract infections. Relieves chronic cough irritation inherent in the common cold, influenza, sinusitis and bronchitis.

Contraindications: In patients with glaucoma or with unusual sensitivity to hydrocodone or to any of the combined components; or to narcotic-containing medications.

Warnings: Hydrocodone may be habit-forming. Since drowsiness may occur, patients should be cautioned against undertaking any hazardous activities requiring alertness or skill. The CNS-depressant effects of narcotic-antitussive agents are enhanced by phenothiazines, other tranquilizers, sedative-hypnotics, narcotic analgesics, alcohol or other CNS-depressants. When such combined therapy is considered, the dose of one or both agents should be reduced.

Precautions: Before prescribing medication to suppress or modify cough, it is important to ascertain that the underlying cause of the cough is identified, that modification of cough does not increase the risk of clinical or physiologic complications, and that appropriate therapy for the primary disease is provided. Usual precautions governing the use of opiates with regard to tolerance and addiction should be observed. Large doses may cause respiratory depression. Also, precautions pertaining to any ingredient combined with hydrocodone should be similarly observed.

Adverse Reactions: Hydrocodone is generally well tolerated, but in some patients drowsiness, dizziness, or nausea may occur; constipation and gastric distress are not ordinarily encountered. Overdosage is characterized by respiratory depression, extreme somnolence which may progress to coma or stupor, skeletal muscle flaccidity, cold and clammy skin, and occasionally bradycardia and hypotension. In severe intoxication, apnea, circulatory collapse, cardiac arrest, and death may occur. Primary attention should be given to the reestablishment of adequate respiratory exchange through provision of a patent airway and the institution of assisted or controlled ventilation. The narcotic antagonists naloxone, nalorphine or levallorphan are specific antidotes against respiratory depression. An appropriate dose should be administered preferably by the intravenous route. Oxygen, intravenous fluids, vasopressors, and other supportive measures should be employed as indicated. For adverse reactions attributable to any additional component, the individual monograph should be consulted.

Dosage and Administration: *Orally* every 4 hours. As an antitussive, 5 mg and as an analgesic, 10 mg. For children, proportionately smaller doses according to age and body weight, and usually ranges from 1/4 to 1 teaspoonful.

Availability:

Hydrocodone Bitartrate

C-II DICODID® Soluble Tablets, 5 mg in bottles of 100. **(Knoll)**

Combinations

C-II or C-III HYCODAN®: **(Endo)**

Each tablet and each 5 ml of syrup contain hydrocodone bitartrate, 5 mg and homatropine methylbromide, 1.5 mg. Each gram of powder contains 770 mg of hydrocodone bitartrate and 230 mg of homatropine methylbromide.

C-III *Oral Tablets* in bottles of 100, 500 and 1000.

C-II *Powder* in bottles of 5 gm.

C-III *Syrup* in pints and gallons.

C-III HYCOTUSS™ Expectorant in bottles of 1 pint. Each 5 ml contains hydrocodone bitartrate, 5 mg, guaifenesin, 100 mg and alcohol, 10% v/v. **(Endo)**

C-III TUSSEND®: **(Dow)**

Expectorant in bottles of 1 pint. Each 5 ml contains hydrocodone bitartrate, 5 mg; pseudoephedrine hydrochloride, 60 mg; guaifenesin, 200 mg and alcohol, 12.5%.

Each tablet and each 5 ml of liquid contain hydrocodone bitartrate, 5 mg and pseudoephedrine hydrochloride, 60 mg. The liquid also contains 5% alcohol.

Liquid in bottles of 1 pint.

Tablets in bottles of 100.

C-III TUSSIONEX®: **(Pennwalt)**

Each capsule and tablet and each 5 ml suspension contain hydrocodone, 5 mg and phenyltoloxamine, 10 mg as cationic exchange resin complexes.

Capsules in bottles of 50.

Suspension in bottles of 1 pint and 900 ml.

Tablets in bottles of 100.

C-III VICODIN Tablets, 5 mg with acetaminophen, 500 mg in bottles of 100 and in unit-dose dispenser packages of 100. **(Knoll)**

HYDROCORTISONE: see The Adrenal Corticosteroids

HYDROFLUMETHIAZIDE: see The Thiazide Diuretics

HYDROMORPHONE HYDROCHLORIDE C-II

Chemical Name: Dihydromorphinone hydrochloride.

Description: Hydromorphone is a hydrogenated ketone of morphine which bears the same chemical relationship to morphine as hydrocodone does to codeine. It occurs as a fine, white, odorless, crystalline powder freely soluble in water and sparingly soluble in alcohol.

Readily absorbed, it begins to exert its effect within 15 minutes following parenteral administration and within 30 minutes following oral use with an analgesic time-span of about 5 to 6 hours. Approximately the same degree of analgesia is provided by 2 mg of hydromorphone as is obtained with 10 to 15 mg of morphine or 100 mg of meperidine, but with significantly less side effects.

Indications: Treatment of all degrees of acute or chronic pain encountered in surgery, myocardial infarction, cancer, pleurisy, colic, fractures, burns and other conditions where a narcotic analgesic is indicated. Combined with guaifenesin for the control of persistent, exhausting cough associated with respiratory infections including the common cold, pulmonary tuberculosis, acute bronchitis, tracheitis and other forms of bronchial irritation.

Contraindications: Intracranial lesions associated with increased intracranial pressure, status asthmaticus, or idiosyncrasy to the drug.

Warnings: Hydromorphone may be habit-forming and may cause respiratory depression. Because rapid intravenous administration increases the possibility of adverse effects such as hypotension and respiratory depression, it is therefore recommended that the injection be given very slowly. Should be used in the first trimester of pregnancy only when the expected benefits outweigh the potential risks.

Precautions: The usual precautions governing opiate analgesics should be observed. Prolonged administration is not recommended.

Adverse Reactions: Nausea, vomiting, dizziness, somnolence, anorexia and constipation, rarely drowsiness. Overdosage may cause respiratory depression; this occurrence may be antagonized by the use of levallorphan tartrate or nalorphine hydrochloride. Subcutaneous administration may cause pain at the injection site, local tissue irritation, and induration, particularly when repeated in the same area.

Dosage and Administration: *Analgesic: Orally* and *parenterally*, 2 mg every 4 to 6 hours initially, increased if necessary. Severe pain can usually be controlled with 3 to 4 mg every 4 to 6 hours. *Rectally*, 1 suppository at night. For postoperative control of pain, particularly following chest surgery, 1 mg parenterally. *Antitussive:* 1 mg orally, increased if necessary, or 1 teaspoonful of cough syrup every 3 or 4 hours. Children, in proportion to age and weight.

Availability:
Ⓒ DILAUDID®: **(Knoll)**
Injection (as hydrochloride): 1, 2, 3, and 4 mg/ml in ampuls of 1 ml in cartons of 10.
Soluble Powder (for compounding) in vials of 1 gm and bottles of 3.5 gm.
Rectal Suppositories, 3 mg in cartons of 6.
Ⓒ DILAUDID Cough Syrup, 1 mg with 100 mg of guaifenesin/5 ml in bottles of 1 pint. **(Knoll)**
Ⓒ HYDROMORPHONE Injection (as hydrochloride), 1, 2, 3 and 4 mg/ml in fill in 2-ml Tubex® (cartridge-needle unit) in Tamp-R-Tel® (tamper-resistant) packages of 10. **(Wyeth)**

HYDROXOCOBALAMIN

Chemical Name: Cobinamide hydroxide phosphate 3'-ester with 5,6-dimethyl-1α-D-ribofuranosylbenzimidazole inner salt.

Description: Hydroxocobalamin, a form of vitamin B-12, is equivalent to cyanocobalamin in vitamin B-12 activity. It differs from cyanocobalamin, however, in that the cyano group of cyanocobalamin has been replaced by a hydroxyl group. Hydroxocobalamin occurs as dark red crystals or as a crystalline powder soluble in water. Its aqueous solutions are deep red in color and are less stable than those of cyanocobalamin.

Absorption from injection sites, liver uptake, serum levels and urinary excretion have been studied in several subjects with 500 and 1000 mcg of radioactive materials. Data indicate that the injected hydroxocobalamin is absorbed more slowly and is taken up by the liver in larger quantities than cyanocobalamin, and they confirm the findings of higher serum levels and slower urinary excretion.

Indications: Therapeutic uses and dosage for hydroxocobalamin are the same as those for cyanocobalamin.

For indications, dosage, adverse reactions, etc., see monograph on cyanocobalamin.

Availability:
AlphaREDISOL® Injection, 1000 mcg/ml in multiple-dose vials of 10 ml. **(Merck Sharp & Dohme)**
NEO-BETALIN® 12 Injection, 1000 mcg/ml in multiple-dose vials of 10 ml. **(Lilly)**
SYTOBEX-H® Injection, 1000 mcg/ml in multiple-dose vials of 10 ml. **(Parke-Davis)**

HYDROXYAMPHETAMINE HYDROBROMIDE

Chemical Name: *dl-p*-(2-Aminopropyl)phenol hydrobromide.

Description: Hydroxyamphetamine hydrobromide is a sympathomimetic amine which indirectly stimulates alpha- and beta-adrenergic receptors by releasing catecholamines from storage sites. It occurs as a white, crystalline powder freely soluble in water and in alcohol. Topically, it is used as a mydriatic. Its function as a mydriatic is probably due to stimulation of the dilatory muscles of the iris. Following instillation, maximal effect usually occurs within 45 to 60 minutes and usually persists for a few hours, with recovery in about 6 hours.

Indications: As a mydriatic.

Contraindications: Narrow-angle glaucoma, and hypersensitivity or idiosyncrasy to the sympathomimetic amines.

Precautions: Use cautiously in patients with hypertension, hyperthyroidism, and diabetes mellitus. Use of any drug in pregnant patients should be undertaken with due consideration to the potential hazard to the fetus.

Adverse Reactions: Reported were increased intraocular pressure, photophobia and blurring of vision. Pupillary dilatation is a symptom of overdosage. Accidental ingestion may result in a marked rise in blood pressure, palpitation, cardiac arrhythmias, substernal discomfort, headache, increased perspiration, nausea, vomiting and gastrointestinal irritation.

Dosage and Administration: *Topically,* Instill 1 or 2 drops into the conjunctival sac.

Availability:
PAREDRINE® Ophthalmic Solution, 1% with 2% boric acid in dropper bottles of 15 ml. **(Smith Kline & French)**

HYDROXYCHLOROQUINE SULFATE

Chemical Name: 2-[[4-[(7-Chloro-4-quinolyl)amino]-pentyl]ethylamino]ethanol sulfate.

Description: Hydroxychloroquine, a 4-aminoquinoline derivative closely related to amodiaquine and chloroquine, is available commercially for oral administration as the sulfate salt. It occurs as a bitter, white or nearly white, crystalline powder freely soluble in water and practically insoluble in alcohol. The 4-aminoquinolines resemble quinine in that they have a quinoline ring structure, an amino group in the number 4 position of the quinoline nucleus and a chlorine atom in the number 7 position. Substitution with a methyl group at position 3 in the nucleus reduces the antimalarial activity and an additional methyl substitution at position 8 completely eliminates antimalarial efficacy.

The precise mechanism of antimalarial activity of the 4-aminoquinolines has not been determined. It has been postulated, however, that this activity is based on their ability to form complexes with deoxyribonucleic acid. It has been shown that these drugs, like quinine, decrease oxygen uptake of the parasites, but the precise metabolic system involved has not been established.

Indications: Treatment and suppression of acute attacks of malaria due to the Plasmodium organisms such as *P. vivax, P. malariae, P. ovale,* and susceptible strains of *P. falciparum.* It is also indicated for the treatment of discoid and systemic lupus erythematosus, and rheumatoid arthritis.

Contraindications: In the presence of retinal or visual field changes attributable to any 4-aminoquinoline compound; in patients with known hypersensitivity to hydroxychloroquine, and for long-term therapy in children.

Warnings: Before administering this drug, the physician should be thoroughly familiar with the contents of the package literature. Also the physician should be aware that some strains of *P. falciparum* are resistant to hydroxychloroquine. Children are especially sensitive to the 4-aminoquinoline compounds. A number of fatalities have been reported following the accidental ingestion of chloroquine, sometimes in relatively small doses (0.75 or 1 gm in one 3-year old child). Patients should be strongly warned to keep these drugs out of the reach of children. A severe attack of psoriasis may be precipitated in patients with this disease; also patients with porphyria may experience an exacerbation of this condition; therefore, the drug should not be used unless in the judgment of the physician the benefits to the patient outweigh the possible adverse effects. Usage of this drug during pregnancy should be avoided except in the suppression or treatment of malaria when, according to the clinician, the benefit outweighs the possible hazards. For additional details, see monograph on Chloroquine.

Precautions: Antimalarial compounds should be used with caution in conjunction with known hepatotoxic drugs, and in alcoholics or in patients with hepatic disease. Periodic blood cell counts are advised for patients on prolonged therapy. If any severe blood disorder appears which is not attributable to the disease under treatment, discontinuation of the drug should be considered. The drug should be administered with caution to patients with G-6-PD (glucose-6-phosphate dehydrogenase) deficiency.

Adverse Reactions: The following reactions have been reported with one or more of the 4-aminoquinoline compounds and should be borne in mind when hydroxychloroquine sulfate is administered. *CNS reactions:* Irritability; nervousness; emotional changes; nightmares; psychosis; headache; dizziness; vertigo; tinnitus; nystagmus; nerve deafness; convulsions; ataxia. *Neuromuscular reactions:* Extraocular muscle palsies; skeletal muscle weakness; absent or hypoactive deep tendon reflexes. *Ocular reactions:* Ciliary body: Disturbance of accommodation with symptoms of blurred vision. This reaction is dose related and reversible with cessation of therapy. Cornea: Transient edema; punctate to lineal opacities; decreased corneal sensitivity. The corneal changes, with or without accompanying symptoms (blurred vision, halos around lights, photophobia), are fairly common, but reversible. Corneal deposits may appear as early as three weeks following initiation of therapy. The incidence of corneal changes and visual side effects appears to be considerably lower with hydroxychloroquine than with chloroquine. Retina: Macula—edema; atrophy; abnormal pigmentation (mild pigment stippling to a "bull's eye" appearance); loss of foveal reflex; increased macular recovery time following exposure to a bright light (photo-stress test); elevated retinal threshold to red light in macular, paramacular and peripheral retinal areas. Other fundus changes—optic disc pallor and atrophy; attenuation of retinal arterioles; fine granular pigmentary disturbances in the peripheral retina; prominent choroidal patterns in advance stage. Visual field defects: Pericentral or paracentral scotoma; central scotoma with decreased visual acuity; rarely, field constriction. The most common visual symptoms attributed to the retinopathy are: reading and seeing difficulties (words, letters, or parts of objects missing); photophobia; blurred distance vision; missing or blacked out areas in the central or peripheral visual field; light flashes and streaks. Retinopathy appears to be dose-related and has occurred within several months (rarely) to several years of daily therapy; a small number of cases have been reported several years after drug therapy was discontinued. It has not been noted during prolonged use of weekly doses of the 4-aminoquinoline compounds for suppression of malaria. Patients with retinal changes may have visual symptoms or may be asymptomatic (with or without visual field changes). Rarely, scotomatous vision or field defects may occur without obvious retinal change. Retinopathy may progress even after the drug is discontinued. In a number of patients, early retinopathy (macular pigmentation sometimes with central field defects) diminished or regressed completely after therapy was discontinued. Paracentral scotoma to red targets ("premaculopathy") is indicative of early retinal dysfunction which is usually reversible with cessation of therapy. A small number of cases of retinal changes have been reported as occurring in patients who received only hydroxychloroquine. These usually consisted of alteration in retinal pigmentation which was detected on periodic ophthalmologic examination; visual field defects were also present in some instances. A case of delayed retinopathy has been reported with loss of vision starting one year after administration of hydroxychloroquine had been discontinued. *Dermatologic reactions:* Bleaching of hair; alopecia; pruritus; skin and mucosal pigmentation; skin eruptions (urticarial, morbilliform, lichenoid, maculopapular, purpuric, erythema annulare centrifugum and exfoliative dermatitis). *Hematologic reactions:* Aplastic anemia; agranulocytosis; leukopenia; thrombocytopenia (hemolysis in individuals with glucose-6-phosphate dehydrogenase (G-6-PD) deficiency). *Gastrointestinal reactions:* Anorexia; nausea; vomiting; diarrhea; abdominal cramps. *Miscellaneous reactions:* Weight loss; lassitude; exacerbation or precipitation of porphyria; nonlight-sensitive psoriasis.

Toxic symptoms may occur within 30 minutes. These consist of headache, drowsiness, visual disturbances, cardiovascular collapse and convulsions, followed by sudden and early respiratory and cardiac arrest. ECG may reveal atrial standstill, nodal rhythm, prolonged intraventricular conduction time, and progressive bradycardia leading to ventricular fibrillation and/or arrest. Treatment is symptomatic and must be prompt, with immediate evacuation of the stomach by emesis (at home) or gastric lavage until completely emptied. Finely powdered activated charcoal, in a dose not less than 5 times the estimated dose ingested, may inhibit further intestinal absorption if introduced by stomach tube after lavage within 30 minutes. Convulsions, if present, should be controlled before attempting gastric lavage. If due to cerebral stimulation, cautious administration of an ultrashort-acting barbiturate may be tried but, if due to anoxia, corrected by oxygen administration, artificial respiration or, in shock with hypotension, by vasopressor therapy. Because of the importance of supporting respiration, tracheal intubation or tracheostomy, followed by gastric lavage, may also be necessary. Exchange transfusions have been used. A patient who survives the acute phase and is asymptomatic should be closely observed for at least 6 hours. Fluids may be forced. Sufficient ammonium chloride (8 gm. daily in divided doses for adults) may be administered for a few days to acidify the urine and help promote urinary excretion.

Dosage and Administration: *Orally.* Dosages are expressed in terms of the sulfate; 200 mg is equivalent to 155 mg of the base. *Malaria: Treatment of an acute attack*—adults, 800 mg initially, followed by 400 mg in 6 to 8 hours and 400 mg on each of 2 consecutive days (total 2 gm). Alternatively, a single dose of 800 mg may be given. Infants up to 1 year of age, 100 mg followed by 3 doses of 100 mg at intervals of 6 or 8 hours (total 400 mg); children 2 to 5 years of age, 400 mg followed by 200 mg 8 hours later (total 600 mg); children 6 to 10 years, 400 mg followed by 2 doses of 200 mg at intervals of 8 hours (total 800 mg); children 11 to 15 years, 600 mg followed by 200 mg 8 hours later and 200 mg 24 hours later (total 1 gm). *Suppression*—adults, 400 mg taken on exactly the same day each week. In infants and children, the weekly suppressive dosage is 5 mg, calculated as the base/kg of body weight, but should not exceed the adult dose regardless of weight. *Lupus erythematosus:* Initially, 400 mg once or twice daily, continued for several weeks or months depending upon the response of the patient. For prolonged maintenance therapy, 200 to 400 mg daily is frequently adequate. *Rheumatoid arthritis:* Adults, initially 400 to 600 mg daily with meals or milk. Following a good response, dosage is reduced by 50% and continued at a usual maintenance level of 200 to 400 mg with meals or with milk. Adrenal corticosteroids and salicylates may be used conjunctively; however, their dosage may be reduced gradually or eliminated after several weeks' use.

Availability:
PLAQUENIL® Tablets, 200 mg in bottles of 100. **(Winthrop)**

HYDROXYPROGESTERONE CAPROATE

Chemical Name: 17-Hydroxypregn-4-ene-3,20-dione hexanoate.

Description: Hydroxyprogesterone is a potent, esterified derivative of the naturally occurring progestational hormone. Although the free compound, 17-α-hydroxyprogesterone, is weak as a progestational agent, esterification of this steroid with caproic acid has resulted in considerable enhancement of both the duration and the degree of progestational activity. A single intramuscular injection of 125 to 250 mg produces a progestational effect on the estrogen-stimulated human endometrium lasting 7 to 14 days.

Hydroxyprogesterone is a long-acting, progestational steroid ester which transforms proliferative endothelium into secretory endothelium, induces mammary gland duct development, and inhibits the production and/or release of gonadotropic hormone; it also shows slight estrogenic, androgenic, or corticoid effects as well, but should not be relied upon for these effects.

Indications: In nonpregnant women, hydroxyprogesterone is indicated for the treatment of advanced adenocarcinoma of the uterine corpus (Stage III or IV), in the management of amenorrhea (primary and secondary) and abnormal uterine bleeding due to hormonal imbalance in the absence of organic pathology, such as submucous fibroids or uterine cancer. It is also indicated for use as a test for endogenous estrogen production, and for the production of secretory endometrium and desquamation.

Contraindications: Hydroxyprogesterone caproate is contraindicated in patients with markedly impaired liver function, carcinoma of the breast, undiagnosed abnormal genital bleeding, missed abortion, and in those with a history of hypersensitivity to the drug. Dosage regimens requiring estrogens are contraindicated in women with a known or suspected genital malignancy, and in patients with thrombophlebitis, thromboembolic disorders, cerebral apoplexy, or a past history of these conditions.

Warnings: The medication should be discontinued pending examination if there is a sudden partial or complete loss of vision, or if there is a sudden onset of proptosis, diplopia, or migraine. Therapy should be terminated if examination reveals papilledema or retinal vascular lesions. Detectable amounts of progestins have been identified in the milk of mothers receiving the drug. The effect of this on the nursing infant has not been determined. Masculinization of the female fetus has occurred when progestins have been used in pregnant women. The physician should observe for the earliest manifestations of thrombotic disorders (thrombophlebitis, cerebrovascular disorders, pulmonary embolism, and retinal thrombosis). If these occur or are suspected the drug should be discontinued immediately.

Precautions: Like other progestogens, hydroxyprogesterone caproate may inhibit production and/or release of gonadotropic hormones, particularly the luteinizing and luteotropic hormones; this action should be considered in the management of sexually-mature women, with regular normal menses, during the first part of the ovarian cycle. Hydroxyprogesterone caproate should be administered with caution to those patients in whom periodic attacks of asthma, migraine, epilepsy, or cardiac or renal dysfunction, are known to be exacerbated by progesterone. The pretreatment physical examination should include examination of the breasts and pelvic organs, and a Papanicolaou smear. In relation to irregular bleeding which does not respond predictably to the hormone therapy, nonfunctional causes should be borne in mind and adequate diagnostic measures instituted. Some compounds with progestational activity may induce fluid retention. Any influence of prolonged sex hormone medication on pituitary, ovarian, adrenal, hepatic or uterine function awaits further study. The pathologist should be advised of progestogen therapy when relevant specimens are submitted. Patients who have a history of psychic depression should be carefully observed and the drug discontinued if the depression recurs to a serious degree. Laboratory test results, particularly of hepatic and endocrine functions, may be affected by progesterone and/or estrogen therapy. Tests to evaluate endocrine and liver function should not be considered definitive unless therapy has been discontinued for at least 60 days.

Adverse Reactions: The following information is pertinent whenever progesterone preparations are used with estrogens; it is not known at the present time if these reactions are applicable to progesterones alone—a statisticallly significant association has been demonstrated between the use of estrogen-progesterone combinations and the occurrence of thrombophlebitis, pulmonary embolism, and cerebrovascular accidents. Also, available evidence is suggestive of an association between the use of progesterones with estrogens and the following untoward effects: neuroocular lesions (e.g., retinal thrombosis and optic neuritis); nausea; vomiting; anorexia; gastrointestinal symptoms (such as abdominal cramps or bloating); edema; breakthrough bleeding, spotting, or withdrawal bleeding; breast tenderness and enlargement; changes in body weight (increase or decrease); headache; increase in cervical mucus; allergic rash; sterile abscess; pain at the injection site; post-injection flare; reactivation of endometriosis; aggravation of migraine headaches; and hepatic cutaneous porphyria becoming manifest. The following adverse reactions are known to occur in patients receiving both progesterones and estrogens: chloasma or melasma, cholestatic jaundice, rise in blood pressure in susceptible individuals, mental depression, and amenorrhea during or after treatment; posttreatment anovulation, cystitis-like syndrome, hirsutism, loss of scalp hair, erythema nodosum, hemorrhagic eruption, premenstrual-like syndrome, changes in libido, changes in appetite, nervousness, dizziness, fatigue, backache, erythema multiforme, itching, and hypomenorrhea, oligomenorrhea, or amenorrhea. The following laboratory tests may give altered results by the concomitant use of progesterones and estrogens: hepatic function (increased sulfobromophthalein retention and other tests); coagulation tests (increase in prothrombin and Factors VII, VIII, IX, and X); metyrapone test; pregnanediol determination; and thyroid function tests (increase in PBI and butanol extractable protein-bound iodine, decrease in T^3 uptake values, and possible diminution in lactation when given immediately postpartum). Female fetal masculinization has been observed in patients who received hydroxyprogesterone caproate. A few instances of coughing, dyspnea, constriction of the chest, and/or allergic-like reactions have occurred following therapy with this drug; the likelihood of these occurring may be increased at higher dosage levels.

Dosage and Administration: *Intramuscularly, deep into the gluteal muscle.* For amenorrhea and abnormal uterine bleeding due to hormonal imbalance in the absence of organic pathology, initially, 375 mg of hydroxyprogesterone is administered at any time. After 4 days of desquamation, or, if there is no bleeding, 21 days after the injection, start cyclic therapy.* Repeat cyclic therapy every 4 weeks for 4 cycles only. For the production of secretory endometrium and desquamation in patients not receiving estrogen therapy, start cyclic therapy* at any time. Repeat cyclic therapy every 4 weeks until no longer required. Patients currently receiving estrogen therapy, initially, 375 mg of hydroxyprogesterone is administered at any time. After 4 days of desquamation, or if there is no bleeding, 21 days after the injection, start cyclic therapy*. Repeat cyclic therapy every 4 weeks until no longer required. For adenocarcinoma of uterine corpus in the advanced stage (Stage III or IV), initially, 1 gm or more of hydroxyprogesterone, 1 or more times each week (usually 1 to 7 gm/week). Treatment should be discontinued if relapse occurs, or, if after 12 weeks of therapy, there is no objective response. The drug should not be used in the early stages (Stage I or II) in place of established anticancer therapy. Test for endogenous estrogen production ("Medical D and C"), inject 250 mg of hydroxyprogesterone at any time. Bleeding in 7 to 14 days indicates endogenous estrogen. The test may be confirmed by a second injection after a 4-week interval.

**Cyclic therapy is a 28-day cycle repeated every 4 weeks. The schedule involves the administration of 20 mg of estradiol valerate on day 1 of each cycle; 2 weeks after day 1, 250 mg of hydroxyprogesterone caproate and 5 mg of estradiol valerate are administered; 4 weeks after day 1 is day 1 of the next cycle.*

Availability:

Hydroxyprogesterone Caproate

Injection, 125 mg/ml in vials of 10 ml; 250 mg/ml in vials of 5 ml. **(Various Mfrs.)**

DELALUTIN® Injection, 125 mg/ml (in sesame oil) in vials of 2 and 10 ml; 250 mg/ml (in castor oil) in vials of 5 ml and in 1-ml Unimatic® (disposable syringes) with needle. **(Squibb)**

HYLUTIN® Injection, 250 mg/ml in vials of 5 ml. **(Key Pharm.)**

HYDROXYUREA

Description: Hydroxyurea is an oral antineoplastic agent, and occurs as a tasteless, white crystalline powder, freely soluble in water and in hot alcohol.

The precise mechanism of action of hydroxyurea is unknown but it appears to exert a cytotoxic effect on tissues with high rates of cellular proliferation. Studies in mouse tumors indicate that the drug inhibits the incorporation of thymidine into DNA. In common with other anti-neoplastic agents, hydroxyurea is teratogenic in animals.

Three mechanisms of action have been postulated for the increased effectiveness of concomitant use of hydroxyurea therapy with irradiation on squamous cell (epidermoid) carcinomas of the head and neck. In vitro studies utilizing Chinese hamster cells suggest that hydroxyurea (1) is lethal to normally radioresistant S-stage cells, and (2) holds other cells of the cell cycle in the G1 or pre-DNA synthesis stage where they are most susceptible to the effects of irradiation. The third mechanism of action has been theorized on the basis of in vitro studies of HeLa cells: it appears that hydroxyurea, by inhibition of DNA synthesis, hinders the normal repair process of cells damaged but not killed by irradiation, thereby decreasing their survival rate; RNA and protein synthesis have shown no alteration.

It is readily absorbed from the gastrointestinal tract. Following oral administration, peak serum concentration is attained within 2 hours, and within 24 hours, the drug is essentially undetectable in the plasma. Over 1/2 of the drug is excrèted in the urine unchanged.

Indications: Treatment of melanoma, resistant chronic myelocytic leukemia, and recurrent, metastatic or inoperable carcinoma of the ovary. Hydroxyurea when used concomitantly with irradiation therapy is intended for use in the local control of primary squamous cell (epidermoid) carcinomas of the head and neck, excluding the lip.

Contraindications: In patients with marked bone marrow depression manifested by acute leukemia, thrombocytopenia or severe anemia.

Warnings: Extreme caution should be exercised to avoid bone marrow depression which may result in leukopenia and eventually thrombocytopenia and bleeding. Severe anemia must be corrected with whole blood replacement before initiating therapy. Since hydroxyurea is excreted primarily by the kidney, it should be used with caution in patients with marked renal dysfunction. Because of the potential mutagenic and teratogenic effects due to the drug's influence on DNA synthesis, use in pregnant women or in women of childbearing age should be undertaken with due consideration to the possible harmful effect to the infant.

Precautions: The drug should be administered only under close medical supervision. The complete status of the blood, including bone marrow examination, as well as kidney and liver function, should be evaluated prior to, and repeatedly, during treatment. Determination of the hemoglobin level, total leukocyte and platelet counts should be made at least once a week throughout the course of therapy. Cautious use of hydroxyurea in patients who have recently received radiation therapy or chemotherapy with other cytotoxic drugs is recommended. Elderly or debilitated patients may require a lower dosage regimen.

Adverse Reactions: Primarily, bone marrow depression (anemia and leukopenia) and abnormal hemopoiesis; less frequently, gastrointestinal disturbances and dermatologic reactions; occasionally, impairment of renal tubular function and, rarely, alopecia and neurologic disturbances. The adverse reactions observed with combined hydroxyurea and irradiation therapy are similar to those reported with the use of hydroxyurea alone. It should be borne in mind that therapeutic doses of irradiation alone produce the same adverse reactions as hydroxyurea; therefore, combined therapy may cause an increase in the incidence and severity of these side effects. Severe mucositis has also been observed.

Dosage and Administration: *Orally.* Dosage should be based on the patient's actual or ideal weight, whichever is less. The recommended dosage regimen, for the treatment of solid tumors, is 80 mg/kg of body weight as a single dose every third day or 20 to 30 mg/kg of body weight as a single daily dose. Dosage for children has not been established. *For carcinoma of the head and neck,* a dose of 80 mg/kg orally administered as a single dose every third day. Therapy with hyroxyurea should be initiated at least 7 days before starting irradiation therapy and should be continued during radiotherapy as well as indefinitely afterwards provided that the patient is kept under adequate observation and there is no evidence of severe reactions. Irradiation should be given at the maximal dose that is considered appropriate for the particular therapeutic situation. *For resistant chronic myelocytic leukemia,* until the intermittent therapy regimen has been evaluated, continuous therapy is recommended (see above). An adequate trial period for determining effectiveness is 6 weeks.

Availability:
HYDREA® Capsules, 500 mg in bottles of 100. **(Squibb)**

HYDROXYZINE

Chemical Name: 1-(*p*-Chloro-α-phenylbenzyl)-4-(2-hydroxyethoxyethyl)piperazine.

Description: Hydroxyzine is a tranquilizing agent pharmacologically related to the antihistamines, and chemically unrelated to phenothiazine, reserpine and meprobamate. Structurally it differs from the antihistamine, chlorcyclizine, in that it has a hydroxyethoxyethyl chain on the piperazine ring instead of a methyl group. Hydroxyzine *hydrochloride* occurs as a bitter, white powder very soluble in water and freely soluble in alcohol. Following oral administration, the *pamoate* salt is thought to be converted to the hydrochloride by gastric hydrochloric acid and its effects are manifested usually within 15 to 30 minutes.

It induces a calming effect in anxious, tense, psychoneurotic adults and also in anxious, hyperkinetic children without impairing mental acuity. It does not depress the cerebral cortex, but its action may be due to suppression of activity in certain key regions of the subcortical area of the CNS. Its antihistaminic and antiemetic effects have been demonstrated experimentally and confirmed clinically. It does not increase gastric secretion or acidity; in most cases, it provides mild antisecretory benefits.

Hydroxyzine has been shown experimentally to possess antispasmodic properties, apparently mediated through interference with the mechanism that responds to spasmogenic agents such as serotonin, acetylcholine, and histamine. Primary skeletal muscle relaxation has been demonstrated experimentally; and secondary skeletal muscle relaxation due to ataraxia should be regarded as additive to this primary effect.

When high clinical doses of hydroxyzine were administered to the pregnant mouse, rat, and rabbit, fetal abnormalities were encountered. Data on clinical studies are insufficient to establish safe use of the drug during early pregnancy.

Indications: Management of anxiety, tension, and psychomotor agitation in conditions of emotional stress. It renders the disturbed patient more amenable to psychotherapy in the long-term treatment of the psychoneurotic and the psychotic, although hydroxyzine should not be used as the sole treatment of psychosis or of clearly demonstrated cases of depression. It has also been found useful in alleviating anxiety and tension in patients undergoing minor surgical procedures; in those with organic disturbances (digestive disorders, dermatosis, senility, the menopausal syndrome, and behavior problems in children); in controlling nausea and vomiting associated with gastritis, gastroenteritis and enteritis; upper respiratory tract infections, influenza and pneumonia; and miscellaneous diseases such as Ménière's syndrome, migraine and vestibulitis; and in patients with cardiac disorders. The drug has not been found to interfere with the action of digitalis and may therefore be used concurrently with it. In addition, it has been recommended as adjunctive therapy in allergic conditions complicated by anxiety and tension as in asthma, chronic urticaria and pruritus. Parenterally, the drug is indicated in the acutely disturbed or hysterical patient; the acute or chronic alcoholic with anxiety withdrawal symptoms or delirium tremens; as preoperative and postoperative and pre- and postpartum adjunctive medication to permit reduction of narcotic dosage, allay anxiety and control emesis.

Contraindications: Hypersensitivity to the drug; during early pregnancy until clinical evidence indicates its safety has been established.

Warnings: The parenteral solution is intended *only* for intramuscular administration; *it should not,* under any circumstances, be injected subcutaneously, intraarterially or intravenously. The preferred site for adults is the upper outer quadrant or the mid-lateral thigh; for children, the mid-lateral thigh, and for infants and small children, the periphery of the upper outer quadrant of the gluteal region. Inadvertent subcutaneous injection may result in significant tissue damage.

Precautions: Patients should be cautioned that in the event of drowsiness, they should not perform any hazardous operations requiring alertness and motor coordination. **Hydroxyzine may potentiate the action of CNS depressants such as barbiturates or narcotic analgesics; when used concomitantly, their dosage should be reduced by at least 50%.**

Adverse Reactions: Drowsiness, rarely impairment of mental acuity, dry mouth and involuntary motor activity, including rare instances of tremor and convulsions. These reactions usually occur with dosages in excess of those recommended.

Dosage and Administration: *Orally.* Adults, from 25 mg 3 times daily to 100 mg 4 times daily. Children under 6 years of age, 50 mg daily in divided doses; over 6 years of age, 50 to 100 mg daily in divided doses. *Parenteral* dosage varies and may range from 25 to 100 mg every 4 to 6 hours. Children over 12 years of age, 0.5 mg/lb *intramuscularly.*

Availability:

Hydroxyzine Hydrochloride

ATARAX®: **(Roerig)**

Syrup, 10 mg/5 ml in bottles of 1 pint.

Tablets: 10, 25 and 50 mg in bottles of 100 and 500; 100 mg in bottles of 100; 25, 50 and 100 mg in unit-dose packages of 100.

VISTARIL® IM Parenteral Solution, 25 and 50 mg/ml in vials of 10 ml and in 1-ml (Isoject®) disposable syringe with needle; 50 mg/ml in vials of 2 ml and in 2-ml disposable syringe with needle. **(Pfizer)**

Hydroxyzine Pamoate

VISTARIL®: **(Pfizer)**

Capsules: 25, 50 and 100 mg in bottles of 100 and 500 and in unit-dose packages of 100 (10 × 10).

Oral Suspension, 25 mg/5 ml in bottles of 120 ml and 1 pint.

l-HYOSCYAMINE SULFATE

Description: Hyoscyamine, as obtained from *Hyoscyamus niger, Atropa belladonna* or *Datura stramonium,* contains variable and substantial amounts of the *dextro*-isomer as well as the *levo*-isomer. This product is pure *levo*-hyoscyamine from which the *d*-isomer has been removed. As a result, the *levo* form represents an extremely potent, accurately standardized anticholinergic and antispasmodic agent. It is said to be twice as potent as atropine, 4 times as potent as methantheline bromide and 20 times as potent as homatropine methylbromide. Atropine owes its parasympatholytic activity chiefly to its content of *levo*-hyoscyamine.

Indications: Whenever antispasmodic or anticholinergic therapy is required. Recommended in conjunction with diet and antacids, for the management of peptic ulcer. As an aid in the control of gastric hypersecretion, intestinal hypermotility and associated abdominal cramps. May be used in functional intestinal disorders to relieve symptoms such as those seen in mild dysenteries and diverticulitis. Also indicated along with morphine or other narcotics in the symptomatic relief of biliary and renal colic; as a "drying agent" in the relief of symptoms of acute rhinitis; in preanesthesia to control salivation and respiratory tract secretions; in the therapy for parkinsonism to reduce rigidity and tremors and to control associated sialorrhea and hyperhidrosis. May be used to reduce pain and hypersecretion in pancreatitis. May also be used in the therapy for poisoning by anticholinesterase agents.

Contraindications: In glaucoma, prostatic hypertrophy and in some cases of cardiac disease and diabetes mellitus.

Precautions: Discontinue if symptoms of hypersensitivity to any component appear.

Adverse Reactions: Reactions may be due to overdosage and may consist of dry mouth and/or nose, urinary difficulty, blurred vision due to mydriasis, and increase in heart rate with subsequent tachycardia. These discomforts can usually be relieved or avoided by decreasing the dosage.

Dosage and Administration: *Orally.* Adults, 0.125 mg to 0.25 mg (1 or 2 tablets) 3 or 4 times daily as needed. Children, proportionately less according to age. Infants weighing 5 lbs, 0.1 ml (3 drops); 7.5 lbs, 0.125 ml (4 drops); 10 lbs, 0.15 ml (5 drops); 15 lbs, 0.2 ml (6 drops); 20 lbs, 0.25 ml (7 drops). Children 1 to 10 years of age, ½ to 1 ml. The adult dosage is 1 to 2 ml. Dosage to be administered at 4-hour intervals. Timecaps, 1 every 12 hours. *Intramuscularly, intravenously* or *subcutaneously,* 1 or 2 ml as indicated. *With barbiturates:* 1 tablet every 3 or 4 hours. *The recommended dosage should not be exceeded.*

Availability:

l-Hyoscyamine Sulfate

ANASPAZ® Tablets, 0.125 mg in bottles of 100 and 500. **(Ascher)**

LEVSIN®: **(Kremers-Urban)**

Drops, 0.125 mg/ml in bottles of 15 ml with dropper.

Elixir, 0.125 mg/5 ml in bottles of 1 pint.

Injection, 0.25 mg/ml in ampuls of 1 ml and in vials of 10 and 30 ml; 0.5 mg/ml in ampuls of 1 ml.

Tablets, 0.125 mg in bottles of 100 and 500 and in unit-dose packages of 100; 0.25 mg (FORTE) in bottles of 100.

LEVSINEX™ Timecaps™ (capsules), 0.375 mg in bottles of 100. **(Kremers-Urban)**

w/Barbiturates (**Warning:** May be habit-forming)

ANASPAZ-PB® Tablets, 0.125 mg with phenobarbital, 15 mg in bottles of 100, 500 and 1000. **(Ascher)**

LEVAMINE® Tablets, 0.125 mg with butabarbital, 15 mg in bottles of 100 and 500. **(Meyer)**
LEVSIN® w/PHENOBARBITAL: **(Kremers-Urban)**
Drops, 0.125 mg with phenobarbital, 15 mg and alcohol, 5%/ml in bottles of 15 ml with dropper.
Elixir, 0.125 mg with phenobarbital, 15 mg/ml in bottles of 1 pint.
Tablets, 0.125 and 0.25 mg (Forte) with phenobarbital, 15 mg in bottles of 100 and 500.
LEVSINEX™ Timecaps™ (capsules), 0.375 mg with phenobarbital, 45 mg in bottles of 100.
(Kremers-Urban)

IBERET-FOLIC-500

Description: Each tablet contains:

Ferrous sulfate (equiv. to 105 mg elemental iron)*	525 mg
Niacinamide	30 mg
Thiamine mononitrate	6 mg
Riboflavin	6 mg
Pyridoxine hydrochloride	5 mg
Ascorbic acid (as sodium ascorbate)	500 mg
Calcium pantothenate	10 mg
Folic acid	0.8 mg
Cobalamin (vitamin B-12)	25 μg

*In a controlled-release form (Gradumet®).

Indications: Prevention and treatment of iron deficiency anemia and prevention of folate and vitamin B deficiency in pregnant and nonpregnant patients.

Contraindications: Patients with pernicious anemia.

Warnings: Folic acid alone is not recommended in the treatment of pernicious anemia and other megaloblastic anemias in which vitamin B-12 is deficient.

Precautions: Where anemia exists, its nature should be established and the underlying causes determined. Folic acid may mask the presence of pernicious anemia by producing reversion of the blood picture to normal but not affecting progression of neurological manifestations. Accordingly, in older patients and those with conditions tending to lead to vitamin B-12 depletion, serum B-12 levels should be regularly assessed during therapy with this product. Concomitant parenteral therapy with vitamin B-12 may be necessary in patients with a deficiency of vitamin B-12. Signs of serious toxicity may be delayed because the iron is in a long-release form. Overdosage may be manifested by increased capillary permeability, reduced plasma volume, increased cardiac output, and sudden cardiovascular collapse. In overdosage, efforts should be made to hasten the elimination of the Gradumet tablets ingested. Treatment involves the use of an emetic followed by gastric lavage if required. Immediately following emesis, a large dose of a saline cathartic should be given to induce active removal of the product from the intestinal tract. This drug should be kept out of reach of children to guard against accidental iron poisoning.

Adverse Reactions: To avoid gastric intolerance (rare), the tablet should be taken after a meal. Allergic sensitization has been reported following both oral and parenteral administration of folic acid.

Dosage and Administration: *Orally.* For treatment and prevention of iron and folate deficiencies, the recommended dosage is 1 tablet daily. May be taken on an empty stomach.

Availability:
IBERET-FOLIC-500® Filmtab® Tablets (red-color) in bottles of 60. **(Abbott)**

IBUPROFEN

Chemical Name: 2-(4-Isobutylphenyl) propionic acid.

Description: Ibuprofen is a synthetic, nonsteroidal drug with antiinflammatory, analgesic and antipyretic properties. It occurs as a white powder that is very slightly soluble in water (less than 1 mg/ml) and is readily soluble in alcohol and in acetone.

Its mode of action, like that of other nonsteroidal antiinflammatory agents, is not known; however, its therapeutic action is not due to pituitary-adrenal stimulation. Clinical studies in rheumatoid arthritis and osteoarthritis have shown that the drug is similar in effectiveness to aspirin, but that ibuprofen was generally found to cause gastrointestinal symptoms in fewer patients. It relieves pain and stiffness, reduces swelling and tenderness, but does not alter the progressive course of the underlying pathology.

It is rapidly absorbed when administered orally, and reaches peak plasma levels in approximately 1 to 2 hours. It is excreted primarily in the urine as unaltered drug and as inactive oxidative metabolites; excretion is virtually complete 24 hours after the last dose. Its half-life has been found to be 2 hours. In preliminary studies, an assay capable of detecting 1 mcg/ml did not show the drug to be present in the milk of lactating women.

Indications: Symptomatic treatment of rheumatoid arthritis and osteoarthritis.

Contraindications: Prior sensitivity reactions to ibuprofen, and in patients with nasal polyps, and angioedema, or in those with a history of aspirin-induced bronchospasm.

Warnings: Gastrointestinal disturbances have been observed in about 15% of the patients. These effects may be reduced by either lowering the dose or by giving the drug with food or milk. Antacids may be tried but there is no adequate evidence that they will control symptoms in these cases. Patients with rheumatoid arthritis complicated by an active peptic ulcer should be treated with an nonulcerogenic drug such as gold. However, if ibuprofen must be given, the patient should be under constant supervision for signs of ulcer perforation or gastrointestinal bleeding. Animal reproduction studies conducted at doses up to ²/₃ that of the maximal clinical dose did not yield evidence of developmental abnormalities, but its effects on labor and parturition are inconclusive. The drug has been shown to inhibit prostaglandin synthesis and release. This effect has been demonstrated by other nonsteroidal antiinflammatory agents and has been associated with an increased incidence of dystocia and delayed parturition when such drugs were administered late in pregnancy. Until clinical data are available to ascertain its safe use during pregnancy, it is not recommended for use in pregnant patients. Also, the use of ibuprofen in children 14 years of age and under should be deferred until safe and effective use has been established.

Precautions: Patients should be instructed to report to their physician any unfavorable gastrointestinal, ocular or dermatological reactions (i.e., gastric irritation, blurred vision, skin rash, etc.). Special attention is advised when this drug is given to patients taking coumarin-type anticoagulant drugs and to those with a history of cardiac decompensation. Ibuprofen has been found to inhibit platelet aggregation, but to a lesser degree than does aspirin or indomethacin. A slight decrease in hemoglobin and hematocrit values was also observed in some patients.

Adverse Reactions: Gastrointestinal reactions (abdominal distress, cramps or pain, indigestion, epigastric pain, heartburn, bloating, flatulence, feeling of fullness, nausea, vomiting, constipation, and diarrhea) were the most frequently noted. A few cases of ulceration, some complicated by bleeding or perforation, have occurred and the clinician should bear in mind that these harmful effects can subsequently lead to a fatal outcome. Other reactions included skin rashes (usually maculopapular and vesiculobullous eruptions, urticaria and erythema multiforme); some patients complained of pruritus but without rash. A few instances of drug-induced toxic ambylopia characterized by reduced visual acuity and difficulty in color discrimination have been reported; therefore, patients who experience any visual disturbances during therapy should report for a complete ophthalmologic examination. One small controlled study demonstrated a slight but statistically significant drug-associated rise in the Ivy bleeding time; the clinical importance of this finding is unknown. Dizziness; fluid retention and edema which may further compromise patients with cardiac decompensation; leukopenia and a mild decrease in hemoglobin and hematocrit have also been noted.

Dosage and Administration: *Orally.* The smallest dose that will yield satisfactory control should be employed. The suggested dosage is 300 to 400 mg 3 or 4 times daily; up to, but not exceeding, 2.4 gm daily may be given. A therapeutic response may be seen in a few days to a week but is most frequently observed in 2 weeks. After a satisfactory response has been achieved, the patient's dose should be reviewed and adjusted accordingly.

Availability:
MOTRIN® Tablets, 300 and 400 mg in bottles of 60 and 500; the 400 mg tablets are also available in unit-dose packages of 100 and in single-unit bottles of 120. **(Upjohn)**

IDOXURIDINE

Chemical Name: 2′-Deoxy-5-iodouridine.

Description: Idoxuridine is a topical antiviral agent used in the treatment of dendritic keratitis. Structurally, it differs from thymidine in that an iodine atom replaces a methyl group of the latter compound. Idoxuridine occurs as a white, crystalline powder slightly soluble in water and in alcohol.

Because of its close structural similarity to thymidine, it is assumed that idoxuridine competitively inhibits uptake of thymidine in viral deoxyribonucleic acid synthesis and/or is itself incorporated into a fraudulent DNA. There is also some evidence that it may act through inhibition of DNA-polymerase, an enzyme required for production of viral DNA. The drug has no effect on ribonucleic acid viruses; however, it has been reported to inhibit bacteria and growth of animal tumors, and it has been employed experimentally in the treatment of human cancers. Additionally, idoxuridine blocks the ability of the herpes simplex virus to infect and reproduce; once the virus is rendered inactive, normal healing processes are allowed to take place; however, it will have no effect on the accumulated scarring, vascularization, or on the resultant progressive loss of vision.

Indications: Treatment of herpes simplex keratitis. Superficial herpes simplex infections respond more favorably than do chronic, deep infections, or those with stromal involvement.

Contraindications: Hypersensitivity to any of the components. Boric acid should not be administered during course of therapy with this drug.

Warnings: Cautious use is advised when administering idoxuridine to pregnant women or to those of childbearing potential.

Precautions: Although corticosteroids may be of benefit in severe infections, they should be used only with caution and the patient observed closely because of the risk of accelerating spread of infections. If there is no response in epithelial infections after 7 or 8 days of treatment, other forms of therapy should be considered. The recommended frequency and duration of administration should not be exceeded. Idoxuridine is not effective in the treatment of corneal inflammation following herpes simplex keratitis in which the virus is not present. To insure that the stability of the preparation is maintained, the ophthalmic solution should not be mixed with other medications.

Adverse Reactions: Irritation, pain, pruritus, inflammation or edema may occur in the eyes or lids. Allergic reactions, although rare, have been reported. Photophobia, occasional appearance of corneal clouding, stippling, and small punctate defects in the corneal epithelium have been observed. However, the punctate defects may be a manifestation of the infection rather than drug-induced since healing usually takes place without interruption of therapy.

Dosage and Administration: *Solution:* Initially, 1 drop in infected eye every hour during the day and every 2 hours at night. Continue this dosage until definite improvement has taken place, as evidenced by loss of staining with fluorescein; then apply 1 drop every 2 hours during the day and every 4 hours at night. Therapy should be continued for 3 to 5 days after disappearance of the lesion. *Ointment:* Apply inside the conjunctival sac of the infected eye 5 times daily, every 4 hours during waking hours and the last application at bedtime. The dosage schedule should not be interrupted. A favorable response is usually evident within 7 to 8 days. If the patient continues to improve, therapy may be continued for up to 21 days. Concomitant use with topical corticosteroids may be employed in the management of herpes simplex with stromal lesions, corneal edema, or iritis. It is important that therapy with idoxuridine be continued for a few days after withdrawal of the steroid.

Availability:
DENDRID® Ophthalmic Solution, 1 mg/ml in dropper bottles of 15 ml. **(Alcon)**
HERPLEX® Ophthalmic Solution, 1 mg/ml in dropper bottles of 15 ml. **(Allergan)**
STOXIL®: **(Smith Kline & French)**
Ophthalmic Ointment, 5 mg/gm in tubes of 4 gm.
Ophthalmic Solution, 1 mg/ml in bottles of 15 ml with dropper. *(Store in refrigerator).*

IMIPRAMINE HYDROCHLORIDE

Chemical Name: 5-(3-Dimethylaminopropyl)-10,11-dihydro-5*H*-dibenz[b,f] azepine monohydrochloride.

Description: Imipramine hydrochloride, a tricyclic antidepressant, is a member of the dibenzazepine group of compounds. It occurs as a white, crystalline substance that turns yellowish or reddish on long exposure to light. It is easily soluble in water, fairly soluble in alcohol and acetone, but is almost insoluble in ether. It differs in structure from promazine by the substitution of ethylene for S binding the two benzene groups.

The manner in which imipramine exerts its antidepressant action is not clear; however, it does not appear to act primarily by stimulating the CNS. The clinical effect is hypothesized as being due to potentiation of adrenergic synapses by blocking the re-uptake of norepinephrine and 5-hydroxytryptamine at the nerve endings. The mode of action of the drug in controlling childhood enuresis is thought to be separate from its antidepressant effect. The effectiveness of treatment may decrease with continued administration.

Following oral administration, imipramine is well absorbed from the gastrointestinal tract. Plasma levels are measurable for only ½ hour in patients who have been given an intramuscular injection of 100 mg, with levels falling below 0.2 mg% a few minutes after administration. About 3% is found in the urine in the form of iminodibenzyl derivatives, some unchanged imipramine, a metabolite and a conjugate.

Independent laboratory studies in 3 species of animals (rat, mouse and rabbit) revealed that when the drug is administered orally in doses up to approximately 2½ times the maximum clinical dose in the rat and mouse and up to 25 times the maximum clinical dose in the rabbit, the drug appears to be essentially free from teratogenic potential. In the 3 species studied, 1 instance (in the rabbit) of fetal abnormality occurred. However, in other studies in rats, systemic and embryotoxic effects were manifested by reduced litter size, slight increase in the rate of stillborn fetuses and reduction in the mean birth weight. Subcutaneous administration of the drug exhibits a slight but definite teratogenic potential manifested, in the rabbit, by higher resorption rates and decrease in mean fetal birth weight; teratogenic findings were noted when the dose was 5 times the maximum clinical dose. In the mouse, teratogenic effects occurred at 1½ and 6½ times the maximum clinical dose, but were not apparent at levels 3 times the maximum clinical dose.

Indications: Relief of symptoms of depression. Endogenous depression is more likely to be alleviated than other depressive states. Also indicated, as temporary adjunctive therapy, in the symptomatic treatment of enuresis in children 6 years of age and older.

Contraindications: Should not be administered concurrently, or for at least 2 weeks after discontinuing the use of an MAO inhibitor, in order to avoid initiating a hyperpyretic crisis or severe convulsive seizures which can be serious, or fatal. The drug is contraindicated during the acute recovery period after a myocardial infarction; also in patients with a known hypersensitivity to imipramine. The possibility of cross-sensitivity to other dibenzazepine compounds should be considered.

Warnings: Pregnant patients, nursing mothers or women of childbearing potential should receive this drug *only* when the potential benefits outweigh the possible hazards to the mother and child. Extreme caution should be exercised when imipramine is used in patients with cardiovascular disease (elderly patients are at special risk of developing cardiotoxic reactions), increased intraocular pressure, a history of narrow-angle glaucoma, or a history of urinary retention. It should be given cautiously to hyperthyroid patients or to those on thyroid medication, to patients with significantly impaired renal or hepatic function or with a history of seizure disorders, and to those receiving guanethidine or similar agents. Patients should be cautioned that their ability to perform tasks requiring alertness or skill may be impaired. **Important Note:** The daily dose for children should not exceed 2.5 mg/kg of body weight, since larger doses have been found to cause ECG changes in pediatric patients. The drug is not recommended for use in children under 6 years of age.

Precautions: Extreme caution is necessary when imipramine is given to seriously depressed patients in whom the possibility of suicide is a major problem. The administration of a tranquilizer with low dosages of imipramine may be required to control hypomanic excitement or psychotic manifestations. The drug should be discontinued as soon as possible prior to surgical procedure. Concurrent administration with anticholinergics, sympathomimetics or with alcohol, or to patients receiving electroconvulsive treatments may result in exaggerated or toxic responses. Imipramine has been noted to alter (lower or raise) blood sugar levels.

Adverse Reactions: The following reactions reported when tricyclic antidepressant drugs were given should be considered when imipramine is administered. These include: *Cardiovascular:* Orthostatic hypotension, hypertension, tachycardia, palpitation, myocardial infarction, arrhythmias, heart block, ECG changes, congestive heart failure, stroke. *Psychiatric:* Confusional states (especially in the elderly) with hallucinations, disorientation, delusions; anxiety, restlessness, agitation; insomnia and nightmares; hypomania; exacerbation of psychosis. *Neurological:* Numbness, tingling, paresthesias of extremities, incoordination, ataxia, tremors; peripheral neuropathy; extrapyramidal symptoms; seizures, alterations in EEG patterns; tinnitus. *Anticholinergic:* Dry mouth, and, rarely, associated sublingual adenitis; blurred vision, disturbances of accommodation, mydriasis; constipation, paralytic ileus; urinary retention, delayed micturition, dilation of the urinary tract. *Allergic:* Skin rash, petechiae, urticaria, itching, photosensitization (avoid excessive exposure to sunlight); edema (general or of face and tongue), drug fever, cross-sensitivity with desipramine. *Hematologic:* Bone marrow depression including agranulocytosis; eosinophilia; purpura; thrombocytopenia. Leukocyte and differential counts should be performed in any patient who develops fever and sore throat during therapy; the drug should be discontinued if there is evidence of pathological neutrophil depression. *Gastrointestinal:* Nausea and vomiting, anorexia, epigastric distress, diarrhea, peculiar taste, stomatitis, abdominal cramps, black tongue. *Endocrine:* Gynecomastia in the male; breast enlargement and galactorrhea in the female; increased or decreased libido, impotence; testicular swelling; elevation or depression of blood sugar levels. *Other:* Jaundice (simulating obstructive); altered liver function; weight gain or loss; perspiration; flushing; urinary frequency; drowsiness, dizziness, weakness and fatigue; headache, parotid swelling, alopecia, proneness to falls. *Withdrawal Symptoms:* Though not indicative of addiction, abrupt cessation of treatment after prolonged therapy may produce nausea, headache and malaise. **Note:** The most common adverse reactions noted in enuretic children are nervousness, sleep disorders, tiredness, and mild gastrointestinal disorders. These usually disappear during continued use of the drug or when the dosage is decreased. Other complications may include constipation, convulsions, anxiety, emotional instability, syncope, and collapse. All of the other reactions reported herein should be considered.

Symptoms of overdosage are manifested by drowsiness, stupor, tachycardia, ataxia, vomiting, respiratory depression, cyanosis, hypotension, shock and/or coma, restlessness, agitation, hyperpyrexia, severe perspiration, hyperactive reflexes, muscle rigidity, athetoid and choreiform movements, convulsions, mydriasis, cardiac arrhythmia, ECG evidence of impaired conduction and signs of congestive heart failure. Since there is no specific antidote, the usual supportive measures (gastric lavage, sedatives, oxygen, etc.) should be initiated and maintained until a favorable clinical response is established.

Dosage and Administration: *Orally. For depression:* Usual adult dose *for hospitalized patients:* initially, 100 mg daily in divided doses, then gradually increased to 200 mg daily as required. If the desired response is not observed after 2 weeks, the dose may be increased to 250 or 300 mg daily. *For outpatients:* initially, 75 mg daily increased to 150 mg daily. Dosages exceeding 200 mg are generally not recommended for outpatients. Maintenance therapy: 50 to 150 mg daily is advised. *Adolescent and geriatric patients:* initially, 30 to 40 mg daily; it is generally not necessary to exceed 100 mg daily. *Intramuscularly.* Initially, up to 100 mg daily in divided doses. From 1 to 3 weeks may pass before the optimal therapeutic effects of the drug are evident. *For enuresis:* Initially, 25 mg daily 1 hour before bedtime. If a satisfactory response does not occur within 1 week, the dose should be increased to 50 mg nightly for children under 12 years of age and up to 75 mg for those 12 years of age or older. A daily dose greater than 75 mg does not enhance efficacy and tends to increase undesirable effects. Evidence suggests that when enuresis occurs during early night, the drug is more effective when given earlier in the day and in divided doses, such as 25 mg in midafternoon and 25 mg at night. Dosage should be gradually tapered off as this may reduce the tendency to relapse. Children who relapse when the drug is discontinued do not always respond to a subsequent course of treatment.

Availability:
ANTIPRESS Tablets, 25 mg in bottles of 100 and 500. **(Lemmon)**
IMAVATE® Tablets, 10 mg in bottles of 100; 25 and 50 mg in bottles of 100 and 1000. **(Robins)**
IMIPRAMINE HYDROCHLORIDE Tablets, 10, 25 and 50 mg in bottles of 100 and 1000 and in unit-dose packages of 100. **(Lederle)**
IMIPRAMINE HYDROCHLORIDE Tablets, 10, 25 and 50 mg in bottles of 100 and 1000 and in unit-dose packages of 100. **(Philips Roxane)**
JANIMINE® Filmtab® (tablets), 10, 25 and 50 mg in bottles of 100 and 1000. **(Abbott)**
PRESAMINE™ Tablets, 10 mg in bottles of 100 and 1000; 25 and 50 mg in bottles of 100, 1000 and 5000. **(USV)**
SK-PRAMINE™ Tablets, 10 mg in bottles of 100; 25 and 50 mg in bottles of 100 and 1000 and in single-unit packages of 100. **(Smith Kline & French)**
TOFRANIL®: **(Geigy)**
Injection, 12.5 mg/ml in ampuls of 2 ml.
Tablets, 10 mg in bottles of 100 and 1000; 25 and 50 mg in bottles of 100, 1000 and 5000, in Dis-Pak (unit-strip packages) of 100 and 1000 and in Gy-Paks of 100 in units of 6.
TOFRANIL-PM® Capsules, 75, 100, 125 and 150 mg in bottles of 30, 100 and 1000; the 75 and 150 mg capsules are also available in unit-dose packages of 100 and 1000. **(Geigy)**

IMMUNE SERUM GLOBULIN, HUMAN

Description: Immune serum globulin is a sterile solution of globulins that contains many antibodies normally present in adult human blood. It contains not less than 15 and not more than 18 gm of protein/100 ml, not less than 90% of which is globulin. It is prepared by pooling solution extracts of human placentas and processed by a modification of the Cohn alcohol fractionation technique. It is an odorless, transparent or slightly opalescent liquid, varying in color from colorless to dark amber. It has a half-life in the body of about 20 days.

It is of particular value, either alone or as an adjuvant, in the prophylaxis and therapy of various infectious diseases, modification of symptoms associated with vaccination with live measles virus, and in the replacement therapy of syndromes of gamma globulin defects.

Indications: In the passive prophylaxis or attenuation of such diseases as measles, poliomyelitis, infectious (epidemic) hepatitis (type A), and in the treatment of dysgammaglobulinemia. Other possible uses are: serum hepatitis, rubella, varicella, and as an adjuvant in refractory infections especially those caused by staphylococci, *Pseudomonas aeruginosa* and Proteus species. In burns, the use of immune globulin in large doses was cited as a valuable adjunct to antibiotic therapy in reducing the incidence of septicemia and possibly deaths.

Precautions: The drug should not be administered intravenously. When injected, every known precaution for the prevention and arrest of untoward reactions should be on hand.

Adverse Reactions: Reactions may be *local* such as pain and tenderness at the injection site, urticaria, angioedema or simple erythema, and *systemic* such as headache, malaise and fever; isosensitization and an anaphylactoid-type reaction may also occur.

Dosage and Administration: *Measles vaccination, modification of symptoms,* 0.02 ml/kg of body weight, injected into the deltoid muscle of one arm immediately after the injection of the attenuated live measles virus vaccine into the opposite arm. *Measles prevention,* 0.22 ml/kg of body weight; *modification* 0.04 ml/kg administered intramuscularly within 6 days after exposure. *Poliomyelitis, prevention,* 0.3 ml/kg intramuscularly or subcutaneously; repeated in 5 weeks if danger of infection continues. *Infectious hepatitis, prevention or modification,* adults, 0.09 to 0.13 ml/kg; children, 0.02 to 0.04 ml/kg intramuscularly; repeated at intervals of 6 weeks, if necessary. *Dysgammaglobulinemia, treatment,* 20 to 50 ml intramuscularly or subcutaneously once a month depending on the severity of the disease or the weight of the patient.

Availability:
GAMASTAN® in vials of 2 and 10 ml. **(Cutter)**
GAMMAGEE® in vials of 2 and 10 ml. **(Merck Sharp & Dohme)**
GAMMAR™ in vials of 2 and 10 ml. **(Armour)**
IMMU-G® in vials of 2 and 10 ml. **(Parke-Davis)**
IMMUNE SERUM GLOBULIN, HUMAN in vials of 2 and 10 ml. **(Hyland)**
IMMUNE SERUM GLOBULIN, HUMAN in Tubex® (cartridge-needle unit) of 2 ml and in vials of 10 ml. **(Wyeth)**

INDIGOTINDISULFONATE SODIUM

Chemical Name: Sodium 5,5′-indigotindisulfonate.

Description: Indigotindisulfonate occurs as a dusky, purplish-blue powder, or blue granules having a coppery luster and is sparingly soluble in water and slightly soluble in alcohol.

The dye is rapidly excreted by the kidneys following intravenous or intramuscular injection, normally appearing within 10 minutes and coloring the urine blue. The sensitivity test requires that 0.1 ml of a 1:100 dilution of the dye be injected intradermally. Sensitive patients will show a clear-cut pseudopodia within 15 to 20 minutes, while at 30 minutes, these will have blended into a more general edema without pseudopodia.

Indications: Used chiefly in localizing the ureteral orifices during cystoscopy and ureteral catheterization, and for determining the appearance time and elimination from each ureter; renal excretion test.

Precautions: Patients with a history of allergy should be tested for sensitivity. An occasional unexplained idiosyncrasy may occur, which may be treated with antihistamines, or if need be with adrenalin.

Dosage and Administration: *Intravenously,* 5 ml of an 0.8% aqueous solution, or more of the solution if given *intramuscularly,* since larger quantities are necessary when given by this route; also appearance time and elimination are slower.

Availability:
INDIGO CARMINE Solution, 8 mg/ml in ampuls and disposable units of 5 ml.
(Hynson, Westcott & Dunning)

INDOCYANINE GREEN

Description: Indocyanine green is a water-soluble, tricarbocyanine dye with a peak spectral absorption at 800 to 810 millimicrons, a wave length equally absorbed by oxygenated and reduced hemoglobin, thus permitting the continuous recording of dilution curves in whole blood without interference from variations in blood oxygen saturation.

When injected intravenously, the dye is rapidly and completely bound to plasma protein, of which albumin is the principal carrier. It is quickly removed from the circulation by the liver, where it is stored and secreted entirely into the bile. It has a hepatic storage capacity of 70 mg/100 ml and excretory time of 7.5 mg/min in healthy individuals.

The dye undergoes no significant extrahepatic or enterohepatic circulation. Blood estimations have shown negligible renal, peripheral, lung or cerebrospinal uptake of the dye. It is nonirritating when inadvertently introduced subcutaneously, and has produced no untoward reactions upon single or repeated intravenous injections or infusions.

The ability of the liver to clear indocyanine green from the circulation, an ability that is considerably slowed by liver disease, provides an accurate index to overall liver function.

Due to its absorption spectrum, changing concentration of the dye in the blood can be monitored by ear densitometry or by obtaining blood specimens at timed intervals.

Indications: As an indicator for the measurement of cardiac output and for the assessment of liver function and hepatic blood flow.

Contraindications: Safe use of this preparation during pregnancy has not been established.

Warnings: Because it is unstable in aqueous solution, the dye should be used on the same day on which it is prepared. The dye, however, is stable in plasma and in whole blood, so that samples obtained in discontinuous sampling techniques may be read hours later. All specimens containing the dye should be read at the same temperature since temperature variation alters the optical density. Sterile techniques should be employed in handling the solution as well as in the performance of the dilution curves. It is recommended that the diluent supplied with this product be used to dissolve the dye because there have been reports of incompatibility with some commercially available water for injection. Heparin preparations containing sodium bisulfite reduce the absorption peak of the dye in blood, and therefore, should be avoided.

Precautions: Probenecid in doses of from 25 to 100 mg/kg of body weight has been shown to affect the hepatic storage and removal of indocyanine green in dogs. Although this occurrence has not been reported in clinical use, it should nevertheless be considered.

Adverse Reactions: Indocyanine green contains a small amount of sodium iodide and should be used with caution in patients who have a history of allergy to iodides. Radioactive-iodine uptake studies should not be performed for at least one week following the use of this preparation.

Dosage and Administration: *Intravenously. Determination of cardiac function:* Usual dose used for dilution curves is: Adults, 5 mg; children, 2.5 mg, and infants, 1.25 mg injected in a 1-ml volume. An average of 5 dilution curves are required for diagnostic cardiac catheterization. The total dose of dye injected should be kept below 2 mg/kg of body weight. *Assessment of liver function:* The patient should be studied in a fasting basal state. After weighing the patient, the dosage is calculated on the basis of 0.5 mg/kg of body weight. When the correct amount of dye has been determined, the dye is injected into an arm vein as rapidly as possible, without allowing the dye to escape outside the vein. For detailed information on technique and dosage, consult package literature.

Availability:
CARDIO-GREEN®: **(Hynson, Westcott & Dunning)**
Injection in disposable, calibrated syringes of 10 and 40 mg.
Sterile Powder in vials of 25 and 50 mg with aqueous solvent.

INDOMETHACIN

Chemical Name: 1-(*p*-Chlorobenzoyl)-5-methoxy-2-methylindole-3-acetic acid.

Description: Indomethacin is a synthetic, nonsteroidal antiinflammatory, analgesic and antipyretic agent with a unique chemical structure which differentiates it from salicylates, corticosteroids, phenylbutazone-like compounds and colchicine. It occurs as a white or nearly white, crystalline powder practically insoluble in water and soluble in alcohol, ether and in acetone. Although its precise mode of action is not known, its therapeutic action is not due to pituitary-adrenal stimulation. The analgesic and antinflammatory actions are thought to be the result of inhibition of the production of prostaglandins in various tissues. It affords relief of symptoms, but does not alter the progressive course of the underlying disease. It relieves pain, reduces fever, swelling and tenderness.

Following the oral administration of a single dose, indomethacin appears to be well absorbed from the gastrointestinal tract, reaches peak plasma levels in ½ to 2 hours, and is excreted primarily in the urine almost entirely as indomethacin glucuronide.

Indications: Rheumatoid arthritis, rheumatoid (ankylosing) spondylitis, degenerative joint disease (osteoarthritis) of the hips, knees and shoulders, and gout. During the interval phase of gouty arthritis, indomethacin together with adequate doses of a uricosuric agent may relieve pain and prevent the recurrence of acute attacks.

Contraindications: In patients who are allergic to indomethacin, or who have nasal polyps associated with angioedema or a bronchospastic reaction to aspirin or to other nonsteroidal antiinflammatory agents.

Warnings: Since gastrointestinal reactions, sometimes severe, have been reported, the physician must be continuously alert for any sign or symptom of an impending gastrointestinal complication. See Adverse Reactions. Should such an event occur, the risk of continuing treatment must be weighed against the possible benefits to the patient. These reactions may be reduced by giving the drug immediately after meals, with food, or with antacids. Examinations for ocular changes, such as corneal deposits and retinal disturbances including those of the macula, should be performed periodically. See Adverse Reactions. The drug is not recommended for pregnant or lactating women or for children 14 years of age and under until safe use has been established. The use of indomethacin in conjunction with aspirin or other salicylates is not advised, also combined use with aspirin does not produce a greater therapeutic effect and may increase the incidence of gastrointestinal complications. Moreover, the chronic concurrent administration of 3.6 gm of aspirin daily may reduce the blood levels of indomethacin by approximately 20%.

Precautions: The physician must avoid undue delay in initiating appropriate treatment of an infection, the signs and symptoms of which may be masked by indomethacin. The patient should be observed carefully for unusual signs of sensitivity to the drug. Although it does not influence hypoprothrombinemia produced by anticoagulants, patients on anticoagulant therapy should be followed carefully in order to detect any alterations in their prothrombin time. When given to patients receiving probenecid, the plasma levels of indomethacin are likely to be increased. Indomethacin has been found to reduce the natriuretic and antihypertensive effects of furosemide, which has been attributed to inhibition of prostaglandin synthesis; therefore, patients receiving both drugs should be observed closely for the desired furosemide effect. It also blocks furosemide-induced increase in plasma renin activity, which may affect evaluation of plasma activity in hypertensive patients. The drug cannot be considered a simple analgesic and should not be used in conditions other than those for which it is indicated. Patients should be cautioned that in the event of dizziness, lightheadedness, blurred vision, or feelings of detachment, they should not perform any hazardous operations requiring alertness or motor coordination. It should be used with considerable care in patients with psychiatric disturbances, epilepsy, or parkinsonism, since the drug may, in some instances, aggravate these conditions.

Adverse Reactions: Careful instructions to, and constant observations of the patient are essential in order to prevent serious and irreversible side effects which may in some instances be fatal. *CNS reactions* may include headache, dizziness, lightheadedness, syncope, drowsiness, convulsions, peripheral neuropathy, coma, depression, psychotic episodes, mental confusion, depersonalization. *Gastrointestinal reactions:* nausea, anorexia, vomiting, epigastric distress, abdominal pain, diarrhea, single or multiple ulcerations, (esophagus, stomach, duodenum or small intestine, including perforation and hemorrhage with a few fatalities), bleeding in gastrointestinal tract without obvious ulcer formation, increased abdominal pain in patients with preexisting ulcerative colitis, stomatitis, gastritis, occult bleeding from the sigmoid colon or from a diverticulum, perforation of preexisting sigmoid lesions (diverticulum, carcinoma), development of ulcerative colitis and regional ileitis. *Hepatic reactions:* jaundice and hepatitis. *Cardiovascular-renal reactions:* edema, elevated blood pressure and hematuria. *Dermatologic-hypersensitivity reactions:* pruritus, urticaria, angioneurotic edema, angiitis, skin rashes, and acute respiratory distress including sudden dyspnea and asthma; also a rapid fall in blood pressure resembling a shock-like state. *Hematologic reactions:* leukopenia, purpura, thrombocytopenia, agranulocytosis, bone marrow depression, anemia secondary to obvious or occult gastrointestinal bleeding. *Eye reactions:* corneal deposits and retinal disturbances, including those of the macula, have been reported in some patients with rheumatoid arthritis taking indomethacin for prolonged periods. Similar ocular changes have been observed in some rheumatoid arthritic patients who had *not* been taking indomethacin. Whether or not the ocular changes are attributable to the drug, it is advisable to discontinue therapy if these changes are observed. Since these changes may be asymptomatic, ophthalmologic examination periodically is desirable in those patients taking the drug for extended periods. *Ear reactions:* tinnitus, and hearing disturbance. *Metabolic reactions:* hyperglycemia, glycosuria, edema, weight gain, and flushing or sweating. *Miscellaneous reactions:* epistaxis, or vaginal bleeding.

Dosage and Administration: *Orally.* In chronic disorders, treatment should be started with a dosage of 25 mg 2 or 3 times daily with food, immediately after meals or with antacids to minimize gastric irritation. Dosage may be increased gradually when necessary but should not exceed 150 to 200 mg daily. Patients with persistant night pain and/or morning stiffness, a large portion (up to a maximum of 100 mg) of the total daily dose at bedtime may be helpful in affording relief. A bedtime dose of either 25, 50 or 100 mg is recommended for such patients. To control acute attacks of gout, 50 mg 3 times daily until all signs and symptoms subside. During the interval phase of gouty arthritis, as little as 25 mg twice daily with adequate amounts of a uricosuric agent such as probenecid will help to prevent an acute attack.

Availability:
INDOCIN® Capsules, 25 mg in bottles of 100 and 1000 and in single-unit packages of 100; 50 mg in bottles of 100 and in single-unit packages of 100. **(Merck Sharp & Dohme)**

INFLUENZA VIRUS VACCINE, MONOVALENT

Description: Influenza virus vaccine, monovalent, ether extracted antigen is composed of the antigen of the strain of type B influenza viruses recommended by the Bureau of Biologics, the Food and Drug Administration, and the Public Health Service. Each 0.5 ml (human dose) is formulated to contain no less than 500 CCA (chick cell agglutination) units of extracted immunizing antigen representative of type B/Hong Kong/5/72. The vaccine contains no more than 1:12,000 formalin added during the process. It does not contain penicillin. Polysorbate 80, U.S.P., 175 mcg/0.5 ml and thiomerosal, 0.01% are added to the refined concentrate.

Indications: For the production of immunity to influenza produced by the strain of virus containing antigens related to those in the vaccine. Prophylaxis is desirable especially for high risk groups such as hospital and health service personnel, those residing in various institutions, the older age groups and individuals with chronic debilitating disease. It is not recommended for routine vaccination of healthy groups of adults and children; however, when a widespread epidemic is forecast, vaccination should be considered. Immunization during pregnancy is not recommended unless the patient is one of the high-risk group.

Contraindications: The use of products prepared from the embryonic fluid of chicken eggs is contraindicated in patients with a history of allergy to eggs, chicken feathers or chicken dander. In those suspected of having an allergic condition, a scratch test or an intradermal injection of 0.05 to 0.1 ml of vaccine diluted 1:100 in sterile saline should precede immunization procedures. Immunization should be deferred in the presence of any acute respiratory disease or other active infection. It should also be deferred in the presence of an epidemic of poliomyelitis unless the risk of influenza represents a greater threat to the patient than the increased possibility of poliomyelitis.

Precautions: Epinephrine should be immediately available for use should an acute anaphylactoid reaction occur in patients having an unsuspected hypersensitivity to any component of the vaccine. Since febrile reactions may occur, the justification for vaccinating individuals with a history of febrile convulsions should be carefully considered.

Adverse Reactions: Local reactions showing varying degrees of tenderness at the injection site, and systemic reactions as evidenced by headache, malaise, nausea, fever, muscle aches, joint pain, chills, fatigue, and anorexia may occur in variable percentages of individuals.

Dosage and Administration: *Intramuscularly* or *subcutaneously.* **Not for intravenous administration.** Injection should be given intramuscularly preferably in the deltoid muscle or the mid-lateral thigh. Intramuscular administration is preferred because it provides a better antigenic response and a lower incidence of local reactions. The recommended dosage schedules are: *Children 3 months to 6 years of age,* 2 injections of 0.05 to 0.1 ml each at intervals of 1 to 2 weeks. *Children 6 to 10 years of age,* 1 injection of 0.25 ml. *Adults and children more than 10 years of age,* 1 injection of 0.5 ml.

Availability:
FLUOGEN®-B Injection in vials of 5 ml. **(Parke-Davis)**

INFLUENZA VIRUS VACCINE, BIVALENT

Description: Influenza virus vaccine, bivalent, ether extracted antigen, types A and B is composed of the antigen of the strains of influenza viruses recommended by the Division of Biologics Standards, the National Institutes of Health, and the Public Health Service. Because both types of influenza virus undergo antigen changes, the vaccine formulation is reviewed periodically and is reformulated when necessary to include the contemporary antigens. The sterile aqueous suspension of inactivated influenza virus is prepared from the extra-embryonic fluid of influenza virus-infected chick embryo. The potency is expressed in terms of chick cell agglutination titer (as CCA units/ml). The vaccine contains a suitable preservative.

Indications: For the production of immunity to influenza produced by the strains of virus containing antigens related to those in the vaccine. Seasonal immunization is recommended for high risk patients especially those suffering from chronic debilitating disease, those residing in various institutions, the older age groups, particularly those over 65 years, and hospital and health service personnel. It is not recommended for routine vaccination of healthy groups of adults and children; however, when a widespread epidemic is forecast, vaccination should be considered. Routine influenza immunization during pregnancy is not recommended unless the patient is in one of the high-risk groups.

Contraindications: The use of products prepared from the embryonic fluid of chicken eggs is contraindicated in patients with a history of allergy to eggs, chicken, chicken feathers or chicken dander. In those suspected of having an allergic condition, a scratch test or an intradermal injection of 0.05 to 0.1 ml of the vaccine diluted 1:100 in sterile saline should precede immunization procedures. Immunization should be deferred in the presence of any acute respiratory disease or other active infection. It should also be deferred in the presence of an epidemic of poliomyelitis unless the risk of influenza represents a greater threat to the patient than the increased possibility of poliomyelitis.

Precautions: Epinephrine should be immediately available for use should an acute anaphylactoid reaction occur in patients having an undisclosed hypersensitivity to any component of the vaccine. Because of the possibility of a febrile reaction following immunization with influenza virus vaccine, the wisdom of attempting to immunize patients with a history of febrile convulsion should be given careful consideration.

Adverse Reactions: Moderate to severe redness, induration and tenderness at the injection site, headache, malaise, nausea, fever, muscle aches, joint pain, chills, fatigue, anorexia, and neurologic disorders have been reported.

Dosage and Administration: *Intramuscularly* or *subcutaneously.* **Not for intravenous administration.** Injections should be given intramuscularly preferably in the deltoid muscle or the midlateral thigh. Intramuscular administration is preferred because it is associated with a lower incidence of local reactions. *Primary immunization:* The optimal primary series consists of 2 doses of vaccine administered 6 to 8 weeks apart. A single dose will afford some degree of protection and a second dose as early as 2 weeks after the first injection will enhance antibody response. *Children 3 months to 6 years of age,* 2 injections of 0.05 to 0.1 ml each, 1 or 2 weeks apart, followed by a third dose of 0.05 to 0.1 ml 2 months later. *Children 6 to 10 years of age,* 2 injections of 0.25 ml each, given at least 2 months apart. *Adults and children over 10 years of age,* 2 injections of 0.5 ml of vaccine given at least 2 months apart. *Booster or recall dose: Children 3 months to 6 years of age,* 1 injection of 0.05 to 0.1 ml; *children 6 to 10 years of age,* 1 injection of 0.25 ml; *adults and children over 10 years of age,* 1 injection of 0.5 ml.

Availability:
FLUAX® Injection in vials of 5 ml and in prefilled disposable syringes of 0.5 ml in packages of 10. **(Merck Sharp & Dohme)**
FLUOGEN® Injection (subvirion) in vials of 5 ml and in vials of 25 ml for jet injector use only. **(Parke-Davis)**

INFLUENZA VIRUS VACCINE, BIVALENT Injection (purified subvirion type) in vials of 5 ml and in Tubex® (cartridge-needle unit) of 0.5 ml. **(Wyeth)**
ZONOMUNE® Injection (zonal centrifuged vaccine) in vials of 2.5 ml. **(Lilly)**

INITIA DROPS W/FLUORIDE: see The Fluoride-Vitamins

THE INSULINS

Description: Insulin is a hormone secreted by the β cells of the islands of Langerhans of the pancreas. Commercially, it is obtained by extracting the pancreas of cattle and hogs; the former may be preferred by some for religious reasons; either may be preferred over the other in cases of hypersensitivity.

Administered parenterally, insulin promotes the oxidation of glucose, lowers the blood-sugar level, and regulates the formation of sugar from noncarbohydrate sources. In the diabetic subject, insulin restores temporarily the ability to utilize carbohydrates and fats in a comparatively satisfactory manner; the concentration of sugar in the blood is confined within normal limits; the urine becomes free of sugar and ketone bodies; and diabetic acidosis and coma are prevented.

Indications: The control of diabetes mellitus which cannot be controlled satisfactorily by dietary regulation alone; to improve appetite and increase weight in selected cases of non-diabetic malnutrition; and, therapeutically, in selected cases of schizophrenia by inducing hypoglycemic shock.

Precautions: It is important that the patient follow carefully a course of diet as prescribed by the physician. Regular insulin is best administered 15 to 30 minutes before a meal. Insulin should be stored in a cool place, but not in a freezer. The expiration date on the package should be observed very carefully.

Adverse Reactions: Overdosage causes weakness, headache and fatigue, nervousness, tremor, nausea, pallor or flushing, and profuse sweating—a characteristic sign of impending or active hypoglycemia. If not treated immediately, the condition may lead to insulin reaction or shock with possible serious consequences. Acute distress with mental disturbances and unconsciousness are manifestations of severe hypoglycemia. Hypoglycemic reactions may be treated by administering some form of carbohydrate. Candy or a lump of sugar is convenient for this purpose and should always be carried by the patient. If the patient becomes delirious or mentally confused, diluted corn syrup or orange juice with sugar should be taken orally. If a mild attack is not immediately relieved or if a sudden or severe attack of hypoglycemia occurs, the physician should be summoned at once. Failure to recover within half an hour is an indication for hospitalization. In severe hypoglycemic reactions, it may be desirable to administer from 10 to 20 gm of dextrose in sterile solution intravenously. Glucagon also is used in the treatment of hypoglycemia (see monograph on Glucagon).

Dosage and Administration: *Parenterally only;* insulin is not effective when taken by mouth. Dosage is always expressed in units; the number of units in a given volume varies with the potency of the preparation employed. It is advisable to keep the volume/injection at 0.25 to 0.75 ml by selecting that potency of insulin which will give the required number of units in this range. There is no average dosage for insulin. The number and size of daily doses and the time of administration, as well as diet and exercise, are problems that require direct and continuous medical supervision. In general, 1 unit of insulin will promote the metabolism of about 1.5 gm of dextrose. Sufficient insulin should be given to keep the fasting blood-sugar at normal levels, but hypoglycemia should be avoided.

For coma or severe diabetic acidosis, 100 to 200 units of regular insulin may be given initially, followed by additional insulin at intervals of 30 minutes. In coma, 1/2 the initial dose may be given *intravenously* and the other half *subcutaneously*. Patients should never be permitted to become hypoglycemic; 1 gm of dextrose is given for each unit of insulin. The urine should be examined every hour for dextrose; if the urine becomes dextrose-free, more dextrose must be given.

The preceding discussion dealt with the insulins as a group. The discussions that follow will deal specifically with each of the following types of insulin, each intended for a particular purpose:

Regular Insulin
Globin Zinc Insulin
Isophane Insulin (NPH)
Protamine Zinc Insulin (PZI)
Zinc Insulin: Lente, Semilente and Ultralente

INSULIN, REGULAR

Description: Regular insulin is an aqueous solution made from the antidiabetic principle of beef and/or pork pancreas, as stated on the label. The insulin is prepared from zinc-insulin crystals (0.45 to 0.9%); each milligram of the crystals contains at least 22 units of insulin. The injection contains about 1.6% glycerin for isotonicity, 0.1 to 0.25% phenol or tricresol as a preservative, and sufficient 0.1*N* hydrochloric acid to yield a pH of 2.5 to 3.5. Following subcutaneous injection, therapeutic effect is evident within ½ to 1 hour, reaching maximum within 2 to 3 hours, with a 6-hour duration of activity.

For indications, precautions, etc., see general statement.

Dosage and Administration: Dosage must be determined for each individual. The solution usually is given *subcutaneously,* 30 minutes before meals. The maximal effect becomes apparent within 2 to 3 hours.

Availability:
ILETIN®: **(Lilly)**
Regular Injection: 40, 80 and 100 units/ml in vials of 10 ml.
Beef Special Injection (made only from beef pancreas), 100 units/ml in vials of 10 ml.
Pork Special Injection (made only from pork pancreas), 100 units/ml in vials of 10 ml; 500 units/ml (concentrated) in vials of 20 ml.
INSULIN Regular Injection: 40, 80 and 100 units/ml in vials of 10 ml. **(Squibb)**

GLOBIN ZINC INSULIN

Description: Globin zinc insulin injection is a sterile solution of insulin modified by the addition of zinc chloride, and globin obtained from globin hydrochloride prepared from the blood of cattle. The globin component has not been found to be allergenic. The amount of insulin used in the preparation of the injectable solution is sufficient to provide either 40, 80 or 100 units per ml.

Globin zinc insulin is an intermediate-acting type; its action ranges somewhere between that of regular insulin and that of protamine zinc insulin. Therapeutic effect is evident in approximately 2 hours, maximum effect is reached between 8 and 16 hours following administration and is almost completely dissipated after 24 hours.

Indications: Treatment of diabetic patients who require an intermediate-acting insulin, it may be used to replace zinc insulin, either wholly or partly, for those who are sensitive to protamine zinc insulin, or who cannot be controlled with other forms of insulin.

Precautions: It is not recommended for the treatment of diabetic coma, and it *should never be given intravenously.*

Dosage and Administration: By *deep subcutaneous injection,* 30 to 60 minutes before breakfast. Dosage should be adjusted to individual requirement for intensity and duration of effect. Initially, dosage usually is about ⅔ to ¾ of the total daily dose of regular insulin and should be administered under the direction of a physician.

For other details as to precautions, adverse reactions, etc., see general statement.

Availability:
GLOBIN ZINC INSULIN Injection, 40, 80 and 100 units/ml in vials of 10 ml. **(Squibb)**

ISOPHANE INSULIN

Synonym: NPH Insulin (Neutral Protamine Hagedorn Insulin).

Description: Isophane insulin is a purified aqueous suspension of minute crystals of insulin, protamine and zinc, buffered to a pH of 7.1 to 7.4. The protamine is one of a series of basic proteins that occurs in the spermatozoa of fish. When brought into a uniform suspension, the preparation contains either 40, 80 or 100 units of insulin per ml together with protamine in appropriate proportions. Isophane insulin is an intermediate-acting form of insulin which combines some of the advantages and eliminates some of the disadvantages of both very short and very long-acting preparations.

Following subcutaneous administration, the onset of action occurs in approximately 1 to 1½ hours, reaches a peak in about 8 to 12 hours and usually persists for as long as 24 hours.

Indications: Management of diabetes which cannot be controlled by diet.

Precautions: Should be administered *subcutaneously* only. Hypoglycemic reactions are similar, but are usually less obvious than those following unmodified insulin.

Adverse Reactions: Hypoglycemia is usually manifested by a feeling of fatigue; also weakness, sweating, tremor or nervousness may be experienced.

For other precautions, adverse reactions, etc., see general statement.

Dosage and Administration: *Subcutaneously only.* Dosage is individualized and should be administered from ½ to 1½ hours before the first meal of the day.

Availability:
ISOPHANE INSULIN Suspension, 40, 80 and 100 units/ml in vials of 10 ml. **(Squibb)**
NPH ILETIN®: **(Lilly)**
Isophane Insulin Suspension, 40, 80 and 100 units/ml in vials of 10 ml.
Beef Special Suspension (made exclusively from beef pancreas), 100 units/ml in vials of 10 ml.
Pork Special Suspension (made exclusively from pork pancreas), 100 units/ml in vials of 10 ml.

PROTAMINE ZINC INSULIN

Synonym: PZI.

Description: Protamine zinc insulin is a cloudy suspension of minute particles which, when brought into uniform suspension, contains either 40 or 80 units of insulin per ml and approximately 1.25 mg of protamine and 0.2 mg of zinc per 100 units of insulin. Protamine zinc insulin is a long-acting form of insulin. Since its action is delayed and prolonged, its effects become evident about 4 to 8 hours following subcutaneous administration, reach a peak in approximately 14 to 20 hours, and persist for as long as 36 hours. Protamine zinc insulin may be mixed with regular insulin.

Indications: Treatment and control of diabetes in patients in whom unmodified insulin fails to provide adequate control unaccompanied by frequent hypoglycemic reactions, ketosis, or evidence of pronounced fluctuations in blood-sugar levels, unless several doses are administered daily.

Precautions: Should be administered *subcutaneously* only. Onset of hypoglycemic reactions may be experienced considerably later than is the case with unmodified insulin.

Adverse Reactions: Hypoglycemia is usually manifested by sweating or by a feeling of fatigue unwarranted by the activities of the patient. Vague symptoms such as lassitude, drowsiness and tremulousness may develop which usually require immediate treatment.

For other precautions, adverse reactions, etc., see general statement.

Dosage and Administration: *Subcutaneously only,* usually once a day from 30 to 90 minutes before breakfast. Because its slow onset of action may lead to glycosuria, it may be best to give a separate dose of unmodified insulin the first few days along with protamine zinc insulin. The two insulins should not be mixed in the same syringe. To circumvent the lowering of blood-sugar levels over a prolonged period, food should be redistributed among various meals. Carbohydrates, in particular, should be divided among other meals in such a manner as to avoid hypoglycemia.

Availability:
PROTAMINE, ZINC & ILETIN®: **(Lilly)**
Suspension, 40, 80 and 100 units/ml in vials of 10 ml.
Beef Special Suspension (made only from beef pancreas), 100 units/ml in vials of 10 ml.
Pork Special Suspension (made only from pork pancreas), 100 units/ml in vials of 10 ml.
PROTAMINE ZINC INSULIN Suspension, 40, 80 and 100 units/ml in vials of 10 ml. **(Squibb)**

ZINC INSULIN

Synonyms: Lente, Semilente and Ultralente Insulin.

Description: Zinc insulin suspension (Lente) is an aqueous, buffered suspension of insulin modified by the addition of zinc chloride so that the solid phase consists of a mixture of crystalline and amorphous insulin in a ratio of about 7 parts of crystals to 3 parts of amorphous material.

Zinc insulin suspension *prompt* (Semilente) is an aqueous, buffered suspension of insulin modified by the addition of zinc chloride so that the solid phase of the suspension is amorphous.

Zinc insulin suspension *extended* (Ultralente) is an aqueous, buffered suspension of insulin modified by the addition of zinc chloride so that the solid phase of the suspension is crystalline.

Sufficient insulin is used in the preparations of these suspensions to provide either 40, 80 or 100 U.S.P. Insulin Units for each ml of the suspension.

Controlling the particle size permits variations in the time of onset and in the duration of action: The *Semilente* has the smaller particle size and the shorter action; duration of effect, about 12 to 16 hours. The *Ultralente* has the larger particle size and a duration of effect in excess of 36 hours. These times are considered average and may vary from patient to patient. The *Lente* has a time action which is intermediate between these; its action falls so close to that of NPH insulin that the two usually can be used interchangeably.

Each ml of these three forms of zinc insulin suspension contains either 40, 80 or 100 units of insulin, with about 0.2 mg of zinc per 100 units of insulin.

Indications: The routine management of diabetic patients, especially those who are allergic to other types of insulin; for those who require separate daily injections of protamine zinc insulin and regular insulin; and for those patients with evidence pointing to thrombotic phenomena in which protamine may be a factor.

Precautions: Zinc insulin suspensions are not adapted for use in place of regular (unmodified) insulin in dealing with acidosis and emergencies. They should not under any circumstances be substituted for another insulin preparation unless directed to do so by the physician.

For other precautions, adverse reactions, etc., see general statement.

Dosage and Administration: *Subcutaneously only,* usually before breakfast. Dosage must be adjusted to suit the needs of each individual patient. A mixture of Semilente and Lente insulins may be indicated when the control of the blood sugar and glycosuria after meals is inadequate with the Lente insulin alone. Ultralente insulin may be mixed with Lente insulin when inadequate control of the blood sugar and glycosuria in the fasting state (before breakfast) is obtained with Lente insulin alone. **Note:** These preparations can be mixed with one another, but must not be mixed with other modified insulins.

Availability:
LENTE ILETIN®: **(Lilly)**
Suspension, 40, 80 and 100 units/ml in vials of 10 ml.
Beef Special Suspension (made only from beef pancreas), 100 units/ml in vials of 10 ml.
Pork Special Suspension (made only from pork pancreas), 100 units/ml in vials of 10 ml.
SEMILENTE ILETIN® Suspension, 40, 80 and 100 units/ml in vials of 10 ml. **(Lilly)**
ULTRALENTE ILETIN® Suspension, 40, 80 and 100 units/ml in vials of 10 ml. **(Lilly)**
LENTE INSULIN Suspension, 40, 80 and 100 units/ml in vials of 10 ml. **(Squibb)**
SEMILENTE INSULIN Suspension, 40, 80 and 100 units/ml in vials of 10 ml. **(Squibb)**
ULTRALENTE INSULIN Suspension, 40, 80 and 100 units/ml in vials of 10 ml. **(Squibb)**

IOCETAMIC ACID

Chemical Name: *N*-Acetyl-N-(3-amino-2, 4, 6-triiodophenyl)-2-methyl-β-alanine.

Description: Iocetamic acid is a water-insoluble compound containing 62% organically bound iodine. It occurs as an off-white, odorless solid, and has a molecular weight of 614. Iocetamic acid is a mixture of 2 racemates which differ slightly in physical properties.

Following oral administration, the drug is rapidly absorbed from the gastrointestinal tract. It provides optimum contrast for cholecystographic studies within 10 to 15 hours. Upon absorption, the drug is conjugated with glucuronic acid in the liver, secreted into the bile as radiopaque glucuronide, which is then concentrated in the functioning gallbladder. These radiopaque conjugates provide contrast density which enables radiographic visualization of the gallbladder. Upon contraction of the gallbladder, it may also provide visualization of the biliary ducts.

Indications: Radiographic visualization of the gallbladder.

Contraindications: In patients with advanced hepatorenal disease, severe renal impairment, and in those known to be hypersensitive to iocetamic acid.

Warnings: Data at present are inadequate to insure safe administration of this product to pregnant or lactating women or to children less than 12 years of age.

Precautions: Care is required in patients with gastrointestinal disorders which may prevent or delay absorption of the medium. Also, severe liver disease may interfere with the metabolism of iocetamic acid or may fail to secrete the contrast material into the bile. These conditions can lead to inadequate radiographic visualization. Therefore, renal and hepatic function should be assessed prior to and for a few days following oral cholecystography. Considerable care is advised in patients with cardiovascular disease, especially those with recent symptoms of coronary artery disease. Prior to administration of iocetamic acid, the physician should determine whether or not the patient has had a previous history of allergy, because a positive history of allergy, such as bronchial asthma or a known sensitivity to iodine-containing compounds, implies greater than usual risk to the patient and calls for extreme caution. Prophylactic administration of an antihistamine to prevent or minimize possible allergic reactions should be considered. Elevation of protein-bound iodine may occur for a prolonged period of time following the ingestion of an iodine-containing medium. However, the successful evaluation of thyroid function can be accomplished using appropriate in vitro radiometric methods. False-positive tests for urine albumin may occur for several days following ingestion of this agent.

Adverse Reactions: The most frequently observed reactions were mild and transient gastrointestinal symptoms such as nausea, vomiting, abdominal cramps, diarrhea, epigastric burning and flatulence. A variety of reactions consisting of frequent or burning micturition, skin rash, pruritus, urticaria, chills, headaches, dizziness, flushing, and heartburn were also noted.

Dosage and Administration: *Orally.* A single dose of 3 gm (4 tablets) or 4.5 gm (6 tablets) is the recommended adult dose. The selection of the proper dose within this range is largely dependent upon the patient's condition and the desired density of the radiographs. In patients with normal liver function and an absence of gastrointestinal symptoms, a 3-gm dose will provide adequate radiographic visualization. In the more difficult patient, in whom it is desired to reduce the incidence of repeat examination, a dose of 4.5 gm should be employed. The package literature should be consulted for additional data.

Availability:
CHOLEBRINE® Tablets, 750 mg in bottles of 100 and in cartons of 5 and 25 strips of 4 or 6 tablets each. **(Mallinckrodt)**

IODINATED GLYCEROL

Chemical Name: 2-(*l*-Iodoethyl)-1,3-dioxolane-4-methanol.

Description: A stable complex of iodinated glyceryl ethers that contains no inorganic iodides or free iodine. Iodinated glyceryl combines the mucolytic properties of glyceryl with those of iodides to produce a marked potentiation of mucolytic activity. It occurs as a pale yellow liquid, with a marked pungent aftertaste, that is miscible with water, with alcohol, and with glycerin. While the iodine contributes to the mucolytic effectiveness, its content is too low to raise the PBI above normal levels in the euthyroid patient. The drug attempts to facilitate easy expectoration by altering sputum viscosity and volume, thereby restoring ciliary action and improving oxygen-carbon dioxide exchange in the respiratory tract.

Indications: Adjunctive treatment of bronchitis, bronchial asthma, pulmonary emphysema, obstructive forms of sinusitis, following surgery or during recovery from pneumonia, and for the management of the pulmonary complications of cystic fibrosis. The product containing phenobarbital has been formulated to provide in addition sedative and antispasmodic action.

Contraindications: Marked sensitivity to iodides.

Warnings: The drug should be discontinued if a skin rash or other evidence of unusual sensitivity appears.

Precautions: The possible effects of the iodine content on patients scheduled for thyroid function tests should be taken into consideration. Although an extremely rare occurrence, iodide-induced goiter with hyperthyroidism in the newborn has been reported with iodide compounds; therefore, cautious use in pregnant patients is indicated.

Adverse Reactions: Gastrointestinal irritation, rash and hypersensitivity have rarely been encountered.

Dosage and Administration: *Orally.* Adults, 20 drops of the 5% solution 4 times daily with liquids or 2 tablets 4 times daily with liquids or 1 teaspoonful of the 1.2% elixir 4 times daily. Children, 5 to 10 drops of the 5% solution 4 times daily with liquids or 1 tablet 4 times daily with liquids or ½ teaspoonful of the 1.2% elixir 4 times daily. Iodinated glycerol-phenobarbital combination: 1 teaspoonful of elixir or 1 tablet every 3 or 4 hours.

Availability:
ORGANIDIN®: **(Wallace)**
Elixir, 1.2% in bottles of 1 pint and 1 gallon. Each 5 ml contains 60 mg of iodinated glycerol (equiv. to 30 mg of organically bound iodine).
Solution, 5% in bottles of 30 ml. Each ml contains 50 mg of iodinated glycerol (equiv. to 25 mg of organically bound iodine).
Tablets in bottles of 100. Each tablet contains 30 mg of iodinated glycerol (equiv. to 15 mg of organically bound iodine).

w/Phenobarbital (**Warning:** May be habit-forming).
ORGAPHEN®: **(Wallace)**
Elixir in bottles of 1 pint. Each 5 ml contains 30 mg of iodinated glycerol (equiv. to 15 mg of organically bound iodine) with phenobarbital, 13 mg and alcohol, 7%.
Tablets in bottles of 100. Each tablet contains 30 mg of iodinated glycerol (equiv. to 15 mg of organically bound iodine) with phenobarbital, 13 mg.

IODIPAMIDE MEGLUMINE

Chemical Name: 3.3′-(Adipolydiimino)*bis*-2,4,6-triiodobenzoic acid.

Description: Meglumine iodipamide injection is a sterile solution of the chemical in water for injection. It occurs as a clear, colorless to light amber, slightly viscous liquid. It is a radiopaque, organic iodine compound containing 26% bound iodine.

Following intravenous administration, meglumine iodipamide is transported to the liver where it is rapidly secreted. It appears in the bile within 10 to 15 minutes following injection, thus permitting visualization of the hepatic and common bile ducts, even in cholecystectomized patients. The biliary ducts are readily visualized in approximately 25 minutes after administration, except in patients with impaired liver function. The contrast media appears in the gallbladder within 1 hour after injection; maximum concentration is reached in 2 to 2½ hours. Following intravenous infusion, the biliary ducts are readily visualized within 20 to 40 minutes after administration with optimum visualization usually occurring within 40 to 80 minutes. The contrast media appears in the gallbladder within 1 hour after completion of the infusion; maximum concentration is reached in 3 or more hours. It is eliminated in the feces without passing through the enterohepatic circulation, except for approximately 10% of the intravenously administered dose which is excreted in the urine.

Indications: For the visualization of the entire biliary tract and the intrahepatic and biliary ducts as well as the intact gallbladder.

Contraindications: In patients hypersensitive to iodipamide salts or who exhibit sensitivity reactions to the test dose, and in those with severe impairment of liver and kidney function.

Warnings: When injected intravenously or intraarterially, the medium has been shown to promote sickling in individuals who are homozygous for sickle cell disease. Since iodine-containing contrast agents may alter the results of thyroid function tests, such tests, if indicated, should be performed prior to the administration of this preparation. A history of sensitivity to iodine implies greater than usual risk to the patient. Safe use of meglumine iodipamide during pregnancy has not been established. Extreme caution is advised in patients with known or suspected pheochromocytoma and the medium [absolute minimum] should be injected only when the intended benefits outweigh the considered risks. Blood pressure should be assessed throughout the procedure and measures to combat a hypertensive crisis should be readily available.

Precautions: Intravenous administration of this agent can produce severe or fatal anaphylactic reactions. This has prompted the use of several pretesting methods, none of which can be relied upon to predict severe reactions. Many authorities question the value of any pretest. A detailed history of allergy of the patient should be taken. A history of bronchial asthma or allergy, or a family history of allergy warrants special attention, and may predict more accurately than pretesting the likelihood of a reaction, although not the severity nor type of reaction in the individual case. The sensitivity test most often performed is accomplished by slowly injecting 0.5 to 1 ml of meglumine iodipamide intravenously. To those patients with strong allergic histories, and to infants and children, successive fractional portions of 1 ml are given. Most hypersensitivity reactions will occur within 15 minutes after injection. If no reaction occurs within this time limit, the full dose may then be given; however, this does not preclude the possibility of a reaction. Patients with previous allergic histories may be premedicated with antihistamines to avoid or ameliorate possible adverse response. Appropriate emergency medication, including a positive-pressure oxygen source, epinephrine, corticosteroids, vasopressors, antihistamines, and suitable intravenous fluids should be immediately on hand, and should be readily available for at least 30 to 60 minutes following completion of the diagnostic procedure, since severe delayed reactions have been known to occur. Some clinicians feel that it may be advisable to have a continuous intravenous infusion running prior to and during administration of the drug. Contrast agents have been found to interfere with some chemical determinations made on urine specimens; therefore, it is recommended that the urine be collected before administration of the medium or two or more days afterwards.

Adverse Reactions: In the recommended doses and with slow injection, meglumine iodipamide is usually well tolerated. Local reactions at the site of injection are not observed, unless excessive amounts are extravasated during administration. Following too rapid injection, mild transient symptoms such as chills, fever, headache, pallor, tremors, restlessness, sensations of warmth, sneezing, perspiration, salivation, flushing, pressure in the upper abdomen, dizziness, nausea, and vomiting may occur. Rarely noted were swollen eyelids, laryngospasm, respiratory difficulties, hypotension, cardiac reactions and cyanosis. These symptoms usually disappear when the injection has been completed. Hypersensitivity reactions may occur. In rare instances, and despite the most careful sensitivity testing, anaphylactoid reactions may occur. Emergency measures must be readily available. Renal function tests may be altered and renal failure may develop.

Dosage and Administration: *Intravenously.* It is important that the preparation be injected slowly over a period of 10 minutes. If the infusion method is used, it is preferable that the medium be infused slowly over a period of 30 to 45 minutes. Cholecystography is preferably carried out in the morning with the patient in a fasting state. The solution should be warmed to body temperature prior to injection, and the patient should be observed closely for untoward reactions. Nausea indicates that the injection rate is too rapid. *For cholecystography,* the usual adult dose is 20 ml of the 52% solution or 100 ml of the 10.3% solution. For infants and children, the suggested dose is 0.3 to 0.6 ml/kg of body weight. Examination of the gallbladder should be started about 2 hours after administration of the drug, and the standard positions in routine examinations of the gallbladder should be used unless otherwise indicated.

Availability:
CHOLOGRAFIN® Injection, 10.3% in single-dose bottles of 100 ml; 52% in single-dose vials of 20 ml and in 20-ml combination packages containing, in addition, a separate ampul for testing. **(Squibb)**

IODOCHLORHYDROXYQUIN

Chemical Name: 5-Chloro-7-iodo-8-quinolinol.

Description: An iodohydroxyquinoline antifungal, antibacterial and amebicidal agent that is closely related both chemically and pharmacologically to diiodohydroxyquin. It occurs as a voluminous, spongy, brownish-yellow, tasteless powder that is practically insoluble in water. It contains approximately 40% iodine and 11% chloride.

In vitro studies have demonstrated that the drug inhibits the growth of various mycotic organisms such as microsporons, trichophytons and *Candida albicans* and gram-positive cocci such as staphylococci and enterococci.

Indications: Treatment of localized dermatophytic infections, especially those complicated by bacteria. Iodochlorhydroxyquin and hydrocortisone combinations are indicated in contact or atopic dermatitis, impetiginized eczema, nummular eczema, infantile eczema, endogenous chronic infectious dermatitis, stasis dermatitis, pyoderma, nuchal eczema, chronic eczematoid otitis externa, acne urticata, localized or disseminated neurodermatitis, lichen simplex chronicus, anogenital pruritus, folliculitis, bacterial dermatoses and mycotic dermatoses such as tinea (capitis, cruris, corporis, pedis), moniliasis, intertrigo and many similar conditions.

Contraindications: Patients with known hypersensitivity to iodine, iodochlorhydroxyquin or hydrocortisone. Hydrocortisone should not be used in the eyes or topically in the presence of tuberculosis, vaccinia, varicella or other viral skin infections.

Warnings: The presence of systemic infections should be treated with the appropriate antibiotic. Safe use in pregnant or lactating women has not been established; therefore, this drug should not be used extensively, in large amounts or for prolonged periods on such patients.

Precautions: May prove irritating to sensitized skin in rare cases; if this should occur, discontinue treatment. May stain hair or fabrics. Although signs and symptoms of systemic toxicity, electrolyte imbalance, or adrenal suppression have not been noted, it should nevertheless be kept in mind that suppression of the pituitary-adrenal system may occur, especially under occlusive dressings for prolonged periods, or when treating extensive areas since significant absorption of the corticosteroid is possible. Iodochlorhydroxyquin may be absorbed through the skin and interfere with thyroid function tests. If such tests are contemplated, a period of one month should elapse between discontinuation of therapy and the performance of these tests.

The ferric chloride test for phenylketonuria (PKU) can yield a false-positive result if iodochlorhydroxyquin is present in the diaper or urine. Prolonged use may result in overgrowth of nonsusceptible organisms requiring appropriate therapy.

Adverse Reactions: Nausea, vomiting, headache, dizziness, pruritus ani have been reported. Rash, hypersensitivity, local burning, irritation, and pruritus may occur, in which case the drug should be withdrawn. In rare instances, topical steroids have been reported to cause striae at the site of applications when used for long periods in intertriginous areas.

Dosage and Administration: *Topically.* Apply a small amount to affected areas 2 to 4 times daily.

Availability:
VIOFORM®: **(Ciba)**
Cream, 3% (OTC) in tubes of 30 gm.
Ointment, 3% (OTC) in tubes of 30 gm.
w/Hydrocortisone
Cream, 3% with hydrocortisone, 1% in tubes of 5 and 20 gm.
Lotion, 3% with hydrocortisone, 1% in squeeze bottles of 15 ml.
Mild Cream, 3% with hydrocortisone, 0.5% in tubes of 15 and 30 gm.
Mild Ointment, 3% with hydrocortisone, 0.5% in tubes of 30 gm.
Ointment, 3% with hydrocortisone, 1% in tubes of 20 gm.
HEXADERM I.Q. Cream, 3% with hydrocortisone, 0.5% in tubes of 30 gm. **(Amfre-Grant)**
RACET® Cream, 3% with hydrocortisone, 0.5% in tubes of 15 and 30 gm and in jars of 1 lb. **(Lemmon)**
RACET®LCD Cream, 3% with hydrocortisone, 0.5% and coal tar solution, 5% in tubes of 30 gm and in jars of 1 lb. **(Lemmon)**

IOPANOIC ACID

Chemical Name: 3-Amino-α-ethyl-2,4,6-triiodohydrocinnamic acid.

Description: Iopanoic acid is a water-insoluble compound containing about 67% organically-bound iodine.

Following oral administration, it is rapidly absorbed from the duodenum and concentrated and stored in the gallbladder. Approximately 50% of the dose is excreted by the liver as a glucuronide within 24 hours and the other 50% within 5 days; ²/₃ of the drug is excreted through the gastrointestinal tract and ¹/₃ through the kidneys. The glucuronide is not reabsorbed, thus there is no enterohepatic recycling; it is visible in the intestinal tract as discrete radiopacities.

The healthy gallbladder concentrates iopanoic acid; faint contrast becomes apparent in about 4 hours, and maximum contrast in about 14 hours. In substantial gallbladder disease, concentration does not take place and no contrast is apparent.

Indications: Radiographic visualization of the gallbladder and bile ducts.

Contraindications: Advanced hepatorenal disease or severe impairment of renal function, severe gastrointestinal disorders that prevent absorption, and in iodine-sensitive patients.

Warnings: When prescribed for pregnant patients or for women of childbearing potential, the physician should carefully consider the benefits versus the possible risks to the fetus.

Precautions: Severe, advanced liver disease may interfere with metabolism of iopanoic acid, thus a greater amount of unchanged medium will be diverted for kidney excretion; also renal function should be assessed before cholecystography in patients with this condition, and renal output and hepatic function should be observed for a few days after the procedure. Patients with preexisting renal disease should not receive high doses of iopanoic acid because possible renal irritation in susceptible individuals could result in reflex vascular spasm with partial or complete renal shutdown. Such patients should be advised to drink liberal amounts of fluids. The fact that this medium has uricosuric activity should be taken into consideration when it is administered to patients with impaired renal function. Caution is advised in patients with coronary disorders, especially those with recent symptoms of coronary artery disease. Blood pressure should be observed after administration of cholecystographic media to these patients. Elevation of PBI for several months, false-positive urine albumin tests for up to three days, and delay in BSP clearance values for up to two days, may occur in patients taking this compound.

Adverse Reactions: The most frequently reported have been mild and transitory nausea, vomiting, cramps, and diarrhea (usually occurring as a few loose stools). Frank diarrhea and cramps have been noted in only a small number of patients and severe diarrhea with prostration is rare. A mild stinging sensation during urination may occur and, rarely, skin and mucous membrane reactions (e.g., skin rash, urticaria with or without pruritus, erythema, and localized areas of edema), and an unusual systemic serum sickness-type reaction with fever, rash, and arthralgia. Occasionally, transitory thrombocytopenia with petechiae have been reported. Miscellaneous subjective complaints are dryness of the throat, burning on swallowing, heartburn, sore throat, dizziness, and headache.

Dosage and Administration: The usual adult dosage is 3 gm *orally,* ingested after a fat-free dinner about 14 hours before the scheduled cholecystography. For repeat examination on the same day as the initial cholecystographic procedure, an additional 3 gm may be given. If repeat examination is to be performed with a double dose, a period of at least 5 to 7 days should intervene between the first and the repeat examinations. No more than a total of 6 gm should be ingested during a period of 24 hours. However, the use of large or repeated doses over a number of days to force visualization of a poorly functioning gallbladder in elderly patients is not recommended. The patient should be given a fat-free meal the evening before roentgenography and allowed nothing by mouth until after the examination has been taken. Shortly before cholecystography the patient should be given an enema to remove any accumulated gas. A fat-containing meal may be given immediately after roentgenography and additional films are obtained to determine the contractile function of the gallbladder; also helps to identify radiopaque or small stones, and to visualize bile ducts.

Availability:
TELEPAQUE® Tablets, 500 mg in envelopes of 6 (the customary adult dose), in cartons of 5 and 25 envelopes and in bottles of 500 tablets with dispensing envelopes. **(Winthrop)**

IOTHALAMATE MEGLUMINE

IOTHALAMATE SODIUM

Description: Both *meglumine* and *sodium iothalamate* are isomers of the respective diatrizoate compounds.

Chemically, *meglumine iothalamate* is 5-acetamido-2,4,6-triiodo-N-methylisophthalamic acid combined with 1-deoxy-1-(methylamino)glucitol (1:). It is an organic iodine preparation which is radiopaque, freely soluble in water and contains 47% iodine.

Sodium iothalamate is the sodium salt of 5-acetamido-2,4,6-triiodo-N-methylisophthalamate. It has similar characteristics to the meglumine preparation but contains 60% iodine.

The extent of roentgenographic definition depends primarily on the site of injection. Intravenous administration results in rapid distribution throughout the circulatory system to the renal area where both preparations are excreted in the urine in unchanged form. The greatest degree of x-ray visualization of the kidney occurs within 3 to 15 minutes but this will be influenced by the status of renal function.

Indications: *Meglumine iothalamate:* diagnostic agent for x-ray definition of the kidneys, bladder and ureters, cerebral and peripheral arteries as well as the peripheral veins. *Sodium iothalamate:* as an x-ray contrast preparation in evaluating the status of the urinary tract by intravenous administration as well as the status of the heart, aorta and its branches. *Sodium iothalamate should not be used for cerebral angiography.*

Contraindications: Hypersensitivity to the preparation. A test dose should always be given. Acute thrombophlebitis is usually a contraindication for venography. Cerebral angiography should be used with caution, if at all, if recent cerebral embolism or thrombosis is suspected.

Warnings: Constant observation and extreme care is necessary in administering this drug to patients with multiple myeloma—some instances of anuria resulting in progressive uremia, renal failure and eventually death have been noted, and to individuals with known or suspected pheochromocytoma—the amount of drug injected should be kept to the absolute minimum, the blood pressure should be assessed throughout the procedure, and measures for treatment of a hypertensive crisis should be available. Particular caution is necessary in those who are homozygous for sickle cell disease since contrast media have been shown to promote sickling when injected intravenously or intraarterially. Data at present are inadequate to insure safe administration of this product to pregnant or lactating women.

Precautions: Fatal anaphylactic reactions may result from administration of these preparations including even a test dose of 1 ml intravenously; therefore, it is essential that the patient be observed for at least 15 minutes following parenteral administration. Prophylactic premedication of allergic patients with antihistamines may be desirable and emergency medication (such as oxygen, vasopressors, barbiturates, antihistamines and adrenocortical steroids) should be immediately available should a reaction occur. These preparations should be utilized cautiously in patients with severe liver or kidney disease, asthmatic patients and in those with a history of iodide sensitivity. In severely ill patients the value of the information to be gained from the diagnostic procedure must be weighed against the possible complications of the procedure. Evaluation of thyroid function, if indicated, should be done prior to administration of these preparations because the iodine in the preparation may interfere with thyroid function tests.

Adverse Reactions: Nonspecific complaints involving the gastrointestinal tract (nausea, vomiting), headache, dizziness, and urticaria have been noted. It is not unusual for the patient to complain of pain at the site of injection or a feeling of warmth. More serious reactions such as temporary blindness, transient hemiplegias, apnea and various neurological reactions occur following cerebral angiography, and abnormalities of cardiac rhythm, including serious ventricular arrhythmias, have occurred during and following angiocardiography.

Dosage and Administration: These diagnostic agents are administered *intravenously* for excretory urography, aortography, angiocardiography, and venography, and *intraarterially* for cerebral angiography, peripheral arteriography, aortography, and for left-sided angiocardiography.

The details of administration and the dose and type of preparation used will depend on the status and size of the patient and the information desired. The physician is referred to the medical literature and the manufacturer's package circular for specific details.

Availability:

Iothalamate Meglumine

CONRAY® Solution, 30% in bottles of 300 ml; 60% in ampuls of 30 ml and in vials of 20, 30, 50 and 100 ml. **(Mallinckrodt)**

CYSTO-CONRAY® Solution, 43% in vials of 50 and 100 ml and in bottles of 250 ml. Dilution units of 250 and 500 ml each containing 100 and 250 ml of meglumine iothalamate respectively. **(Mallinckrodt)**

CYSTO-CONRAY® II Solution, 17.2% in bottles of 250 and 500 ml. **(Mallinckrodt)**

Iothalamate Sodium

ANGIO-CONRAY® Solution, 80% in vials of 50 ml. **(Mallinckrodt)**

CONRAY-400% Solution, 66.8% in vials of 25 and 50 ml. **(Mallinckrodt)**

Iothalamate Meglumine and Sodium

VASCORAY® Solution, 520 mg (52%) meglumine iothalamate and 260 mg (26%) sodium iothalamate in vials of 25 and 50 ml and in bottles of 200 ml. **(Mallinckrodt)**

IPODATE CALCIUM

IPODATE SODIUM

Chemical Name: Calcium and sodium salts, respectively, of 3-(dimethylaminomethyleneamino)-2,4,6-triiodophenyl-propionic acid.

Description: Both salts are oral radiopaque contrast media for cholangiography and cholecystography. The iodine content of calcium ipodate is 61.7%; that of sodium ipodate, 61.4%. The calcium salt is practically insoluble in water, while the sodium salt is very soluble in water.

Both salts are rapidly absorbed from the gastrointestinal tract, and begin to appear in the bile within 30 minutes; optimal concentration in the hepatic and biliary ducts occurs within 1 to 3 hours. Adequate opacification of the ducts, which usually persists for about 45 minutes, permits rapid, diagnostically satisfactory visualization, even after cholecystectomy. The gallbladder is optimally opacified approximately 10 hours after ingestion of either salt. Diagnostically adequate filling, however, often takes place within 5 hours or less, particularly with the calcium salt. Both salts visualize the gallbladder; contrast density is said to be excellent even in obese patients, and the ability of the gallbladder to concentrate and then expel bile may be readily observed. Nonopaque stones may be visualized and radiodense calculi and papillomata are not obscured. Since the shadow obtained is usually homogeneous, layering of the contrast agent is not likely to be a problem.

Indications: For cholecystography; also may be used for cholangiography although they are not considered the drugs of choice.

Contraindications: Hypersensitivity to ipodate salts.

Warnings: A history of sensitivity to iodine or other iodinated compounds is not an absolute contraindication to the use of these preparations, but calls for extreme caution in administration. The safe use of these preparations during pregnancy has not been established; therefore, their use in pregnant patients is warranted only when in the judgment of the physician their use is deemed essential to the welfare of the patient.

Precautions: Anuria may result in the presence of combined renal and hepatic disease or severe renal impairment. Also renal toxicity has been reported in a few patients with liver dysfunction who were given oral cholecystographic agents followed by urographic agents. Administration of urographic agents should therefore be postponed in any patient with a known or suspected hepatic or biliary disorder who has recently taken a cholecystographic contrast agent. Gastrointestinal disorders which might interfere with absorption or liver dysfunction which might result in inadequate biliary secretion of the medium are likely to result in unsatisfactory visualization. Thyroid function, if indicated, should be performed prior to the administration of these preparations since iodine containing contrast agents may alter the results of these tests. Increasing the dosage above that recommended increases the possibility of hypotension. Contrast agents may interfere with some chemical determinations made on urine specimens; therefore, urine should be collected before administration of the contrast medium or two or more days afterwards.

Adverse Reactions: Mild and transient nausea, vomiting or diarrhea sometimes occurs but the incidence can be reduced by restricting the dosage to 3 gm, and administering only the granules to patients who may be prone to gastrointestinal reactions. Headache, dysuria, or abdominal pain may occur infrequently as transient disturbances. Hypersensitivity reactions may include urticaria, serum sickness-like reactions (fever, rash, arthralgia), other skin rashes, and, rarely, anaphylactoid shock. These are more likely to occur in individuals with a history of allergy, asthma, hay fever or urticaria, and in those who have previously demonstrated hypersensitivity to iodine compounds. Urticarial, serum sickness-like and other skin rash reactions may be controlled by antihistamines and, if necessary, corticosteroids. Serious anaphylactoid reactions are not controlled by antihistamines, and require such measures as the immediate use of epinephrine or phenylephrine, oxygen, and intravenous corticosteroids.

Dosage and Administration: *Orally.* The capsules should be taken with as little water as possible, and the granules should be stirred vigorously into a small amount of water and swallowed immediately. *For routine cholecystography,* 3 gm (6 capsules or 1 or 2 packets) is given in the evening, 2 hours after a routine or fat-free meal. The contrast agent should be administered 10 to 12 hours before the roentgenologic examination. An additional 3 gm of calcium ipodate is administered the following day 2 or 3 hours before cholecystography if the initial dose must be augmented so that a satisfactory cholecystogram may be obtained. *For cholangiography,* no prior preparation of the patient is necessary. Roentgenograms are made at intervals of 15 minutes, beginning 1 hour after administration of the medium. Optimal visualization of the ducts is generally achieved between 1½ to 2½ hours following ingestion of calcium ipodate. A total of 6 gm/24-hour period should not be exceeded. For additional details, see package literature.

Availability:
ORAGRAFIN®: **(Squibb)**
Capsules (sodium salt), 500 mg in vials of 6, in bottles of 100 and in Unimatic®s (single-dose) cartons of 100.
Granules (calcium salt), 3 gm/8 gm foil packet in cartons of 25.

IRCON-FA

Description: Each tablet contains ferrous fumarate, 250 mg (approx. 82 mg of elemental iron) and folic acid, 1 mg.

Indications: To prevent the development of anemia during pregnancy. It is not intended for the treatment of fully developed anemias.

Contraindications: In the presence of pernicious anemia and in anemias not due to iron deficiency.

Warnings: Folic acid alone is not a reliable agent in the treatment of pernicious anemia and other megaloblastic anemias where vitamin B-12 is deficient.

Precautions: It is advised that periodic blood studies be performed to ascertain whether or not therapy is adequate. Use with care in the presence of peptic ulcer, regional enteritis and ulcerative colitis. Folic acid, especially in doses of more than 1 mg daily, may obscure pernicious anemia, in that hematologic remission may occur while neurologic involvement progresses.

Adverse Reactions: Gastric distress, abdominal cramps, and diarrhea may occur in iron-sensitive patients. Allergic sensitization has been reported following both oral and parenteral administration of folic acid.

Dosage and Administration: *Orally.* The usual dose in the 2nd and 3rd trimesters of pregnancy is 1 tablet daily, taken in the morning between breakfast and lunch with a glass of water or milk. If severe vomiting is a problem, the dose may be taken in midafternoon.

Availability:
IRCON®-FA Tablets (red film-coated) in bottles of 100. **(Key Pharm.)**

IRON DEXTRAN

Description: Iron dextran is a combination of ferric hydroxide in complex with partially hydrolyzed dextran of low molecular weight. This dextran is pharmacologically distinct from the high molecular weight dextran used as a blood volume expander.

It is absorbed from the site of injection primarily through the lymphatic system with 1 to 15% being absorbed within 2 hours and 60 to 68% being absorbed within several days; the remainder is gradually absorbed over a period of several months or longer. Serum iron increases gradually, following intramuscular injection, while the iron is slowly cleared from the blood and within 12 hours hemosiderin may appear in the bone marrow. Sixteen to 60% of iron administered as iron dextran is utilized for hemoglobin synthesis with utilization being greater in iron-deficient than in normal or mildly anemic individuals. The greatest rise in hemoglobin occurs within 14 to 21 days after therapy is initiated; however, maximum utilization may not occur for 50 to 120 days. Iron dextran which is not immediately utilized for hemoglobin synthesis is stored chiefly in the liver. Some iron may diffuse into tissue fluids or may be utilized for synthesis of myoglobin or nonhemoglobin heme enzymes.

Indications: *For specifically-diagnosed cases of iron-deficiency anemia and then only when oral administration of iron is ineffective or impractical.* Such anemia may include: patients in the last trimester of pregnancy; patients with gastrointestinal diseases, or those recovering from gastrointestinal surgery; patients with chronic bleeding with continual and extensive iron losses not rapidly replenishable with oral iron; patients intolerant to blood transfusion as a source of iron; infants with hypochromic anemia, and patients who cannot be relied upon to take oral iron.

Contraindications: In hypersensitive patients; and in all anemias other than iron-deficiency anemia.

Warnings: Severe anaphylactic reactions have occurred with the use of iron dextran injection, and some fatalities have been reported. Thus, it should be used only in the treatment of definitely established cases of iron deficiency anemia, confirmed by appropriate laboratory investigation, and in those patients for whom oral therapy is not amenable. Although iron dextran has been reported to be carcinogenic in experimental animals, the risk of this occurrence in clinical use, following recommended dosage, appears to be extremely remote. Safe use of iron dextran during pregnancy has not been established with respect to adverse effects on human fetal development; therefore, it should not be used in the first trimester of pregnancy, and should be used in women of childbearing potential only when, in the judgment of the physician, the potential benefits outweigh the possible risks. Use with exceptional care in the presence of severe hepatic dysfunction.

Precautions: Unwarranted therapy with parenteral iron will cause excess storage of iron with the consequent possibility of exogenous hemosiderosis. Such iron overload is particularly likely to occur in patients with hemoglobinopathies and other refractory anemias that might be erroneously diagnosed as iron deficiency anemia. Patients with iron deficiency anemia and rheumatoid arthritis may experience an acute exacerbation of joint pain and swelling following intravenous administration of iron dextran. Therapy should be guided by periodic hematologic determinations.

Adverse Reactions: Anaphylactoid including fatal anaphylaxis; severe febrile reactions; arthralgia and myalgia; local discomfort (soreness, inflammation, phlebitis) and brown staining at the injection site; peripheral vascular "flushing" with rapid intravenous administration; hypotensive reaction; possible arthritic reactivation in patients with quiescent rheumatoid arthritis, and minor reactions that may include headache, transitory paresthesias, nausea, shivering, itching, and rash have been noted.

Dosage and Administration: *Intramuscularly;* only into the upper outer quadrant of the buttock, *never* into the arm or other exposed area. Dosage is based upon body weight and gm Hb/ml of blood and ranges from 0.5 ml in infants to 5 ml in adults daily, every other day or weekly. *Intravenously,* initially, 0.5 ml; if no reaction occurs then 2 ml daily may be given after a lapse of 2 or 3 days. The preparation should be given at the rate of 1 ml/minute.

Availability:
IMFERON® Solution (Colloidal), 50 mg/ml in ampuls of 2 and 5 ml (IV only) and in multiple-dose vials of 10 ml (IM only). **(Merrell-National)**

ISOCARBOXAZID

Chemical Name: 5-Methyl-3-isoxazolecarboxylic acid 2-benzylhydrazide.

Description: Isocarboxazid is a monoamine oxidase inhibitor of the hydrazine group which is structurally and pharmacologically related to other compounds of this group. It occurs as a colorless, crystalline solid very slightly soluble in water and sparingly soluble in alcohol.

Monoamine oxidase, an enzyme found primarily in nerve tissue, liver and lungs, catalyzes the oxidative deamination of various amines, including epinephrine, norepinephrine and serotonin. Inhibition of this enzyme results in an increase in the concentration of these amines in the brain stem. It has been assumed that an increase in free serotonin and norepinephrine is responsible for the therapeutic effect produced by the monoamine oxidase inhibitors. However, the precise mode of action of these compounds has not been established.

They block the detoxification of many drugs by the liver and this may be the reason for their potentiation of such agents as general anesthetics, barbiturates, morphine, alcohol, corticosteroids, and atropine. The action of the monoamine oxidase inhibitors is cumulative; a latent period of a few days to several months may occur before the onset of activity, and effects may persist for up to 3 weeks after therapy is discontinued.

Indications: In the management of depression that is unresponsive to electroconvulsive therapy or to tricyclic antidepressants and in cases where tricyclic agents are contraindicated.

Contraindications: In hypersensitive patients, severe impairment of kidney or liver function, congestive heart failure, or pheochromocytoma. Concomitant use with sympathomimetic drugs, with foods having a high concentration of tryptophan (broad beans) or tyramine (cheese, beers, wines, pickled herring, chicken livers, yeast extract), with excessive caffeine, and with other MAO inhibitors is contraindicated. At least 10 days should elapse between the discontinuance of isocarboxazid and institution of another MAO inhibitor or antidepressant drug. Such combinations can produce a hypertensive crisis in addition to fever, marked sweating, excitation, delirium, tremor, twitching, convulsions, coma, and circulatory collapse. Isocarboxazid should not be used in combination with CNS depressants such as narcotics and alcohol. Circulatory collapse and death have been reported when administered with meperidine. Isocarboxazid should be discontinued at least 10 days prior to elective surgery.

Warnings: Because of the drug's effect on blood pressure, it should not be administered to elderly or debilitated patients, or in the presence of hypertension, cardiovascular or cerebrovascular disease, or to patients with severe or frequent headaches. Particular care should be exercised when used in combination with antihypertensive drugs including thiazide diuretics since hypotension may result. Strict supervision, and preferably hospitalization, is advised when patients with potential suicidal tendencies begin to respond to the drug, as the risk of suicide is frequently greatest near the end of the depressive cycle. Isocarboxazid is not recommended for use in patients under 16 years of age. Safe use during pregnancy or lactation, or in women of childbearing age has not been established; therefore, the potential benefits of the drug must be weighed against the possible hazard to the mother and fetus.

Precautions: Concomitant use of this drug and other psychotropic agents should be avoided because of the possibility of potentiation and lowering of the margin of safety. The effects of isocarboxazid may persist for a substantial period after discontinuance of the drug and this should be borne in mind when other drugs are prescribed following therapy with this compound. Use with caution in overactive, stimulated or agitated patients, as well as in schizophrenic and manic-depressive patients since there may be a tendency for patients to swing from a depressive to manic phase. If jaundice or impaired liver function occurs, discontinue therapy. Periodic liver function tests are advised during therapy. Isocarboxazid appears to have varying effects in epileptic patients; consideration must be given to the possibility of increased frequency of seizures if the drug is prescribed for such patients. All patients should be observed for symptoms of postural hypotension; if this occurs, the dose should be reduced or the drug discontinued. MAO inhibitors may affect glucose metabolism or potentiate hypoglycemic agents; this should be considered if administered to diabetic patients.

Adverse Reactions: Orthostatic hypotension, disturbances in cardiac rate and rhythm, dizziness, vertigo, constipation, headache, overactivity, hyperreflexia, tremors, muscle twitching, mania, hypomania, jitteriness, confusion and memory impairment, insomnia, peripheral edema, weakness, fatigue, dry mouth, blurred vision, hyperhidrosis, anorexia, and body weight changes, gastrointestinal disturbances, and minor sensitivity reactions such as skin rashes; rarely, akathisia, ataxia, black tongue, coma, dysuria, euphoria, hematologic changes, incontinence, neuritis, photosensitivity, sexual disturbances, spider telangiectases and urinary retention; hallucinations; toxic ambylopia have been reported.

Dosage and Administration: *Orally.* Initial adult dosage is 30 mg daily, given in single or divided doses. As soon as clinical improvement is observed, a reduced maintenance dosage of 10 to 20 mg (or less) daily should be instituted. The physician is urged to read carefully the package literature for the management of overdosage.

Availability:
MARPLAN® Tablets, 10 mg (peach-colored) in bottles of 100 and 1000. **(Roche)**

ISOETHARINE

Chemical Name: 1-(3,4-Dihydroxyphenyl)-2-isopropylamino-1-butanol.

Description: Isoetharine is an adrenergic (sympathomimetic) amine with $beta_2$ selectivity. It acts directly on the $beta_2$ receptors of the bronchial smooth muscle to produce dilatation and relaxation of the bronchi and arterioles. It possesses minor $beta_1$ (cardiogenic) activity.

Bronchometer is formulated as isoetharine mesylate, 0.61% w/w in a solution containing saccharin, menthol, alcohol, 30% w/w and fluorochlorohydrocarbons as gaseous propellants. It is preserved with ascorbic acid, 0.1% w/w. Bronkosol is formulated as isoetharine hydrochloride, 1% w/w in an aqueous-glycerin solution containing sodium chloride, citric acid, sodium hydroxide with methylparaben, propylparaben and acetone sodium bisulfite.

Indications: Symptomatic relief of bronchial asthma and other conditions in which bronchospasm may be a complicating factor such as emphysema, bronchitis and other bronchopulmonary disorders.

Contraindications: Hypersensitivity to any of the components.

Warnings: Occasionally, a severe paradoxical airway resistance (cause unknown) has been reported with repeated excessive use. Cardiac arrest has occurred in several instances. It is therefore advisable that the use of the drug be discontinued and alternative therapy instituted if such resistance develops. Concurrent administration with epinephrine or other sympathomimetic amines should be avoided as they are direct cardiac stimulants and may cause excessive tachycardia. However, they may be alternated if desired. Although there has been no evidence of teratogenic effects with these drugs, their use during pregnancy or lactation or in women of childbearing potential requires that the expected benefits be weighed against the possible hazards to the mother and child.

Precautions: Dosage must be adjusted carefully in patients with hyperthyroidism, hypertension, acute coronary disease, cardiac asthma, limited cardiac reserve and in individuals sensitive to sympathomimetic amines, since overdosage may result in tachycardia, palpitation, nausea, headache, or epinephrine-like side effects. The nebulizer should be kept away from extreme heat and should not be incinerated.

Adverse Reactions: Although relatively free from toxic side effects, too frequent use—as with other sympathomimetic amines—may cause tachycardia, palpitation, nausea, headache, changes in blood pressure, anxiety, tension, restlessness, insomnia, tremor, weakness, dizziness and excitement. For this reason, patients should follow dosage instructions exactly.

Dosage and Administration: *Bronkometer:* The average adult dose is 1 or 2 *inhalations.* Occasionally, more may be required. It is important, however, to wait 1 full minute after the first 1 or 2 inhalations in order to be certain that another is necessary. In most cases, inhalations need not be repeated more often than every 4 hours, although more frequent administration may be necessary in severe cases. Instructions for administration are enclosed in each package. Briefly, the patient should inhale deeply while pressing firmly on the nebulizer. This releases 1 measured oral dose. **Note:** Each ml delivers 20 metered doses in a fine aerosol mist of controlled, uniform particle size of 560 mcg (340 mcg of isoetharine). Warm or cold water should be run through the mouthpiece once daily to cleanse it. May be sanitized by immersion in alcohol. *Bronkosol: Oral Inhalation.* The average adult dose is 3 to 7 inhalations. Can be administered by hand nebulizer, oxygen aerosolization or intermittent positive pressure breathing (IPPB). Usually treatment need not be repeated more often than every 4 hours, although more frequent administration may be necessary in severe cases.

Availability:

BRONKOMETER® Aerosol (as the mesylate) tpr actuator with 10 ml refill; 10 ml refill only; 10 ml vial with oral nebulizer for desk or bedside; 20 ml refill. **(Breon)**

BRONKOSOL® Aerosol (as the hydrochloride) for inhalation in bottles of 10 and 30 ml. **(Breon)**

ISOFLUROPHATE

Description: Isoflurophate is an oily, colorless liquid unstable in aqueous solutions in which it forms hydrofluoric acid; however, it is stable in alcohol and in vegetable oils.

Isoflurophate is a parasympathomimetic agent that reduces intraocular tension and produces a relatively prolonged miotic action and spasm of the muscles of accommodation. It inhibits cholinesterase irreversibly; its action on the enzyme is more prolonged than that of physostigmine and similar drugs whose action is reversible. However, when used as directed with local corneal instillation of isoflurophate, the decrease in plasma cholinesterase is so slight that systemic side effects are extremely rare. The action of this compound is inhibited by prior use of other drugs which also inactivate cholinesterase, such as physostigmine.

Indications: In the evaluation and treatment of accommodative convergent strabismus, in primary open-angle glaucoma, in conditions obstructing aqueous outflow, such as synechial formation that are amenable to miotic therapy, and following iridectomy.

Contraindications: In acute congestive (narrow-angle) glaucoma, in glaucoma associated with iridocyclitis, in active uveal inflammation, and in those hypersensitive to isoflurophate or to any of the components. It should be used with extreme caution, if at all, in the presence of marked vagotonia, bronchial asthma, spastic gastrointestinal disturbances, peptic ulcer, pronounced bradycardia and hypotension, recent myocardial infarction, epilepsy, parkinsonism, or any other disorder that may respond adversely to vagotonic effects.

Warnings: Patients receiving this drug should not be given succinylcholine prior to or during general anesthesia because of possible respiratory and cardiovascular collapse. Due to potential adverse additive effects, administer with considerable caution to patients with myasthenia gravis who are receiving systemic anticholinesterase therapy; conversely, considerable caution should also be exercised in the use of anticholinesterase medications for the treatment of patients with myasthenia gravis who are undergoing topical therapy with cholinesterase inhibitors. Safe use during pregnancy has not been established; therefore, its potential benefits must be weighed against the possible hazards to the mother and fetus.

Precautions: With the exception of patients with aphakia, isoflurophate should be used in glaucoma only when shorter-acting miotics have proved inadequate. Gonioscopy is recommended prior to medication. It is advised that the drug be discontinued before undergoing ophthalmologic surgery. It should be used with caution in ocular hypertension accompanied by intraocular inflammatory processes. Systemic effects are rare when the drug is administered topically by the proper technique in recommended doses. However, despite all precautions, there is some evidence that repeated administration of the drug may cause depression of the concentration of cholinesterase in the serum and erythrocytes, with resultant systemic effects. As systemic absorption may occur through the skin, any isoflurophate that might touch the skin should be thoroughly washed away with large volumes of water. The drug should be discontinued if salivation, urinary incontinence, diarrhea, profuse sweating, muscle weakness, respiratory difficulties, shock or cardiac irregularities occur. Patients receiving this drug who are exposed to organophosphate-type insecticides and pesticides should be cautioned of the added systemic effects from absorption through the respiratory tract or skin. Wearing of respiratory masks, frequent washing, and clothing changes may be advisable.

Adverse Reactions: Those that may occur include stinging, burning, lacrimation, muscular twitching of the eyelids, conjunctival and ciliary hyperemia, browache, headache, induced myopia, activation of latent iritis or uveitis, and occasionally, retinal detachment. Prolonged use may result in the development of iris cysts, particularly in children, conjunctival thickening and obstruction of nasolacrimal canals. Should systemic effects occur, manifested by nausea, vomiting, abdominal cramps, diarrhea, urinary incontinence, salivation, dyspnea, bradycardia, or cardiac irregularities, the parenteral administration of atropine sulfate, 0.4 to 0.6 mg or more for adults and proportionately less for children is indicated. Pralidoxime chloride, in addition to atropine, may be considered, and artificial respiration may be necessary. Lens opacities have been noted in patients on anticholinesterase therapy. Therefore, routine slit-lamp examinations, including the lens, should accompany prolonged and frequent use of this drug. A rise in intraocular pressure may occur in the treatment of wide- or open-angle glaucoma; this occurrence may be critical and seriously damaging to the eye.

Dosage and Administration: *Topically,* for ophthalmic use only. *For the treatment of glaucoma:* initially, 1/4 inch strip of ointment is placed in the eye every 8 to 72 hours. A decrease in intraocular pressure should occur within a few hours. Tonometric examinations should be performed at least hourly for 3 or 4 hours, to ascertain that no immediate rise in pressure occurs. *For the treatment of strabismus:* 1/4 inch strip of ointment is administered every night for 2 weeks. *For accommodative esotropia:* initially, 1/4 inch strip of ointment every night for 2 weeks, then reduced to from 1/4 inch strip every other day to 1/4 inch strip once a week for 2 months.

Availability:
FLOROPRYL® Ophthalmic Ointment, 0.025% in tubes of 3.5 gm. **(Merck Sharp & Dohme)**

ISOMETHEPTENE

Chemical Name: N,1,5,-Trimethyl-4-hexenylamine.

Description: Isometheptene is a smooth muscle relaxant, and exerts its antispasmodic effect by stimulating the sympathetic inhibitory fibers and by a direct musculotropic action, thus reducing spasm without disturbing normal functions. The vasoconstricting effect of the drug is exerted mainly on the dilated carotid and cerebral vessels; however, it does not produce ergot-like effects.

Indications: May be effective in the prevention and relief of migraine, migraine variants, and tension headache. The addition of an analgesic [acetaminophen] and a sedative [dichloralphenazone] helps to elevate the patient's threshold to pain and to alleviate the emotional overtones.

Contraindications: In patients taking MAO inhibitors, and in those with severe renal, hepatic or organic heart disease, severe hypertension or glaucoma.

Precautions: Caution should be observed in patients with hypertension or peripheral vascular disease and after recent cardiovascular attacks.

Adverse Reactions: Elevated blood pressure, transient dizziness, lassitude, cold sweats, and skin rash are usually mild and can be controlled or eliminated by reducing the dose.

Dosage and Administration: *Orally. For migraine headache,* initially for adults, 2 capsules followed by 1 capsule every hour until relief is obtained. Up to 5 capsules may be given within a 12-hour period. *For tension headache,* the usual adult dose is 1 or 2 capsules every 4 hours. Up to 8 capsules may be given within a 24-hour period.

Availability:
MIDRIN® Capsules (as mucate), 65 mg with dichloralphenazone, 100 mg and acetaminophen, 325 mg in bottles of 50, 100 and 500. **(Carnrick)**

ISONIAZID

Chemical Name: Isonicotinic acid hydrazide (INH).

Description: Isoniazid occurs as colorless or white crystals or as a crystalline powder freely soluble in water and sparingly soluble in alcohol.

It is active against human, bovine, and B.C.G. strains of *Mycobacterium tuberculosis.* A highly specific agent, it is ineffective against other microorganisms. The mode of action is unknown but the drug is firmly bound to actively growing, sensitive, tubercle bacilli and does not affect these organisms when they are in the metabolic resting state. When used alone, resistant strains emerge very rapidly; when combined with other tuberculostatic drugs, the emergence of resistant strains is delayed. It is rapidly and almost completely absorbed, when administered either orally or parenterally, and peak blood levels are reached in about 1 to 2 hours and decline to 50% or less within 6 hours. It diffuses readily into all body fluids (cerebrospinal, pleural, and ascitic), tissues, organs, and excreta (saliva, sputum and feces). The drug also passes through the placental barrier and into milk in concentrations comparable to those in the plasma. From 50 to 70% of a dose of isoniazid is excreted in the urine in 24 hours.

Isoniazid is metabolized primarily by acetylation and dehydrazination. The rate of acetylation is genetically determined. Approximately 50% of Negroes and Caucasians are "slow inactivators;" while the majority of Eskimos and Orientals are "rapid inactivators." The rate of acetylation does not significantly alter the effectiveness of isoniazid. However, slow acetylation may lead to higher blood levels of the drug and thus an increase in toxic reactions.

Pyridoxine (B-6) deficiency is sometimes observed in adults receiving high doses of isoniazid and is considered due to its competition with pyridoxal phosphate for the enzyme apotryptophanase.

Indications: Treatment of all forms of active tuberculosis, preferably in conjunction with other antituberculous drugs. It is recommended for oral prophylactic use in individuals who have a high risk of developing active tuberculosis, in all infants and children under 3 years of age who exhibit positive reactions to either the Mantoux or the tuberculin patch test, and to all children and adults who have recently converted from a negative to a positive tuberculin reaction.

Contraindications: In patients who develop severe hypersensitivity reactions, including drug-induced hepatitis and acute liver disease of any etiology.

Warnings: Severe and sometimes fatal hepatitis associated with isoniazid therapy has been reported. Individuals on isoniazid preventive treatment should be carefully monitored and interviewed at monthly intervals, and should be well-informed that the daily consumption of alcohol may increase the risk of isoniazd-related hepatitis. Also, patients should be instructed to report immediately any of the prodromal symptoms of hepatitis such as fatigue, weakness, malaise, anorexia, nausea or vomiting. If symptoms and signs suggestive of hepatic damage are detected, the drug should be discontinued promptly and patients should be followed closely. Preventive treatment should be deferred in individuals with acute hepatic diseases. Isoniazid has been reported to induce pulmonary tumors in a number of strains of mice. Although no isoniazid-related congenital anomalies have been found in reproduction studies in mammalian species (mice, rats and rabbits), it has been reported that in both rats and rabbits, isoniazid may exert an embryocidal effect when administered orally during pregnancy. Therefore, it should be given to pregnant women only when therapeutically necessary. Since isoniazid has been found to cross the placental barrier and to pass into breast milk, neonates and breast-fed infants of isoniazid-treated mothers should be carefully observed for any evidence of adverse effects.

Precautions: Should be administered cautiously in patients with epilepsy and only when the condition has been controlled with appropriate medication. In some slow inactivators, the effects of phenytoin may be potentiated since isoniazid interferes with the metabolism of this drug. This may result in phenytoin intoxication which is characterized by nystagmus, ataxia and lethargy. Therefore, an adjustment in the dosage of phenytoin is necessary. Also should be given with caution and in the lowest effective doses where renal damage is suspected or known to exist. It should not be used in the treatment of renal tuberculosis unless adequate facilities for the estimation of isoniazid blood levels are available. All drugs should be discontinued at the first signs of hypersensitivity reaction. If isoniazid is reinstituted, it should be in very small and gradually increasing doses to determine whether the manifestations are drug-induced. Use of isoniazid should be carefully monitored in patients with convulsive disorders, preexisting hepatic diseases, and in those who are alcoholic, or who are receiving concurrent medication on a long-term basis. Periodic ophthalmoscopic examination during isoniazid therapy is recommended when visual symptoms occur. Pyridoxine administration is recomended in individuals likely to develop neuropathies secondary to isoniazid therapy.

Adverse Reactions: Toxic effects are usually encountered only with high doses of isoniazid and the incidence is reportedly higher in "slow inactivators." These include: *Nervous system reactions:* Peripheral neuropathy occurs most often in the malnourished and is usually preceded by paresthesias in the feet and hands. Convulsions, toxic encephalopathy, optic neuritis and atrophy, memory impairment, and toxic psychosis have also been reported. *Gastrointestinal and hepatic reactions:* Nausea, vomiting, epigastric distress, elevated serum transaminases (SGOT and SGPT), bilirubinemia, bilirubinuria, hepatitis with or without jaundice. The common presenting symptoms are anorexia, nausea, vomiting, fatigue, malaise, and weakness. Isoniazid-associated hepatitis is generally considered a hypersensitivity reaction. *Hematologic reactions:* Agranulocytosis, hemolytic, sideroblastic or aplastic anemia, thrombocytopenia, and eosinophilia. *Hypersensitivity reactions:* Fever, skin eruptions (morbilliform, maculopapular, purpuric or exfoliative), lymphadenopathy and vasculitis, and a local reaction at the site of injection. *Metabolic and endocrine reactions:* Pyridoxine deficiency, pellagra, hyperglycemia, metabolic acidosis, and gynecomastia. *Miscellaneous reactions:* Rheumatic syndrome and systemic lupus erythematosus-like syndrome. Acute isoniazid poisoning is characterized by coma, intractable seizures, respiratory distress, metabolic acidosis, hyperglycemia, and acetonuria.

Dosage and Administration: *Orally or parenterally* as a single dose. Oral dosage should be given with meals. *In the treatment of active tuberculosis,* 5 mg/kg of body weight daily (up to 300 mg). Infants and children, 10 to 20 mg/kg daily (up to 300 to 500 mg). Preventive treatment, adults, 300 mg daily; infants and children, 10 mg/kg daily (up to 300 mg). Concomitant administration of pyridoxine is recommended, particularly in pediatric patients.

Availability:
Isoniazid
DOW-ISONIAZID™ Tablets, 100 and 300 mg in unit-dose cartons of 100. **(Dow)**
ISONIAZID Tablets, 100 mg in bottles of 100 and 1000. **(ICN)**
ISONIAZID Tablets, 100 mg in bottles of 100 and 1000; 300 mg in bottles of 100. **(Lilly)**
NICONYL® Tablets, 100 mg in bottles of 1000. **(Parke-Davis)**
NYDRAZID®: **(Squibb)**
Injection, 100 mg/ml in vials of 10 ml.
Syrup, 10 mg/ml in bottles of 1 pint.
Tablets, 100 mg in bottles of 100 and 1000.

ISOPHANE INSULIN (NPH): see The Insulins

ISOPROPAMIDE IODIDE

Chemical Name: (3-Carbamoyl-3,3-diphenylpropyl)diisopropylmethyl ammonium iodide.

Description: Isopropamide is a quaternary ammonium compound available as the iodide. It is a long-acting anticholinergic, producing an effective 10- to 12-hour basal antisecretory-antispasmodic response at low, oral, dosage levels. The effects of the drug are similar to the peripheral effects produced by the belladonna alkaloids. It does not exert sympathetic ganglionic blockade unless therapeutic doses are exceeded.

Indications: Adjunctive therapy in the treatment of peptic ulcer. Also, may be useful in the irritable bowel syndrome (irritable colon, spastic colon, mucous colitis, acute enterocolitis, and functional gastrointestinal disorders). Whether or not the drug heals the ulcer, decreases the rate of recurrences or prevents complications has not been concluded.

Contraindications: Glaucoma; obstructive uropathy (e.g., bladder neck obstruction due to prostatic hypertrophy); obstructive disease of the gastrointestinal tract (as in achalasia, pyloroduodenal stenosis, etc.); obstructive or paralytic ileus, intestinal atony of the elderly or debilitated patients; unstable cardiovascular status in acute hemorrhage; severe ulcerative colitis; toxic megacolon complicating ulcerative colitis; and myasthenia gravis.

Warnings: Heat prostration (fever and heat stroke due to decreased sweating) may occur in the presence of a high environmental temperature. Treatment with this drug in patients with diarrhea due to incomplete intestinal obstruction, especially those with ileostomy or colostomy would be inappropriate and possibly harmful. Since drowsiness or blurred vision may occur, the patient should be cautioned not to engage in activities requiring alertness or motor coordination. When used in pregnant or lactating women or in women of childbearing potential, the anticipated therapeutic benefits must be weighed against the possible hazards to the mother and fetus.

Precautions: Since the iodine in isopropamide iodide may alter PBI tests results and will suppress I^{131} uptake, it is advised that therapy be discontinued one week prior to these tests. Although rare, an iodine skin rash may occur. Cautious use is required in elderly patients, in the presence of autonomic neuropathy, hepatic or renal disease, ulcerative colitis, hyperthyroidism, coronary heart disease, congestive heart failure, cardiac arrhythmia, hypertension, nonobstructing prostatic hypertrophy, and hiatal hernia associated with reflux esophagitis. It should be noted that the use of anticholinergic drugs in the treatment of gastric ulcer may produce a delay in gastric emptying time (antral stasis) and, thus, complicate therapy. This drug may not be effective in the presence of complications due to biliary tract disease. Tachycardia should be ruled out before giving this drug since an increase in heart rate may result. Overdosage may produce a curare-like action.

Adverse Reactions: Those usually observed were xerostomia (dry mouth); urinary hesitancy and retention; blurred vision; tachycardia; palpitations; mydriasis; cycloplegia; constipation; bloated feeling; nausea; dysphagia; fever; and nasal congestion. Other adverse reactions possible with anticholinergic agents include: increased ocular tension; loss of taste; headaches; nervousness; drowsiness; weakness; dizziness; insomnia; vomiting; impotence; suppression of lactation; severe allergic reaction or drug idiosyncrasies including anaphylaxis; urticaria and other dermal manifestations; some degree of mental confusion and/or excitement, especially in elderly patients. Decreased sweating may occur. It should be noted that adrenergic innervation of the eccrine sweat glands on the palms of the hands and soles of the feet makes complete control of sweating impossible. Complete anhidrosis cannot occur because large doses of the drug would be required, and this would produce severe side effects from parasympathetic paralysis. Overdosage involves the cardiovascular, respiratory, gastrointestinal, central and peripheral nervous systems. Symptoms may include dryness of the mouth, dysphagia, thirst, blurred vision, dilated pupils, photophobia, fever, rapid pulse and respiratory rate, and disorientation. Depression and circulatory collapse may result from severe overdosage.

Dosage and Administration: *Orally.* Adults and children over 12 years of age, 5 mg every 12 hours. Some patients with severe symptoms may require 10 mg or more every 12 hours. The usual supportive measures, such as diet, antacids, sedatives, rest and psychotherapy, are recommended to assure maximal benefits.

Availability:
DARBID® Tablets, 5 mg in bottles of 50. **(Smith Kline & French)**

ISOPROTERENOL
METAPROTERENOL

Chemical Name: Isoproterenol: 3,4-Dihydroxy-α-[(isopropylamino)methyl] benzyl alcohol.

Chemical Name: Metaproterenol: 1-(3,5-Dihydroxyphenyl)-2-isopropylaminoethanol sulfate.

Description: *Isoproterenol* is a synthetic, beta-sympathomimetic amine structurally related to epinephrine. The hydrochloride and sulfate share the same actions and uses. The hydrochloride occurs as a white to nearly white, odorless, crystalline powder freely soluble in water and sparingly soluble in alcohol. *Metaproterenol sulfate* is a potent beta-adrenergic stimulator with rapid onset of action. It occurs as a white, crystalline, racemic mixture of 2 optically active isomers. Its chemical structure differs from that of isoproterenol in that its 2 hydroxy groups are attached at the meta position on the benzene ring instead of 1 at the meta and 1 at the para position.

It has been postulated that beta-adrenergic stimulating agents produce many of their pharmacological effects by activating the enzyme adenyl cyclase which catalyzes the conversion of adenosine triphosphate to cyclic adenosine monophosphate. Acting almost exclusively on beta receptors, *isoproterenol* increases cardiac output (positive inotropic and chronotropic effects), decreases peripheral vascular resistance, increases venous return to the heart, and relaxes most smooth muscles, primarily those of the bronchial and gastrointestinal tracts. Excessive doses can produce a sharp drop in blood pressure and repeated large doses may result in cardiac enlargement and focal myocarditis. Its duration of action and calorigenic effects are similar to those of epinephrine; however, it causes less hyperglycemia. *Isoproterenol* can also cause CNS excitation. Clinical studies have revealed that when *metaproterenol* is administered orally approximately 40% of the compound is absorbed and is excreted primarily as glucuronic acid conjugates. No studies to date have been performed on the absorption, biotransformation and excretion of the drug following inhalation administration.

Oral inhalation of these drugs is the preferred route of administration for the treatment of asthmatic attacks. They provide relaxation of the smooth muscle of the bronchioles thus preventing and relieving bronchoconstriction.

Indications: Orally, for the management of bronchial asthma, allergic coughs and the chronic bronchitis usually associated with these conditions. Sublingually, for the treatment of carotid sinus hypersensitivity; ventricular tachycardia and ventricular arrhythmias; Adams-Stokes syndrome and atrioventricular heart block. May also be used as a bronchodilator in the management of patients with bronchopulmonary disease. Oral inhalation, for the treatment of bronchospasm associated with acute and chronic bronchial asthma, pulmonary emphysema, bronchitis, and bronchiectasis. Parenterally, for the management of bronchospasm during anesthesia and of shock (hypofusion syndrome) and in the treatment of cardiac standstill or arrest as an adjunctive measure.

Contraindications: In patients with tachycardia caused by digitalis intoxication. Its use in patients with preexisting cardiac arrhythmias associated with tachycardia generally is considered contraindicated because the stimulating effect on the heart may aggravate such disorders. Contraindicated also in those patients hypersensitive to the drug or to any of the drugs combined with isoproterenol or metaproterenol.

Warnings: Frequent or continuous use for prolonged periods of time is not recommended. Deaths have been reported following excessive use, and cardiac arrest was noted in several instances. Also, a few patients have been reported to develop severe paradoxical airway resistance with repeated use of these inhalation preparations. Facilities for administering oxygen mixtures and respiratory assistance should be immediately available. As with all potent drugs use in pregnant or lactating women or in women of childbearing potential requires that the expected benefits of the drug outweigh the possible hazards to the mother and child.

Precautions: These compounds and epinephrine should not be used together, since both are direct cardiac stimulants and their combined effects may induce serious arrhythmia. However, they may be used alternately. Dosage should be adjusted carefully for patients with coronary insufficiency, hypertension, congestive heart failure, coronary artery disease, diabetes mellitus, or hyperthyroidism, and in those sensitive to sympathomimetic amines. Caution is also recommended when used in patients with prostatic hypertrophy or glaucoma. Large doses of iodides (component of an elixir) may elevate protein-bound iodine values, and should not be given during pregnancy since goiter may be induced in the fetus. For precautions to be exercised in the hypoperfusion syndrome, in cardiac arrest and arrhythmias, and bronchospasm during anesthesia, the package literature should be consulted.

Adverse Reactions: Reported reactions are similar to those usually occurring with sympathomimetic agents, and are usually dose-related. These include flushed skin, sweating, mild tremors, nervousness, restlessness, headache, weakness, dizziness, tachycardia with palpitations, hypertension, pulmonary edema, precipitation of Adams-Stokes seizures during normal sinus rhythm or transient heart block, throat irritation due to the alcohol in the aerosol preparation and nausea and vomiting [overdosage with sublingual tablets], and bad taste. Reactions to iodides include metallic taste, acneiform eruptions, erythema of face and chest, gastric distress, and painful swelling of the salivary glands. Patients should be evaluated periodically for possible depression of thyroid function. Theophylline may cause gastric intolerance such as nausea and vomiting.

Dosage and Administration: *Oral Inhalation:* To control an acute attack of asthma, a single deep inhalation, followed by another if necessary. Or 5 to 15 deep inhalations using the 1:200 solution; 7 deep inhalations using 5 drops of the 1:100 solution or 2 or 3 inhalations using the micronized powder (usually treatment need not be repeated more often than every 3 to 4 hours). Patients should not exceed a total of 12 inhalations a day. *Not recommended for children under 12 years of age. Sublingually,* 10 to 20 mg depending upon the patient's response. Dosage should not exceed 60 mg/day. *Orally:* adults, 30 ml or one 20-mg tablet 3 or 4 times daily; children, 1 to 3 years of age, 5 to 10 ml; 3 to 6 years, 10 to 15 ml; 6 to 12 years, 15 to 30 ml; children 9 years of age and over, one 20-mg tablet; 6 to 9 years, one 10-mg tablet. The tablets are not recommended for children under 6 years of age. For cardiac standstill and heart block, Isuprel Injection: *Intravenously,* the initial dose range is 0.02 to 0.06 mg (1 to 3 ml of diluted solution, 1:50,000); subsequent dose range is 0.01 to 0.2 mg (0.5 to 10 ml of diluted solution). *Intravenous infusion,* the initial dose range is 5 mcg/minute (1.25 ml of diluted solution 1:250,000/minute). *Intramuscularly,* 0.2 mg (1 ml); subsequent dose range is 0.02 to 1 mg (0.1 to 5 ml). *Subcutaneously,* 0.2 mg (1 ml); subsequent dose range is 0.15 to 0.2 mg (0.75 to 1 ml). *Intracardiac,* 0.02 mg (0.1 ml). Isuprel Glossets: *Sublingually,* the initial dose is 10 mg; subsequent dose range is 5 to 50 mg.

Availability:

Isoproterenol Hydrochloride

DUO-MEDIHALER® Solution, 4 mg with phenylephrine bitartrate, 6 mg/ml in vials of 15 and 22.5 ml with or without oral adapter. **(Riker)**

ISUPREL®: **(Breon)**

Glossets®, 10 and 15 mg (for sublingual use) in bottles of 50.

Injection, 0.2 mg/ml (1:5000) in ampuls of 1 and 5 ml.

Mistometer® Solution, 2.8 mg/ml (1:400) in aerosol vials of 15 ml.

Solution for Nebulization, 1:100 in bottles of 10 ml; 1:200 in bottles of 10 and 60 ml.

Compound Elixir: Each 15 ml contains isoproterenol hydrochloride, 2.5 mg with phenobarbital, 6 mg (**Warning:** May be habit-forming); ephedrine sulfate, 12 mg; theophylline, 45 mg; potassium iodide, 150 mg and alcohol, 19% in bottles of 1 pint and 1 gallon.

NORISODRINE® Aerotrol® (controlled-dose nebulizer), 0.25% in containers of 15 ml. **(Abbott)**

VAPO-ISO® Solution, 0.5% (1:200) in vials of 10 ml with dropper. **(Fisons)**

Isoproterenol Sulfate

MEDIHALER-ISO® Suspension, 2 mg/ml in vials of 15 and 22.5 ml with or without oral adapter. **(Riker)**

NORISODRINE®: **(Abbott)**

Oral Inhalation, 10 mg (10%) and 25 mg (25%)/Aerohaler® cartridge in cartons of 4 vials of 3 sifter cartridges. Each metered dose expressed from the inhaler delivers 0.045 and 0.11 mg, respectively of isoproterenol sulfate.

Syrup with Calcium Iodide, 3 mg with calcium iodide, 150 mg/5 ml in bottles of 1 pint and 1 gallon and in Abbo-Pac® (unit-dose) containers of 5 ml.

Metaproterenol Sulfate

ALUPENT®: **(Boehringer Ingelheim)**

Powder (micronized), 225 mg in metered-dose vials of 15 ml with mouth piece. Each metered dose expressed from the inhaler delivers approximately 0.65 mg of metaproterenol.

Syrup, 10 mg/5 ml in bottles of 1 pint.

Tablets, 10 and 20 mg in bottles of 100.

METAPREL®: **(Dorsey)**

Powder (micronized), 225 mg in metered-dose vials of 15 ml with mouth piece. Each metered dose expressed from the inhaler delivers approximately 0.65 mg of metaproterenol.

Syrup, 10 mg/5 ml in bottles of 1 pint.

Tablets, 10 and 20 mg in bottles of 100.

ISOSORBIDE DINITRATE

Chemical Name: 1,4:3,6-Dianhydrosorbitol-2,5 dinitrate.

Description: Isosorbide dinitrate, an organic nitrate, occurs as a white, crystalline powder slightly soluble in water. Its mechanism of action in the relief of angina pectoris is unknown at this time, although the basic pharmacologic action is to relax smooth muscle.

Since therapy, currently, is essentially empirical, clinical improvement is generally measured by a decrease in the severity of the symptoms of angina and the need for medication. Specifically, a reduction in number, intensity and duration of anginal attacks and a reduction in usage of nitroglycerin (prophylactic or therapeutic) have been used as a yardstick for measuring clinical improvement. It should be emphasized that in evaluating isosorbide dinitrate, clinical improvement has been measured subjectively.

Indications: Sublingually, for the prevention and treatment of angina pectoris. Orally, for the relief of angina pectoris. It is not intended to abort the acute episode, but is regarded as useful in the prophylactic treatment of angina. The addition of phenobarbital is indicated for those patients in whom the anginal attack is accompanied by anxiety or its related symptoms.

Contraindications: Hypersensitivity to the drug or to phenobarbital.

Warnings: Data supporting the use of nitrites during the early days of the acute phase of myocardial infarction are insufficient to establish safety. Phenobarbital may be habit-forming.

Precautions: Should be used with caution in patients with glaucoma. Tolerance to this drug and cross tolerance to other nitrites and nitrates may occur.

Adverse Reactions: Headache is the most common adverse reaction and may be severe and persistent. Lowering the dose and the use of analgesics usually help in controlling this complication which will eventually diminish or disappear as therapy is continued. Cutaneous vasodilation with flushing; dizziness and weakness as well as other signs of cerebral ischemia associated with postural hypotension; drug rash and/or exfoliative dermatitis have been noted. An occasional patient exhibits marked sensitivity to the hypotensive effects of nitrites and severe responses (nausea, vomiting, weakness, restlessness, pallor, perspiration and collapse) can occur even with the usual therapeutic dose. Alcohol may enhance this effect. This drug can act as a physiological antagonist to norepinephrine, acetylcholine, histamine, and many other agents.

Dosage and Administration: The prevention and treatment of an anginal attack, 2.5 to 10 mg *orally* or *sublingually* 3 or 4 times daily or 1 sustained-action capsule every 12 hours. Oral dosage should be taken when the stomach is empty. If vascular headache cannot be controlled effectively by ordinary measures, the drug may be taken with meals to minimize this effect. Chewable or sublingual administration begins to exert its effect within 2 to 5 minutes and persists for 1 to 2 hours. Oral and sustained-action administration begins to exert its effect within 15 to 30 minutes and persists for up to 12 hours.

Availability:
ISORDIL®: **(Ives)**
Chewable Tablets, 10 mg in bottles of 100 and in Clinipak® (unit-dose packages) of 100.
Tetradose® Oral Tablets, (E.Z. Split®), 5 and 10 mg in bottles of 100, 500 and 1000 and in Clinipaks® of 100; 20 mg in bottles of 100 and 500 and in Clinipaks of 100; 30 mg in bottles of 100.
Sublingual Tablets, 2.5 mg in bottles of 100 and 500 and in Clinipaks of 100; 5 mg in bottles of 100, 250 and 500 and in Clinipaks® of 100.
Tembids® (sustained-action tablets), 40 mg in bottles of 100, 500 and 1000; (sustained-action capsules), 40 mg in bottles of 100 and 500.
w/Phenobarbital Tablets, 10 mg with phenobarbital, 15 mg in bottles of 100 and 500.
ISOSORBIDE DINITRATE: **(Lederle)**
Sublingual Tablets, 2.5 and 5 mg in bottles of 1000.
Tablets, 5 and 10 mg in bottles of 1000.
SORBITRATE®: **(Stuart)**
Chewable Tablets, 5 mg in bottles of 100 and 500 and in unit-dose packages of 100; 10 mg in bottles of 100.
Oral Tablets, 5 and 10 mg in bottles of 100 and 500 and in unit-dose packages of 100; 20 mg in bottles of 100.
S.A. Tablets (sustained action), 40 mg in bottles of 100 and 500.
Sublingual Tablets, 2.5 and 5 mg in bottles of 100 and 500; the 5 mg tablets are also available in unit-dose packages of 100.
w/Phenobarbital Tablets, 10 mg with phenobarbital, 15 mg in bottles of 100.

ISOXSUPRINE HYDROCHLORIDE

Chemical Name: *p*-Hydroxy-α-[1-[(1-methyl-2-phenoxyethyl)amino]ethyl]benzyl hydrochloride.

Description: Isoxsuprine hydrochloride, a beta-adrenergic stimulant, occurs as a white, odorless, bitter, crystalline substance sparingly soluble in water.

Isoxsuprine increases peripheral vascular and cerebrovascular blood flow by directly relaxing the vascular musculature, and relaxes the uterine muscles by acting directly on the myometrium. It acts without ganglionic blockade, neural mediation, hormonal or other undesirable effects. Rapidly absorbed from the gastrointestinal tract, therapeutic blood levels are attained within 1 hour and persist for about 3 hours.

Indications: As a vasodilator in peripheral vascular disease and cerebrovascular insufficiency. It may be used in the management of thromboangiitis obliterans (Buerger's disease), Raynaud's disease and threatened abortion.

Contraindications: Parenterally in the presence of hypotension or tachycardia. Intravenous administration is not recommended because of the increased likelihood of adverse reactions. There are no known contraindications to oral administration at recommended dosage levels.

Precautions: Do not give immediately postpartum or in the presence of arterial bleeding.

Adverse Reactions: Adverse effects usually are due to overdosage and may consist of transient palpitation or dizziness as well as nausea, vomiting, and abdominal distress. Single intramuscular doses of 10 mg may result in hypotension and tachycardia becoming more pronounced as the dosage is increased. Single intramuscular doses in excess of 10 mg are therefore not recommended. Although rarely occurring, the appearance of a severe rash following oral administration warrants immediate withdrawal of the drug.

Dosage and Administration: *Orally,* 10 to 20 mg 3 or 4 times daily. *Intramuscularly,* 5 to 10 mg 2 or 3 times daily. Intramuscular administration may be used initially in severe or acute conditions.

Availability:
ISOLAIT Tablets, 10 mg in bottles of 1000. **(Elder)**
VASODILAN®: **(Mead Johnson)**
Injection, 5 mg/ml in ampuls of 2 ml.
Tablets, 10 mg in bottles of 100, 1000 and 5000 and in unit-dose packages of 100; 20 mg in bottles of 100, 500, 1000 and 5000 and in unit-dose packages of 100.

KANAMYCIN SULFATE

Description: Kanamycin is an aminoglycoside antibiotic produced by the fermentation of cultures of *Streptomyces kanamyceticus.* The antibiotic is composed of 2 amino sugars (hexosamines) glycosidically linked to deoxystreptamine, and is similar to neomycin and to streptomycin, both structurally and pharmacologically. The sulfate salt of kanamycin occurs as a white, odorless, crystalline powder freely soluble in water and insoluble in alcohol.

Kanamycin sulfate is rapidly absorbed following intramuscular injection—little or none is absorbed following oral administration—reaches peak serum levels within 1 hour and is almost completely dissipated by the 12th hour. The drug diffuses rapidly into most body fluids including synovial and peritoneal fluids as well as bile, but significant amounts do not diffuse into the amniotic fluid or into spinal fluid through uninflamed meninges, or into the saliva or bronchial secretions. The drug is excreted almost entirely by glomerular filtration and is not reabsorbed by the renal tubules. Hence, high concentrations are reached in the nephron and the urine may contain levels 10 to 20 times higher than those in serum. Renal excretion is extremely rapid. Approximately ½ of the injected dose is excreted within 4 hours in patients with normal renal function and excretion is complete within 24 to 48 hours. Patients with impaired renal function or with diminished glomerular filtration pressure excrete kanamycin much more slowly. Such patients may build up excessively high blood levels which greatly increase the risk of ototoxic reactions. Following oral administration, most of the intestinal bacteria are rapidly eliminated with bacterial suppression lasting for 48 to 72 hours. The unabsorbed portion of the drug is excreted unchanged in the feces.

Kanamycin is active in vitro against many strains of *Staphylococcus aureus, Staphylococcus epidermidis, Neisseria gonorrhoeae, H. influenzae, E. coli, Enterobacter aerogenes, Shi-*

gella, Salmonella, K. pneumoniae, Serratia marcescens, Mima-Herellea, and many strains of *Proteus* that are frequently resistant to other antibiotics. The invading organism should be cultured and its sensitivity demonstrated as a guide to therapy. If the Kirby-Bauer method of disc sensitivity is used, a 30-mcg kanamycin disc should give a zone of over 17 mm when tested against a kanamycin-sensitive bacterial strain. Although most strains of *Salmonella typhosa* are sensitive in vitro to kanamycin, the clinical efficacy of the drug in acute typhoid fever or for the relief of the typhoid carrier state has not been established.

Indications: *Oral kanamycin:* Suppression of intestinal bacteria for short-term adjunctive therapy, and for preoperative sterilization of the bowel, treatment of intestinal infections due to sensitive organisms (including *Shigella* and *Salmonella*), and conjunctively with parenteral kanamycin in the adjunctive treatment of neurologic manifestations associated with severe liver damage (coma). *Parenteral kanamycin:* The treatment of the following bacterial infections due to sensitive organisms: acute and chronic pyelonephritis, cystitis, prostatitis, tracheitis, pneumonia, lung abscess, pleuritis, pulmonary complications of cystic fibrosis, abscesses, wound infections, infected grafts, cellulitis, lymphangitis, pyoderma, anthrax, osteomyelitis, periostitis, septicemia, bacteremia, amebiasis, salmonellosis, shigellosis, gastroenteritis, staphylococcal enterocolitis, and conjunctively with other antibacterial agents in the treatment of mixed infections and superinfections.

Contraindications: A history of hypersensitivity to kanamycin sulfate is a contraindication to its use. Prior administration of kanamycin sulfate or other ototoxic agents which may have induced subclinical damage to the eighth nerve may contraindicate kanamycin sulfate if effective alternative therapy is available. **This drug is not indicated in long-term therapy** (e.g., tuberculosis) **because of the ototoxic hazard with extended administration.**

Warnings: The major toxic effect of parenterally administered kanamycin sulfate is its action on the auditory portion of the eighth nerve. High frequency deafness usually occurs first and can be detected by audiometric testing. Tinnitus or vertigo may occur and are evidence of vestibular injury and impending bilateral, irreversible deafness. In patients with impaired kidney function, the risk of severe ototoxic reactions and permanent deafness is sharply increased. In such cases, the daily dosage should be reduced and the interval between doses lengthened. If there is evidence of progressive renal dysfunction (increasing NPN, BUN, creatinine or oliguria) during therapy, audiometric tests are advised and discontinuation of the drug should be considered. Older patients and patients receiving a total dose of more than 15 gm of kanamycin sulfate should be carefully observed for signs of eighth nerve damage. Infants and children generally tolerate the drug well; and when the recommended precautions are followed, the incidence of toxic reactions is low. Although there have been isolated reports of respiratory depression following intraperitoneal instillation of kanamycin, there is no conclusive proof that this side-effect can be produced with recommended doses of the drug. The concurrent systemic use of other ototoxic and/or nephrotoxic drugs, particularly streptomycin, polymyxin B, polymyxin E (colistin), neomycin, gentamicin, and viomycin, should be avoided. The administration of kanamycin sulfate and rapid-acting diuretic agents, e.g., ethacrynic acid, furosemide, meralluride sodium, mercaptomerin sodium, and mannitol (particularly when the diuretic is given intravenously) may cause irreversible deafness. Therefore, concurrent use of these agents should be avoided. Safe use of this drug during pregnancy has not been established.

Precautions: Because of the high concentration of kanamycin in the urinary excretory system, patients should be well hydrated to prevent chemical irritation of the renal tubules. Kidney function should be assessed prior to initiating therapy and periodically during the course of treatment. The drug should be discontinued at the first sign of renal damage or auditory nerve damage. The risk of ototoxicity is increased when kanamycin is used in conjunction with ethacrynic acid, and irreversible deafness may result. Neuromuscular paralysis with respiratory depression may occur when this drug is administered intraperitoneally concomitantly with anesthesia and muscle-relaxing drugs such as ether, tubocurarine, succinylcholine, decamethonium, and sodium citrate. In such instances, patients should be observed carefully for signs of respiratory depression. The overgrowth of resistant organisms, such as bacteroides, some strains of *Clostridia,* enterococci and yeasts, has been observed. If superinfection appears, the drug should be discontinued and appropriate therapy instituted. The preoperative use of oral kanamycin is contraindicated in the presence of intestinal obstruction. Although negligible amounts of oral kanamycin are absorbed from intact intestinal mucosa, the possibility of increased absorption from ulcerated or denuded areas should be considered. Parenteral kanamycin should *not* be mixed with other antibacterial agents; each should be given separately according to its recommended route of administration and dosage.

Adverse Reactions: *Nephrotoxicity*—Including albuminuria, presence of red and white cells, and granular casts; azotemia and oliguria have been reported. *Ototoxicity*—Tinnitus, vertigo, and partially reversible to irreversible deafness have been reported, usually associated with higher than recommended dosage. Rapid development of hearing loss has been reported in patients with poor kidney function treated concurrently with kanamycin and one of the rapid-acting diuretic agents given intravenously. These have included ethacrynic acid, furosemide, and mannitol. *Other*—Some local irritation or pain may follow intramuscular injection. In addition to the serious toxic effects described above, other adverse reactions of the drug observed on rare occasions are skin rash, drug fever, headache, and paresthesia. The most common adverse reactions to oral administration are nausea, vomiting and diarrhea. The "Malabsorption Syndrome" characterized by increased fecal fat, decreased serum carotene, and a fall in xylose absorption has been reported with prolonged therapy.

Dosage and Administration: *Orally. Preoperative sterilization of the bowel:* 1 gm every hour for 4 hours, followed by 1 gm every 6 hours for 36 to 72 hours. *Intestinal infections:* adults, 3 to 4 gm/day in divided doses for 5 to 7 days. Infants and children, 50 mg/kg/day in 4 to 6 divided doses for 5 to 7 days. *Hepatic coma:* 8 to 12 gm/day in divided doses. *Intramuscularly.* The usual dosage for adults or children is 15 mg/kg/day—not to exceed 1.5 gm/day—in divided doses every 6 to 8 hours, or every 12 hours if continuously high blood levels are desired. *Intravenously.* This route is recommended only when the intramuscular route is not feasible, but *never* in patients with severe renal insufficiency. Adults and children, 15 to 30 mg/kg/day in 2 or 3 divided doses, diluted with sodium chloride injection or 5% dextrose in water injection. Dissolving the contents of one 0.5-gm vial in 200 ml or the contents of one 1-gm vial in 400 ml of sterile diluent will yield a concentration of 2.5 mg/ml. The resultant solution should be given by slow intravenous infusion at the rate of 60 to 80 drops/minute. For other routes of administration and dosages employed, consult the package literature.

Availability:
KANTREX®: **(Bristol)**
Capsules, 0.5 gm in bottles of 20 and 100.
Injection, 0.5 gm/2 ml in ampuls of 2 ml; 1 gm/3 ml in ampuls of 3 ml.
Pediatric Injection, 75 mg/2 ml in ampuls of 2 ml.

KERALYT

Description: Contains salicylic acid, 6% in a gel containing propylene glycol, 60% and ethyl alcohol, 19.4%.

Indications: For removal of excessive keratin in hyperkeratotic skin disorders including ichthyoses (vulgaris, sex-linked and lamellar), keratosis palmaris, plantaris and pilaris, pityriasis rubra pilaris, psoriasis of the body, scalp, palms, and soles of feet. Has been found helpful as adjunctive therapy for fungal infections and for verruca plantaris (a viral epidermal tumor of the sole of the foot).

Contraindications: Hypersensitivity to any of the components.

Precautions: Due to the salicylic acid content, use in children under 12 years of age should be limited to no more than 1 tube (28.4 gm) in 24 hours. Contact with eyes and mucous membranes should be avoided, and should be kept out of reach of children. *Recommended for external use only.*

Dosage and Administration: *Topically.* Before bedtime, hydrate the skin by soaking or by applications of hot packs for at least 5 minutes, then apply gel to the affected area and place under occlusion. The medication is washed off in the morning, and if excessive drying and/or irritation is noted, a bland cream or lotion may be applied. Once clearing is apparent, an occasional application will usually maintain the remission. In those areas where occlusion is difficult or impossible, more frequent applications may be made. Unless hands are being treated, they should be washed thoroughly after each application.

Availability:
KERALYT® Gel in tubes of 28.4 gm. **(Westwood)**

KETAMINE HYDROCHLORIDE

Chemical Name: dl 2-(*o*-Chlorophenyl)-2-(methylamino)cyclohexanone hydrochloride.

Description: Ketamine hydrochloride, a cyclohexanone agent that is chemically related to phencyclidine, is a rapid-acting, nonbarbiturate, general anesthetic that produces anesthesia characterized by profound analgesia, normal pharyngeal-laryngeal reflexes, normal or slightly enhanced skeletal muscle tone, cardiovascular and respiratory stimulation, and occasionally a transient and minimal respiratory depression.

Animal studies have shown that the drug is rapidly absorbed following parenteral administration and that it is rapidly distributed into body tissues, with relatively high concentrations appearing in body fat, liver, lung and brain; lower concentrations have been found in the heart, skeletal muscle and blood plasma. Placental transfer of the drug occurred in dogs and monkeys. No significant degree of binding to serum albumin has been found.

Immediately following injection, blood pressure begins to rise reaching a maximum within a few minutes, and generally returning to preanesthetic values within 15 minutes; the median peak rise ranges from 20 to 25% of the preanesthetic level.

The clinical anesthetic state produced has been termed "dissociative anesthesia" In that it appears to interrupt selectively association pathways of the brain before producing somesthetic sensory blockade. It may selectively depress the thalamoneocortical system before significantly obtunding the more primitive cerebral centers and pathways (reticular activating and limbic systems).

Indications: As the sole anesthetic agent for diagnostic and surgical procedures of short duration; with additional doses, it can be used in procedures requiring anesthesia for periods of 6 hours or longer. If skeletal muscle relaxation is desired, a muscle relaxant should be used. The drug is also recommended for the induction of anesthesia prior to the administration of other general anesthetic agents, and to supplement low potency agents such as nitrous oxide. Specific areas of application are described fully in the package literature.

Contraindications: Patients with significant elevation of blood pressure, and those known to be hypersensitive to the drug.

Warnings: The drug should be used by or under the direction of an anesthesiologist. Cardiac function should be monitored continually during the procedure in patients with hypertension or cardiac decompensation. Because of chemical interaction (precipitate formation), barbiturates and ketamine hydrochloride *should not* be mixed in the same syringe. Recovery time may be prolonged if barbiturates or narcotics, or both, are used concomitantly with ketamine. Postoperative confusional states may occur during the recovery period. Overdosage or a too rapid rate of administration of ketamine may cause respiratory depression, in which case supportive ventilation should be employed. Mechanical support of respiration is preferred to the administration of analeptic agents. Safe use during pregnancy has not been established.

Precautions: Resuscitative equipment should be available and ready to use. Emergence reactions, which occur in about 12% of the patients, can be highly disturbing. Vivid dreams, usually unpleasant, may occur during the recovery period. Psychic changes are manifested by hallucinations and delirium, and may be accompanied by confusion, excitement and irrational behavior. These may persist for a few hours; however, recurrences have taken place up to 24 hours postoperatively. Emergence reactions have been reported to occur more frequently in adults (except for those over 65 years of age) than in children, thus establishing the fact that these reactions are not so closely related to dosage but bear a definite relation to the age of the patient. They are also less frequent when the drug is given intramuscularly. The incidence of these reactions may be reduced if verbal and tactile stimulation of the patient is minimized during the recovery period. This does not preclude the monitoring of vital signs. In addition, the use of a small hypnotic dose of a short-acting or ultrashort-acting barbiturate or other agent such as diazepam may be required to terminate a severe emergence reaction. Mechanical stimulation of the pharynx should be avoided whenever possible if ketamine is used alone. In pharyngeal, laryngeal or bronchial procedures, adequate muscle relaxants are required because of active reflexes. In surgical procedures involving visceral pain pathways, ketamine should be supplemented with a drug that dulls sensibility to pain. Utmost care should be exercised in chronic alcoholics and in the acute alcoholic-intoxicated patient. An increase in cerebrospinal fluid pressure has been reported following administration of ketamine. Use with extreme caution in patients with preanesthetic elevated cerebrospinal fluid pressure.

Adverse Reactions: *Cardiovascular:* Blood pressure and pulse rate are frequently elevated following administration of ketamine. However, hypotension and bradycardia have been observed. Arrhythmia has been noted. *Respiration:* Although respiration is frequently stimulated, severe depression of respiration or apnea may occur following rapid intravenous administration of high doses of this anesthetic. Laryngospasm and other forms of airway obstruction have occurred during ketamine anesthesia. *Eye:* Diplopia and nystagmus have been noted following administration. It also may cause a slight elevation in intraocular pressure measurement. *Psychological:* Emergence reactions manifested by hallucinations and delirium which may be accompanied by confusion, excitement, and irritational behavior. *Neurological:* In some patients, enhanced skeletal muscle tone may be manifested by tonic and clonic movements sometimes resembling seizures. *Gastrointestinal:* Anorexia, nausea, and vomiting have been observed; however, these are not usually severe and allow the great majority of patients to take liquids by mouth shortly after regaining consciousness. *General:* Local pain and exanthema at the injection site have infrequently been reported. Transient erythema and/or morbilliform rash have also been reported.

Dosage and Administration: Because of rapid induction following the initial intravenous injection, the patient should be in a supported position during administration. The initial *intravenous* dose may range from 1 to 4.5 mg/kg of body weight. The average amount required to produce 5 to 10 minutes of surgical anesthesia has been 2 mg/kg of body weight. Anesthesia is achieved within 30 seconds after injection. The dose should be given slowly over a period of 1 minute. More rapid administration may result in respiratory depression and enhanced pressor response. The initial *intramuscular* dose may range from 6.5 to 13 mg/kg of body weight. A dose of 10 mg/kg usually produces surgical anesthesia for 12 to 25 minutes. Increments of 1/2 to the full induction dose may be repeated as needed for the maintenance of anesthesia.

Availability:
KETAJECT® Solution (as hydrochloride equivalent to ketamine base), 10 mg/ml in vials of 20 and 50 ml; 50 mg/ml in vials of 10 ml; 100 mg/ml in vials of 5 ml. **(Bristol)**
KETALAR® Solution (as hydrochloride equivalent to ketamine base), 10 mg/ml in vials of 20 and 50 ml; 50 mg/ml in vials of 10 ml; 100 mg/ml in vials of 5 ml. **(Parke-Davis)**

K-LYTE
K-LYTE/CL

Description: Each effervescent tablet and each measured dose of powder supplies 25 mEq of elemental potassium. Each DS effervescent tablet supplies 50 mEq of elemental potassium. The tablets also contain citric acid, 2.1 gm, cylamic acid, artificial flavor and color. In water the tablets become: potassium citrate, potassium bicarbonate and potassium cyclamate.

Indications: Prevention and treatment of hypokalemia which may occur secondary to diuretic or corticosteroid administration, in the presence of severe vomiting and diarrhea, or when dietary potassium is low. Carefully monitored, they may be used in the treatment of cardiac arrhythmias due to digitalis intoxication.

Contraindications: Impaired renal function with oliguria or azotemia; Addison's disease; hyperkalemia from any cause.

Warnings: High serum concentrations of potassium may cause death through cardiac depression, arrhythmias or arrest. Considerable caution is therefore advised in patients with cardiac disorders.

Precautions: Should not be used in patients with low urinary output unless under the direct supervision of a physician. Frequent checks of the clinical status of the patient, and periodic ECG and/or serum potassium levels should be performed. In established hypokalemia, attention should be directed toward correction of the frequently associated hypochloremic alkalosis and other potential electrolyte disturbances. Potassium supplements should be given cautiously to patients receiving digitalis. To minimize the possibility of gastrointestinal irritation associated with the oral ingestion of concentrated potassium salt preparations, patients should be carefully directed to dissolve each dose completely in the stated amount of water. Since each dose of K-Lyte/Cl contains about 20 to 25 calories of sucrose, this should be considered for patients who must restrict their caloric intake.

Adverse Reactions: Nausea, vomiting, diarrhea and abdominal discomfort may occur. Potassium intoxication is usually manifested by listlessness, mental confusion, tingling of the extremities and other symptoms associated with hyperkalemia.

Dosage and Administration: *Orally,* 1 tablet dissolved in ½ glass of water or 1 dose of powder dissolved in ¾ glass of water 2 to 4 times daily or 1 DS tablet in ½ glass of water 1 or 2 times daily. Generally, 2 tablets supply the daily requirement for the normal adult. **Note:** To reduce the chance of gastrointestinal upset or a too rapid absorption of potassium, it is suggested that these products be taken with meals and sipped slowly over a period of 5 to 10 minutes.

Availability:
K-LYTE® (as bicarbonate and citrate) Effervescent Tablets in cartons of 30 and 250. **(Mead Johnson)**
K-LYTE DS (as bicarbonate and citrate) Effervescent Tablets in cartons of 30. **(Mead Johnson)**
K-LYTE/Cl (as chloride) Powder in containers of 225 gm (30 individual-measured doses) and in cartons of 30 and 250 packets. **(Mead Johnson)**

KOMED HC

Description: A nonstaining, nonoily and nontacky lotion containing micronized particles of hydrocortisone acetate, 0.5%; sodium thiosulfate, 8%; salicylic acid, 2%; isopropyl alcohol, 25%; menthol, camphor, colloidal alumina, disodium edetate and purified water.

Indications: Topical treatment of acne conditions accompanied by inflammation.

Contraindications: Topical steroids are contraindicated in vaccinia, varicella, and in those patients with a history of hypersensitivity to any of the components in the preparation. Not for ophthalmic use.

Precautions: If signs of irritation or sensitivity develop, discontinue use. If bacterial or fungal infections appear during therapy, appropriate measures should be taken. Observe usual precautions attendant upon the use of topical corticosteroids.

Adverse Reactions: Burning, itching, irritation, dryness of skin, folliculitis, hypertrichosis, acneform eruptions, and hypopigmentation have been observed following topical application of corticosteroids, and maceration of the skin, secondary infection, skin atrophy, striae, and miliaria following occlusive dressings.

Dosage and Administration: *Topically.* Wash the affected area thoroughly and apply a thin film twice daily or as directed.

Availability:
KOMED® HC Lotion in squeeze bottles of 60 ml. **(Barnes-Hind)**

KUTAPRESSIN

Description: A liver derivative complex prepared by fractionation and purification in which the more common ingredients of liver extracts are eliminated. The product contains no protein —although numerous amino acids are present—is virtually nonallergenic, and does not exhibit any antianemia activity. It acts specifically to enhance the resolution of inflammation and edema.

Indications: Reduction of inflammation and edema associated with such skin conditions as acne (all forms including acne rosacea), herpes zoster, pityriasis rosea, seborrheic dermatitis, urticaria, severe sunburn, eczemas, and contact dermatitis including poison ivy and poison oak.

Contraindications: Hypersensitivity or intolerance to liver.

Precautions: Not for intravenous administration. Should be used with caution in patients known to be sensitive to liver or to other allergic diatheses.

Adverse Reactions: No serious reactions have been reported; an occasional mild allergic response may occur.

Dosage and Administration: *Subcutaneously* or *intramuscularly,* 2 ml 3 times weekly.

Availability:
KUTAPRESSIN® Injection in ampuls of 2 ml and in vials of 10 and 20 ml. **(Kremers-Urban)**

KUTRASE

KU-ZYME

Description: An enzymatic digestant to help digest proteins, carbohydrates, cellulose and fats. The addition of phenyltoloxamine and *l*-hyoscyamine, provides calmative and antispasmodic action for functional indigestion. Each capsule contains:

	Kutrase	*Ku-Zyme*
Amylolytic enzyme	30 mg	30 mg
Proteolytic enzyme	6 mg	6 mg
Lipolytic enzyme	75 mg	75 mg
Cellulolytic enzyme	2 mg	2 mg
Phenyltoloxamine citrate	15 mg	—
l-Hyoscyamine	0.0625 mg	—

Each Ku-Zyme HP capsule contains lipase, 8000 NF units; protease, 30,000 NF units and amylase, 30,000 NF units.

Indications: As an aid to patients with reduced digestive enzyme capacities and for functional indigestion in which the symptoms include gas, bloating, nervous stomach, and other anxiety-induced gastric symptoms. Ku-Zyme HP capsules are indicated as enzyme replacement therapy in such conditions as cystic fibrosis, chronic pancreatitis, postpancreatectomy, in obstruction of the pancreatic ducts caused by cancer, pancreatic insufficiency and for steatorrhea of malabsorption syndrome and postgastrectomy (Bilroth II and total). May also be employed as a presumptive test of pancreatic function, especially chronic pancreatitis-induced insufficiency.

Contraindications: Hypersensitivity to pork proteins.

Precautions: Not indicated for use in children. Caution is advised in patients with glaucoma, prostatic hypertrophy or heart disease. Phenyltoloxamine may cause drowsiness; therefore, the patient should be cautioned not to perform any hazardous operation requiring alertness or skill.

Adverse Reactions: Occasionally, slightly loose stools may occur. Possibly, an allergic reaction to one of the enzymes may develop, although this has not been reported.

Dosage and Administration: *Orally,* 1 or 2 capsules with each meal. Maximal dosage of Kutrase is 6 capsules daily. HP capsules, generally 1 to 3 capsules with each meal.

Availability:
KUTRASE® Capsules (green and white) in bottles of 50 and 500. **(Kremers-Urban)**
KU-ZYME® Capsules (yellow and white) in bottles of 50 and 500 and in unit-dose packages of 100. **(Kremers-Urban)**
KU-ZYME HP Capsules in bottles of 100. **(Kremers-Urban)**

LACTULOSE

Chemical Name: 4-0-β-Galactopyranosyl-D-fructofuranose.

Description: A synthetic disaccharide with a molecular weight of 342.3 for use in the treatment of hepatic encephalopathy. The commercial preparation contains in each 15 ml of solution 10 gm of lactulose, less than 2.2 gm of galactose, less than 1.2 gm of lactose and 1.2 gm or less of other sugars.

Controlled studies have revealed that the digestive tract does not contain enzymes which can split lactulose into its component monosaccharides, hence virtually all ingested lactulose reaches the colon unhydrolyzed. Only about 0.4 to 2% of the compound is absorbed intact, and is excreted unchanged in the urine within a time-span of 24 hours. Although its precise mechanism of action is still under discussion, it has been proposed that acidification of colonic contents by the breakdown products of lactulose causes decreased passage of ammonia from the colon into the circulation and increased passage of ammonia from the circulation into the intestinal lumen, thus reducing blood ammonia levels by 25 to 50%.

Following an oral dose, the drug undergoes bacterial fermentation in the cecum (small intestine). This action causes it to be broken down into acids of smaller molecular weight, primarily lactic acid and to a lesser extent acetic acid, which significantly lower stool pH, thus enabling the ammonia to be excreted in the feces as ammonium salts. The dose is adjusted to give the patient 2 or 3 semisolid stools daily. Beneficial effects are usually observed within 24 to 48 hours, and maximal improvement is generally seen after a week or more of therapy. Further clinical experience is necessary to decide whether or not lactulose should replace neomycin or be used in combination with it.

Indications: Prevention and treatment of portal-systemic encephalopathy, including the stages of hepatic precoma and coma.

Contraindications: Patients who require a low galactose diet.

Warnings: Although laboratory studies with pregnant animals did not reveal a teratogenic potential, the drug should not be given during pregnancy unless, in the judgment of the physician, the therapeutic benefits outweigh the possible hazards to the fetus.

Precautions: Lactulose should be used with caution in diabetic patients. Patients receiving the drug in conjuction with neomycin or other antiinfective agents should be closely monitored since these agents may eliminate certain colonic bacteria, and thus interfere with the desired degradation of lactulose, thereby preventing the acidification of colonic contents. Other laxatives should not be used, especially during the initial phase of therapy, because the loose stools resulting from their use may falsely suggest that adequate lactulose dosage has been achieved. In the overall management of portal systemic encephalopathy, it should be recognized that there is a serious underlying liver disease with complications such as electrolyte disturbance (e.g. hypokalemia) for which other specific therapy may be required.

Adverse Reactions: Lactulose may produce gaseous distention with flatulence or belching and abdominal discomfort such as cramping in about 20% of patients. Infrequently reported were nausea and vomiting. Excessive dosage can lead to diarrhea. In the event of overdosage, it is expected that diarrhea and abdominal cramps would be the major symptoms.

Dosage and Administration: *Orally.* The usual dosage is 2 to 3 tablespoonsful 3 or 4 times daily. The dosage may be adjusted every day or every other day to produce 2 or 3 soft stools daily. In the initial phase of therapy, 2 to 3 tablespoonsful every hour may be given to induce rapid laxation.

Availability:
CEPHULAC® Syrup in bottles of 1 pint and 2 quarts and in unit-dose bottles of 15, 30 and 45 ml in cartons of 100 (4 x 25). **(Merrell-National)**
DUPHALAC® Syrup in bottles of 1 pint and 2 quarts and in unit-dose bottles of 30 and 45 ml in cartons of 25. **(Philips Roxane)**

LANATOSIDE C
DESLANOSIDE

Description: Lanatoside C is one of the cardioactive glycosides derived from *Digitalis lanata*. It is not found in the *Digitalis purpurea* group. It is used orally.

Deslanoside is prepared by alkaline hydrolysis of lanatoside C and has the same cardiac actions as the parent glycoside. It is prepared in a solution for parenteral administration.

Both glycosides have actions and indications similar to the general group of cardiac glycosides including a positive inotropic effect to increase the force of contraction in the failing heart. Deslanoside has a rapid onset and a relatively short duration of action making it efficacious for rapid digitalization. Lanatoside C, the oral form, is useful for maintenance therapy.

Indications: Treatment of congestive heart failure amenable to digitalis therapy; in cardiac arrhythmias, such as atrial fibrillation or flutter and paroxysmal atrial tachycardia. May be of value in cardiogenic shock.

Contraindications: Toxic effects induced by any digitalis preparation; hypersensitivity to the drug; ventricular fibrillation or tachycardia.

Warnings: Many of the arrhythmias for which digitalis is advised are identical to those reflecting digitalis intoxication. Clinical determination of the cause of these irregularities should be attempted before drug administration. The occurrence of nausea and vomiting may be a reflection of the underlying condition or of digitalis intoxication; therefore, it is necessary to establish their fundamental cause before continuing digitalis therapy.

Precautions: If serum potassium levels are low, the cardiotoxic action of these agents is increased and disturbances in rhythm are likely to occur; therefore, serum potassium concentrations should be measured and hypokalemia corrected, if present, prior to initiating therapy. Considerable caution should be exercised when administering to patients under the influence of digitalis from previous medication. Parenteral administration of calcium to digitalized patients is hazardous since it may produce serious cardiac arrhythmias. Dosage should be carefully adjusted in cases involving myxedema, renal insufficiency, potassium administration, and electrical conversion of arrhythmias. Patients with chronic constrictive pericarditis are apt to respond unfavorably to these drugs. Unless cardiac failure is severe, it is doubtful whether digitalis should be employed for idiopathic hypertrophic subaortic stenosis. Other measures should be employed to control heart failure in patients with incomplete AV block, especially patients who are subject to Stokes-Adams syndrome.

Adverse Reactions: Every form of arrhythmia and conduction disturbance can occur as a result of digitalis toxicity. Common symptoms of digitalis overdosage are anorexia, nausea and vomiting, diarrhea, blurred vision, flickering objects of yellow and green color, disorientation, headache, weakness and apathy. Gynecomastia is an uncommon effect of deslanoside.

Dosage and Administration: *Lanatoside C: Orally.* The average, total digitalizing dosage is 10 mg (20 tablets), divided as follows: first day, 7 tablets; second day, 5 tablets; third day, 4 tablets; thereafter, 3 tablets daily until full digitalization is achieved. Maintenance, 1 to 3 tablets daily. *Deslanoside: Intramuscularly or intravenously.* Parenteral administration should be employed only when the drug cannot be taken orally or when rapid digitalization is extremely urgent. Rapid digitalization can be obtained within 12 hours by giving 8 ml (1.6 mg) either I.M. or I.V. Intravenously, the dose may be given as a single dose or in 2 doses of 4 ml each. Intramuscularly, doses of 4 ml are injected at each of 2 sites.

Availability:
CEDILANID® (lanatoside C) Tablets, 0.5 mg in bottles of 100. **(Sandoz)**
CEDILANID-D (deslanoside) Injection, 0.2 mg/ml in ampuls of 2 ml. **(Sandoz)**

LAROBEC

Description: Each tablet contains:

Thiamine mononitrate	15 mg
Riboflavin	15 mg
Niacinamide	100 mg
Calcium pantothenate	20 mg
Cyanocobalamin	5 μg
Folic acid	0.5 mg
Ascorbic acid	500 mg

A prophylactic or therapeutic nutritional supplement specific to the needs of patients with Parkinson's disease and syndrome who are receiving levodopa therapy.

Indications: Supportive nutritional supplementation in patients under treatment with levodopa and requiring water-soluble vitamins.

Warnings: Administration of vitamin B-6 may be required if signs of pyridoxine deficiency develop. This product is not intended for treatment of pernicious anemia or other primary or secondary anemias. Neurologic involvement may develop or progress, despite temporary remission of anemia, in patients with pernicious anemia who receive more than 0.1 mg of folic acid daily and who are inadequately treated with vitamin B-12.

Dosage and Administration: *Orally,* 1 or 2 tablets daily, or as indicated by the patient's needs. To be administered concomitantly with levodopa.

Availability:
LAROBEC® Tablets (orange) in bottles of 100. **(Roche)**

LEVALLORPHAN TARTRATE

Chemical Name: (-)-N-Allyl-3-hydroxymorphinan tartrate.

Description: Levallorphan tartrate is a narcotic antagonist that is chemically related to levorphanol tartrate from which it differs in the replacement of the methyl group on the nitrogen atom by an allyl group. It occurs as a white or practically white, odorless, crystalline powder that is soluble in water and sparingly soluble in alcohol.

Levallorphan *is not a narcotic,* but acts as a narcotic antagonist in the presence of a strong narcotic effect. In appropriate dosage, it prevents or relieves narcotic-induced respiratory depression. If used in the absence of such a narcotic effect, it may cause respiratory depression and other undesirable effects. Following administration, it usually acts within 1 minute, its effect lasting for 2 to 5 hours.

Indications: Treatment of significant narcotic-induced respiratory depression.

Contraindications: Mild respiratory depression; narcotic addicts in whom it may produce withdrawal symptoms.

Warnings: Levallorphan is not effective against respiratory depression due to barbiturates, anesthetics, other non narcotic agents or pathologic causes, and should not be employed in such instances, since it may increase respiratory depression.

Precautions: In the excessively narcotized patient, artificial respiration with oxygen and other supportive measures should be employed in conjunction with levallorphan. This drug does not counteract mild respiratory depression *and may increase it.* Repeated doses decrease the effectiveness of levallorphan and may eventually produce respiratory depression equal to or greater than that produced by narcotics. It should be kept in mind that narcotic antagonists may precipitate violent withdrawal symptoms in patients strongly addicted to narcotics.

Adverse Reactions: Dysphoria, miosis, pseudoptosis, lethargy, dizziness, drowsiness, gastric upset, sweating, pallor, nausea and a sense of heaviness in the limbs may occur. In high dosage, levallorphan may produce psychotomimetic manifestations such as weird dreams, visual hallucinations, disorientation and feelings of unreality. In asphyxia neonatorum, irritability and a tendency to increased crying may occur. In the event of overdosage assisted respiration including maintenance of a patent airway, the administration of oxygen and other supportive measures should be instituted.

Dosage and Administration: *Parenterally.* To reverse respiratory depression from narcotic overdosage inject 1 mg *intravenously;* may be followed, if required, by 1 or 2 additional doses of 0.5 mg at intervals of 10 to 15 minutes. The initial dose should not exceed 1 mg and the total dose should not exceed 3 mg. In asphyxia neonatorum, inject 0.05 to 0.1 mg into the umbilical cord vein immediately following delivery. If this vein cannot be used, injection may be made *intramuscularly* or *subcutaneously.*

Availability:
LORFAN® Injection, 1 mg/ml in ampuls of 1 ml and in vials of 10 ml. **(Roche)**

LEVARTERENOL BITARTRATE

Chemical Name: l-α-(Aminomethyl)-3,4-dihydroxybenzyl alcohol bitartrate.

Description: Levarterenol is a sympathetic stimulant closely related to epinephrine, chemically and pharmacologically; it differs chemically only in the absence of a methyl group on the nitrogen atom. However, its clinical action differs by its overall vasoconstrictor influence and its marked slowing of the pulse rate in recumbent individuals. Levarterenol increases blood pressure through its inotropic effect and its influence as a mediator of peripheral vasoconstriction. It also improves coronary blood flow and is less likely to induce fibrillation than is epinephrine.

Levarterenol functions as a powerful peripheral vasoconstrictor (alpha-adrenergic action) and as a potent inotropic stimulator of the heart and dilator of coronary arteries (beta-adrenergic action). Both of these actions result in an increase in systemic blood pressure and coronary artery blood flow. Cardiac output will vary reflexly in response to systemic hypertension, but is usually increased in hypotensive individuals when the blood pressure is raised to an optimal level. In myocardial infarction accompanied by hypotension, levarterenol bitartrate usually increases aortic blood pressure, coronary artery blood flow, and myocardial oxygenation, thereby helping to limit the area of myocardial ischemia and infarction. Venous return is increased and the heart tends to resume a more normal rate and rhythm than in the hypotensive state. In hypotension that persists after correction of blood volume deficits, levarterenol helps raise the blood pressure to an optimal level and establish a more adequate circulation.

Indications: Restoration of blood pressure in controlling certain acute hypotensive states (e.g., pheochromocytomectomy, sympathectomy, poliomyelitis, spinal anesthesia, myocardial infarction, septicemia, blood transfusions, and drug reactions). As an adjunctive aid in the treatment of cardiac arrest and profound hypertension.

Contraindications: Levarterenol bitartrate should not be given to patients who are hypotensive from blood volume deficits except as an emergency measure to maintain coronary and cerebral artery perfusion until blood volume replacement therapy can be completed. If the drug is continuously administered to maintain blood pressure in the absence of blood volume replacement, the following may occur: severe peripheral and visceral vasoconstriction, decreased renal perfusion and urine output, poor systemic blood flow despite "normal" blood pressure, tissue hypoxia, and lactate acidosis. Levarterenol also should not be given to patients with mesenteric or peripheral vascular thrombosis (because of the risk of increasing ischemia and extending the area of infarction) unless, in the opinion of the attending physician, the administration of the drug is necessary as a life-saving procedure. Cyclopropane and halothane anesthetics increase cardiac autonomic irritability and therefore seem to sensitize the myocardium to the action of intravenously administered epinephrine or levarterenol. Hence, the use of levarterenol during cyclopropane and halothane anesthesia is generally considered contraindicated because of the risk of producing ventricular tachycardia or fibrillation. The same type of cardiac arrhythmias may result from the use of levarterenol in patients with profound hypoxia or hypercarbia.

Warnings: Due caution is advised in patients taking monoamine oxidase (MAO) inhibitors or antidepressants of the triptyline or imipramine types since a severe, prolonged hypertension may occur.

Precautions: Blood pressure should be checked every 2 minutes from the onset of therapy until the desired blood pressure (low normal) is obtained, then every 5 minutes thereafter if administration is to be continued. Careful attention to the rate of flow and to the patient's response is advised. Whenever possible, the drug should be injected into a large vein, particularly into the antecubital vein. Care should be taken to avoid extravasation of the solution into tissue. To prevent sloughing and necrosis in areas in which extravasation has taken place, the area should be infiltrated immediately or as soon as possible with 10 to 15 ml of saline solution containing from 5 to 10 mg of an adrenergic blocking agent (e.g., phentolamine).

Adverse Reactions: Bradycardia sometimes occurs, probably as a reflex result of a rise in blood pressure. Headache may indicate overdosage and extreme hypertension. Overdosage with levarterenol may also result in severe hypertension, reflex bradycardia, marked increase in peripheral resistance, and decreased cardiac output. Prolonged administration of any potent vasopressor may result in plasma volume depletion which should be continuously corrected by appropriate fluid and electrolyte replacement therapy. If plasma volumes are not corrected, hypotension may recur when levarterenol is discontinued or blood pressure may be maintained at the risk of severe peripheral vasoconstriction with diminution in blood flow and tissue perfusion.

Dosage and Administration: *Intravenous infusion.* Add 4 ml of the 0.1% solution to 1000 ml of a 5% dextrose solution (1 ml of dilution contains 4 mcg of levarterenol base). Inject intravenously (preferably through polyethylene tubing) through a drip bulb. Adjust the flow to establish and maintain low normal blood pressure, which usually is from 80 to 100 mm Hg systolic (and even lower in patients in hemorrhagic or hypovolemic shock, pending replacement of circulating blood volume). In previously hypertensive patients, a somewhat higher systolic blood pressure may be maintained. The average maintenance dose ranges from 0.5 to 1 ml (2 to 4 mcg base)/minute. Occasionally, larger or even enormous daily doses (up to 68 mg base) may be necessary if the patient remains hypotensive. If large volumes of fluid are needed, administer a more dilute solution than 4 mcg/ml. Conversely, when the fluid volume should be restricted, higher concentrations than 4 mcg/ml may be used. Therapy should be continued until adequate blood pressure and tissue perfusion are maintained without therapy. Before administering this drug, refer to the package literature for detailed information.

Availability:
LEVOPHED® Injection, 1 mg/ml (as base) in ampuls of 4 ml (must be diluted). **(Breon)**

LEVODOPA
CARBIDOPA

Chemical Name: Levodopa (—)-3-(3,4-Dihydroxyphenyl)-L-alanine.

Chemical Name: Carbidopa (—)-L-α-hydrazino-α-methyl-β-(3,4-dihydroxybenzene) propanoic acid monohydrate.

Description: *Levodopa* is a naturally occurring amino acid. The commercial product occurs as a colorless, crystalline compound slightly soluble in water and insoluble in alcohol. Its molecular weight is 197.2.

The symptoms of Parkinson's disease (parkinsonism, or Parkinson's syndrome) evidently involve the depletion of striatal dopamine. Since dopamine apparently does not cross the blood-brain barrier, its administration is not effective in the treatment of Parkinson's disease, whereas levodopa (the *levo*rotatary isomer of dopa), the metabolic precursor of dopamine, does in fact cross the blood-brain barrier. Presumably it is converted into dopamine in the basal ganglia. This theoretically is the mechanism by which oral levodopa acts to ameliorate the symptoms of the disease. The major urinary metabolites are dopamine and homovanillic acid (HVA). Of these, HVA is found in the largest quantities. In 24-hour urinary samples, HVA accounts for 13 to 42% of the ingested dose of levodopa.

Results of studies in dogs and in cats suggest that the cardiovascular effects of levodopa are attributable largely to the action of dopamine as well as to its conversion to norepinephrine. Acute drug-interaction studies in rats and in mice reveal that levodopa increases the pharmacologic effects and toxicity of monoamine oxidase inhibitors (MAOI). Laboratory studies with rodents have indicated that levodopa at dosages in excess of 200 mg/kg/day have an adverse effect on fetal and postnatal growth and viability.

Carbidopa, an inhibitor of aromatic amino acid decarboxylation, inhibits the extracerebral decarboxylation of levodopa thus reducing the amount of levodopa required to treat Parkinson's disease by about 75%. As a result, the nausea and vomiting, often a problem when levodopa is used alone, is reduced. Since it does not cross the blood-brain barrier, it therefore does not affect the metabolism of levodopa within the CNS. It occurs as a white, crystalline compound that is slightly soluble in water; its molecular weight is 244.3. When administered with levodopa, it increases both plasma levels and the plasma half-life of levodopa and decreases the plasma and urinary levels of dopamine and homovanillic acid (HVA). In clinical pharmacologic studies, the simultaneous administration of carbidopa and levodopa produced greater urinary excretion of levodopa in proportion to the excretion of dopamine than the administration of the two drugs at separate times. Pyridoxine hydrochloride, in oral doses of 10 to 25 mg, may reverse the effects of levodopa by increasing the rate of aromatic amino acid decarboxylation. Carbidopa inhibits this action of pyridoxine. The 10 to 1 proportion of levodopa and carbidopa is based on evidence that the peripheral dopa decarboxylase is saturated by carbidopa at doses of approximately 70 to 100 mg daily.

Indications: Treatment of Parkinson's disease (paralysis agitans) and syndrome. It is helpful in relieving many of the symptoms and improving functional capacity in patients with this disorder. Pyridoxine may be added to the regimen when the combination product is employed.

Contraindications: Known hypersensitivity to the drug; when sympathomimetic amines are contraindicated; concomitant administration with MAOI in which case the inhibitor should be discontinued 2 weeks before initiating therapy with levodopa; concomitant administration with phenytoin or papaverine since the beneficial effects of levodopa in Parkinson's disease may be reversed; in patients with clinical or laboratory evidence of *uncompensated* endocrine, renal, hepatic, cardiovascular or pulmonary disease; in patients with narrow-angle glaucoma or blood dyscrasias; and in nursing mothers. Because levodopa may activate a malignant melanoma, it should not be given to patients with a suspicious, undiagnosed skin lesion or a history of melanoma.

Warnings: Because of the high incidence of adverse reactions and the need to individualize therapy, the physician should be thoroughly familiar with the contents of the package literature before commencing therapy. Since evidence is lacking that levodopa is indeed effective in neurologic diseases other than paralysis agitans and parkinsonism, accurate diagnosis is considered mandatory. Adequate clinical and laboratory facilities should be readily available so that treatment can be monitored properly. Long-term safety and efficacy of the drug has not been established.

Levodopa should be given with extreme caution to (1) patients with bronchial asthma or emphysema who may require sympathomimetic agents; (2) patients with a history of myocardial infarction who have residual atrial, nodal or ventricular arrhythmias (therapy should be initiated with extreme caution, and in a facility where antiarrhythmic and intensive coronary care facilities are available); (3) patients with active peptic ulcer (facilities for treatment of gastrointestinal hemorrhage should be available); and (4) patients with psychoses or severe psychoneuroses. All patients should be observed carefully for the development of mental changes, depression with suicidal tendencies, or other serious antisocial behavior. Levodopa must be discontinued at least 8 hours before the patient is started on the combination product.

Pyridoxine hydrochloride, 10 to 25 mg orally, reportedly reverses rapidly the antiparkinson effects of levodopa when it is used alone. This should be considered before recommending multivitamin preparations containing pyridoxine.

Since safe use has not been established, the drug(s) should be given to women of child-bearing potential only when the anticipated benefits outweigh the potential hazards to mother and child. Not recommended for use in children under 12 years of age.

Precautions: Hepatic, hematopoietic, cardiovascular and renal function should be evaluated periodically when therapy is extended. The control of the diabetic patient with hypoglycemia may be affected adversely as the result of levodopa. Its use in diabetics therefore should be accompanied by frequent monitoring of the patient and proper adjustment of the antidiabetic regimen. Routine caution is advised when tricyclic antidepressants are given in conjunction with levodopa. Since levodopa may potentiate the effects of sympathomimetic drugs, a reduction in the dosage of these drugs may be necessary. Patients with open-angle (chronic wide-angle) glaucoma may be given levodopa—but with caution—provided the intraocular pressure is well controlled and the patient observed carefully for changes in intraocular pressure during therapy. Careful observation is also required of patients taking antihypertensive drugs, particularly methyldopa, reserpine, or ganglionic blocking agents to avoid precipitating a postural hypotensive episode. If the concomitant administration of psychoactive drugs is deemed necessary, such drugs should be given cautiously and the patient should be observed carefully for unusual side effects. Levodopa reportedly is ineffective in the treatment of drug-induced extrapyramidalism. Patients with a history of convulsions should be treated with caution. While no untoward reactions from general anesthesia have been encountered to date, it is suggested that local or regional anesthesia be used whenever possible. Where general anesthesia is unavoidable, cardiorespiratory functions should be evaluated carefully. Patients who improve on therapy with levodopa should resume normal activities gradually and cautiously, consistent with other medical considerations such as the presence of osteoporosis or phlebothrombosis. Levodopa may be used concomitantly with other antiparkinson drugs such as benztropine mesylate, trihexyphenidyl hydrochloride or procyclidine hydrochloride, in which cases the usual dose of each may require reduction.

Adverse Reactions: Most frequent: nausea, anorexia, vomiting, cardiac irregularities, orthostatic hypotension; choreiform, dystonic and other adventitious movements; dizziness, sedation, dyskinesia; such psychiatric symptoms as agitation, anxiety, confusion, depression, hallucinations, delusions, insomnia, nightmares, and mental changes including paranoid ideation and psychotic episodes. Less frequent—*psychiatric:* suicidal tendencies, increased libido with possible antisocial behavior, euphoria, lethargy, fatigue, stimulation, malaise, dementia; *neurologic:* ataxia, convulsions, faintness, impaired gait, headache, increased hand tremor, akinetic episodes, torticollis, trismus, oculogyric crisis, weakness, numbness, gnashing of teeth; *gastrointestinal:* constipation, diarrhea, epigastric and abdominal distress and pain, flatulence, eructation, hiccups, sialorrhea, dysphagia, bitter taste, dry mouth, tight mouth, lips or tongue, duodenal ulcer, gastrointestinal bleeding, burning sensation of the tongue; *cardiovascular:* nonspecific ECG changes, palpitations, hypertension, flushing, phlebitis; *hematologic:* one case of hemolytic anemia; *dermatologic:* sweating, edema, loss of hair, pallor, rash, malodor; *musculoskeletal:* low back pain, muscle spasm and twitching, blepharospasm, musculoskeletal pain; *respiratory:* feeling of pressure in chest, cough, hoarseness, bizarre breathing pattern, postnasal drip; *urogenital:* urinary frequency, retention, incontinence, hematuria, nocturia, and one report of interstitial nephritis; *special senses:* blurred vision, diplopia, mydriasis, activation of latent Horner's syndrome; *other:* fever, hot flushes, weight gain or loss. If cardiac arrhythmias occur, they should be treated appropriately and consideration given to withdrawing levodopa and substituting other antiparkinsonian therapy. Other reactions reported include elevated BUN, SGOT, SGPT, lactic dehydrogenase, bilirubin, alkaline phosphatase or PBI, occasional reductions in white blood cells, hemoglobin and hematocrit. Elevated uric acid has been noted with the colorimetric method, but not with uricase. Rarely, a positive Coombs' test with prolonged therapy. Dark sweat and urine also have been reported, but discontinuing therapy with levodopa is not considered necessary.

The management of overdosage involves general supportive measures, including immediate gastric lavage. Intravenous fluids should be administered and an adequate airway maintained. Electrocardiographic monitoring should be instituted, and the patient carefully observed for the development of arrhythmias; if required, appropriate antiarrhythmic therapy should be given. That the patient may have taken several drugs should be considered. The value of dialysis has not been determined. Although pyridoxine reportedly has reversed the antiparkinsonian effects of levodopa, its usefulness in the management of overdosage has not been established.

Dosage and Administration: *Orally.* The daily dosage producing maximal improvement with tolerated reactions must be determined and titrated carefully for each patient. The usual initial dosage is 0.5 to 1 gm daily, divided into 2 or more doses. The daily dosage should then be increased gradually in increments of 125 to 750 mg every 2 or 3 days as tolerated. The usual daily dosage ranges from 4 to 6 gm in 3 or more divided doses with food, but should not exceed 8 gm. Optimal therapeutic dosage usually is reached in 6 to 8 weeks.

If general anesthesia is to be used, levodopa should be discontinued 24 hours before a surgical procedure and reinstituted as soon as the patient can take medication orally. Whenever therapy is interrupted briefly, dosage should again be adjusted gradually; however, in many cases the patient can be titrated rapidly to his previous therapeutic dosage.

Levodopa with carbidopa: *Patients presently receiving levodopa:* The usual dosage is 3 to 6 (250/25) tablets daily given in divided doses. Up to, but no more than, 8 tablets should be given since experience with carbidopa in daily dosages greater than 200 mg is limited. *Patients not presently receiving levodopa:* Initially, 1 (100/10) tablet 3 times daily, then increased by 1 tablet every day or every other day until a dosage of 6 tablets daily is reached. If still further titration is necessary, ½ or 1 (250/25) tablet is given every day or every other day until a dosage of 8 tablets daily is reached. Alternately, dosage may be titrated to 6 (250/25) tablets daily and further adjusted with increments of levodopa.

Availability:
BENDOPA® Capsules, 250 and 500 mg in bottles of 100, 500 and 1000. **(ICN)**
DOPAR® Capsules, 100 and 250 mg in bottles of 100; 500 mg in bottles of 100 and 1000. **(Norwich-Eaton)**
LARODOPA®: **(Roche)**
Capsules, 100 mg in bottles of 100; 250 and 500 mg in bottles of 100 and 500.
Tablets, 100 mg in bottles of 100; 250 and 500 mg in bottles of 100 and 500.
w/Carbidopa
SINEMET® Tablets, 100 and 250 mg with carbidopa, 10 and 25 mg respectively in bottles of 100. **(Merck Sharp & Dohme)**

LEVOPROPOXYPHENE

Chemical Name: α-*l*-4-Dimethylamino-3-methyl-1,2-diphenyl-2-butanol propionate.

Description: Levopropoxyphene, as the napsylate, is a salt of the *levo* isomer of propoxyphene and structurally is related to methadone. It occurs as a white, slightly bitter, crystalline powder slightly soluble in water and soluble in alcohol. In contrast to the *dextro* isomer of propoxyphene, the *levo* isomer possesses no analgesic properties, but is antitussive by its action on the CNS without altering respiratory tract fluid or interfering with expectoration. The drug is not a cure for any pulmonary disorder, but it is a valuable adjunct to other forms of therapy and will provide symptomatic relief.

Indications: Symptomatic treatment of cough. It decreases the frequency and intensity of cough associated with acute and chronic respiratory diseases and other conditions.

Contraindications: In patients hypersensitive to levopropoxyphene. None that are considered absolute have been reported.

Precautions: In some cases, it may not be advisable to decrease the frequency or intensity of cough in order to insure adequate pulmonary function. If symptoms of CNS stimulation or sedation develop, the dosage should be reduced or the medication discontinued. It is essential to caution patients that the drug may impair their mental and/or physical abilities required for the performance of potentially hazardous tasks, such as driving a car or operating dangerous machinery.

Adverse Reactions: Reports include nausea, epigastric burning, skin rash, urticaria, drowsiness, nervousness, or dizziness. Symptoms of overdosage include uncontrollable muscle tremor, agitation and vomiting, followed by sedation. Recommended treatment is gastric lavage along with symptomatic and supportive measures. No specific antagonists are known. According to animal data, nalorphine is contraindicated in the treatment of overdosage.

Dosage and Administration: *Orally.* Adults, 100 mg every 4 hours. Children, 0.5 mg/lb of body weight every 4 hours. Dosage may be adjusted in either direction, depending upon the results.

Availability:
NOVRAD®: **(Lilly)**
Capsules (Pulvules®), 100 mg in bottles of 50.
Oral Suspension, 50 mg/5 ml in bottles of 120 ml. *(Avoid freezing.)*

LEVORPHANOL TARTRATE Ⓒ II

Chemical Name: *l*-3′-Hydroxy-*N*-methylmorphinan tartrate.

Description: Levorphanol is a synthetic narcotic analgesic chemically and pharmacologically related to morphine. It produces an intensity of analgesia equal to that of morphine (but less likely to produce nausea, vomiting and constipation) and greater than that of meperidine, in doses far smaller than those required for either. It provides relief of pain up to 8 hours whether given orally or parenterally.

Indications: Relief of moderate to severe pain in such conditions as severe trauma, renal or biliary colic, myocardial infarction, and intractable pain of cancer or other tumors. Also as preoperative medication and for postoperative relief of pain.

Contraindications: Acute alcoholism, bronchial asthma, increased intracranial pressure, respiratory depression and anoxia.

Warnings: May be habit-forming. The same degree of care should be taken when administering this drug as with morphine. It should be used during the first trimester of pregnancy only when the expected benefits outweigh the potential risks to the mother or fetus.

Precautions: It has been suggested that this drug be administered with a narcotic antagonist to prevent or to counteract narcotic-induced respiratory depression particularly in parturients and neonates, or during nitrous oxide-oxygen anesthesia with narcotic supplementation.

Adverse Reactions: Nausea, vomiting, dizziness. Infrequently reported were respiratory depression, hypotension, urinary retention and cardiac arrhythmias; occasionally skin rash, urticaria, rarely pruritus or sweating have been noted.

Dosage and Administration: *Orally or subcutaneously,* 2 mg; may be increased to 3 mg if necessary.

Availability:
Ⓒ II LEVO DROMORAN®: **(Roche)**
Injection, 2 mg/ml in ampuls of 1 ml and in vials of 10 ml.
Tablets, 2 mg in bottles of 100.

LEVOTHYROXINE SODIUM

Chemical Name: Sodium L-3,3′, 5,5′-tetraiodothyroxine.

Description: Sodium levothyroxine is the monosodium salt of the *levo* isomer of thyroxine, the principal secretion of the thyroid gland. It occurs as a hygroscopic, cream-color, odorless, tasteless, micronized, crystalline powder slightly soluble in water and in alcohol.

After absorption, *l*-thyroxine is firmly and almost completely bound to a plasma protein fraction. From this union it is gradually released into the tissue cells where it exerts its characteristic effect of producing an increased metabolic rate—usually after a lapse of 12 to 48 hours. One milligram causes an increase in heat production of about 1000 calories.

Indications: Specific replacement or substitution therapy for diminished or absent thyroid function resulting from primary or secondary atrophy of the gland, congenital defect, surgery, excessive radiation, or antithyroid drugs. May be administered orally for conditions of the hypothyroid state such as myxedema, cretinism, simple nontoxic goiter and in hypothyroidism generally, including the hypothyroid state in children, in pregnancy and in the elderly, and parenterally in myxedematous coma or other thyroid dysfunctions where rapid replacement of the hormone is required or when a patient does not respond to oral therapy.

Contraindications: In the presence of thyrotoxicosis, acute myocardial infarction, and adrenal insufficiency as in Addison's disease.

Warnings: Levothyroxine should be used with caution in patients with cardiovascular disease, including hypertension. The development of chest pain or other aggravation of cardiovascular disease will require a decrease in dosage. Injection of epinephrine in patients with coronary artery disease may precipitate an episode of coronary insufficiency. This may be enhanced in patients receiving thyroid preparations. Careful observation is required if catecholamines are administered to patients in this category. Patients with coronary artery disease should be carefully observed during surgery, since the possibility of precipitating cardiac arrhythmias may be greater in those treated with thyroid hormones. Thyroid replacement may potentiate anticoagulant effects with agents such as warfarin or bishydroxycoumarin and reduction of one-third in anticoagulant dosage should be undertaken upon initiation of levothyroxine therapy. Subsequent anticoagulant dosage adjustment should be made on the basis of frequent prothrombin determinations. In patients whose hypothyroidism is secondary to hypopituitarism, adrenal insufficiency will probably also be present. When adrenal insufficiency and hypothyroidism coexist, the adrenal insufficiency should be corrected by corticosteroids before administering thyroid hormones.

Precautions: Patients with hypothyroidism, and especially myxedema, are particularly sensitive to thyroid preparations so that treatment should begin with small doses and increments should be gradual. In patients with diabetes mellitus, addition of thyroid hormone therapy may cause an increase in the required dosage of insulin or oral hypoglycemic agents. Conversely, decreasing the dose of thyroid hormone may possibly cause hypoglycemic reactions if the dosage of insulin or oral hypoglycemic agents is not adjusted.

Adverse Reactions: Excessive dosage of thyroid medication may result in symptoms of hyperthyroidism. Since, however, the effects do not appear at once, the symptoms may not appear for 1 to 3 weeks after the dosage regimen is begun. The most common signs and symptoms of overdosage are continued weight loss, heart palpitations with or without pain, leg cramps, nervousness, vomiting, diarrhea or abdominal cramps, sweating, tachycardia, cardiac arrhythmias, angina pectoris, tremors, headache, insomnia, intolerance to heat, and fever. If symptoms of overdosage appear, discontinue medication for several days and reinstitute treatment at a lower dosage level.

Dosage and Administration: *Orally.* As with any type of thyroid therapy, dosage must be adjusted to approximate the deficit in the patient's thyroid secretion. *Adults:* generally, the initial dose is 0.1 mg daily. Daily dosage may be increased gradually in increments of 0.05 to 0.1 mg every 1 to 3 weeks until the desired response is obtained; total daily dosage is given once daily. *Children:* the initial dosage should not exceed 0.05 mg daily. Increments of 0.025 to 0.05 mg daily may be added in the same manner as with adults to establish maintenance levels. *Intravenously.* For myxedematous coma or stupor with no evidence of severe heart disease, the adult dose is 0.2 to 0.4 mg utilizing a solution containing 0.1 mg/ml. Detectable effects are usually observed 6 hours after injection and are fully appreciated during the following day. A repeat injection of 0.1 to 0.2 mg may be given on the 2nd day if significant improvement has not occurred. May also be given *intramuscularly* when the oral route is not feasible and a rapid onset of effect is not desired. Consult package literature for additional information on dosage schedules.

Availability:
LETTER® Tablets: 0.025, 0.05, 0.1, 0.15, 0.2, 0.3 and 0.5 mg in bottles of 100 and 1000; the 0.05, 0.1, 0.15, 0.2 and 0.3 mg tablets are also available in Armadose® (unit-dose) packages of 100. **(Armour)**

SYNTHROID®: **(Flint)**
Injectable, 0.5 mg (lyophilized) in single-dose vials of 10 ml with a 5-ml vial of diluent.
Tablets: 0.025, 0.05, 0.1, 0.15, 0.2 and 0.3 mg in bottles of 100 and 1000; the 0.05, 0.1, 0.15, 0.2 and 0.3 mg tablets are also available in unit-dose packages of 100.

LEXAVITE

Description: Each ml contains:

Vitamin B-12 activity equiv. (derived from liver)	2 μg
Cyanocobalamin (crystalline)	8 μg
Thiamine hydrochloride	10 mg
Riboflavin (as riboflavin 5′ phosphate sodium)	5 mg
Niacinamide	150 mg
Pyridoxine hydrochloride	5 mg
Sodium pantothenate	5 mg
Benzyl alcohol	2%

Indications: Treatment of liver disease; also pernicious anemia and other macrocytic anemias with associated vitamin B complex deficiency.

Contraindications: Hypersensitivity to any of the components.

Precautions: Discontinue therapy if a local or generalized reaction occurs.

Adverse Reactions: Pain and tenderness at site of injection, slight fever; weakness, increased pulse rate, perspiration, a drop in systolic blood pressure, pruritus or urticaria; rarely a severe reaction (anaphylactoid) to thiamine hydrochloride.

Dosage and Administration: *Intramuscularly* only. Treatment of pernicious anemia, 1 to 3 ml daily for 2 or 3 successive days, then 1 to 2 ml weekly until the blood has returned to normal. Maintenance dose, 1 ml every 10 days. Vitamin B deficiencies, 2 ml 3 times weekly; this dosage is decreased or increased as dictated by the patient's condition and response to therapy. Children require proportionately less.

Availability:
LEXAVITE® Injection in ampuls of 10 ml. **(Lilly)**

LEXTRON

Description: Each pulvule contains:

Liver-stomach concentrate (as intrinsic powder)	50 mg
Iron, elemental (as iron and ammonium citrates)	30 mg
Vitamin B-12 (activity equiv.)	2 μg
Thiamine hydrochloride	1 mg
Riboflavin	0.25 mg

Lextron Ferrous and Lextron F.G. are identical in composition to Lextron except for the amount and form of iron: each Lextron Ferrous Pulvule supplies 35 mg of elemental iron as ferrous sulfate and each Lextron F.G. Pulvule supplies 20 mg of elemental iron as ferrous gluconate.

Indications: Treatment of anemias that respond to liver and iron.

Contraindications: Hemochromatosis, hemosiderosis, and hypersensitivity to any of the components.

Precautions: Periodic clinical and laboratory studies to determine the cause and extent of the anemia are essential and recommended.

Adverse Reactions: Skin rash (rare), diarrhea or constipation. Pallor and cyanosis, vomiting, hematemesis, diarrhea, melena, shock, drowsiness, and coma are symptoms of iron intoxication, and are generally treated by exchange transfusion and chelating agents. General management consists of gastric and rectal lavage with sodium bicarbonate solution or milk, administration of intravenous fluids and electrolytes, and the use of oxygen.

Dosage and Administration: *Orally,* 3 or 4 pulvules 3 times daily. In the average case of pernicious anemia, 12 pulvules daily will produce a standard response.

Availability:
LEXTRON®/LEXTRON FERROUS/LEXTRON F.G. Pulvules® (Capsules) in bottles of 84 and 500. **(Lilly)**

LIDOCAINE HYDROCHLORIDE

Chemical Name: 2-(Diethylamino)-N-(2,6-dimethylphenyl)acetamide hydrochloride.

Description: Lidocaine hydrochloride, an aminoethyl amide type of local anesthetic, occurs as a white, odorless, crystalline powder very soluble in water and in alcohol.

Lidocaine apparently blocks transmission of nerve impulses by stabilizing the potential of nerve membrane or by elevating the threshold of excitability through chemical combination with polar groups in the lipoprotein film of the nerve membrane. Local anesthetics may also interfere with oxidative processes within the nerve.

Lidocaine appears to have 2 to 3 times the anesthetic potency of procaine and about the same potency as mepivacaine and prilocaine. It produces some degree of vasodilation requiring the addition of epinephrine to retard vascular absorption of the anesthetic.

Lidocaine has also been reported to increase the electrical stimulation threshold of the ventricle during diastole and thereby exerts an antiarrhythmic effect. In recommended dosage, it produces no change in systolic arterial blood pressure, absolute refractory period, or myocardial contractility. Following intramuscular (deltoid) injection, effective antiarrhythmic blood levels are usually attained within 5 to 15 minutes and the therapeutic action is sustained for approximately 60 to 90 minutes.

The drug is absorbed slowly from the injection site and removed slowly from the blood. It is distributed to almost all body tissues, is metabolized mainly in the liver and excreted via the kidneys. Approximately 90% of lidocaine administered is excreted in the form of various metabolites, while less than 10% is excreted unchanged.

Indications: Lidocaine hydrochloride 0.5%, 1%, and 2% solutions with and without epinephrine are used for infiltration, caudal and epidural anesthesia and for field block and regional nerve block. The 5% solution with glucose 7.5% is used for spinal anesthesia. The 4% sterile solution is indicated for the production of local anesthesia of the mucous membranes of the respiratory tract or the genitourinary tract. It may be injected transtracheally to anesthetize the larynx and trachea. It may also be administered by retrobulbar injection to provide anesthesia for ophthalmic surgery. The 4% topical solution is to be used only for the production of *topical* anesthesia of accessible mucous membranes of the oral and nasal cavities and proximal portions of the digestive tract. The 3% creme is recommended for relief of pain, soreness and the discomfort of itching due to anal and vulvar pruritus, pruritic eczemas, abrasions, hemorrhoids and fissures, minor burns and similar conditions of the skin and mucous membranes. The 5% ointment is recommended for the production of anesthesia of accessible mucous membranes of the oropharynx and for the temporary relief of pain associated with minor abrasions of the skin and for topical anesthesia of the anorectal tissues in the treatment of conditions such as anal fissures. It is also useful as an anesthetic lubricant for endotracheal intubation. The 2.5% ointment is recommended for the temporary relief of pain associated with minor abrasions of the skin. The viscous solution may be used for the production of topical anesthesia of irritated or inflamed mucous membranes of the mouth and pharynx. The jelly is used for the prevention and control of pain in procedures involving the male and female urethra and for topical treatment of painful urethritis. Lidocaine suppositories provide temporary relief of pain and discomfort associated with inoperable, irritative or inflammatory anorectal conditions such as hemorrhoids and postoperative edema. They may also be employed pre- and postoperatively in hemorrhoidectomy and sclerosing therapy, and in conjunction with proctoscopic and sigmoidoscopic examinations. The lidocaine solutions packaged especially for intravenous or intramuscular use are specifically indicated in the acute management of ventricular arrhythmias occurring during cardiac manipulation and in life-threatening arrhythmias, particularly those which are ventricular in origin, such as occur during acute myocardial infarction.

Contraindications: Lidocaine is contraindicated in patients with a known history of hypersensitivity to local anesthetics of the amide type. Local anesthetic agents should not be used in patients in severe shock or with heart block. Local anesthetic procedures should not be used when there is sepsis in the region of the proposed injection or application. In addition, the following conditions preclude the use of spinal anesthesia: severe hemorrhage and septicemia. Lidocaine should not be used intravenously for the treatment of cardiac arrhythmias in patients with Adams-Stokes syndrome, Wolff-Parkinson-White syndrome, or with severe degrees of sinoatrial, atrioventricular or intraventricular block. Traumatized mucosa and secondary bacterial infection of the area of proposed application are contraindications for topical use.

Warnings: Resuscitative equipment and drugs should be immediately available when any local anesthetic is used. The safe use of lidocaine has not been established with respect to adverse effects upon fetal development. Careful consideration should be given to this fact before administering this drug to women of childbearing potential, particularly during early pregnancy. This does not exclude the use of the drug at term for obstetrical analgesia because lidocaine has been used effectively in such instances. Adverse effects on the fetus, course of labor, or delivery have rarely been observed when proper dosage and proper technique have been employed. Solutions which contain a vasoconstrictor should be used with extreme caution in patients receiving drugs known to produce blood pressure alterations (i.e., MAO inhibitors, tricyclic antidepressants, phenothiazines, etc.) as either severe and sustained hypotension or hypertension may occur. Vasopressor agents (administered for the treatment of hypotension related to caudal or other epidural blocks or spinal anesthesia) should not be used in the presence of oxytocic drugs, as a severe persistent hypertension and even rupture of cerebral blood vessels may occur. Constant monitoring with an electrocardiograph is essential in the proper administration of lidocaine intravenously. Signs of excessive depression of cardiac conductivity, such as prolongation of PR interval and QRS complex and the appearance or aggravation of arrhythmias, should be followed by prompt cessation of the intravenous infusion of this agent. Patients with atrial fibrillation may experience an occasional acceleration of ventricular rate. If irritation or sensitivity occurs or infection appears, lidocaine should be discontinued and appropriate therapy instituted. The drug should be administered with considerable caution in the presence of hypovolemia and shock and all forms of heart block.

Precautions: The safety and effectiveness of lidocaine hydrochloride depend on proper dosage, correct technique, adequate precautions, and readiness for emergencies. The lowest dosage that results in effective anesthesia should be used to avoid high plasma levels and serious adverse effects. Injection of repeated doses of lidocaine may cause significant increases in blood levels with each repeated dose due to slow accumulation of the drug or its metabolites. Tolerance varies with the status of the patient, especially if liver and kidney function is impaired. Debilitated and elderly patients, acutely ill patients, and children should be given reduced doses commensurate with their age and physical status. **Injections should always be made slowly and with frequent aspirations.** Aspiration is advisable since it reduces the possibility of intravascular injection, thereby keeping the incidence of adverse effects and anesthetic failures to a minimum. Epidural anesthesia and caudal anesthesia should be administered with utmost care in patients with the following conditions: existing neurological disease, spinal deformities, septicemia and severe hypertension and in the very young. Fetal bradycardia frequently follows paracervical block and may be associated with fetal acidosis; therefore, fetal heart rate should always be monitored during paracervical anesthesia. Added risk appears to be present in prematurity, toxemia of pregnancy, and fetal distress. The physician should weigh the possible advantages against the hazards when considering paracervical block in these conditions. When the recommended dose is exceeded, the incidence of fetal bradycardia increases. Solutions which contain a vasoconstrictor should be used with caution in the presence of diseases which may adversely affect the patient's cardiovascular system. Serious cardiac arrhythmias may occur if preparations containing a vasoconstrictor are employed in patients during or following the administration of chloroform, halothane, cyclopropane, trichlorethylene, or other related agents. The use of any vasoconstrictor drug is not recommended in surgery involving the digits, nose, ear, or penis. The drug should be used with caution in patients with severely traumatized mucosa and in individuals with known drug sensitivities. Patients allergic to para-aminobenzoic acid derivatives (procaine, tetracaine, benzocaine, etc.) have not shown cross sensitivity to lidocaine. Local anesthetics react with certain metals and cause the release of their respective ions which, if injected, may cause severe local irritation. Adequate precaution should be taken to avoid this type of interaction.

Adverse Reactions: Adverse reactions may result from high plasma levels due to excessive dosage, rapid absorption or inadvertent intravascular injection, or may result from a hypersensitivity, idiosyncrasy or diminished tolerance on the part of the patient. Such reactions are systemic in nature and involve the CNS and/or the cardiovascular system. CNS reactions are excitatory and/or depressant, and may be characterized by nervousness, dizziness, lightheadedness, apprehension, euphoria, tinnitus, vomiting, sensation of heat, cold or numbness, twitching, blurred or double vision and tremors, followed by drowsiness, convulsions, unconsciousness, respiratory depression, and possibly respiratory arrest. The excitatory reactions may be very brief or may not occur at all, in which case the first manifestations of toxicity may be drowsiness, merging into unconsciousness and respiratory arrest. Cardiovascular reactions are depressant, and may be characterized by hypotension, myocardial depression, bradycardia and possibly cardiac arrest. Allergic reactions are characterized by cutaneous lesions, urticaria, edema or anaphylactoid reactions. The detection of sensitivity by skin testing is of doubtful value.

Treatment of toxic manifestations consists of assuring and maintaining a patent airway and supporting ventilation using oxygen and assisted or controlled respiration as required. This usually will be sufficient in the management of most reactions. Should circulatory depression occur, vasopressors, such as ephedrine or metaraminol, and intravenous fluids may be used. The effects of central stimulation, including convulsions, are best counteracted by intravenous administration of small increments of an ultra-short acting barbiturate (thiopental or thiamylal) or a short-acting barbiturate (pentobarbital or secobarbital).

Dosage and Administration: It is important not to exceed the smallest dose necessary to produce the desired results. Dosages should be reduced for children and for elderly and debilitated patients. *Parenterally.* In normal healthy adults, the individual dose of lidocaine hydrochloride with epinephrine should be kept below 500 mg and in any case should not exceed 7 mg/kg (3.5 mg/lb) of body weight. When used without epinephrine, the amount of lidocaine hydrochloride administered should be kept below 300 mg and in any case should not exceed 4.5 mg/kg (2 mg/lb) of body weight. For continuous epidural or caudal anesthesia, the maximum recommended dosage should not be administered at intervals of less than 2 hours. For children of less than 10 years who have a normal lean body mass and normal body development, the maximal dose may be determined by the application of one of the standard pediatric drug formulas (e.g. Clark's rule or Young's rule). In order to minimize the possibility of toxic reactions in children, the use of 0.5 or 1% concentrations of lidocaine hydrochloride is recommended. *Intravenously (for cardiac arrhythmias).* The usual dose is 50 to 100 mg delivered at the rate of 25 to 50 mg/minute; may be repeated after 5 minutes if the desired response is not obtained. However, no more than 200 to 300 mg of lidocaine should be administered during a 1-hour period. Experience with the drug for intravenous use in children is limited. *Intramuscularly,* usually 300 mg administered into the deltoid muscle; may be repeated after an interval of 60 to 90 minutes if the clinical situation warrants. *Intraspinally.* Obstetrical low spinal or "saddle block" anesthesia: The dosage recommended for normal vaginal delivery is approximately 1 ml (50 mg). For Cesarean section and those deliveries requiring intrauterine manipulations, 1.5 ml (75 mg) is usually adequate. Surgical anesthesia: The dosage recommended for abdominal surgical anesthesia is 1.5 to 2 ml (75 to 100 mg). *Rectally.* Insert 1 suppository after each bowel movement and before retiring, or as required for the control of symptoms. The recommended dose of no more than 5 suppositories in 24 hours should not be exceeded. **Note:** In the event of rectal bleeding, or if a rash, irritation, or other signs of sensitivity develop, discontinue use. Also, not recommended for patients under 12 years of age. *Topically.* Apply the ointment in liberal amounts for adequate control of symptoms. *Intraorally.* Usually 1 tablespoonful of the viscous solution undiluted is recommended. The solution should be swished around in the mouth and can be swallowed without water. May be repeated at intervals of 3 hours. **Note:** No more than 120 ml (approximately 8 tablespoonsful) should be administered in a 24-hour period.

See package literature for complete details of precautions, adverse reactions, contraindications and dosage regimens.

Availability:

Lidocaine Hydrochloride

Injection, 1 and 2% in Abboject® syringes of 5 ml. **(Abbott)**

Injection, 1% in Bristoject® syringes of 5 and 10 ml; 2% in Bristoject syringes of 5 ml; 4% in Diiject® syringes of 25 and 50 ml. **(Bristol)**

Injection, 1 and 2% in Tubex® (sterile cartridge-needle unit) of 2.5 ml. **(Wyeth)**

XYLOCAINE® (as hydrochloride): **(Astra)**

Injection, 0.5% in single-dose and multi-dose vials of 50 ml.

Injection, 1% in multi-dose vials of 20 and 50 ml, in single-dose vials of 30 ml, in ampuls of 2, 5 and 30 ml and in prefilled syringes of 5 ml.

Injection, 1.5% in ampuls of 20 ml and in single-dose vials of 20 ml.

Injection, 1.5% (for saddle block) with dextrose, 7.5% in ampuls of 2 ml.

Injection, 2% in multi-dose vials of 20 and 50 ml, in prefilled syringes of 5 ml, in dental cartridges of 1.8 ml and in ampuls of 2 and 10 ml. Also in single-dose containers of 5 and 50 ml for intravenous use in cardiac arrhythmias.

Injection, 4% in ampuls of 5 ml and in bottles of 50 ml.

Injection, 5% (for spinal block) with glucose, 7.5% in ampuls of 2 ml.

Injection, 10% (for IV use in cardiac arrhythmias) in ampuls of 5 ml.

Jelly, 2% in tubes of 30 ml.

Topical Solution, 4% in screw-cap bottles of 50 ml.

Viscous Solution, 2% in plastic bottles of 100 and 450 ml.

w/Epinephrine

Injection, 0.5% with epinephrine 1:200,000 in vials of 50 ml.

Injection, 1% with epinephrine 1:100,000 in vials of 20 and 50 ml and with epinephrine 1:200,000 in ampuls of 30 ml.

Injection, 1.5% with epinephrine 1:200,000 in ampuls of 30 ml and in single-dose vials of 30 ml.

Injection, 2% with epinephrine 1:50,000 in dental cartridges of 1.8 ml; with epinephrine 1:100,000 in dental cartridges of 1.8 ml, in multi-dose vials of 20 and 50 ml and in ampuls of 2 ml; with epinephrine 1:200,000 in single-dose vials of 20 ml.

Lidocaine (as base)

LIDA-MANTLE® Creme, 3% in tubes of 15 and 30 gm. **(Dome)**

XYLOCAINE: **(Astra)**

Ointment, 2.5% (OTC) in tubes of 35 gm.

Ointment, 5% in tubes of 15 and 35 gm.

Ointment, 5% (flavored) in tubes of 3.5 gm.

Suppositories, 100 mg with bismuth subgallate, 115 mg; zinc oxide, 375 mg; aluminum subacetate, 75 mg; Peruvian balsam, 100 mg and neutral glycerides of saturated vegetable fatty acids, q.s.ad 2.6 gm in cartons of 5.

LINCOMYCIN

Description: Lincomycin is an antibiotic obtained from cultures of *Streptomyces lincolnensis* and is available as the hydrochloride monohydrate. It occurs as a white, crystalline powder freely soluble in water and soluble in alcohol.

Lincomycin has been shown to be effective against most of the common gram-positive pathogens. Depending on the sensitivity of the organism and concentration of the antibiotic, it may be either bactericidal or bacteriostatic. Cross resistance has not been demonstrated with penicillin, chloramphenicol, ampicillin, cephalosporins or the tetracyclines. Despite chemical differences, lincomycin exhibits antibacterial activity similar to but not identical with the macrolide antibiotics (e.g. erythromycin). Some cross resistance (with erythromycin) including a phenomenon known as dissociated cross resistance or macrolide effect has been reported. Microorganisms have not developed resistance to lincomycin rapidly when tested by in vitro or in vivo methods. Staphylococci develop resistance to this antibiotic in a slow, stepwise manner based on in vitro, serial subculture experiments. This pattern of resistance development is unlike that shown for streptomycin. Studies indicate that lincomycin does not share antigenicity with penicillin compounds. In vitro studies indicate that the spectrum of activity includes *Micrococcus (Staphylococcus) aureus, Staphylococcus albus, β hemolytic Streptococcus, Streptococcus viridans, Diplococcus pneumoniae, Clostridium tetani, Clostridium perfringens, Corynebacterium diphtheriae and Corynebacterium acnes.* The drug is not active against most strains of *Streptococcus faecalis,* nor against *Neisseria gonorrhoeae, Haemophilus influenzae,* or other gram-negative organisms or yeasts.

Lincomycin is absorbed rapidly following a 500-mg oral dose, reaching peak levels in 2 to 4 hours. Levels are maintained above the minimum inhibitory concentration for most gram-positive organisms for 6 to 8 hours. Urinary recovery of the drug in a 24-hour period ranges from 1 to 31% (mean: 4) after a single oral dose of 500 mg. Tissue level studies indicate that bile is an important route of excretion. Significant levels have been demonstrated in the majority of body tissues. Although the drug is not present in significant amounts in the spinal fluid of normal volunteers, it has been demonstrated in the spinal fluid of one patient with pneumococcal meningitis. Intramuscular administration of a single dose of 600 mg produces a peak serum level at 30 minutes with detectable levels persisting for 24 hours. Urinary excretion after this dose ranges from 1.8 to 24.8% (mean: 17.3). The intravenous infusion over a 2-hour interval of 600 mg of lincomycin in 500 ml of 5% glucose in distilled water yields therapeutic levels for 14 hours. Urinary excretion ranges from 4.9 to 30.3% (mean: 13.8). The biological half-life after oral, intramuscular or intravenous administration is 5.4 ± 1 hour. **Note:** Hemodialysis and peritoneal dialysis do not effectively remove lincomycin from the blood.

Indications: In infections caused by susceptible gram-positive pathogens, particularly streptococci, pneumococci and staphylococci, resistant to other antibiotics. Lincomycin may be given together with other antimicrobial agents when indicated.

Contraindications: Hypersensitive patients, minor bacterial infections or viral infections, and newborn infants.

Warnings: The drug has been responsible for severe and persistent diarrhea, occasionally with blood and mucus in the stools, that has at times resulted in an acute colitis. A few fatalities have been reported. If this occurs, the drug should be withdrawn or, if necessary, continued only with close observation of the patient. Moderate to severe cases should be managed with fluid, electrolyte and protein supplementations. Treatment with corticoids, either systemically or by retention enemas, may relieve the colitis. The physician should be aware that diarrhea has been observed to begin up to several weeks following cessation of therapy with this drug.

Precautions: Should be used with caution in patients with a history of asthma or significant allergies. The use of antibiotics occasionally results in the overgrowth of nonsusceptible organisms, particularly yeasts. If superinfection occurs, appropriate measures should be taken. When patients with preexisting monilial infections require lincomycin, concomitant antimonilial treatment should be given. During prolonged therapy, liver function studies and blood counts should be performed periodically. Safe use during pregnancy and effectiveness in the prophylactic treatment of rheumatic fever have not been established. For the present, lincomycin should not be used in patients with preexisting liver disease unless clinical circumstances so indicate. Lincomycin has neuromuscular blocking properties and may, therefore, enhance the action of other neuromuscular blocking agents.

Adverse Reactions: *Gastrointestinal:* glossitis, stomatitis, nausea, vomiting, persistent diarrhea, enterocolitis and pruritus ani. *Hemopoietic:* neutropenia, leukopenia, agranulocytosis, and thrombocytopenic purpura; rarely, aplastic anemia and pancytopenia. *Hypersensitivity:* angioneurotic edema, serum sickness and anaphylaxis. *Skin and mucous membranes:* skin rashes, urticaria, vaginitis, and rare instances of exfoliative and vesiculobullous dermatitis, and erythema multiforme, some resembling the Stevens-Johnson syndrome. *Liver:* abnormal findings in liver function tests, particularly elevated serum transaminase. *Cardiovascular:* Instances of hypotension and cardiopulmonary arrest (rare) have been reported following rapid intravenous administration. *Miscellaneous:* No serious renal or neurologic abnormalities and no ototoxicity have been reported. Occasionally, pain at the injection (IM) site.

Dosage and Administration: *Orally.* Dosage should be adjusted according to the severity of the infection. Adults, 500 mg or more every 6 to 8 hours; children over 1 month of age, 10 to 20 mg/kg 3 or 4 times daily. Nothing should be taken by mouth except water for 1 to 2 hours before and after oral administration. *Intramuscularly.* Adults, 600 mg every 12 or 24 hours; children over 1 month of age, 10 mg/kg every 12 or 24 hours. *Intravenously.* Adults, 600 mg to 1 gm added to 250 ml or more of 5% glucose in water or normal saline and given as an infusion every 8 to 12 hours. Children over 1 month of age, 10 to 20 mg/kg/day divided into 2 or 3 doses and given as an infusion every 8 to 12 hours. Should be diluted in the same manner as for adults. Lincomycin has also been administered *subconjunctively* (0.25 ml) and *topically* to treat corneal ulcers. Patients with severely impaired renal function should be given about 25 to 30% of the dose recommended for patients with normally functioning kidneys.

Availability:
LINCOCIN®: **(Upjohn)**
Capsules, 500 mg in bottles of 24 and 100.
Injection, 300 mg/ml in vials of 2 and 10 ml and in 2-ml U-Ject® (disposable syringes).
Pediatric Capsules, 250 mg in bottles of 24.
Syrup, 250 mg/5 ml in bottles of 60 ml.

LIOTHYRONINE SODIUM

Chemical Name: Sodium L-3[4-(4-Hydroxy-3-iodophenoxy)-3,5-diiodophenyl]alanine.

Description: Sodium liothyronine is the sodium salt of the L-isomer of 3,3',5-triiodothyronine and occurs as a light-tan, crystalline powder very slightly soluble in water and in alcohol. Structurally, it differs from sodium levothyroxine in that an iodine atom is absent in the 5 position. Twenty-five micrograms of liothyronine is equivalent to about 65 mg of desiccated thyroid or thyroglobulin and 0.1 mg of L-thyroxine. Its onset of action is faster than that of other thyroid substances, and has a more rapid cutoff permitting quicker dosage adjustments and easier control of the effects of overdosage. Since it is not firmly bound to serum protein, it is readily available to body tissues with a biological half-life of 2½ hours.

Indications: In conditions where thyroid-replacement therapy is indicated. Among these are hypothyroidism, ranging from mild hypothyroidism to frank myxedema; cretinism; simple (non-toxic) goiter; male infertility due to hypothyroidism. It is useful in patients with gastrointestinal disturbances that can interfere with absorption of nonsynthetic thyroid. It is also useful in patients who are allergic to desiccated thyroid or thyroid extract derived from pork or beef. May be used in the T_3 suppression test to differentiate suspected *hyper*thyroidism from euthyroidism.

Contraindications: Uncorrected adrenal insufficiency.

Warnings: The drug should not be used in the presence of cardiovascular disease unless thyroid-replacement therapy is clearly indicated. In such cases, it should be used with caution and initiated at a low dosage, with due consideration for its relatively rapid onset of action. The starting dosage should never exceed 5 mcg daily, increased if necessary by increments of 5 mcg daily at intervals of 2 weeks. Morphologic hypogonadism and nephrosis should be ruled out before this drug is given. If hypopituitarism is present, the adrenal insufficiency must be corrected before the drug is given. Since myxedematous patients are very sensitive to thyroid, dosage should be initiated at a very low level and increased gradually. Severe and prolonged hypothyroidism can lead to a decreased level of adrenocortical activity commensurate with a lowered metabolic state. When thyroid-replacement therapy is administered, the metabolism increases at a greater rate than adrenocortical activity. This action can precipitate adrenocortical insufficiency. Therefore, in severe and prolonged hypothyroidism, supplemental adrenocortical steroids may be necessary. In rare instances, the administration of thyroid may precipitate a hyperthyroid state or may aggravate existing hyperthyroidism.

Precautions: Since sodium liothyronine is not as firmly bound to serum protein as is thyroxine, the PBI may remain at hypothyroid levels even though the patient is euthyroid. The drug may lower the PBI when given to normal patients. The drug may depress thyroid function, particularly when the daily dosage exceeds 75 mcg. This effect disappears rapidly, usually within 2 weeks after the drug has been discontinued.

Adverse Reactions: In rare instances, allergic skin reactions have been noted. Abnormally high BMR levels, tachycardia, excitability, headache, irritability, increased bowel motility, excessive perspiration, and menstrual irregularities are signs of overdosage. Angina pectoris or congestive heart failure may be induced or aggravated. Shock may also develop. Therapy should be interrupted until symptoms disappear, then resumed with smaller doses, usually after 1 or 2 days.

Dosage and Administration: *Orally.* Dosage should be adjusted according to the severity of the condition and the patient's response. Most patients should be started on 25 mcg daily, increased by 12.5 or 25 mcg daily every week or two. Dosages of 100 mcg daily, and higher, may be required. In myxedema and simple goiter, 5 mcg daily, increased by 5 to 10 mcg daily every week or two until a dosage of 25 mcg daily is reached at which time dosage may be increased every week or two by 12.5 or 25 mcg; usual maintenance dose is 50 to 100 mcg daily. For male infertility due to hypothyroidism, the recommended initial dosage is 5 mcg daily. Based on sperm count and motility, daily dosage may be increased by 5 or 10 mcg every 2 to 4 weeks. Daily dosage will usually not exceed 25 mcg, and rarely should dosage exceed 50 mcg daily. In geriatric patients or in children, 5 mcg daily initially, increased by increments of no more than 5 mcg. Infant cretins, 5 mcg daily initially, increased by increments of 5 mcg every 3 or 4 days until the desired response is achieved. Infants a few months old may require 20 mcg daily for maintenance. At 1 year, 50 mcg daily may be required. Above 3 years, full adult dosage may be required.

Availability:
CYTOMEL® Tablets, 5 and 50 mcg in bottles of 100; 25 mcg in bottles of 100 and 1000.

(Smith Kline & French)

LIOTRIX

Description: A combination of synthetic thyroactive fractions, sodium levothyroxine and sodium liothyronine, in a ratio of 4:1 that closely resembles the effects of endogenous secretion. For example, a combination of 60 mcg of T_4 (sodium levothyroxine) and 15 mcg of T_3 (sodium liothyronine) represents the approximate activity of 65 mg of desiccated thyroid. The ratio of these thyroactive hormones is such that it closely simulates the clinical and biochemical effects of desiccated thyroid and of the natural endogenous thyroid secretion.

With this combination, the most widely used parameter of thyroid function—the PBI (protein-bound iodine)—may be used to aid in the assessment of the response since, when the euthyroid state is achieved, the values may ordinarily be expected to fall within the normal range.

Indications: Treatment of hypothyroidism regardless of the etiology. Use of this product for suppression therapy in simple (nontoxic) goiter promptly results in reducing the size of the thyroid gland.

Contraindications: Thyrotoxicosis, acute myocardial infarction, uncorrected adrenal insufficiency, and hypersensitivity to any of the components.

Warnings: Should be used with extreme caution, and only if thyroid-replacement therapy is clearly indicated, in the presence of cardiovascular disease, including hypertension in which case, dosage of thyroid should be reduced. Morphologic hypogonadism and nephroses should be ruled out before this drug is given. When adrenal insufficiency and hypothyroidism coexist, the former should be corrected by corticosteroids before administering thyroid hormones. Patients undergoing surgery require special attention since the possibility of precipitating cardiac arrhythmias may be greater in patients treated with thyroid hormones. Patients taking anticoagulant medication such as warfarin or bishydroxycoumarin may need to have the anticoagulant dosage reduced by ⅓ with subsequent adjustment of dosage made on the basis of frequent prothrombin determinations.

Precautions: The treatment of patients with hypothyroidism and especially myxedema should begin with small doses and increments should be gradual. Thyroid hormone therapy in diabetic patients may cause an increase in the required dosage of insulin or oral hypoglycemic agents. Conversely, reducing the dosage of thyroid hormone may possibly cause hypoglycemic reactions if the dosage of insulin or oral hypoglycemic agents is not adjusted. As with all thyroid preparations, this drug will alter the results of thyroid function tests.

Adverse Reactions: Excessive dosage may result in symptoms of hyperthyroidism appearing within 1 to 3 weeks after initiation of therapy. The most common signs and symptoms of overdosage are loss of weight, palpitation, menstrual irregularities, nervousness, diarrhea or abdominal cramps, sweating, tachycardia, cardiac arrhythmias, angina pectoris, congestive heart failure, tremors, headache, insomnia, intolerance to heat and fever. If symptoms of overdosage appear, discontinue medication for several days and reinstitute treatment at a lower dosage level. Dosage should be reduced if headache appears in those individuals who are euthyroid while taking this product. However, if headache persists or the patient develops signs of hypothyroidism at the lower dosage, another thyroid preparation should be substituted.

Dosage and Administration: *Orally,* as a single daily dose preferably before breakfast. For most patients, a single daily dose of 32, 65 or 130 mg will maintain euthyroidism. For newly diagnosed or untreated hypothyroidism, therapy may be initiated with a 16- or 32-mg tablet daily depending on the patient's status, and increased gradually every 1 or 2 weeks. In children, dosage increments should be made every 2 weeks. For unstabilized hypothyroid patients receiving some form of thyroid therapy, direct substitution of liotrix for the current dose of the other hormonal product can be made plus the increments of 32 to 65 mg equivalent every 2 weeks. In patients previously rendered euthyroid with desiccated thyroid, sodium levothyroxine or sodium liothyronine, each 65-mg tablet of liotrix usually will replace 65 mg of desiccated thyroid, 0.1 mg of sodium levothyroxine or 25 mcg of sodium liothyronine. Dosage adjustments other than those routinely necessary with any thyroid therapy are seldom necessary.

Availability:
EUTHROID® Tablets, ½, 1, 2 and 3, approximately equivalent to 32, 65, 130 and 200 mg of desiccated thyroid respectively in bottles of 100 and 1000. **(Warner-Chilcott)**
THYROLAR® Tablets, ¼, ½, 1, 2, 3, and 5 approximately equivalent to 16, 32, 65, 130, 200 and 325 mg of desiccated thyroid respectively in bottles of 100 and 1000. **(Armour)**

LITHIUM CARBONATE

Description: Lithium ion is an element of the alkali-metal group with the atomic number 3, atomic weight 6.94 and an emission line at 671 mu on the flame photometer. Lithium carbonate occurs as a white, light, alkaline powder sparingly soluble in cold water, slightly soluble in boiling water, insoluble in alcohol and soluble in dilute acids.

Readily absorbed following oral administration, it reaches peak plasma levels within 1 to 3 hours, then rapidly decreases within 5 to 6 hours followed by a slower decline over the next 24 hours or more. There is no evidence of binding to plasma proteins, therefore, it is available for tissue use; concentration in cerebrospinal fluid represents approximately 40% that of plasma. The drug is excreted primarily in the urine; fecal excretion is insignificant. Renal excretion is proportional to plasma concentration.

Studies have shown that lithium alters sodium transport in nerve and muscle cells and brings about a shift toward intraneuronal metabolism of catecholamines. Its specific mechanism in treating mania is unknown; however, normalization of the patient generally occurs within 1 to 3 weeks.

Indications: Treatment of manic episodes in manic-depressive psychotics.

Warnings: Lithium should generally not be given to patients with significant renal or cardiovascular disease, severe debilitation or dehydration, or sodium depletion, and to those receiving diuretics, since the risk of toxicity is very high in such patients. If the psychiatric indication is life-threatening, and if such a patient fails to respond to other measures, lithium treatment may be undertaken with extreme caution, including daily serum determinations and adjustment to the usually low doses tolerated by these individuals. In such instances, hospitalization of the patient is advised. *Since lithium toxicity is closely related to serum lithium levels, unfavorable reactions can occur at doses close to therapeutic levels. Facilities for prompt and accurate serum determinations should be readily available before initiating therapy.* Therapy must be discontinued if clinical signs of toxicity occur, e.g., diarrhea, vomiting, tremor, mild ataxia, drowsiness, muscular weakness. Patients should be cautioned that the drug may impair their mental and physical abilities and should, therefore, refrain from engaging in any hazardous activity. Reproduction studies with animals have indicated that the drug exhibits a toxic effect on the fetuses of some species. In addition, individual cases of lithium intoxication in both mother and infant at the time of delivery have been reported. Therefore, if lithium is considered for use in pregnant or lactating women or women of childbearing potential, the possibility of risk to the fetus or infant should be weighed against the anticipated therapeutic benefits. Until further clinical studies substantiate its safe and effective use in children under 12 years of age, its use in such patients is not recommended.

Precautions: Lithium tolerance increases considerably during acute mania and decreases when symptoms subside. Since lithium reduces sodium reabsorption by the renal tubule which could lead to hyponatremia, the patient should maintain a normal diet, including salt, and adequate fluid intake (2500 to 3000 ml) at least during the initial stabilization period. Decreased tolerance reportedly has followed protracted sweating or diarrhea, in which case supplemental fluid and salt should be administered. Diuretics should not be used concomitantly with lithium carbonate. Diffuse nontoxic goiter has been reported in some patients on maintenance therapy with lithium and in one infant born to a lithium-treated mother.

Adverse Reactions: Reactions are rare at serum lithium levels below 1.5 mEq/L, except in the patient sensitive to lithium. Fine hand tremor, polyuria and mild thirst may occur during therapy for the acute manic phase, and may persist throughout treatment. Transient, mild nausea and general discomfort may appear during the first few days of therapy.

Toxic reactions may occur at serum levels ranging from 1.5 to 3 mEq of lithium/liter. Serum levels should not exceed 2 mEq/L during the acute treatment phase, or 1.5 mEq/L during maintenance therapy. The following reactions have been reported and appear to be related to serum lithium levels: *Neuromuscular:* tremor, muscle hyperirritability (fasciculations, twitching, clonic movements of limbs), ataxia, choreo-athetotic movements, hyperactive deep tendon reflexes. *CNS:* blackouts, seizures, slurred speech, dizziness, vertigo, urinary and fecal incontinence, somnolence, psychomotor retardation, restlessness, confusion, stupor, coma. *Cardiovascular:* cardiac arrhythmia, hypotension, peripheral circulatory collapse. *Gastrointestinal:* anorexia, nausea, vomiting, diarrhea. *Genitourinary:* albuminuria, oliguria, polyuria, glycosuria. *Dermatologic:* drying and thinning of hair, anesthesia of skin, chronic folliculitis. *Autonomic nervous system:* blurred vision, dry mouth. *Miscellaneous:* fatigue, lethargy, tendency to sleep, dehydration, weight loss, allergic vasculitis, transient scotomata.

Adverse reactions apparently unrelated to dosage include *thyroid abnormalities:* nontoxic goiter, hypothyroidism, lowered PBI (protein-bound iodine), increased I^{131} uptake; *electroencephalographic changes:* diffuse slowing, widening of frequency spectrum, potentiation and disorganization of background rhythm; *electrocardiographic changes:* reversible flattening, isoelectricity or inversion of T-waves; *miscellaneous:* thirst, leg ulcers, headache, leukocytosis, transient hyperglycemia, generalized pruritus with or without rash, swelling of ankles or wrists, lowered glucose tolerance, weight gain, metallic taste. **Note:** blood for serum lithium determinations should be drawn 8 to 12 hours after the previous dose, a time when lithium concentrations are relatively stable. Serum levels alone should not be the sole determining factor. Accurate evaluation requires both clinical and laboratory analysis. Toxic levels for lithium approximate therapeutic levels. For this reason, patients should be under close medical supervision, and blood levels should be monitored twice weekly during the stabilization period and monthly after the maintenance dosage has been established. At the present time, no specific antidote for lithium poisoning is known. Gastric suction and replacement of fluids and electrolytes have been suggested. Urea, sodium bicarbonate, acetazolamide and aminophylline increase excretion of lithium significantly.

Dosage and Administration: *Orally.* Initially, 600 mg 3 times daily. This regimen should produce the desired serum level of 1 to 1.5 mEq/liter. For maintenance, 300 mg 3 or 4 times daily should maintain a serum level of 0.6 to 1.2 mEq/liter. If serum level exceeds 2 mEq/liter the drug should be discontinued; may be reinstated at a lower dosage after a lapse of 24 or more hours. Patients in acute mania can tolerate and often need high doses of lithium to achieve therapeutic effect, and to attain desirable serum concentration. However, the dosage should be reduced rapidly to maintenance levels when the acute attack subsides in order to avoid excessive serum concentrations and the resultant toxic reactions.

Availability:
ESKALITH® Capsules, 300 mg in bottles of 100 and 500. **(Smith Kline & French)**
LITHANE® Tablets, 300 mg in bottles of 100, 500 and 1000. **(Roerig)**
LITHIUM CARBONATE: **(Philips Roxane)**
Capsules, 300 mg in bottles of 100 and in unit-dose packages of 100.
Tablets, 300 mg in bottles of 100 and 1000.
LITHONATE® Capsules, 300 mg in bottles of 100 and 1000 and in unit-dose packages of 100. **(Rowell)**
LITHONATE-S™ Syrup (as citrate), 300 mg/5 ml (8 mEq) in bottles of 480 ml. *Contains no sugar.* **(Rowell)**
LITHOTABS™ Tablets, 300 mg in bottles of 100 and 1000. **(Rowell)**

LIVER INJECTION(S)

Description: *Liver injection* is a sterile solution in water for injection of that soluble thermostable fraction of mammalian livers which increases the number of red corpuscles in the blood of individuals affected with pernicious anemia. Each ml of liver injection has a vitamin B-12 activity equivalent to either 10 or 20 mcg of cyanocobalamin. Liver injection formerly was standardized in terms of U.S.P. units, but since 1952 it is standardized on the basis of vitamin B-12 content. Thus, liver injection containing 20 mcg/ml of vitamin B-12 is considered therapeutically equivalent to preparations formerly labeled 15 U.S.P. units/ml.

Liver injection, crude, is prepared in the same manner but the process of extraction is stopped at an earlier stage. Each ml has a vitamin B-12 activity equivalent to either 1 or 2 mcg of cyanocobalamin.

Indications: Treatment of pernicious anemia, tropical and nontropical sprue, and certain cases of megaloblastic anemia of infancy, achrestic anemia, and nutritional macrocytic anemia.

Precautions: DO NOT INJECT INTRAVENOUSLY. Intramuscular administration should be preceded by every known precaution for the prevention and arrest of allergic and other untoward reactions. A careful history should review possible sensitivity. A separate heat-sterilized syringe and needle should be used for each patient to prevent the transmission of homologous serum hepatitis and other infections from one patient to another.

Adverse Reactions: Local or generalized allergic reactons may occur. There may be pain and tenderness at the injection site and even slight fever. Generalized systemic reactions may include weakness, increased pulse rate and perspiration, reduced systolic blood pressure, pruritus or urticaria.

Dosage and Administration: *Intramuscularly* only. Initially in pernicious anemia, 5 to 20 mcg daily for the first 2 or 3 days, followed by 7 to 15 mcg weekly until clinical and hematologic improvement has occurred. To maintain clinical and hematologic remission, 10 mcg every 10 to 15 days or longer. Patients exhibiting extensive neurologic involvement or other degenerative changes often require more than this average dose.

Availability:
LIVER INJECTION, CRUDE:
Injection, 2 mcg/ml in vials of 10 and 30 ml. **(Lilly)**
LIVER INJECTION:
Injection, 20 mcg/ml in vials of 10 ml. **(Lederle)**
Injection, 10 and 20 mcg/ml in vials of 10 ml. **(Lilly)**
Injection (PERNAEMON®), 20 mcg/ml in vials of 10 ml. **(Organon)**
Injection, 10 and 20 mcg/ml in Steri-Vials® of 10 ml. **(Parke-Davis)**

LIVITAMIN with INTRINSIC FACTOR

Description: Each capsule contains:

Thiamine mononitrate	3 mg

Riboflavin	3 mg
Niacinamide	10 mg
Pyridoxine hydrochloride	3 mg
Cyanocobalamin	5 μg
Ascorbic acid	100 mg
Ferrous fumerate (elemental iron 33 mg)	100 mg
Copper sulfate	0.66 mg
Calcium pantothenate	2 mg
Desiccated liver	150 mg
Vitamin B-12 with intrinsic factor conc.*	1/3 OU

*N.F. oral unit.

Indications: Treatment of macrocytic and microcytic anemias, and in those anemias associated with dietary inadequacy attending convalescence, pregnancy, and those encountered in late childhood and early adolescence. Also in anemias due to iron deficiency, particularly when there is a deficiency of vitamin B complex, and in uncomplicated cases of pernicious anemia in which the intrinsic factor is essential.

Contraindications: In the presence of hemochromatosis and hemosiderosis.

Warnings: Overdosage may result in iron toxication or gastrointestinal disturbances.

Precautions: Not all patients with pernicious anemia show satisfactory therapeutic response to oral vitamin B-12 with intrinsic factor. In addition, some patients with an initially good response appear to become refractory to intrinsic factor after varying periods of oral therapy. Periodic examinations and laboratory studies of pernicious anemia patients are essential and recommended. Failure of response, or inadequate response, is an indication for parenteral vitamin B-12, generally recognized as the preferred treatment.

Adverse Reactions: Occasionally gastrointestinal intolerance to iron salts may be encountered; usually minimized by taking the medication immediately after meals. No toxic effects have been reported for vitamin B-12 with intrinsic factor; nevertheless, the possibility of gastrointestinal allergy to the animal protein from liver or intrinsic factor should be considered.

Dosage and Administration: *Orally,* 1 tablet 3 times daily taken immediately after meals.

Availability:
LIVITAMIN® with INTRINSIC FACTOR Capsules in bottles of 100 and 1000. **(Beecham)**

LOMUSTINE (CCNU)

Chemical Name: [1-(2-Chloroethyl)-3-cyclohexyl-1-nitrosourea].

Description: Lomustine, a nitrosourea chemotherapeutic agent, is used primarily for the treatment of brain tumors and Hodgkin's disease. The drug appears to act as an alkylating agent, but as with other nitrosoureas, it may also inhibit several key enzymatic processes. In common with other members of this group, it is highly lipid soluble. Nitrosourea compounds have been found to be active against experimental tumors, and to inhibit DNA, RNA, and protein synthesis. Lomustine occurs as a yellow powder that is soluble in water, alcohol, and in saline solutions. Molecular weight has been reported to be 233.71, and the drug to be relatively un-ionized at a physiological pH.

Following oral administration of radioactive drug, in doses ranging from 30 to 100 mg/M², approximately 50% of the drug has been found to be excreted in the urine within 24 hours. When administered intravenously, tissue levels are comparable to plasma levels at 15 minutes. The serum half-life of free drug and/or its metabolites tends to range from 16 to 48 hours. Because of its high lipid solubility and relative lack of ionization at a physiological pH, lomustine readily crosses the blood brain barrier and the level of a radio-labeled dose in the cerebral spinal fluid is 50% or greater than that present in the plasma. Animal studies have revealed that the drug can cause embryotoxic, teratogenic, and carcinogenic effects, and to affect fertility in male rats when they were given doses somewhat higher than the clinical dose.

Indications: Palliative treatment of brain tumors and Hodgkin's disease. The drug is generally used concurrently with other standard modalities of therapy or in combination with approved cancer chemotherapeutic agents.

Contraindications: Patients with known hypersensitivity to the drug.

Warnings: Safe use in pregnant patients has not been established. Because of the potential severity of reactions to lomustine, the drug should be administered only by clinicians experienced in the use of antineoplastic chemotherapy. Bone marrow depression, which may be delayed, is the most serious toxic effect; therefore, it is advised that blood counts be conducted every week for at least 6 weeks following administration of the drug. Periodic liver function tests are also advised.

Precautions: Special care is recommended in patients whose circulating platelets, leukocytes, or erythrocytes are below normal.

Adverse Reactions: Nausea and vomiting may occur 3 to 6 hours after an oral dose and usually last less than 24 hours. The frequency and duration of these reactions may be reduced by the use of antiemetics prior to administration, and by giving the drug to fasting patients. Thrombocytopenia usually occurs in about 4 weeks and may persist for 1 to 2 weeks. Approximately 65% of the patients develop white blood cell counts below 5000/mm³ and 36% below 3000/mm³. Repeated doses may produce cumulative bone marrow depression; therefore, subsequent courses of therapy should not be undertaken until bone marrow function has recovered. Usually, courses of treatment should not be repeated at intervals of less than 6 weeks. Infrequently reported reactions include stomatitis, alopecia, anemia, and hepatic toxicity manifested by transient reversible elevation of liver function tests. Neurological reactions such as disorientation, lethargy, ataxia, and dysarthria have occurred in some patients, but whether or not these were drug-induced has not been established.

Dosage and Administration: *Orally,* as a single dose every 6 weeks. For adults and children with normal bone marrow function, 130 mg/M²; those with compromised bone marrow function, 100 mg/M². Subsequent doses should be adjusted according to the hematologic response of the patient to the preceding dose. When programmed to be used in combination with other myelosuppressive agents, the dose of each drug should be adjusted accordingly.

Availability:
CeeNU® Capsules in vials containing 2 capsules each and in individual bottles containing 20 capsules each of 100 mg (green/green), 40 mg (purple/green) and 10 mg (purple/purple).

(Bristol)

LOPERAMIDE HYDROCHLORIDE Ⓒ

Chemical Name: 4-(p-Chlorophenyl)-4-hydroxy-N,N-dimethyl-α,α-diphenyl-1-piperidinebutyramide monohydrochloride.

Description: Loperamide is a synthetic antidiarrheal medication that inhibits peristaltic activity by exerting a direct effect on the circular and longitudinal muscles of the intestinal wall. A derivative of both haloperidol and diphenoxylate, its action has been found to be more specific, more potent and of longer duration than diphenoxylate. Clinical trials have demonstrated that the drug prolongs the transit time of the intestinal contents, reduces the daily fecal volume, increases the consistency of the stools and diminishes the loss of fluid and electrolytes. Moreover, tolerance to the antidiarrheal effect has not been observed. The major advantages of loperamide have been reported to be due to a lack of drug interaction with various medications (antibiotics, sulfonamides, corticosteroids, antihypertensives, barbiturates and tranquilizers) and a lack of detectable CNS effect or addictive characteristics in patients, although physical dependence of the morphine-type was observed in monkeys given higher doses than the prescribed clinical regimen. Also helpful is the fact that when biochemical and hematological parameters were monitored during clinical trials, no trends toward abnormality during therapy were noted. Similarly, urinalyses, EKG and clinical ophthalmological examinations did not show any significant alterations.

Following oral administration, peak plasma levels are attained in 4 hours, and the plasma half-life persists for about 40 hours. Unchanged drug remains below 2 ng/ml after the intake of a 2-mg dose, and most of the administered drug is excreted in the feces.

Indications: Control and symptomatic relief of acute, nonspecific diarrhea and of chronic diarrhea associated with inflammatory bowel disease. May also be used for reducing the volume of discharge from ileostomies. It is not recommended for use in patients with acute diarrhea caused by toxigenic organisms (*E. coli, Salmonella, Shigella*) or with pseudomembranous colitis due to broad-spectrum antibiotics.

Contraindications: Patients with known hypersensitivity to loperamide and those in whom constipation must be avoided.

Warnings: Dehydration subsequent to diarrhea may develop; should this occur, appropriate therapy to counteract fluid loss and electrolyte imbalance are indicated. Drugs which inhibit intestinal motility or delay intestinal transit time have been reported to induce toxic megacolon in patients with ulcerative colitis. In such instances, therapy should be discontinued immediately if abdominal distention or other untoward symptoms occur.

Precautions: In acute diarrhea, if clinical improvement is not apparent in 48 hours, the medication should be withdrawn. Although impaired fertility or harm to the fetus has not been observed when loperamide was given to rats and rabbits in doses 30 times the human therapeutic dose, it is not advocated for administration during pregnancy unless the clinical situation clearly warrants its use. Lactating women should not nurse their babies until it has been fully established whether or not the drug is excreted in human milk. Safe and effective use in children under 12 years of age has not been confirmed.

Adverse Reactions: Among the possible side effects, some of which may be expressions of the disease itself, are abdominal pain, distention or discomfort; constipation; drowsiness or dizziness; dry mouth; nausea and vomiting; skin rash and tiredness.

Dosage and Administration: *Orally.* The recommended initial dosage is 2 capsules followed by 1 capsule after each unformed stool, but not exceeding 8 capsules a day. When control is achieved in chronic diarrhea, the dosage should be reduced to meet the individual requirements. The average daily maintenance dosage is 2 to 4 capsules.

Availability:
C-V IMODIUM® Capsules, 2 mg (light and dark green) in bottles of 100. **(Ortho)**

LORAZEPAM C-IV

Chemical Name: 7-Chloro-5-(o-chlorophenyl)-1,3-dihydro-3-hydroxy-2H-1,4-benzodiazepin-2-one.

Description: Lorazepam is an anxiolytic drug that is chemically and pharmacologically related to oxazepam and other benzodiazepines. Studies in healthy individuals have demonstrated that the drug produces a tranquilizing effect on the CNS with no appreciable effect on the respiratory or cardiovascular systems. It has been found useful for the symptomatic relief of anxiety associated with functional or organic disorders. Generally, it has been claimed to have little or no clinical merit in the treatment of primary depressive disorders or psychosis. It occurs as a nearly white powder that is almost insoluble in water.

Following oral administration, lorazepam is readily and almost completely absorbed from the gastrointestinal tract and is promptly eliminated by the kidneys. A 2-mg dose produces peak plasma concentrations of 20 ng/ml in approximately 2 hours; and studies have shown that about 85% of the plasma content is bound to protein. The drug is rapidly conjugated at its 3-hydroxy group to its major metabolite lorazepam glucuronide which has shown no demonstrable CNS activity in animals. The mean half-life of the unconjugated drug is about 12 hours and of the glucuronide metabolite about 18 hours. When administered for periods lasting up to 6 months, no evidence of drug accumulation has been observed. The effectiveness of the drug following prolonged use (exceeding 4 months) has not been clinically evaluated. Reproduction studies in animals have demonstrated a potential for embryotoxicity and increased neonatal mortality. However, no evidence of carcinogenic potential emerged in rats during an 18-month study with lorazepam. No studies regarding mutagenesis have been undertaken.

Indications: Symptomatic relief of anxiety, tension, agitation, irritability, and insomnia associated with anxiety neuroses and transient situational disturbances; anxiety associated with depressive symptoms and as a treatment for symptoms of anxiety if such symptoms are a significant feature of functional or organic disorders, particularly those involving the gastrointestinal or cardiovascular systems.

Contraindications: Known hypersensitivity to benzodiazepine compounds, and acute narrow-angle glaucoma.

Warnings: Because sedation is the most common reaction produced by the antianxiety agents, patients should be specifically warned to avoid activities that require alertness and physical coordination, such as operating motor vehicles or dangerous machinery; also that their tolerance to alcohol and other CNS-depressant drugs will be diminished. Withdrawal reactions may occur if the drug is discontinued abruptly. These reactions are similar to those produced by barbiturates and alcohol and are usually characterized by convulsions, tremor, abdominal and/or muscle cramps, vomiting and sweating. Addiction-prone individuals should be under careful surveillance when receiving benzodiazepines because of the predisposition of such patients to habituation and dependence.

Precautions: Particular attention should be given to patients whose anxiety is accompanied by depression, since suicidal impulses may be present. In order to avoid oversedation in elderly or debilitated patients, the initial daily dosage should not exceed 2 mg. Dosage should be terminated gradually, because abrupt withdrawal of lorazepam may result in symptoms similar to those for which the patients are being treated. The usual precautions should be observed in patients with impaired renal or hepatic function. The drug is of no significant benefit in treating gastrointestinal or cardiovascular disorders which may coexist with the anxiety. Because of the possibility of esophageal dilatation, special care is advised when the drug is used for prolonged periods or in geriatric patients, and treatment should be accompanied by frequent monitoring of the upper gastrointestinal tract. Leukopenia and elevations of LDH (lactic dehydrogenase) may develop; therefore, periodic blood counts and liver-function tests are recommended in patients on long-term therapy. If lorazepam is considered for use in pregnant patients, the possibility of risk to the fetus must be weighed against the expected therapeutic benefits. As a general rule, nursing should not be undertaken while the patient is taking this drug until it has been confirmed that it is not excreted in breast milk. Safe and effective use in children under 12 years of age has not been established.

Adverse Reactions: Those that do occur are generally observed at the beginning of therapy and usually disappear on continued medication or upon decreasing the dose. The most frequently observed was sedation, followed by dizziness, weakness, and unsteadiness. The incidence of sedation and unsteadiness increased as the age of the patients increased. Less frequently observed were disorientation, depression, nausea, change in appetite, headache, sleep disturbance, agitation, dermatologic symptoms, disturbance of eye function, together with various gastrointestinal symptoms and autonomic manifestations. Small decreases in blood pressure have been noted but are not clinically significant, probably being related to the relief of anxiety produced by the drug. Manifestations of overdosage include somnolence, confusion, and coma. Induced vomiting and/or gastric lavage should be undertaken, followed by general supportive care, monitoring of vital signs, and close observation of the patient. Hypotension, although unlikely, usually may be controlled with levarterenol bitartrate injection, USP. Caffeine and sodium benzoate injection, USP may be used to counteract CNS-depressant effects. The usefulness of dialysis has not been determined.

Dosage and Administration: *Orally.* The usual range is 2 to 6 mg daily in divided doses, the largest dose being taken before bedtime. However, the daily dosage may vary from 1 to 10 mg. *For anxiety,* most patients require an initial dosage of 2 to 3 mg daily divided into 2 or 3 doses. *For insomnia due to anxiety or transient situational stress,* a single daily dose of 2 to 4 mg may be given, usually at bedtime. For elderly or debilitated patients, an initial dosage of 1 to 2 mg daily in divided doses is recommended, to be adjusted as needed and tolerated. When a higher dosage is indicated, the evening dose should be increased before the daytime dose.

Availability:

Ⓒ IV ATIVAN® Tablets, 0.5, 1 and 2 mg in bottles of 100 and 500 and in Redipak® (strip-packs) of 25. **(Wyeth)**

LOXAPINE SUCCINATE

Chemical Name: 2-Chloro-11-(4-methyl-1-piperazinyl) dibenz [b, f,] [1, 4] oxazepine.

Description: A dibenzoxazepine compound that represents a new subclass of tricyclic antipsychotic agents. It is chemically distinct from the thioxanthenes, butyrophenones, and phenothiazines.

Although the exact mode of action has not been determined, animal studies involving several species showed that the drug exerts its influence by acting on the subcortical inhibitory areas of the brain to stabilize emotional circuits. Orally administered, the drug is readily and almost completely absorbed from the gastrointestinal tract. Tranquilizing action appears within 20 to 30 minutes, reaches maximum within 1½ to 3 hours and usually lasts for 24 hours. It is rapidly absorbed from the plasma, is extensively metabolized, and is excreted mainly within 24 hours. Metabolites are excreted in the urine in the form of conjugated and in the feces as unconjugated compounds.

In experimental studies with rats, rabbits and dogs given up to twice the maximal clinical dose, no embryotoxic or teratogenic effects were observed. However, rats treated from mid-pregnancy to term with doses of 0.6 to 1.8 mg/kg of body weight (which approximates the usual clinical dose but which are considerably below the maximum recommended dose) have shown renal papillary abnormalities in the offspring.

Indications: Treatment of the manifestations of schizophrenia. Its use in the management of behavioral complications in mentally deficient patients is not recommended.

Contraindications: Known hypersensitivity to the drug, in severe drug-induced depression of the CNS (barbiturates, narcotics, alcohol, tranquilizers, analgesics, antihistamines), and in comatose states.

Warnings: Safe use during pregnancy or lactation has not been established; therefore, its use in pregnant or lactating women or in those of childbearing potential requires that the benefits derived from treatment be weighed against the possible hazards to the mother and fetus. Until further clinical experience is gained, loxapine is not recommended for children under 16 years of age. The tranquilizing effects of the drug may impair mental and/or physical abilities, especially during the first few days of treatment; thus, ambulatory patients should be forewarned about engaging in activities requiring alertness or physical coordination; also about the drug's capability of increasing the effects of alcohol and other CNS-depressant agents.

Precautions: Considerable care is essential in patients with a history of convulsive disorders, those taking anticonvulsant drugs, or those who have cardiovascular disease. Increased pulse rates have been reported in the majority of patients receiving antipsychotic doses; also, transient hypotension has been noted. If severe hypotension develops, vasopressors such as norepinephrine and angiotension may be indicated. The usual doses of epinephrine may not be effective because its vasopressor activity is inhibited by loxapine. The clinician should be alert for signs of pigmentary retinopathy and lenticular pigmentation. The usual care is required in patients with glaucoma or a tendency to urinary retention, particularly when this medication is given concomitantly with anticholinergic or antispasmodic drugs. Because of a potential antiemetic effect, loxapine may mask signs of overdosage of toxic drugs and may obscure conditions such as intestinal obstruction or brain tumor.

Adverse Reactions: Those noted were generally manifestations of CNS involvement. Drowsiness may occur at the beginning of therapy or when dosage is increased, but it usually subsides with continued therapy. Sedation has been found to be less than that of certain aliphatic phenothiazines and slightly more than that seen with the piperazine phenothiazines. Dizziness, faintness, staggering gait, muscle twitching, weakness, and confusional states have been reported. Frequently noted, especially during the first few days of treatment, were extrapyramidal reactions which in most patients involved Parkinson-like symptoms (tremor, rigidity, excessive salivation, and masked facies); also akathisia (motor restlessness). These symptoms are usually not severe and can be controlled by reduction of dosage or by administration of antiparkinsonism drugs. Less frequently noted were dystonic and dyskinetic reactions; however, these may be more severe. Dystonic reactions were manifested by muscle spasm of neck and face, tongue protrusion, and oculogyric movement, and dyskinetic reaction by choreo-athetoid movements. These reactions may require reduction of dosage or temporary withdrawal of the drug in addition to appropriate countermeasures.

Tardive dyskinesia may appear in some patients on long-term therapy or may occur after drug therapy has been discontinued. The risk appears to be greater in elderly patients on high-dose therapy, especially female patients. The symptoms are persistent and in some patients appear to be irreversible. The syndrome is characterized by rhythmical involuntary movement of the tongue, face, mouth, or jaw (e.g., protrusion of tongue, puffing of cheeks, puckering of mouth, chewing movements). These may be accompanied by involuntary movements of the extremeties. There is no known treatment for this condition; antiparkinsonism agents usually do not alleviate the symptoms, and it is advised that the drug be withdrawn if the above phenomena appear. If treatment is reinstituted, or dosage of loxapine increased, or another drug substituted, the syndrome may be masked. It has been reported that fine vermicular movements of the tongue may be an early sign of the syndrome, and if therapy is discontinued at that time this reaction may not develop.

Tachycardia, hypotension, hypertension, lightheadedness, syncope, and a few cases of ECG changes similar to those seen with phenothiazines have been reported. It is not known whether or not these were drug-induced. Dermatitis, edema (puffiness of face), pruritus, and seborrhea have also been reported. The development of skin rashes (etiology uncertain) during the summer months in a few patients may indicate a possible photosensitive and/or phototoxic reaction. Other side effects noted were dry mouth, nasal congestion, constipation, and blurred vision; these are more likely to occur with concomitant use of antiparkinsonism agents. Rarely, galactorrhea and menstrual irregularities of uncertain etiology have been reported. Some patients experienced nausea, vomiting, loss or gain in weight, dyspnea, ptosis, hyperpyrexia, flushed facies, headache, paresthesia, and polydipsia. The signs and symptoms of overdosage may range from mild depression of the CNS and cardiovascular system to profound hypotension, respiratory depression, and unconsciousness. The possible occurrence of extrapyramidal symptoms and/or convulsive seizures should be kept in mind. Treatment is essentially symptomatic and supportive and generally involves those measures that facilitate elimination of the drug from the body and reverse the undesirable effects.

Dosage and Administration: *Orally* usually in divided doses 2 to 4 times daily. The recommended initial dosage is 10 mg twice daily; for severely disturbed patients up to a total of 50 mg may be required. The amount may be increased fairly rapidly over the first 7 to 10 days until effective control of symptoms is achieved. The therapeutic and maintenance dosage usually ranges from 60 to 100 mg daily; however, amounts up to a maximal of 250 mg may be given. Daily dosages over 250 mg are not recommended. For maintenance therapy, dosage should be reduced to lowest level compatible with therapeutic response; many patients have been maintained satisfactorily at dosages in the range of 20 to 60 mg daily.

Availability:
DAXOLIN™ Capsules, 10, 25 and 50 mg in bottles of 100 and 1000. **(Dome)**
DAXOLIN C Oral Concentrate, 25 mg/ml in bottles of 120 ml with calibrated dropper. **(Dome)**
LOXITANE® Capsules, 5, 10, 50 and 100 mg in bottles of 100 and 1000 and in Lox-A-Pac® (unit-dose) packages of 100. **(Lederle)**
LOXITANE C Oral Concentrate, 25 mg/ml in bottles of 120 ml with calibrated dropper. **(Lederle)**

LUFTODIL

Description: Each tablet contains:

Theophylline	100 mg
Ephedrine hydrochloride	24 mg
Guaifenesin	200 mg
Phenobarbital	16 mg

Indications: Symptomatic treatment of bronchial asthma, asthmatic and chronic bronchitis and pulmonary emphysema.

Contraindications: Idiosyncrasy, renal disease and Addison's disease.

Warnings: Phenobarbital may be habit-forming. Should be used with care in the presence of cardiovascular disease, diabetes, thyroid disease, cerebral arteriosclerosis or mental disturbance.

Adverse Reactions: Occasionally nervousness, apprehension, restlessness and gastric irritation with possible abdominal discomfort, nausea and vomiting may occur. Administration with or after meals may help to avoid these symptoms; if not, the dosage should be reduced or the drug discontinued.

Dosage and Administration: *Orally.* Adults, 1 tablet 3 or 4 times daily and at bedtime if necessary. Children 6 to 12 years of age, 1/2 the adult dosage.

Availability:
LUFTODIL® Tablets in bottles of 100. **(Mallinckrodt)**

MAFENIDE

Chemical Name: α-Amino-*p*-toluenesulfonamide.

Description: Mafenide is a bactericidal agent for a wide range of bacteria, including various gram-negative and gram-positive organisms particularly *Pseudomonas aeruginosa;* also for certain strains of anaerobes that cause gas gangrene. It is active in the presence of pus and blood, is not affected by changes in pH, nor inhibited by *para*-aminobenzoic acid. It is readily absorbed when applied topically, and rapidly converted to a metabolite (*p*-carboxybenzene-sulfonamide) which is excreted by the kidneys.

Indications: Treatment of second and third degree burns.

Warnings: Should be administered with caution to patients with a history of hypersensitivity to mafenide. It is not known whether or not there is cross sensitivity to other sulfonamides. Safe use of mafenide during pregnancy has not been established. Therefore, the preparation is not recommended for the treatment of women of childbearing potential, *unless* the burned area covers more than 20% of the total body surface, or the need for the therapeutic benefit is greater than the possible risk to the fetus.

Precautions: Fungal dissemination through the infected burn may occur concomitantly with reduction of bacterial growth. If acidosis occurs, particularly in patients with pulmonary or renal dysfunction, therapy should be discontinued for 24 to 48 hours and fluid therapy continued in order to restore the acid-base balance. A syndrome of marked hyperventilation with resulting respiratory alkalosis has been reported to occur in some patients. Mafenide should be used with caution in burn patients with acute renal failure.

Adverse Reactions: The most frequently reported reaction was pain or a burning sensation. Allergic manifestations included rash, itching, facial edema, swelling, hives, blisters, erythema, and eosinophilia. Other reactions, which have occurred rarely, are tachypnea or hyperventilation, acidosis, increase in serum chloride, decrease in arterial pCO_2, excoriation of new skin, and bleeding of skin. A single case of bone marrow depression has been reported following mafenide therapy. Also fatal hemolytic anemia with disseminated intravascular coagulation, presumably related to a glucose-6-phosphate dehydrogenase deficiency. Accidental ingestion of mafenide has been found to cause diarrhea.

Dosage and Administration: *Topically.* Prompt institution of the appropriate measures for controlling shock and pain is of prime importance. The burn wounds are then cleansed and debrided and the cream is applied 1 or 2 times daily in 1/16-inch thickness with a sterile gloved hand; the burned areas should be covered with the cream at all times. If a dressing is required, only a thin layer should be used.

Availability:
SULFAMYLON® Cream (as acetate equiv. to 85 mg/gm of base) in tubes of 56.7 and 113.4 gm and in cans of 411 gm. **(Winthrop)**

MAGNESIUM SULFATE

Description: For systemic action, magnesium sulfate must be administered parenterally. It is employed in this way for its depressant effect on the CNS and, via the peripheral neuromuscular junction, on muscle. The nature of this depression is not fully known. In addition, it is a direct antagonist of calcium with reference to the CNS and muscle.

Indications: Magnesium sulfate may be of therapeutic value in the following conditions: convulsive states, particularly eclampsia, but also in uterine tetany, especially that from oxytocic agents, in which it acts as a myometrial relaxant; barium poisoning, in which it antagonizes the general muscle stimulation characteristic of this condition; hypertension or encephalopathy secondary to acute nephritis in children; and intravenously as an osmotic agent in the management of cerebral edema.

Contraindications: In patients with heart block or myocardial damage.

Precautions: Since magnesium sulfate is excreted almost entirely by the kidneys, it should be given very cautiously in the presence of serious impairment of renal function. The patient should be observed carefully during therapy; calcium gluconate or calcium gluceptate should be ready for intravenous administration as an antidote in case of abnormally high plasma levels of magnesium. In the presence of severe renal insufficiency, no more than 20 gm of magnesium should be given within a 48-hour period. In eclampsia, however, renal function usually is not seriously impaired, and magnesium may be excreted more rapidly. The dosage of concomitantly administered barbiturates, narcotics or other hypnotics (or systemic anesthetics) should be adjusted with caution because of the additive central depressive effects of magnesium. Parenteral magnesium should be administered with extreme caution to patients receiving digitalis preparations. Treating magnesium toxicity with calcium in the digitalized patient is hazardous because serious alterations in cardiac conduction and heart block may result.

Adverse Reactions: Flushing, sweating, hypotension, circulatory collapse, and depression of cardiac and CNS function are symptoms of abnormally high levels of magnesium in plasma. The most immediate danger to life is respiratory depression.

Dosage and Administration: *Intramuscularly* or *intravenously,* depending upon the speed of action desired. The rate of intravenous injection should not exceed 1.5 ml of a 10% solution (or equivalent)/minute, and administration should be discontinued as soon as the desired therapeutic effect has been obtained. The effect following intramuscular injection is slower in onset but may persist for several hours. The following are average adult doses: As an *anticonvulsant,* 1 gm. *In magnesium deficiency states,* 1 to 2 gm. *In uterine tetany,* 1 to 2 gm intravenously. In *paroxysmal atrial tachycardia,* 30 to 40 ml of a 10% solution administered intravenously in 30 seconds (*with care*). In *barium poisoning,* 1 to 2 gm intravenously. For *reduction of cerebral edema,* 25 ml of a 10% solution intravenously.

Availability:
MAGNESIUM SULFATE:
Injection, 10% in ampuls of 10 and 20 ml; 25% in ampuls of 10 ml; 50% in ampuls of 2, 5, 10, 20 and 30 ml. **(Various Mfrs.)**
Injection, 12.5% in Pintop® vials of 20 ml containing 8 ml; 50% in ampuls of 2 ml and in Abbo-Ject® (disposable syringes) of 5 and 10 ml. **(Abbott)**
Injection, 50% in Bristoject® (prefilled disposable syringes) of 10 ml. **(Bristol)**
Injection, 10% (I.V.) in ampuls of 20 ml, 50% (I.M.) in ampuls of 2 ml. **(Lilly)**
Injection, 50% in ampuls of 2 ml. **(Parke-Davis)**

MANNITOL

Description: Mannitol is an unmetabolizable hexahydroxy alcohol and occurs as a white, crystalline, odorless powder freely soluble in water and slightly soluble in alcohol.

Mannitol traditionally is used as a diagnostic agent to measure glomerular filtration rates. It is filtered by the glomeruli, and only negligible amounts are reabsorbed by the renal tubules. Mannitol clearance is slightly less than that of inulin.

The precise mode of action of intravenously administered mannitol has not been fully determined. It is metabolized only to a limited extent, is rapidly filtered by the glomeruli, and is *not* significantly reabsorbed from the renal tubules. A relatively rapid increase in the volume of renal tubular fluid and an increase in urine flow usually occur following administration. Approximately 80% of a 100-gm dose appears in the urine in about 3 hours. Intravenous infusion of mannitol solutions expands the plasma volume, decreases the hematocrit, decreases vascular resistance and increases renal blood flow. The decreased hematocrit is associated with marked alterations in shape and diminution in the size of the red blood cells. When hypertonic solutions of mannitol are infused, the osmotic pressure gradient of the blood is markedly increased. This action results in movement of water from the cells and tissues into the blood vessels. Mannitol distributes throughout the body fluids and a state of equilibrium in these fluids is reached about 30 minutes after a single injection.

Reduction of intraocular pressure following infusion of the drug is dependent upon establishing an increase in plasma osmotic pressure. Achievement of this is dependent upon adequate dosage, speed of administration, degree of loss from the capillaries, intracapillary pressure, and rate of elimination of this compound.

Indications: As a therapeutic agent for the promotion of diuresis, in the prevention or treatment of the oliguric phase of acute renal failure before irreversible renal damage becomes established. Also, to reduce intracranial pressure and to treat cerebral edema by reducing brain mass; to reduce elevated intraocular pressure when the elevated pressure is not amenable to reduction by other means and to promote urinary excretion of toxic substances. As a diagnostic agent for the measurement of glomerular filtration rate.

Contraindications: Severely impaired renal function that fails to respond to the test dose of mannitol; severe dehydration; active intracranial bleeding except during craniotomy; severe congestive heart failure, and pulmonary edema associated with abnormal capillary fragility or membrane permeability. It should not be given to patients whose kidney function does not respond to the test dose within 3 to 5 minutes.

Warnings: Mannitol must be administered with caution to patients with doubtful renal reserve. If increasing oliguria or azotemia develops after institution of mannitol therapy, the patient's clinical status should be carefully reviewed and the infusion stopped if necessary. Large doses may increase the risk of circulatory overload. Water intoxication may occur when large amounts are given to patients unable to excrete the drug, or to excrete the drug rapidly. The diuretic response following rapid infusion of 15% or 20% mannitol injection may further aggravate preexisting hemoconcentration. Excessive loss of water and electrolytes may lead to serious imbalances. By sustaining diuresis, mannitol administration may obscure and intensify inadequate hydration and hypovolemia. Serum sodium and potassium levels should be carefully monitored during mannitol administration. It should also be administered with extreme caution to patients with head injury where the possibility of intracranial bleeding exists, since reduction of intracranial pressure might aggravate intracranial bleeding. Safe use of mannitol has not been established with respect to adverse effects upon fetal development. Therefore, the drug should not be used in women of childbearing potential and particularly early in pregnancy unless in the judgment of the physician the potential benefits outweigh the hazards. Dosage requirements for patients 12 years of age and under have not been established.

Precautions: The clinical condition of the patient should be evaluated periodically during and after mannitol infusion along with necessary laboratory determinations to assess renal and cardiovascular function and state of hydration. Electrolyte values should be determined as necessary to prevent significant imbalances. Solutions of mannitol should not be infused simultaneously with whole blood because of the possibility that agglutination of the erythrocytes may occur in the tubing. However, if it is essential that blood be given with the infusion, at least 20 mEq of sodium chloride should be added to each liter of mannitol solution to avoid this complication. Care should be taken to avoid extravasation at site of vein puncture. In cases of oliguria, an extra-renal precipitating factor may be responsible. While mannitol infusions can be used in such cases to establish urinary output, therapy also should be directed to alleviating the precipitating factor. Not to be administered unless the solution is clear and a vacuum is present. If crystals are observed in the solution, the bottle and contents should be warmed to 50° C in a water bath, and cooled to body temperature before infusion. When infusing mannitol 20%, the administration set should include a filter.

Adverse Reactions: The adverse effects reported seem to be related to rapid infusion of large doses resulting in circulatory overload, water intoxication, and changes in levels of electrolytes. A syndrome resembling water intoxication has been reported with large doses of mannitol infused in a short period of time such as 200 gm in 8 hours. An acute transient rise in plasma volume reportedly followed a mannitol infusion of 100 gm in 1.5 hours. Loss of sodium and chloride in the urine may occur in patients who receive large doses over a prolonged period of time. The following adverse reactions have been reported: acute renal tubular changes (osmotic nephrosis), convulsions ending in death, thirst, headache, transient chest pains, chilliness, pulmonary congestion, acidosis, marked diuresis, urinary retention, edema, blurred vision, nausea, vomiting, rhinitis, arm pain, skin necrosis, thrombophlebitis, urticaria, dehydration, hypotension, hypertension, dizziness, tachycardia, and fever.

Dosage and Administration: By *intravenous infusion only.* The percentage of the solution used, the dosage and rate of administration vary depending upon the clinical situation. The usual adult dosage ranges from 50 to 200 gm in a 24-hour period, but in most instances an adequate response will be achieved at a dosage of approximately 100 gm/24 hours. The rate of administration is usually adjusted to maintain a urine flow of at least 30 to 50 ml/hour. A test dose of 12.5 gm (about 100 ml of a 15% solution) may be given in 3 to 5 minutes to test renal response. If adequate, the recommended dose may be given. *For cardiovascular and other types of surgery and trauma producing renal insufficiency,* 50 to 100 gm as a 5, 10, or 15% solution may be given. The usual dose for treatment of oliguria is 100 gm administered as a 15 or 20% solution. *Adjunctive therapy in neurosurgery and ophthalmology,* 1.5 to 2 gm/kg of body weight as a 15 or 20% solution is recommended since its effectiveness in reducing elevated pressure depends on establishing intravascular hyperosmolarity. The total dose can be given over a period of 30 to 60 minutes or more, and can be used before and after surgery. *Promotion of diuresis in the treatment of intoxications,* a 5, 10, 15 or 20% solution may be given for as long as it may be needed or until a maximum of 200 gm has been infused. *To measure glomerular filtration rate,* 100 ml of a 20% solution should be diluted with 180 ml of normal saline solution. Normal clearance rates are approximately 125 ml/minute for males and 116 ml/minute for females.

Availability:
MANNITOL Injection, 5 and 10% in containers of 500 ml; 15 and 20% in containers of 1000 ml. **(Various Mfrs.)**
MANNITOL Injection, 5 and 10% in Abbo-Vac® (single-dose) containers of 1000 ml; 15 and 20% in Abbo-Vac containers of 500 ml. **(Abbott)**
MANNITOL Injection, 10% in containers of 1000 ml; 15 and 20% in containers of 500 ml. **(Cutter)**
MANNITOL Injection, 25% in ampuls of 50 ml. **(Merck Sharp & Dohme)**

MANNITOL HEXANITRATE

Description: Mannitol hexanitrate is an organic nitrate rendered nonexplosive by admixture with carbohydrate. A vasodilator of the nitrite type, it causes gradual and relatively persistent vasodilation of the smaller blood vessels, including the coronary arteries, accompanied by a fall in blood pressure within 30 to 60 minutes. May be combined with reserpine for additional hypotensive effects and with phenobarbital to help calm the patient.

The pharmacologic actions of powdered whole root rauwolfia serpentina are essentially those of its major alkaloid, reserpine. For further information on the actions, indications, and cautions associated with preparations containing rauwolfia, see monograph on Reserpine.

Indications: Treatment of moderate to mildly severe labile hypertension; not for severe types of hypertension or those with renal involvement. Used prophylactically in anginal syndrome; however, it is not intended to abort the acute anginal episode.

Contraindications: Glaucoma, debility, in patients with a history of or with active peptic ulcer or colitis, and in those who are hypersensitive to any of the components. Also those patients in whom hypotensive effects would be dangerous; this should be considered when treating patients with coronary and cerebral arteriosclerosis.

Precautions: Tolerance to the drug develops quickly and blood pressure is not permanently lowered. Prolonged use may result in methemoglobinemia; therefore, it should not be given to patients with anemia. Overdosage may lead to cardiovascular collapse.

Adverse Reactions: Nasal congestion, anorexia, drowsiness, loose stools, dizziness, bizarre dreams, headache, weight gain, paradoxical effect (agitated or paranoid depression), parkinsonism and postural hypotension.

Dosage and Administration: *Orally,* 1 tablet 4 times daily; if the hypotensive effects are not apparent within 7 days, the dosage may be safely increased to 2 tablets 4 times daily. For the management of angina pectoris, 1 or 2 tablets every 4 to 6 hours.

Availability:
Mannitol Hexanitrate
Tablets, 32 mg in bottles of 100 and 1000. **(Various Mfrs.)**
Combinations
Tablets, 32 mg with phenobarbital, 16 mg (**Warning:** May be habit-forming) in bottles of 100, 1000 and 5000. **(Various Mfrs.)**
RUHEXATAL with RESERPINE Tablets, 30 mg with reserpine, 0.1 mg in bottles of 100 and 1000. **(Lemmon)**

MAZINDOL Ⓒ III

Chemical Name: 5-*p*-Chlorophenyl-5-hydroxy-2,3-dihydro-5*H*-imidazo (2, 1-a) isoindole, a tautomeric form of 2-[2′-(*p*-chlorobenzoyl) phenyl]-2-imidazoline.

Description: Mazindol is an imidazo-isoindole anorectic agent possessing pharmacologic activity similar to the amphetamines in the treatment of obesity. However, it is very different in its chemical structure and does not contain the phenethylamine chain. In both animal and clinical studies, the compound has proved to be active in reducing body weight. It is reported to produce moderate CNS stimulation and appetite suppression in mice, rats and monkeys.

Mazindol differs from other commonly known appetite suppressants in that its effects appear to be due, at least in part, to its ability to facilitate electrical activity in the septal area of the brain which is known to influence the appetite regulating centers of the hypothalamus—the phenethylamine compounds do not significantly alter septal activity but are thought to provide their effects through a direct action on the hypothalamus—and to its effects on norepinephrine metabolism in the CNS. Mazindol's action differs from that of *d*-amphetamine in 4 ways—it does *not:* (1) block norepinephrine synthesis in the afferent neuron; (2) increase the release of norepinephrine; or (3) deplete available norepinephrine; and (4) in its major action it blocks the re-uptake of norepinephrine to the afferent neuron. Consequently, more epinephrine is ultimately available to act on the receptor neuron.

Further studies with animals showed that the drug produces a transient increase in blood pressure with no significant alterations in cardiac rate or pulmonary hemodynamics; minor elevations in pulse rate have been reported, but true tachycardia occurs infrequently. No alterations in gastrointestinal propulsion rate was noted. In rats mazindol showed an ability to lower plasma triglycerides and to partially inhibit absorption of glucose from the gastrointestinal tract.

Following oral administration, the drug was found to be well absorbed in a number of animals. At anorectic doses, the effect is somewhat delayed in onset but prolonged in duration. Although tolerance has been demonstrated with anorectic agents, clinical studies lasting 24 weeks showed that tolerance to this compound did not develop and weight loss continued throughout the trial. The amount of weight loss associated with the use of mazindol varies from trial to trial, and the increased weight loss appears to be related in part to variables other than the use of this drug.

Indications: Management of exogenous obesity as a short-term (a few weeks) adjunct in a regimen of weight reduction based on caloric restriction.

Contraindications: Glaucoma, agitated states, known hypersensitivity or idiosyncrasy to mazindol, patients with a history of drug abuse, and during or within 14 days following the administration of monoamine oxidase inhibitors (a hypertensive crisis may result).

Warnings: Tolerance to the anorectic effect may develop within a few weeks. If this occurs, the recommended dose should not be exceeded in an attempt to increase the effect; rather, the drug should be discontinued. Patients should be cautioned that the drug may impair their ability to engage in potentially hazardous activities such as operating machinery or driving a motor vehicle. Mazindol may also decrease the hypotensive effect of guanethidine. The pressor effect of exogenous catecholamines such as levarterenol or isoproterenol may be markedly potentiated in patients who are or who have recently been taking this drug; therefore, should it be necessary to give a pressor amine to such a patient in shock (e.g., from a myocardial infarction), extreme care is advised in monitoring blood pressure at frequent intervals and initiating pressor therapy with a low initial dose and careful titration.

Since mazindol shares important pharmacologic properties with amphetamines, the possibility of abuse and addiction to the drug should be considered. Only limited data are available concerning the clinical effects and management of overdosage; therefore, the monograph on Amphetamine should be consulted. Abstinence effects have been observed in dogs after abrupt cessation following prolonged periods of treatment and "liking" scores in human subjects yielded equivocal results.

Safe use during pregnancy has not been established; it should therefore not be given to women who are or may become pregnant unless, in the opinion of the physician, the potential benefits outweigh the possible hazards to the mother and fetus. Mazindol is not recommended for use in children under 12 years of age.

Precautions: Insulin requirements in diabetes mellitus may be altered in association with the use of anorexigenic drugs and the concomitant dietary regimen. To minimize the possibility of overdosage, the smallest amount feasible should be prescribed or dispensed at one time. Cautious use and monitoring of blood pressure are required in mild hypertension; the drug is not recommended in severe hypertension or in symptomatic cardiovascular disease including arrhythmias.

Adverse Reactions: The most common are dry mouth, tachycardia, constipation, nervousness, and insomnia. Other secondary reactions reported were: *Cardiovascular:* Palpitation and tachycardia. *CNS:* Overstimulation, restlessness, dizziness, insomnia, dysphoria, tremor, headache, depression, drowsiness, and weakness. *Gastrointestinal:* Dryness of mouth, unpleasant taste, diarrhea, constipation, nausea, and other gastrointestinal disturbances. *Skin:* Rash, excessive sweating, and clamminess. *Endocrine:* Impotence and, rarely, changes in libido. *Eye:* Treatment of dogs with high doses of the drug for prolonged periods resulted in some corneal opacities which were reversible on cessation of medication. No such effect has been observed clinically. Acute overdosage may be additionally manifested by rapid breathing, fatigue, hypertension, and circulatory collapse.

Dosage and Administration: *Orally.* One tablet (1 mg) 3 times daily 1 hour before meals, or one 2-mg tablet daily 1 hour before lunch.

Availability:
(C-III) SANOREX® Tablets, 1 and 2 mg in bottles of 100. **(Sandoz)**

MEASLES AND RUBELLA VIRUS VACCINE, LIVE

Description: A combination of live, attenuated measles and rubella viruses that provide active immunization following a single injection. The vaccine is prepared from the Moraten attenuated line of measles virus derived from Ender's attenuated Edmonston strain and grown in cell cultures of chick embryo free of avian leukosis, and from Meyer and Parkman's attenuated strain of rubella virus (HPV-77) adapted to and propagated in duck embryo cell culture. The two viruses are mixed before being lyophilized.

Indications: For simultaneous immunization against measles and rubella in children from 15 months of age to puberty; however, the safety and efficacy of this product in individuals over 7 years of age has not been firmly established, but it has been proposed that the immune response should in no way differ from those to be expected following administration of either component vaccine alone. The vaccine is not recommended for infants less than 15 months of age because of the possible retention of maternal neutralizing antibodies that may interfere with the immune response. It is also recommended for individuals living in isolated communities; and in high-risk areas where infection may occur in a significant proportion of infants before 15 months. The advantage of early protection must be weighed against the chance for failure of response; infants vaccinated under these conditions should be revaccinated after reaching 15 months of age for optimal protection.

Contraindications: In pregnant women or in those women who might become pregnant within 3 months following vaccination. In patients who are known to be highly allergic to chicken or duck, or to chicken or duck eggs or feathers, or to neomycin (each dose of reconstituted vaccine contains approximately 25 mcg of neomycin). It is also contraindicated in the presence of an upper respiratory tract infection or other febrile illness; in untreated active tuberculosis; in patients being treated with agents that are known to depress resistence—these include steroids (ACTH, corticosteroids), irradiation, alkylating agents, and antimetabolites. It should not be given to individuals with blood dyscrasias, leukemia, lymphomas of any type, or other malignancies affecting the bone marrow or lymphatic systems, or to those who have a gamma globulin deficiency such as agammaglobulinemia, hypogammaglobulinemia or dysgammaglobulinemia.

Precautions: This vaccine should be administered subcutaneously *only*. Epinephrine should be readily available for immediate use in the event of an anaphylactoid reaction. Vaccination should be withheld 1 month before or 1 month after immunization with other live virus vaccines. Since temperature elevation may occur following vaccination, caution is necessary especially in those children with a history of febrile convulsions, cerebral injury, or with any condition in which stress due to fever should be avoided. Immunization with this vaccine should be deferred if the child has received more than 0.02 ml of immune serum globulin (human)/pound of body weight, or if whole blood or plasma has been administered, during the preceding 6 weeks, since exogenous antibodies may interfere with the response to this vaccine. Excretion of live, attenuated rubella virus from the throat of a majority of susceptible individuals has occurred; therefore, the possible danger of transmission of this virus to nonvaccinated or susceptible individuals must be considered. However, to date, transmission of the virus has not been regarded to be a significant risk. There have been no reports of transmission of live attenuated measles virus. Since the vaccine may temporarily depress tuberculin skin sensitivity, and thus produce a false-negative test, the tuberculin test should be scheduled before administering the vaccine. **Note: This preparation is intended for use with jet injector or syringe in large scale programs. It must be used within 8 hours of reconstitution.**

Adverse Reactions: The occurrence of fever and occasionally febrile convulsions; rash; mild local reactions such as erythema, induration, tenderness, and regional lymphadenopathy; thrombocytopenia and purpura; allergic reactions such as urticaria; arthritis, arthralgia and polyneuritis have been reported. Rarely noted were subacute sclerosing panencephalitis and other CNS reactions. Local reactions characterized by marked swelling, redness, and vesiculation at the injection site have occurred. Symptoms relating to joints (pain, swelling, stiffness, etc.) and to the peripheral nerves (pain, numbness, and tingling, etc.) occurring within 2 months after immunization should be considered as possibly vaccine-related.

Dosage and Administration: *Subcutaneously* only. A single dose of 0.5 ml of the reconstituted vaccine should be administered preferably into the outer aspect of the upper arm. The vaccine is *not* to be injected intravenously.

Availability:
M-R-VAX® Vaccine (lyophilized) in single-dose vials with disposable syringe containing diluent and in multiple-dose vials of 10 and 50 doses with diluent. Each dose of reconstituted vaccine contains not less than 1000 $TCID_{50}$ of Measles Virus Vaccine, Live, Attenuated and 1000 $TCID_{50}$ of Rubella Virus Vaccine, Live, expressed in terms of the assigned titer of the NIH Reference measles and rubella viruses. **(Merck Sharp & Dohme)**

MEASLES, MUMPS AND RUBELLA VIRUS VACCINE, LIVE

Description: A combination of live, attenuated measles, mumps and rubella viruses that provides active immunization following a single injection. The vaccine is prepared from the Moraten further-attenuated line of measles virus derived from Ender's attenuated Edmonston strain; the Jeryl Lynn (B level) mumps strain (these strains are grown in cell cultures of chick embryo free of avian leukosis), and Meyer and Parkman's attenuated strain of rubella virus

(HPV-77) adapted to and propagated in duck embryo cell culture. The three viruses are mixed before being lyophilized.

Indications: For simultaneous immunization against measles, mumps, and rubella in children from 15 months of age to puberty; however, the safety and efficacy of this product in individuals over 8 years of age has not been established. The vaccine is not recommended for infants less than 15 months of age because of the possible retention of maternal antibodies that may interfere with the immune response. It is also recommended for individuals living in isolated communities; and in high-risk areas where infection may occur in a significant proportion of infants before 15 months. The advantage of early protection must be weighed against the chance for failure or response; infants vaccinated under these conditions should be revaccinated after reaching 15 months of age for maximal protection.

Contraindications: In pregnant women or in those women who might become pregnant within 3 months following vaccination. In patients who are known to be highly allergic to chicken or duck, or to chicken or duck eggs or feathers, or to neomycin (each dose of reconstituted vaccine contains approximately 25 mcg of neomycin). It is also contraindicated in the presence of an upper respiratory tract infection, or other febrile illness; in untreated active tuberculosis; in patients being treated with agents that are known to depress resistance—these include steroids (ACTH, corticosteroids), irradiation, alkylating agents, and antimetabolites. It should not be given to individuals with blood dyscrasias, leukemia, lymphomas or other generalized malignancies, or to those who have a gamma globulin deficiency such as agammaglobulinemia, hypogammaglobulinemia or dysgammaglobulinemia.

Precautions: This vaccine should be administered subcutaneously *only*. Patients must be carefully observed for signs of sensitivity and appropriate precautionary measures should be available in the event of an anaphylactoid reaction. Vaccination should be withheld 1 month before or 1 month after immunization with other live virus vaccines. Since temperature elevation may occur following vaccination, caution is necessary especially in those children with a history of febrile convulsions, cerebral injury, or with any condition in which stress due to fever should be avoided. Immunization with this vaccine should be deferred if the child has received more than 0.02 ml of immune serum globulin (human)/pound of body weight or if whole blood or plasma has been administered during the preceding 6 weeks, since exogenous antibodies may interfere with the response to this vaccine. Excretion of live, attenuated rubella virus from the throat of a majority of susceptible individuals has occurred; therefore, the possible danger of transmission of this virus to nonvaccinated or susceptible individuals must be considered. However, to date, transmission of the virus has not been regarded to be a significant risk. There have been no reports of transmission of live, attenuated measles or mumps viruses. Since the vaccine may temporarily depress tuberculin skin sensitivity, and thus produce a false-negative test, the tuberculin test should be scheduled before administering the vaccine.

Adverse Reactions: The incidence of fever and occasionally febrile convulsion; rash; mild local reactions such as erythema, induration, tenderness, and regional lymphadenopathy; thrombocytopenia and purpura; allergic reactions such as urticaria; arthritis, arthralgia, and polyneuritis have been noted. Rarely noted were subacute sclerosing panencephalitis and other CNS reactions. Local reactions characterized by marked swelling, redness, and vesiculation at the injection site have occurred. Symptoms relating to the joints (pain, swelling, stiffness, etc.) and to the peripheral nerves (pain, numbness, and tingling, etc.) occurring within 2 months after immunization should be considered as possibly vaccine-related.

Dosage and Administration: *Subcutaneously* only. A single dose of the reconstituted vaccine should be administered preferably into the outer aspect of the upper arm. The vaccine is *not* to be injected intravenously.

Availability:
M-M-R® Vaccine (lyophilized) in single-dose vials with a disposable syringe containing diluent. Each dose of reconstituted vaccine contains not less than 1000 $TCID_{50}$ of Measles Virus Vaccine, Live, Attenuated; 5000 $TCID_{50}$ of Mumps Virus Vaccine, Live and 1000 $TCID_{50}$ of Rubella Virus Vaccine, Live, expressed in terms of the assigned titer of NIH Reference measles, mumps, and rubella viruses. **(Merck Sharp & Dohme)**

MEASLES VIRUS VACCINE, LIVE, ATTENUATED

Description: The vaccine is a lyophilized suspension of the attenuated Edmonston strain of rubeola virus. It is prepared by growing the virus in chick-embryo, or canine-renal tissue culture maintained in a nutrient fluid medium. To prevent bacterial contamination, neomycin sulfate, or dihydrostreptomycin sulfate and polymyxin B sulfate, are added during processing. The virus-containing fluid is filtered into vials and then frozen and dried from the frozen state. Potency of the vaccine is standardized according to the specifications of the U.S. Public Health Service. Each dose of reconstituted vaccine is equivalent to not less than 1000 $TCID_{50}$ (Tissue Culture Infective Dose) of NIH Reference Measles Vaccine. Various test systems are employed to exclude possible bacterial or viral contaminants.

Indications: For active immunization of children 15 months of age and older. The vaccine is not recommended for infants less than 15 months because of the possible retention of maternal antibodies that may interfere with the immune response. It is also recommended for individuals, adults included, living in isolated communities where measles is not endemic, and in high-risk areas where measles infection may occur in a significant proportion of infants before 15 months of age. The advantage of early protection must be weighed against the chance for failure of response; infants vaccinated under these conditions or if administered with immune serum globulin or measles immune globulin should be revaccinated after reaching 15 months of age for optimal protection. Inoculation a few days before exposure confers substantial protection, but given immediately after provides little or no protection. Despite the risk of local reaction, children who have previously been given inactivated vaccine alone or followed by live vaccine within 3 months should be revaccinated with live vaccine to avoid the severe atypical form of natural measles that may occur.

Contraindications: In pregnant women, in patients who are known to be highly sensitive to egg, chicken, chicken feathers, or to neomycin (each dose of reconstituted vaccine contains approximately 25 mcg of neomycin). It is also contraindicated in the presence of upper respiratory tract infection, or other febrile illness; untreated active tuberculosis; in patients being treated with agents that are known to depress resistance—these include ACTH, corticosteroids, except those patients who are receiving corticosteroids as replacement therapy, irradiation, alkylating agents or antimetabolites. It should not be administered to individuals with blood dyscrasias, leukemia, lymphomas of any type, or other malignant neoplasms affecting the bone marrow or lymphatic systems, or to those who have a gamma globulin deficiency such as agammaglobulinemia, hypogammaglobulinemia or dysgammaglobulinemia.

Precautions: This vaccination should be administered subcutaneously *only*. Epinephrine should be available for immediate use should an anaphylactoid reaction occur. Vaccination should be withheld 1 month before and 1 month after immunization with other live virus vaccines with the exception of monovalent or trivalent poliovirus, live, oral, which may be administered simultaneously. Since temperature elevation may occur following vaccination, caution is essential especially in those children with a history of febrile convulsion, cerebral injury, or with any condition in which stress due to fever should be avoided. Although extremely rare, thrombocytopenia and purpura associated with live virus measles vaccines have been known to occur. Vaccination should be deferred for 3 months or longer following receipt of immune serum globulin (human) or whole blood or plasma. Since the vaccine may temporarily depress tuberculin skin sensitivity, and thus produce a false-negative test, the tuberculin test should be scheduled before administering the vaccine. Children under treatment for tuberculosis have not experienced exacerbation of the disease when immunized with live measles virus vaccine; no studies have been reported to date of the effect of measles virus vaccines on untreated tuberculous children.

Adverse Reactions: Although rare, localized erythema, tenderness and vesiculation may occur at the injection site. Fever and/or rash usually are seen about 5 to 12 days after an injection; rarely, febrile convulsions. Significant CNS reactions such as encephalitis and encephalopathy have been noted to occur within 30 days following vaccination; rarely, subacute sclerosing panencephalitis. Preexisting infections such as otitis or tonsilitis may be exacerbated and may require specific treatment.

Dosage and Administration: *Subcutaneously* only. The recommended immunizing dose is a single injection of 0.5 ml administered preferably into the outer aspect of the upper arm.

Availability:
ATTENUVAX® in combination package consisting of a single-dose vial of lyophilized vaccine and 1 disposable syringe containing sterile diluent. The vaccine is prepared by using a more attenuated line of measles virus derived from Ender's attenuated Edmonston strain. The further modification of the virus was achieved by multiple passage of Edmonston virus in cell cultures of chick embryo at low temperature. **(Merck Sharp & Dohme)**
M-VAC® in a combination package consisting of a single-dose vial of vaccine (chick embryo origin) and 1 Lederject® (disposable syringe) containing the diluent. **(Lederle)**

MEBENDAZOLE

Chemical Name: Methyl 5-benzoylbenzimidazole-2-carbamate.

Description: A broad-spectrum anthelmintic drug that has been found effective in the treatment of infection caused by susceptible worm infestation. Mebendazole appears to exert its activity by preventing the parasite from absorbing exogenous glucose, thereby depleting its endogenous reserves to such a degree that it becomes inadequate for survival. Cure rates reported range from 61 to 75% in trichuriasis (whipworm), 91 to 100% in ascariasis (roundworm), 96 to 98% in ancylostomiasis (hookworm), and 90 to 100% in enterobiasis (pinworm). Following oral administration, an insignificant amount is absorbed from the gastrointestinal tract. Most of this is excreted in the urine within 3 days either as unchanged drug or as metabolites.

Experimental studies with pregnant rats that were given single oral doses as low as 10 mg/kg of body weight revealed embryotoxic and teratogenic activity.

Indications: Treatment of *Trichuris trichiura* (whipworm). *Enterobius vermicularis* (pinworm), *Ascaris lumbricoides* (roundworm), *Ancylostoma duodenale* (common hookworm), *Necator americanus* (American hookworm) in single or mixed infections. Therapy should be accompanied by the usual hygienic precautions for prevention of reinfection or cross-infection.

Contraindications: In pregnant women and in patients with known hypersensitivity to the drug.

Precautions: Due to insufficient experience with this drug in children under 2 years of age, the relative benefits versus the risks should be considered when treating patients in this age group. **Note:** Mebendazole is nonstaining.

Adverse Reactions: Transient symptoms of abdominal pain and diarrhea have occurred in cases of massive infection and expulsion of worms.

Dosage and Admininistration: *Orally.* The same dosage schedule applies to both adults and children. *For control of whipworm, roundworm, and hookworm infection,* 1 tablet twice daily (morning and evening) for 3 consecutive days. *For control of pinworm infection,* 1 tablet as a single dose. If necessary, the course may be repeated in 3 weeks. No special procedures, such as fasting or purging, are required.

Availability:
VERMOX® Tablets, 100 mg in cartons of 12. **(Ortho)**

MECAMYLAMINE HYDROCHLORIDE

Chemical Name: 3-Methylaminoisocamphane hydrochloride.

Description: Mecamylamine hydrochloride is a secondary amine possessing the properties of a ganglionic blocking agent. Unlike most ganglionic blockers, it possesses no quaternary nitrogen atoms in its molecular structure.

It is a potent antihypertensive agent when administered orally, and is almost completely absorbed from the gastrointestinal tract.

Mecamylamine reduces blood pressure in both normotensive and hypertensive individuals, the onset of action being gradual (½ to 2 hours) and of long duration (at least 6 to 12 hours). The blood pressure in supine patients is also reduced although the antihypertensive effect is predominantly orthostatic.

Indications: Management of moderately severe to severe essential hypertension; also uncomplicated cases of malignant hypertension.

Contraindications: Mecamylamine should be administered only when a potent ganglionic blocking agent is indicated as noted above. It should not be used in mild, labile essential hypertension or in unreliable, uncooperative patients. Coronary insufficiency, uremia, and a recent myocardial infarction are absolute contraindications. It should be used with extreme caution, if at all, in the presence of a rising or elevated BUN and in the absence of frank uremia. Ganglionic blocking agents should not be given to patients with chronic pyelonephritis that is being treated with antibiotics and sulfonamides. Glaucoma and pyloric stenosis are other contraindications.

Warnings: Tremor, convulsions, mental changes and choreiform movements may occasionally occur, most frequently when large doses of mecamylamine are administered, especially to patients with cerebral or renal insufficiency. Rebound hypertension may occur in patients when ganglionic blocking agents are discontinued abruptly; cerebral vascular accidents or acute congestive heart failure may result. Withdrawal of mecamylamine should be done gradually while other types of antihypertensive therapy are initiated.

Precautions: The patient's condition should be evaluated carefully, particularly renal and cardiovascular function. When renal, cerebral or coronary blood flow is deficient, any additional impairment which might result from added hypotension must be avoided. Utmost care is needed in patients with marked cerebral and coronary arteriosclerosis or after a recent cerebral accident. The action of mecamylamine may be potentiated by excessive heat, fever, infection, hemorrhage, pregnancy, anesthesia, surgery, vigorous exercise, other antihypertensive drugs, alcohol, and salt depletion resulting from diminished intake or increased excretion due to diarrhea, vomiting, excessive sweating or diuretics. During therapy, sodium intake should not be restricted but, if necessary, the dosage of the ganglion blocker must be adjusted. Since urinary retention may occur in patients taking this drug, caution is advised in the presence of prostatic hypertrophy, bladder neck obstruction, and urethral stricture.

Adverse Reactions: Anorexia, dryness of the mouth, glossitis, nausea, vomiting, constipation (sometimes preceded by small, frequent liquid stools), ileus, weakness, fatigue, sedation, orthostatic dizziness and syncope, paresthesias, dilated pupils, blurred vision, decreased libido, urinary retention, and interstitial pulmonary edema and fibrosis. Pressor amines should be employed to counteract excessive hypotension. Rare instances of tremor, choreiform movements, mental abberations, and convulsions have been noted.

Dosage and Administration: *Orally.* Dosage must be individualized. Initial dose is 2.5 mg twice daily after meals. Increments of 2.5 mg at intervals of no less than 2 days until desired response is obtained may be necessary. The average total daily dosage is 25 mg in 3 equally divided doses, preferably taken after meals. However, some patients may respond sufficiently to a daily dose of no more than 2.5 mg. When given with other antihypertensive medication, the dosage of both drugs should be reduced to avoid excessive hypotension. Adjunctive therapy with reserpine or hydrochlorothiazide may be indicated. Consult package literature for complete dosage information.

Availability:
INVERSINE® Tablets, 2.5 and 10 mg in bottles of 100. **(Merck Sharp & Dohme)**

MECHLORETHAMINE HYDROCHLORIDE

Chemical Name: 2,2′-Dichloro-N-methyldiethylamine hydrochloride.

Description: Mechlorethamine hydrochloride is a nitrogen analog of sulfur mustard, and occurs as a white, hygroscopic, crystalline powder very soluble in water and soluble in alcohol.

A polyfunctional alkylating agent that forms highly reactive carbonium ions which react with a number of essential cellular components, thereby altering their normal biological function. Alkalinization results in a covalent bond between the drug and a macromolecule in the tissue. The ability of the alkylating agents to interfere with DNA function, primarily through reactions with guanine, is assumed to be the most important site of action. The resultant defective DNA molecules are unable to carry out normal cellular reproductive functions. These agents are capable of reacting with cellular components at any time during the cell cycle and therefore have some advantages over other agents which act only during specific phases of the cell cycle. Its cytotoxic effect is manifest primarily in rapidly proliferating cells, including those of the lymphatic and hematopoietic systems, gonads, intestinal and corneal epithelium and certain neoplasms. Bone marrow and lymphoid tissues usually are the only normal tissues significantly affected by the drug. Toxic effects, biologic changes, and therapeutic results effected by mechlorethamine in many ways resemble those produced by total body roentgen irradiation. There is pharmacologic evidence that the nitrogen mustards have induced fetal abnormalities in pregnant mammals. Following injection, it combines with reactive groups so rapidly that it becomes inactive within a few minutes.

Indications: Intravenous administration in the palliative treatment of generalized Hodgkin's disease (Stages III and IV). Response can be improved by using the drug with other cancer chemotherapeutic agents. Useful in generalized lymphosarcoma, mycosis fungoides, polycythema vera, and in selected cases of bronchogenic carcinoma. Beneficial palliative effects have been obtained in epidermoid carcinoma of the lung, but was found to be ineffective in anaplastic and oat cell carcinoma of the lung. Although patients with chronic myelocytic leukemia, chronic lymphocytic leukemia and the acute leukemias will show an antitumor response, it is not the drug of choice for these conditions and its use should be restricted to those emergency situations when a rapid reduction in significantly high white blood cell count is required. Intracavitary administration may be useful in controlling pleural, peritoneal, or pericardial malignant effusions.

Contraindications: Pregnancy; indiscriminate trial in patients with inoperable cancer or those in the terminal stage of cancer, or those with known infectious diseases. It is contraindicated in patients with severe leukopenia, thrombocytopenia, anemia due to generalized invasion of bone marrow, and in coexistent or suspected infectious granuloma. Results are unpredictable in disseminated and malignant tumors of different types.

Warnings: Before using mechlorethamine, an accurate histologic diagnosis of the disease, a knowledge of its natural course, and an adequate clinical history are important. The hematologic status of the patient must first be determined. It is essential to understand the hazards and therapeutic effects to be expected. Careful clinical judgment must be exercised in selecting patients; if the indication is not well defined, the drug should not be employed. Extensive and rapid development of amyloidosis may occur in the presence of acute and chronic suppurative inflammation. The possible therapeutic benefits of the drug in pregnant women or in women of childbearing potential must be weighed against the considered risks to the fetus.

Precautions: The powder or its solution is a vesicant. If contamination of skin, mucous membranes or eyes occurs accidentally, wash with clean, running water for at least 15 minutes followed by 2% solution of sodium thiosulfate. If the eyes become involved, medical attention should be sought immediately. Extravasation into tissues outside a vein may cause pain, swelling and, occasionally, sloughing. Hematologic function is characteristically depressed and therapy with this drug should be discontinued until bone marrow function has recovered. Hyperuricemia may develop during therapy, particularly in the treatment of lymphomas. Urate precipitation may be minimized by maintaining an adequate fluid intake.

Adverse Reactions: The drug frequently causes unpleasant and sometimes serious adverse effects. Between 1 to 3 hours after an injection, nausea may occur and 50% of patients vomit. Antiemetics or sedatives, parenterally or orally, 30 minutes after injection may alleviate this effect. The usual course (0.1 mg/kg of body weight for 4 doses) produces moderate leukopenia (2000 to 3000 cells) within 1 to 3 weeks; larger doses may produce severe, possibly fatal, leukopenia, anemia, thrombocytopenia and a hemorrhagic diathesis with subsequent delayed bleeding. Antibiotics to protect against infection and blood transfusions to combat marked hematopoietic depression, supplemented with general supportive measures may be necessary. Other systemic effects noted were drowsiness, headache, fever, a metallic taste following injection, anorexia, weakness and diarrhea. Infrequently noted were jaundice, alopecia, vertigo, tinnitus, and impaired hearing; rarely, hemolytic anemia associated with lymphomas and chronic lymphocytic leukemia. Occasionally, a maculopapular skin eruption occurs, but this may be idiosyncratic and does not necessarily recur with subsequent courses of the drug. In one patient erythema multiforme has been observed. Herpes zoster, probably due to a latent herpes infection, has followed treatment with mechlorethamine. Further treatment should be discontinued during the acute phase of this illness to avoid progression to generalized herpes zoster. Since the gonads are susceptible to the drug, treatment may be followed by delayed menstruation or ameorrhea of several months duration. Impaired spermatogenesis may also occur; therefore, patients should be warned of the potential risk to their reproductive capacity. Thrombosis and thrombophlebitis may result from direct contact of the drug with the intima of the injected vein.

Dosage and Administration: *Intravenously.* For each course of therapy a total dose of 0.4 mg/kg of body weight is given preferably as a single dose. This total dose may also be given in amounts of 0.1 or 0.2 mg/kg each day for 2 or 4 consecutive days. Subsequent courses may be given only after bone-marrow function has recovered; this is best ascertained by repeated studies of the peripheral blood elements. However, it is often possible to give repeated courses as early as 3 weeks after the previous treatment. Patients whose bone marrow is not compromised may tolerate a total dose of 0.6 or 0.8 mg/kg of body weight, but dangerous degrees of leukopenia and thrombocytopenia are likely to occur if doses of this magnitude are employed. *Direct intracavity administration.* For malignant effusions, particularly of pleural origin, 0.2 to 0.4 mg/kg of body weight generally provides sufficient palliation. Complete directions for administration and dosage accompany the package literature.

Availability:
MUSTARGEN® in vials of 20 ml containing 10 mg of the drug extended with 90 mg of sodium chloride in cartons of 4 vials. **(Merck Sharp & Dohme)**

MECLIZINE HYDROCHLORIDE

Chemical Name: 1-(*p*-Chloro-α-phenylbenzyl)-4-(*m*-methylbenzyl)piperazine hydrochloride.

Description: Meclizine hydrochloride is an antihistamine structurally and pharmacologically related to cyclizine and to chlorocyclizine. It occurs as a white or slightly yellowish, crystalline powder slightly soluble in water and soluble in alcohol.

In common with other similar drugs, meclizine exhibits CNS depressant, anticholinergic, antiemetic, antispasmodic and local anesthetic effects, in addition to antihistaminic activity. Meclizine has a pronounced depressant action on labyrinthine excitability and on conduction in vestibular-cerebellar pathways. Following oral administration, the effects of the drug persist for 8 to 24 hours; its metabolic fate is unknown.

Indications: Management of nausea, vomiting, and dizziness associated with motion sickness; also vertigo associated with diseases affecting the vestibular system.

Contraindications: Administration of meclizine during pregnancy or to women of childbearing potential is contraindicated in view of the teratogenic effect of the drug in animal studies. It is also contraindicated in individuals who have shown a previous hypersensitivity to this drug.

Warnings: Since drowsiness may occur, patients should be warned not to engage in activities requiring alertness or skill. Safe use of this drug in children has not been established.

Adverse Reactions: Drowsiness, dry mouth and on rare occasions, blurred vision, have been reported.

Dosage and Administration: *Orally.* For motion sickness, the initial dose is 25 to 50 mg taken 1 hour before leaving on a trip. Thereafter, the dose may be repeated every 24 hours for the duration of the journey. For control of vertigo associated with disorders of the vestibular system, the recommended dosage is 25 to 100 mg daily in divided doses, depending upon the clinical response.

Availability:
Meclizine Hydrochloride
ANTIVERT®: **(Roerig)**
Chewable Tablets, 25 mg in bottles of 100 and 500.
Tablets, 12.5 and 25 mg in bottles of 100, 500 and 1000 and in unit-dose packages of 100.
BONINE® (OTC) Chewable Tablets, 25 mg in bottles of 100 and 500. **(Pfipharmecs)**
MECLIZINE HYDROCHLORIDE: **(Lederle)**
Chewable Tablets, 25 mg in bottles of 100 and 1000.
Tablets, 12.5 and 25 mg in bottles of 100 and 1000 and in single-unit packages of 100.

MEDIATRIC (CIII)

Description: Each capsule or tablet contains:

Conjugated estrogens equine (Premarin®)	0.25 mg
Methyltestosterone	2.5 mg
Ascorbic acid (vitamin C)*	100 mg
Cyanocobalamin	2.5 μg
Thiamine mononitrate	10 mg
Riboflavin	5 mg
Niacinamide	50 mg
Pyridoxine hydrochloride	3 mg
Calcium pantothenate	20 mg
Ferrous sulfate exsic	30 mg
Methamphetamine hydrochloride	1 mg

**For capsules,* provided as ascorbic acid, 70 mg and as sodium ascorbate, 30 mg.

Each 15 ml of liquid contains:

Conjugated estrogens equine (Premarin®)	0.25 mg
Methyltestosterone	2.5 mg
Thiamine hydrochloride	5 mg
Cyanocobalamin	1.5 μg
Methamphetamine hydrochloride	1 mg
Alcohol	15%

Indications: Preventive geriatrics in both male and female patients.

Contraindications: Carcinoma of the prostate.

Precautions: A careful check should be made on the status of the prostate gland when therapy is given for protracted intervals.

Adverse Reactions: Withdrawal bleeding, breast tenderness or hirsutism may occur.

For complete data on contraindications, warnings, precautions and adverse reactions, refer to monographs on The Estrogens and Testosterone.

Dosage and Administration: *Orally. Men,* 1 capsule, tablet or 3 teaspoonsful of liquid daily or as required. *Women,* 1 capsule, tablet or 3 teaspoonsful of liquid daily, or more, taken in courses of 21 days with a rest period of 1 week between courses.

Availability:
(CIII) MEDIATRIC®: **(Ayerst)**
Capsules in bottles of 100 and 1000.
Liquid in bottles of 1 pint.
Tablets in bottles of 100 and 1000.

MEDROXYPROGESTERONE ACETATE

Chemical Name: 17-Hydroxy-6α-methylpregn-4-ene-3,20-dione acetate.

Description: Medroxyprogesterone acetate is a synthetic, orally potent progestogen, with actions and uses similar to other progestogens. It occurs as a nearly white, odorless, crystalline powder practically insoluble in water and sparingly soluble in alcohol.

The drug shows exceptionally high progestational activity, whether taken orally or administered intramuscularly. Its duration of activity when taken orally is relatively short whereas its duration of activity is prolonged considerably when given intramuscularly. Because of this prolonged action and the resulting difficulty in predicting the time of withdrawal bleeding following injection, the repository injection form is not recommended in secondary amenorrhea, or functional uterine bleeding. In these conditions, oral therapy is recommended.

Indications: Intramuscular medroxyprogesterone is indicated as adjunctive therapy and palliative treatment of inoperable, recurrent and metastatic endometrial carcinoma. Orally, it is indicated in secondary amenorrhea and abnormal uterine bleeding, due to hormonal imbalance in the absence of organic pathology.

Contraindications: Thrombophlebitis, thromboembolic disorders, cerebral apoplexy or patients with a history of these conditions; liver dysfunction or disease; known or suspected malignancy of breast or genitalia; undiagnosed vaginal bleeding; missed abortion; as a diagnostic test for pregnancy; known sensitivity to the drug.

Warnings: The drug should be discontinued immediately upon manifestations of thrombotic disorders (thrombophlebitis, pulmonary embolism, and cerebral thrombosis and embolism), sudden partial or complete loss of vision, or if there is a sudden onset of proptosis, diplopia, migraine, papilledema or retinal vascular lesions. Use of the drug during the first 4 months of pregnancy in an attempt to prevent habitual or threatened abortion is not justified because of possible congenital heart defects and limb reduction defects occurring in the offspring. In addition, the use of progestational agents, with their uterine-relaxant properties, may delay spontaneous abortion of a fertilized defective ova. Detectable amounts of progestogens have been identified in the milk of mothers receiving this drug; however, the effect on the nursing infant has not been determined. Following repeated injections, amenorrhea and infertility may persist for periods up to 18 months and occasionally longer.

Precautions: Pretreatment examination should include breasts and pelvic organs, as well as a Papanicolau smear. The possible occurrence of mammary nodules which may become malignant should be kept in mind. Endocrine and liver function studies, if they become abnormal, should be repeated 2 months after the drug has been withdrawn. Patients should be observed for signs of fluid retention and conditions which might be influenced by this factor. Adequate diagnostic measures are indicated in cases of undiagnosed vaginal bleeding. Patients with a history of psychic depression should be observed and the drug discontinued if the depression recurs to a serious degree. Because of a decrease in glucose tolerance in some patients on estrogen-progestogen combinations, diabetics should be carefully observed during therapy. The pathologist should be advised of progestogen therapy when relevant specimens are submitted.

Adverse Reactions: Sensitivity reactions consisting of urticaria, angioneurotic edema, pruritus and generalized rash; acne, mild alopecia and hirsutism; prolonged postpartum bleeding in patients receiving the drug parenterally during pregnancy; and occasional thromboembolic phenomena. Also noted were breakthrough bleeding, spotting, change in menstrual flow, amenorrhea, breast tenderness, galactorrhea; change in weight (increase or decrease); changes in cervical erosion and cervical secretion; and mental depression. The following complications have been observed in patients taking estrogen-progestin combination drugs: rise in blood pressure in susceptible individuals; premenstrual-like syndrome; changes in libido; changes in appetite; cystitis-like syndrome; headache; nervousness; insomnia; somnolence; occasionally jaundice; dizziness; fatigue; backache; erythema multiforme; erythrema nodosum; hemorrhagic eruption; and itching. The following laboratory results may be altered by the use of estrogen-progestin combination drugs: increased sulfobromophthalein and other hepatic function tests; coagulation tests (increase in prothrombin factors VII, VIII, IX and X); metyrapone test; pregnanediol determination, and thyroid function (increase in PBI, and butanol extractable protein bound iodine and decrease in T^3 uptake values).

Dosage and Administration: *Orally. For secondary amenorrhea,* the usual dosage ranges from 5 to 10 mg daily for 5 to 10 days. Withdrawal bleeding generally occurs within 3 to 7 days after discontinuing the medication. *For abnormal uterine bleeding,* the recommended dosage is 5 to 10 mg administered on the 16th to the 21st day of the menstrual cycle. If bleeding is satisfactorily controlled, 2 subsequent courses of treatment should be given. *Intramuscularly. For endometrial carcinoma,* the recommended initial dosage ranges from 400 to 1000 mg once weekly administered as long as beneficial results are obtained.

Availability:
AMEN® Tablets, 10 mg in bottles of 50 and 1000. **(Carnrick)**
DEPO-PROVERA® Suspension, 100 mg/ml in vials of 5 ml; 400 mg/ml in U-Jects® of 1 ml and in vials of 2.5 and 10 ml. **(Upjohn)**
PROVERA® Tablets, 2.5 mg in bottles of 25; 10 mg in bottles of 25 and 100 and in Dosepak®s (unit-dose packages) of 100. **(Upjohn)**

MEDRYSONE: see The Adrenal Corticosteroids

MEFENAMIC ACID

Chemical Name: *N*-(2,3-Xylyl)-anthranilic acid.

Description: Mefenamic acid is a synthetic, non-narcotic analgesic structurally unrelated to other analgesics. It occurs as an off-white, crystalline powder insoluble in water and slightly soluble in alcohol.

Laboratory studies indicate that the drug possesses antipyretic-analgesic and antiinflammatory activity. The drug is devoid of any capacity to relieve morphine abstinence signs in abstinent, morphine-habituated monkeys. Although no fetal anomalies were induced in animals, decrease in fertility and increase in stillbirths or resorption were observed.

Gradually absorbed from the gastrointestinal tract, it reaches peak plasma levels in 2 to 4 hours, and its duration of action persists for about 6 hours. It is strongly bound to plasma proteins and is distributed unevenly in various tissues. Clinical studies have shown that 50% of a single oral dose is excreted in the urine and feces, both as free drug and as metabolites, within 24 hours.

Indications: Short term (1 week) administration for the relief of mild to moderate pain.

Contraindications: In patients hypersensitive to mefenamic acid, in those with ulceration or chronic inflammation of either the upper or lower gastrointestinal tract, and in children under 14 years of age.

Warnings: Safe use during pregnancy has not been established. Administration of mefenamic acid for periods exceeding 1 week is not recommended. If diarrhea occurs, therapy should be promptly discontinued. The patient so affected is usually unable to tolerate the drug thereafter. Cautious use of the drug in patients with a history of kidney or liver disease is advised; BUN values may rise during therapy. Microscopic examination in dogs given 100 or 200 mg/kg revealed slight centrolobular hepatocellular vacuolation. Also, there was some evidence of edema and blunting of renal papilla in dogs administered 200 mg/kg. Rats given 100 mg/kg showed microscopic evidence of renal papillary necrosis with epithelial cell degeneration.

Precautions: Administer with caution to patients with abnormal renal function or inflammatory disease of the gastrointestinal tract. In animal toxicity studies, rats given 100 mg/kg of the drug have been known to develop small intestinal mucosal erosions and ulcers. If a rash occurs, promptly withdraw the drug. Mefenamic acid may also prolong prothrombin time. Therefore, when the drug is administered to patients receiving oral anticoagulant drugs, frequent monitoring of prothrombin time is necessary. Caution is also advised when giving the drug to asthmatics, since an acute exacerbation of their condition may occur. A false-positive reaction for urinary bile, using the diazo tablet test, may result after mefenamic acid administration. If biliuria is suspected, other diagnostic procedures, such as the Harrison test, should be performed.

Adverse Reactions: Diarrhea, which may be severe and is at times associated with inflammation of the bowel or hemorrhage, may occur in patients taking mefenamic acid. There is a low but definite incidence of severe auto-immune hemolytic anemia in patients given this drug for prolonged periods of time. Thrombocytopenic purpura, leukopenia, eosinophilia, pancytopenia, agranulocytosis, and bone marrow hypoplasia have been reported in association with mefenamic acid therapy. Minor reactions occurring more frequently during this drug therapy are drowsiness, nausea, gastrointestinal discomfort, dizziness, "nervousness," and headache. Less commonly, vomiting, "gas," urticaria, rash, blurred vision, insomnia, and perspiration have occurred. There have been rare reports of palpitations, facial edema, dyspnea, eye irritation, ear pain, dysuria, hematuria, reversible loss of color vision, and increased need for insulin in a diabetic. There has been inconsistent evidence from laboratory studies of mild renal and hepatic toxicity.

Dosage and Administration: *Orally.* Adults and children over 14 years of age, 500 mg initially followed by 250 mg every 6 hours as needed. Therapy should not be continued beyond 1 week, because the margin of safety is reduced at higher doses and for longer periods of administration.

Availability:
PONSTEL® Kapseals® (capsules), 250 mg in bottles of 100. **(Parke-Davis)**

MEGESTROL ACETATE

Chemical Name: 17α-Acetoxy-6-methylpregna-4,6-diene-3,20-dione.

Description: Megestrol acetate is a potent orally effective progestational agent with antineoplastic activity against endometrial carcinoma. It occurs as a white, crystalline solid with a molecular weight of 384.5.

While the precise mechanism by which megestrol produces its antineoplastic effects against endometrial carcinoma is unknown, an antiluteinizing effect mediated by way of the pituitary has been postulated. Also, present evidence suggests a local effect as a result of the marked changes brought about by the direct instillation of progestational agents into the endometrial cavity.

In clinical studies, plasma levels of titrated drug and metabolites reach a peak within 1 to 3 hours following oral administration. About 16% of the radioactive dose was excreted in the urine within 48 hours. Animal studies showed that megestrol tends to concentrate in the liver, fat tissue, and adrenals.

In a clinical trial with 77 patients, 27 (35%) showed objective response as manifested by cessation of vaginal bleeding, cessation of ascites, or regression of tumor masses. The longest duration of continuing objective response is now more than 5 years. Studies with rats showed that megestrol had no significant effect on mammary fibroadenoma or adenocarcinoma, methylcholanthrene carcinoma, acute leukemia and Dunning leukemia, and spontaneous leiomyosarcoma. However, malignant lymphoma in mice may have been stimulated. Female dogs receiving the drug for up to 7 years showed an increased incidence of both benign and malignant breast tumors.

Indications: Adjunctive or palliative treatment of recurrent or metastatic breast or endometrial carcinoma. It should not replace currently accepted procedures such as surgery, radiation, etc.

Contraindications: None known when used as recommended.

Warnings: Not recommended for other types of neoplastic diseases.

Precautions: Generally, no specific precautions were noted when megestrol was used as suggested, but close surveillance of the patient is advised. To be used cautiously in patients with a history of thrombophlebitis.

Adverse Reactions: Two reports of a feeling of coldness.

Dosage and Administration: *Orally. Breast cancer:* The recommended dosage is 40 mg 4 times daily. *Endometrial carcinoma:* The dosage ranges from 40 to 320 mg daily in divided doses. Two months of continuous treatment is considered an adequate trial period.

Availability:
MEGACE® Tablets, 20 and 40 mg in bottles of 100. **(Mead Johnson)**

MELPHALAN

Chemical Name: L-3-[*p*-[*Bis*(2-chloroethyl)amino]phenyl]alanine.

Description: Melphalan, the L-isomer of the phenylalanine derivative of mechlorethamine, appears to be more active than medphalan, the D-isomer. Melphalan occurs as a white powder very slightly soluble in water and in propylene glycol.

Melphalan is an alkylating agent that seems to be equally effective whether given orally or intravenously. It has the general pharmacologic properties of nitrogen mustard compounds. It has been found to remain active in the blood longer (2 to 6 hours) than nitrogen mustard (10 minutes). The drug is said to exert its cytotoxic action by the cross-linking of DNA of cells in the resting stage. Since response may be gradual, it is important that repeated courses or continuous therapy be given so that improvement may continue slowly over many months. The maximal benefit may be missed if treatment is abandoned prematurely.

Indications: Treatment of multiple myeloma.

Contraindications: Should not be given if other similar chemotherapeutic agents or radiation has been administered in the recent past, or if the neutrophil and/or platelet counts are depressed; also it should not be given concurrently with radiation.

Warnings: As with other nitrogen mustard drugs excessive dosage will produce marked bone marrow depression. Frequent blood counts are essential to determine optimal dosage and to avoid toxicity. The drug should be discontinued or the dosage reduced upon evidence of abnormal depression of the bone marrow. Safe use of melphalan during pregnancy has not been established with respect to adverse effects on fetal development. Therefore, it should be used in women of childbearing potential and particularly during the first trimester of pregnancy only when, in the judgment of the physician, the potential benefits outweigh the possible hazards.

Precautions: If the leukocyte count falls below 3000 cells/cu mm, or the platelet count below 100,000/cu mm, the drug should be discontinued until the blood picture has had a chance to recover.

Adverse Reactions: Nausea and vomiting have been noted with the use of high doses. Also, dose-related bone marrow depression produces anemia, neutropenia, and thrombocytopenia.

Dosage and Administration: *Orally.* Usual dosage is 6 mg daily which may be given as a single dose. The dosage schedule should be adjusted on the basis of blood counts done at weekly intervals; after 2 or 3 weeks of treatment, the drug should be discontinued for up to 4 weeks during which time the blood count should be carefully followed. When the white blood cell and platelet counts are rising, a maintenance dose of 2 mg daily may be instituted. For additional dosage regimens, refer to the package literature.

Availability:
ALKERAN® Tablets, 2 mg in bottles of 50. **(Burroughs Wellcome)**

MENADIOL SODIUM DIPHOSPHATE

Chemical Name: 2-Methyl-1,4-naphthalenediol diphosphoric acid ester tetrasodium salt.

Description: Menadiol is a potent, synthetic, water-soluble analog of vitamin K. Its potency is approximately ½ that of menadione. It occurs as a white to pink, hygroscopic powder very soluble in water, forming solutions with a pH between 7 and 9.

It is readily absorbed and promptly utilized by the liver for the production of prothrombin and other essential clotting factors. The action of menadiol is generally detectable within 1 to 2 hours. Vitamin K, as it occurs in nature, is fat soluble and not well absorbed from the intestine unless bile salts are present. Deficiency may result from lack of vitamin K, inadequate intestinal absorption, or, in the presence of severe liver damage, failure in utilization. It is manifested by hemorrhage due to hypoprothrombinemia.

In vitamin K deficiency, the blood prothrombin time is prolonged. This test is used to detect deficiencies before hemorrhage occurs, to determine the effect of treatment, and to differentiate hemorrhage caused by vitamin K deficiency from hemorrhage of other etiology.

Indications: Treatment of hypoprothrombinemia secondary to factors limiting absorption or synthesis of vitamin K, such as obstructive jaundice, biliary fistula, sprue, ulcerative colitis, celiac disease, intestinal resection, cystic fibrosis of the pancreas, regional enteritis and antibacterial therapy. It is also indicated in hypoprothrombinemia secondary to administration of salicylates. May also be used to test liver function.

Contraindications: Should not be administered to women during the last few weeks of pregnancy as a prophylactic measure against physiological hypoprothrombinemia or hemorrhagic disease of the newborn. Contraindicated in those patients hypersensitive to this agent.

Warnings: Phytonadione is generally the preferred vitamin K preparation in the treatment of hemorrhage due to anticoagulant-induced hypoprothrombinemia, and in the prophylaxis and treatment of hemorrhagic disease of the newborn because of its greater margin of safety. Menadiol sodium diphosphate also does not counteract the anticoagulant action of heparin. Safe use of this drug in pregnant women with respect to adverse effects on the fetus has not been established, nor has it been definitely confirmed as to whether or not the drug may affect fertility.

Precautions: Large doses may result in a temporary resistance to prothrombin-depressing anticoagulant agents. When anticoagulant therapy is reinstituted following high doses of menadiol sodium diphosphate, it may be necessary to administer somewhat larger doses of the prothrombin-depressing anticoagulant or to use a drug (e.g., heparin) that acts on a different principle. When hypothrombinemia results from extensive liver damage, vitamin K therapy cannot be expected to be effective except to the extent of improving the function of the undamaged hepatic tissue. Also repeated large doses of vitamin K are not warranted in liver disease if the initial response to the vitamin is unsatisfactory. In patients with severe hepatic disease, large doses of synthetic vitamin K may further depress liver function. Lack of response may indicate that there is a coagulation defect or that the condition being treated is unresponsive to vitamin K. This drug can induce erythrocyte hemolysis in patients with relatively low levels of glucose-6-phosphate dehydrogenase.

Adverse Reactions: In adults, toxic manifestations are extremely uncommon, but bromsulphalein retention and prolongation of prothrombin time have been reported following maximal doses. Occasional occurrences of allergic reactions, such as skin rash and urticaria, also minor instances of gastric upset, have been reported. In infants excessive doses of vitamin K analogs may cause increased bilirubinemia that may result in kernicterus which may lead to brain damage or even death.

Dosage and Administration: *Orally, intramuscularly, intravenously* or *subcutaneously.* Adult dosage ranges from 5 to 15 mg and children 5 to 10 mg once or twice daily. Duration of treatment and frequency of dosage should be governed by blood prothrombin-time determinations. As a liver function test, 75 mg *intravenously.*

Availability:

KAPPADIONE® Injection, 10 mg/ml in ampuls of 1 ml in cartons of 25. **(Lilly)**

SYNKAYVITE®: **(Roche)**

Injection, 5 and 10 mg/ml in ampuls of 1 ml; 75 mg/2 ml in ampuls of 2 ml.

Tablets, 5 mg in bottles of 100.

MENADIONE

Chemical Name: 2-Methyl-1,4-naphthoquinone, and as sodium bisulfite.

Description: Menadione is a synthetic, fat-soluble, analog of vitamin K which, in the presence of bile salts, is readily absorbed from the gastrointestinal tract following oral administration and is promptly utilized by the liver for the production of prothrombin and other essential clotting factors.

Menadione sodium bisulfite is the solubilized form of menadione which can be administered parenterally. Because of its solubility, it is effective without bile salts in conditions where the flow of bile is obstructed. It shares the actions and uses of menadione and menadiol.

Indications: Treatment of vitamin K deficiency secondary to the administration of antibacterial therapy; hypoprothrombinemia secondary to factors limiting absorption or synthesis of vitamin K such as obstructive jaundice, biliary fistula, sprue, ulcerative colitis, celiac disease, intestinal resection, cystic fibrosis of the pancreas, regional enteritis, and antibacterial therapy. It is also indicated in hypoprothrombinemia secondary to administration of salicylates.

Contraindications: The risks associated with the use of water-soluble or synthetic vitamin K derivatives do not justify administration of this drug to the newborn or to the mother during the last few weeks of pregnancy. Hypoprothrombinemia following hepatocellular disease is usually not favorably influenced, and may be further augmented by the administration of vitamin K. Also contraindicated in patients hypersensitive to menadione.

Warnings: Menadione can hemolyze red blood cells in patients deficient in glucose-6-phosphate dehydrogenase, as well as in the newborn, especially premature infants. Since this drug does not counteract the anticoagulant action of heparin, phytonadione is the preferred treatment of hemorrhage due to anticoagulant-induced hypoprothrombinemia. There is no adequate information available at the present time as to whether this drug may affect fertility or have a teratogenic potential or other adverse effect on the fetus.

Precautions: Large doses may result in a temporary resistance to prothrombin-depressing anticoagulant agents. When anticoagulant therapy is reinstituted following high doses of menadione, it may be necessary to administer somewhat larger doses of the prothrombin-depressing anticoagulant or to use a drug (e.g., heparin) that acts on a different principle. When hypoprothrombinemia results from extensive liver damage, vitamin K therapy cannot be expected to be effective except to the extent of improving the function of the undamaged hepatic tissue. Also, repeated large doses of vitamin K are not warranted in liver disease if the initial response to the vitamin is unsatisfactory. In patients with severe liver disease, large doses of synthetic vitamin K may further depress liver function. Lack of response may indicate that there is a coagulation defect or that the condition being treated is unresponsive to vitamin K. Menadione may induce erythrocyte hemolysis in patients with relatively low levels of glucose-6-phosphate dehydrogenase.

Adverse Reactions: Nausea, vomiting and headache have been reported after doses of 5 mg. Prolonged prothrombin time has been observed after massive parenteral doses of vitamin K analogs. Sensitivity reactions, such as dermatitis and anaphylactoid symptoms, have been observed. In infants, particularly premature infants, excessive doses of vitamin K analogs may cause increased bilirubinemia which in turn can lead to brain damage or even death.

Dosage and Administration: *Orally.* The usual dosage ranges from 2.5 to 5 mg daily. Larger doses may be needed in patients with severe vitamin K deficiency. In obstructive jaundice and other conditions interfering with the absorption of vitamin K, dosage ranges from 5 to 10 mg daily. *Intramuscularly* or *intravenously,* 2.5 to 10 mg depending upon the indication for which it is used.

Availability:

MENADIONE Tablets, 5 mg in bottles of 100. **(Lilly)**

Menadione Sodium Bisulfite

HYKINONE® Injection, 5 and 10 mg/ml in ampuls of 1 ml. **(Abbott)**

MENOTROPINS

Abbreviations:

LH = Luteinizing hormone.

IU = International unit. One unit of LH for the IRP for HMG is biologically equivalent to approximately 1/2 unit of HCG.

FSH = Follicle-stimulating hormone.
HCG = Human chorionic gonadotropin (anterior pituitary-like sex hormone).
HMG = Human menopausal gonadotropins.
IRP = International Reference Preparation of the World Health Organization.
ICSH = Interstitial cell-stimulating hormone from the anterior lobe of the pituitary gland.

Description: Menotropins is a purified preparation of gonadotropins extracted from the urine of postmenopausal women. It is standardized biologically for FSH and LH (ICSH) gonadotropic activities in terms of the IRP for HMG established by the World Health Organization.

Taken as directed, menotropins promotes the growth of the graafian follicles in women in whom the cause of anovulation is secondary rather than primary ovarian failure. Treatment in most instances results only in ovarian follicular growth and maturation. To effect ovulation, HCG must be given following the administration of menotropins when clinical assessment of the patient indicates that the follicles have indeed matured sufficiently.

Indications: To induce ovulation in selected anovulatory women who wish to become pregnant. Infertility may be treated in women with primary amenorrhea, secondary amenorrhea with or without galactorrhea, polycystic ovary syndrome, anovulatory cycles, irregular menses. Package literature should be consulted for the criteria used in selecting patients for treatment.

Contraindications: A high urinary gonadotropin level indicating primary ovarian failure; overt thyroid and adrenal dysfunction; an organic intracranial lesion such as a pituitary tumor; infertility due to any cause other than secondary ovarian failure; abnormal vaginal bleeding of undetermined origin; ovarian cysts or enlargement due to any cause other than polycystic ovary syndrome; and pregnancy.

Warnings: Menotropins is a potent gonadotropic substance capable of causing mild to severe adverse reactions. It should be used only by physicians who are thoroughly familiar with infertility problems.

Precautions: Careful diagnosis is essential in selecting patients for therapy. To minimize the hazards associated with abnormal ovarian enlargement, which may result from therapy, the lowest effective dose should be used. Mild to moderate uncomplicated ovarian enlargement if it occurs, generally regresses without treatment within 2 or 3 weeks. The hyperstimulation syndrome, characterized by sudden ovarian enlargement accompanied by ascites with or without pain and/or pleural effusion, occurs in a very small percentage of patients in which case treatment should be terminated and the patient hospitalized. The occurrence of hemoconcentration associated with fluid loss into the abdominal cavity should be thoroughly assessed in the following manner: daily determinations—more often if needed—of fluid intake and output, body weight, hematocrit, serum and urinary electrolytes, and urinary specific gravity. The ascitic fluid should never be removed because of the potential danger of injury to the ovary. Ruptured ovarian cysts, usually resulting from pelvic examination, may cause hemoperitoneum. If this occurs, and if bleeding is of such a nature that surgical intervention is required, the conservative approach with partial resection of the enlarged ovary or ovaries is generally considered adequate. Patients with significant enlargement of the ovaries following ovulation should refrain from sexual intercourse because of the danger of hemoperitoneum resulting from ruptured ovarian cysts. Before initiating treatment with menotropins, the patient and her husband should be informed of the frequency and the potential hazards of multiple births.

Adverse Reactions: Ovarian enlargement; hyperstimulation syndrome; hemoperitoneum; arterial thromboembolism; febrile reactions of undetermined origin; and defects at birth including congenital anatomic defects and mongolism.

Dosage and Administration: The contents of 1 vial is dissolved in 1 to 2 ml of sterile saline solution and administered *intramuscularly* immediately. Any unused reconstituted material should be discarded. The recommended dosage initially is the contents of 1 ampul daily for 9 to 12 days, followed 1 day after the last dose by 10,000 units of chorionic gonadotropin (HCG). Therapy should not continue beyond 12 days. If there is evidence of ovulation but no pregnancy, this dosage regimen should be repeated for at least 2 more courses before increasing the dosage to 2 ampuls daily for 9 to 12 days, along with 10,000 I.U. of HCG 24 hours after the last dose of menotropins. If evidence of ovulation is manifested, but pregnancy does not ensue, the same dosage should be repeated for 2 more courses. Doses larger than this are not recommended. Package literature should be consulted for more detailed information.

Availability:
PERGONAL® for Injection (lyophilized) in 2-ml vials containing 75 IU each of FSH and LH and 10 mg of lactose. **(Serono)**

MEPENZOLATE BROMIDE

Chemical Name: *N*-methyl-3-hydroxypiperidine benzilate methobromide.

Description: Mepenzolate bromide is a synthetic, anticholinergic quaternary ammonium compound closely related, chemically and pharmacologically, to pipenzolate. It differs from pipenzolate only in that it has a methyl group in place of an ethyl group attached to the nitrogen atom. It occurs as a white, crystalline powder sparingly soluble in water.

In common with other parasympatholytic drugs, the effects produced by mepenzolate are similar to those of atropine. As with other quaternary anticholinergics, it has little or no direct spasmolytic action on smooth muscle; high doses may block ganglionic and skeletal neuromuscular transmission. To date, there has been no conclusive evidence as to whether this drug is useful in healing the peptic ulcer, decreasing the rate of recurrences or preventing complications.

Following oral administration, gastrointestinal absorption is poor and irregular, effects appear in about 1 hour and persist for 3 to 4 hours. The drug is excreted primarily in the urine and bile, and as unabsorbed drug in feces.

Indications: Adjunctive therapy in the treatment of peptic ulcer, the irritable bowel syndrome (irritable colon, spastic colon, mucous colitis, acute enterocolitis and functional gastrointestinal disorders), neurogenic bowel disturbances including the splenic flexure syndrome and neurogenic colon. Formulated with phenobarbital for adjunctive therapy in the treatment of diverticulitis, mild ulcerative colitis and diarrheas such as functional diarrheas, loose stools, postgastrectomy syndrome, dumping syndrome, drug-induced diarrheas, acute enteritis, intestinal viral infection, colitis, ileocolitis and diarrheas due to ileostomies and ileoanal anastamoses.

Contraindications: Intolerance or hypersensitivity to the drug, in glaucoma (particularly narrow-angle), in obstructive disease of either the genitourinary or gastrointestinal tract, in toxic megacolon, in intestinal atony of the elderly or debilitated patient, in acute hemorrhage where the cardiovascular status is unstable, and in myasthenia gravis. Phenobarbital is contraindicated in acute intermittent porphyria, in patients hypersensitive to it, and in those in whom it produces restlessness and/or excitement.

Warnings: Should be used with extreme caution in advanced, severe ulcerative colitis; however, as noted earlier, it is contraindicated in the extreme stage of this disorder (toxic megacolon). Treatment with this drug in diarrhea due to incomplete intestinal obstruction, especially in patients with ileostomy or colostomy would be inappropriate and possibly harmful. Heat prostration (fever and heat stroke due to decreased sweating) may occur in the presence of high environmental temperatures. Since drowsiness and blurred vision may occur, patients should be cautioned not to engage in activities requiring alertness and motor coordination. Safe use of this drug during pregnancy with regard to adverse effects on the fetus has not been established. Phenobarbital may be habit-forming. See monograph on Phenobarbital for additional warnings.

Precautions: Mepenzolate must be used as an adjunct to, not as replacement for, therapy while determining and correcting the underlying causative factors of diarrhea and other signs of intestinal dyskinesia. Should be used with caution in open-angle glaucoma (contraindicated in narrow-angle glaucoma), ulcerative colitis, nonobstructing prostatic hypertrophy, hiatal hernia associated with reflux esophagitis, urinary retention, and other conditions adversely affected by atropine-like drugs. In the treatment of gastric ulcer the use of anticholinergic agents may produce a delay in gastric emptying time and may complicate such therapy (antral stasis). This drug may not be effective in the presence of biliary tract complications. Special care is required in patients with hyperthyroidism, coronary heart disease, congestive heart failure, cardiac arrhythmias, and hypertension. It should be kept in mind that a curare-like action may occur with excessive dosages. Concomitant administration of anticholinergic drugs and any other agents which would increase the anticholinergic effects of mepenzolate should be avoided.

Adverse Reactions: These may include dry mouth; urinary hesitancy and retention; blurred vision and tachycardia; palpitation; mydriasis; dilation of the pupil; cycloplegia; increased ocular tension; loss of taste; headaches; nervousness; drowsiness; weakness; dizziness; insomnia; nausea; vomiting; impotency; suppression of lactation; constipation; bloated feeling; severe allergic reaction or drug idiosyncrasies, including anaphylaxis, urticaria and other dermal manifestations; some degree of mental confusion and/or excitement especially in elderly patients; and decreased perspiration. See monograph on Phenobarbital for additional adverse reactions.

Dosage and Administration: *Orally.* One or 2 tablets or teaspoonsful 3 times daily with meals and 1 or 2 tablets or teaspoonsful at bedtime. The lower dosage should be instituted initially and then adjusted subsequently according to the patient's response. Phenobarbital has been added for those patients who may require sedation.

Availability:
CANTIL®: **(Merrell-National)**
Liquid, 25 mg/5 ml in bottles of 60 ml and 1 pint.
Tablets, 25 mg in bottles of 100, 250 and 1000.
CANTIL-PHB: **(Merrell-National)**
Liquid, 25 mg/5 ml with phenobarbital, 16 mg in bottles of 60 ml and 1 pint.
Tablets, 25 mg with phenobarbital, 16 mg in bottles of 100, 250 and 1000.

MEPERIDINE HYDROCHLORIDE Ⓒ II

Chemical Name: Ethyl 1-methyl-4-phenyl isonipecotate hydrochloride.

Description: Meperidine is a synthetic narcotic analgesic, spasmolytic and sedative. Its degree of analgesia is said to be somewhere between that of codeine and morphine. Following an intramuscular injection, the analgesic effect peaks in about 45 minutes and persists for 2 to 4 hours and, perhaps, 6 hours with larger than usual doses. Its sedative effect is slight, has no antitussive properties, and is not constipating.

The drug owes its spasmolytic action on the smooth muscles of the lower gastrointestinal tract, the uterus, bronchial tree, and the urinary bladder, somewhat to its parasympatholytic effect, but for the most part to its papaverine-like depression of muscle fibers.

There is some evidence that suggests that meperidine may produce less smooth muscle spasm, constipation, and depression of the cough reflex than equianalgesic doses of morphine. Meperidine, in 60- to 80-mg parenteral doses, is approximately equivalent in analgesic effect to 10 mg of morphine. The onset of action is slightly more rapid and the duration of action is slightly shorter than that of morphine. Meperidine is significantly less effective by the oral rather than by the parenteral route, but the exact ratio of oral to parenteral effectiveness is not known.

Indications: Relief of moderate to severe pain, for preoperative medication, for support of anesthesia, and for obstetrical analgesia. Meperidine is combined with APC or acetaminophen to provide additive analgesic effect in addition to antipyretic action and with promethazine to provide enhanced analgesic and sedative effects.

Contraindications: Hypersensitivity to meperidine. In patients who are receiving monoamine oxidase inhibitors (MAOI) or those who have received such agents within 14 days, the action of meperidine is greatly, and even dangerously, potentiated and resembles the syndrome of acute narcotic overdosage (coma, severe respiratory depression, cyanosis, and hypotension). In others, the predominant manifestations have been hyperexcitability, convulsions, tachycardia, hyperpyrexia, and hypertension. The mechanism of these reactions is unclear, but may be related to preexisting hyperphenylalaninemia. If a narcotic is indicated in such patients, a sensitivity test should be performed before administering meperidine. Intravenous hydrocortisone or prednisolone has been used to treat severe reactions, with the addition of intravenous chlorpromazine in those individuals exhibiting hypertension and hyperpyrexia. The usefulness and safety of narcotic antagonists in the treatment of these reactions is not known.

Warnings: Meperidine can produce drug dependence of the morphine type and therefore has the potential for being abused. Psychic dependence, physical dependence, and tolerance may develop upon repeated administration, and it should, therefore, be prescribed and administered with the same degree of caution appropriate to the use of morphine. Meperidine should be used with utmost caution and in reduced dosage in patients who are concurrently receiving other narcotic analgesics, general anesthetics, phenothiazines, other tranquilizers, sedative-hypnotics (including barbiturates), tricyclic antidepressants, and other CNS depressants (including alcohol). Respiratory depression, hypotension, and profound sedation or coma may result. The respiratory depressant effects of meperidine and its capacity to elevate cerebrospinal fluid pressure may be markedly exaggerated in the presence of head injury, other intracranial lesions, or a preexisting increase in intracranial pressure. Furthermore, narcotics produce adverse reactions which may obscure the clinical course of patients with head injuries. In such patients, meperidine must be used with extreme caution and only if its use is deemed essential. If necessary, the drug may be given intravenously, but the injection should be given very slowly, preferably in the form of a diluted solution. Rapid intravenous injection of meperidine, increases the incidence of adverse reactions; severe respiratory depression, apnea, hypotension, peripheral circulatory collapse, and cardiac arrest have occurred. It should not be administered intravenously unless a narcotic antagonist (nalorphine hydrochloride and levallorphan tartrate are considered to be specific antidotes against respiratory depression) and the facilities for assisted or controlled respiration are immediately available. When administered parenterally, especially intravenously, the patient should be lying down.

Meperidine should be used with extreme caution in patients having an acute asthmatic attack, in those with chronic obstructive pulmonary disease or cor pulmonale, in patients having a substantially decreased respiratory reserve, or with preexisting respiratory depression, hypoxia, or hypercapnia. In such patients, even usual therapeutic doses may decrease respiratory drive while simultaneously increasing airway resistance to the point of apnea. The administration of meperidine may result in severe hypotension in an individual whose ability to maintain his blood pressure has already been compromised by a depleted blood volume or concurrent administration of drugs such as the phenothiazines or certain anesthetics. It may also impair the mental and/or physical abilities required for the performance of potentially hazardous tasks such as driving a car or operating machinery. The patient should be cautioned accordingly.

Meperidine, as with other narcotics, may produce orthostatic hypotension in ambulatory patients. It should not be used in pregnant women prior to the labor period, unless in the judgment of the physician the potential benefits outweigh the possible hazards, because safe use during pregnancy prior to labor has not been established relative to possible adverse effects on fetal development. When used as an obstetrical analgesic, meperidine crosses the placental barrier and can produce respiratory depression and psychophysiologic functions in the newborn; resuscitation may be required. It appears in the milk of nursing mothers receiving the drug.

Precautions: Meperidine should be used with caution in patients with atrial flutter and other supraventricular tachycardias because of a possible vagolytic action which may produce a significant increase in the ventricular response rate. It may also aggravate preexisting convulsions in patients with convulsive disorders. If dosage is escalated substantially above recommended levels because of tolerance development, convulsions may occur in individuals without a history of convulsive disorders. The administration of meperidine may obscure the diagnosis or clinical course in patients with acute abdominal conditions. The drug should be given with caution and the initial dose should be reduced in certain patients such as the elderly or debilitated, and those with severe impairment of hepatic or renal function, hypothyroidism, Addison's disease, and prostatic hypertrophy or urethral stricture.

Adverse Reactions: The major hazards of meperidine, as with other narcotic analgesics, are respiratory depression and, to a lesser degree, circulatory depression; respiratory arrest, shock, and cardiac arrest have occurred. The most frequently observed adverse reactions include lightheadedness, dizziness, sedation, nausea, vomiting, and sweating. These effects seem to be more prominent in ambulatory patients and in those who are not experiencing severe pain. In such individuals, lower doses are advisable. Some adverse reaction in ambulatory patients may be alleviated if the patient lies down. Other adverse reactions include: *Nervous system:* Euphoria, dysphoria, weakness, headache, agitation, tremor, uncoordinated muscle movements, transient hallucinations and disorientation, visual disturbances. Inadvertent injection near a nerve trunk may result in sensory-motor paralysis which is usually, though not always, transitory. *Gastrointestinal:* Dry mouth, constipation, biliary tract spasm. *Cardiovascular:* Flushing of the face, tachycardia, bradycardia, palpitation, syncope, phlebitis following intravenous injection. *Genitourinary:* Urinary retention. *Allergic:* Pruritus, urticaria, other skin rashes, wheal and flare over the vein with intravenous injection. *Other:* Pain at injection site; local tissue irritation and induration following subcutaneous injection, particularly when repeated; antidiuretic effect.

The major symptoms of overdosage are respiratory depression (a decrease in respiratory rate and/or tidal volume, Cheyne-Stokes respiration, cyanosis), extreme somnolence progressing to stupor or coma, skeletal muscle flaccidity, cold and clammy skin, and occasionally bradycardia and hypotension. Severe overdosage may result in apnea, circulatory collapse, cardiac arrest, and death. Primary attention should be given to the reestablishment of adequate respiratory exchange. Measures essential for supportive care include intravenous naloxone hydrochloride (specific antidote), oxygen, intravenous fluids, vasopressors, etc.; these should be readily available and employed as indicated. The stomach should be evacuated by emesis or gastric lavage.

Dosage and Administration: Adults, from 50 to 150 mg *orally, intramuscularly* or *subcutaneously* every 3 or 4 hours as needed. For women in labor, 50 to 100 mg *intramuscularly* or *subcutaneously* when pains become regular, repeated 3 or 4 times at intervals of 1 to 3 hours as needed. Children, 0.5 to 0.8 mg/lb of body weight *orally, intramuscularly* or *subcutaneously,* at intervals of 3 or 4 hours. The dose of meperidine should be reduced by 1/4 to 1/2 when administered together with phenothiazines and similar agents that potentiate the action of this drug.

Availability:

Meperidine Hydrochloride

C-II DEMEROL®: **(Winthrop)**
Injection, 25 mg/ml in half-filled disposable syringes (Carpujects®) of 2 ml and in ampuls and Uni-Amp® (unit-dose) ampuls of 0.5 ml; 50 mg/ml in Uni-Amp® (unit-dose) ampuls of 1 ml, in vials of 30 ml and in half-filled disposable syringes (Carpujects) of 2 ml. (The half-filled syringe permits mixture with other compatible medication.)
Injection, 75 mg/ml in half-filled disposable syringes (Carpujects) of 2 ml and in ampuls and Uni-Amp (unit-dose) ampuls of 1.5 ml.
Injection, 100 mg/ml in ampuls of 1 and 20 ml and in half-filled disposable syringes (Carpujects) of 2 ml and Uni-Amp (unit-dose) ampuls of 1 ml.
Syrup, 50 mg/5 ml in bottles of 1 pint.
Tablets, 50 and 100 mg in bottles of 100 and 500.

C-II MEPERIDINE HYDROCHLORIDE Injection, 25 and 75 mg/ml in ampuls of 1 ml; 50 mg/ml in ampuls of 1 and 2 ml. **(Knoll)**

C-II MEPERIDINE HYDROCHLORIDE Injection, 50, 75 and 100 mg/ml in half-filled disposable syringes (Steri-Dose®) of 2 ml. (The half-filled syringe permits mixture with other compatible medication.) **(Parke-Davis)**

C-II MEPERIDINE HYDROCHLORIDE: **(Wyeth)**
Injection, 25 mg/ml in half-filled disposable syringes of 2 ml; 50 mg/ml in disposable syringes of 1 ml, in half-filled disposable syringes of 2 ml and in multiple-dose vials of 30 ml; 75 mg/ml in disposable syringes of 1 ml and in half-filled disposable syringes of 2 ml; 100 mg/ml in disposable syringes of 1 ml, in half-filled disposable syringes of 2 ml and in multiple-dose vials of 20 ml. (The half-filled syringe permits mixture with other compatible medication.) All potencies are available in Tamp-R-Tel® (tamper-resistant) packages of 10.
Tablets, 50 mg in Redipak® (unit-dose) cartons of 25.

Combinations

C-II A.P.C. with DEMEROL Tablets, 30 mg with aspirin, 200 mg; phenacetin, 150 mg and caffeine, 30 mg in bottles of 100. **(Winthrop)**

A.P.C. with MEPERIDINE Tablets, 30 mg with aspirin, 200 mg; phenacetin, 150 mg and caffeine, 30 mg in Redipak® (unit-dose) cartons of 25. **(Wyeth)**

Ⓒ II DEMEROL® APAP Tablets, 50 mg with acetaminophen, 300 mg in bottles of 100. **(Breon)**
Ⓒ II MEPERGAN®: **(Wyeth)**
Fortis Capsules, 50 mg with promethazine hydrochloride, 25 mg in bottles of 100.
Injection, 25 mg/ml each of meperidine and promethazine in multiple-dose vials of 10 ml; 50 mg each in 2-ml disposable syringes (Tubex®), in Tamp-R-Tel® (tamper-resistant) packages of 10.

MEPHENTERMINE

Chemical Name: *N*,α,α,-Trimethylphenethylamine.

Description: Mephentermine differs from most sympathomimetic amines in that its amino group is attached to a tertiary carbon atom which is not asymmetric. It is administered as the water-soluble sulfate. The drug is a cerebral metabolic stimulant but has no cerebral vasoconstrictor action, differing in this respect from levarterenol. It enhances and prolongs the pressor response of subsequently injected epinephrine. Dibenamine blocks the effect of this drug. Also, it is an indirectly acting sympathomimetic amine in that it effects the release of norepinephrine. It has sympathomimetic properties similar to those of other *p*-phenylethylamines.

The drug increases the blood pressure in patients probably by enhancing cardiac contraction thereby increasing cardiac output. To a lesser degree, an increase in peripheral resistance, due to peripheral vasoconstriction, may contribute to the elevation of blood pressure. It produces cerebral stimulation, but the degree is not as great as that of the amphetamines. The pharmacologic effects of mephentermine on the cardiovascular system result from the direct action on the myocardium, on the conduction system of the heart, and on the small blood vessels. An increase in force of myocardial contraction is the mechanism by which it produces a pressor response, since it has little effect on total peripheral resistance. During surgery, a positive inotropic effect, which preceded and accompanied an adequate pressor response, was observed. Mephentermine is effective in controlling and correcting hypotension secondary to ganglionic blockade. As with ephedrine, it will not correct, but will potentiate the hypotension secondary to the adrenolytic effects of chlorpromazine. In laboratory studies with cats and dogs, cerebral stimulation induced by mephentermine appeared to be about 1/3 to 1/2 as great as that produced by amphetamine. Although utilization of cerebral oxygen is increased following pressor doses of the drug, there is no change in cerebral vascular resistance or cerebral blood flow.

Indications: Treatment of hypotension secondary to ganglionic blockade and that occurring with spinal anesthesia. Although not recommended as corrective therapy for shock of hypotension secondary to hemorrhage, mephentermine may be used as an emergency measure to maintain blood pressure in such cases until blood or blood substitutes become available.

Contraindications: Hypotension induced by chlorpromazine; in combination with monoamine oxidase inhibitors, and in patients with a history of sensitivity to the drug.

Warnings: Persistent hypotension during or after surgery usually indicates hypovolemia and should be treated by replacement of the circulating blood volume. Serious ventricular arrhythmias may occur in patients under general anesthesia with either cyclopropane or halothane if mephentermine is administered to control hypotension. The drug must be used with caution in patients with known cardiovascular disease, and in chronically ill patients since its action on the cardiovascular system may be profound. It should not be administered to patients who are receiving reserpine, guanethidine or tricyclic antidepressants. If vasopressor drugs are intended for use in correcting hypotension during parturition, the obstetrician should bear in mind that some oxytocic drugs may cause severe hypertension which may result in cerebral hemorrhage during the postpartum period. Use of the drug during pregnancy, lactation or in women of childbearing potential requires that the therapeutic benefits of the drug be weighed against the possible hazards to the mother and child.

Precautions: Use with caution in the treatment of shock secondary to hemorrhage; however, an infusion of 300 to 600 mg of mephentermine in a 5% dextrose solution, to maintain blood pressure until whole blood replacement is accomplished, is effective emergency therapy. Patients with hyperthyroidism may show an increased responsiveness to mephentermine. The rate of infusion should be carefully regulated in order to avoid an excessive blood pressure response, since a rapidly induced hypertensive response has been reported to cause acute pulmonary edema, cardiac arrhythmias and cardiac arrest. Fatal ventricular arrhythmia has been reported to occur in one patient with Laennec's cirrhosis. When vasopressor amines are used for long periods, the resulting vasoconstriction may prevent adequate expansion of circulating volume and may cause perpetuation of the shock state. There is evidence that plasma volume may be reduced in all types of shock, and that the measurement of central venous pressure is the most useful means of assessing the adequacy of the circulating blood volume. Therefore, blood or plasma volume expanders should be employed when the principal reason for hypotension or shock is decreased circulating volume. Cautious use is advised in patients with heart or thyroid disease, hypertension, or diabetes, Also, it should be known that sympathomimetic agents may provoke a relapse in patients with a history of malaria.

Adverse Reactions: Side effects are usually minimal and result from stimulation of the CNS. Following administration of recommended doses, an occasional patient may display signs of anxiety. Cardiac arrhythmias may occur and the blood pressure may be raised excessively, particularly in patients with heart disease. There have been no reports of toxic reactions to this drug.

Dosage and Administration: *Hypotension during surgery, after spinal anesthesia, or in severe illness:* 30 to 45 mg *intravenously* in a single injection with repeated doses of 30 mg as necessary, or continuous *intravenous infusion* of 0.1% mephentermine sulfate in 5% dextrose in water. *Hypotension secondary to spinal anesthesia in cesarean section:* 15 mg *intravenously* repeated if necessary. To prevent hypotension in spinal anesthesia, during or after surgery: 30 to 45 mg *intramuscularly* 10 to 20 minutes before anesthesia, operation or termination of operation. *Shock accompanying myocardial infarction:* 60 mg *intravenously* in a single 2-ml injection, followed by continuous *intravenous infusion* of 0.1% mephentermine sulfate in 5% dextrose in water, or 15 to 45 mg serial doses *intravenously* supplemented with 30 to 45 mg *intramuscularly.*

Availability:
WYAMINE® SULFATE Injection, 15 mg/ml in vials of 1 and 10 ml and ampuls of 2 ml; 30 mg/ml in vials of 1 and 10 ml and in disposable syringes (Tubex®) of 1 ml. **(Wyeth)**

MEPHENYTOIN

Chemical Name: 3-Methyl-5,5-phenylethylhydantoin.

Description: Mephenytoin is an anticonvulsant drug that exhibits pharmacologic effects similar to both phenytoin and the barbiturates. It occurs as a white, crystalline powder very slightly soluble in water.

Indications: Control of grand mal epilepsy and other convulsive states, including focal, Jacksonian and psychomotor seizures. It is not effective in petit mal epilepsy.

Contraindications: Hypersensitivity to hydantoin compounds.

Warnings: There have been reports suggesting an association between the use of anticonvulsant drugs in women with epilepsy and an increase in the incidence of birth defects in infants born to these women. While a definite cause and effect relationship has not been firmly established, it is advised that the medication be discontinued prior to and during pregnancy, primarily in patients in whom withdrawal would not pose a serious threat. However, these drugs should not be suspended in patients inclined to major seizures because of the strong possibility of precipitating status epilepticus with its attendant hypoxia and risk to both the mother and unborn child. At present, it is not known whether or not even minor seizures impart some risk to the developing embryo or fetus. This drug should be reserved for patients who do not respond to other anticonvulsant medications. Gradual reduction of dosage is advised in order to minimize the risk of precipitating seizures. The monograph on Phenytoin should be consulted for possible drug interactions.

Precautions: Because of the possibility of serious toxic effects, the patient must be kept under close medical supervision at all times. Before initiating treatment with this drug, it is advisable to obtain baseline liver function studies, and patients should be instructed to report promptly any symptoms of hepatitis such as jaundice, dark urine, anorexia, abdominal discomfort, or other gastrointestinal symptoms. White blood cell, differential and neutrophil counts should be determined frequently during the initial phase of therapy and at least every month thereafter. If the neutrophils fall to between 2500 and 1600/cu mm, blood counts should be done every 2 weeks; discontinue use of the drug if the count drops to 1600. The drug should be withdrawn at the first sign of a blood dyscrasia. Patients should be advised that if any unusual symptoms develop (sore throat, fever, bleeding from mucous membranes, glandular swelling, skin reaction), they must discontinue use of the drug and report immediately for examination.

Adverse Reactions: A number of side effects and toxic reactions have been reported with mephenytoin as well as with other hydantoin compounds. Many of these appear to be dose-related while others seem to be a manifestation of a hypersensitivity reaction to these drugs. *Blood dyscrasias:* Leukopenia, neutropenia, agranulocytosis, thrombocytopenia and pancytopenia have occurred. Eosinophilia, monocytosis, and leukocytosis have been described. Simple anemia, hemolytic anemia, megaloblastic anemia and aplastic anemia have occurred but are uncommon. *Skin and mucous membrane manifestations:* Maculopapular, morbilliform, scarlatiniform, urticarial, purpuric (associated with thrombocytopenia) and nonspecific skin rashes have been reported. Exfoliative dermatitis, erythema multiforme (Stevens-Johnson Syndrome), toxic epidermal necrolysis and fatal dermatitides have been described on rare occasions. Skin pigmentation and rashes associated with a lupus erythematosus syndrome have also been reported. *Central effects:* Drowsiness is frequently related to overdosage and may, in many instances, be reduced or alleviated by a reduction in dosage. Ataxia, diplopia, nystagmus, dysarthria, fatigue, irritability, choreiform movements, depression and tremor have been encountered on occasions. Nervousness, nausea, vomiting, sleeplessness and dizziness may occur during the initial stages of therapy. Generally these symptoms are transient, often disappearing even with continued treatment. Mental confusion and psychotic disturbances and increased seizures have been reported, but a definite causal relationship to the drug is uncertain. *Miscellaneous:* Hepatitis, jaundice and nephrosis have also been reported but whether or not these were drug-induced has not been established. Alopecia, weight gain, edema, photophobia, conjunctivitis and gum hyperplasia have been encountered infrequently. Polyarthropathy, pulmonary fibrosis, lupus erythematosus syndrome and lymphadenopathy which simulates Hodgkin's disease have also been observed but are extremely rare.

Dosage and Administration: *Orally.* Dosage should be adjusted to the needs of the individual patient. Optimum dosage is attained by starting with $^1/_2$ or 1 tablet daily during the first week and increasing thereafter by $^1/_2$ or 1 tablet at weekly intervals. No dose should be increased until it has been taken for at least 1 week. The average adult dosage is 2 to 6 tablets daily. Some patients may require 8 tablets or more in order to obtain full seizure control. Children, 1 to 4 tablets daily.

Availability:
MESANTOIN® Tablets, 100 mg (scored) in bottles of 100 and 1000 and in Sando-Pak®s (unit-dose packages) of 100. **(Sandoz)**

MEPHOBARBITAL C-IV

Chemical Name: 5-Ethyl-1-methyl-5-phenylbarbituric acid.

Description: Mephobarbital is an antiepileptic and sedative drug that occurs as a white, nearly odorless, tasteless powder slightly soluble in cold water, freely soluble in hot water and in alcohol.

Mephobarbital exerts a strong sedative, anticonvulsive, and antispasmodic action but has a relatively mild hypnotic effect. The conversion of the drug to phenobarbital by the hepatic microsomal enzymes confers the same pharmacologic properties, toxicity and clinical uses as those associated with phenobarbital. However, because of incomplete absorption following oral administration, the dose is approximately twice that of phenobarbital. It reduces the incidence of epileptic seizures in grand mal, petit mal and psychomotor seizures. When mephobarbital is combined with phenytoin, the two drugs act synergistically thus providing a more potent sedative, anticonvulsant and antispasmodic effect.

Indications: Treatment of grand and petit mal epilepsy, tension and anxiety states.

Contraindications: Hypersensitivity to mephobarbital or to barbiturates, and in the presence of porphyria.

Warnings: Mephobarbital may be habit-forming, therefore the same degree of care should be taken when administering this drug as with other barbiturates. Refer to monograph on Phenobarbital. Concomitant use with other CNS depressant agents such as alcohol, strong analgesics, tranquilizers, etc., may result in additive effects including severe CNS depression. Since barbiturates stimulate the activity of hepatic enzymes responsible for drug metabolism, they may decrease the blood concentration and clinical effectiveness of these drugs when given concurrently. They have also been reported to accelerate the metabolism of certain antihistamines, steroids, anticonvulsants, vitamin D, and other drugs. Also they may lower the blood level of coumarin anticoagulants and thus shorten prothrombin time. To avoid precipitating status epilepticus, the drug should not be abruptly withdrawn, but should be discontinued gradually.

Precautions: Dosage should be carefully regulated in senile or debilitated patients, in those with impaired hepatic, renal, cardiac or respiratory function, and in individuals with myasthenia gravis and myxedema. Mephobarbital may impair mental or physical abilities required in the performance of hazardous tasks. Use of any drug in pregnant patients should be undertaken with due consideration to the potential hazards to the fetus. Since blood dyscrasias may occur, periodic blood examinations are advisable.

Adverse Reactions: *CNS effects* are generally manifested by dizziness, headache, "hangover," confusion, especially in elderly patients, paradoxical excitation, and exacerbation of existing pain; *gastrointestinal effects* by nausea, vomiting, and epigastric distress; *cardiovascular effects* by hypotension; *allergic effects* by facial edema, skin rash, bullae and vesicles, purpura, erythema multiforme, and rarely, exfoliative dermatitis; severe allergic reactions may result in degenerative changes in the liver; *hematologic effects* by megaloblastic anemia, agranulocytosis, and thrombocytopenia. For the management and treatment of overdosage, refer to the monograph on Phenobarbital. Combined with phenytoin, side effects noted were tremor, dizziness, restlessness, ataxia, skin reactions, gastrointestinal symptoms, hypertrophy of the gums, hepatitis, hirsutism, blood dyscrasias, pseudolymphoma; and severe ataxia which may develop in some patients after prolonged use.

Dosage and Administration: *Orally. Epilepsy:* Average adult dosage, 400 to 600 mg daily. Children under 5 years of age, 16 to 32 mg; children over 5 years of age, 32 to 64 mg 3 or 4 times daily. *As sedative:* Adults, 32 to 100 mg (optimal dose 50 mg) 3 or 4 times daily. *In incipient or active delirium tremens,* 200 mg 3 times daily for adults and 16 to 32 mg 3 or 4 times daily for children. *Combined with phenytoin:* Adults, 1 or 2 tablets 3 times daily. Children over 6 years of age, 2 or 3 tablets daily; children under 6 years of age, ½ tablet once or twice daily; infants from birth to 12 months of age, ¼ tablet once or twice daily. Initial dose should be small with gradual increments until the optimal dosage is determined.

Availability:
C-IV MEBARAL® Tablets, 32, 50, 100 and 200 mg in bottles of 250. **(Breon)**
C-IV MEBROIN® Tablets, 90 mg with phenytoin, 60 mg in bottles of 250. **(Winthrop)**

MEPIVACAINE HYDROCHLORIDE

Chemical Name: 1-Methyl-2′,6′-pipecoloxylidide monohydrochloride.

Description: Mepivacaine is a local anesthetic structurally similar to lidocaine. It occurs as a white powder that is soluble in both water and alcohol.

The drug apparently produces its anesthetic effect by stabilizing the neuronal membrane, preventing the initiation and transmission of nerve impulses. The onset of anesthetic action is rapid and its duration is prolonged, sometimes lasting for several hours. The duration of action can be further prolonged by the addition of a vasoconstricting agent such as epinephrine. It does not ordinarily produce tissue damage or irritation. Its amide structure secures it from detoxification by the circulating plasma esterases.

Indications: Mepivacaine is indicated to produce local anesthesia by infiltration injection, nerve block, caudal or other epidural block. It is not intended for routine spinal anesthesia or dental use.

Contraindications: Known hypersensitivity to the amide group of local anesthetics or to methylparaben which is added to the multiple dose vials. In addition, spinal anesthesia should be performed only by those familiar with the technique and disease of the cerebrospinal system. Infection at the site of puncture and sepsis with positive blood cultures are also contraindications.

Large doses of local anesthetics are contraindicated in patients with heart block. Also, local anesthesia should not be attempted alone in patients who are emotionally upset or uncooperative. Caudal anesthesia is contraindicated in uncontrollable hysteria and in extremely obese persons in whom the sacral hiatus cannot be palpated. Paracervical block is contraindicated in the presence of fetal distress or whenever predisposing factors causative of fetal distress are present such as prematurity, postmaturity, toxemia and diabetes. Fetal heart rate should be monitored carefully following paracervical block and appropriate therapy should be instituted promptly if fetal bradycardia should occur. Local anesthetics containing epinephrine or other vasoconstrictors should not be used during the first 15 minutes following administration of cyclopropane, chloroform, halothane, or other related drugs, since such concomitant use may produce cardiac arrhythmias.

Warnings: Resuscitative equipment and drugs, including short-acting barbiturates, should be immediately available when a local anesthetic agent is used. The physician should be aware that a severe prolonged hypertensive action may occur when solutions to which a vasoconstrictor, particularly epinephrine or norepinephrine, have been added are given to patients receiving antidepressants of the triptyline or imipramine types or monoamine oxidase (MAO) inhibitors. Safe use during pregnancy has not been established with respect to adverse effects on fetal development; therefore, careful consideration should be given to this fact when intended for use in pregnant patients.

Precautions: The normal precautions observed with all local anesthetics also apply to mepivacaine. Solution to which epinephrine has been added should be used with caution in elderly patients or in those with diabetes mellitus, elevation of blood pressure, cardiac disease and hyperthyroidism. In obstetrics, if vasopressor drugs are used during caudal analgesia either to correct hypotension or to add to the local anesthetic solution, the obstetrician should be cautioned that if an oxytocic drug is employed, severe persistent hypertension and even rupture of a cerebral blood vessel may occur during the postpartum period; hence oxytocic drugs should not be used. Epinephrine should not be added to solutions of the anesthetic to be administered to patients in labor. Since toxic reactions may occur, close familiarity with the various techniques and readiness to use known precautionary and emergency measures are mandatory. Excessive premedication with sedatives, tranquilizers and antiemetic agents prior to local anesthesia should be avoided, especially in infants, small children and the elderly. Injections into an inflamed or infected area should be avoided, as well as inadvertent intravascular injection which may cause serious complications.

Adverse Reactions: Systemic reactions, usually involving the CNS and cardiovascular system due to overdosage (high plasma levels), rapid absorption or inadvertent intravascular injection, characterized by excitement and/or depression and including, nervousness, dizziness, blurred vision, drowsiness, convulsions, coma, respiratory arrest, bradycardia, hypotension, cardiac failure and cardiac arrest. In obstetrics, instances of fetal bradycardia have been noted. Allergic reactions involving the skin such as urticaria and edema; rarely, hypersensitivity, idiosyncrasy and anaphylactoid have been reported. Reactions following epidural or caudal anesthesia may also include high or total spinal block; urinary retention; fecal incontinence; loss of perineal sensation and sexual function; persistent analgesia, paresthesia, and paralysis of the lower extremities; headache and backache; and slowing of labor and increased incidence of forceps delivery. Toxic effects of local anesthetics require symptomatic treatment since there is no specific cure. The physician should be prepared to maintain a patent airway and to support ventilation with oxygen and assisted or controlled respiration. Supportive treatment of the cardiovascular system includes intravenous fluids and when appropriate, vasopressors, preferably those that stimulate the myocardium. Convulsions may be controlled with oxygen and intravenous administration, in small increments, of a barbiturate such as an ultrashort-acting barbiturate (thiopental or thiamylal), and if not available, a short-acting barbiturate (secobarbital or pentobarbital) or a short-acting muscle relaxant (succinylcholine).

Dosage and Administration: The dosage varies considerably and depends upon the surgical procedure, body area, individual response and anesthetic technique. The following dosages generally have proved satisfactory and are therefore suggested as a guide. *For nerve block* (cervical, brachial, intercostal, pudendal), from 5 to 20 ml of a 1 or 2% solution, depending on the area and extent of block (in pudendal and paracervical block, ½ of the total amount is injected on each side). *For transvaginal block* (paracervical plus pudendal) up to 40 ml of a 1% solution (½ the total amount is injected on each side). *For caudal and epidural block,* from 15 to 30 ml of a 1% solution, from 10 to 25 ml of a 1.5% solution, from 10 to 20 ml of a 2% solution. *For infiltration,* up to 40 ml of a 1% solution (or an equivalent amount of an 0.5% solution, depending on the area of the operative field; dilute with Sodium Chloride Injection, U.S.P.). *For therapeutic block,* from 1 to 5 ml of a 1 or 2% solution. Dosages should be reduced for elderly or debilitated patients and for children. The total dose should not exceed 1 gm in any 24-hour period. For complete dosage schedule and administrative techniques, consult package literature.

Availability:
CARBOCAINE®: **(Breon)**
Solution, 1 and 2% in saline with preservative in multiple-dose vials of 50 ml. *For infiltration and nerve block.*
Solution, 1 and 1.5% in modified Ringer's Solution without preservative in single-dose vials of 30 ml; 2% in same vehicle as 1 and 1.5% in single-dose vials of 20 ml. *For nerve block, caudal, epidural and infiltration anesthesia.*

MEPREDNISONE: see The Adrenal Corticosteroids

MEPROBAMATE Ⓒ IV

Chemical Name: Carbamic acid 2-methyl-2-propyltrimethylene ester.

Description: Meprobamate is a central depressant drug of the propanediol series. It occurs as a bitter, white powder slightly soluble in water and freely soluble in alcohol.

It exhibits a blocking action on certain central internuncial neurons and inhibits the electrical activity of the thalamus. The fact that doses required to produce significant thalamic-inhibition have no effect on the cortical areas suggests that blockage of cortical-thalamic impulses occurs. It also produces mild skeletal muscle relaxation incidental to its central depressant activity.

Following oral administration, meprobamate is rapidly absorbed from the gastrointestinal tract with peak blood levels appearing in about 2 hours. The drug is metabolized by the liver and excreted in the urine within 24 hours.

Indications: Orally, for the relief of anxiety and tension; as an adjunct in the treatment of various disease states in which anxiety and tension are manifested; and to promote sleep in anxious, tense patients. Intramuscularly, for the treatment of tetanus in addition to other suitable measures.

Contraindications: Acute intermittent porphyria and allergic or idiosyncratic reactions to meprobamate. The polyethylene glycol component in the parenteral solution is contraindicated in patients with renal damage.

Warnings: Physical and psychological dependence and abuse have been reported with meprobamate. Therefore, careful supervision of dose and amounts prescribed is advised, particularly in addiction-prone individuals. When chronic intoxication from prolonged use does occur, it usually involves ingestion of greater than recommended doses and is manifested by ataxia, slurred speech, and vertigo. It has been suggested that when administration of excessive dosage has continued for weeks or months, the medication should not be discontinued abruptly but should be reduced gradually over a period of 1 to 2 weeks. Alternately, a short-acting barbiturate may be substituted, then gradually withdrawn. Sudden withdrawal of the drug after prolonged and excessive use may be followed by recurrence of preexisting symptoms, such as anxiety, anorexia, or insomnia, or by withdrawal reactions such as vomiting, ataxia, tremors, muscle twitching, confusional states, hallucinosis, and in rare instances, convulsions. Such seizures are more likely to occur in patients with CNS damage or with preexistent or latent convulsive disorders. Onset of withdrawal symptoms occurs usually within 12 to 48 hours after discontinuation of medication, but these usually cease within the next 12 to 48 hours.

Patients should be warned that meprobamate may impair the mental and physical abilities required for performance of potentially hazardous tasks such as driving or operating machinery. Since the effects of the concomitant use of meprobamate with alcohol or with other CNS depressants may be additive, appropriate caution should be exercised with patients who take more than one of these agents simultaneously. There have been reports concerning the relationship between the increased risk of congenital malformations and the use of meprobamate during the first trimester of pregnancy; therefore, its use in pregnant women or in women of childbearing potential should be avoided if possible. Meprobamate passes the placental barrier, and has been found to be present not only in umbilical cord blood at or near maternal plasma levels but also in breast milk of lactating mothers at concentrations 2 to 4 times that of maternal plasma. This factor should be taken into account when the use of the drug is contemplated in nursing mothers. The parenteral solution should *not* be given intravenously because the vehicle used may cause thrombosis or hemolysis.

Precautions: The least effective dose should be administered, particularly to elderly or debilitated patients, in order to prevent oversedation. Caution should be exercised in the administration of meprobamate to patients with impaired liver or kidney function; to epileptic patients, and to those with suicidal tendencies.

Adverse Reactions: Drowsiness, ataxia, dizziness, slurred speech, headache, vertigo, weakness, paresthesias, impairment of visual accommodation, euphoria, overstimulation, paradoxical excitement, fast EEG activity; nausea, vomiting, diarrhea; palpitation, tachycardia, various forms of cardiac arrhythmia, transient ECG changes; syncope, hypotensive crisis. Milder reactions are characterized by an itchy, urticarial, or erythematous maculopapular rash which may be generalized or confined to the groin. Other reactions have included leukopenia, acute nonthrombocytopenic purpura, petechiae, ecchymosis, eosinophilia, adenopathy, fever, fixed drug eruption with cross reaction to carisoprodol, and cross sensitivity between meprobamate and mebutamate or carbromal. Rarely reported are hyperpyrexia, chills, angioneurotic edema, bronchospasm, oliguria, anuria, anaphylaxis, erythema multiforme, exfoliative dermatitis, stomatitis, proctitis, Stevens-Johnson syndrome, bullous dermatitis, agranulocytosis, aplastic anemia, thrombocytopenia purpura, and exacerbation of porphyric symptoms.

Dosage and Administration: *Orally.* The usual adult dosage is 400 mg 3 or 4 times daily; dosage may be increased but should not exceed 2.4 gm daily. The usual dosage for children 6 to 12 years of age is 100 to 200 mg 2 or 3 times daily. *Intramuscularly* only. The usual dosage for adults is 400 mg and for children 200 mg every 3 or 4 hours. The usual dosage for infants is 125 mg every 6 hours.

Availability:

C-IV EQUANIL®: **(Wyeth)**

L-A Capsules (long-acting), 400 mg in bottles of 50.

Tablets, 200 and 400 mg in bottles of 50, 100, 500 and 1000 and in Redipak®s (unit-dose) packages of 25 and 100 (5 and 20 strips of 5 tablets each).

Wyseals® (specially coated tablets), 400 mg in bottles of 50 and 500.

C-IV KESSO-BAMATE® Tablets, 200 and 400 mg in bottles of 100 and 1000. **(McKesson)**

C-IV MEPRIAM™ Tablets, 400 mg in bottles of 1000. **(Lemmon)**

C-IV MEPROBAMATE Tablets, 400 mg in bottles of 1000. **(Elder)**

C-IV MEPROBAMATE Tablets, 400 mg in bottles of 100 and 1000. **(Lederle)**

C-IV MEPROBAMATE Tablets, 400 mg in bottles of 1000 and in unit-dose packages of 100 (10 × 10). **(Parke-Davis)**

C-IV MEPROBAMATE Tablets, 200 mg in bottles of 100 and 1000 and in unit-dose cartons of 100; 400 mg in bottles of 100, 1000 and 5000 and in unit-dose cartons of 100 and 250. **(Philips Roxane)**
C-IV MEPROSPAN® Capsules (sustained-release), 200 and 400 mg in bottles of 100. **(Wallace)**
C-IV MILTOWN® Tablets, 200 mg in bottles of 100; 400 mg in bottles of 100, 500 and 1000 and in unit-dose packages of 500 and 1000; 600 mg in bottles of 100. **(Wallace)**
C-IV SK-BAMATE™ Tablets, 200 mg in bottles of 100; 400 mg in bottles of 100 and 1000. **(Smith Kline & French)**

MERCAPTOMERIN SODIUM

Chemical Name: *N*-(γ-Carboxymethylmercaptomercuri-β-methoxy)-propylcamphoramic acid disodium salt.

Description: Mercaptomerin sodium, a mercaptide, is an organomercurial compound in which the xanthine has been replaced by sodium thioglycollate—one of the monothiols. It occurs as a hygroscopic, white powder that is freely soluble in water and soluble in alcohol.

Its diuretic action is due to the release of small concentrations of mercuric ions which reduce tubular reabsorption of fluid; the resulting diuresis eliminates water and sodium. In laboratory studies with animals, these substances have been shown to reduce the cardiotoxic effects of organic mercury while preserving the diuretic action.

Following subcutaneous injection of a 2-ml dose in patients with edema, urinary flow usually began in approximately 2 hours, and reached a sustained diuresis of over 5 ml/minute in about 3 hours. In another series diuresis reached a maximum in 12 to 18 hours and gradually subsided over the subsequent 48 hours; in some patients the diuresis lasted up to 3 days. Conditions such as hypochloremic alkalosis, potassium deficiency, low-salt syndrome, reduced glomerular filtration rate, and muscular activity may render the patient refractory to mercurial diuretics becuase the amount of chloride available for excretion is reduced. On correcting the hypochloremia, diuresis ensues.

Indications: Treatment of edema secondary to congestive heart failure, the nephrotic syndrome, the nephrotic stage of glomerulonephritis, and hepatic cirrhosis or portal obstruction.

Contraindications: Not to be used in advanced chronic nephritis and acute renal disease, ulcerative colitis, signs of dehydration, or intravenously. Discontinue if symptoms of mercury sensitivity appear.

Warnings: A few instances of anaphylactic reactions have been reported. Safe use during gestation and lactation has not been established.

Precautions: Patients should be observed carefully for signs of salt depletion, especially in hot weather. Excessive dehydration is more likely to occur in elderly than in young patients, particularly in long-standing cases treated with prolonged salt restriction and frequent diuresis. The physician should be aware that certain factors leading to sodium retention in congestive heart failure such as impaired cardiovascular-renal hemodynamics, elevated venous pressure, altered serum electrolytes, increased adrenocortical activity, stimulation of volume receptors may contribute to the failure of certain cardiac patients to respond to mercurial diuretics. The hypokalemia produced by the action of diuretics can sensitize or exaggerate the response of the heart to the toxic effects of digitalis manifested by increased ventricular irritability. In view of the potential electrolyte and volume disturbances common to all diuretic agents, it is recommended that serum electrolytes (Na, K, Cl) be determined periodically, especially in patients on prolonged therapy. The development of albuminuria, hematuria, or oliguria warrants immediate withdrawal of the drug. Overdosage or too rapid administration may lead to muscle cramps and shock.

Adverse Reactions: Rarely, an idiosyncrasy to the mercurials may occur as indicated by flushing of the face, fever, chills, gastrointestinal disturbances, cutaneous eruptions, pruritus and urticaria. These symptoms are generally of an allergic nature and are not in themselves serious, but serve as warning signals of more serious reactions that may develop if the drug is continued. Therefore, it is well-advised to withdraw treatment in the presence of such symptoms. Weakness, somnolence, muscle pains and shock secondary to depletion of extracellular electrolytes have occurred following excessive or injudicious use.

Dosage and Administration: *Intramuscularly* or *subcutaneously,* 0.2 to 2 ml daily, preferably by subcutaneous injection, to achieve and maintain dry weight.

Availability:
THIOMERIN® Solution, 125 mg/ml (equiv. to 40 mg mercury) in vials of 2 and 10 ml and in 2-ml Tubex® (cartridge-needle units). **(Wyeth)**

MERCAPTOPURINE

Chemical Name: 6-Purinethiol.

Description: Mercaptopurine is a chemical analog of the nucleic acid constituent adenine and the physiological purine base hypoxanthine.

This compound is a purine antagonist. It is a highly reactive chemical that combines with cellular components in internucleotide linkages; it thereby prevents cell division and new protein synthesis. A large part of mercaptopurine is converted in the body by xanthine oxidase to 6-thiouric acid, but a small fraction is converted to its nucleotide, 6-mercaptopurine ribotide, which is a structural analog of inosinic acid, and interferes with the conversion of inosinic to adenylic acid, an essential component of nucleic acid. Tumors that develop resistance or tolerance to the drug result from the loss by the tumor cell of its capacity to convert mercaptopurine to its therapeutically active riboside.

Following oral administration, it is readily absorbed from the intestinal tract, and approximately 50% of the dose can be accounted for as urinary excretion products within 24 hours. The half-life in the blood lasts about 1½ hours. It is excreted by the kidneys both unchanged and as various metabolites.

Indications: Primarily for the treatment of acute leukemia. In general it appears that a higher proportion of children than adults respond favorably to the drug. Temporary remission may be obtained in cases of chronic myelocytic leukemia. Mercaptopurine is not indicated in the treatment of Hodgkin's disease, chronic lymphatic leukemia or solid tumors.

Warnings: When cytotoxic drugs are to be used during pregnancy, the possible effect on the fetus should be kept in mind. It is therefore advisable to defer treatment with these drugs as long as possible, or until after the first trimester of pregnancy.

Precautions: Caution must be exercised to avoid toxicity (bone marrow depression resulting in leukopenia and eventually thrombocytopenia and bleeding). Blood counts should be taken frequently, preferably on a weekly basis. Since the drug may have a delayed action, it is important to withdraw the medication temporarily at the first sign of an abnormally large fall in the white cell count, or of abnormal depression of the bone marrow. Therapy should be initiated with smaller doses in patients with impaired renal function because slower elimination and greater cumulation of the drug may result. Jaundice has been observed, and it is recommended that mercaptopurine be withheld if there is evidence of toxic hepatitis or biliary stasis, as the jaundice may disappear. Hyperuricemia and hyperuricosuria may develop during treatment, reflecting the destruction of cells with release of purines. This circumstance may lead to impairment of renal function with oliguria. The concurrent administration of allopurinol in doses of 300 to 600 mg daily will require a reduction in dose to approximately ⅓ to ¼ of the usual dose of mercaptopurine. Subsequent adjustment of doses of mercaptopurine should be made on the basis of therapeutic response and any toxic effects.

Adverse Reactions: The most significant toxic manifestation is hematologic with leukopenia, and, with excessive dosage, thrombocytopenia and bleeding. If oral lesions, which are rarely seen, do occur, they resemble thrush rather than antifolic ulcerations. Nausea, vomiting and anorexia may occur as the result of overdosage. Jaundice has been observed in some instances, suggesting possible liver damage or biliary stasis; also drug fever has been noted on occasion. Other complications occasionally noted were mild diarrhea and sprue-like symptoms; however, it has not been established whether or not these were drug-related.

Dosage and Administration: *Orally.* The dosage varies from patient to patient. Initial doses usually range from 100 to 200 mg daily. The average daily dose is about 2.5 mg/kg/day for adults and children 5 years of age and older given in single or divided doses. Most patients tolerate this dose for several weeks. If no clinical improvement is seen after 4 weeks, the dose may be increased to 5 mg/kg/day. The appearance of serious toxic manifestations warrants withdrawal of the drug; may be reinstated at ½ the previous dosage when these symptoms disappear. A suitable maintenance dose should be established if early relapse is to be avoided.

Availability:
PURINETHOL® Tablets, 50 mg in bottles of 25 and 250. **(Burroughs Wellcome)**

MERETHOXYLLINE

Chemical Name: *o*-(*N*-γ-Hydroxymercuri-β-hydroxyethoxypropylcarbamido) phenoxyacetic acid, procaine salt, with theophylline.

Description: Each ml contains merethoxylline procaine, 100 mg (equiv. to 39.3 mg of mercury and 45 mg of procaine base) and theophylline (anhydrous), 50 mg.

In common with other organomercurial diuretics, the drug acts by depressing the renal tubular reabsorption of sodium, chloride, and water. Urinary potassium is increased or decreased, depending upon whether the initial secretory rate is low or high. The addition of theophylline is responsible also for the rise in cardiac output and fall in right auricular pressure which follows administration in patients with congestive heart failure.

Indications: Treatment of edema secondary to congestive heart failure, the nephrotic syndrome, the nephrotic stage of glomerulonephritis, and hepatic cirrhosis or portal obstruction.

Contraindications: Sensitivity to mercury or to drugs containing the *p*-aminobenonzoic acid group (benzocaine, tetracaine, butacaine, etc.), procaine, or theophylline; acute glomerulonephritis; ulcerative colitis; gouty diathesis.

Warnings: Anaphylactic reactions have been reported. Safe use of merethoxylline during pregnancy, lactation, or in women of childbearing potential has not been established; therefore, it should be used in such patients only when it is deemed essential to the patient's welfare. *Not for intravenous use.*

Precautions: Extreme caution should be exercised in the presence of benign prostatic hypertrophy; distention of the bladder may precipitate obstruction. Use with caution if the BUN level is more than 60 mg/100 ml. The drug should be discontinued if albuminuria, hematuria, or oliguria is noted. Lack of response may be due to insufficient restriction of the patient's activity, inadequate dosage of cardiac glycosides, underlying renal disease or electrolyte imbalance. Frequent or injudicious use of the drug may result in dehydration and electrolyte depletion, especially if restriction of salt intake has been rigid and prolonged. In edematous patients who are heavily digitalized; rapid mobilization of large quantities of fluid may be followed by symptoms of digitalis overdosage. The drug should not be used as a substitute for digitalis or other therapeutic measures in the treatment of diseases associated with edema. The necessary precautions should be undertaken when giving the drug to patients who are on sulfonamide therapy.

Adverse Reactions: *Hypersensitivity reactions:* flushing, pruritus, urticaria, cutaneous rash (which may become exfoliative), and occasionally anaphylactic reactions. *Gastrointestinal reactions:* nausea, vomiting, diarrhea, and abdominal pain. *Bone-marrow depression:* neutropenia and agranulocytosis. Stomatitis, marginal gingivitis, metallic taste, diarrhea, and proteinuria may result from excessive parenteral therapy or in patients with advanced renal disease. *Local reactions:* ecchymoses and induration. *Genitourinary reactions:* transient azotemia or an increase in preexistent azotemia, acute urinary retention, rarely, hyperuricemia.

Dosage and Administration: *Deep subcutaneous* or *intramuscular* administration in doses of 0.5 to 2 ml as needed to produce diuresis or maintain an edema-free state. The diuretic effect is potentiated by ammonium chloride, theophylline preparations and bed rest.

Availability:
DICURIN® PROCAINE Injection in ampuls of 10 ml. **(Lilly)**

MERSALYL & THEOPHYLLINE

Chemical Name: Mersalyl: *o*-[[3-(Hydroxymercuri)-2-methoxypropyl]carbamoyl] phenoxyacetic acid sodium salt.

Description: Mersalyl is a mercurial diuretic and occurs as a white, crystalline powder freely soluble in water, containing not less than 39.6% of mercury in nonionizable form. It is usually given with theophylline in a 2:1 ratio. If the solution is discolored or contains a precipitate, it should not be used.

The compound exerts a powerful diuretic effect by withdrawing fluid and salt from edematous tissues and by directly stimulating kidney function. The addition of theophylline increases absorption of the mercurial component from the muscle by more than 300% in 1 hour, with almost complete disappearance of the injected dose (97%) within this period.

Indications: Treatment of edema and ascites in cardiac and cardiorenal diseases, nephrosis, cirrhosis of the liver, thrombophlebitic and thyrocardiac edema.

Contraindications: Acute nephritis, advanced chronic kidney disease with nitrogen retention, or urine of fixed specific gravity, severe liver disease, colitis with bloody stools or mercury idiosyncrasy, and subcutaneous administration.

Precautions: Use with caution in patients likely to be subject to ventricular arrhythmias, such as those having frequent ventricular extrasystoles, receiving digitalis, or having suffered recent myocardial infarction. Care should be taken not to restrict the intake of salt so that hypochloremia and its associated symptoms (weakness, collapse, hypotension, hemoconcentration, and azotemia) may be avoided. Particular caution is advised in treating children; a small test dose may be given initially and increased gradually only if untoward effects such as chills, febrile reactions, malaise, morbilliform rash, vomiting, or convulsive seizures do not occur. During prolonged treatment, the urine should be examined regularly for albumin, casts and blood cells.

Adverse Reactions: Stomatitis, gastric disturbance, severe diarrhea (sometimes with bloody stools), vertigo, headache, febrile reaction and cutaneous eruptions. Rare instances of idiosyncrasy to mercurial diuretics have been reported, characterized by symptoms of anaphylactic shock and attributable to ventricular arrhythmia. A few cases have terminated fatally. Other reactions generally noted with mercurial diuretics and which may possibly occur with the use of this drug include flushing, pruritus, urticaria, cutaneous rash (may become exfoliative); nausea, vomiting, and abdominal pain; ecchymosis and induration; transient azotemia or an increase in preexistent azotemia, acute urinary retention; bone marrow depression characterized by neutropenia and agranulocytosis; and rarely, hyperuricemia. Stomatitis, marginal gingivitis, metallic taste, diarrhea, and proteinuria may arise from excessive parenteral therapy or in patients with advanced renal disease.

Dosage and Administration: Deep *intramuscular* or slow *intravenous (never subcutaneous).* The intramuscular route is the preferred method of administration. Intravenous injections are advisable in the presence of marked general edema, and should be made *very slowly* to reduce the risk of producing shock-like symptoms. The solution may be diluted with 5 or 10 ml of water for injection. Adults, a test dose of 0.5 ml the first day, if well-tolerated, the dose may be increased to 1 ml, rarely 2 ml, on the following day. The usual dose is 1 or 2 ml once or twice weekly administered early in the morning so that most of the diuresis may be accomplished before bedtime; however, 0.5 to 1 ml may be administered daily or every other day. Children, 0.25 ml to test susceptibility, followed by 0.5 or 1 ml on the following day. As an auxiliary measure, 6 to 10 gm of ammonium chloride or ammonium nitrate may be given orally each day.

Availability:
SALYRGAN®-THEOPHYLLINE Injection, 100 mg/ml with theophylline, 50 mg/ml in ampuls of 2 ml.
(Winthrop)

MESORIDAZINE: see The Phenothiazines

MESTRANOL + ETHYNODIOL DIACETATE

Chemical Name: Ethynodiol—19-nor-17α-pregn-4-en-20-yne-3β,17-diol.

Description: Ethynodiol diacetate is a synthetic progestogen, structurally related to norethindrone, which is a 19-nor steroid derivative possessing androgenic qualities. It antagonizes some uterine effects of progesterone and estrone, but lacks significant androgenic activity. In common with norethynodrel, norethindrone and chlormadinone, ethynodiol alone is effective in suppressing ovulation. Ethynodiol-mestranol minimizes breakthrough bleeding and provides adequate cyclic control.

Indications: Ovulation control.

Contraindications: In patients with undiagnosed abnormal vaginal bleeding, known or suspected carcinoma of the breast or estrogen-dependent neoplasia, markedly impaired liver function, missed abortion, or in those with thrombophlebitis, thromboembolic disorders, cerebral apoplexy or a past history of these conditions, and in known or suspected pregnancy.

Warnings: The physician should be alert to the earliest manifestations of thrombotic disorders (thrombophlebitis, coronary thrombosis, cerebrovascular disorders, pulmonary embolism, and retinal thrombosis). Should any of these occur or be suspected, the drug should be discontinued immediately. Retrospective studies have reported an increased risk of thromboembolic complications following surgery; therefore, it is recommended that the drug be discontinued at least 1 month prior to any surgical procedure. The hazard of developing coronary artery disease (fatal or nonfatal myocardial infarction) appears to be greater in women who are over 40 years of age, and in those who smoke (women should be strongly advised not to smoke) or who have a history of preeclamptic toxemia, hypercholestrolemia, diabetes, hypertension or obesity. Other retrospective studies have shown a statistically significant association between thrombophlebitis, pulmonary embolism, and cerebral thrombosis and embolism with the use of oral contraceptives. Studies also indicated that the risk did not persist after discontinuation of the drug, and that it was not enhanced by long continued administration. However, it was suggested that there might be an increased risk of thromboembolic disease when sequential products were used. The occurrence of a sudden, partial or complete loss of vision or a sudden onset of proptosis, diplopia, migraine, or papilledema warrants immediate withdrawal of the drug. Additionally, hepatic lesions (adenomas, hepatomas, hamartomas, regenerating nodules, etc.) occasionally fatal, have been reported in women on short-term as well as long-term therapy. Such lesions may be present as an abdominal mass or with signs and symptoms of severe abdominal distress; these should be considered if the patient has abdominal pain or evidence of intraabdominal bleeding. Since safe use during pregnancy has not been established, it is suggested that patients, who have missed 2 consecutive periods, have pregnancy ruled out before continuing the contraceptive regimen. Also, if the patient has not adhered to the prescribed schedule, the possibility of pregnancy should be considered at the time of the first missed period. The drug should not be given to nursing mothers because of the possible estrogenic responses in the infant.

Precautions: Before initiating therapy, a thorough history and physical examination should be performed with special reference to breast and pelvic organs and a Papanicolaou smear should be performed. Treatment should be discontinued for 2 months before endocrine and liver function tests are undertaken. A decrease in glucose tolerance has been observed in a significant percentage of patients on estrogen-progestogen combination drugs; therefore, patients, especially diabetic patients, should be carefully observed while taking this drug. Use with caution in patients with a history of psychic depression, and in those with a history of metabolic disease or conditions that might be aggravated by possible estrogen-induced fluid retention, such as epilepsy, migraine, asthma, and cardiac and renal dysfunctions. Preexisting uterine fibromyomas may increase in size during therapy and patients with these tumors should be examined periodically. If breakthrough bleeding persists, nonfunctional causes should be considered. Women should be advised of the possibility of an increase in the amount of estrogen-induced cervical mucus. Susceptible individuals may experience an increase in blood pressure; also progestogens may mask the onset of the menopause. It should be used judiciously in young patients in whom bone growth is not complete.

Adverse Reactions: A statistically significant association has been demonstrated between the use of oral contraceptives and the following serious adverse reactions: Thrombophlebitis, pulmonary embolism, cerebrovascular accidents, retinal thrombosis and optic neuritis, hepatic adenoma, hypertension, congenital anomalies, gallbladder disease, nausea, vomiting, gastrointestinal symptoms such as abdominal cramps and bloating, breakthrough bleeding, spotting, change in menstrual flow, amenorrhea during and after treatment, edema, chloasma or melasma, which may persist, breast changes (tenderness, enlargement, and secretion), decrease or increase in weight, changes in cervical erosion and cervical secretions, suppression of lactation when given immediately postpartum, cholestatic jaundice, migraine, rash (allergic), rise in blood pressure, mental depression, anovulation post-treatment, premenstrual-like syndrome, changes in libido, changes in appetite, cystitis-like syndrome, headache, intolerance to contact lenses, nervousness, dizziness, fatigue, backache, hirsutism, loss of scalp hair, erythema multiforme, erythema nodosum, hemorrhagic eruption, itching, vaginitis. The following laboratory tests may be altered by the use of this drug: liver function (increased BSP and other values); increased prothrombin, Factors VII, VIII, IX and X; decrease in antithrombin III; increase in platelet aggregability; increase in PBI and butanol-extractable PBI and decreased T^3 values; metyrapone test and the pregnanediol determination.

Dosage and Administration: *Orally,* 1 tablet daily for 20 consecutive days, beginning on day 5 of the menstrual cycle; the first day of menstruation is considered day 1. Medication is then discontinued. Withdrawal bleeding usually begins 2 or 3 days after therapy has been discontinued. This regimen is repeated; if withdrawal flow does not occur, or if it occurs on the fourth day or later after the cycle of tablets has been completed, another regimen is begun on the eighth day after the last tablet has been taken in the previous cycle. A simplified dosage schedule for Ovulen-21 is 3 weeks on and 1 week off. For example, the patient takes 1 tablet daily for 21 consecutive days beginning on day 5 of the menstrual cycle, takes nothing for 7 days before starting a new cycle.

Availability:
OVULEN® Tablets, ethynodiol diacetate, 1 mg and mestranol, 0.1 mg in Compack® tablet dispensers of 20 in cartons of 120 (6 × 20) and refills in cartons of 240 (12 × 20). **(Searle)**
OVULEN-21® Tablets, ethynodiol diacetate, 1 mg and mestranol, 0.1 mg in Compack® tablet dispensers of 21 in cartons of 126 (6 × 21) and refills in cartons of 252 (12 × 21) and 1008 (48 x 21). Also available in cartons of 10 and 100 Triopak™ containers (630 and 6300 tablets); each Triopak has 1 Compack and 2 refills. **(Searle)**
OVULEN-28® Tablets (21 white and 7 pink placebo), ethynodiol diacetate, 1 mg and mestranol, 0.1 mg in Compack® dispensers of 28 tablets in cartons of 168 (6 × 28) and Compack refills in cartons of 336 (12 × 28). Also available in cartons of 10 Triopak™ containers (840 tablets); each Triopak has 1 Compack and 2 refills (84 tablets). **(Searle)**

MESTRANOL + NORETHINDRONE

Chemical Name: Norethindrone: 17-Hydroxy-19-nor-17α-pregn-4-en-20-yn-3-one.

Description: Norethindrone, a synthetic progestogen, differs structurally from norethynodrel only in the position of the double bond in ring A of the steroid nucleus.

Norethindrone possesses some inherent estrogenic and androgenic activity. Masculinization of the female fetus has been reported following administration of this compound during pregnancy; therefore, its use in threatened or recurrent abortion is not advised. The combination of norethindrone and mestranol provides contraceptive action by inhibiting the pituitary, reducing the amount of gonadotropin thus preventing ovulation.

For Indications, Contraindications, Warnings, Precautions, Adverse Reactions, see monograph on Mestranol + Ethynodiol Diacetate.

Dosage and Administration: *Orally,* 1 white tablet daily at bedtime, for 14 days, starting on day 5 of the menstrual cycle and continuing through day 18; then 1 blue tablet daily at bedtime, for 6 days, starting on day 19 and continuing through day 24. The first day of the menstrual cycle is day 1. Withdrawal bleeding usually begins within 4 days after the last tablet has been taken. In those cases where withdrawal bleeding may be delayed until 4 to 6 days after the 20-day course of therapy, the patient should still start the next course of medication on the seventh day following completion of the previous 20-day course.

Availability:
NORINYL®-2 Tablets, norethindrone, 2 mg with mestranol, 0.1 mg in dispenser compacks (Memorette®) of 20 and in refill folders of 20 tablets. **(Syntex)**
NORINYL 1 + 50 Tablets (21-day), norethindrone, 1 mg with mestranol, 0.05 mg in dispenser compacks (Memorette) of 21 and in refill folders of 21 tablets. **(Syntex)**
NORINYL 1 + 50 Tablets (28-day), norethindrone, 1 mg with mestranol, 0.05 mg in dispenser compacks (Memorette) of 28 and in folders of 28 tablets, consisting of 21 tablets active ingredients and 7 tablets inert material. **(Syntex)**
NORINYL 1 + 80 Tablets (21-day), norethindrone, 1 mg with mestranol, 0.08 mg in dispenser compacks (Memorette) of 21 and in refill folders of 21 tablets. **(Syntex)**
NORINYL 1 + 80 Tablets (28-day), norethindrone, 1 mg with mestranol, 0.08 mg in dispenser compacks (Memorette) of 28 and in refill folders of 28 tablets each consisting of 21 tablets active ingredients and 7 tablets inert material. **(Syntex)**
ORTHO-NOVUM 1/50®-21 Tablets, 1 mg norethindrone with mestranol, 0.05 mg in Dialpak® tablet dispensers of 21 and in 3-cycle dispensers of 63. **(Ortho)**
ORTHO-NOVUM 1/50-28 Tablets, 1 mg norethindrone with mestranol, 0.05 mg in Dialpak® tablet dispensers of 28 consisting of 21 tablets active ingredients and 7 tablets inert material. **(Ortho)**
ORTHO-NOVUM 1/80®-21 Tablets 1 mg norethindrone with mestranol, 0.08 mg in Dialpak tablet dispensers of 21 and in 3-cycle dispensers of 63. **(Ortho)**
ORTHO-NOVUM 1/80®-28 Tablets, 1 mg norethindrone with mestranol 0.08 mg in Dialpak tablet dispensers of 28 consisting of 21 tablets active ingredients and 7 tablets inert material. **(Ortho)**
ORTHO-NOVUM® 2 mg-21 Tablets, 2 mg norethindrone with mestranol, 0.1 mg in Dialpak tablet dispensers of 21 and in 3-cycle dispensers of 63. **(Ortho)**
ORTHO-NOVUM® 10 mg-20 Tablets, 10 mg norethindrone with mestranol, 0.06 in Dialpak tablet dispensers of 20. **(Ortho)**

MESTRANOL + NORETHYNODREL

Chemical Name: Norethynodrel: 17-Hydroxy-19-nor-17α-pregn-5(10)-en-20-yn-3-one.

Description: Norethynodrel, a synthetic progestogen, differs structurally from norethindrone in that the C=C double bond is in the 5-10 position in ring A of the steroid nucleus. It possesses estrogenic as well as progestational properties. The combination of norethynodrel with mestranol is used to minimize breakthrough bleeding and to provide adequate cyclic control.

For Indications, Contraindications, Warnings, Precautions, Adverse Reactions, see monograph on Mestranol + Ethynodiol Diacetate.

Dosage and Administration: *Orally,* 2.5 or 5 mg daily for 20 consecutive days beginning on day 5 of the cycle, counting the first day of menstruation as day 1 or on the first Sunday after the onset of menstruation. Withdrawal bleeding will usually start within 3 days after taking the last tablet.

Availability:
ENOVID® Tablets, 5 mg (pink) norethynodrel and mestranol, 0.075 mg in bottles of 100 and 500 and in Calendar-Pack™ of 20 in cartons of 120 (6 × 20) and 600 (30 × 20). Also available with 10 mg of norethynodrel and 0.15 mg of mestranol in bottles of 50 and 500. **(Searle)**
ENOVID-E® Tablets, 2.5 mg (pale pink) norethynodrel and mestranol, 0.1 mg in bottles of 250 and in Compack tablet dispensers of 20 in cartons of 6 and refills in cartons of 240 (12 × 20). **(Searle)**
ENOVID-E 21 Tablets, 2.5 mg in Compack tablet dispensers of 21 tablets arranged in 3 numbered rows of 7 tablets each in cartons of 6, in cartons of 12 refills and in Triopak® tablet containers each containing 1 Compack tablet dispenser and 2 refills in cartons of 10.

METAPROTERENOL: see Isoproterenol

METARAMINOL BITARTRATE

Chemical Name: *l*-1-(m-Hydroxyphenyl)-2-amino-1-propanol hydrogen D-tartrate.

Description: Metaraminol bitartrate is a sympathomimetic amine which acts primarily on the α-receptors increasing both systolic and diastolic blood pressure due to vasoconstriction and generally accompanied by a marked reflex bradycardia. As a pressor agent its action is similar to norepinephrine. Although it has a more prolonged effect, its potency is less than that of norepinephrine. It occurs as a white, crystalline powder that is freely soluble in water, slightly soluble in alcohol, and practically insoluble in chloroform and in ether.

Metaraminol is used for the management of hypotension; its action is a direct one on both the heart and blood vessels, producing peripheral vasoconstriction and a positive inotropic effect on the heart. Adrenolytic agents decrease, but do not reverse, its pressor effects.

While metaraminol is absorbed from the gastrointestinal tract after oral administration, its pharmacological effect by that route is feeble. Therefore, the parenteral form is used clinically where a pressor response is noted within 1 to 2 minutes after intravenous infusion, about 10 minutes after intramuscular injection and about 5 to 20 minutes after subcutaneous injection. Depending upon the dose and the clinical condition, the pressor response may remain for 20 to 60 minutes.

Indications: Prevention and treatment of the acute hypotensive state that sometimes occurs with spinal anesthesia; adjunctively to treat hypotension due to hemorrhage, reactions to medications, surgical complications, and shock associated with brain damage due to trauma or tumor. It may also be useful as an adjunct in the treatment of hypotension due to cardiogenic shock and septicemia.

Contraindications: Hypersensitivity or idiosyncrasy to metaraminol.

Warnings: Because of the danger of excessive cardiac irritability, metaraminol should be avoided when anesthetics, such as cyclopropane, which increase the responsiveness of the myocardium, are used. Safe use during pregnancy has not been established.

Precautions: Vasopressor drugs should be used cautiously in patients with coronary artery disease, hyperthyroidism, hypertension, and diabetes mellitus. Careful attention to the rate of flow and the patient's response is advised since rapidly induced hypertensive responses have been reported to cause acute pulmonary edema, cardiac arrhythmias, and cardiac arrest. In several instances, ventricular extrasystoles that appeared during infusion subsided promptly when the rate of infusion was reduced. Concomitant use with digitalis may increase the risk of ectopic arrhythmias, and MAO inhibitors may enhance the action of metaraminol. Sympathomimetic amines may also provoke a relapse in patients with a history of malaria. When vasopressor amines are used for long periods, the resulting vasoconstriction may prevent adequate expansion of circulating volume and may cause continuation of the shock state. There is evidence that plasma volume may be reduced in all types of shock, and that the measurement of central venous pressure is the most useful means of assessing the adequacy of the circulating blood volume. Therefore, blood or plasma volume expanders should be employed when the principal reason for hypotension or shock is decreased circulating volume. Patients with cirrhosis should be treated with caution, and with adequate restoration of electrolytes if diuresis ensues.

Adverse Reactions: Sinus or ventricular tachycardia, or other arrhythmias, particularly in patients with myocardial infarction. Care should be taken in administering metaraminol since abscess formation, tissue necrosis and sloughing may be seen following administration. In choosing the site of injection, it is important to avoid those areas recognized as unsuitable for use of any pressor agent and to discontinue the infusion immediately if infiltration or thrombosis occurs. The larger veins of the antecubital fossa or the thigh are preferred to veins in the dorsum of the hand or ankle, particularly in patients with peripheral vascular disease, diabetes mellitus, Buerger's disease, or conditions with coexistent hypercoagulability.

Dosage and Administration: *Intramuscularly, intravenously* or *subcutaneously*. The route of administration and the dosage used will depend on the situation encountered. A dose of 5 to 10 mg is usually administered *intramuscularly* initially with subsequent doses dependent upon the response. After suitable dilution with 500 ml of 5% glucose alone or in isotonic saline, 15 to 100 mg of metaraminol is utilized for *intravenous infusion;* the rate being determined by that necessary to maintain the blood pressure. An excessive elevation of blood pressure should be avoided.

Availability:
ARAMINE® Injection, 10 mg/ml in ampuls of 1 ml and in vials of 10 ml.
(Merck Sharp & Dohme)

METAXALONE

Chemical Name: 5-(3,5-Dimethylphenoxymethyl)-2-oxazolidinone.

Description: Metaxalone is a cyclic carbamate compound of the propanediol series which is pharmacologically related to meprobamate and similar drugs. Structurally and pharmacologically, it is most closely related to mephenoxalone, its structure differing only in the groups present in the benzene ring. It occurs as a white, crystalline powder practically insoluble in water and soluble in alcohol.

Metaxalone appears to block reflex spasm through suppression of nerve impulses in the polysynaptic pathways, primarily in the spinal cord and to a lesser extent at supraspinal levels. This action restores muscle tone without altering normal posture or gait.

Indications: Relief of discomfort associated with acute, painful musculoskeletal conditions as an adjunctive aid to rest, physical therapy and other helpful measures. The drug does not directly relax tense skeletal muscles.

Contraindications: Known hypersensitivity to the drug, in patients with a known tendency to drug-induced hemolytic or other anemias, and in those with significantly impaired renal or hepatic function.

Precautions: Variations in white cell count and hemoglobin levels have been reported in a few patients; until the significance of these variations can be determined, therapy for more than 10 days is not recommended. Administer with utmost care to patients with preexisting liver damage; serial studies of liver function are recommended. False-positive Benedict's tests, due to an unknown reducing substance, have been noted; a glucose-specific test will differentiate findings. Safe use in pregnant and lactating women or in children under 12 years of age awaits further studies.

Adverse Reactions: Nausea, vomiting, gastrointestinal upset, drowsiness, dizziness, headache, nervousness, irritability, hypersensitivity reaction characterized by rash with or without pruritus; leukopenia, hemolytic anemia, and jaundice.

Dosage and Administration: *Orally,* 2 tablets 3 or 4 times daily, for up to but not exceeding 10 consecutive days.

Availability:
SKELAXIN® Tablets, 400 mg in bottles of 100 and 500. **(Robins)**

METHACYCLINE

Chemical Name: 4-Dimethylamino-1,4,4α,5,5α,6,11,12α-octahydro-3,5,10,12,12α-pentahydroxy-6-methylene-1, 11-dioxo-2-naphthacenecarboxamide.

Description: Methacycline, a synthetic broad-spectrum antibiotic, occurs as a light-yellow, crystalline powder soluble in water and sparingly soluble in alcohol. It is prepared by removal of hydroxyl and hydrogen from the sixth position of the oxytetracycline molecule. The hydrochloride salt of methacycline is freely soluble in water. It is readily absorbed and is bound to plasma proteins, concentrated by the liver in the bile, excreted in the urine and feces at high concentration and in a biologically active form. Cross-resistance among the tetracyclines is common. A tetracycline disc may be used to determine microbial susceptibility. If the Kirby-Bauer method of disc susceptibility testing is used, a 30 mcg tetracycline disc should give a zone of at least 19 mm when tested against a tetracycline-susceptible bacterial strain. Since it is a member of the tetracycline series of antibiotics, it may be expected to be useful in the treatment of infections which respond to the tetracyclines.

Indications: Primarily in the treatment of infections caused by Rickettsiae (Rocky mountain spotted fever, typhus fever, Q fever, richettsialpox, and tick fevers), *Mycoplasma pneumoniae* (PPLO, Eaton agent), psittacosis and ornithosis, lymphogranuloma venereum, granuloma inguinale, and *Borrelia recurrentis.* Additionally, infections that generally respond to treatment include those due to *Haemophilus ducreyi* (chancroid), *Pasteurella pestis and Pasteurella tularensis, Bartonella bacilliformis, Bacteroides, Vibrio comma, Vibro fetus,* and *Brucella* (in conjunction with streptomycin). *Escherichia coli, Enterobacter aerogenes* (formerly *Aerobacter aerogenes), Shigella, Mima, Herellea, Haemophilus influenzae, Klebsiella* and *Streptococcus* can be treated with methacycline when sensitivity tests indicate the presence of susceptible strains. For upper respiratory tract infections due to group A beta-hemolytic streptococci, penicillin is the usual drug of choice, including prophylaxis of rheumatic fever. *Diplococcus pneumoniae, Staphylococci aureus,* skin and soft tissue infections usually respond to methacycline, although it is not the primary drug in the treatment of any type of staphylococcal infections. Similarly, this drug may be used when penicillin cannot be given to patients with *Neisseria gonorrhoeae, Treponema pallidum* and *Treponema pertenue* (syphilis and yaws), *Listeria monocytogenes, Clostridium, Bacillus anthracis, Fusobacterium fusiforme* (Vincent's infection) and *Actinomyces.* Methacycline has been found useful as adjunctive therapy in the treatment of acute intestinal amebiasis and severe acne. May be used in the treatment of trachoma, although the infection is not always eliminated, as judged by immunofluorescense. May also be used in the treatment of trachoma and inclusion conjunctivitis.

Contraindications: Hypersensitivity to the drug.

Warnings: In renal impairment, lower than usual doses should be given and, if treatment is prolonged, serum level determinations are advised. May form a stable calcium complex in bone-forming tissues. Use of this drug during tooth development (last trimester of pregnancy, neonatal period, and early childhood) may cause discoloration of the teeth (yellow-gray-brownish). Individuals with a history of photosensitivity reactions should be instructed to avoid exposure to direct sunlight; treatment should be discontinued at the first sign of skin discomfort. The antianabolic action of methacycline may cause an increase in BUN. While this is not a problem in those with normal renal function, in patients with significantly impaired function, higher serum levels of the drug may lead to azotemia, hyperphosphatemia, and acidosis. Results of animal studies indicate that tetracyclines cross the placenta, are found in fetal tissues and can have toxic effects on the developing fetus usually manifested by delayed bone growth. Evidence of embryotoxicity has also been noted in animals treated early in pregnancy. Premature infants given oral doses of 25 mg/kg of body weight every 6 hours showed a decrease in the fibula growth rate. This was attributed to the drug's capability of forming a stable calcium complex in any bone-forming tissue. However, this reaction was shown to be reversible when the drug was discontinued. It should be noted that methacycline has been found to be present in the milk of lactating women.

Precautions: There may be an overgrowth of monilia and resistant staphylococci, in which case the drug should be discontinued and appropriate therapy instituted. When treating gonorrhea in which lesions of primary or secondary syphilis are suspected, proper diagnostic procedures including dark-field examination are in order. In all cases in which concomitant syphilis is suspected, monthly serology should be undertaken for at least four months. Increased intracranial pressure with bulging fontanelles has been observed in infants receiving this drug; these symptoms disappeared when therapy was discontinued. Because methacycline has been shown to depress plasma prothrombin activity, patients who are on anticoagulant therapy may require a downward adjustment of their anticoagulant dosage. When therapy is prolonged, periodic laboratory evaluation of organ systems, including hematopoietic, renal and hepatic studies should be performed. Concomitant use with penicillin should be avoided.

Adverse Reactions: *Gastrointestinal:* anorexia, nausea, vomiting, diarrhea, glossitis, dysphagia, enterocolitis and inflammatory lesions (with monilial overgrowth) in the anogenital region. These reactions have been caused by both the oral and parenteral administration of tetracyclines. *Skin:* maculopapular and erythematous rashes, exfoliative dermatitis (uncommon) and photosensitivity. *Renal:* rise in BUN. *Hypersensitivity reactions:* urticaria, angioneurotic edema, anaphylaxis, anaphylactoid purpura, pericarditis and exacerbation of systemic lupus erythematosus. *Blood:* hemolytic anemia, thrombocytopenia, neutropenia and eosinophilia. Prolonged use may produce brown-black microscopic discoloration of the thyroid but no abnormalities of thyroid function studies have been known to occur.

Dosage and Administration: *Orally.* Usually, 600 mg daily, divided into 2 or 4 equal doses; may be doubled in case of severe infection. *Treatment of uncomplicated gonorrhea,* 900 mg initially, followed by 300 mg 4 times daily for a total of 5.4 gm. *Treatment of syphilis,* a total of 18 to 24 gm in equally divided doses over a period of 10 to 15 days is recommended and should be accompanied by laboratory tests. *Treatment of Eaton Agent pneumonia,* the usual adult dosage is 900 mg daily for 6 days. Children, 3 to 6 mg/lb of body weight in 2 or 4 equally divided doses. Therapy should be continued for at least 24 to 48 hours after symptoms and fever have subsided. In the treatment of streptococcal infections, a therapeutic dosage regimen should be continued for at least 10 days. Taking the drug at least 1 hour before, or 2 hours after meals will facilitate absorption. Pediatric dosages should not be given with milk or other calcium-containing foods. Aluminum hydroxide gel decreases the absorption of antibotics and is therefore contraindicated.

Availability:
RONDOMYCIN®: **(Wallace)**
Capsules, 150 mg (equiv. to 140 mg base) in bottles of 100; 300 mg (equiv. to 280 mg base) in bottles of 50.
Syrup, 75 mg/5 ml (equiv. to 70 mg/5 ml base) in bottles of 60 ml and 1 pint.

METHADONE HYDROCHLORIDE Ⓒ II

Chemical Name: 6-(Dimethylamino)-4,4-diphenyl-3-heptanone hydrochloride.

Description: Methadone is a synthetic narcotic analgesic similar in effect to morphine, but because of greater lipid solubility its duration of effect is more prolonged than that of morphine. It occurs as a white, crystalline material soluble in water, freely soluble in alcohol and in chloroform, and practically insoluble in ether and in glycerin.

Like morphine, methadone in full therapeutic doses depresses respiration and the cough reflex, increases intestinal tone and the amplitude of contractions, and produces miosis. Sedation and narcosis are less significant than with morphine and is, therefore, inferior to morphine as a preanesthetic medication. It has been found useful as a replacement agent in the management of morphine and heroin addiction. It can prevent or relieve acute withdrawal symptoms. The methadone abstinence syndrome, although qualitatively similar to that of morphine, differs in that the onset of action is slower, duration of effect is more prolonged, and the symptoms are less severe. When administered orally, methadone is approximately 1/2 as potent as when given parenterally. Oral administration results in a delay of the onset of action, a lowering of the peak effect, and an increase in the duration of analgesic effect.

Indications: When an analgesic effect is required, especially for the relief of postoperative pain, and pain associated with renal colic, metastatic lesions of malignant tumors, fractures, etc. Methadone is preferable to morphine for prolonged use, since it induces less physical dependence. It is also used in detoxification and temporary maintenance treatment of narcotic addiction.

Contraindications: Hypersensitivity to methadone.

Warnings: Methadone can produce drug dependence of the morphine type and, therefore, has the potential for being abused. Because psychic dependence, physical dependence and tolerance may develop following repeated administration, methadone should be prescribed and administered with the same degree of caution appropriate to the use of morphine. This drug should be used with considerable caution and in reduced dosage in patients who are concurrently receiving other narcotic analgesics, general anesthetics, phenothiazines, other tranquilizers, sedative-hypnotics, tricyclic antidepressants and other CNS depressants (including alcohol). Respiratory depression, hypotension, and profound sedation or coma may result. The physician should be on guard not to confuse symptoms of anxiety with those of narcotic abstinence and should not attempt to treat such symptoms by increasing the dosage of methadone. The capacity of methadone to depress respiration and elevate cerebrospinal-fluid pressure may be markedly exaggerated in the presence of increased intracranial pressure. Furthermore, narcotics produce side-effects that may obscure the clinical course of patients with head injuries. In such individuals, methadone must be used with extreme caution and only if it is deemed essential. It should be used with extreme caution in patients having an acute asthmatic attack, in those with chronic obstructive pulmonary disease or cor pulmonale, and in individuals with a substantially decreased respiratory reserve, preexisting respiratory depression, hypoxia, or hypercapnia. In such patients, even usual therapeutic doses of methadone may decrease respiratory drive while simultaneously increasing airway resistance to the point of apnea.

The administration of methadone may result in severe hypotension in an individual whose ability to maintain his blood pressure has already been compromised by a depleted blood volume or concurrent administration of such drugs as the phenothiazines or certain anesthetics. Methadone may impair the mental and/or physical abilities required for the performance of potentially hazardous tasks, such as driving a car or operating machinery. The patient should be cautioned accordingly. It may also produce orthostatic hypotension in ambulatory patients. Safe use during pregnancy has not been established in relation to possible adverse effects on fetal development. Therefore, methadone should not be used in pregnant women unless, in the judgment of the physician, the potential benefits outweigh the possible hazards. It is not recommended for obstetric analgesia because its long duration of action increases the probability of respiratory depression in the newborn. Methadone is not recommended for use as an analgesic in children, since documented clinical experience has been insufficient to establish a suitable dosage regimen for the pediatric age group.

Precautions: Therapeutic doses of meperidine have precipitated severe reactions in patients concurrently receiving monoamine oxidase inhibitors or in those having received such agents within the previous 14 days. Similar reactions have not, thus far, been reported with methadone; but if the use of methadone is necessary in such patients, a sensitivity test should be performed in which repeated small incremental doses are administered over the course of several hours while the patient's condition and vital signs are under careful observation. Additionally, patients who are addicted to heroin or who are on the methadone maintenance program may experience withdrawal symptoms when given pentazocine. The administration of methadone or other narcotics may obscure the diagnosis of acute abdominal conditions or their clinical course. Methadone should be given with caution and the initial dose should be reduced in elderly or debilitated patients and in those with severe impairment of hepatic or renal function, hypothyroidism, Addison's disease, prostatic hypertrophy or urethral stricture.

Adverse Reactions: The major hazards of methadone are respiratory depression and, to a lesser degree, circulatory depression; respiratory arrest, shock, and cardiac arrest have occurred. The most frequently observed adverse reactions include lightheadedness, dizziness, sedation, nausea, vomiting, and sweating. These effects seem to be more prominent in ambulatory patients, and in those who are not suffering severe pain. In such individuals, lower doses are advisable. Other adverse reactions include the following: *CNS:* Euphoria, dysphoria, weakness, headache, insomnia, agitation, disorientation, and visual disturbances. *Gastrointestinal:* Dry mouth, anorexia, constipation, and biliary tract spasm. *Cardiovascular:* Flushing of the face, bradycardia, palpitation, faintness, and syncope. *Genitourinary:* Urinary retention or hesitancy, antidiuretic effect, and reduced libido and/or potency. *Allergic:* Pruritus, urticaria, other skin rashes, edema, and, rarely, hemorrhagic urticaria.

Serious overdosage of methadone is characterized by respiratory depression (a decrease in respiratory rate and/or tidal volume, Cheyne-Stokes respiration, cyanosis), extreme somnolence progressing to stupor or coma, maximally constricted pupils, skeletal-muscle flaccidity, cold and clammy skin, and, sometimes, bradycardia and hypotension. In severe overdosage, particularly by the intravenous route, apnea, circulatory collapse, cardiac arrest, and death may occur. Primary attention should be given to the reestablishment of adequate respiratory exchange through provision of a patent airway and institution of assisted or controlled ventilation. **The physician must remember, however, that methadone is a long-acting depressant (36 to 48 hours), whereas the antagonists act for much shorter periods (1 to 3 hours).** The patient must, therefore, be monitored continuously for recurrence of respiratory depression and treated repeatedly with the narcotic antagonist as needed. If the diagnosis is correct and respiratory depression is due only to overdosage of methadone, the use of other respiratory stimulants is not indicated. An antagonist should not be administered in the absence of clinically significant respiratory or cardiovascular depression. Nalorphine hydrochloride (0.1 mg/kg) or levallorphan tartrate (0.02 mg/kg) should be given intravenously as soon as possible. Repeat, if necessary, every 15 minutes. Oxygen, intravenous fluids, vasopressors, and other supportive measures should be employed as indicated. **Note:** In an individual physically dependent on narcotics, the administration of the usual dose of a narcotic antagonist will precipitate an acute withdrawal syndrome. The severity of this syndrome will depend on the degree of physical dependence and the dose of the antagonist administered. The use of a narcotic antagonist in such a patient should be avoided if possible. If it must be used to treat serious respiratory depression in the physically dependent patient, the antagonist should be administered with extreme care.

Dosage and Administration: *Intramuscularly* or *subcutaneously,* 2.5 to 10 mg according to the severity of pain, repeated only when pain returns. *Orally.* As an analgesic for adults, 2.5 mg every 6 to 8 hours for moderate pain; 5 mg every 6 to 8 hours for more severe pain; and 10 mg every 4 to 6 hours for very severe pain. The treatment course for detoxification should not exceed 21 days (3 weeks) and should not be repeated until after an elapse of 28 days (4 weeks) following completion of the preceding course. Initially, 15 to 20 mg given in a single dose is usually sufficient to suppress withdrawal symptoms. Patients heavily addicted may be given 40 mg either as a single dose or in 2 equally divided doses at an interval of 4 to 8 hours, with additional 10-mg doses as the clinical situation warrants; however, some patients may require up to 120 mg daily. Stabilization may be continued for 2 to 3 days and then the dose decreased on a daily or every other day basis. In hospitalized patients, a daily reduction of 20% of the total daily dose may be tolerated; ambulatory patients will require a proportionately slower schedule. Dosage levels for pregnant patients should be kept as low as possible and they should be made fully aware of the possible risks to themselves or the fetus. **Note: To be dispensed only by physicians affiliated with federally approved addiction-treatment programs or for analgesic use in hospitals.**

Availability:
C-II DOLOPHINE®: **(Lilly)**
Injection, 10 mg/ml in ampuls of 1 ml and in vials of 20 ml.
Tablets, 5 mg in bottles of 100 and 1000; 10 mg in bottles of 100.
C-II METHADONE HYDROCHLORIDE Dispersable Tablets (Diskets®), 40 mg in bottles of 100. **(Lilly)**

METHAMPHETAMINE HYDROCHLORIDE C-II

Synonym: Desoxyephedrine hydrochloride.

Chemical Name: *N*, α-Dimethylphenethylamine hydrochloride.

Description: Methamphetamine hydrochloride is the *dextro*rotatory isomer of phenylisopropyl-methylamine. It occurs as a white, crystalline powder freely soluble in water and in alcohol.

Readily absorbed from the gastrointestinal tract, the effects of the drug persist for 6 to 12 hours, but, with large doses, may continue up to 24 hours. The anorectic effect diminishes after a few weeks.

Pharmacologically, methamphetamine is qualitatively similar to amphetamine and ephedrine including CNS and respiratory stimulation, and in sympathomimetic activity including pressor response, mydriasis, bronchodilation, and contraction of the urinary-bladder sphincter.

Indications: Short-term (a few weeks) adjunctive agent in the management of exogenous obesity in a regimen of weight reduction based primarily on caloric restriction. Also useful as an adjunct to other remedial measures (psychological, educational, or social) in the management of children with minimal brain dysfunction. However, this form of therapy is not intended for use in children who exhibit symptoms secondary to environmental factors and/or primary psychiatric disorders, including psychosis.

Contraindications: During or within 14 days following the administration of monoamine oxidase inhibitors (MAOI); hypertensive crises may result. It is also contraindicated in patients with glaucoma, advanced arteriosclerosis, symptomatic cardiovascular disease, moderate to severe hypertension, hyperthyroidism, or known hypersensitivity or idiosyncrasy to sympathomimetic amines. Amphetamines should not be given to patients who are in an agitated state, or who have a history of drug abuse.

Warnings: Amphetamines have a significant potential for abuse. In view of their limited short-term anorectic effect and rapid development of tolerance, they should be used with extreme caution and only for limited periods of time in weight reduction programs. Tolerance to the anorectic effect usually develops within a few weeks. When this occurs, the recommended dose should not be exceeded in an attempt to increase the effect; rather, the drug should be discontinued. Methamphetamine may impair the ability of the patient to engage in potentially hazardous activities such as operating machinery or driving a motor vehicle; the patient should therefore be cautioned accordingly. Since this drug has a significant potential for abuse, tolerance and extreme psychological dependence have occurred; there are reports of patients who have increased the dosage to many times that recommended. Abrupt cessation following prolonged high dosage administration results in extreme fatigue and mental depression; changes are also noted on the sleep EEG. Manifestations of chronic intoxication with amphetamines include severe dermatoses, marked insomnia, irritability, hyperactivity, and personality changes. The most severe manifestation of chronic intoxication is psychosis, often clinically indistinguishable from schizophrenia. Safe use during pregnancy has not been established. Reproduction studies in mammals at high multiples of the human dose have suggested both an embryotoxic and a teratogenic potential. Use of amphetamines by women who are or who may become pregnant, and especially those in the first trimester of pregnancy, requires that the potential benefit be weighed against the possible hazard to mother and infant. Amphetamines are not recommended for use as anorectic agents in children under 12 years of age.

Precautions: Methamphetamine should be used with caution in patients with even mild hypertension. The drug should not be employed to combat fatigue or to replace rest in normal individuals. Insulin requirements in diabetes mellitus may be altered in association with the use of amphetamines and the concomitant dietary regimen. Amphetamines may decrease the hypotensive effect of guanethidine. Prescribing and dispensing these drugs should be limited to the smallest amount that is feasible at one time in order to minimize the possibility of overdosage.

Adverse Reactions: *Cardiovascular:* Palpitation, tachycardia, elevation of blood pressure. *CNS:* Overstimulation, restlessness, dizziness, insomnia, euphoria, dysphoria, tremor, headache; rarely, psychotic episodes at recommended doses. *Gastrointestinal:* Dryness of mouth, unpleasant taste, diarrhea, other gastrointestinal disturbances. *Allergic:* Urticaria. *Endocrine:* Impotence, changes in libido. Manifestations of acute overdosage with amphetamines include restlessness, tremor, hyperreflexia, rapid breathing, confusion, assaultiveness, hallucinations, and panic states. Fatigue and depression usually follow the central stimulation. *Cardiovascular* effects include arrhythmias, hypertension or hypotension, and circulatory collapse. *Gastrointestinal* symptoms include nausea, vomiting, diarrhea, and abdominal cramps. Fatal poisoning usually terminates in convulsions and coma. Management of acute intoxication is primarily symptomatic and includes gastric lavage, and sedation with a barbiturate. Experience with hemodialysis or peritoneal dialysis is inadequate to permit recommendations in this regard.

Dosage and Administration: *Orally.* For obesity: Usually, 2.5 to 5 mg daily, taken ½ hour before each meal. The Gradumet or long-acting tablets are usually taken once daily in the morning. For adjunctive treatment of minimal brain dysfunction: Initially, 2.5 to 5 mg once or twice daily; increased in increments of 5 mg at weekly intervals until optimal clinical response is achieved. The usual effective dose is 20 to 25 mg daily.

Availability:

Methamphetamine Hydrochloride

(C-II) DESOXYN®: **(Abbott)**

Gradumet® (long-release tablets), 5 mg in bottles of 100; 10 and 15 mg in bottles of 100 and 500.

Tablets, 2.5 mg in bottles of 100; 5 mg in bottles of 100 and 1000.

(C-II) METHAMPEX™ Tablets, 10 mg (pink) in bottles of 100 and 1000. **(Lemmon)**

METHANDROSTENOLONE

Chemical Name: 17β-Hydroxy-17α-methylandrosta-1,4-diene-3-one.

Description: Methandrostenolone is a synthetic steroidal hormone structurally and pharmacologically related to other androgenic-anabolic steroids.

Methandrostenolone improves nitrogen balance but only when there is sufficient intake of calories and protein. Whether this positive nitrogen balance is of primary benefit in the utilization of protein-building dietary substances has not been established. The action of anabolic steroids are similar to those of male sex hormones with the possibility of causing serious disturbances of growth and sexual development if given to young children. They suppress the gonadotropic functions of the pituitary gland and may exert a direct effect upon the testes.

Human growth hormone is the preferred treatment of pituitary dwarfism. If this hormone is not available, anabolic agents may be used to treat this condition.

Indications: Treatment of senile and postmenopausal osteoporosis as adjunctive therapy; considered to be of no value as primary therapy. Equal or greater consideration should be given to diet, calcium balance, physiotherapy, and other general health-promoting measures. Also, for pituitary dwarfism when growth hormone is not available.

Contraindications: Hypersensitivity to methandrostenolone; male patients with carcinoma of the prostate or breast; carcinoma of the breast in some females; pregnancy because of masculinization of the fetus, and nephrosis or the nephrotic phase of nephritis.

Warnings: Methandrostenolone will not enhance athletic ability.

Precautions: Hypercalcemia may develop both spontaneously and as a result of hormonal therapy in women with disseminated breast carcinoma. If it develops during treatment with this agent, the drug should be withdrawn. Since edema may occur, caution is required in administering methandrostenolone to patients with cardiac, renal, or hepatic disease. Concomitant administration with adrenal steroids or ACTH may add to the edema. If amenorrhea or menstrual irregularities develop, the drug should be discontinued until the etiology is determined. Anabolic steroids are known to increase sensitivity to anticoagulants; therefore, dosage of the anticoagulant may have to be decreased in order to maintain the prothrombin time at the desired therapeutic level. Also, they have been shown to alter glucose tolerance tests; diabetics should be followed carefully and an adjustment of the insulin or oral hypoglycemic dosage should be instituted. It is advised that liver function be checked at regular intervals in patients receiving this drug. Methandrostenolone should be used with utmost care in patients with a history of benign prostatic hypertrophy, myocardial infarction or coronary artery disease. Serial determinations of serum cholesterol should be made, and if an increase is noted during therapy, the dosage of this agent should be adjusted accordingly.

Adverse Reactions: In males, *prepubertal:* phallic enlargement, and increased frequency of erections; *postpubertal:* inhibition of testicular function, oligospermia, and gynecomastia. **In females,** hirsutism, male pattern baldness, deepening of the voice, clitoral enlargement. These changes are usually irreversible even after prompt discontinuance of therapy and are not prevented by concomitant use of estrogens. In addition the following may occur: menstrual irregularities, and masculinization of the fetus. **In both sexes,** nausea, a feeling of fullness, loss of appetite, burning of the tongue, increased or decreased libido, acne (especially in females and prepubertal males), inhibition of gonadotropin secretion, bleeding in patients on concomitant anticoagulant therapy, premature closure of epiphyses in children, vomiting, and jaundice. There have been rare reports of hepatocellular carcinoma, particularly in association with long-term therapy in patients receiving androgenic and anabolic steroids. Alterations may occur in the following tests: metyrapone test, glucose tolerance test, thyroid function tests (decrease in protein bound iodine, thyroxine-binding capacity, and radioactive iodine uptake), electrolytes (retention of sodium, chloride, water, potassium, phosphates, and calcium), hepatic function tests (increased bromsulphalein, serum cholesterol, SGOT, serum bilirubin, and alkaline phosphatase), blood coagulation tests (suppression of clotting factors II, V, VII, and X) and decreased 17-ketosteroid excretion.

Dosage and Administration: *Orally.* Therapy should be intermittent and no longer than is necessary for optimal results. Initially, 5 mg daily. In severe debilitated states, 10 mg daily for up to 3 weeks. For maintenance, 2.5 to 5 mg daily. Dosage for children should not exceed 0.05 mg/kg/day. A proper diet, particularly adequate protein intake, is necessary to assure the full anabolic benefits.

Availability:
DIANABOL® Tablets, 2.5 mg (pale yellow) in bottles of 100; 5 mg (blue) in bottles of 100 and 1000. **(Ciba)**

METHANTHELINE BROMIDE

Chemical Name: Diethyl(2-hydroxyethyl)methylammonium bromide xanthene-9-carboxylate.

Description: Methantheline bromide is a synthetic anticholinergic quaternary ammonium compound which differs structurally from propantheline bromide in that 2 ethyl groups replace 2 isopropyl groups in the nitrogen atom of propantheline. It is a very bitter, white powder very soluble in water and freely soluble in alcohol.

Methantheline bromide acts as a ganglionic-blocking agent on the sympathetic and the parasympathetic autonomic nervous systems. It also exerts an atropine-like action at the postganglionic nerve endings of the parasympathetic system. Its therapeutic effect is due to slowing of gastrointestinal propulsion and diminishing of gastric acid secretion.

Indications: Treatment of peptic ulcer as adjunctive therapy, and for the treatment of uninhibited hypertonic bladder. The parenteral form is indicated for use as a preanesthetic drying medication.

Contraindications: Glaucoma, obstructive disease of the gastrointestinal tract (pyloroduodenal stenosis, achalasia, paralytic ileus, etc.), obstructive uropathy (bladder neck obstruction due to prostatic hypertrophy), intestinal atony of the elderly or debilitated patient, megacolon complicating ulcerative colitis, hiatal hernia associated with reflux esophagitis, unstable cardiovascular status in acute hemorrhage, and myasthenia gravis.

Warnings: Methantheline should be used with considerable care in patients with severe cardiac disease. Patients should be made aware that fever and heat stroke may occur due to anhidrosis, particularly when the environmental temperature is elevated. Diarrhea may be an early symptom of incomplete intestinal obstruction, especially in patients with ileostomy or colostomy; in this instance treatment with this drug would be inappropriate and possibly harmful. Overdosage may cause a curare-like action manifested by loss of control of voluntary muscles, particularly respiratory muscles. Therefore, such patients should receive prompt and continuing artificial respiration until the drug effect has been exhausted.

Precautions: Urinary retention may be avoided in elderly patients with prostatic hypertrophy, if they are advised to micturate at the time of taking the medication. Overdosage should be avoided in patients severely ill with ulcerative colitis. As with any drug its use during pregnancy or in women of childbearing potential should be undertaken with due consideration to the potential hazards to the unborn child. May have an inhibitory effect of lactation.

Adverse Reactions: Dry mouth, blurred vision; overdosage may produce a curare-like reaction.

Dosage and Administration: *Orally, intramuscularly* or *intravenously*. Peptic ulcer, initially, 50 to 100 mg every 6 hours day and night. Uninhibited hypertonic neurogenic bladder, initially, 50 to 100 mg 4 times daily. Dosages should be subsequently adjusted to the patient's needs and tolerance. Newborn infants, 12.5 mg twice daily then 3 times daily. Infants from 1 to 12 months of age, 12.5 mg 4 times daily, increased gradually to 25 mg 4 times daily. Children more than 1 year of age, 12.5 to 50 mg 4 times daily. Parenterally, ½ the oral dose.

Availability:
BANTHINE®: **(Searle)**
Injection (serum type) in vials of 50 mg.
Tablets, 50 mg (pink) in bottles of 100 and 500.

METHAPYRILENE HYDROCHLORIDE

Chemical Name: N, N-Dimethyl-N′ (2-thenyl)-N′-(2-pyridyl)-ethylenediamine hydrochloride.

Description: Methapyrilene is an antihistamine and an analog of tripelennamine and pyrilamine. It occurs as a white, crystalline powder very soluble in water and freely soluble in alcohol. Onset of action is rapid but its duration is short.

Indications: *Orally* for the symptomatic treatment of seasonal and perennial allergic rhinitis, vasomotor rhinitis, allergic conjunctivitis due to inhalant allergens and foods, mild uncomplicated allergic skin manifestations of urticaria and angioedema; dermatographia. *Parenterally* for the amelioration and prevention of allergic reactions to blood or plasma in patients with a known history of such reactions, and in anaphylaxis as an adjunct to epinephrine and other standard measures. May be combined with sympathomimetic amines when asthma is an inconstant complicating symptom. Analgesic-antipyretics may be added to combat fever accompanying the common cold with allergic overtones.

Contraindications: Hypersensitivity to methapyrilene or to any compound formulated with the drug; in newborn or premature infants; in nursing mothers; in patients receiving monoamine oxidase inhibitors (MAOI); in those with lower respiratory tract disease, including asthma; narrow-angle glaucoma; stenosing peptic ulcer; symptomatic prostatic hypertrophy; bladder neck obstruction; or pyloroduodenal obstruction.

Warnings: Dosages for infants and children should be carefully regulated since overdosage may result in hallucinations, convulsions, and possibly death. Since antihistamines may cause drowsiness and/or mental sluggishness, patients should be cautioned not to engage in occupations requiring alertness or motor coordination until their response to the drug has been deteminined. In very young children a paradoxical excitation may occur. Elderly patients are more likely to respond to antihistamines with dizziness, sedation and hypotension. Patients receiving antihistamines should be warned against the concomitant use of alcoholic beverages or other drugs (e.g., hypnotics, sedatives, tranquilizers, antianxiety agents, etc.) that depress the CNS. The drug should not be administered to patients receiving MAO inhibitors since these agents prolong and intensify the anticholinergic effects of antihistamines. There is insufficient data as to whether this drug may reduce fertility in both male and female patients or have teratogenic or other adverse effects on the fetus. The phenacetin component may damage the kidneys when used in large amounts or for prolonged periods; therefore, patients should be advised not to exceed the recommended dose or to take the drug for more than three days without consulting the physician.

Precautions: Due to its atropine-like action, routine precautions should be followed when the drug is used in patients with a history of bronchial asthma, increased intraocular pressure, hyperthyroidism, cardiovascular-renal disease, hypertension, or diabetes. Salicylate-containing compounds should be used with considerable care in patients with peptic ulcer, and in those with nasal polyps and asthma. Phenacetin should not be administered repeatedly to patients with anemia or with cardiac, pulmonary, or hepatic disease. The prolonged and excessive use of phenacetin-containing products may aggravate renal disease. Caffeine should not be given to patients who are extremely sensitive to its CNS-stimulating action. In the presence of prostatism, the administration of a sympathomimetic drug (cyclopentamine) may cause urinary retention; therefore, the maximum dosage of 2 pulvules 5 times daily should not be exceeded.

Adverse Reactions: Those frequently encountered are sedation; drowsiness; dryness of mouth, nose, and throat; thickening of bronchial secretions; dizziness; epigastric distress; and disturbed coordination. Those rarely encountered unless large doses are used include fatigue, confusion, restlessness, excitation, nervousness, insomnia, euphoria, anorexia, nausea, vomiting, diarrhea, constipation, hypotension, tightness of chest and wheezing, urticaria, drug rash, anaphylactic shock, blurred vision, diplopia, vertigo, tinnitus, headache, palpitation, tachycardia, nasal stuffiness, urinary frequency, urinary retention, difficult urination, photosensitivity, hemolytic anemia, leukopenia, agranulocytosis, irritability, tremor, convulsions, neuritis, acute labyrinthitis, and hysteria. Complications due to phenacetin are usually the result of toxic doses and may include cyanosis, acute hemolytic anemia, skin lesions, and fever. Those due to caffeine overdosage are manifested by insomnia, restlessness, excitement, diuresis, tachycardia, and extrasystoles. Combining cyclopentamine and methapyrilene tends to counteract the adverse effects of each other.

Dosage and Administration: *Orally.* Adults, 25 to 50 mg 4 or 5 times daily. Children and infants, 0.4 to 0.6 mg/lb of body weight 5 times daily if needed. *Parenterally.* Initially, 0.5 to 1 ml (10 to 20 mg), increased to 2 ml if feasible. Dosage for children is proportionately smaller. Oral dosage should not exceed 250 mg/day.

Availability:
HISTADYL®: **(Lilly)**
Capsules (Pulvules®), 25 mg (OTC) and 50 mg in bottles of 100.
Injection, 20 mg/ml in vials of 10 ml.
Syrup, 30 mg/5 ml (as the fumarate) in bottles of 1 pint.
HISTA-CLOPANE® Capsules, 25 mg with cyclopentamine hydrochloride, 12.5 mg in bottles of 100. **(Lilly)**
HISTADYL® and A.S.A.® Compound Capsules, 25 mg (as hydroxybenzoyl benzoate) with aspirin, 227 mg; phenacetin, 160 mg, and caffeine, 32.5 mg in bottles of 100 and 1000. **(Lilly)**
Ⓒ V HISTADYL E. C. Syrup in bottles of 120 ml and 1 pint and 1 gallon. Each 30 ml contains 81 mg with codeine phosphate, 60 mg (**Warning:** May be habit-forming); ephedrine hydrochloride, 30 mg, ammonium chloride, 660 mg; menthol, 3.9 mg and alcohol, 5%. **(Lilly)**

METHAQUALONE Ⓒ II

Chemical Name: 2-Methyl-3-*o*-tolyl-4(3*H*)-quinazolinone.

Description: Methaqualone, a synthetic CNS-depressant compound, is similar to the barbiturates in its sedative and hypnotic action. It has been found useful in individuals who cannot tolerate barbituric acid derivatives. It occurs as white crystals that are sparingly soluble in water and in alcohol and practically insoluble in ether.

The precise mode of action of methaqualone is not known. Its central effects in animals indicate that the drug acts on a different CNS site from that of barbiturates or glutethimide. In clinical studies, low doses appear to depress the sensory area of the cortex, larger doses to reduce motor activity, and high doses to exert a selective depressant effect on polysynaptic spinal reflexes. Laboratory studies have also demonstrated that methaqualone produces skeletal muscle relaxant, weak antihistaminic, antispasmodic, antitussive and strong local anesthetic effects; however, these have not been noted clinically. Studies with pregnant rats revealed that high doses produced skeletal abnormalities in the offspring.

It is readily absorbed from the gastrointestinal tract. Following an oral dose of 300 mg, the soporific effect usually occurs within 10 to 30 minutes and lasts for approximately 6 to 10 hours. The drug is metabolized in the liver and excreted in the urine and feces chiefly as the glucuronide.

Indications: To produce sleep and to provide daytime sedation.

Contraindications: In patients with known hypersensitivity to methaqualone, and in women who are or may become pregnant. Also in children less than 14 years of age.

Warnings: The hypnotic dose should be taken *only* at bedtime, immediately before retiring. Patients taking methaqualone should not be permitted to undertake hazardous tasks requiring alertness or physical coordination. The drug may potentiate the action of other CNS depressants including sedatives, analgesic, or psychotropic drugs and alcohol because of an additive effect. It should not be used continuously for periods exceeding 3 months. Although patient dependence has rarely been reported, the possible development of severe psychological and physical dependence should be considered, particularly if the drug is administered to individuals known to be addiction-prone, to those whose history suggests that they may increase the dosage on their own initiative, and also to those who may use the drug for nontherapeutic purposes.

Precautions: Extreme caution is required when administering methaqualone to patients with anxiety states when evidence of impending depression or suicidal tendencies exists. Because the drug is metabolized in the liver, the usual precautions should be observed in the presence of impaired hepatic function.

Adverse Reactions: *Neuropsychiatric:* headache, hangover, fatigue, dizziness, torpor, transient paresthesia of the extremities. An occasional patient has experienced restlessness or anxiety. *Hematologic:* aplastic anemia (rare). *Gastrointestinal:* dry mouth, anorexia, nausea, emesis, epigastric discomfort, and diarrhea. *Dermatologic:* diaphoresis, bromhidrosis, exanthema, and urticaria.

Acute overdosage may result in delirium and coma, with restlessness and hypertonia, progressing to convulsions. Spontaneous vomiting and increased secretion are common and may lead to aspiration pneumonitis or respiratory obstruction. Large overdoses have been accompanied by cutaneous edema, pulmonary edema, hepatic damage, renal insufficiency, and bleeding. Overdoses of methaqualone appear to be less often associated with cardiac or respiratory depression than are overdoses of the oral barbiturates, but shock and respiratory arrest may occasionally occur. Coma has occurred with acute overdosage averaging 2.4 gm and deaths have been reported following ingestion of 8 gm. However, in other instances, patients have survived ingestion of the drug up to 22 gm. Most fatal cases occur when ingestion of an overdose of methaqualone is accompanied by alcohol.

Dosage and Administration: *Orally.* As a hypnotic, 200 to 400 mg at bedtime. For sedation, 200 mg after each meal and at bedtime. Should not be used in children less than 14 years of age. Dosage for aged, debilitated or highly agitated patients should be individualized according to requirements and tolerances.

Availability:

(C-II) PAREST®-200 Capsules, 200 mg in bottles of 100. **(Parke-Davis)**

(C-II) PAREST-400 Capsules, 400 mg in bottles of 100. **(Parke-Davis)**

(C-II) QUAALUDE®-150 Tablets, 150 mg in bottles of 100. **(Lemmon)**

(C-II) QUAALUDE-300 Tablets, 300 mg in bottles of 100 and 500. **(Lemmon)**

(C-II) SOPOR™ Tablets, 150 and 300 mg in bottles of 100 and 500 and in unit-dose packages of 100. **(Arnar-Stone)**

METHARBITAL (C-III)

Chemical Name: 5,5-Diethyl-1-methylbarbituric acid.

Description: Metharbital is the *N*-methyl congener of barbital and is largely demethylated to barbital in the body. It occurs as a white, crystalline, faintly aromatic powder slightly soluble in water and soluble in alcohol.

The drug produces anticonvulsant effects which are similar to those produced by phenobarbital and mephobarbital. In experimental animals metharbital has been shown to be unusually effective against pentylenetetrazol-induced convulsions. It is less effective against convulsions induced by electroshock. Toxicity studies in laboratory animals indicate that the drug is less toxic and has less sedative effect than phenobarbital.

Metharbital is adequately absorbed from the gastrointestinal tract following oral administration. It is demethylated in the liver to barbital, and is excreted largely in this form by the kidneys.

Recent reports have suggested that some anticonvulsant drugs, especially barbiturates, may be associated with neonatal hemorrhage in infants born to mothers treated with these drugs during pregnancy. Such drug therapy appears to reduce the levels of vitamin K-dependent clotting factors in the infant, causing an increased tendency to hemorrhage in the neonatal period. It has been suggested that vitamin K be given prophylactically to such infants at birth.

Indications: Treatment of grand mal, petit mal, myoclonic epilepsy and mixed types of seizures. It may be used in conjunction with other antiepileptic drugs.

Contraindications: In patients with known hypersensitivity to barbiturates, and in those with a history of manifest or latent porphyria.

Warnings: Metharbital may be habit-forming. May cause neonatal coagulation defects in infants born to mothers treated with metharbital during pregnancy. There is strongly suggestive evidence that a teratogenic potential exists; therefore, its use in the gravid patient must be carefully weighed in terms of benefit-to-risk to the patient as well as the fetus.

Precautions: Use with caution in patients receiving coumarin or coumarin-type drugs. Metharbital should be used with caution in patients with hepatic impairment. Abrupt withdrawal of the drug may result in status epilepticus in epileptic patients who have been on regular daily doses.

Adverse Reactions: Gastric distress, dizziness, increased irritability, skin rash and drowsiness; large doses may cause loss of consciousness and coma. The usual supportive measures for barbiturate intoxication should be employed.

Dosage and Administration: *Orally.* Initially, 1 tablet 1 to 3 times daily. Initial pediatric dosage is ½ tablet 1 to 3 times daily, depending on the age and weight of the patient. A dose of 5 to 15 mg/kg/day has been recommended for children. Dosage must be adjusted to each patient for optimal effect. When added to an established regimen to replace or supplement other anticonvulsant therapy, the dosage of other medication should be gradually reduced while increasing that of metharbital so as to avoid or minimize recurrence of seizures.

Availability:
Ⓒ III GEMONIL® Tablets, 100 mg in bottles of 100. **(Abbott)**

METHAZOLAMIDE

Chemical Name: *N*-(4-Methyl-2-sulfamoyl-Δ^2-1,3,4-thiadiazolin-5-ylidene)acetamide.

Description: Methazolamide is a carbonic anhydrase inhibitor structurally and physiologically related to acetazolamide. It occurs as a white or yellowish-white, crystalline powder soluble in hot water and in alcohol.

In common with other carbonic anhydrase inhibitors, methazolamide inhibits formation of hydrogen and bicarbonate ions from carbon dioxide and water. This action results in increased excretion of bicarbonate, sodium and potassium from the renal tubules thus producing diuresis; however, it is less active than acetazolamide. In addition, methazolamide inhibits ocular carbonic anhydrase and lowers intraocular pressure, probably by decreasing formation of aqueous humor.

The onset and duration of action of methazolamide are more prolonged than those of acetazolamide. Following oral ingestion, the onset of fall in intraocular pressure occurs within 2 to 4 hours, reaches a peak in 6 to 8 hours and persists for about 10 hours or more. The complete distribution pattern and metabolic fate of the drug are unknown.

Indications: Adjunctive treatment of chronic simple (open-angle) glaucoma, secondary glaucoma, and preoperatively in acute angle-closure glaucoma where delay of surgery is desired in order to lower intraocular pressure. Its use in glaucoma due to severe peripheral anterior synechiae or hemorrhage is of doubtful value.

Contraindications: Severe or absolute glaucoma, or chronic noncongestive angle-closure glaucoma. Also contraindicated in patients with adrenocortical, hepatic or renal insufficiency, or with hyperchloremic acidosis and a depletion of sodium and potassium ions.

Warnings: The drug should not be used in women of childbearing age or during pregnancy, especially in the first trimester, unless the benefits to be gained in the control of glaucoma outweigh potential adverse effects.

Precautions: Methazolamide should be administered with caution to patients with hepatic cirrhosis, or with respiratory disorders associated with severe loss of pulmonary ventilation, and to those on steroid medication because of the potentiality of a hypokalemic state developing. Blood dyscrasias and renal or hepatic damage, reported with other sulfonamide derivatives, have not been observed with methazolamide but the possibility of their occurrence should be borne in mind.

Adverse Reactions: Anorexia, nausea, vomiting; malaise, fatigue, drowsiness, headache;

vertigo, mental confusion, depression, paresthesias of the extremities and at the mucocutaneous junction of the lips, mouth and anus. These reactions are relatively mild in character and usually disappear upon withdrawal of the drug. A decrease in urinary citrate excretion as well as uric acid output has also been noted, but drug-induced urinary calculi have not been reported.

Dosage and Administration: *Orally.* Dosage varies from 50 to 100 mg 2 or 3 times daily. May be used concomitantly with miotic and osmotic agents.

Availability:
NEPTAZANE® Tablets, 50 mg in bottles of 100. **(Lederle)**

METHDILAZINE HYDROCHLORIDE: see The Phenothiazines

METHENAMINE

Chemical Name: Hexamethylenetetramine.

Description: Methenamine hippurate, the hippuric acid salt of methenamine, contains approximately 44% methenamine and 56% hippuric acid.

Methenamine mandelate is a chemical combination of approximately 48% methenamine and 52% mandelic acid.

Since urine is a good culture medium for many urinary pathogens, invasion by a few organisms may lead to bacteriuria in susceptible individuals. The rationale for therapy in urinary tract infection (bacteriuria) is to change the urine from a growth-supporting to a growth-inhibiting medium. The antibacterial effect of methenamine and its salts depends upon the formation of formaldehyde in an acid medium. Methenamine is readily absorbed but remains essentially inactive until it is excreted by the kidney and concentrated in the urine where, in an acid medium, the drug is hydrolyzed to ammonia and the bactericidal agent, formaldehyde. Symptomatic relief generally occurs within 24 to 72 hours.

Methenamine mandelate has been combined with the urinary analgesic, phenazopyridine hydrochloride, which is also excreted in the urine where it exerts a topical analgesic effect on the mucosa of the urinary tract, hopefully, to obviate the need for systemic analgesics or narcotics.

Indications: Suppression or elimination of bacteriuria associated with pyelonephritis, pyelitis, pyelocystitis, urethritis, ureteritis, cystitis, trigonitis and other urinary tract infections; and for infected residual urine sometimes accompanying neurologic diseases. When used as recommended, the drug is particularly suitable for long-term therapy.

Contraindications: In patients hypersensitive to any of the components, in those with renal and/or hepatic insufficiency, or severe hydration. It is also contraindicated as the sole therapeutic agent in acute parenchymal infections causing systemic symptoms.

Warnings: In early pregnancy the safe use of methenamine has not been established; in the last trimester of pregnancy, safe use is suggested, but has not been definitely proven. Combined therapy with sulfamethiazole or sulfathiazole is not recommended since these drugs will precipitate with formaldehyde in the urine.

Precautions: Larger than recommended dosage may cause bladder irritation, painful and frequent micturition, albuminuria, and hematuria. The drug should not be used when acidification of urine is contraindicated or unattainable, as with some urea-splitting bacteria. Because slightly elevated serum transaminase levels have been seen in a few instances, liver function should be evaluated in patients on long-term therapy. Adequate hydration must be maintained. Since the oral suspension formulations have a vegetable oil base, they should be administered with particular care to elderly, debilitated or otherwise susceptable patients in order to avoid inducing lipid pneumonia.

Adverse Reactions: Occasionally, gastrointestinal manifestations or dermatological complaints such as nausea, upset stomach, dysuria, and skin rash and itching.

Dosage and Administration: *Orally. Methenamine:* The usual dosage is 1 gm 4 times daily. *Methenamine hippurate:* The average dose is 1 gm twice daily for adults and children over 12 years of age. Children 6 to 12 years of age, 0.5 to 1 gm twice daily. *Methenamine mandelate:* Adults and children over 12 years of age, 1 gm 4 times daily. Children 6 to 12, half the adult dosage; children 5 years or younger, 250 mg/30 lbs of body weight 4 times daily. The contents of a packet of granules should be dissolved in 60 to 120 ml of water immediately before using. Alkalinizing foods and medication should be restricted so that the urinary pH can be maintained at 5.5 or less. *With phenazopyridine hydrochloride:* The usual adult dose is 2 tablets 4 times daily. Children over 60 lbs of body weight usually 1 tablet/15 lbs daily in divided doses.

Availability:

Methenamine

METHENAMINE Tablets, 500 mg in bottles of 100. **(Lilly)**

Combinations

METHENAMINE and SODIUM BIPHOSPHATE, 325 mg with sodium biphosphate, 325 mg in bottles of 100 and 1000. **(Lilly)**

Methenamine Hippurate

HIPREX® Tablets, 1 gm in bottles of 100 and 500. **(Merrell-National)**

UREX® Tablets, 1 gm in bottles of 100 and 500. **(Riker)**

Methenamine Mandelate

MANDELAMINE®: **(Warner-Chilcott)**

Granules in packets of 0.5 and 1 gm.

Suspension, 50 mg/ml in bottles of 120 ml and 1 pint; 100 mg/ml (Forte) in bottles of 240 ml and 1 pint.

Tablets, 250 mg (E.C.), 0.5 gm (Hafgrams®) and 1 gm in bottles of 100 and 1000 and in unit-dose packages of 100.

METHENAMINE MANDELATE: **(Lederle)**

Suspension, 500 mg/5 ml in bottles of 120 ml and 1 pint.

Tablets, 0.5 and 1 gm in bottles of 1000.

w/Phenazopyridine Hydrochloride

AZOLATE Tablets, 0.5 gm with phenazopyridine hydrochloride, 50 mg in bottles of 50, 100 and 1000. **(Amfre-Grant)**

AZO-MANDELAMINE® Tablets, 0.5 gm with phenazopyridine hydrochloride, 50 mg in bottles of 100. **(Warner-Chilcott)**

METHICILLIN: see The Penicillins

METHIMAZOLE

Chemical Name: 1-Methyl-2-mercaptoimidazole.

Description: Methimazole is an antithyroid drug that is related chemically to propylthiouracil and other thiouracil derivatives; it differs primarily in that it has a 5 instead of a 6-membered ring. It occurs as a white to pale buff, crystalline powder freely soluble in water and in alcohol.

Methimazole inhibits the synthesis of thyroid hormones and thus is effective in the treatment of hyperthyroidism. The onset of action and degree of response vary directly with dosage. It does not inactivate existing thyroxine and triiodothyronine which is stored in colloid or is circulating in the blood, nor does it interfere with the effectiveness of thyroid hormones administered either orally or parenterally.

Indications: Treatment of hyperthyroidism, preoperatively, or when thyroidectomy is contraindicated or not advisable; may also be used to ameliorate hyperthyroidism in preparation for subtotal thyroidectomy or radioactive iodine therapy.

Contraindications: Hypersensitivity or idiosyncrasy to methimazole.

Warnings: Judicious use of the drug, with or without thyroid, is recommended in pregnant patients. Since methimazole readily crosses the placental barrier and may induce goiter and even cretinism in the developing fetus, the avoidence of hypothyroidism in both the mother and child is essential. Postpartum patients taking this drug should not nurse their babies.

Precautions: Patients should be under close observation, and should be instructed to report immediately any evidence of illness, particularly sore throat, skin eruptions, fever, headache, or general malaise. In such instances, white blood cell and differential counts should be made to determine whether agranulocytosis has developed. Particular care should be exercised with patients who are receiving additional drugs known to cause agranulocytosis.

Adverse Reactions: Minor reactions include skin rash, urticaria, nausea, vomiting, epigastric distress, arthralgia, paresthesia, loss of taste, abnormal loss of hair, myalgia, headache, pruritus, drowsiness, neuritis, edema, vertigo, skin pigmentation, jaundice, sialadenopathy, and lymphadenopathy. Major reactions include inhibition of myelopoiesis (agranulocytosis, granulopenia, and thrombocytopenia), drug fever, a lupus-like syndrome, hepatitis, periateritis, and hypoprothrombinemia. Excessive dosages may cause agranulocytosis; rarely, exfoliative dermatitis, hepatitis, neuropathies, or CNS stimulation or depression. The drug should be discontinued upon the development of agranulocytosis, pancytopenia, hepatitis, fever, or exfoliative dermatitis. Prolonged use may result in hypothyroidism. For bone marrow depression, use of an antibiotic, transfusions of fresh whole blood, and a corticosteroid should be considered. For hepatitis, rest and an adequate diet and, in severe cases, corticosteroid therapy may be indicated. General management may consist of symptomatic and supportive therapy, including rest, analgesics, gastric lavage, intravenous fluids, and mild sedation.

Dosage and Administration: *Orally.* Initially, 15 to 40 mg daily, divided into 3 doses at intervals of 8 hours. Patients with severe hyperthyroidism may require 60 mg or more daily for adequate control. Maintenance dosage of 5 to 15 mg daily divided into 2 or 3 doses. For pediatric patients, initially, 0.4 mg/kg of body weight divided into 3 doses at intervals of 8 hours. Maintenance dose is approximately 1/2 the initial dose.

Availability:
TAPAZOLE® Tablets, 5 and 10 mg in bottles of 100 and 1000. **(Lilly)**

METHIODAL SODIUM

Chemical Name: Monoiodomethanesulfonic acid sodium salt.

Description: Methiodal sodium is prepared by the action of sodium sulfite on methylene iodide, or sodium sulfite on iodoform. Sodium iodomethanesulfonate contains 52% iodine firmly bound in organic form.

Indications: For retrograde pyelography.

Contraindications: Intravascular administration.

Precautions: Although rare, the possibility of acute renal shutdown exists; therefore, it is advised that the study be performed on only one side at a time.

Adverse Reactions: The medium is well tolerated, thus minimizing the likelihood of ureteropelvic spasm. Minor side reactions of retrograde pyelography, which occasionally occur, consist of nausea, vomiting, excessive salivation, and sweating. Rarely, mucosal edema caused by the medium or instrumentation can result in usually reversible oliguria or anuria. Reactions attributable to allergy or idiosyncrasy have been sneezing, coughing, nasal stuffiness, rhinitis, conjunctival symptoms, dermal reactions such as urticaria or pruritus, laryngospasm, angioneurotic edema, bronchospasm, anxiety, dyspnea, dizziness, convulsions, and rarely, anaphylactoid shock with cardiovascular collapse. Reactions have been serious and sometimes fatal.

Dosage and Administration: *Retrograde pyelography* in adults, 5 to 11 ml (average 7.5 ml) of a 15 or 20% solution for a unilateral study. Children under 1 year of age, less than 1.5 ml; 1 to 5 years of age, 1.5 to 3 ml; over 5 years, 4 to 5 ml. The amounts will vary according to the number of exposures taken and to the disorder under examination.

Availability:
SKIODAN®: **(Winthrop)**
Solution, 40% in bottles of 100 ml.
Solution, 20% in bottles of 50 ml.

METHIXENE HYDROCHLORIDE

Chemical Name: 1-Methyl-3-(thioxanthen-9-ylmethyl) piperidine hydrochloride.

Description: Methixene hydrochloride, a synthetic, tertiary amine anticholinergic drug, occurs as a bitter, white, crystalline powder readily soluble in water, alcohol, and chloroform and insoluble in ether.

In common with other parasympatholytic agents, methixene produces an atropine-like blocking action on parasympathetic-innervated peripheral structures including smooth muscle. It exerts its influence by acting primarily on the gastrointestinal tract and, in the recommended dosage, does not produce characteristic atropine-like side effects.

Following oral administration, methixene is readily absorbed from the gastrointestinal tract, is metabolized in the liver, and excreted in the urine as unchanged drug and its stereoisomeric sulfoxides.

Indications: Adjunctive management of gastrointestinal disorders associated with hypermotility or spasm such as biliary dyskinesia, duodenal ulcer, duodenitis, epigastric distress, functional bowel distress, gastric ulcer, gastritis, gastroenteritis, irritable bowel, pylorospasm, rapid transit syndrome, spastic colon, ulcer distress.

Contraindications: In patients with glaucoma (particularly narrow-angle); obstructive uropathy as in bladder neck obstruction due to prostatic hypertrophy, obstructive disease of the gastrointestinal tract as in achalasia, paralytic ileus, pyloroduodenal stenosis; intestinal atony of the elderly or debilitated; unstable cardiovascular status in acute hemorrhage; toxic megacolon complicating ulcerative colitis, and in myasthenia gravis.

Warnings: Use of the drug during pregnancy, lactation, or in women of childbearing potential requires that the therapeutic benefits be weighted against the possible hazards to the mother and child. In the presence of a high environmental temperature, heat prostration due to anhidrosis can occur with the use of this drug. Diarrhea may be an early symptom of incomplete intestinal obstruction, especially in patients with ileostomy or colostomy. In this instance treatment with methixene would be inappropriate and possibly harmful.

Precautions: A curare-like action may occur with overdosage. Tachycardia should be ruled out before administering this preparation. Use with caution in patients with hyperthyroidism, coronary heart disease, congestive heart failure, cardiac arrhythmias, hypertension, and nonobstructing prostatic hypertrophy. Routine caution is also required in patients with hiatal hernia associated with reflux esophagitis, in those with advanced hepatic or renal disease, gastric ulcer, ulcerative colitis, and autonomic neuropathy. This drug may not be effective in the presence of complicating biliary tract disease. Patients should be cautioned not to engage in hazardous tasks if they experience drowsiness or dizziness.

Adverse Reactions: These may include xerostomia, urinary hesitancy and retention, blurred vision and drowsiness (patients should be cautioned not to engage in activities requiring alertness or skill), tachycardia, decreased sweating, palpitations, mydriasis, dilatation of the pupil, cycloplegia, increased ocular tension, loss of taste, headaches, nervousness, weakness, dizziness, insomnia, nausea, vomiting, impotence, suppression of lactation, constipation, bloated feeling, severe allergic reactions or drug idiosyncrasias including anaphylaxis, urticaria and other dermal manifestations, some degree of mental confusion and/or excitement especially in the geriatric patient.

Dosage and Administration: *Orally,* 1 or 2 tablets 3 times daily. Pediatric dosage has not been determined.

Availability:
TREST® Tablets, 1 mg (white) in bottles of 100. **(Dorsey)**

METHOCARBAMOL

Chemical Name: 3-(*o*-Methoxyphenoxy)-2-propanediol-1-carbamate.

Description: Methocarbamol is a guaiacol glyceryl derivative, skeletal muscle relaxant. Animal studies have shown that methocarbamol acts primarily on the internuncial neurons of the spinal cord. It exerts a prolonged blocking effect on polysynaptic reflex pathways at dosages which do not significantly alter transmission through monosynaptic reflex arcs, and interrupts abnormal impulses from areas of disturbed muscle. It has no direct action on the contractile mechanism of striated muscle, the motor end-plate or the nerve fiber. However, the exact mechanism of action of methocarbamol in clinical use has not been established, but may be due to general CNS depression.

Following parenteral administration, effects of the drug may be noted within 10 minutes, whereas the effects following oral administration may be apparent for 24 hours.

Indications: Relief of discomfort associated with acute musculoskeletal disorders, and other traumatic injuries, acute strains and sprains, myositis, and arthritis as adjunctive aid to rest, physical therapy and other supportive measures. Combined with aspirin to provide antiinflammatory, antipyretic and mild analgesic action.

Contraindications: Because polyethylene glycol-300 is the vehicle for the injectable form, the drug is contraindicated in patients with known or suspected renal pathology. The vehicle is known to have increased preexisting acidosis and urea retention in patients with renal impairment. Hypersensitivity to the ingredients also is a contraindication.

Warnings: Safe use of this medication has not been established with regard to possible adverse effects upon fetal development. Therefore, this drug should not be used in women who are or may become pregnant and particularly during the first trimester of pregnancy unless in the judgment of the physician the potential benefits outweigh the possible hazards.

Precautions: Rate of injection should not exceed 3 ml/min, and extravasation must be avoided. Total dosage should not exceed 30 ml (3 ampuls) daily for more than 3 consecutive days except in the treatment of tetanus. Caution should be observed in using the injectable form in suspected or known epileptic patients. Safe and effective use in children under 12 years of age has not been established. Since the drug appears in breast milk, lactating women should be instructed not to nurse their babies while taking this medication. Methocarbamol may cause a color interference in certain screening tests for 5-hydoxyindoleacetic acid and vanilmandelic acid. *The drug is not recommended for subcutaneous administration.*

Adverse Reactions: *Injectable:* Dizziness, lightheadedness, drowsiness, vertigo, fainting, syncope, hypotension, gastrointestinal upset, metallic taste, thrombophlebitis, sloughing and/or pain at the site of injection, anaphylactic reaction, urticaria, pruritus, rash, conjunctivitis with nasal congestion, flushing, nystagmus, diplopia, mild muscular incoordination, bradycardia, blurred vision, headache, fever. In most cases of syncope there was spontaneous recovery. In others, epinephrine, injectable steroids and/or injectable antihistamines were employed to hasten recovery. Certain of these reactions may have been due to an overly rapid rate of intravenous injection. The onset of convulsive seizures during intravenous administration has been reported, including instances in known epileptics. The psychic trauma of the procedure may have been a contributing factor. Although several observers have reported success in terminating epileptiform seizures with injectable methocarbamol, its administration to patients with epilepsy is not recommended. *Tablets:* Lightheadedness, dizziness, drowsiness, nausea, allergic manifestations such as urticaria, pruritus, rash, conjunctivitis with nasal congestion, blurred vision, headache, fever.

Dosage and Administration: *Orally.* For the relief of acute sketetal muscle spasm, adults, 6 gm daily for 2 or 3 days; children, 27 to 33.5 mg/lb of body weight daily divided into 4 to 6 equal doses. *Intravenously* or *intramuscularly.* For the relief of moderate skeletal muscle spasm, 1 gm followed by oral administration for maintenance. For severe cases or in postoperative conditions in which oral administration is not feasible, 2 to 3 gm may be required; children, initially 15 mg/kg repeated every 6 hours. (See Precautions.) Package literature should be consulted for special directions for use in tetanus, and directions for intravenous and intramuscular use.

Availability:
Methocarbamol
Tablets, 500 and 750 mg in bottles of 100 and 500. **(Lederle)**
ROBAXIN® **(Robins)**
Injection, 100 mg/ml in ampuls of 10 ml.
Tablets, 500 and 750 mg in bottles of 100 and 500 and in Dis-Co® packs (unit-dose) packages of 100 in cartons of 5.
ROBAXISAL® Tablets, 400 mg with aspirin, 325 mg in bottles of 100 and 500. **(Robins)**

METHOHEXITAL SODIUM Ⓒ

Chemical Name: Sodium α-*dl*-1-methyl-5-allyl-5-(1-methyl-2-pentynyl) barbiturate.

Description: Methohexital is a rapid, ultra short-acting barbiturate anesthetic that differs chemically from related agents in that its molecule contains no sulfur. Methohexital sodium occurs as a white, crystalline powder freely soluble in water.

It is similar in action to sodium thiopental, but is more potent and consequently produces the same degree of anesthesia with smaller doses. Although its metabolic fate in the body is not clear, methohexital does not appear to concentrate in fat tissue as much as other barbiturate anesthetics; therefore, its cumulative effects are less and recovery is more rapid.

Indications: For induction of anesthesia, for supplementing other anesthetic agents, as intravenous anesthesia for short surgical procedures, or as an agent for inducing a hypnotic state.

Contraindications: Should not be used when general anesthesia is contraindicated, in patients with latent or manifest porphyria, or with known hypersensitivity to barbiturates.

Warnings: Methohexital should be administered only by clinicians experienced in intravenous anesthesia or under the supervision of such an individual. Appropriate equipment should be on hand for the prevention and treatment of anesthetic emergencies. Methohexital sodium may be habit-forming. Repeated or continuous infusion may cause cumulative effects that may result in prolonged somnolence and respiratory and circulatory depression. The additive action of this agent and other CNS depressants such as alcohol or opiates may cause respiratory arrest with possible fatal results. Although studies with animals produced no teratogenic effects on fetal development, it should nevertheless be used with caution in pregnant women and only when in the judgment of the physician, the benefits outweigh the possible hazards to the fetus.

Precautions: Respiratory depression, apnea, or hypotension may occur with the use of this drug. Special care should be exercised in debilitated patients and in those with impaired function of respiratory, circulatory, renal, hepatic or endocrine systems. Extreme caution is required in patients in status asthmaticus. Extravascular injection may cause pain, swelling, ulceration, and necrosis. Intraarterial injection is dangerous and may produce gangrene of an extremity.

Adverse Reactions: Intravenous administration of methohexital may produce laryngospasm, salivation, cough, sneezing, or hiccups. Pulmonary ventilation should be maintained as transient apnea may occur during induction. Skin rashes, urticaria, pain at the site of injection, and a burning sensation along the course of the vein have been reported. If extravascular leakage should occur, moist heat to the infiltrated area is indicated. Other reactions reported were circulatory depression, thrombophlebitis, bronchospasm, skeletal-muscle hyperactivity (twitching to convulsive-like movements), emergence delirium, headache, injury to nerves adjacent to injection site, nausea and emesis. Acute allergic reactions, such as erythema, pruritus, urticaria, rhinitis, dyspnea, hypotension, restlessness, anxiety, abdominal pain, and peripheral vascular collapse have also been noted.

Dosage and Administration: *Intravenously.* For the introduction of anesthesia, a 1% solution is given at the rate of 1 ml in 5 seconds. A dose of 5 to 12 ml is usually sufficient. For intermittent administration to maintain general anesthesia, 2 to 4 ml will be required every 4 to 7 minutes. When given by continuous intravenous drip, an 0.2% solution at the rate of 1 drop/second may be used. The drug should not be mixed with acid solutions such as atropine sulfate, dimethyltubocurarine iodide, or succinylcholine chloride; also, because it is incompatible with silicone, the drug should not be permitted to come in contact with rubber stoppers or parts of disposable syringes that have been treated with silicone.

Availability:
Ⓒ BREVITAL® SODIUM Powder for injection, 500 mg in ampuls of 50 ml with or without water for injection; 2.5 gm in ampuls of 250 ml; 5 gm in ampuls of 500 ml. **(Lilly)**

METHOTREXATE

Chemical Name: N-[*p*-[[(2,4-Diamino-6-pteridinyl)methyl]-methylamino]benzoyl] glutamic acid.

Description: Methotrexate is a folic acid antagonist differing structurally from aminopterin by the presence of a methyl group in the 10-position. It occurs as an orange-brown, crystalline powder practically insoluble in water and in alcohol.

The drug elicits its antimetabolic action by interfering with the participation of folinic acid (the active principle of folic acid) in nucleic acid synthesis, thus disrupting the mitotic process.

In most instances it is readily absorbed from the gastrointestinal tract and reaches peak activity within 1 to 2 hours. Following parenteral administration peak serum levels are reached within ½ to 1 hour, and the mean plasma half-life has been found to be about 2 hours. Approximately ½ of the absorbed drug is reversibly bound to serum protein, and there is evidence that it may be displaced by a number of drugs, including sulfonamides and salicylates (see Precautions). Excretion of single daily doses occurs in the urine in amounts from 55 to 88% or higher within 24 hours. Because methotrexate's passage through the blood-brain barrier is very limited, any neoplastic cells that have entered the CNS probably are not affected by tolerated concentrations of the drug in the plasma.

Indications: Treatment of uterine choriocarcinoma, chorioma, chorioadenoma destruens and hydatidiform mole; in the suppression of acute and subacute leukemias and leukemic meningitis, especially in children. Greatest effect has been observed in acute leukemia characterized by blast forms in bone marrow or blood. May also be used in lymphosarcoma, in certain inoperable tumors of the head, neck and pelvis, and in mycosis fungoides. Methotrexate has been suggested for use in the treatment of severe, recalcitrant, disabling psoriasis that does not adequately respond to other form of therapy.

Contraindications: Psoriatic patients, who are pregnant, or who have severe renal or hepatic disorders, or preexisting blood dyscrasias, such as bone marrow hypoplasia, leukopenia, thrombocytopenia or anemia.

Warnings: Methotrexate must be used only by physicians experienced in antimetabolite chemotherapy. Patients should be fully informed that fatal and severe toxic reactions may occur, and it is essential that they be under the constant supervision of the physician. It has been reported that deaths have occurred when the drug was employed in the treatment of psoriasis; therefore, the drug should be restricted to severe, recalcitrant and disabling psoriasis which does not adequately respond to other forms of therapy, and only when diagnosis has been established by either biopsy or dermatological examination or both. Careful consideration should be given to the fact that methotrexate may cause marked depression of bone marrow, anemia, leukopenia, thrombocytopenia, and bleeding; liver atrophy, necrosis, cirrhosis, fatty changes, and periportal fibrosis. Since changes may occur without previous signs of gastrointestinal or hematologic toxicity, it is imperative that hepatic function be determined prior to initiation of treatment and monitored regularly throughout therapy. Special caution is indicated in the presence of preexisting liver damage or impaired liver function. Concomitant use of drugs that possess hepatotoxic potential, including alcohol, should be avoided. Methotrexate has caused fetal death, and congenital anomalies, therefore, it is not recommended in women of childbearing potential unless there is appropriate medical evidence that the benefits can be expected to outweigh the considered risks.

Precautions: Methotrexate should be used with caution in the presence of infections, or in patients with malignant disease who have preexisting bone marrow aplasia, leukopenia, thrombocytopenia or anemia. Concomitant use with drugs known to have a depressing effect on the hematopoietic system should be avoided. Dosage should be discontinued at the first sign of oral erythema, ulceration, bleeding, chills, fever, or hematologic depression. Because methotrexate is largely eliminated in the urine, the patient's renal status should be determined before treatment. In general, the following laboratory tests are recommended as part of essential clinical evaluation and appropriate monitoring of patients who are taking this drug: complete hemogram; hematocrit; urinalysis; and hepatic and renal function tests. The tests should be performed prior to, during and after therapy has been discontinued. It may also be essential to perform liver biopsy or bone marrow aspiration studies in cases in which high doses or long-term treatment is necessary. A chest roentgenogram is also indicated. Since the drug is used in doses that are nearly toxic, such drugs as salicylates, sulfonamides, phenytoin, and some antibacterials as tetracycline, chloramphenicol and *p*-aminobenzoic acid may displace methotrexate from its binding sites, thus increasing its toxic potential. These drugs, especially sulfonamides (whether antibacterial, hypoglycemic or diuretic) and salicylates should not be given concurrently until the significance of these findings is established. Additionally, probenecid has been found to increase the plasma levels of methotrexate. Vitamin preparations containing folic acid or its derivatives may alter responses to the drug. Should be used with extreme caution in the presence of infection, peptic ulcer, ulcerative colitis, debility, and in extreme youth and old age. If profound leukopenia occurs, bacterial infection may appear or become a threat. Cessation of therapy and appropriate antibiotic therapy is indicated. In severe bone marrow depression, blood or platelet transfusions may be necessary. The immuno-suppressive action of the drug must be taken into account in evaluating the use of this drug where immune responses in the patient may be important or essential.

Adverse Reactions: The most common adverse reactions include ulcerative stomatitis, leukopenia, nausea and abdominal distress. Others reported are malaise, undue fatigue, chills and fever, dizziness and decreased resistance to infection. In general, the incidence and severity of side effects are considered to be dose-related. Adverse reactions as reported for the various systems are as follows: *Skin:* erythematous rashes, pruritus, urticaria, photosensitivity, depigmentation, alopecia, ecchymosis, telangiectasia, acne, furunculosis. Lesions of psoriasis may be aggravated by concomitant exposure to ultraviolet radiation. *Blood:* bone marrow depression, leukopenia, thrombocytopenia, anemia, hypogammaglobulinemia, hemorrhage from various sites, septicemia. *Alimentary System:* gingivitis, pharyngitis, stomatitis, anorexia, vomiting, diarrhea, hematemesis, melena, gastrointestinal ulceration and bleeding, enteritis, hepatic toxicity resulting in acute liver atrophy, necrosis, fatty metamorphosis, periportal fibrosis or hepatic cirrhosis. *Urogenital System:* renal failure, azotemia, cystitis, hematuria; defective oogenesis or spermatogenesis, transient oligospermia, menstrual dysfunction; infertility, abortion, fetal defects, severe nephropathy. *CNS:* headaches, drowsiness, blurred vision. Aphasia, hemiparesis, paresis and convulsions have occurred, possibly related to hemorrhage or to complications from intraarterial catheterization. Convulsion, paresis and Guillain-Barre syndrome, increased cerebrospinal-fluid pressures have followed intrathecal administration. *Other reactions:* related to or attributed to the use of methotrexate such as pneumonitis; metabolic changes, precipitating diabetes; osteoporotic effects, abnormal tissue-cell changes, and even sudden death have been reported.

Dosage and Administration: It is preferred to administer methotrexate *orally* inasmuch as the drug is rapidly and nearly completely absorbed. The *parenteral* form has been given by *intramuscular, intravenous, intraarterial* or *intrathecal* routes. The parenteral form should be reconstituted with water for injection, as addition of other diluents will render the resulting solution hypertonic. Each 5 mg vial should be reconstituted with 2 ml of water for injection and each 50 mg vial with 20 ml of water for injection, which results in a concentration of 2.5 mg of methotrexate/ml. *For choriocarcinoma,* 15 to 30 mg daily for 5 days *orally* or *intramuscularly.* May be repeated 3 to 5 times as required with rest periods of 1 or more weeks, or until the manifesting toxic symptoms subside. One or 2 courses are given after reducing chorionic gonadotropin titers to less than 50 IU/24 hours. *For acute leukemia in children,* methotrexate is administered either alone or in combination with steroids. May be given *orally* or *intravenously* in doses of 3.3 mg/M^2 of methotrexate and 60 mg/M^2 of prednisone daily. Remission occurs in about 50% of patients usually within 4 to 6 weeks. When remission is achieved methotrexate is then administered twice weekly in doses of 30 mg/M^2 *orally* or *intramuscularly,* or every 2 weeks in doses of 2.5 mg/kg of body weight *intravenously.* Intrathecal administration in doses of 0.2 to 0.5 mg/kg of body weight may be given at intervals of 2 to 5 days. This course of treatment is usually repeated until the cell count and the cerebrospinal fluid pressure return to normal. At this point an additional dose is advised. May also be administered in doses of 12 mg/M² once weekly for 2 weeks, then once monthly; larger doses may cause convulsions. *For lymphomas,* the recommended oral dosage is 10 to 25 mg daily for 4 to 8 days. In severe stages, the drug is generally administered concomitantly with other antitumor agents. Treatment usually requires several courses interposed with 7 to 10 days of rest period. *For mycosis fungoides,* the usual oral dose is 2.5 to 10 mg daily; may also be given *intramuscularly* in doses of 50 mg once weekly or 25 mg twice weekly. Therapy may take weeks or months before remission is achieved. The treatment regimen is guided by patient response and hematologic monitoring. *For the treatment of psoriasis:* There are 3 commonly used general types of dosage schedules: 1) weekly oral or parenteral intermittent large doses; 2) divided dose intermittent oral schedule over a 36-hour period; 3) daily oral dose with a rest period. All schedules should be continually tailored to the individual patient. The following dose schedules pertain to an average 70-kg adult. An initial test dose 1 week prior to initiation of therapy is recommended to detect any idiosyncrasy. A suggested dose range is 5 to 10 mg parenterally. *Recommended starting dose schedules:* 1) weekly single oral, intramuscular or intravenous dose schedule: 10 to 25 mg/week until adequate response is achieved. With this dosage schedule, 50 mg/week should ordinarily not be exceeded; 2) divided oral dose schedule: 2.5 mg at 12-hour intervals for 3 doses or at 8-hour intervals for 4 doses each week. With this dosage schedule, 30 mg/week should not be exceeded; 3) daily oral dose schedule: 2.5 mg daily for 5 days followed by at least a 2-day rest period. With each dosage schedule, 6.25 mg/day should not be exceeded. Dosages in each schedule may be gradually adjusted to achieve optimal clinical response, but not to exceed the maximum stated for each schedule. Once optimal clinical response has been achieved each dosage schedule should be reduced to the lowest possible amount of drug and to the lowest possible rest period. The use of methotrexate may permit the return to conventional topical therapy, which should be encouraged. See package literature for further dosage instructions.

Availability:
METHOTREXATE: **(Lederle)**
Powder for injection (as sodium salt) in vials of 5, 20 and 50 mg.
Tablets, 2.5 mg in bottles of 100.

METHOTRIMEPRAZINE HYDROCHLORIDE: see The Phenothiazines

METHOXAMINE HYDROCHLORIDE

Chemical Name: α-(1-Aminoethyl)-2,5-dimethoxybenzyl alcohol hydrochloride.

Description: Methoxamine hydrochloride is a sympathomimetic amine related to phenylephrine in pharmacologic action. It occurs as colorless or white crystals or as a white, crystalline powder having a bitter taste, is freely soluble in water and soluble in alcohol.

The pressor action of methoxamine is due primarily to direct peripheral vasoconstriction; it produces a prompt and prolonged rise in blood pressure following parenteral administration. It also elicits an atropine-reversible bradycardia by reflex vagal mediation. It does not produce cerebral stimulation, tachycardia, cardiac arrhythmias, even when used in conjunction with cyclopropane anesthesia.

When injected intravenously, the pressor effect occurs almost immediately and lasts for about 1 hour; the onset of action after intramuscular injection occurs within 15 minutes and persists for about 90 minutes.

Indications: To support, restore or maintain normal blood pressure during surgery; for preoperative use in patients with low blood pressure who are poor surgical risks, especially when emergency operations are involved. It is helpful in postoperative collapse, during surgery, particularly when spinal anesthesia is used, and for relieving supraventricular tachycardia.

Contraindications: Methoxamine is not indicated for combination with local anesthetics to prolong their action at the local sites.

Precautions: It should be borne in mind that the use of methoxamine injections is not a substitute for the replacement of blood, plasma, fluids and electrolytes. Caution should be observed when used closely following the parenteral administration of ergot alkaloids, to prevent excessive rise in blood pressure. It should be administered with extreme care to patients with hyperthyroidism or severe hypertension. The physician should take into consideration that the drug-induced increase in peripheral resistance may cause or exacerbate heart failure associated with a diseased mycardium.

Adverse Reactions: Higher than recommended dosages may produce excessive blood pressure which may be accompanied by severe headache, pilomotor response, a desire to void, and forceful vomiting.

Dosage and Administration: *Intramuscularly* or *intravenously.* Dosage must be well-regulated and given according to the need and direction of the physician. The usual intramuscular dose is 10 to 15 mg; may be given immediately prior to or at the time of administering spinal anesthesia. This dose may also be given to correct a fall in blood pressure. The usual intravenous dose for emergencies is 3 to 5 mg injected slowly. The intravenous injection may be supplemented by intramuscular injection to provide a more sustained effect. For preoperative and postoperative treatment of only moderate hypertension, 5 to 10 mg intramuscularly. In paroxysmal supraventricular tachycardia, the average dose is 10 mg injected slowly by the intravenous route.

Availability:
VASOXYL® Injection, 10 mg/ml with preservative in vials of 10 ml; 20 mg/ml with preservative in ampuls of 1 ml. **(Burroughs Wellcome)**

METHOXSALEN

Chemical Name: 6-Hydroxy-7-methoxy-5-benzofuranacrylic acid.

Description: Methoxsalen is a methoxypsoralen derivative obtained in pure crystalline form from the active principle contained in the fruit of Ammi majus Linn, a plant once used to induce pigmentation in vitiliginous skin areas.

Methoxsalen is a photodynamic agent and as such it augments the normal response of the skin (i.e. increases melanin pigment) to ultraviolet light. Exposure to ultraviolet light in patients who have received this drug causes a thickening of the stratum corneum, initiates an inflammatory reaction in the skin, and increases the amount of melanin in the exposed area. However, the exact mechanism of action in the process of melanogenesis is not known.

Following oral ingestion, increased sensitivity appears in 1 hour, attains a peak in 2 hours, and disappears in approximately 8 hours.

Indications: Repigmentation of idiopathic vitiligo, as a suntan accelerator and a sunburn protector. Topical application is indicated for the treatment of vitiligo only.

Contraindications: In hepatic insufficiency, and in those diseases associated with photosensitivity such as porphyria, acute lupus erythematosus, hydroa, and polymorphic light eruptions. In leukoderma of infectious origin and in albinism, methoxsalen increases tolerance to sunlight but has no effect on pigmentation. Prior clinical and investigative use has not been sufficient to establish safe use in children under 12 years of age. Concomitant use with other photosensitizing drugs, whether for local or systemic use, is contraindicated.

Warnings: The drug should be used with extreme caution and only under close medical supervision.

Precautions: Since methoxsalen can produce intense photosensitivity which may result in serious burning and blistering, strict adherence to dosage is mandatory, and the dose should NOT be increased because severe burning may occur. When used to increase tolerance to sunlight or to accelerate tanning, the total dosage should not exceed 28 capsules, nor should it be administered for periods exceeding 2 weeks. The dosage should be on a continuous regimen. Patients should be instructed to adhere to the prescribed dosage schedule and procedure. Patients taking the drug for vitiligo should have liver function tests performed monthly for the first few months and occasionally thereafter. Dosages should be reduced or the drug discontinued if impairment of liver function is suspected. Topical use of the drug can cause acute vesicular cutaneous photosensitization. Severe erythema and blistering are usually due to high concentrations of the drug and overexposure to long-wave ultraviolet radiation. Diluting the lotion to concentrations of 1:10,000 or 1:1000 is helpful in avoiding excessive reaction. The chance of overexposure can be minimized by topical application of sunscreens containing benzophenone derivatives or by washing the treated area after exposure to sunlight.

Adverse Reactions: Gastric distress, nausea, diarrhea, nervousness, insomnia and depression may occur with oral administration, and severe erythema, blistering, and pain may follow topical application.

Dosage and Administration: *Orally.* Recommended dosage to protect against sunburn and enhance pigmentation: Adults, 2 capsules approximately 2 hours before exposure to sunlight. Taking the drug after meals or with a glass of milk appears to minimize any gastrointestinal discomfort. The exposure time during the first 3 or 4 days of the procedure should be limited to 30 minutes or less, thereafter the exposure time may be increased. *The dosage should not be increased.* To repigment vitiliginous areas: Adults and children over 12 years of age, 2 capsules daily. Doses should be followed in 2 to 4 hours by exposure to ultraviolet radiation. *Topically.* Low concentrations of the lotion are applied daily to the affected area (50 to 200 mcg/inch^2). After an interval of 2 hours, the treated area is exposed to sunlight or long-wave ultraviolet light for 30 to 60 seconds. The initial time exposure may be increased gradually but should not exceed 1/2 the minimal erythemic dose.

Availability:
OXSORALEN: **(Elder)**
Capsules, 10 mg in bottles of 28 and 100.
Lotion, 1% (10 mg/ml) in bottles of 30 ml.

METHOXYFLURANE

Chemical Name: 2.2-Dichloro-1, 1-difluoroethyl methyl ether.

Description: Methoxyflurane is a halogenated, volatile liquid with potent anesthetic properties. It is of extremely low toxicity and is pharmacologically compatible with those drugs ordinarily employed in preoperative medication and during surgery. At room temperature, the recommended concentrations of methoxyflurane are nonflammable and nonexplosive in air, oxygen or nitrous oxide mixtures; therefore, it is safe when electrocautery, electronic monitors, or radiologic equipment is used. It occurs as a clear, colorless liquid with a characteristic fruity odor. An antioxidant, butylated hydroxytoluene, 0.01% is added to retard decomposition. The clinical signs of anesthesia resemble those of halothane, except that respiratory depression and muscular relaxation are more prominent and it possesses a higher blood:gas partition ratio than does halothane which accounts for the relatively long induction time and for an emergence that is remarkably slow.

It provides adequate analgesia and muscle relaxation for most surgical procedures; however, it is generally used with nitrous oxide-oxygen mixture and a neuromuscular blocking agent to limit the need for high concentrations of the drug which can cause unfavorable cardiovascular and renal effects. Following surgical anesthesia, drowsiness and analgesia generally persist after consciousness has been regained, thus obviating or reducing the need for narcotics in the immediate postoperative period.

Indications: Induction and maintenance of analgesia and general anesthesia in all types of surgery, particularly minor surgical procedures. It may be used in obstetrics as an effective analgesic in the management of labor and as a suitable anesthetic during delivery.

Contraindications: Should not be used in patients in whom a previous exposure to a halogenated anesthetic was followed by unexplained fever with or without jaundice. It should not be used in concentrations that will provide skeletal muscle relaxation.

Warnings: All patients who undergo anesthesia with this anesthetic should be monitored for urinary output and possible signs of renal impairment. Methoxyflurane may cause renal tubular dysfunction especially high output renal failure which can lead to death. Special care to avoid unnecessarily deep anesthesia is required, especially in aged or obese patients, in surgical procedures of long duration, and during assisted or controlled ventilation. It should be noted that absence of hypotension cannot be relied upon as evidence that dosage has not been excessive. The symptoms of renal dysfunction include a large urinary output with a low specific gravity, with a volume equivalent to or in excess of intake. This usually results in a negative fluid balance, pronounced weight loss, elevation of serum electrolytes, osmolality, BUN and uric acid. When impaired renal function is present preoperatively, the benefits-to-risks ratio must be carefully considered and serial tests of renal function and fluid-electrolyte status should be obtained. Clinical evidence suggests that methoxyflurane should not be administered with tetracyclines because concurrent administration of these agents may seriously impair renal function and death can occur. Also, the possibility exists that it may enhance the adverse renal effects of other drugs including certain antibiotics of known nephrotoxic potential such as gentamicin, kanamycin, colistin, polymyxin B, and amphotericin B. This should be carefully considered when prescribing such drugs during the preoperative, operative, and postoperative periods. Since the major factors contributing to nephrotoxicity are thought to be high concentrations of the anesthetic and prolonged anesthesia, it should not be used in procedures that may extend beyond 4 hours or where profound anesthesia is indicated. To avoid possible cumulative effects, general anesthesia with this agent should not be repeated within an interval of less than one month. Safe use during pregnancy has not been established, therefore, it should not be used in women of childbearing potential, and particularly during the first trimester of pregnancy, unless in the judgment of the physician, the potential benefits outweigh the unknown hazards to the fetus.

Precautions: Cirrhosis, a history of viral hepatitis or other abnormalities involving liver dysfunction may be the basis for selecting an anesthetic other than a halogenated agent. It can possibly superimpose renal impairment in diabetic patients with renal dysfunction, polyuria, or obesity, or who are not adequately controlled. Ventilation should be assessed carefully, and should, if depressed, be augmented to insure adequate oxygenation and carbon dioxide removal. Barbiturates and narcotics, used as adjuncts, should be administered in conservative doses to avoid ventilatory depression. A sufficient reduction in respiratory minute volume occurs during deep anesthesia to produce a significant respiratory acidosis if ventilation is not adequately assisted. Methoxyflurane causes a slight metabolic acidosis. This anesthetic agent augments the effect of nonpolarizing muscle relaxants so that their usual dosage should be reduced by approximately one-half. Epinephrine or levarterenol (norepinephrine) may be employed cautiously during anesthesia with this agent.

Adverse Reactions: Renal and hepatic dysfunction and fatal hepatic necrosis have been reported. Such reactions appear to represent a sensitivity response to halogenated anesthetics. Transient alterations in liver function tests may follow its use. Other reactions noted include cardiac arrest, malignant hyperpyrexia, prolonged postoperative somnolence, respiratory depression, laryngospasm, bronchospasm, nausea, vomiting, postoperative headache, hypotension, and emergence delirium.

Dosage and Administration: *Inhalation,* by closed, semi-closed, or open drop technique, as directed. Lid reflex, skin color, capillary refill time, pulse rate and pupillary reaction to light should be used as a guide to dosage. For maintenance of clinical anesthesia or for administration of analgesia, concentrations in the range of 0.3 to 0.8% are useful.

Availability:
PENTHRANE® Liquid in bottles of 15 and 125 ml. **(Abbott)**

METHOXYPHENAMINE HYDROCHLORIDE

Chemical Name: *O*-Methoxy-*N*, α-dimethylphenethylamine.

Description: Methoxyphenamine is a synthetic sympathomimetic amine with direct action on beta-adrenergic receptors of smooth muscles, thus relieving broncho-constriction with resulting increase in vital capacity. Unlike ephedrine, the effect of the drug in stimulating the CNS, or producing elevated blood pressure, digestive disorders, insomnia, irritability and nervousness is minimal. The combination of methoxyphenamine and aminophyline potentiates the bronchodilator effect and may be employed to control mild to moderately severe asthmatic attacks without the necessity of administering barbiturates. Following oral administration, relief is obtained within 20 to 30 minutes and therapeutic benefit continues for 3 to 4 hours.

Indications: Symptomatic relief of seasonal and generalized asthma and perennial rhinitis, urticaria, gastrointestinal allergy. Combination of methoxyphenamine and aminophylline for the management of bronchial asthma.

Contraindications: Hypersensitivity to methoxyphenamine or to any compound formulated with it.

Precautions: Use with caution in elderly patients and in those with hypertension, thyrotoxicosis, acute coronary disease, cardiac decompensation and diabetes mellitus.

Adverse Reactions: The distressing side effects common to the sympathomimetic amines are related to or associated with their pressor activity. These include elevated blood pressure and pulse rate, cardiac palpitation, psychomotor stimulation, anxiety, nervousness, wakefulness, dry mouth, nausea, paradoxical drowsiness, and faintness. Aminophylline may produce gastric discomfort.

Dosage and Administration: *Orally. Tablets:* 50 to 100 mg repeated in intervals of 4 hours as needed. *Syrup:* 1 or 2 teaspoonsful every 3 to 4 hours. Children, ½ to teaspoonful. *Capsules with aminophylline:* 1 every 4 to 6 hours. Average total daily dosage range is from 1 to 6 capsules.

Availability:
ORTHOXINE®: **(Upjohn)**
Syrup, 10 mg/ml in bottles of 1 pint.
Tablets, 100 mg in bottles of 100 and 500.
ORTHOXINE and AMINOPHYLLINE Capsules, 50 mg with aminophylline (hydrous), 100 mg in bottles of 100.

METHSCOPOLAMINE BROMIDE

Chemical Name: *N*-Methylscopolammonium bromide.

Description: Methscopolamine bromide, an anticholinergic agent, inhibits gastric secretions and decreases gastrointestinal motility without significantly affecting the CNS. It occurs as white crystals or as a white odorless, crystalline powder that is freely soluble in water, slightly soluble in alcohol, and insoluble in chloroform.

Indications: Adjunctive measure in the treatment of peptic ulcer and gastric disorders associated with hyperacidity and hypermotility. May also be useful as adjunctive therapy in the management of the postgastrectomy-dumping syndrome, gastrointestinal dysfunction characterized by hypermobility (diarrhea due to irritable colon, to chronic ulcerative colitis or to extensive intestinal resections and ileostomies), excessive perspiration which aggravates certain dermatoses, and excessive salivation. May also prove useful in the symptomatic relief of hyperemesis gravidarum, functional nausea and vomiting, ureteral and vesical spasms, acute nonspecific diarrhea, and diarrhea associated with certain antibiotics. The addition of phenobarbital provides sedation and relieves anxiety and tension.

Contraindications: Glaucoma; obstructive uropathy (e.g., bladder neck obstruction due to prostatic hypertrophy); obstructive disorders of the gastrointestinal tract as in achalasia, paralytic ileus, pyloroduodenal stenosis; intestinal atony of the elderly or debilitated patients; unstable cardiovascular status in acute hemorrhage; severe ulcerative colitis; toxic megacolon complicating ulcerative colitis; myasthenia gravis, and patients with a known history of allergy or hypersensitivity to atropine or its analogues.

Warnings: Heat prostration manifested by fever and heat stroke due to decreased sweating may occur in the presence of high environmental temperature. The drug should not be used if diarrhea exists since it may be an early symptom of incomplete intestinal obstruction, especially in patients with ileostomy or colostomy. Patients should be cautioned that if they experience drowsiness or blurred vision, they should not engage in activities requiring alertness and skill. Safe use during pregnancy has not been established.

Precautions: Use with considerable caution, if at all, in patients with autonomic neuropathy, hepatic or renal disease, early evidence of ileus as in peritonitis, ulcerative colitis (since large doses may suppress intestinal motility to the point of producing a paralytic ileus and thus may precipitate or aggravate the serious complication of toxic megacolon), hyperthyroidism, coronary heart disease, congestive heart failure, cardiac arrhythmias, hypertension, nonobstructing prostatic hypertrophy, and hiatnal hernia associated with reflux esophagitis since anticholinergic drugs may aggravate this condition. The use of anticholinergic drugs in the treatment of gastric ulcer may produce a delay in gastric emptying time and thus may complicate such therapy (antral stasis). This drug may not be useful in the presence of biliary tract disease. Extreme caution is indicated when prescribing this product in the presence of tachycardia since heart rate may be increased. Overdosage may produce a curare-like action. The recommended dosage should not be exceeded. An occasional infant (most frequently infants less than 1 month of age) may react with flushing and fever. The Pamine PB drops should be given with caution, in low dosage and only when close observation of the infant is possible.

Adverse Reactions: Those generally associated with anticholinergic agents, and which may occur with methscopolamine include xerostomia; urinary hesitance and retention; blurred vision; tachycardia; palpitations; mydriasis; cycloplegia; increased ocular tension; loss of taste; headaches, nervousness; drowsiness; weakness; dizziness; insomnia; nausea; vomiting; impotence; suppression of lactation; constipation; bloated feeling; severe allergic reaction or drug idiosyncrasies including anaphylaxis; urticaria and other skin manifestation; some degree of mental confusion and/or excitement especially in elderly patients; decreased sweating. It should be noted that adrenergic innervation of the eccrine sweat glands on the palms and soles make complete control of sweating impossible. An end-point of complete anhidrosis cannot occur because large doses of the drug would be required and this would produce severe untoward effects from parasympathetic paralysis. Acute overdosage may cause dry mouth, difficulty in swallowing; severe thirst; blurred vision, photophobia; flushed, hot, dry skin; rash; hyperthermia; palpitations, tachycardia and weak pulse, elevated blood pressure; urinary urgency with difficulty in micturition; abdominal distention; restlessness, confusion, delirium and other signs suggestive of an acute organic psychosis.

Dosage and Administration: *Orally.* Average adult dosage is 2.5 mg ½ hour before meals and 2.5 to 5 mg at bedtime. An initial dosage of 12.5 mg daily may be sufficient. The dosage for children should be proportionately less depending upon the patient's age and weight. A recommended schedule is 0.2 mg/kg of body weight daily divided into 4 doses. After acute symptoms are controlled, therapy may be continued with the tablets. For effective therapeutic results, the dosage must always be titrated to the individual patient's response.

Availability:

Methscopolamine Bromide

PAMINE® Tablets, 2.5 mg in bottles of 100 and 500. **(Upjohn)**

w/Phenobarbital (**Warning:** May be habit-forming.)

PAMINE PB Tablets, 2.5 mg with phenobarbital, 15 mg in bottles of 100 and 500. **(Upjohn)**

METHSUXIMIDE

Chemical Name: *N*,2-Dimethyl-2-phenylsuccinimide.

Description: Methsuximide is an anticonvulsant drug structurally and pharmacologically related to phensuximide.

Methsuximide suppresses the paroxysmal spike and wave pattern which is common in petit mal seizures. The frequency of epileptiform attacks is reduced, apparently by depression of the motor cortex and elevation of the threshold of the CNS to convulsive stimuli.

Rapidly absorbed and metabolized following ingestion, methsuximide does not bind readily to plasma proteins. Less than 1% is excreted unchanged in the urine; the remainder is metabolized by the hepatic microsomal enzymes to N-demethyl and parahydroxyphenyl derivatives and their glucuronides. A much higher plasma concentration of the N-demethyl derivative than that of the parent compound has been detected in patients on prolonged therapy; also this metabolite has been implicated in the production of delayed coma following acute overdosage of methsuximide.

Animal reproduction studies have shown an increase in the number of stillbirths and ossification defects in neonatal rats.

Indications: Control of petit mal seizures that are refractory to other drugs.

Contraindications: In patients with a history of hypersensitivity to succinimides.

Warnings: Periodic blood counts, urinalysis and liver function studies are advised for all patients receiving this drug since blood dyscrasias (some with a fatal outcome), renal and liver impairment have been reported. The physician should be aware that systemic lupus erythematosus can occur with methsuximide. Clinical reports suggest that the use of anticonvulsant drugs in pregnant women may have a teratogenic effect on the unborn child. While a definite cause and effect relationship has not been firmly established, it is recommended that the medication be discontinued prior to and during pregnancy, primarily in patients in whom withdrawal would not pose a serious threat. However, these drugs should not be suspended in individuals susceptible to major seizures because of the strong possibility of precipitating status epilepticus with its attendant hypoxia and risk to both the mother and fetus. It is not known whether or not even minor seizures constitute some risk to the developing embryo or fetus. The drug may impair the mental and physical abilities required for the performance of potentially hazardous tasks, such as driving a motor vehicle or other such activity requiring alertness; therefore, the patients should be cautioned accordingly.

Precautions: Slow withdrawal of methsuximide is advised when signs of unusual depression, aggressiveness, or other behavioral alterations appear. It is important to proceed slowly when increasing or decreasing the dosage, as well as when adding or eliminating other medication. Abrupt withdrawal of the medication may precipitate petit mal status. When used alone in mixed types of epilepsy, it may increase the frequency of grand mal seizures in some patients.

Adverse Reactions: *Gastrointestinal System:* Gastrointestinal symptoms occur frequently and have included nausea or vomiting, anorexia, diarrhea, weight loss, epigastric and abdominal pain, and constipation. *Hemopoietic System:* Hemopoietic complications associated with the administration of methsuximide have included eosinophilia, leukopenia, monocytosis, and pancytopenia. *CNS:* Neurologic and sensory reactions reported during therapy with this drug have included drowsiness, ataxia or dizziness, irritability and nervousness, headache, blurred vision, photophobia, hiccups, and insomnia. Drowsiness, ataxia, and dizziness have been the most frequent side effects noted. Psychologic abnormalities have included confusion, instability, mental slowness, depression, hypochondriacal behavior, and aggressiveness. There have been rare reports of psychosis, suicidal behavior, and auditory hallucinations. *Integumentary System:* Dermatologic manifestations which have occurred with the administration of methsuximide have included urticaria, Stevens-Johnson syndrome, and pruritic erythematous rashes. *Other:* Miscellaneous reactions reported include periorbital edema and hyperemia.

Dosage and Administration: *Orally,* 300 mg daily the first week, increased if necessary by weekly increments of 300 mg daily for 3 weeks until a daily dosage of 1.2 gm has been reached. For children, the dosage should be reduced proportionately.

Availability:

CELONTIN® Kapseals® (capsules), 150 (Half-Strength) and 300 mg in bottles of 100.

(Parke-Davis)

METHYCLOTHIAZIDE: see The Thiazide Diuretics

METHYLDOPA

Chemical Name: L-3-(3, 4-Dihydroxyphenyl)-2-methylalanine.

Description: Methyldopa is an antihypertensive agent structurally unrelated to previously available drugs. It occurs as a white, odorless powder sparingly soluble in water and very slightly soluble in alcohol. Methyldopate hydrochloride is the ethyl ester of the hydrochloride salt of methyldopa, and is freely soluble in water and in alcohol.

Following oral administration, methyldopa is well absorbed from the gastrointestinal tract; effects are apparent within 1 to 2 hours, reach maximal within 4 to 6 hours and persist for up to 24 hours; the drug is excreted by the kidneys. Following intravenous administration, methyldopate hydrochloride is rapidly hydrolyzed to methyldopa, and has a similar onset and duration of action.

The drug is capable of inhibiting the enzyme responsible for decarboxylation of dopa thereby interfering with the formation of dihydroxyphenethylamine (dopamine) the precursor of norepinephrine, and of 5-hydroxytryptophan (5-HTP), the precursor of serotonin. Its mechanism of action is uncertain, but the antihypertensive effect may be associated with its metabolism to alpha-methylnorepinephrine. This metabolite probably lowers blood pressure by stimulation of central inhibitory alpha-adrenergic receptors, by acting as a false neurotransmitter and/or by decreasing plasma renin activity. Methyldopa has been shown to cause a net reduction in the tissue concentration of serotonin, dopamine, norepinephrine, and epinephrine. The drug has been reported to have no direct effect on cardiac function, and usually does not reduce glomerular filtration rate, renal blood flow, or filtration fraction.

Indications: Sustained moderate to severe hypertension. It is not recommended for patients with pheochromocytoma or for those with mild or labile hypertension amenable to treatment with mild sedatives or thiazide diuretics. The treatment of acute hypertensive crises may be initiated with injectable methyldopate hydrochloride. Chlorothiazide or hydrochlorothiazide complements the action of methyldopa and the use of these agents frequently produces a more pronounced antihypertensive response than when either methyldopa or a thiazide diuretic is the sole therapeutic agent.

Contraindications: Hypersensitivity to the compound, in pheochromocytoma, or in active liver disease such as acute hepatitis and active cirrhosis. It should be used with caution in patients with a history of previous liver disease or dysfunction. In common with all diuretics, chlorothiazide and hydrochlorothiazide are contraindicated in patients with anuria. See general statement on Thiazide Diuretics and monograph on Chlorothiazide and Hydrochlorothiazide for additional contraindications, precautions and adverse reactions.

Warnings: Suspicion of acquired hemolytic anemia should be followed by hemoglobin and/or hematocrit determinations. If anemia is present, laboratory studies should be performed to determine the presence of hemolysis. Evidence of hemolytic anemia is an indication for withdrawal of the drug. Discontinuation of methyldopa alone or the initiation of adrenocortical steroids usually results in a prompt remission; however, the physician should recognize that hemolytic anemia could lead to potentially fatal complications. Some patients on continued therapy with methyldopa develop a positive direct Coombs test. The incidence averages between 10 to 20%, and rarely occurs during the first 6 months of therapy. If it is not encountered within 12 months of therapy it is unlikely to develop with continued administration of this medication. This phenomenon is also dose-related with the lowest incidence occurring in patients receiving 1 gm or less daily. Reversal of the positive Coombs test occurs within weeks to months after the drug has been withdrawn. Should the need for transfusion arise, prior knowledge of a positive Coombs reaction will aid in evaluating the cross match. Patients with a positive Coombs test at the time of cross match may exhibit an incompatible minor cross match. When this occurs, an indirect Coombs test should be performed. If the results are negative, transfusion with such blood which is otherwise compatible in the major cross match may be carried out. If positive, the advisability of transfusion with blood compatible in the major cross match should be determined by a hematologist. Occasionally, fever has occurred within the first 3 weeks of therapy associated in some instances with eosinophilia or abnormalities in one or more liver function tests, such as serum alkaline phosphatase, serum transaminases (SGOT, SGPT), bilirubin, cephalin cholesterol flocculation, prothrombin time, and bromsulphalein retention. Jaundice, with or without fever, may develop usually within the first 2 or 3 months of therapy. In some patients these complications resemble those due to cholestasis. Safe use of methyldopa during pregnancy or in women of childbearing potential has not been established.

Precautions: Determination of liver function and a white cell and differential blood count should be made at intervals during the first 6 to 8 weeks of therapy, or whenever an unexplained fever occurs. If fever does occur in the absence of infection, therapy should be terminated. A paradoxical pressor response has been reported with intravenous administration of the drug. Methyldopa may potentiate the antihypertensive action of other similarly acting drugs. Spuriously high concentrations of catecholamines in the urine will interfere with the diagnosis of pheochromocytoma. Patients with severe bilateral cerebrovascular disease may experience involuntary choreoathetotic movements. Also, patients may require reduced doses of anesthetics when taking this drug. If hypotension does occur during anesthesia, it usually can be controlled by vasopressors. It should be considered that dialysis may cause hypertension since the drug is removed by this procedure. Methyldopa will not provide a diagnostic test for pheochromocytoma. It may interfere with the measurement of creatinine by the alkaline picrate method and of the uric acid by the phosphotungstate method.

Adverse Reactions: Those reported were transient sedation initially or with increased dosage, headache, asthenia, weakness, symptoms associated with reduction of blood pressure such as dizziness, lightheadedness and symptoms of cerebrovascular insufficiency. Aggravation of angina, symptoms of orthostatic hypotension, bradycardia, stuffed nose, dry mouth, abdominal distention, constipation, flatus, diarrhea, nausea, vomiting, sore tongue ("black tongue"), weight gain, edema, darkened urine after voiding, breast enlargement, lactation, impotence, skin rash, mild arthralgia, myalgia, paresthesias, parkinsonism, psychic disturbances (nightmares and mild psychoses or depression), reversible thrombocytopenia, fever, abnormal liver function, mild and reversible jaundice, elevated BUN, bilateral Bell's palsy also have been reported.

Dosage and Administration: *Orally.* Initially, 250 mg 2 or 3 times daily for 2 days. Thereafter, daily dosage may be adjusted by adding or deleting 250 mg, preferably at intervals of not less than 2 days until an adequate response has been achieved. Daily dosage should not exceed 3 gm. Children, initially, 10 mg/kg of body weight daily divided into 2 or 4 doses. The daily dosage is then increased or decreased until an adequate response is achieved. The maximum daily dose is 6.5 mg/kg or 3 gm whichever is less. *Intravenously,* 250 to 500 mg every 6 hours as required; doses in excess of 1 gm every 6 hours are not recommended. Children, 20 to 40 mg/kg of body weight daily divided into 4 doses. The desired dose should be added to 100 ml of 5% dextrose injection and infused slowly over a period of 30 to 60 minutes. Once under control, oral methyldopa may be substituted, starting with the same dosage schedule used parenterally.

Availability:

Methyldopa

ALDOMET®: **(Merck Sharp & Dohme)**

Injection, 50 mg/ml (methyldopate hydrochloride) in ampuls of 5 ml.

Tablets, 125 mg in bottles of 100; 250 mg in bottles of 100 and 1000 and in single-unit packages of 100; 500 mg in bottles of 100 and 500 and in single-unit packages of 100.

w/Chlorothiazide

ALDOCLOR® Tablets, 250 mg with either 150 or 250 mg of chlorothiazide in bottles of 100. **(Merck Sharp & Dohme)**

w/Hydrochlorothiazide

ALDORIL® Tablets, 250 mg with either 15 or 25 mg of hydrochlorothiazide in bottles of 100 and 1000. **(Merck Sharp & Dohme)**

ALDORIL D30/D50 Tablets, 500 mg with either 30 or 50 mg of hydrochlorothiazide in bottles of 100. **(Merck Sharp & Dohme)**

METHYLPHENIDATE HYDROCHLORIDE Ⓒ II

Chemical Name: α-Phenyl-2-piperidineacetic acid methyl ester hydrochloride.

Description: Methylphenidate hydrochloride is a piperidine derivative that is structurally related to amphetamine. It is a mild stimulant and antidepressant drug which brightens mood and improves performance without causing excessive stimulation or jitteriness. It occurs as a white, odorless, fine crystalline powder that is freely soluble in water.

The mode of action of methylphenidate is not completely understood, but the drug presumably activates the brain stem arousal system and cortex to produce its stimulant effect.

Indications: Treatment of minimal brain dysfunction in children as adjunctive therapy when remedial measures alone are insufficient. It also has been found useful in the treatment of narcolepsy. It may also be effective in the treatment of drug-induced lethargy, mild depression, and apathetic or withdrawn senile behavior.

Contraindications: Should not be given to anxious, tense or agitated patients, or to those with glaucoma, or who are hypersensitive to the drug.

Warnings: Methylphenidate is not intended for use in children under 6 years of age; for the treatment of severe depression of either exogenous or endogenous origin, or for the prevention or treatment or normal fatigue states. Patients requiring long-term therapy should be carefully monitored. Safe concomitant use of methylphenidate and anticonvulsants has not been established, and the drug should be withdrawn in the presence of epileptic seizures. Cautious use and monitoring of blood pressure at suitable intervals are required in patients with hypertension. Methylphenidate may potentiate the effects of pressor agents and MAO inhibitors, and may decrease the effect of guanethidine. Clinical studies have revealed that the drug may inhibit the metabolism of coumarin, phenobarbital, phenytoin, primidone, phenylbutazone, imipramine, and desipramine; therefore, a downward adjustment of the dosage of these drugs may be required when given concurrently with methylphenidate. Safe use in pregnant or in lactating women has not been established; therefore, the benefits must be weighed against the potential hazards to the fetus or child. It should be administered with extreme caution to emotionally unstable patients, especially those with a history of drug dependence or alcoholism. Chronic use can lead to marked tolerance and psychic dependence which can result in frank psychotic episodes. Careful supervision is required during drug withdrawal, and long-term follow-up may be necessary because of the patient's basic personality disturbances.

Precautions: Therapy should be discontinued if exacerbation of an agitated state occurs. Periodic blood, differential and platelet counts are advised during prolonged therapy.

Adverse Reactions: The most commonly noted were nervousness and insomnia. Other reactions included hypersensitivity (including skin rash, urticaria, arthralgia, exfoliative dermatitis, erythema multiforme with histopathological findings of necrotizing vasculitis and thrombocytopenic purpura), anorexia, nausea, dizziness, palpitations, headache, dyskinesia, drowsiness, increase and/or decrease in blood pressure and pulse rate, tachycardia, angina, cardiac arrhythmia, abdominal pain, weight loss during prolonged therapy. In children, loss of appetite, abdominal pain, weight loss during long-term therapy, insomnia, and tachycardia usually occur more frequently. Toxic psychosis has also been noted. Leukopenia and/or anemia, and a few instances of scalp hair loss have been reported, but it could not be established whether or not these were drug-related. Overdosage may produce vomiting, agitation, tremors, hyperreflexia, muscle twitching, convulsions (may be followed by coma), euphoria, confusion, hallucination, delirium, sweating, flushing, headache, hyperpyrexia, tachycardia, palpitation, cardiac arrhythmias, hypertension, mydriasis, and dryness of the mucous membranes. Treatment consists of the standard procedures applicable to amphetamine overdose.

Dosage and Administration: *Orally.* The average dose is 20 to 30 mg daily divided into 2 or 3 doses, preferably 30 to 45 minutes before meals. Some patients may require 40 to 60 mg daily; in others 10 to 15 mg will be adequate. *Children with minimal brain damage,* the initial dosage is 5 mg twice daily with gradual weekly increments of 5 to 10 mg. Daily dosages above 60 mg are not recommended.

Availability:
CII RITALIN® Tablets, 5 mg in bottles of 100, 500 and 1000; 10 mg in bottles of 100, 500, 1000 and in Accu-Pak® blister-units of 100; 20 mg in bottles of 100 and 1000. **(Ciba)**

METHYLPREDNISOLONE: see The Adrenal Corticosteroids

METHYLTESTOSTERONE: see Testosterone

METHYPRYLON Ⓒ III

Chemical Name: 3, 3-Diethyl-5-methyl-2, 4-piperidinedione.

Description: Methyprylon is a nonbarbiturate sedative-hypnotic agent. It occurs as a white, crystalline powder, freely soluble in water; possesses a molecular weight of 183.25. In animal studies, methyprylon has been shown to increase the threshold of the arousal centers in the brain stem. When taken at bedtime, sleep usually occurs within 45 minutes and lasts from 5 to 8 hours.

The hypnotic effect of a 300-mg dose is equivalent to that of a 200-mg dose of secobarbital. Rapidly metabolized and excreted, onset of action occurs within ½ hour and the sedative effect lasts for 6 to 7 hours. In normal individuals the plasma half-life is approximately 4 hours. About 97% of the drug is excreted in the urine as various metabolites and glucuronides with only 3% as unchanged drug.

Indications: Relief of insomnia of varied etiology.

Contraindications: Hypersensitivity to methyprylon.

Warnings: Patients should be cautioned about the possible combined effects with alcohol and other CNS depressant drugs, also against hazardous occupations requiring complete alertness such as operating machinery or driving a motor vehicle. Because of possible physical and psychological dependence, the customary precautions must be exercised in administering the drug to individuals known to be addiction-prone, or to those whose history suggests they may increase the dosage on their own initiative. Withdrawal symptoms, when they occur, tend to resemble those associated with the withdrawal of barbiturates, and therefore require the same means of therapy. Use of this drug during pregnancy, lactation or in women of childbearing age requires that the potential benefit be weighed against its possible hazards to the mother and child.

Precautions: The usual precautions should be observed in the presence of hepatic or renal disorders. Total daily intake should not exceed 400 mg. If used repeatedly or for prolonged periods, blood counts should be made at regular intervals.

Adverse Reactions: Drowsiness, dizziness, mild to moderate gastric upset (diarrhea, esophagitis, nausea, vomiting), headache, paradoxical excitation, skin rash, rarely neutropenia and thrombocytopenia have been noted. Overdosage is usually manifested by somnolence, confusion, coma, constricted pupils, respiratory depression and hypotension. Respiratory rate, pulse rate and blood pressure should be monitored in addition to instituting supportive care. Immediate gastric lavage with precautions to prevent pulmonary aspiration, administration of appropriate intravenous fluids and maintenance of an adequate airway are complements to the management program.

Dosage and Administration: *Orally.* Dosage should be individualized for maximum beneficial effects. The usual adult dosage is 1 capsule (300 mg) or 1 or 2 tablets (200 or 400 mg) before retiring. Children, dosage should be adjusted according to age and weight; 50 mg increased up to 200 mg if required, given at bedtime. *Not recommended for children under 3 months of age.*

Availability:
Ⓒ III NOLUDAR®: **(Roche)**
Capsules, 300 mg in bottles of 100 and 500.
Tablets, 50 mg in bottles of 100; 200 mg in bottles of 100 and 500.

METHYSERGIDE

Chemical Name: 1-Methyl-lysergic acid butanolamide maleate.

Description: Methysergide is a partially synthetic compound structurally related to lysergic acid butanolamide.

Methysergide has been shown, in vitro and in vivo, to inhibit or block the effects of serotonin, a substance which may be involved in the mechanism of vascular headaches. Serotonin has been variously described as a central neurohumoral agent or chemical mediator, as a "headache substance" acting directly or indirectly to lower pain threshold (others in this category include tyramine; polypeptides, such as bradykinin; histamine, and acetylcholine), as an intrinsic "motor hormone" of the gastrointestinal tract, and as a "hormone" involved in connective tissue reparative processes. Suggestions have been made by investigators as to the mechanism whereby methysergide produces its clinical effects, but this has not been finally established.

Indications: Prophylactic treatment of vascular headaches, notably migraine and cluster headaches. It is specifically indicated for those patients whose headaches are of sufficient frequency and severity to warrant preventive therapy. It is not indicated for the management of acute attacks.

Contraindications: Pregnancy, peripheral vascular disease, severe arteriosclerosis, severe hypertension, coronary artery disease, phlebitis or cellulitis of the lower limbs, pulmonary or collagen disease, fibrotic conditions, impaired liver or renal function, valvular heart disease, debilitated states, and serious infections.

Warnings: With long-term, uninterrupted administration, retroperitoneal fibrosis or related conditions—pleuropulmonary fibrosis and cardiovascular disorders with murmurs or vascular bruits—have been reported. Patients must be warned to report immediately the following symptoms: cold, numb, and painful hands and feet; leg cramps on walking; any type of girdle; flank, or chest pain, or any associated symptomatology. Should any of these symptoms develop, methysergide should be discontinued. Continuous administration should not exceed 6 months. There must be a drug-free interval of from 3 to 4 weeks after each 6-month course of treatment. The dosage should be reduced gradually during the last 2 to 3 weeks of each treatment course to avoid "headache rebound." The drug is not recommended for use in children.

Precautions: All patients receiving methysergide should remain under constant supervision of the physician and be examined regularly for the development of fibrotic or vascular complications. The manifestations of retroperitoneal fibrosis, pleuropulmonary fibrosis, and vascular shutdown have shown a high incidence of regression once the drug is withdrawn. These facts should be borne in mind to avoid unnecessary surgical intervention. Cardiac murmurs, which may indicate endocardial fibrosis, have shown varying degrees of regression, with complete disappearance in some and persistence in others. This drug has been specifically designed for the prophylaxis of vascular headache and has no place in the management of the acute attack.

Adverse Reactions: Within the recommended dose levels, the following side effects have been reported: *Fibrotic Complications:* Fibrotic changes have been observed in the retroperitoneal, pleuropulmonary, cardiac, and other tissues, either singly or, very rarely, in combination. *Retroperitoneal Fibrosis:* This nonspecific fibrotic process is usually confined to the retroperitoneal connective tissue above the pelvic brim and may present clinically with one or more symptoms such as general malaise, fatigue, weight loss, backache, low grade fever (elevated sedimentation rate), urinary obstruction (girdle or flank pain, dysuria, polyuria, oliguria, elevated BUN), vascular insufficiency of the lower limbs (leg pain, Leriche syndrome, edema of legs, thrombophlebitis). The single most useful diagnostic procedure in suspected cases of retroperitoneal fibrosis is intravenous pyelography. Typical deviation and obstruction of one or both ureters may be observed. *Pleuropulmonary Complications:* A similar nonspecific fibrotic process, limited to the pleural and immediately subjacent pulmonary tissues, usually presents clinically with dyspnea, tightness and pain in the chest, pleural friction rubs, and pleural effusion. These findings may be confirmed by chest roentgenograms. *Cardiac Complications:* Nonrheumatic fibrotic thickenings of the aortic root and of the aortic and mitral valves usually present clinically with cardiac murmurs and dyspnea. *Other Fibrotic Complications:* Several cases of fibrotic plaques simulating Peyronie's disease have been described. *Cardiovascular Complications:* Encroachment of retroperitoneal fibrosis on the aorta, inferior vena cava and their common iliac branches may result in vascular insufficiency of the lower limbs, the presenting features of which are mentioned under retroperitoneal fibrosis. Intrinsic vasoconstriction of large and small arteries, involving one or more vessels or merely a segment of a vessel, may occur at any stage of therapy. Depending on the vessel involved, this complication may present with chest pain, abdominal pain, or cold, numb, painful extremities with or without paresthesias and diminished or absent pulses. Progression to ischemic tissue damage has rarely been reported. Prompt withdrawal of the drug at the first signs of impaired circulation is recommended to obviate such effects. Postural hypotension and tachycardia have also been observed. Gastrointestinal Symptoms: Nausea, vomiting, diarrhea, heartburn, abdominal pain. These effects tend to appear early and can frequently be obviated by gradual introduction of the medication and by administration of the drug with meals. Constipation and elevation of gastric hydrochloride have also been reported. CNS Symptoms: Insomnia, drowsiness, mild euphoria, dizziness, ataxia, lightheadedness, hyperesthesia, unworldly feelings (described variously as "dissociation," "hallucinatory experiences," etc.). Some of these symptoms may be associated with vascular headaches, per se, and may, therefore, be unrelated to the drug. Dermatological Manifestations: Facial flush, telangiectasia, and nonspecific rashes have rarely been reported. Increased hair loss may occur, but in many instances the tendency has abated despite continued therapy. Edema: Peripheral edema, and more rarely, localized brawny edema may occur. Dependent edema has responded to lowered doses, salt restriction, or diuretics. Weight Gain: Weight gain may be a reason to caution patients regarding their caloric intake. Hematological Manifestations: Neutropenia, eosinophilia. Miscellaneous: Weakness, arthralgia, myalgia.

Dosage and Administration: *Orally,* 2 to 4 tablets, preferably 1 tablet with each meal. No pediatric dosage has been established. A trial period of 3 weeks should be instituted to evaluate response to the drug. **Important Note:** There must be a medication-free interval of 3 to 4 weeks after every 6-month course of treatment.

Availability:
SANSERT® Tablets, 2 mg in bottles of 100. **(Sandoz)**

METOLAZONE

Chemical Name: 7-Chloro-1,2,3,4-tetrahydro-2-methyl-4-oxo-3-o-tolyl-6-quinazoline-sulfonamide.

Description: Metolazone is an oral diuretic-saluretic and antihypertensive agent of the quinazoline-sulfonamide group of compounds. It is sparingly soluble in water, but is more soluble in plasma, blood, alkali, and organic solvents.

At maximum therapeutic dosage, metolazone is about equal to the thiazides in diuretic potency. It also shares a common mechanism of action with these compounds in that it produces diuresis by decreasing the tubular reabsorption of electrolytes. This action results in a marked increase in urinary excretion of sodium and chloride (saluresis) while potassium is excreted to a lesser degree. Potassium salts may be added to the regimen of patients receiving therapy for prolonged periods, and to guard against excessive potassium depletion in patients known to be prone to hypokalemia.

Metolazone acts primarily to inhibit sodium reabsorption at the renal cortical diluting site and in the proximal convoluted tubule. In clinical usage the drug does not appear to inhibit carbonic anhydrase. Its proximal action has been manifested, clinically, by increased excretion of phosphate and magnesium ions; by markedly increased fractional excretion of sodium in patients with severely compromised glomerular filtration (below 20 ml/min), and in animals by the results of micropuncture studies. A decrease in calcium ion excretion has not been noted.

Metolazone is readily absorbed from the gastrointestinal tract. Diuresis usually occurs within 1 hour, reaches a peak in 2 hours, and persists for 12 to 24 hours or more depending upon the dosage. *A single daily dose is recommended.* The prolonged duration of action is attributed to protein-binding and enterohepatic recycling. It is excreted largely unchanged in the urine.

Although the mechanism of antihypertensive action has not been established, it probably is due either to diuresis and sodium loss or to an effect on vascular function to reduce peripheral resistance or both. An antihypertensive action may be apparent in 3 or 4 days; however, administration for 3 to 4 weeks is usually required for optimum effect.

In animals pretreated with metolazone, the drug did not alter the characteristic effect of heparin on clotting time nor protamine antagonism, dicumarol on prothrombin time nor vitamin K antagonism, the response of guanethidine, reserpine and hydralazine to cardiovascular parameters or the pressor response of the subsequent dose of norepinephrine.

Indications: A saluretic-diuretic agent for the treatment and control of edema associated with congestive heart failure, and the nephrotic syndrome. Indicated as a primary measure in the treatment of mild to moderate hypertension. In severe hypertension it may be used as an adjunct to other agents.

Contraindications: Anuria, hepatic coma or precoma, and idiosyncrasy or hypersensitivity to metolazone. The routine use of diuretics in otherwise healthy pregnant women, with or without mild edema, is contraindicated and possibly hazardous. This drug is not recommended for use in pediatric patients. Potassium supplementation is contraindicated when metolazone is given with potassium-sparing diuretics.

Warnings: A cross-sensitivity reaction should be considered in patients with a history of allergy to sulfonamide-derived drugs, thiazides or quinethazone. Loss of potassium may cause weakness, cramps, and cardiac irritability. The development of hypokalemia in patients under treatment with digitalis may precipitate severe and even fatal cardiac arrhythmias. Use with caution in the presence of severe renal dysfunction to avoid inducing azotemia, hyperuricemia, oliguria, and acute attacks of gout in susceptible individuals. On occasion, considerable potentiation with furosemide has been noted which resulted in massive diuresis and severe electrolyte imbalance. Therapy should always be initiated cautiously in patients receiving other antihypertensive or ganglionic blocking agents, and reduction of the dosage of these agents may be advisable while the patient is kept under careful and continuous supervision. Reduction in dosage is also required when metolazone is given with a potassium-sparing diuretic to avoid developing potassium retention and hyperkalemia. Frequent determination of serum potassium is required and potassium supplementation should be instituted whenever indicated. Hypokalemia will be more common in association with intensive or prolonged diuretic therapy. with concomitant steroid or ACTH therapy, and with inadequate electrolyte intake. Metolazone should be used with caution in pregnant patients since the drug crosses the placental barrier and may result in fetal or neonatal jaundice, thrombocytopenia, and possibly other adverse reactions which have occurred in the adult. However, teratologic studies in mice, rats and rabbits have not shown teratogenic effects in these animals. Since the drug also appears in breast milk, mothers should be cautioned not to breast feed their babies while they are taking this drug.

Precautions: Serum potassium, BUN, uric acid and blood sugar determinations should be performed prior to and at appropriate intervals during therapy. All patients should be observed for clinical signs of fluid or electrolyte imbalance namely: hyponatremia, hypochloremic alkalosis and hypokalemia. Serum and urine electrolyte determinations are particularly important when the patient is vomiting excessively or receiving parenteral fluids. Medications such as digitalis may also influence serum electrolytes. Warning signs, irrespective of cause, are dryness of mouth, thirst, weakness, lethargy, drowsiness, restlessness, muscle pains or cramps, muscular fatigue, hypotension, oliguria, tachycardia, and gastrointestinal disturbances such as nausea and vomiting. While not reported to date for metolazone, related diuretics have increased responsiveness to tubocurarine and decreased arterial responsiveness to norepinephrine; therefore, it may be advisable to discontinue therapy with this drug 3 days prior to elective surgery. Because the drug exerts an effect on glucose metabolism, insulin requirements may be altered in diabetics, and hyperglycemia and glycosuria may occur in the presence of latent diabetes. Any chloride deficit should be corrected; if dietary salt is unduly restricted, especially during hot weather, in severely edematous patients with cardiac failure or renal disease, a low salt syndrome may complicate therapy. Caution should be observed in patients with severely impaired renal function to avoid cumulative effects, and in those with a susceptibility to hyperuricemia or gout. Orthostatic hypotension may occur and may be potentiated by alcohol, barbiturates, narcotics, or concurrent therapy with other antihypertensive drugs. Although not reported to date, the possible development of pathological changes in the parathyroid glands with hypercalcemia and hypophosphatemia should be kept in mind.

Adverse Reactions: Complications which have been noted with metolazone include constipation; syncope, drowsiness, and dizziness; orthostatic hypotension, excessive volume depletion, hemoconcentration, and venous thrombosis; dryness of mouth, symptomatic and asymptomatic hypokalemia, hyponatremia, hypochloremia, hypochloremic alkalosis, hyperuricemia, hyperglycemia, glycosuria, increase in BUN or creatinine levels, fatigue, muscle cramps or spasm, weakness, and restlessness. Reactions which may occur include nausea, vomiting, anorexia, diarrhea, abdominal bloating, epigastric distress, intrahepatic cholestatic jaundice, and hepatitis; vertigo, and headache; leukopenia; urticaria, and other skin rashes; palpitation, chest pain; chills, and acute gouty attacks. Adverse reactions which have occurred with other diuretics but have not, as yet, been reported with this drug include pancreatitis, paresthesias, xanthopsia, agranulocytosis, thrombocytopenia, aplastic anemia, purpura, photosensitivity, and necrotizing angiitis (cutaneous vasculitis). Whenever adverse reactions are moderate or severe, the dosage should be reduced or the drug withdrawn.

Dosage and Administration: *Orally.* Therapy should be titrated to gain the maximal initial therapeutic response, and to determine the minimal dose possible to maintain this response. For the initiation of diuresis, 5 to 20 mg once daily. For mild to moderate hypertension, 2.5 to 5 mg once daily. For patients with congestive cardiac failure who tend to experience paroxysmal nocturnal dyspnea, it is advisable to employ a dosage near the upper end of the range, to ensure prolongation of diuresis and saluresis for a full 24-hour period.

Availability:
DIULO™ Tablets, 2.5 mg (pink), 5 mg (blue) amd 10 mg (yellow) in bottles of 100. **(Searle)**
ZAROXOLYN® Tablets 2.5 mg (pink), 5 mg (blue) and 10 mg (yellow) in bottles of 100 and 1000. **(Pennwalt)**

METOPROLOL TARTRATE

Chemical Name: 1-Isopropylamino-3-[p-(2-methoxyethyl)-phenoxy]-2-propanol *dextro*-tartrate.

Description: Metoprolol is a synthetic, beta-adrenergic-receptor blocking agent with predominant blocking effects on $beta_1$ receptors. The drug's major advantage in the treatment of hypertension is its cardio-selective activity. It preferentially focuses its action on $beta_1$ receptors in the heart muscle while leaving $beta_2$ receptors comparatively, but not completely, unaffected. Since these events are dose-related, smaller doses of metoprolol are less likely to provoke bronchospasm, particularly in susceptible patients and in those with bronchial asthma or chronic bronchitis. Although the precise mechanism of antihypertensive action has not been clearly defined, it has been suggested that the following factors may be involved: competitive ability to antagonize catecholamines at peripheral (especially cardiac) adrenergic neuron sites, resulting in a decrease in cardiac output; inhibition of the vasomotor centers leading to a reduced sympathetic outflow to the periphery; and suppression of renin activity by the kidney. Pharmacologic studies have established that it reduces heart rate and cardiac output at rest and on exercise, reduces systolic blood pressure on exercise, inhibits isoproterenol-induced tachycardia, and reduces reflex orthostatic tachycardia. Confirmation of cardio-selective $beta_1$ activity is due to the drug's inability to reverse the $beta_2$-mediated vasodilating effects of epinephrine, in contrast to nonselective beta-blocking agents which completely reverse this effect. In addition to its lack of intrinsic sympathomimetic activity, it also causes a significantly less reduction in FEV_1 and FVC, and only weak membrane stabilizing activity. The drug readily crosses the blood brain barrier and appears in CSF in excess (78%) of the simultaneous plasma concentration. It occurs as a white, crystalline solid that is soluble in water.

Orally administered metoprolol is rapidly and almost completely absorbed with significant beta-blocking effect apparent within 1 hour while the duration of pharmacologic effect, as measured by reduction of exercise heart rate, is related to the amount given. The time for a 50% reduction of the maximum registered effect after single oral doses of 20, 50 and 100 mg was 3.3, 5 and 6.4 hours respectively in normal subjects. Only a small fraction of the drug (about 12%) is bound to serum albumin. Elimination is mainly by biotransformation in the liver and the plasma half-life range is 3 to 4 hours. Because of variable plasma levels attained with a given dose and the lack of a consistent relationship of antihypertensive activity to a particular dose, selection of the proper dosage requires individual titration. While there is a linear relationship between plasma levels and reduction of exercise heart rate, antihypertensive activity does not appear to be related to plasma levels of metoprolol.

Indications: Management of hypertension. May be used as the sole agent or in combination with other antihypertensive medications, especially thiazide-type diuretics.

Contraindications: Sinus bradycardia, heart block greater than first degree, cardiogenic shock, overt cardiac failure, and hypersensitivity to the drug.

Warnings: Patients requiring utmost care are those with cardiac failure, ischemic heart disease, bronchospastic diseases, diabetes mellitus, thyrotoxicosis, and those undergoing major surgery. Continuous depression of the myocardium with beta-blocking agents over a period of time can, in some instances, lead to cardiac failure. Therefore, it is imperative to use extreme care in hypertensive patients with congestive heart failure controlled by digitalis and diuretics, since both digitalis and metoprolol slow AV conduction. At the first sign of impending cardiac failure, patients should be fully digitalized and/or be given a diuretic, and the response closely observed. If cardiac failure continues despite adequate measures, metoprolol should be withdrawn. Abrupt cessation of therapy in patients with angina pectoris may produce an exacerbation of their condition, and in some, may cause myocardial infarction. All patients, with or without angina, should be strongly cautioned not to interrupt treatment without the consent of their physician. Generally, beta-blocking drugs should not be given to patients with bronchospastic disease, but because of metoprolol's relatively mild $beta_2$ effect, it may be used with caution and at the *lowest* dose possible, preferably in combination with another $beta_2$-stimulating agent. To maintain adequate antihypertensive control, the dosage for such patients should be extended to 3 times instead of 2 times daily. It may be judicious to withdraw the drug prior to major surgery, since the heart's ability to respond to reflex adrenergic stimuli may be impaired and may thus augment the risk of general anesthesia and surgical procedures. Because it is a competitive inhibitor of beta-receptor agonists, its effects can be reversed by the administration of such agents (dobutamine or isoproterenol). Such patients may develop protracted severe hypotension. Difficulty in restarting and maintaining the heart beat has also been reported with beta-blocking agents. The drug may mask the signs and symptoms of hyperthyroidism and hypoglycemia, and may potentiate insulin-induced hypoglycemia. Therefore, special care should be exercised in patients with diabetes, particularly individuals with labile diabetes, and in those suspected of developing thyrotoxicosis, since abrupt withdrawal of the medication might precipitate a thyroid storm.

Precautions: Special care is also advised in patients with impaired hepatic or renal function. Catecholamine-depleting drugs (reserpine) may have an additive effect when given with beta-blocking agents. Patients receiving such combined medication should be closely observed for evidence of hypotension and/or marked bradycardia which may cause vertigo, syncope, or postural hypotension. The drug should be given to pregnant patients only when the clinical situation clearly indicates its use. It is advised that nursing not be undertaken while the patient is taking this drug. Safe and effective use in children has not been established.

Adverse Reactions: Most side effects have been mild and transient. Tiredness and dizziness have occurred in 10% of patients, depression in 5%; headache, nightmares and insomnia; shortness of breath and bradycardia in 3%, cold extremities, Raynaud's disease, palpitation, congestive heart failure; wheezing; diarrhea in 5%, nausea, gastric pain, constipation, flatulence, and heartburn in 1%; pruritus in less than 1%, and Peyronie's disease (extremely rare). Oculomucocutaneous syndrome, associated with another beta-blocking agent was not observed with this drug. The following adverse effects that have occurred with other similarly acting drugs and may possibly occur with metoprolol include reversible mental depression, progressing to catatonia; visual disturbances; hallucinations; an acute reversible syndrome characterized by disorientation for time and place, short-term memory loss, emotional lability, slightly clouded sensorium, and decreased performance on neuropsychometrics; AV block; agranulocytosis, nonthrombocytopenic purpura, thrombocytopenic purpura; erythematous rash, fever combined with aching and sore throat, laryngospasm and respiratory distress; reversible alopecia; elevated blood urea levels in patients with severe heart disease, elevated serum transaminase, alkaline phosphatase, and lactic dehydrogenase.

Dosage and Administration: *Orally.* The usual initial dose is 50 mg twice daily whether used alone or added to a diuretic. Dosage may be increased at weekly intervals (or longer) until optimal blood pressure reduction has been achieved. Maximum effect is usually apparent after 1 week of therapy. The usual maintenance dosage is 100 mg twice daily, but may range from 100 to 450 mg daily. Dosages above 450 mg have not been evaluated.

Availability:
LOPRESSOR™ Tablets, 50 and 100 mg in bottles of 100 and 1000 and in unit-dosage packages of 100. **(Geigy)**

METRIZAMIDE

Chemical Name: 2-[3-Acetamido-2,4,6-triiodo-5-(N-methylacetamido)benzamido]-2-deoxy-D-glucopyranose.

Description: Metrizamide is a radiopaque diagnostic medium used primarily for specific myelographic procedures and total spinal column radiography. The medium's significant clinical feature is that it does not have to be removed by lumbar puncture from the cerebrospinal fluid, since it is absorbed into the blood stream, thus reducing painful side effects as well as the time necessary for the procedure. Approximately 60% of the administered dose is excreted unchanged through the kidneys within 48 hours. Derived from metrizoic acid and glucosamine, it occurs as a water-soluble, nonionic, white powder with a molecular weight of 789 and an iodine content of 48.25%. Each 20-ml vial contains 3.75 gm of metrizamide (1.81 gm of organically bound iodine) and 1.2 mg of edetate calcium disodium. Each 50-ml vial contains 6.75 mg of metrizamide (3.26 gm of organically bound iodine) and 2.16 mg of edetate calcium disodium. pH is adjusted with carbon dioxide. When reconstituted to the lowest recommended concentration (170 mg of iodine/ml), it has a specific gravity of 1.184 at 37° C, is hyperbaric to and isotonic with cerebrospinal fluid, and has a pH of about 7.4.

The initial concentration and volume of the medium, in conjunction with appropriate patient manipulation, will determine the extent of the diagnostic contrast that can be achieved; this can be monitored by fluoroscopy. Optimal visualization is dependent upon the specific technique employed as well as the region under observation.

Indications: Metrizamide is specifically indicated for lumbar, thoracic, cervical, and total columnar myelography and for use in computerized tomography of the intracranial subarachnoid spaces following spinal subarachnoid injection.

Contraindications: Known hypersensitivity to the medium.

Warnings: Fatal reactions, although not reported in clinical use with metrizamide, have accompanied the administration of radiopaque contrast media; it is therefore of utmost importance that a course of action be carefully planned for the immediate treatment of serious reactions, and that adequate and appropriate facilities and experienced personnel be readily available in the event a severe reaction occurs. The inherent risks of myelography in patients whose cerebrospinal fluid is found to contain an excessive amount of blood must be weighed against the necessity of performing this procedure. Although no teratogenic effects attributable to metrizamide have been observed in reproduction studies in animals, the benefits to be gained in pregnant patients must be weighed against the possible adverse effects on fetal development. Its use in children under 12 years of age is not recommended until further clinical experience is achieved.

Precautions: Special care is advised in patients with a history of epilepsy, severe cardiovascular disease, chronic alcoholism, multiple sclerosis, or with a history of bronchial asthma or other allergic manifestations. Prior to injection of any contrast medium, patients should be questioned in regard to a history of allergy or asthma. While a positive history does not arbitrarily contraindicate the use of the agent, it does emphasize the need for extra caution and preparedness to treat any reaction; premedication with antihistamines for the purpose of avoiding or minimizing possible allergic reaction may be considered. No conclusive relationship between severe reactions and antigen-antibody reactions or other manifestations of allergy has been established. Epileptic patients should be maintained on their anticonvulsant medication, and should a seizure occur, intravenous diazepam or sodium phenobarbital is recommended. Prophylactic anticonvulsant treatment with barbiturates or diazepam orally for 24 to 48 hours should be considered in patients with evidence of inadvertent intracranial entry of a large or concentrated bolus of the contrast medium since there is an increased risk of seizures in such cases. Drugs, such as neuroleptics including the phenothiazines derivatives, which lower the seizure threshold should be avoided. If possible, they should be withdrawn at least 48 hours before and not be reinstated for at least 12 hours after the examination. Patients with hepatorenal insufficiency or renal failure should receive this agent only when the need for the examination dictates a need since excretion of this material may be severely limited. Reexamination should then be delayed for 5 to 7 days.

Adverse Reactions: In general, complications following subarachnoid injection of metrizamide are not substantially different from those observed after lumbar puncture alone. The most frequently occurring adverse reactions are headache, nausea, and vomiting. These reactions occur 3 to 8 hours postinjection, almost all occurring within 24 hours. They are usually mild to moderate in degree, generally lasting for a few hours and disappearing within 24 hours. Rarely have the headaches been severe or persisted beyond 24 hours. Backache, neck stiffness, numbness, and paresthesias, leg or sciatic-type pain occurred less frequently, often in the form of a transient exacerbation of preexisting symptomatology. Temperature elevations and dizziness have also been reported. Infrequently, muscle spasm or generalized convulsions have occurred 4 to 8 hours following injection and in some cases were attributed to a history of epilepsy, medication with neuroleptic drugs, or inadvertent overdose. In all cases, treatment with intravenous diazepam or sodium phenobarbital has provided rapid control. Transient alterations in vital signs may occur, the significance of which is difficult to assess, since these parameters may be affected by the procedure or by the patient's physical or emotional state. Other rarely occurring adverse reactions include chills, pruritus, urticaria, nasal congestion, and dyspnea; mild and transitory perceptual aberrations such as hallucinations, depersonalization, anxiety, depression, hyperesthesia, visual and speech disturbances, confusion and disorientation, malaise, weakness, EEG changes, and meningismus; chest pain, tachycardia, bradycardia, and other arrhythmias; and diarrhea.

Dosage and Administration: *Intraspinal.* The dosage and concentration of the radiopaque medium will depend upon the degree and extent of contrast required in the area(s) under examination and on the equipment and technique employed. Concentrations which are approximately isotonic (170 to 190 mg iodine/ml) are recommended for examination in the lumbar region. For movement of the medium to distant target areas, higher concentrations are recommended to compensate for dilution of metrizamide with cerebrospinal fluid. A total dose of 3 gm of iodine should not be exceeded. The procedure can be performed without the use of anesthesia, and premedication with sedatives or tranquilizers are usually not needed. For complete information on precise methods and general procedures, refer to the package literature.

Availability:
AMIPAQUE® Injection, 3.75 gm in single-dose vials of 20 ml; 6.75 gm in single-dose vials of 50 ml in packages containing 1 vial with 1 vial of diluent or in combination packages containing 5 vials with 5 vials of diluent. **(Winthrop)**

METRIZOATES MEGLUMINE AND CALCIUM
METRIZOATES MEGLUMINE, SODIUM, CALCIUM AND MAGNESIUM

Chemical Name: 3-Acetamido-2,4,6-triiodo-5-(*N*-methylacetamido) benzoic acid salts.

Description: Clear, aqueous solutions of salts of metrizoic acid that are used in diagnostic roentogenography. Each ml of the *280* solution contains 140.1 mg of meglumine, 0.35 mg of calcium, and 461.8 mg of metrizoic acid; total salt concentration is 60.2% w/v, and the iodine concentration is 28%. Each ml of the *440* solution contains 75.9 mg of meglumine, 16.6 mg (0.7 mEq) of sodium, 0.78 mg of calcium, 0.15 mg of magnesium, and 730 mg of metrizoic acid. The total salt concentration is 82.3% w/v, and the iodine concentration is 44%. The pH is adjusted with metrizoic acid or meglumine. The solutions may be autoclaved and should be protected from light.

Following intravenous injection, excretion is rapid when renal function is normal. Approximately 86% of the administered dose is recovered in the urine in unchanged form in 6 hours and 95% in 24 hours, with about 1.6% in the feces.

Indications: Both solutions may be used in selective angiographic procedures of cerebral angiography and peripheral arteriography. The *280* solution is also indicated for excretory urography and the *440* solution for angiocardiography in adults and children and for aortography including visualization of the branches of the aorta.

Contraindications: For excretory urography in patients with anuria. Epidural injection is also contraindicated as well in myelography or for examination of dorsal cysts or sinuses which might communicate with the subarachnoid space. Injection of even a small amount into the subarachnoid space can cause convulsions which may be fatal. During the progressive period of stroke, carotid angiography should be avoided because of the increased risk of cerebral complications. Hypersensitivity to metrizoic acid salts is also a contraindication. Additionally, the *440 solution* is contraindicated in selective spinal arteriography, or arteriography of trunks providing spinal branches (usually the thyrocervical, costocervical, subclavian, vertebral, bronchial, intercostal), since mild to severe muscle spasm and serious neurologic sequelae including permanent paralysis have occurred. Administration of the medium in the presence of advanced renal disease associated with severe uremia as well as direct injection into the carotid or vertebral arteries should be avoided.

Warnings: Since radiopaque materials have caused serious and fatal reactions in some patients, it is important to plan a course of action, and to have the necessary facilities on hand in the event a reaction occurs. The benefit-to-risk ratio should be evaluated before administering these solutions in patients with recent myocardial infarction. Intravascular administration of contrast media may promote sickling in patients who are susceptible to sickle cell disease. The results of PBI and RAI uptake studies, which depend on iodine estimations, will not accurately reflect thyroid function for up to 16 days following administration of angiographic media. However, function tests not depending on iodine estimations, e.g., T_3 resin uptake or direct thyroxine assays, are not affected. Administration of radiopaque materials in patients known or suspected to have pheochromocytoma should be performed with extreme caution. If, in the opinion of the physician, the possible benefits of such procedures outweigh the considered risk, the amount of the medium injected should be kept to an absolute minimum. Blood pressure should be monitored throughout the procedure, and measures for treatment of a hypertensive crisis should be readily available. No teratogenic effects attributable to either solution have been observed in reproduction studies in animals. However, before administering to women of childbearing potential, the physician should carefully consider the possible risk to the fetus. In addition, most clinicians consider elective contrast radiography of the abdomen contraindicated during pregnancy. When performing aortography by the translumbar technique, utmost care should be taken to avoid inadvertent intrathecal injection (see Contraindications). If convulsions occur, the patient should be placed in an upright position in order to confine the hyperbaric solution to the lower portion of the body; if necessary an anesthetic may be given. If a large dose has been administered, exchange of the cerebrospinal fluid with a proper vehicle should be considered. Although visualization of any branch of the aorta may be achieved by intraaortic injection of the 440 solution, selective (catheter) arteriographic procedures such as coronary arteriography are not recommended at the present time due to inadequate clinical experience.

Precautions: A history of allergy may be useful in predicting reactions of a mild, intermediate or serious nature, and may imply a greater than usual risk; however, it does not necessarily contraindicate use of the medium. Routine caution is advised in patients with asthma and in those sensitive to iodine-containing compounds. Antihistamines may be given prior to the procedure in order to avoid or minimize possible allergic reactions. A test dose of 0.5 to 1 ml of the contrast medium administered intravenously before injecting the full dose has been employed. However, this does not assure that a serious or even a fatal response will not occur, since severe reactions and fatalities have been reported with both the test dose alone, or with the full dose after a nonreactive test dose in patients with or without a history of allergy. No conclusive relationship between severe or fatal reactions such as anaphylactoid reactions or laryngospasm, and antigen-antibody reactions has been established. The patient's vital signs should be monitored when large doses of the 440 solution are being administered; also large doses may aggravate preexisting incipient heart failure. Hypotension should be corrected promptly since it may induce serious cardiac arrhythmias. Because of the hemodynamic changes which may occur on injection into the right heart outflow tract, special care, especially in regard to dosage, should be observed in patients with right ventricular failure, pulmonary hypertension or obliterated pulmonary vascular beds. In cyanotic infants, apnea, bradycardia, and other cardiac arrhythmias, lethargy and depression, and a tendency to acidosis are more likely to occur; therefore, they should be carefully observed for any delayed adverse effects such as cardiac arrhythmias, electrolyte imbalance or hemodynamic disturbances. Unlike the adult, the amount of the total dosage in young infants is of considerable importance, since they are more prone to convulsions. Before initiating the procedure, the minimum amount necessary for adequate contrast should be determined. With each repeat dose, the hazard of adverse reactions is increased. In the presence of thromboangiitis obliterans, or ascending infection associated with severe ischemia, angiography should be performed with extreme caution, if at all. A vigorous pulsatile flow should be established before using a catheter or pressure injecton technique. A screening dose of about 2 ml, in order to locate the exact site of the needle or catheter tip, will aid in preventing injection of the main dose into a branch of the aorta or intramurally. In the translumbar technique, severe pain during injection may indicate intramural placement, and abdominal or back pain after the procedure may indicate hemorrhage from the injection site. Following catheter procedures, a gentle pressure hemostasis for 5 to 10 minutes is suggested, followed by observation of the patient for 30 to 60 minutes and immobilization of the limb for several hours to prevent hemorrhage from the site of arterial puncture. Under conditions of slowed aortic circulation, there is an increased likelihood of aortography causing muscle spasm. Occasional serious neurologic complications, including paraplegia, have also been reported to occur in patients who had aortic-iliac or even femoral artery bed obstruction, abdominal compression, hypotension, hypertension, spinal anesthesia, injection of vasopressors to increase contrast, or low injection sites. In these patients the concentration, dose, and number of repeat injection of the medium should be maintained at a minimum with appropriate intervals between injections. The position of the patient and catheter tip should be carefully evaluated.

Adverse Reactions: Those most frequently encountered are urticaria with or without pruritus, erythema, dermatitis, and maculopapular rash; less frequent are coughing, sneezing, nasal stuffiness, rhinitis and anxiety, and, rarely, dry mouth, chills, sweating, edema, dyspnea, dizziness, angioneurotic edema, bronchospasm, or laryngospasm. In most patients, these reactions usually clear up rapidly and spontaneously. Serious reactions such as cardiovascular disturbances including shock or cardiac arrest may occur but are rare. Visual and speech disturbances, vertigo, weakness or paralysis, convulsions, nervousness, lightheadedness, headache, and tremor were also infrequently reported. Complications due to technical procedures may include thrombosis, thrombophlebitis, hemorrhage from the puncture site, and hematomas, or ecchymoses following extravasation or subintimal injection. Brachial plexus injury (usually transient) is often due to an incorrect injection procedure (patients will usually complain of pain or paresthesia), or prolonged incorrect placement of the arm. Loss or weakness of pulse rate and a fall in blood pressure in a catheterized artery may occur and usually requires no treatment. Pain or burning sensation with some spasm may occur, and is more marked in patients with arterial insufficiency. Therefore, the procedure is more satisfactorily performed under general or spinal anesthesia depending on location. Arterial thrombosis, displacement of arterial plaques, and ipsilateral venous thrombosis are very rare complications. Pain at the injection site, facial flushing or a feeling of body warmth, and nausea and vomiting may occur during or immediately following injection and may be related to the physical nature of the medium or to an abrupt hemodynamic change induced by the medium.

For additional contraindications, warnings, precautions and adverse reactions, see the monograph on the Diatrizoates.

Dosage and Administration: *Intraarterially* or *intravenously*. *For cerebral angiography:* the usual dosage for visualization of the cerebral vasculature varies with the site and method of administration, as well as the age and condition of the patient. *For carotid and vertebral angiography:* in adults, the single injection dose is 6 to 10 ml of the *280* solution. For brachial or axillary retrograde catheter or cannulation techniques, the single injection dose is 35 to 75 ml of the *280* solution. Dosage for children is proportional to age and weight. *For peripheral arteriography:* the usual single injection dose in adults is 20 to 40 ml of the *280* solution. *For excretory urography:* the usual adult dose is 30 to 60 ml administered *intravenously*. These doses may be repeated as indicated. For optimal results with minimal reactions, the entire dose should be injected within 1 to 3 minutes. The suggested dose for children up to 12 years of age is as follows: Up to 10 lbs, 5 to 10 ml; 10 to 30 lbs. 10 to 15 ml; 30 to 60 lbs. 15 to 30 ml. Children older than 12 years of age and weighing more than 60 lbs may be given an adult dose. *For angiocardiography:* the usual adult dose is a single injection of 40 to 50 ml of the

440 solution, with a range varying from 20 to 60 ml, and a maximum of up to 200 ml. Children, 0.88 to 1.32 mg/kg of body weight with a range varying from 0.44 to 1.76 mg/kg. For patients with stenotic lesions, the lower limits are employed whereas in children with cardiomegaly or with large volume shunts or where right chamber injection is also intended to opacify the left chamber, the upper limits may be required. In young infants, however, the total dosage administered should be maintained below 3 ml/kg in those under 2 months of age in any single procedure. *For aortography:* the usual single adult dose is 40 ml of the *440* solution with a range of 20 to 60 ml; up to 200 ml has been used in multiple injections. In infants and children, sodium diatrizoate, 50% is advised in doses of 0.5 ml/kg of body weight. *For peripheral arteriography:* the usual adult dose is 10 to 25 ml of the *440* solution; repeat doses may be given, if necessary.

Availability:
ISOPAQUE®: **(Winthrop)**
280 Aqueous Solution in vials of 20, 30 and 50 ml.
440 Aqueous Solution in vials of 50 ml.

METRONIDAZOLE

Chemical Name: 2-Methyl-5-nitroimidazole-1-ethanol.

Description: Metronidazole has direct trichomonacidal and amebicidal activity. Because it acts systemically, it is effective against trichomonads harbored in intravaginal and extravaginal sites in the female and in the genitourinary tract of the male. It is also effective against intestinal and liver infestations of *Entamoeba histolytica*. It occurs as pale yellow crystals that are slightly soluble in water and in alcohol.

Metronidazole is well absorbed following oral administration. The peak serum levels are attained in about 1 hour. Both unchanged drug and several metabolites are excreted in the urine in various proportions. The metabolites result from oxidation of side chains and glucuronide formation. Because the potential teratogenicity of the drug is unknown, it is best to avoid use during pregnancy since the drug is known to cross the placenta and to appear in breast milk. Also, low concentrations appear in the saliva during treatment.

In studies with Swiss mice, metronidazole was reported to increase the incidence of lung tumors (primarily adenomas) over those found in control animals. It was also reported that an increase in malignant lymphomas occurred in female mice. In two long-term studies with Sprague-Dawley female rats that were given this drug, increases in the incidence of mammary tumors were also noted; however, it has been found that mammary tumors occur readily in female rats of this strain.

Indications: Treatment of trichomoniasis in male and female patients when the presence of the trichomonad has been demonstrated by wet smear or culture, or when associated with endocervicitis, cervicitis, or cervical erosion, and for the sexual partners of those patients who have a recurrence of the infection provided trichomonal infection is demonstrated in the urogenital tract of the consort. It is also indicated in the treatment of both acute intestinal amebiasis (amebic dysentery) and amebic liver abscess.

Contraindications: Blood dyscrasias, active organic disease of the CNS, during the first trimester of pregnancy, and hypersensitivity to the drug.

Warnings: Results of studies with rats and mice have shown that metronidazole has tumorigenic activity, especially pulmonary tumorigenesis, following prolonged oral administration. Also noted were increases in the incidence of various neoplasms, particularly mammary tumors in female rats.

Precautions: Use during the second and third trimesters of pregnancy and during lactation should be restricted to those patients in whom topical measures have proved inadequate. Mild leukopenia has been reported, and it is recommended that total and differential leukocyte counts be made before and after treatment, especially if a second course of therapy is necessary. Patients should be advised not to take alcoholic beverages while on medication because abdominal cramps, nausea, headache, vomiting and flushing may occur. Because metronidazole may potentiate the hypothrombinemic effect of coumarin and warfarin, a reduction in the dose of these agents may be necessary. Additionally, certain chemical analyses for serum glutamic oxaloacetic transaminase may be altered. The appearance of abnormal neurologic signs demands prompt cessation of therapy. The physician should be alert to symptoms of an overgrowth of Monilia in patients taking this drug. In the treatment of amebic liver abscess, the pus should be aspirated during therapy.

Adverse Reactions: Nausea, headache, anorexia, vomiting, diarrhea, epigastric distress, abdominal cramping, constipation, a metallic, sharp and unpleasant taste, furry tongue, glossitis, stomatitis, leukopenia, dizziness, vertigo, incoordination, ataxia, convulsive seizures, numbness or paresthesia of extremities, fleeting joint pains, confusion, irritability, depression, insomnia, mild erythematous eruption, weakness, urticaria, flushing, dryness of the mouth, vagina or vulva, pruritus, dysuria, cystitis, sense of pelvic pressure, dyspareunia, fever, polyuria, incontinence, decrease of libido, nasal congestion, proctitis, pyuria, and rarely, an unexplained darkening in the color of the urine have been reported. Flattening of the T wave may be seen in electrocardiographic tracings.

Dosage and Administration: *Orally.* Trichomoniasis, *in both the male and female,* 1 tablet 3 times daily for 7 consecutive days. Should repeat courses be required, an interval of 4 to 6 weeks should elapse between courses. Total and differential leukocyte counts should be made before, during and after retreatment. Should partners show signs of trichomonad infestation, it is important that they be treated concurrently to avoid reinfestation. Amebiasis, *Adults: For acute intestinal amebiasis,* 750 mg 3 times daily for 5 to 10 days. *For amebic liver abscess,* 500 to 750 mg 3 times daily for 5 to 10 days. Children: 35 to 50 mg/kg of body weight/day, divided into 3 doses, for 10 days.

Availability:
FLAGYL® Tablets, 250 mg (white) in bottles of 100, 250 and 1000 and in patient pack tablet dispensers of 21. **(Searle)**

METYRAPONE

Chemical Name: 2-Methyl-1,2-di-3-pyridyl-1-propanone.

Description: Metyrapone is a synthetic compound possessing the unique facility for selective inhibition of 11-beta hydroxylation in the adrenal cortex. It occurs as a nearly white to light amber, crystalline powder soluble in alcohol.

The inhibition of cortisol (hydrocortisone), corticosterone and aldosterone synthesis is followed by a compensatory increase in ACTH secretion by the anterior pituitary of the patient with adequate pituitary-adrenal function. This rise in ACTH stimulates the adrenal cortex, and increased amounts of 17-ketosteroids and 17-hydroxycorticosteroids appear in the urine. Since this increase in ACTH secretion does not occur in patients with poor pituitary reserve, there is no significant increase in the excretion of corticoid precursors following the administration of metyrapone.

Indications: A diagnostic test for hypothalamico-pituitary function which may be of value in assessing the patient's ability to withstand surgical procedures and other stresses.

Contraindications: Adrenal cortical insufficiency; hypersensitivity to metyrapone.

Warnings: Safe use in pregnant women or in women of childbearing potential has not been established.

Precautions: All therapy with corticosteroids must be discontinued prior to and during testing with this drug. The ability of the adrenals to respond to exogenous ACTH should be demonstrated before this agent is employed as a test. Metyrapone may induce acute adrenal insufficiency in patients with reduced adrenal secretory capacity. Erroneous results in pituitary function as determined by this test may occur in patients taking phenytoin for as long as 2 weeks following cessation of therapy. A subnormal response may also occur in pregnant patients and in those on estrogen therapy.

Adverse Reactions: Nausea, abdominal discomfort, dizziness, headache, sedation, and allergic rash. Occasionally thrombophlebitis has occurred following intravenous administration.

Dosage and Administration: *Orally.* Adults, 750 mg every 4 hours for 6 doses. Children, 15 mg/kg of body weight every 4 hours for 6 doses. A minimal single dose of 250 mg is recommended. *Intravenously.* Adults and children, 30 mg/kg of body weight in 1000 ml saline solution or 5% dextrose solution administered by intravenous infusion over a period of 4 hours beginning between 8 and 10 a.m. The 24-hour urine collection should begin at the start of the test. For further details, consult package literature.

Availability:
METOPIRONE®: **(Ciba)**
Injection (as ditartrate), 100 mg/ml (equivalent to 43.8 mg metyrapone base and 56.2 mg tartaric acid) in ampuls of 10 ml.
Tablets, 250 mg in bottles of 18.

MICONAZOLE NITRATE

Chemical Name: 1-[2,4-Dichloro-*β*-(2, 4-dichlorobenzyloxy) phenethyl] imidazole nitrate.

Description: Miconazole nitrate is a synthetic antifungal agent that is chemically unrelated to other fungicidal compounds. It occurs as a white to off-white, crystalline powder that is very soluble in water and only slightly soluble in most organic solvents and in diluted solutions of inorganic acids. Molecular weight is 479.16. Although its pharmacologic mode of action has not been established, in vitro studies show that it possesses fungicidal action against Candida albicans and other species of this genus. It has also been found to inhibit the growth of the common dermatophytes *Trichophyton rubrum, Trichophyton mentagrophytes,* and *Epidermophyton floccosum,* and the organism responsible for tinea versicolor (*Malassezia furfur*). Its therapeutic value appears to be due to its action primarily on the yeast cell membrane resulting in selective inhibition of the uptake of those components necessary for cell reproduction and growth. Clinical trials have shown it to be well-tolerated and effective in both pregnant and nonpregnant women as well as those taking oral contraceptives. Follow-up reports on 117 pregnant patients revealed no adverse effects or complications attributable to miconazole in infants born to these women.

Indications: Treatment of vulvovaginal candidiasis (moniliasis). Since it is effective only for candidal infections of the vulvovaginal area, other pathogens commonly associated with vulvovaginitis (Trichomonas and *Haemophilus vaginalis*) should be ruled out by appropriate laboratory methods (KOH smears and/or cultures). Also for the treatment of tinea pedis (athlete's foot), tinea cruris, tinea corporis and tinea versicolor caused by dermatophytes.

Contraindications: Known hypersensitivity to miconazole nitrate.

Precautions: Discontinue use upon the appearance of any symptoms suggesting sensitivity or irritation. Since small amounts of the drug are absorbed from the vagina, it should be used in the first trimester of pregnancy only when the physician considers it essential to the welfare of the patient. Avoid contact with eyes.

Adverse Reactions: Those that occurred were usually reported during the first week of therapy. Vulvovaginal burning, itching or irritation occurred in 6.6% of 528 patients, while other complications such as vaginal burning, pelvic cramps, hives, skin rash and headache rarely occurred (each less than 0.2%).

Dosage and Administration: *Intravaginally.* Insert 1 applicatorful into the vagina once daily at bedtime for 7 days. The course of therapy may be repeated after other pathogens have been ruled out. *Topically.* Sufficient cream should be applied to cover the affected areas twice daily, morning and evening and once daily in patients with tinea versicolor. Candida infections should be treated for 2 weeks and dermatophyte infections for 1 month in order to reduce the possibility of recurrence. Massage treated area gently until cream disappears. In intertriginous areas, the cream should be applied sparingly.

Availability:
MICATIN: **(Johnson & Johnson)**
Cream, 2% in tubes of 15 and 30 gm.
Lotion, 2% in bottles of 12 and 30 ml.
MONISTAT® 7 Cream, 2% in tubes of 47 gm with measured-dose applicator. **(Ortho)**

MINOCYCLINE HYDROCHLORIDE

Chemical Name: 7-Dimethylamino-6-deoxy-6-demethyl tetracycline hydrochloride.

Description: Minocycline hydrochloride is a semi-synthetic derivative of tetracycline. Its antibacterial action is similar to that of other tetracyclines with activity against a wide range of gram-negative and gram-positive organisms; however, its therapeutic effectiveness is achieved at lower dosages. It is active against gonorrhea organisms, and shows moderate in vitro activity against certain strains of staphylococci which have been found resistant to other tetracyclines. A minocycline-susceptibility powder may be used for additional susceptibility testing. In tube dilution testing, microorganisms may be considered susceptible (likely to respond to minocycline therapy) if the minimum inhibitory concentration (M.I.C.) is not more than 4 mcg/ml. Microorganisms may be considered intermediate (harboring partial resistance) if the M.I.C. is 4 to 12.5 mcg/ml and resistant (not likely to respond to minocycline therapy) if the M.I.C. is greater than 12.5 mcg/ml. In susceptibility plate testing, if the Kirby-Bauer method of susceptibility testing (using a 30 mcg tetracycline disc) gives a zone of 18 mm or greater, the bacterial strain is considered to be susceptible to any tetracycline.

Studies to date have indicated that the absorption of minocycline from the gastrointestinal tract is not notably affected by the presence of foods and dairy products. Absorption is impaired when minocycline is administered concomitantly with antacids containing aluminum, calcium or magnesium. Oral administration of the C-labeled drug in dogs produced high blood concentration and extensive distribution to all tissues. When given to rats and dogs, minocycline has been found to produce discoloration of the thyroid gland with changes in thyroid function; however, no change in thyroid function has been observed in patients treated with this antibiotic.

Following a single oral dose of 200 mg administered to 10 normal individuals, serum levels ranged from 0.74 to 4.45 mcg/ml (average 2.24) in 1 hour, and from 0.34 to 2.36 mcg/ml (average 1.25) in 12 hours. The serum half-life following a single 200-mg dose in 12 essentially normal individuals ranged from 11 to 17 hours, in 7 patients with hepatic dysfunction from 11 to 16 hours, in 5 patients with renal dysfunction from 18 to 69 hours. The urinary and fecal recovery of minocycline when administered to 12 normal individuals is ½ to ⅓ that of other tetracyclines.

For Indications, Contraindications, Warnings, Precautions and Adverse Reactions, see monograph on Tetracycline Hydrochloride.

Dosage and Administration: *Orally* or *intravenously.* The usual dosage for adults is 200 mg initially followed by 100 mg every 12 hours and for children, 4 mg/kg of body weight initially followed by 2 mg/kg every 12 hours. Therapy should be continued for at least 24 to 48 hours after symptoms and fever have subsided. For the treatment of syphilis, the usual dosage should be administered over a period of 10 to 15 days. Close follow-up, including laboratory tests, is recommended. For treatment of gonorrhea in patients in whom penicillin is contraindicated, a dose of 200 mg initially followed by 100 mg every 12 hours for a minimum of 4 days; post-therapy cultures should be undertaken within 2 to 3 days. In the treatment of meningococcal carrier state, the recommended dosage is 100 mg every 12 hours for 5 days.

Availability:

MINOCIN®: **(Lederle)**

Capsules, 50 mg in bottles of 100 and in unit-dose strips of 10 in packages of 10; 100 mg in bottles of 50 and 100 and in unit-dose strips of 10 in packages of 10.

Injection (IV) in vials of 100 mg.

Syrup, 50 mg/5 ml (yellow, custard-flavored) in bottles of 60 ml.

VECTRIN®: **(Parke-Davis)**

Capsules, 50 and 100 mg in bottles of 50 and in unit-dose packages of 100.

Injection (IV) in Steri-Vial®'s of 100 mg.

Syrup, 50 mg/5 ml in bottles of 60 ml.

MITHRAMYCIN

Description: Mithramycin is a potent antineoplastic agent and occurs as a yellow, crystalline compound produced by a microorganism, *Streptomyces plicatus.*

Although the exact mechanism by which mithramycin inhibits tumors is not known, studies have shown that it forms a complex with deoxyribonucleic acid (DNA) and inhibits the synthesis of cellular and enzymic ribonucleic acid (RNA). The binding of mithramycin to DNA in the presence of magnesium (or other bivalent cations) is responsible for the inhibition of DNA-dependent or DNA-directed synthesis of RNA. This action presumably accounts for the biological properties of this drug.

Mithramycin shows potent cytotoxicity against malignant cells of human origin (Hela cells) growing in tissue culture; it is lethal to Hela cells in 48 hours at concentrations as low as 0.5 mcg/ml of tissue culture medium. It also shows significant antitumor activity against experimental leukemia in mice when administered intraperitoneally.

Indications: Treatment of carefully selected hospitalized patients with malignant testicular tumors resistant to surgical intervention or radiation therapy, or both. On the basis of limited clinical experience to date, the drug may also be considered for the treatment of certain symptomatic patients with hypercalcemia and hypercalciuria associated with a variety of advanced neoplasms. The use of mithramycin in other types of neoplastic diseases is not recommended at the present time.

Contraindications: Thrombocytopenia, thrombocytopathy, coagulation disorders, or an increased susceptibility to bleeding due to other causes, impaired bone-marrow function. The drug should not be used initially to treat ambulatory patients or those who cannot be observed carefully and frequently during and after therapy. Appropriate laboratory facilities are mandatory.

Warnings: Patients should be given the drug only when in a hospital where necessary laboratory facilities are readily available, and by or under the supervision of a physician who is experienced in the use of chemotherapy for cancer; these precautions are deemed essential because of the possibility of serious adverse reactions. Severe thrombocytopenia, tendency to bleed and even death may result from the use of mithramycin. Although severe toxicity is more apt to occur in patients with advanced disease or who are otherwise considered poor risks for therapy, serious toxicity may also occur occasionally even in patients who are in relatively good condition. Each patient should be evaluated carefully with regard to the potential benefits versus the risk of toxicity with this drug.

Precautions: *See Warnings also.* Electrolyte imbalance, especially hypocalcemia, hypokalemia and hypophosphatemia, should be corrected before initiating therapy with mithramycin. The drug should be used with extreme caution in patients with significant impairment of renal or hepatic function. Platelet count, prothrombin and bleeding times should be determined frequently during therapy and for several days after the last dose. Thrombocytopenia or significantly prolonged prothrombin or bleeding time is an indication for terminating therapy.

Adverse Reactions: The most important manifestation of toxicity consists of a bleeding syndrome that usually begins in the nose. In some cases, however, this hemorrhagic syndrome can start with hematemesis which may progress to more widespread hemorrhage in the gastrointestinal tract or to a generalized tendency to bleed. This predisposition to abnormal hemostasis is probably due to abnormalities in multiple clotting factors. Evidence suggests that this hemorrhagic syndrome is related to dosage and duration of treatment. The most common reactions (nonhemorrhagic) consist of gastrointestinal symptoms such as anorexia, nausea, vomiting, diarrhea and stomatitis. Other less frequently reported reactions include fever, drowsiness, weakness, lethargy, malaise, headache, depression, phlebitis, flushed face and skin rash. The following laboratory abnormalities have been reported during therapy, and in most instances were reversible following withdrawal of the drug: *Hematologic:* depression of platelet count, white cell count, hemoglobin and prothrombin content, elevated clotting and bleeding times; abnormal clot retraction; rare instances of leukopenia. *Liver Function:* increased levels of SGOT, SGPT, lactic dehydrogenase, alkaline phosphatase, serum bilirubin, ornithine carbamyl transferase, isocitric dehydrogenase, and increased retention of bromsulphalein. *Renal Function:* increased BUN and serum creatinine; proteinuria. *Electrolyte concentrations:* depressed serum calcium, phosphorus and potassium. Extravasation of the solution may result in local irritation and cellulitis at the injection site. Should thrombophlebitis or perivascular cellulitis occur, the infusion should be terminated and reinstituted at another site. The application of moderate heat to the site of extravasation may help to disperse the compound and minimize discomfort and local tissue irritation. The use of antiemetic agents prior to and during treatment may be helpful in relieving nausea and vomiting.

Dosage and Administration: *Intravenously.* The appropriate daily dose should be diluted in 1 liter of 5% glucose in water and infused slowly over a period of 4 to 6 hours. *Treatment of testicular tumors:* The recommended daily dose is 25 mcg, but not more than 30 mcg/kg of body weight, for a period of 8 to 10 days provided significant side effects or evidence of toxicity are not manifest during therapy. In the absence of a favorable response, additional courses of therapy at monthly intervals are warranted. *Treatment of hypercalcemia and hypercalciuria associated with neoplasia:* The recommended daily dose is 25 mcg/kg of body weight for 3 or 4 days. Additional courses of therapy may be given at intervals of 1 week or more to achieve the desired result or to maintain serum and urinary calcium excretion at normal levels. Renal function should be monitored carefully before, during and after treatment. When used during pregnancy or in women of childbearing potential, the anticipated benefits should be weighed against the potential hazards to embryo or fetus.

To reconstitute, add aseptically 4.9 ml of sterile water for injection to the contents of the vial and shake to effect solution. Each ml of the resultant solution will contain 500 mcg of mithramycin. Unused portions of the solution must be discarded. Fresh solutions must be prepared in the above manner each day of therapy.

Availability:
MITHRACIN® (freeze-dried) for injection in vials of 2.5 mg (2500 mcg) with 100 mg of mannitol and disodium phosphate to adjust to pH 7. These vials must be stored in a refrigerator (below 10° C). **(Pfizer)**

MITOMYCIN

Description: Mitomycin is a potent antineoplastic agent and occurs as a deep blue-violet crystalline compound produced by the microorganism *Streptomyces caespitosus.* It also possesses a wide range of antibacterial activity.

Although the exact mechanism by which mitomycin inhibits tumor growth is not fully understood, studies have shown that it forms a complex with deoxyribonucleic acid (DNA)—guanine and cytosine content correlates with the degree of mitomycin-induced cross-linking—and in high concentrations it suppresses cellular and enzymatic ribonucleic acid (RNA) synthesis and protein synthesis.

Following intravenous injection in dogs, mitomycin appeared in the urine within 5 to 6 minutes, and approximately 18 to 29% was recovered within 1 hour. Simultaneous creatinine clearance studies revealed that excretion is primarily by glomerular filtration. In children given intravenous doses, the urinary recovery was about 5 to 20% within 1 hour and practically all of the drug was recovered in 2 hours.

Patients receiving this drug must be selected on the basis of possible therapeutic benefit versus the inherent risk since this drug has been found to be carcinogenic in mice and rats. Mitomycin produced a greater than 100% increase in tumor incidence in male Sprague-Dawley rats and a greater than 50% increase in tumor development in female Swiss mice. The animals were given the maximum tolerated doses intraperitoneally 3 times a week for 6 months and were observed for a 12-month period. These doses approximate those recommended for clinical use.

Indications: As a palliative form of therapy or as a component of various approved chemotherapeutic agents for the treatment of disseminated adenocarcinoma of the stomach or pancreas as an adjunctive measure to surgery and radiation.

Contraindications: Prior hypersensitivity to mitomycin, thrombocytopenia, coagulation disorders, or an increased susceptibility to bleeding due to other causes.

Warnings: It is recommended that mitomycin be administered preferably to hospitalized patients who can be observed carefully and frequently during and after treatment, and where the necessary laboratory facilities are readily available. It should be administered under the supervision of a physician who is experienced in the use of chemotherapy for cancer; these precautions are deemed essential because of the possibility of undesirable effects, especially those associated with the high incidence of bone marrow depression, and renal toxicity. Severe thrombocytopenia and leukopenia, a tendency to bleed, and even death may result—poor-risk patients are especially vulnerable—from the use of this drug. Each patient should be carefully evaluated with regard to the potential benefits versus the risk of toxicity of mitomycin. Safe use in pregnant women has not been established.

Precautions: *See Warnings also.* The drug should be used with care in patients with significant impairment of renal function, or with any evidence of bone marrow depression. Platelet count, prothrombin and bleeding times, differential and hemoglobin studies should be performed frequently during and for at least 7 weeks following therapy. Treatment should be suspended or modified when drug-induced bone marrow depression has resulted in a platelet count below 75,000 and a white blood cell count below 4000, or a significant prolongation of prothrombin or bleeding time. Patients should also be observed for any evidence of renal toxicity.

Adverse Reactions: The most common and serious complication resulting from the use of mitomycin is bone marrow toxicity characterized by thrombocytopenia and/or leukopenia. These may occur any time within 8 weeks after onset of therapy with an average of 4 weeks. It was observed that in 25% of patients treated with this drug, bone marrow function did not return to pretreatment status. The highest incidence of bone marrow toxicity appears to occur when the drug is administered daily for 6 or more days followed by alternate day therapy. The lowest incidence occurred when doses were given daily for 2 to 5 days, followed thereafter by a weekly or twice weekly dosage schedule. There appears to be no correlation between the total dose administered and bone marrow toxicity. Other acute side effects consisted of fever, anorexia, nausea, and vomiting. Alopecia, desquamation, induration, pruritus, pain on injection, cellulitis, ulceration and sloughing at the injection site which may result from extravasation of the drug, hemoptysis, dyspnea, coughing, pneumonia, and a significant rise in BUN in a few patients were also noted. The following conditions occurred but it has not been decided whether or not they were drug-induced: headache, blurring of vision, confusion, drowsiness, syncope, fatigue, edema, thrombophlebitis, anemia, hematemesis, diarrhea, and pain.

Dosage and Administration: *Intravenously* only. The recommended course of therapy is 20 mg/square meter of body surface as a single dose administered by means of a functioning catheter or 2 mg/M² daily for 5 days, followed by a drug-free interval of 2 days, and then 2 mg/M² daily for an additional 5 days (total initial dose is 20 mg/M² given over a period of 10 days). Doses exceeding 20 mg/M² have not been shown to be more effective and are more toxic than lower doses. If the disease continues to progress after 2 courses, therapy should be terminated since the probability of a response is minimal. When combined with other myelosuppressant agents, the dose of mitomycin should be individualized and adjusted appropriately.

Availability:
MUTAMYCIN® Injection in vials of 5 and 20 mg. **(Bristol)**

MITOTANE

Chemical Name: 1,1-Dichloro-2-(*o*-chlorophenyl)-2-(*p*-chlorophenyl)-ethane.

Description: Mitotane is the *ortho, para* isomer of the insecticide DDD (dichlorodiphenyldichloroethane), which is why it is frequently referred to as o,p'-DDD. It occurs as a white, granular, crystalline substance insoluble in water, slightly soluble in alcohol and in acetone, and soluble in chloroform.

The precise mechanism by which the drug is adrenotoxic is unknown. However, it has been postulated that it acts directly upon the cells of the adrenal cortex causing necrosis and atrophy. Available data suggest that o,p'-DDD modifies the peripheral metabolism of steroids and that it directly suppresses the adrenal cortex. The drug has been shown to alter the extra-adrenal metabolism of cortisol, leading to a reduction in measurable 17-hydroxycorticosteroids (17-OHCS) without an accompanying fall in plasma steroid levels. The drug apparently increases the formation of 6-β hydroxycortisol.

Clinical studies have shown that approximately 40% of an oral dose is absorbed, and about 10% is recovered in the urine as a water-soluble metabolite, a small amount of a metabolite is recovered in the bile, and that the balance of the ingested dose is found in most body tissues, fatty tissue being the primary repository.

Indications: Treatment of inoperable cases of functioning and nonfunctioning types of adrenocortical carcinoma.

Contraindications: Hypersensitivity to the drug.

Warnings: Treatment should be initiated in a hospital until a stable dosage schedule has been reached. The drug should be temporarily discontinued immediately following shock or severe trauma because of the drug's potential for inhibiting adrenal function. Replacement therapy with steroids should be instituted in these patients, since the depressed adrenals may take some time to overcome inertia before secreting endogenous corticosteroids. Because it is metabolized in the liver and excreted in the bile, o,p'-DDD should be given cautiously to patients with hepatic disease other than metastasis from the adrenal cortex. Since the drug's safety still is questionable, it should be used in women of childbearing potential and in nursing mothers only after considering the drug's anticipated benefits and its potential hazards to mother and child.

Precautions: To minimize the possibility of infarction and hemorrhage in a tumor due to a rapid, positive effect of the drug, all tumor tissue should be surgically removed, if possible, from large metastatic lesions before commencing therapy with o,p'-DDD. Long-term, continuous administration of high doses may lead to brain damage and its sequelae. Behavioral and neurologic studies should be undertaken at regular intervals when therapy is continued beyond 2 years. Treated patients may develop adrenal insufficiency, in which case consideration should be given to replacement therapy with adrenocortical steroids (see Warnings). Sedation, lethargy, vertigo and other CNS effects can occur. Ambulatory patients should therefore be cautioned not to drive or otherwise engage in any hazardous occupation requiring alertness or skill.

Adverse Reactions: Gastrointestinal disturbances (80%) usually consisted of anorexia, nausea or vomiting and, less frequently, diarrhea. CNS depression, manifested as lethargy and somnolence, was the most common (25%), while dizziness or vertigo was reported in about 15% of treated patients. Cutaneous eruptions were seen in about 15% of cases, although they did not appear to be dose-related in all instances. Infrequently occurring effects involved the eye (blurred vision, diplopia, lens opacity, toxic retinopathy); genitourinary system (hematuria, hemorrhagic cystitis and albuminuria), cardiovascular system (hypertension, orthostatic hypotension and flushing); and generalized aching, elevated temperature and lowered protein-bound iodine (PBI).

Dosage and Administration: *Orally.* Initially, 9 to 10 gm daily, divided into 3 or 4 equal doses, reduced to the lowest effective dose if side effects appear. If the patient can tolerate higher doses and improved clinical response is in sight, the dosage should be increased until adverse reactions occur. The highest tolerated dosage may vary from 2 to 16 gm daily, but usually ranges from 8 to 10 gm daily. Therapy should be continued so long as clinical benefits are observed. Maintenance of clinical status or retarded growth of metastatic lesions can be regarded as clinical benefits if they are undeniably apparent. If no clinical benefits are seen after 3 months at the maximal tolerated dosage (MTD), the case may be considered a clinical failure. However, 10% of the patients who showed a measurable response required more than 3 months at the MTD. Early diagnosis and prompt institution of treatment improve the probability of a positive response.

Availability:
LYSODREN® Tablets, 0.5 gm in bottles of 100. **(Calbiochem)**

MOLINDONE HYDROCHLORIDE

Chemical Name: 3-Ethyl-6,7-dihydro-2-methyl-5-(morpholinomethyl) indol-4(5*H*)-one hydrochloride.

Description: Molindone hydrochloride, an antipsychotic drug, is a dihydroindolone compound that is *not* structurally related to the phenothiazines, the butyrophenones or the thioxanthenes. It occurs as a white, crystalline powder, that is freely soluble in water and in alcohol. Its molecular weight is 312.67.

Preclinical studies have shown that the pharmacological actions of molindone predominantly resemble those of the major tranquilizers. It reduces spontaneous locomotion and aggressiveness, suppresses conditional response, counteracts the bizarre stereotyped behavior and hyperactivity induced by amphetamines, and the depression caused by tetrabenazine, a tranquilizing agent. In clinical studies, tranquilization is achieved without producing muscle relaxation or incoordinating effects. Based on EEG studies, molindone exerts its effect on the ascending reticular activating system. Metabolic studies have shown that the drug reaches peak blood levels within 1 hour, and that tranquilization is achieved without compromising alertness.

Indications: Management of the manifestations of schizophrenia.

Contraindications: Severe CNS depression due to alcohol, barbiturates, narcotics, or other centrally-acting depressants; comatose states; and known hypersensitivity to the drug.

Warnings: Although evidence of teratogenesis has not been observed in animal reproduction studies, the anticipated benefits must nevertheless be weighed against the potential hazards to the fetus. Since no data are available on its appearance in the milk of lactating mothers, routine precautions are advised when the drug is given to such patients. Use of molindone in children under 12 years of age is not recommended because safe and effective conditions for its usage have not been established.

Precautions: Since drowsiness may occur, especially during the early period of dosage adjustment, patients should be cautioned not to engage in activities that require alertness, judgment, and physical coordination. The physician should be aware that an antiemetic potential exists that may obscure signs of intestinal obstruction or brain tumor and that the calcium ions (calcium sulfate) in the formulation may interfere with the absorption of phenytoin sodium and tetracyclines.

Adverse Reactions: The most frequently noted was transient drowsiness. Less frequently noted were Parkinsonian reactions (akinesia characterized by rigidity, immobility, reduction of voluntary movement and tremor), akathisia, restlessness, insomnia, depression, dizziness, blurred vision, hyperactivity, euphoria, dry mouth, headache, nausea, tachycardia, weight gain or loss, thoughts of suicide, postural hypotension, initial heavy menses, amenorrhea, lactation, rash, spasticity, dystonia, oculogyric crisis, gastrointestinal upset, increased libido, leukopenia, and nonspecific EKG changes. Abrupt withdrawal of the drug after prolonged high dosage did not produce an abstinence syndrome. No increased toxicity has been observed when molindone was given concurrently with chloral hydrate, barbiturates, and antiparkinsonian drugs. It should be kept in mind that the adverse reactions that have been observed with the phenothiazines may possibly occur with this drug.

Dosage and Administration: *Orally.* Dosage is based on the severity of symptoms and may range from 15 to 60 mg daily in mild cases to 225 mg daily in severe cases. The initial dosage is 50 to 75 mg daily, increased to 100 mg daily in 3 or 4 days, then adjusted according to the clinical response. However, patients who are chronically resistent to the drug may require up to 400 mg daily to achieve a satisfactory response. Elderly and debilitated patients should be started on a lower dosage schedule. The usual maintenance dosage for mild symptoms is 5 to 15 mg and for moderate symptoms is 10 to 25 mg 3 or 4 times daily; for severe symptoms 225 mg daily. Dosages may be administered once daily.

Availability:
LIDONE™ Capsules, 5, 10 and 25 g in bottles of 100. **(Abbott)**
MOBAN® Tablets, 5 mg (orange), 10 mg (lavender) and 25 mg (light green) in bottles of 100 and 1000. **(Endo)**

MONOBENZONE

Chemical Name: *p*-(Benzylopy)phenol.

Description: Monobenzone, the monobenzyl ether of hydroquinone, is an antioxidant agent that is used to inhibit melanin production. It is practically insoluble in cold water but is very soluble in alcohol and ether. The process by which it produces its amelanotic activity is due to inhibition of tyrosinase, an enzyme responsible for the conversion of tyrosine to dihydroxyphenylalanine which is a precursor of melanin. Response to therapy may be delayed for at least a month since the drug neither destroys melanocytes nor facilitates the loss of previously synthesized melanin.

Indications: A potent depigmenting agent that is recommended only for total, irreversible (final) depigmentation in disseminated vitiligo.

Contraindications: Hypersensitivity to monobenzone.

Warnings: Depigmentation is usually observed within 1 to 4 months; therefore, if satisfactory results have not been obtained within this period, treatment should be regarded as a failure and should be discontinued. It is not recommended for such conditions as freckling, hyperpigmentation due to photosensitization following use of certain perfumes (berlock dermatitis), melasma (cholasma) of pregnancy, and hyperpigmentation following inflammation of the skin. It is of no value in the treatment of cafe-au-lait spots, pigmented nevi, malignant melanoma, or any pigmentation resulting from pigments other than melanin, including bile, silver, and artificial pigments.

Precautions: Avoid use if early vitiligo is suspected. Sunlight exposure to treated areas tends to neutralize the depigmenting effect.

Adverse Reactions: In non-Caucasians, undesirable depigmentation can result. Discontinue use if irritation, burning sensation or dermatitis occurs.

Dosage and Administration: *Topically.* Apply 2 or 3 times daily until the desired results are achieved, and then twice weekly to maintain the effect.

Availability:
BENOQUIN Ointment, 20% in tubes of 15 and 38 gm and in jars of 453.6 gm. **(Elder)**

MORPHINE Ⓒ

Description: Morphine, a narcotic analgesic, is the principal alkaloid of opium. It is a complex derivative of phenanthrene containing a lactam ether linkage between carbons 4 and 5 of the phenanthrene group. Its analgesic and narcotic properties are due chiefly to a phenolic OH group at position 3 and an alcoholic OH group at C-6. Morphine sulfate occurs as white crystals or as a white, crystalline powder that is soluble in water, slightly soluble in alcohol and insoluble in chloroform and ether. Although it is readily absorbed from the gastrointestinal tract, parenteral administration assures more reliable activity.

The precise mechanism of action is unknown but it is assumed to act on basic enzymes systems. Physiologic studies suggest that there are specific receptors in the brain. The dominant feature of the drug is its descending depression of the CNS. Its apparent stimulant effects have been found to be attributable to depression of inhibitory mechanisms. Morphine depresses the cerebral cortex and medullary centers after initially stimulating them. The reflexes and spinal functions are predominantly stimulated. The drug depresses the respiratory center and the cough reflex, stimulates the vomiting center, constricts the pupils, increases the smooth muscle tone of the gastrointestinal and genitourinary tracts, and produces mild vasodilatation. Morphine exerts its analgesic action primarily by increasing the pain threshold and by dulling the sensibility or reaction to pain. Euphoria is frequently experienced as a result of the relief obtained. Tolerance may develop so that increasingly larger doses are needed to relieve a given degree of pain, and addiction ordinarily develops following prolonged administration.

The maximal analgesic effect occurs in 20 minutes after intravenous injection, in 30 to 60 minutes after intramuscular injection, and in 60 to 90 minutes after subcutaneous injection. Analgesia usually persists for 4 hours, but in some patients it may last up to 7 hours. In the liver, morphine is conjugated with glucuronic acid to form 3-glucuronide which passes into the bile and is reabsorbed and excreted in the urine. Small amounts of free morphine are also excreted in the urine. Approximately 90% of the total excretion occurs within the first 24 hours.

Indications: Symptomatic relief of severe pain, as a preanesthetic medication, and as a soporific in selected cases. For the relief of acute visceral pain, atropine is added to the regimen to counteract the spasmodic effect of morphine.

Contraindications: Bronchial asthma, respiratory depression, idiosyncrasy or hypersensitivity to the drug.

Warnings: Morphine may be habit-forming and has the potential for being abused. Psychic dependence, physical dependence, and tolerance may develop upon repeated administration. Utmost caution is advised when the drug is administered to patients with increased intracranial pressure, an acute asthmatic attack, chronic obstructive pulmonary disease or cor pulmonale, since fatalities have occurred, and to those with preexisting respiratory depression, hypoxia, or hypercapnia. Severe hypotension may occur in any individual whose ability to maintain blood pressure has already been compromised by a depleted blood volume or by the concurrent administration of drugs such as the phenothiazines or certain anesthetics. Ambulatory patients may experience orthostatic hypotension, and syncope may occur due primarily to peripheral vasodilatation. Because rapid intravenous administration increases the possible occurrence of severe respiratory depression or hypotension, it is recommended that the injection be given very slowly. Patients should be cautioned that the sedative effect of morphine may impair their alertness and physical coordination required for hazardous tasks. As with any drug, its use during pregnancy requires careful consideration of the benefits versus the risks to the mother and fetus.

Precautions: Morphine produces adverse reactions which may obscure the diagnosis or clinical course of acute abdominal conditions or head injuries. Particular caution is advised and the initial dose reduced when the drug is given to elderly or debilitated patients, to infants, and to those with severe impairment of hepatic or renal function, to patients with asthma, hypothyroidism, toxic psychoses, Addison's disease, prostatic hypertrophy or urethral stricture. Patients with supraventricular tachycardias require special care because of a possible vagolytic action which may produce a significant increase in the rate of ventricular response. Morphine may aggravate preexisting convulsions in patients with convulsive disorders, and if the dosage is escalated substantially above those recommended, convulsions may occur in those individuals who have no history of such disorders. The drug should be used with caution and in reduced dosage in patients who are concurrently receiving other narcotic analgesics, general anesthetics, phenothiazines, other tranquilizers, sedative-hypnotics, tricyclic antidepressants and other CNS depressants including alcohol. Morphine sulfate should not be added to intravenous fluids. It has been found to be incompatible with aminophylline, sulfisoxazole diolamine, meperidine hydrochloride, and with the sodium salts of amobarbital, chlorothiazide, phenytoin, heparin, methicillin, nitrofurantoin, novobiocin, phenobarbital, bicarbonate, iodide, sulfadiazine, and thiopental. It may on occasion be injected through the Y-tube of administration sets.

Adverse Reactions: The major hazards are respiratory depression, and to a lesser degree, circulatory depression, since respiratory arrest, shock and cardiac arrest have occurred. The most frequently observed untoward effects include lightheadedness, dizziness, sedation, nausea, vomiting, and sweating. These seem to be more prominent in ambulatory patients and in those who are not experiencing severe pain. In such individuals, lower doses are advisable. Some adverse reactions in ambulatory patients may be alleviated if the patient lies down. Other reactions include euphoria, dysphoria, weakness, headache, agitation, tremor, uncoordinated muscle movements, transient hallucinations, disorientation and visual disturbances; dry mouth, constipation, and biliary tract spasm; flushing of the face, tachycardia, bradycardia, palpitation, faintness and syncope; urinary retention; antidiuretic effect; pruritus, urticaria, other skin rashes, rarely hemorrhagic urticaria. Wheal and flare over the vein with intravenous injection may occur. Pain at the injection site, local tissue irritation and induration following subcutaneous injection, particularly when repeated, have also been noted. A suitable narcotic antagonist such as nalorphine should be readily available to counteract toxic effects.

Dosage and Administration: *Subcutaneously, intramuscularly* or *intravenously* (very slowly). The usual range is from 5 to 20 mg every 4 hours as needed.

Availability:

C-II Morphine Sulfate

Injection, 8, 10 and 15 mg/ml in ampuls of 1 ml. **(Knoll)**

Injection, 15 mg/ml in ampuls of 20 ml. **(Lilly)**

Injection, 15 mg/ml in Steri-Dose® (disposable syringes) of 1 ml in packages of 10. **(Parke-Davis)**

Injection, 10 and 15 mg/ml in Carpujects® (half-filled syringes) of 2 ml. **(Winthrop)**
Injection, 2 and 4 mg/ml in Tubex® sterile cartridge-needle units of 1 ml; 8, 10 and 15 mg/ml in Tubex(s) of 1 ml and in half-filled containers of 2 ml. **(Wyeth)**
Tablets (hypodermic), 10 mg in bottles of 100; 15 and 30 mg in bottles of 100 and 500. **(Lilly)**

w/Atropine Sulfate
Injection in vials of 30 ml. Each ml contains morphine sulfate, 16 mg and atropine sulfate, 0.4 mg. **(Beecham)**
Injection in ampuls of 20 ml. Each ml contains morphine sulfate, 15 mg and atropine sulfate, 0.4 mg. **(Lilly)**
Tablets (hypodermic) in bottles of 100. Each tablet contains morphine sulfate, 15 mg and atropine sulfate, 0.4 mg. **(Lilly)**

MSC TRIAMINIC

Description: Each timed-release tablet contains phenylpropanolamine hydrochloride, 50 mg; pheniramine maleate, 25 mg; pyrilamine maleate, 25 mg and methscopolamine nitrate, 4 mg.

Indications: Relief from symptoms of nasal congestion especially when associated with excessive secretion such as profuse nasal discharge or postnasal drip that frequently occurs in common colds, sinusitis and nasal allergy.

Contraindications: Glaucoma and prostatic hypertrophy.

Precautions: Since drowsiness may occur, patients should be warned against operating dangerous machinery requiring alertness or motor coordination. Use with caution in the presence of hypertension, hyperthyroidism, cardiovascular disease or diabetes.

Adverse Reactions: Occasional drowsiness, blurred vision, cardiac palpitations, flushing, dizziness, nervousness or gastrointestinal upsets.

Dosage and Administration: *Orally.* Adults and children over 12 years of age, 1 tablet 3 times daily, in morning, midafternoon and at bedtime. Tablets should be swallowed whole.

Availability:
MSC TRIAMINIC® Tablets in bottles of 50. **(Dorsey)**

MULVIDREN-F: see The Fluoride-Vitamins

MUMPS IMMUNE GLOBULIN, HUMAN

Description: A solution containing about 16.5% of the gamma globulin fraction of the serum of healthy adults who have been hyperimmunized with mumps virus vaccine. The antibody content, as determined by complement fixation tests, is approximately 20 times that of the unconcentrated human hyperimmune serum.

Indications: Conferring passive immunity upon individuals exposed to mumps. The protection of adults who have been exposed to mumps but who never had the disease during childhood is of particular importance because of the serious nature of complications which often follow mumps. There is evidence that the globulin is effective in the treatment and reduction of complications when adequate dosage is used sufficiently early.

Adverse Reactions: Some slight soreness may be expected at the injection site, but systemic reactions to human gamma globulin preparations are very rare.

Dosage and Administration: *Intramuscularly,* preferably in the gluteal muscle. *Should not be administered intravenously. Prophylaxis:* For individuals up to 90 lbs, 1.5 ml; between 90 and

140 lbs, 3 ml; over 140 lbs, 4.5 ml. The full dose should be given at once within 1 week after exposure. If exposure continues or recurs, the dose should be repeated at intervals of 1 to 2 weeks as long as exposure continues. *Treatment:* Administration must be started as early as possible. The dose must be larger than for prophylaxis, or repeated after 24 to 48 hours, with further dosage if mumps reappears or fails to disappear.

Availability:
HYPAROTIN® in vials of 1.5 and 4.5 ml. **(Cutter)**

MUMPS VIRUS VACCINE, LIVE, ATTENUATED

Description: This vaccine is prepared from the Jeryl Lynn (B Level) strain, named after the patient from whom the virus was initially recovered. According to the general procedures of Enders, the virus used to prepare the vaccine is grown in cell cultures of chick embryos which were free of avian leukosis, and thoroughly tested for safety and efficacy.

Clinical studies in susceptible children and adults have shown that a single dose induced an effective antibody response in about 98% of cases. Evidence also indicates that the infection induced by the vaccine is not contagious. Antibodies induced by the vaccine persist for at least 6 years without substantial decline, and the pattern of antibody closely resembles that observed for natural mumps although the antibody level is significantly lower than that following the natural infection. If this pattern continues, permanent immunization is to be expected; nevertheless, continued surveillance is still required.

Indications: Immunization against mumps in children 15 months of age and older (but may be given as early as 12 months), and in adolescents and adults who have not had mumps, or who are not sure that they have had mumps.

Contraindications: Sensitivity to eggs, chicken, chicken feathers, or neomycin (25 mcg), primary immuno-deficiency states, including cellular immune deficiencies, hypogammaglobulinemic and dysgammaglobulinemic states, in patients with blood dyscrasias, leukemia, lymphomas of any type, or other malignancies affecting the bone marrow or lymphatic systems, or those receiving corticosteroids, irradiation, alkylating agents or antimetabolites, pregnancy, in patients with an active infection, unless the chance of clinical mumps involves greater risk.

Precautions: *For subcutaneous administration only.* Do not administer with other vaccines; allow 1 month to elapse between elective immunizations with the exception of monovalent or trivalent poliovirus vaccine, live, oral, which may be administered simultaneously. Vaccination should be deferred for at least 3 months following blood transfusions, or the administration of human plasma or more than 0.02 ml/lb of body weight of human immune serum globulin. The tuberculin test should be scheduled 4 weeks or more before immunization in order to prevent a false-negative response. At the time of vaccination pregnancy should be ruled out, and women should be cautioned not to become pregnant within the 3 months following vaccination, since the potential unfavorable effects of the vaccine on fetal development are not known.

Adverse Reactions: Mild fever occurs occasionally. Parotitis, purpura and allergic reactions such as urticaria have been rarely reported. Epinephrine should be available for immediate use if needed.

Dosage and Administration: The total volume of reconstituted vaccine, containing not less than 5000 $TCID_{50}$ (tissue culture infectious doses), is injected *subcutaneously* into the outer aspect of the upper arm.

Availability:
MUMPSVAX® (lyophilized), in single-dose vials containing 5000 $TCID_{50}$ with disposable syringe containing diluent. **(Merck Sharp & Dohme)**

M.V.I.

Description: M.V.I. (Multi-Vitamin Infusion) is a solution of water-solubilized vitamins A, D and

E together with vitamin B complex and vitamin C. The solution is ready for use when added directly to any infusion fluid. Each 10-ml ampul or 5-ml vial (concentrate) provides:

Ascorbic acid		500 mg
Vitamin A	(10,000 U.S.P. units)	3 mg
Ergocalciferol	(1000 U.S.P. units)	25 μg
Thiamine hydrochloride		50 mg
Riboflavin		10 mg
Niacinamide		100 mg
Pyridoxine hydrochloride		15 mg
Dexpanthenol		25 mg
dl-α-tocopheryl acetate		5 IU

Each 10 ml ampul also contains sorethytan laurate, 1%; sodium hydroxide, 1% and gentisic acid ethanolamide, 2% as preservative. Each 5 ml concentrate also contains propylene glycol, 30%; sodium hydroxide for pH adjustment, and sorethytan laurate, 1.6%; the riboflavin in Concentrate as riboflavin-5-phosphate.

Indications: Emergency feedings in stress situations with profound alterations in the body's metabolic demands and consequent tissue depletion of nutrients. These situations may be provoked by surgery, extensive burns, fractures and other trauma, severe infectious diseases, comatose states, etc.

Precautions: Intravenous administration of thiamine has been known to cause allergic reactions. Should not be injected directly into a vein, undiluted, as it may give rise to dizziness, faintness, etc. Intravenous use should be discontinued as early as practical in favor of intramuscular or oral vitamins.

Dosage and Administration: *For dilution in intravenous infusions only.* One daily dose of 10 ml of M.V.I. solution or 5 ml of M.V.I Concentrate added directly to not less than 500 ml, preferably 1000 ml, of intravenous dextrose, saline, or similar infusion solutions (plasma, protein hydrolysates).

Availability:
M.V.I.® CONCENTRATE in vials of 5 ml. **(USV)**
M.V.I.® Solution in ampuls of 10 ml. **(USV)**

MYRINGACAINE

Description: Myringacaine is an otic solution possessing vasoconstrictor, analgesic and hygroscopic properties. Each ml in a base of glycerin and propylene glycol contains:

Benzocaine	4%
Ephedrine hydrochloride	0.44%
Orthohydroxyphenylmercuric chloride	0.05%

Indications: Adjunct to antibiotics for the relief of pain associated with myringitis (inflammation of the ear drum) which may be secondary to external otitis or otitis media.

Precautions: Since this product fundamentally is palliative, it should not be relied upon as the sole treatment in infections of the external auditory canal or of the middle ear. Treatment of these infections should include concurrent administration of appropriate antibiotic or chemotherapeutic agents.

Adverse Reactions: Occasional sensitivity to one of the components, in which case therapy should be discontinued and appropriate therapy instituted.

Dosage and Administration: *Topically.* Instill into the external ear canal every 1 to 3 hours, and retain with a tampon.

Availability:
MYRINGACAINE® Otic Solution in bottles of 15 ml with dropper. **(Upjohn)**

NAFCILLIN: see The Penicillins

NALDECON

Description: Each sustained-action tablet, 5 ml of syrup or 1 ml of drops contains:

	Tablets	*Syrup*	*Pediatric Syrup or Drops*
Phenylpropanolamine hydrochloride	40 mg	20 mg	5 mg
Phenylephrine hydrochloride	10 mg	5 mg	1.25 mg
Phenyltoloxamine citrate	15 mg	7.5 mg	2 mg
Chlorpheniramine maleate	5 mg	2.5 mg	0.5 mg

Indications: Relief of distressing symptoms of colds and other upper respiratory infections, acute and chronic sinusitis, hay fever, and other pollen allergies such as rhinorrhea, postnasal drip, nasal and/or sinus congestion, lacrimation, sneezing, itching of eyes and nose, and head stuffiness.

Contraindications: Unusual sensitivity to any of the ingredients.

Precautions: Drowsiness may occur; therefore, patients should be cautioned not to drive or to engage in activities requiring alertness or skill. Patients with high blood pressure, heart disease, diabetes mellitus, thyroid disease, glaucoma, peripheral vascular disorders or prostatic hypertrophy should be cautioned to use only as directed by the physician.

Dosage and Administration: *Orally. Tablets:* Adults and children over 12 years of age, 1 tablet 3 times daily (morning, midafternoon and at bedtime). Children 6 to 12 years of age, ½ tablet on the same schedule. *Syrup:* Adults and children 12 years of age and over, 1 teaspoonful (5 ml) every 3 or 4 hours. Dosage should not exceed 4 teaspoonsful (20 ml) in 24 hours. Children 6 to 12 years of age, ½ teaspoonful every 3 or 4 hours. Dosage should not exceed 2 teaspoonsful (10 ml) in 24 hours. *Pediatric drops and syrup:* Children 3 to 6 months of age, ¼ dropper (0.25 ml) of drops; 6 to 12 months, ½ dropper (0.5 ml) of drops or ½ teaspoon of syrup; 1 to 6 years, 1 dropperful (1 ml) of drops or 1 teaspoonful (5 ml) of syrup; 6 to 12 years, 2 teaspoonsful (10 ml) of syrup. Doses should be administered every 3 to 4 hours and should not exceed 4 doses in a 24-hour period.

Availability:
NALDECON®: **(Bristol)**
Pediatric Drops in bottles of 20 ml.
Pediatric Syrup in bottles of 1 pint.
Syrup in bottles of 1 pint.
Tablets in bottles of 100 and 500.

NALIDIXIC ACID

Chemical Name: 1-Ethyl-1, 4-dihydro-7-methyl-4-oxo-1, 8-naphthyridine-3-carboxylic acid.

Description: Nalidixic acid, a naphthyridine derivative, is an antibacterial agent unrelated to sulfonamides, antibiotics or nitrofurans. It occurs as a pale yellow crystalline substance that is soluble in highly alkaline solutions and in chloroform and practically insoluble in alcohol.

This drug has marked antibacterial activity against gram-negative bacteria including *Proteus mirabilis, P. morganii, P. vulgaris,* and *P. rettgeri; Escherichia coli;* Aerobacter; and Klebsiella. Pseudomonas strains are generally resistant to the drug. It is bactericidal and is effective over the entire urinary pH range. Cross resistance between nalidixic acid and oxolinic acid has been observed. Fungal overgrowth during administration of this agent has not been reported.

Following oral administration, it is rapidly absorbed from the gastrointestinal tract, partially metabolized in the liver, and rapidly excreted through the kidneys. Unchanged nalidixic acid appears in the urine along with an active metabolite, hydroxynalidixic acid, which has antibacterial activity similar to that of nalidixic acid. Other metabolites include glucuronic acid conjugates of nalidixic acid and hydroxynalidixic acid, and the dicarboxylic acid derivative.

The hydroxy metabolite represents 30% of the biologically active drug in the blood and 85% in the urine. Peak serum levels of active drug average approximately 20 to 40 mcg/ml (90% protein bound) 1 to 2 hours after administration of a 1-gm dose to a fasting normal individual. The half-life is about 90 minutes. Peak urine levels of active drug average approximately 150 to 200 mcg/ml 3 to 4 hours after administration, with a half-life of about 6 hours. Approximately 4% of the drug is excreted in the feces. Traces of nalidixic acid were found in the blood and urine of infants whose mothers had received the drug during the last trimester of pregnancy.

Indications: Treatment of acute and chronic genitourinary tract infections caused by sensitive gram-negative bacteria including Proteus, *E. coli,* Aerobacter and Klebsiella, and certain strains of Pseudomonas. Disc susceptibility testing with the 30-mcg disc should be performed prior to administration of the drug, and during treatment if clinical response warrants.

Contraindications: In patients with known hypersensitivity to the drug, and in those with a history of convulsive disorders.

Warnings: Nalidixic acid is not recommended in the first trimester of pregnancy; however, it has been used during the last 2 trimesters without producing apparent ill effects in either mother or fetus. Toxic psychosis, convulsions, and increased intracranial pressure may develop in patients taking more than the recommended dosage. (see Adverse Reactions).

Precautions: Periodic blood, renal and liver function tests are advisable if treatment lasts more than 1 or 2 weeks. The dosage recommended should not be arbitrarily doubled unless under the careful supervision of a physician. It should be used with caution in patients with liver disease, epilepsy, or severe cerebral arteriosclerosis, and in those with severely impaired kidney function. Patients should be cautioned to avoid unnecessary exposure to direct sunlight and, if a photosensitivity reaction occurs, therapy should be discontinued. Bacteria may develop resistance to the drug, or resistant organisms, not previously present or identified, may emerge. Periodic cultures and bacterial sensitivity tests are advisable, particularly if the response is unsatisfactory or if relapse occurs. Nalidixic acid may enhance the effects of oral anticoagulants, warfarin or bishydroxycoumarin, by displacing significant amounts from serum albumin binding sites. When Benedict's or Fehling's solutions or Clinitest® Reagent Tablets are used to test the urine of patients taking nalidixic acid, a false-positive reaction for glucose may be obtained, due to the liberation of glucuronic acid from the metabolites excreted. However, a colorimetric test for glucose based on an enzyme reaction (e.g., with Clinistix® Reagent Strips or Tes-Tape®) does not give a false-positive reaction to the liberated glucuronic acid. Incorrect values may be obtained for urinary 17-keto and ketogenic steroids in patients receiving this drug, because of an interaction between nalidixic acid and the *m*-dinitrobenzene used in the usual assay method. In such cases, the Porter-Silber test for 17-hydroxycorticoids may be used.

Adverse Reactions: Reactions reported following therapeutic doses include *CNS effects:* drowsiness, weakness, headache, dizziness and vertigo. Reversible subjective visual disturbances without objective findings have occurred infrequently (generally with each dose during the first few days of treatment). These reactions include overbrightness of lights, change in color perception, difficulty in focusing, decrease in visual acuity, and double vision. They usually disappeared promptly when dosage was reduced or therapy was discontinued. Toxic psychosis or brief convulsions have been reported rarely, usually following excessive doses. In general, the convulsions have occurred in patients with predisposing factors such as epilepsy or cerebral arteriosclerosis. In infants and children receiving therapeutic doses of nalidixic acid, increased intracranial pressure with bulging anterior fontanel, papilledema, and headache has occasionally been observed. A few cases of 6th cranial nerve palsy have been reported. Although the mechanisms of these reactions are unknown, the signs and symptoms usually disappeared rapidly with no sequelae when treatment was discontinued. *Gastrointestinal:* abdominal pain, nausea, vomiting, and diarrhea. *Allergic:* rash, pruritus, urticaria, angioedema, eosinophilia, arthralgia with joint stiffness and swelling, and rarely, anaphylactoid reaction. Photosensitivity reactions consisting of erythema and bullae on exposed skin surfaces usually resolve in 2 weeks to 2 months after therapy has been discontinued; however, bullae may continue to appear with successive exposures to sunlight or with mild skin trauma for up to 3 months after the drug has been withdrawn. *Other:* rarely, cholestasis, paresthesia, metabolic acidosis, thrombocytopenia, leukopenia, or hemolytic anemia which in some patients may have been associated with a deficiency in activity of glucose-6-phosphate dehydrogenase.

Dosage and Administration: *Orally.* Adults, 4 gm daily (1 gm 4 times daily) for 1 to 2 weeks; thereafter, the dosage may be reduced to 2 gm daily. Children, according to age and weight (approximately 25 mg/lb of body weight daily), administered in 4 equally divided doses; thereafter, 15 mg/lb/day may be given. Until further experience is gained, infants under 1 month should *not* be given this drug.

Availability:
NegGRAM®: **(Winthrop)**
Capsules (Caplets®) 250 mg in bottles of 56; 500 mg in bottles of 56, 500 and 1000 and in unit-dose packages of 100 and 250; 1 gm in bottles of 100.
Suspension, 250 mg/5 ml in bottles of 1 pint.

NALOXONE HYDROCHLORIDE

Chemical Name: N-allyl-nor-oxymorphone hydrochloride.

Description: Naloxone hydrochloride, a narcotic antagonist, is a synthetic congener of oxymorphone. It differs from oxymorphone merely by replacement of the methyl radical attached to the nitrogen atom with an allyl group. It occurs as slightly off-white crystals that are soluble in water, slightly soluble in alcohol and practically insoluble in ether.

The action of naloxone is similar to that of other narcotic antagonists, but differs in that it does not share some of their morphine-like physiologic properties, i.e., respiratory depression, psychotomimetic effects or pupillary constriction. No pharmacological activity is noted when naloxone is administered in the absence of narcotic-type drugs. However, in the presence of physical dependence on narcotics, naloxone will precipitate withdrawal symptoms, although it has *not* been shown to produce tolerance nor to cause physical or psychologic dependence.

The onset of action occurs within 2 minutes after intravenous injection and it is only slightly less rapid when administered subcutaneously or intramuscularly. The drug is extensively and rapidly metabolized. The major urinary metabolite is naloxone-3-glucuronide and the minor ones are the glucuronides of the N-dealkylated analog and the 6-hydroxy analog of naloxine hydrochloride.

Results of studies with mice and rats given 10 mg/kg/day for 3 weeks did not disclose any abnormality in fertility, general reproductive performance, or lactation, or any adverse or teratogenic effects on the fetus. The only prominent sign of toxicity in newborn and young rats was cyanosis and in young adult rats was convulsions.

Indications: Primarily for the complete or partial reversal of respiratory depression induced by natural or synthetic narcotics, by propoxyphene, or by pentazocine; also for the diagnosis of narcotic addiction; it is not effective against respiratory depression due to non-narcotic drugs or to other causes.

Contraindications: Hypersensitivity to naloxone.

Warnings: Cautious administration is advisable since this drug is capable of precipitating an acute withdrawal syndrome in addicted individuals. Because the duration of action of some narcotics may exceed that of naloxone, patients should be under constant surveillance since repeated doses may be necessary. It should be given to pregnant patients only when the potential benefits outweigh the possible hazards to mother and fetus.

Precautions: In addition to naloxone, other resuscitative measures should be readily available in the event of acute narcotic intoxication. If bleeding occurs, as has been rarely observed, complete blood coagulation studies, including thromboplastin time, are indicated. Cautious administration is recommended in patients with cardiac irritability.

Adverse Reactions: Noted rarely were nausea and vomiting.

Dosage and Administration: *Intravenously, intramuscularly* or *subcutaneously.* The usual initial adult dose is 0.4 mg, and the neonatal dose is 0.01 mg/kg of body weight; may be administered at 2- to 3-minute intervals until the desired degree of respiratory recovery has been achieved. If required, repeat doses may be given within 1- to 2-hour intervals. Supplemental intramuscular doses have been shown to produce a longer lasting effect. Because of its rapid onset of action, intravenous administration is recommended in emergency situations.

Availability:
NARCAN® **(Endo)**
Injection, 0.4 mg/ml in ampuls of 1 ml
Neonatal Injection, 0.02 mg/ml in ampuls of 2 ml in cartons of 10.

NANDROLONE

Chemical Name: 17-β-Hydroxyestr-4-en-3-one decanoate and phenpropionate esters.

Description: Nandrolone is a synthetic steroid structurally and pharmacologically related to norethandrolone and other androgenic anabolic steroids.

Both esters share the same actions and uses. However, because of its slower rate of hydrolysis, the decanoate ester has a duration of action lasting 3 or 4 weeks, whereas the phenpropionate ester will continue to exert its anabolic effect for 1 to 3 weeks, depending upon the dosage employed. They promote body tissue-building processes and reverse catabolic or tissue-depleting processes. Nitrogen balance is improved but only if there is sufficient intake of calories and protein. Whether or not this positive nitrogen balance is of primary benefit in the utilization of protein-building dietary substances has not been confirmed. The elimination of a methyl group from the C-19 position has resulted in reduction of the androgenic properties and a retention and enhancement of its anabolic, tissue-building properties. Thus such doses can be utilized that provide significant anabolic effects without undesired androgenic effects; however, complete dissociation of anabolic and androgenic effects has not been achieved. The actions of anabolic steroids are therefore similar to those of male sex hormones with the possibility of causing serious disturbances of growth and sexual development if given to young children. These steroids suppress the gonadotropic functions of the pituitary and may exert a direct effect upon the testes.

Indications: Control of metastatic breast cancer. As adjuvant therapy in senile and postmenopausal osteoporosis; equal or greater consideration should be given to diet, calcium balance, physiotherapy and good health-promoting measures. In pituitary dwarfism anabolic agents may be used with care until growth hormone is available. Also in the treatment of those conditions in which a potent tissue-building or protein-sparing action is desired such as pre- and postoperative care, burns, uremia and as adjuvant therapy for certain types of refractory anemia.

Contraindications: Carcinoma of the prostate or breast in male patients, carcinoma of the breast in some female patients, during pregnancy, and in the presence of nephrosis or the nephrotic phase of nephritis.

Warnings: Anabolic steroids do not enhance athletic ability.

Precautions: Patients with inoperable mammary cancer may develop hypercalcemia and exaggerated hypercalciuria. Therefore, serum and urinary calcium levels should be determined to evaluate treatment. Routine caution is advocated when administrating nandrolone to patients with cardiac, renal or hepatic disease since edema may occur which may be further provoked by the concomitant administration of adrenal corticosteroids or ACTH. The occurrence of amenorrhea or menstrual irregularities warrants discontinuation of therapy until the etiology has been established. Since anabolic steroids have been reported to increase prothrombin-time response in patients receiving anticoagulants and may thus precipitate hemorrhagic complications, the dosage of the anticoagulant may have to be decreased in order to maintain the prothrombin time at the desired therapeutic level. They have also been reported to alter glucose tolerance test. Diabetic patients should be followed carefully and their insulin or oral hypoglycemic dosage adjusted accordingly. Cautious use is advised in patients with benign prostatic hypertrophy and in those with a history of myocardial infarction or coronary artery disease. Serial determinations of serum cholesterol should be made at regular intervals and therapy adjusted accordingly in patients with cardiovascular complications.

Adverse Reactions: Typical androgenic effects are rare, and are generally mild and usually reversible. *In prepubital males,* phallic enlargement and increased frequency of erections have been noted. *In postpubertal males,* inhibition of testicular function, oligospermia and gynecomastia. *In females,* hirsutism, male pattern baldness, deepening of the voice and clitoral enlargement have been reported. These changes are usually irreversible even after prompt discontinuance of therapy and are not prevented by concomitant use of estrogens. Also reported were menstrual irregularities, and masculinization of the fetus. *In both sexes,* nausea, increased or decreased libido, acne (especially in females and prepubertal males), inhibition of gonadotropin secretion, bleeding in patients on concomitant anticoagulant therapy, premature closure of epiphyses in children, and alteration in the following clinical laboratory tests: The metyrapone test, glucose tolerance test, the thyroid function tests (a decrease in the PBI, in thyroxine-binding capacity and radioactive iodine uptake), the electrolyte retention of sodium, chlorides, water, potassium, phosphates and calcium, and liver function tests (increased serum cholesterol, and suppression of clotting factors II, V, VII, and X).

Dosage and Administration: *Intramuscularly.* Adults, 50 to 100 mg of the *decanoate* every 3 to 4 weeks, or 25 to 50 mg of the *phenpropionate* weekly. Children 2 to 13 years of age, the average dose is 25 to 50 mg (decanoate) every 3 to 4 weeks, or 25 mg (phenpropionate) every 2 to 4 weeks. If possible, repeat courses of therapy should follow a rest period of 4 weeks.

Availability:
DECA-DURABOLIN® Injection (decanoate), 50 mg/ml in ampuls of 1 ml and in vials of 2 ml; 100 mg/ml in vials of 2 ml. **(Organon)**
DURABOLIN® Injection (phenpropionate), 25 mg/ml in ampuls of 1 ml and in vials of 5 ml; 50 mg/ml in vials of 2 ml. **(Organon)**

NAPHAZOLINE HYDROCHLORIDE

Chemical Name: 2-(1-Naphthylmethyl)imidazoline hydrochloride.

Description: Naphazoline hydrochloride is a sympathomimetic agent which, when applied to nasal or ocular mucous membranes, produces vasoconstriction and reduces local congestion for prolonged periods. Its mode of action appears to be due to its direct effect on the alpha (excitatory) receptors of the vascular smooth muscle.

Indications: For prompt, prolonged relief of nasal congestion due to the common cold, sinusitis, hay fever, etc. Also for the symptomatic relief of minor ocular irritation and allergic manifestations. It relieves such symptoms as itching, smarting or redness. Also useful as an ocular vasoconstrictor and decongestant.

Contraindications: In narrow-angle glaucoma, and hypersensitivity to naphazoline or to any compound formulated with it.

Warnings: Extreme caution is advised in patients who are receiving MAO inhibitors, since a severe hypertensive crisis may ensue. Adequate clinical studies to determine whether or not this drug may affect fertility, or have a teratogenic potential or other adverse effect on the fetus have not been performed.

Precautions: Excessive, prolonged or frequent use may be harmful to the nasal mucous membranes. Only 2 drops of the nasal solution should be used and no more often than every 3 hours. If congestion persists after 5 days' use, the solution should be discontinued. Overdosage in young children may cause marked sedation and, if severe, emergency treatment may be necessary. Cautious use is advised in the presence of hypertension, cardiac irregularities, hyperglycemia (diabetes), or hyperthyroidism.

Adverse Reactions: Occasionally, transient stinging and hypersensitivity reactions may occur. Also noted were pupillary dilation with increased intraocular pressure; systemic effects due to absorption of the drug (hypertension, cardiac irregularities, hyperglycemia). Accidental ingestion, especially in children, may produce marked sedation which may result in coma and marked reduction in body temperature.

Dosage and Administration: *Nasal solution:* instill only 2 drops into each nostril every 3 hours; solution may be used in an atomizer, but not in one made of aluminum or with aluminum parts. *Nasal spray:* 2 sprays into each nostril every 4 to 6 hours. *Ophthalmic solution:* instill 1 to 3 drops into the conjunctival sac; this usually is sufficient for almost immediate decongestion.

Availability:
ALBALON® Ophthalmic Solution, 0.1% with polyvinyl alcohol, 1.4% (Liquifilm®) in dropper bottles of 15 ml. **(Allergan)**
ALBALON-A Ophthalmic Solution, 0.05% with antazoline phosphate, 0.5% in bottles of 15 ml with dropper. **(Allergan)**
DEGEST 2 (OTC) Ophthalmic Solution, 0.012% with antipyrine, 0.1% in plastic dropper bottles of 15 ml. **(Barnes-Hind)**
NAPHCON® Ophthalmic Solution, 0.012% (OTC) in Drop-Tainers® of 15 ml; *Forte* Solution, 0.1% (Rx) in Drop-Tainers of 15 ml. **(Alcon)**
PRIVINE® Hydrochloride: **(Ciba)**
Nasal Solution, 0.05% (OTC) in bottles of 30 ml and 1 pint.
Nasal Spray, 0.05% (OTC) in plastic squeeze bottles of 20 ml.
VASOCON Ophthalmic Solution, 0.1% in bottles of 15 ml with dropper tip. **(Smith, Miller & Patch)**
VASOCON-A Ophthalmic Solution, 0.05% with antazoline phosphate, 0.5% in bottles of 15 ml with dropper tip. **(Smith, Miller & Patch)**

NAPRIL

Description: Each capsule contains:

For immediate release
Phenylephrine hydrochloride .... 15 mg
For sustained release
Phenylpropanolamine hydrochloride .... 25 mg
Pyrilamine maleate .... 25 mg
Chlorpheniramine maleate .... 4 mg

Provides prompt and continuous relief of nasal congestion for up to 12 hours. The two antihistamines, pyrilamine maleate and chlorpheniramine maleate, help to alleviate sneezing, rhinorrhea and itching of the eyes.

Indications: Recommended for the symptomatic relief of sinus and nasal congestion associated with coryza, rhinorrhea, and allergic manifestations.

Contraindications: Hypersensitivity to any of the components.

Precautions: Since drowsiness is a possibility, patients should be cautioned not to engage in activities requiring alertness or physical coordination. Routine caution is necessary in patients with hypertension, heart disease, diabetes, or thyrotoxicosis.

Adverse Reactions: Drowsiness, nervousness and rapid pulse may occur in susceptible patients or in extreme overdose.

Dosage and Administration: *Orally.* Adults and children 12 years of age and over, 1 capsule twice daily, morning and evening.

Availability:
NAPRIL® Plateau Caps® (sustained-release capsules) in bottles of 50. **(Marion)**

NAPROXEN

Chemical Name: (+)-6-Methoxy-α-methyl-2-naphthaleneacetic acid.

Description: A synthetic, nonsteroidal, antiarthritic drug that is chemically related to the arylacetic acid class of compounds. Naproxen exerts its antiinflammatory, analgesic and antipyretic effects independently of pituitary-adrenal function. It occurs as a white to off-white, crystalline substance that is highly lipid soluble, is sparingly soluble in highly acetic solutions but freely soluble in highly alkaline solutions.

The mode of action, like that of other nonsteroidal antiinflammatory agents, has not been determined; however, naproxen has been found to inhibit prostaglandin synthesis. Patients with rheumatoid arthritis usually experienced a significant decrease in pain, fever, swelling, stiffness and tenderness and increased mobility, but showed no apparent alteration in the progressive course of the underlying disease. Therapeutic effectiveness is similar to that of aspirin, but the frequency and severity of gastrointestinal adverse effects (nausea, dyspepsia, heartburn) and CNS involvement (tinnitus, dizziness, lightheadedness) were less in naproxen-treated patients. Whether or not it causes less peptic ulceration than does aspirin is not known.

Reproduction studies in rats have shown the drug to be associated with prolonged labor and difficult parturition when given during late pregnancy. Evidence suggests that this may be due to decreased uterine contractility probably resulting from the inhibition of prostaglandin synthesis. Clinical studies have revealed that the drug readily crosses the placental barrier, and has also been found in the milk of lactating women at a concentration of approximately 1% of that found in the plasma.

Well absorbed after oral administration, it reaches peak plasma levels within 2 to 4 hours, and a 13-hour half-life ensures a sustained antiinflammatory effect. Steady-state conditions are normally achieved after 4 or 5 doses. At therapeutic levels, the drug is bound to serum albumin to the extent of over 99%, and approximately 95% is excreted in the urine, primarily as unchanged drug and metabolites. The rate of excretion has been found to coincide closely with the rate of drug clearance from the plasma.

Because of its strong affinity for albumin-binding sites, naproxen may displace from their binding sites other drugs with albumin-binding activity, and consequently may provoke significant drug interactions. Likewise, naproxen itself could be displaced thus making increased quantities of the free drug available which could cause serious complications. The drug is capable of displacing bishydroxycoumarin or warfarin from their binding sites. In this situation the activity of the anticoagulant is increased whereupon prothrombin time is prolonged, and hemorrhage may occur. Naproxen may also potentiate the pharmacologic action of hydantoin, sulfonamide or sulfonylurea; therefore, patients receiving such concomitant therapy should be carefully observed for this effect.

Indications: Relief of the signs and symptoms of rheumatoid arthritis. May be used alone or in combination with gold salts and/or adrenal corticosteroids.

Contraindications: Patients with known hypersensitivity to the drug. Since cross-sensitivity has been demonstrated, naproxen should not be given to patients in whom aspirin or other nonsteroidal antiinflammatory agents induce the syndrome of asthma, rhinitis or urticaria.

Warnings: Patients prone to gastrointestinal tract irritation or those with a history of peptic ulcer should be under close supervision since perforation of the ulcer and gastrointestinal bleeding, sometimes severe, and occasionally fatal, have been reported. In these cases attempts should be made to treat the arthritis with nonulcerogenic drugs such as gold salts.

Precautions: Naproxen is not recommended for use in pregnant or lactating women or in children under 16 years of age until safe and effective use has been established. Caution should be exercised by patients whose activities require alertness and physical coordination if they experience drowsiness, dizziness, vertigo, or depression. It is advised to monitor the serum creatinine and/or creatinine clearance in patients with diminished renal function; mild elevations in BUN occurred in a few cases, but it has not been determined if this was due to the drug. If concurrent steroid dosage is reduced or eliminated during naproxen therapy, the steroid dosage should be reduced slowly and the patient observed for signs of adrenal insufficiency and exacerbation of rheumatoid arthritis or other adverse reactions. Although there have been no reports of drug-induced eye complications, it is recommended that ophthalmologic examinations be carried out shortly after therapy has been initiated and at periodic intervals thereafter. The possibility of fluid retention and edema should be considered especially when treating patients with questionable or compromised cardiac function. It should be kept in mind when bleeding times are determined that the drug decreases platelet aggregation and prolongs bleeding time. Also, patients with initial hemoglobin values of 10 gm or less who are to receive long-term therapy should have their hemoglobin values determined frequently . Because naproxen may increase urinary values for 17-ketogenic steroids due to interaction between the drug or its metabolites and m-dinitrobenzene used in the assay, it is therefore advised to discontinue the drug 72 hours prior to performing adrenal function tests.

Adverse Reactions: Complications related to the gastrointestinal tract were infrequent bleeding with or without ulceration. In some cases the relationship to naproxen was difficult to assess. Other adverse reactions, in decreasing order of prevalence, were heartburn, nausea, dyspepsia, abdominal pain, constipation, stomatitis, diarrhea, vomiting, melena. Those related to the CNS were headache, drowsiness, dizziness, lightheadedness, vertigo, inability to concentrate, depression; to the skin were pruritus, skin eruptions, sweating, ecchymoses, skin rashes, urticaria, purpura; to special senses were tinnitus, visual disturbances, hearing disturbances; to the cardiovascular system were edema, palpitations, dyspnea. Occasionally reported was thirst. Rarely reported were angioneurotic edema, thrombocytopenia, agranulocytosis, jaundice.

Dosage and Administration: *Orally.* The usual daily dosage is 500 mg in divided doses. This may be increased to 750 mg or decreased, depending on the response of the patient. Daily doses above 750 mg, and administration more frequently than twice daily are not recommended.

Availability:
NAPROSYN® Tablets (scored), 250 mg in bottles of 100 and 500. **(Syntex)**

NATABEC w/FLUORIDE: see the Fluoride-Vitamins

NATABEC Rx

Description: Each capsule contains:

Vitamin A (as acetate)	(4000 units)	1.2 mg
Vitamin D (ergocalciferol)	(400 units)	10 μg
Ascorbic acid		50 mg
Thiamine mononitrate		3 mg
Riboflavin		2 mg
Pyridoxine hydrochloride		3 mg
Cyanocobalamin		5 μg
Niacinamide		10 mg
Ferrous sulfate		150 mg
Calcium carbonate		600 mg
Folic acid		1 mg

Indications: Nutritional support of pregnancy and lactation. The addition of folic acid helps to prevent megaloblastic anemia of pregnancy.

Precautions: Folic acid may obscure pernicious anemia in that the peripheral blood picture may revert to normal while the neurological manifestations remain progressive.

Adverse Reactions: No undesirable side effects have been reported to date.

Dosage and Administration: *Orally.* One capsule daily, or as directed by the physician.

Availability:
NATABEC Rx® Kapseals® in bottles of 100. **(Parke-Davis)**

NATAFORT

Description: Each tablet provides:

Vitamin A (as acetate)	(6000 units)	1.8 mg
Vitamin D (ergocalciferol)	(400 units)	10 μg
Ascorbic acid		100 mg
Thiamine mononitrate		3 mg
Riboflavin		2 mg
Pyridoxine hydrochloride		15 mg
Cyanocobalamin		5 μg
Folic acid		1 mg
Niacinamide		15 mg
Vitamin E (*dl*-alpha-tocopheryl acetate, 30 mg)		30 IU
Calcium carbonate		350 mg
Magnesium oxide		1.7 mg
Potassium iodide		0.15 mg
Ferrous fumerate		65 mg

Indications: Prenatal vitamin and mineral supplement. The addition of folic acid helps to prevent megaloblastic anemia of pregnancy.

Precautions: The use of folic acid in patients with pernicious anemia may mask this condition in that the peripheral blood picture may return to normal while the neurological manifestations may progress.

Adverse Reactions: No undesirable adverse effects have been reported to date.

Dosage and Administration: *Orally.* The usual daily dose is 1 tablet.

Availability:
NATAFORT® Filmseal® (tablets) in bottles of 100. **(Parke-Davis)**

NATALINS Rx

Description: Each tablet contains:

Vitamin A (as acetate)	(8000 U.S.P. units)	2.4 mg
Vitamin D (ergocalciferol)	(400 U.S.P. units)	10 μg
Vitamin E (dl-alpha tocopheryl acetate)		30 IU
Ascorbic acid (as sodium ascorbate)		90 mg
Thiamine mononitrate		2.55 mg
Riboflavin		3 mg
Pyridoxine hydrochloride		10 mg
Cyanocobalamin		8 μg
Niacinamide		20 mg
Folic acid		1 mg
Pantothenic acid		15 mg
Biotin		0.05 mg
Calcium carbonate		200 mg
Iron (from 132 mg ferrous fumerate)		60 mg
Magnesium hydroxide		100 mg
Calcium iodate		150 μg
Cupric oxide		2 mg
Zinc oxide		15 mg

Indications: Dietary supplement, particularly indicated during pregnancy and lactation. The folic acid helps prevent the development of megaloblastic anemia during pregnancy.

Contraindications: In patients with hemochromatosis or those with Wilson's disease.

Precautions: Pernicious anemia should be excluded before initiating treatment. Folic acid may mask the symptoms of pernicious anemia by correcting the hematological picture while the neurological manifestations remain progressive. In patients with kidney stones, the calcium content of this product should be considered before prescribing. Also, the recommended dose should not be exceeded.

Adverse Reactions: No undesirable side effects have been reported to date.

Dosage and Administration: *Orally.* One tablet daily, or as prescribed by the physician.

Availability:
NATALINS® Rx Tablets in bottles of 100 and 1000. **(Mead Johnson)**

NEOMYCIN SULFATE

Description: Neomycin sulfate is a salt of a bactericidal antibiotic obtained from the metabolic products of the actinomycete *Streptomyces fradiae.* The antibiotic is stable over a pH range of 2 to 9 and is not inactivated by exudate, enzymes, or by-products of bacterial growth.

Neomycin is effective against the majority of pathogenic gram-positive and gram-negative bacilli, including the organisms that are known inhabitants of the intestinal tract, as well as most strains of *Staphylococcus aureus.* Growth of most intestinal bacteria is rapidly suppressed following oral administration of neomycin, and the suppression persists for 48 to 72 hours. Nonpathogenic yeasts and, occasionally, resistant strains of *Enterobacter aerogenes* (formerly *Aerobacter aerogenes*) replace the intestinal bacteria. Neomycin is ineffective against *Pseudomonas* organisms, fungi and viruses. The antibiotic is not destroyed or reduced in activity by gastric acid. Because of its poor absorption from the gastrointestinal tract, neomycin, rarely produces systemic or toxic effects when given orally. The small absorbed fraction (3%) is rapidly excreted with normal kidney function. The unabsorbed portion of the drug (approximately 97%) is eliminated unchanged in the feces. From 30 to 50% of a parenteral dose is excreted in the urine. If the Kirby-Bauer method of disc sensitivity is used, a 30 mcg disc should give a zone of 16 mm or more when the organism is sensitive to neomycin.

Indications: Orally, neomycin is used in the treatment of infectious diarrheas due to susceptible organisms. It is also valuable in the "sterilization" of the intestinal tract before abdominal surgery, particularly when partial or complete resections of the intestine or colon are contemplated. Parenterally, it is useful in the treatment of urinary tract infections caused by *Kl. pneumoniae, Escherichia coli, Enterobacter aerogenes, Pr. vulgaris, Ps. aeruginosa,* and in enteropathogenic organisms. Because of its potential toxicity it should be reserved for hospitalized patients in whom no other antimicrobial agent is effective. In hepatic coma, prolonged administration of neomycin has been shown to be effective adjunctive therapy by reducing ammonia-forming bacteria in the intestinal tract. The subsequent reduction in blood ammonia has resulted in neurologic improvement.

Contraindications: In hypersensitive patients; intestinal obstruction.

Warnings: Patients treated with neomycin should be under close clinical observation because of the potential hazard of nephrotoxic and ototoxic effects. Such effects are usually dose-related. Patients with renal insufficiency may develop toxic blood levels of the drug unless doses are properly regulated. If renal insufficiency develops during treatment, the dosage should be reduced or the antibiotic discontinued. Urine and blood examinations and audiometric tests should be given prior to and during extended therapy in individuals with hepatic and/or renal disease to avoid nephrotoxicity and eighth nerve damage from improper dosage. The possibility of acute toxicity increases in premature and newborn infants. Oral neomycin has also been reported to produce a transient and reversible gastrointestinal malabsorption of certain nutrients and potassium penicillin V. The underlying mechanism which causes the malabsorption, and the effect of neomycin on intestinal absorption of other antibiotics, are not yet known. It is suggested that when concomitant systemic penicillin therapy is indicated in patients receiving neomycin orally, parenteral penicillin should be administered in order to insure its full effectiveness. Safe use of neomycin during pregnancy has not been established.

Precautions: Caution should be taken in concurrent use of other ototoxic and/or nephrotoxic antimicrobial drugs while neomycin is administered orally. These include streptomycin, kanamycin, polymyxin B, colistin, viomycin, gentamicin, and cephaloridine. Because it produces a neuromuscular blocking effect, neomycin enhances the action of other neuromuscular blocking agents, anesthetics, parenterally administered magnesium and other drugs with muscle-relaxant properties. If signs of respiratory paralysis appear, respiration should be assisted and the drug discontinued. The concurrent use of potent diuretics such as ethacrynic acid, furosemide, urea and mannitol (particularly when the diuretics are given intravenously) should be avoided. They may cause cumulative adverse effects of the neomycin on the kidney and auditory nerve. Prolonged use of oral neomycin may result in overgrowth of nonsusceptible organisms, particularly fungi. If this occurs, appropriate therapy should be instituted. The drug should be used with caution in patients with extensive ulceration of the bowel. Because of the possibility of increased absorption following oral administration in patients with poor renal function, high serum levels may occur. Therefore, prolonged administration of large oral doses should be avoided. There are reports in current medical literature indicating that there is an increase in the prevalence of individuals sensitive to neomycin.

Adverse Reactions: Diarrhea, nausea and vomiting are the most common side effects. The malabsorption syndrome characterized by increased fecal fat, decreased serum carotene, and a fall in xylose absorption has also been reported. In addition, irreversible damage to the auditory branch of the eighth cranial nerve, renal failure and respiratory depression following intramuscular administration, transient rise in nonpathogenic yeasts, overgrowth of monilia following prolonged oral therapy, and hypersensitivity reactions, primarily skin rashes, have been reported.

Dosage and Administration: *Orally* In bacterial diarrheas, 0.5 to 1 gm every 6 hours for 2 to 3 days. To rid carriers of *Salmonella* or *Shigella,* 0.5 gm 4 times daily for 10 days. To sterilize the bowel, 1 gm every hour for 4 doses, followed by 1 gm every 4 hours for 4 doses. *Intramuscularly* for systemic infections, 10 to 15 mg/kg of body weight daily in divided doses every 6 hours. Not more than 1 gm should be given in 1 day and for not more than 10 days. For *intraperitoneal instillation,* 100 ml of an 0.5% solution or 500 mg of the drug/24-hour day and for not more than 3 days. Dosage for children should be reduced proportionately. *Topically.* Insert a small amount into the conjunctival sac 3 or 4 times daily. When a favorable response is observed, the number of daily applications may be reduced until the disorder is under control. In deep-seated infections, local application of neomycin should be supplemented by systemic therapy with other chemotherapeutic agents.

Availability:
MYCIFRADIN®: **(Upjohn)**
Oral Solution, 125 mg/5 ml in bottles of 60 ml and 1 pint.
Sterile Powder in vials of 0.5 gm (intramuscular use in solution).
Tablets, 0.5 gm in bottles of 20, 100 and 500.
MYCIGUENT®: **(Upjohn)**
Cream, 5 mg/gm in tubes of 15 gm.
Ointment, 5 mg/gm in tubes of 15, 30 and 120 gm.
Ophthalmic Ointment (sterile), 5 mg/gm in tubes of 3.5 gm with applicator tip.
NEOBIOTIC® Tablets, 0.5 gm in bottles of 100. **(Pfipharmecs)**
NEOMYCIN SULFATE Tablets, 0.5 gm in bottles of 100. **(Lederle)**
NEOMYCIN SULFATE Ointment, 5 mg/gm in tubes of 15 and 30 gm. **(Lilly)**
NEOMYCIN SULFATE Tablets, 0.5 gm in bottles of 20 and 100 and in 10 strips of 10 individually labeled blisters each containing 1 tablet. **(Lilly)**
NEOMYCIN SULFATE Sterile Powder in vials of 0.5 gm. **(Squibb)**
NEOMYCIN SULFATE Tablets, 0.5 gm in bottles of 100. **(Squibb)**
NEOMYCIN SULFATE Nonsterile Powder for compounding in bottles of 100 gm. **(Upjohn)**

NEO-POLYCIN

Description: A combination of antibiotics that are effective in treating a wide range of gram-negative and gram-positive organisms, and many strains of *Proteus* and *Pseudomonas aeruginosa.*

Indications: The ophthalmic preparations are indicated for short-term treatment of superficial external eye infections, and the topical preparation for treatment of all types of bacterial infections of the skin and mucous membranes. These include such conditions as pyoderma, folliculitis, paronychia, sycosis barbae and impetigo. It may also be used in controlling secondary bacterial infections in skin carcinoma, burns, eczemas, contact dermatitis, fungal infections, acne, psoriasis, varicose ulcers and neurodermatitis, and for the prevention of bacterial infections due to traumatic lesions and surgical incisions.

Contraindications: Hypersensitivity to any of the components.

Warnings: Since neomycin is known to be nephrotoxic and ototoxic, special care is advised when treating extensive burns, trophic ulceration, and other such conditions in which absorption of the drug is possible. No more than one application daily is recommended where widespread body surfaces are affected, especially if the patient has impaired renal function or is receiving other aminoglycoside antibiotics concurrently. Prolonged use may result in overgrowth of nonsusceptible organisms including fungi. Ophthalmic ointments may retard corneal healing. *The topical ointment should not be used in the eyes or in the external ear canal if the eardrum is perforated.*

Precautions: The drug should be discontinued if itching, burning or inflammation occurs. Patients should be observed closely for overgrowth of nonsusceptible organisms and, if symptoms of new infections appear, appropriate measures should be instituted. Culture and susceptibility testing should be performed during treatment. Allergic cross-reactions with kanamycin, paromomycin, streptomycin, and possibly gentamicin may occur. Application of the ophthalmic solution may produce a transient mild, stinging sensation. There are reports in current medical literature indicating that there is an increase in the prevalence of individuals sensitive to neomycin.

Dosage and Administration: *Topically.* Spread the ointment thinly over the infected area 1 to 3 times daily as required. The ophthalmic ointment is introduced into the conjunctival sac of the eye 2 or more times daily. Instill 1 or 2 drops of the ophthalmic solution into the conjunctival sac every 3 or 4 hours; in severe infection, use every 15 minutes to ½ hour.

Availability:
NEO-POLYCIN®: **(Dow)**
Ophthalmic Ointment in tubes of 3.5 gm with applicator tip. Each gm contains neomycin sulfate, equivalent to neomycin, 3.5 mg; zinc bacitracin, 500 units; polymyxin B sulfate, 10,000 units.
Ophthalmic Solution in bottles of 10 ml with sterile dropper. Each ml contains neomycin sulfate, equivalent to neomycin, 1.75 mg; polymyxin B sulfate, 5000 units; gramicidin, 0.025 mg.
Topical Ointment in tubes of 15 and 30 gm and in unit-dose packs of 1 gm in cartons of 144. Each gm contains neomycin sulfate, equivalent to neomycin, 3.5 mg; zinc bacitracin, 400 units; polymyxin B sulfate, 5000 units in a Fuzene® ointment base.

NEOSTIGMINE

Chemical Name: (*m*-Hydroxyphenyl)trimethylammonium dimethylcarbamate.

Description: Neostigmine is a cholinergic stimulant that enhances cholinergic action by facilitating the transmission of impulses across the myoneural junction. It is a synthetic compound closely related to physostigmine (eserine) but is more stable and better tolerated. It occurs as a white, crystalline, odorless powder of bitter taste that is soluble in water (1:10). It is available as the methylsulfate for parenteral use and as the bromide for oral use.

Studies have shown that the drug inhibits or inactivates acetylcholine esterases and thus allows the accumulation of acetylcholine at cholinergic sites. It also has a direct effect on voluntary muscle fibers, and possibly on autonomic ganglion cells and neurons of the CNS.

Following injection, peak concentration in the liver occurs in about 2 hours and is equivalent to 2% of the dose. Approximately 50% of the dose is excreted in the feces in 24 hours; 10% is excreted in the urine in 5 hours and 20% after 24 hours.

Indications: Prevention and treatment of postoperative abdominal distention and urinary retention; as a screening test for early pregnancy; the treatment of delayed menstruation; as a diagnostic test for, and in the symptomatic control of myasthenia gravis. However, edrophonium chloride usually is recommended as a better diagnostic test for myasthenia gravis because of its more rapid onset and brief duration of action. Neostigmine can also be used as an antidote for tubocurarine.

Contraindications: In patients hypersensitive to the drug; in those with mechanical obstruction of the intestine or genitourinary tract or with urinary tract infections; and in patients known to be sensitive to bromides.

Warnings: Because of the presence of the bromide ion, the oral form should be used with caution in asthmatic patients, and concomitantly with anticholinergic drugs that may retard intestinal motility.

Precautions: When large doses are administered, the prior or simultaneous injection of atropine sulfate may be advisable. Overdosage may result in a cholinergic crisis which should be differentiated from a myasthenic crisis due to an increase in the severity of the disease. Certain antibiotics, especially neomycin, streptomycin and kanamycin, have a mild but definite nondepolarizing blocking action which may accentuate neuromuscular block. These antibiotics should only be used in the myasthenic patient where definitely indicated, and then careful adjustment should be made of adjunctive anticholinesterase dosage.

Adverse Reactions: Reactions are most commonly related to overdosage and may include nausea, vomiting, diarrhea, abdominal cramps, increased salivation, increased bronchial secretions, miosis, diaphoresis, muscle cramps, weakness and fasciculation.

Dosage and Administration: *Subcutaneously* or *intramuscularly. For prevention of postoperative distention and urinary retention,* 1 ml of the 1:4000 solution (0.25 mg) immediately after operation, and repeat every 4 to 6 hours for 2 or 3 days. *For treatment of established atony,* 1 ml of a 1:2000 solution (0.5 mg) as required. If urination does not occur within an hour, the patient should be catheterized. After the patient has voided, or the bladder has been emptied, continue with 0.5 mg every 3 hours for at least 5 injections. *For diagnosis of pregnancy and treatment of delayed menstruation,* 1 ml of the 1:1000 solution (1 mg) *intramuscularly* daily for 3 consecutive days. Absence of uterine bleeding is regarded as presumptive evidence of pregnancy, provided local pelvic lesions, systemic disease and endocrine disorders have been ruled out. If the patient is not pregnant, bleeding usually occurs within 72 hours after the 3rd injection. *For symptomatic control of myasthenia gravis,* 1 ml of the 1:2000 solution (0.5 mg) initially; subsequent doses are based on individual patient's response. *Orally.* In most patients treatment in dosages ranging from 15 mg to as much as 375 mg daily has been utilized. The average dosage, however, of 150 mg daily divided into equal doses over a period of 24 hours is usually adequate for the control of symptoms. *As an antidote for tubocurarine,* 0.5 to 1 mg *intravenously.*

Availability:
PROSTIGMIN®: **(Roche)**
Injectable (methylsulfate), 0.25 mg/ml (1:4000) in ampuls of 1 ml; 0.5 mg/ml (1:2000) in ampuls of 1 ml and in vials of 10 ml; 1 mg/ml (1:1000) in vials of 10 ml.
Tablets (bromide), 15 mg in bottles of 100 and 1000.

NIACIN

Synonym: Nicotinic acid.

Chemical Name: 3-Pyridine carboxylic acid.

Description: Niacin occurs as a fine, white, crystalline, odorless powder or as white crystals, sparingly soluble in water, but freely soluble in boiling water and in boiling alcohol. It is insoluble in ether and in chloroform.

In the body niacin is converted to niacinamide, which is an essential constituent of coenzymes I and II that occur in enzyme systems involved in the oxidation of carbohydrates.

It is readily absorbed from the gastrointestinal tract, and large doses may be given either orally or parenterally with equal effect. It exerts its action directly on the musculature of the peripheral vessels, and when given in adequate dosage produces cutaneous vasodilatation and increased blood flow. These effects occur in a few minutes and usually last up to an hour, and are evidenced by symptoms of flushing, itching and tingling sensations, with an increase in skin temperature and increased motility and secretion of the stomach. When given in large doses, niacin has also been reported to reduce elevated serum cholesterol and total lipid levels in hypercholesterolemic and hyperlipemic states; however, the precise mode of action has not been established. Since the drug reduces prebeta lipoproteins, it may therefore be effective in all types of hyperlipoproteinemia except type I. Essential triglyceridemia type IV and mixed hyperlipidemia type V respond rapidly with a reported reduction in triglyceride levels of up to 68%. Clinical studies have shown that when patients were given a full dose of niacin, the average triglyceride level was reduced from the first day of treatment, and a significant reduction of cholesterol levels was noted after the fourth or fifth day of therapy. **Important Note:** There is as yet no evidence that drug-induced lowering of plasma lipoprotein concentration has a detrimental, beneficial or any effect on the morbidity due to atherosclerosis or coronary heart disease. Niacin is excreted in the urine as *N*-methylnicotinamide, a fluorescent compound formed in the liver.

Indications: Prophylaxis and treatment of pellagra, and of those conditions associated with circulatory deficiency. Niacin is also indicated in the treatment of hypercholesterolemia and hyperbetalipoproteinemia as an adjuvant to diet and other measures.

Contraindications: In patients with a known hypersensitivity or idiosyncrasy to niacin, or in those with arterial bleeding, severe hypotension, hemorrhaging, hepatic dysfunction, or an active acute peptic ulcer.

Warnings: Use of niacin in pregnant and lactating women or in women of childbearing potential requires that the therapeutic benefits be weighed against the possible hazards to the mother and child. Until further clinical trials substantiate its safe and effective use, it is not recommended for use in pediatric patients.

Precautions: Patients with gallbladder disease, or those with a past history of jaundice, liver disorders or peptic ulcer should be under close medical supervision while taking this drug. Frequent monitoring of liver function tests and blood glucose levels should be performed, especially in the initial stage of therapy. Diabetic patients may require adjustment of diet and insulin dosage in the event of decreased tolerance. Due to an additive vasodilating effect, postural hypotension may occur when niacin is added to the therapeutic regimen of patients taking antihypertensive drugs of the adrenal blocking type. Since elevated uric acid levels have occurred, this drug should be used with caution in patients predisposed to gout. Large doses may be attended by some degree of liver impairment including an abnormal glucose tolerance curve.

Adverse Reactions: Transient flushing and a feeling of warmth may occur; however, these effects seldom reach undesirable levels so as to necessitate discontinuation of the drug. Other complications that were noted include decreased glucose tolerance, activation of peptic ulcer, abnormalities of hepatic function test, jaundice, gastrointestinal disorders, dryness of skin, keratosis nigricans, pruritus, headache, tingling of the skin, skin rash, allergies, hyperuricemia, toxic amblyopia, and hypotension.

Dosage and Administration: *Orally.* Initially, small doses should be given in order to avoid or minimize the distressing symptoms of intolerance manifested by flushing, pruritus and gastrointestinal disorders. *For circulatory disorders,* the usual adult dosage is 125 to 250 mg twice daily (morning and evening). *For hyperlipidemic states,* 1 to 2 gm daily taken with or immediately after meals, or as directed by the physician.

Availability:

DIACIN Capsules (timed-release), 200 mg in bottles of 100. **(Lemmon)**

NICO-400® Capsules (sustained-release), 400 mg in bottles of 100. **(Marion)**

NICOBID® Tempules® (long-acting, timed-release capsules), 125 and 250 mg in bottles of 100 and 500; 500 mg in bottles of 100. **(Armour)**

NICOCAP® Capsules (sustained-release), 400 mg in bottles of 50. **(ICN)**

NICOLAR® Tablets, 500 mg in bottles of 100. **(Armour)**
NICOSPAN Capsules (timed-release), 400 mg in bottles of 100, 500 and 1000. **(Key Pharm.)**
WAMPOCAP™ Capsules, 500 mg in bottles of 100. **(Wallace)**

NIACIN + GLYCINE

Description: The combination provides the vasodilating properties of niacin with the vasodilating and thermogenic properties of aminoacetic acid (glycine). This action produces sustained heat production which cannot be used by the body but is radiated peripherally by way of increased cardiac output and increased peripheral vascular flow, thus eliciting a feeling of warmth and tingling of the skin.

Indications: To relieve pain, dizziness and faintness, and to increase tolerance to cold and sudden changes in temperature, especially in the hands and feet.

Precautions: Caution is advised when given concomitantly with a coronary vasodilator.

Adverse Reactions: Hepatic damage, hyperglycemia, hyperuricemia, acanthosis nigricans, toxic amblyopia, transient itching, flushing.

Dosage and Administration: *Orally,* 1 or 2 teaspoonsful 3 times daily before meals. The recommended dosage should not be exceeded.

Availability:
GERILIQUID® in bottles of 1 pint. Each 5 ml (teaspoonful) contains niacin, 75 mg, aminoacetic acid (glycine), 750 mg and alcohol, 5% in a sherry-wine base. **(Key Pharm.)**

NICOTINYL ALCOHOL

Description: Nicotinyl alcohol is a vasodilator which produces a direct relaxing effect on peripheral blood vessels; therapeutic action is more prolonged than that of niacin, and it is less likely to produce severe flushing and other distressing side effects.

Indications: May be of use in conditions associated with deficient circulation such as peripheral vascular disease, vascular spasm, varicose ulcers, decubital ulcers, chilblains, Meniere's syndrome and vertigo.

Precautions: Nicotinyl alcohol should be used with caution in pregnant patients.

Adverse Reactions: Transient flushing, gastric disturbances, minor skin rashes and allergies may occur but seldom require withdrawal of the drug.

Dosage and Administration: *Orally,* 1 or 2 Timespan tablets morning and night, or 1 or 2 tablets or teaspoonsful of elixir 3 times daily.

Availability:
RONIACOL®: **(Roche)**
Elixir, 50 mg/5 ml in bottles of 1 pint.
Tablets (as the tartrate), 50 mg in bottles of 100 and 500.
Timespan® Tablets (sustained-release tablets) as the tartrate, 150 mg in bottles of 100 and 500.

NIDAR (C-II)

Description: Each tablet contains:

Pentobarbital sodium	25 mg
Secobarbital sodium	25 mg
Butabarbital sodium	7.5 mg
Phenobarbital	7.5 mg

Indications: For nighttime sedation and refreshing sleep up to 8 hours.

Contraindications: In patients hypersensitive to barbiturates, severe hepatic disease, uncontrolled pain, latent or manifest porphyria or a familial history of porphyria, severe respiratory disease, and in addiction-prone individuals.

Warnings: Barbiturates may be habit-forming. Evidence has been produced that barbiturates stimulate hepatic microsomal enzymes and therefore may increase the metabolism of some drugs, including the coumarin anticoagulants, thus lowering their blood concentration and clinical effectiveness. Judicious use of this drug is required during pregnancy especially in the first trimester. Barbiturates readily cross the placental barrier and if administered during labor may have a depressant effect on the fetus. They also appear in the milk of lactating women.

Precautions: Considerable care is required in patients with renal or hepatic impairment when excretion may be delayed; in elderly patients who may experience accentuated nocturnal confusion and restlessness under barbiturate therapy; in patients previously addicted to barbiturates and in patients with fever, hyperthyroidism, diabetes mellitus, severe anemia, and congestive heart failure. Occasional "hangover" may occur. Hypersensitive patients may experience restlessness, excitement, skin rashes, fever, and collapse. Overdosage may result in stupor, lowered body temperature, feeble heart action, depression or paralysis of the respiratory centers. Barbiturates may have an additive effect with other CNS depressants such as other sedatives, tranquilizers, alcohol, centrally-acting analgesics, hypnotics, and anesthetics and can result in excessive depression when administered concurrently with any of these drugs. Prolonged use of barbiturates, even in therapeutic doses, may result in psychic or physical dependence, and in susceptible individuals, continued uncontrolled use may lead to habituation. Ambulatory patients should be specifically warned not to engage in activities that require alertness, judgment or physical coordination.

Adverse Reactions: Lassitude, morbilliform rash and urticaria, vertigo, "hangover," nausea, vomiting, diarrhea, excitement, fever and delirium, stupor and ataxia may occur with prolonged use.

Dosage and Administration: *Orally. For insomnia,* 1 or 2 tablets ½ hour before bedtime. *For sedation,* 1 tablet 2 or 3 times daily.

Availability:
Ⓒ NIDAR® Tablets in bottles of 100. **(Armour)**

NIKETHAMIDE

Chemical Name: *N,N*-Diethylnicotinamide.

Description: Nikethamide is a CNS stimulant which acts principally on the medullary centers increasing the rate and depth of respiration and producing peripheral vasoconstriction. It presumably acts by enhancing excitation rather than by blocking central inhibition.

Indications: Treatment of CNS depression, respiratory depression and circulatory failure, particularly when due to the effects of CNS-depressant drugs. Also used as combined nikethamide-electroconvulsive therapy for acute mania.

Contraindications: Hypersensitivity to nikethamide or related compounds.

Warnings: *Do not inject intraarterially.* Since safe use during pregnancy has not been established; it should be given only when its use is deemed essential to the welfare of the patient.

Adverse Reactions: Most common is an unpleasant feeling of burning or itching, especially at the back of the nose. Occasionally noted were flushing, or a feeling of warmth, sneezing, coughing, sweating, nausea, vomiting, restlessness, a feeling of fear, changing depth and frequency of respiration, tachycardia, elevated blood pressure, muscle twitching (especially facial), and convulsions. Muscle spasms and convulsions may develop with severe overdosage; the use of a short-acting barbiturate is usually effective in relieving these complications.

Dosage and Administration: Anesthetic overdosage: *to shorten narcosis,* 4 ml *intravenously* or *intramuscularly. To increase amplitude of respiration,* 2 to 5 ml *intravenously. To overcome* *respiratory depression,* 5 to 10 ml *intravenously,* repeated as necessary. *To combat respiratory paralysis,* 15 ml *intravenously* as minimum initial dose, repeated as required. Other methods of resuscitation, including assisted respiration, should also be employed. Asphyxia in newborn: After the air passages have been cleared, 1.5 ml into umbilical vein. In the event of cardiac arrest, 0.5 to 1 ml may be administered *intracardially.* Narcotic, hypnotic and carbon monoxide poisoning: Initial dose of 5 to 10 ml *intravenously,* followed by 5 ml every 5 minutes for first hour, then booster dosages of 5 ml on the hour or, in more serious cases, as often as every half-hour. Artificial respiration, gastric lavage, oxygen and other means of stimulation should be employed. Cardiac decompensation and coronary occlusion: For maintenance therapy, 3 to 5 ml *orally* 3 to 5 times daily. In emergencies, 5 to 10 ml *intravenously* or *intramuscularly.* Shock: 10 to 15 ml *intravenously.* Size and frequency of dose depend upon the response of the patient. In absence of whole blood or plasma, dosages of 10 to 15 ml every 2 to 3 hours are of value in compensating peripheral circulation until blood or plasma is available. Acute alcoholism: Initially, 5 to 20 ml *intravenously* to overcome central depression. Electroconvulsive therapy: Recommended dosage is 5 ml *intravenously* 1 minute before the electric stimulus is applied. For maintenance therapy, 3 to 5 ml of the oral solution every 4 to 6 hours when necessary.

Availability:
CORAMINE®: **(Ciba)**
Aqueous Solution, 25% in ampuls of 1.5 ml.
Oral Solution, 25% in bottles of 90 ml and 1 pint.

NILCOL

Description: Each tablet and each tablespoonful (15 ml) of elixir contain:

	Tablet	*Elixir*
Phenylpropanolamine hydrochloride	50 mg	25 mg
Chlorpheniramine maleate	4 mg	2 mg
Guaifenesin	200 mg	100 mg
Dextromethorphan hydrobromide	30 mg	15 mg
Alcohol	—	10%

Indications: Symptomatic relief of nasal and bronchial congestion and respiratory infections (coughs, influenza, common cold, sinusitis, allergic rhinitis or hay fever).

Contraindications: Hypersensitivity to any of the components.

Precautions: Because of the possibility of drowsiness, patients should be cautioned against driving or operating machinery. Should be used cautiously in patients with hyperthyroidism, hypertension and hypertensive-cardiovascular disease, diabetes mellitus, and liver disease. Use during pregnancy is not recommended.

Adverse Reactions: Anxiety, restlessness, tension, insomnia, tremor, weakness, headache, vertigo, sweating, nausea, and vomiting may occur.

Dosage and Administration: *Orally. Adults*—1 tablet or 2 tablespoonsful of elixir 3 or 4 times daily. *Children 6 to 12 years of age*—½ tablet or 1 tablespoonful of elixir 3 or 4 times daily; *4 to 6 years of age*—2 teaspoonsful of elixir 3 or 4 times daily; *2 to 4 years of age*—1 teaspoonful 3 or 4 times daily.

Availability:
NILCOL®: **(Warner-Chilcott)**
Elixir in bottles of 1 quart with dosage cups.
Tablets in bottles of 100.

NITROFURANTOIN

Chemical Name: 1-[(5-Nitrofurfurylidene)amino]hydantoin.

Description: Nitrofurantoin is a synthetic, antibacterial nitrofuran derivative, and occurs as a solid or as bitter, orange-yellow crystals or fine powder that is very slightly soluble in water and in alcohol.

It is bacteriostatic in low concentration and activity in vitro; it is considered to be bactericidal in higher concentration. Nitrofurantoin's presumed mode of action is based upon its interference with several bacterial enzyme systems. It appears that bacteria develop only a limited resistance to furan derivatives. About 45% of the drug is rapidly excreted unchanged in the urine in which it reaches a high concentration. It is highly soluble in the urine, to which it may impart a brown color.

The large crystal size of Macrodantin® is said to improve gastrointestinal tolerance while providing relatively slower absorption and excretion without a reduction in clinical effectiveness. Some patients who cannot tolerate the tablets are able to take the macrocrystalline capsules without experiencing nausea and vomiting.

Indications: Treatment of infections of the genitourinary tract, i.e., pyelonephritis, pyelitis and cystitis, when due to susceptible organisms, as shown by culture and sensitivity testing. It is not intended to replace surgical procedures when mechanical obstruction or stasis is present. It is not indicated for therapy of any systemic infections or for use in prostatitis or in any genitourinary tract infections other than pyelonephritis, pyelitis and cystitis.

Contraindications: In the presence of anuria or oliguria; in significant impairment of renal function; in patients who are hypersensitive to the drug; at term in pregnancy and in infants under 1 month of age.

Warnings: Certain ethnic groups of people of Mediterranean and Near-Eastern origin and Negroes who exhibit a deficiency of glucose-6-phosphate dehydrogenase in their red blood cells should be observed closely for the possible development of hemolytic anemia, and the drug discontinued if there is any evidence of hemolysis. *Pseudomonas* is the organism most commonly implicated in superinfection in patients treated with this drug. Routine caution is essential in women of childbearing potential and in lactating women. The drug should be used only when the potential benefits outweigh the possible risks to mother and child. Safe use in children under 12 years of age has not been established.

Precautions: Should be used with caution in the presence of mild renal impairment, accompanied by frequent chemical and cellular blood evaluations, and blood and urine assays for nitrofurantoin. Patients with renal impairment, anemia, diabetes, electrolyte imbalance, deficiency of vitamin B, or a debilitating disease, have been predisposed to peripheral neuropathy. In these patients, the drug should be used only when indicated specifically by in vitro sensitivity tests. If numbness or tingling occurs, the drug should be withdrawn. Nitrofurantoin should not be given concomitantly with drugs that may cause impairment of renal function. Acute, subacute or chronic pulmonary reaction has been observed in patients treated with nitrofurantoin. If these reactions develop, therapy should be discontinued and appropriate measures taken. Patients on long-term therapy should be closely observed for the onset of pulmonary reactions such as diffuse interstitial pneumonitis and/or pulmonary fibrosis.

Adverse Reactions: *Gastrointestinal reactions:* Anorexia, nausea, emesis are the most frequent reactions; less frequently, abdominal pain and diarrhea; rarely, hepatitis. This dose-related toxicity reaction can be minimized by reduction of dosage, especially in the female patient. *Hypersensitivity reactions:* Pulmonary sensitivity reactions, which can be acute, subacute, or chronic. Acute reactions are commonly manifested by fever, chills, cough, chest pain, dyspnea, pulmonary infiltration with consolidation of pleural effusion on roentgenogram and eosinophilia. The acute reactions usually occur within the 1st week of therapy and resolve with cessation of drug therapy. Subacute or chronic pulmonary reaction is associated with prolonged therapy. Insidious onset of malaise, dyspnea on exertion, cough, altered pulmonary function, and roentgenographic and histologic findings of diffuse interstitial pneumonitis or fibrosis or both are common manifestations. Impaired pulmonary function may result even after cessation of drug therapy. *Dermatologic reactions:* Maculopapular, erythematous, or eczematous eruption, pruritus, urticaria, and angioedema. *Other sensitivity reactions:* Anaphylaxis, asthmatic attack in patients with a history of asthma, cholestatic jaundice, drug fever, and arthralgia. *Hematologic reactions:* Hemolytic anemia, granulocytopenia, eosinophilia, and megaloblastic anemia. *Neurological reactions:* Peripheral neuropathy, headache, dizziness, nystagmus, and drowsiness. *Miscellaneous reactions:* Transient alopecia, superinfections in the genitourinary tract by resistant organisms, and tooth staining from direct contact with the oral suspension.

Dosage and Administration: *Orally.* Depending upon severity of infection, the average dosage ranges from 50 to 100 mg 4 times daily, not to exceed 400 mg daily. Therapy may be continued for 10 to 14 days, and dosage should be reduced by 25 to 50% if therapy is to be continued for prolonged periods. Children, 15 to 89 lbs, 1/2 to 3 teaspoonsful of the oral suspension 4 times daily. Children under 15 lbs, 5 to 7 mg/kg (2.2 to 3.2 mg/lb) /day, divided into 4 equal doses. The drug may be given with food or milk to minimize gastric upset.

Availability:

Nitrofurantoin

CYANTIN® Tablets, 50 mg in bottles of 100 and 1000 and in unit-dose packages of 100 (20 x 5); 100 mg in bottles of 100 and 1000 and in unit-dose packages of 100 (20 x 5). **(Lederle)**

FURADANTIN® **(Norwich-Eaton)**

Oral Suspension, 25 mg/5 ml in bottles of 60 ml and 1 pint.

Tablets, 50 and 100 mg in bottles of 25, 100 and 500 and in hospital unit-dose packages of 100.

MACRODANTIN® Capsules, 25 mg (macrocrystals) in bottles of 100; 50 and 100 mg (macrocrystals) in bottles of 30, 100, 500 and 1000 and in hospital unit-dose packages of 100 (10 x 10). **(Norwich-Eaton)**

TRANTOIN® Tablets, 50 and 100 mg in bottles of 100 and 1000 and in unit-dose cartons of 100. **(McKesson)**

NITROFURAZONE

Chemical Name: 5-Nitro-2-furaldehyde semicarbazone.

Description: Nitrofurazone is an antibacterial substance synthesized from furfural, and occurs as an odorless, lemon-yellow, crystalline powder very slightly soluble in water and slightly soluble in alcohol.

The drug is bactericidal in concentrations of 1:75,000 to 1:50,000 and inhibitory in concentrations of 1:200,000 to 1:100,000. It is said to be effective against a variety of gram-positive and gram-negative bacteria; however, it is not particularly effective against *Ps. aeruginosa* or *D. pneumoniae.* The drug acts by inhibiting the enzymes required for carboyhydrate metabolism in bacteria. This enzymatic inhibition occurs in both the aerobic and anaerobic cycles of carboyhydrate metabolism, which explains its bactericidal effect in these organisms.

The oral administration of nitrofurazone to rats for 7 days at extremely high dosage levels of 240 mg/kg/day produced severe hepatorenal lesions whereas only renal changes were seen when the dosage level was reduced to 60 mg/kg/day for 60 days. Dosage levels of 30 to 60 mg/kg/day shortened the time of appearance of the typical mammary gland tumor associated with older female rats. These tumors exhibited the same histological characteristics seen in the spontaneously occurring tumors and were seen only in the female animals. Mammary tumors were not found in rats treated with nitrofurazone orally for 1 year at levels of approximately 11 mg/kg/day. Spermatogenic arrest was noted in the male rats at dosage levels of 30 mg/kg/day and above. Dogs treated orally with nitrofurazone for 400 days at levels of 11 mg/kg/day showed no toxic effects. A single intravenous dose of 20, 35, or 75 mg/kg in dogs produced clinical signs of lacrimation, salivation, emesis, diarrhea, excitation, weakness, ataxia and weight loss, whereas 100 mg/kg produced convulsions and death. There was no evidence of toxicosis in rhesus monkeys treated with doses of nitrofurazone as high as 58 mg/kg/day for 10 weeks and 23 mg/kg/day for 63 weeks. Finally, when 30 mg/kg of nitrofurazone was administered to pregnant rabbits once daily on days 7 through 15 of pregnancy there was a slight increase in the frequency of stillbirths, but no teratogenic effects were noted.

Indications: Adjunctive therapy of patients with second- and third-degree burns when bacterial resistance to other drugs is a real or potential problem, and in skin grafting when bacterial contamination may cause graft rejection and/or donor site infection.

Contraindications: Known prior sensitization to nitrofurazone.

Warnings: Nitrofurazone has been shown to produce mammary tumors in female rats that were fed high doses of the drug. Safe use of this agent in pregnant women has not been established, and its use should therefore be restricted to those cases in which the need justifies the possible hazards to the unborn child.

Precautions: Occasionally, overgrowth of nonsusceptible organisms including fungi may occur; therefore, if irritation, sensitization, or superinfections develop, the drug should be withdrawn and appropriate measures instituted. Sensitization may be minimized by less frequent applications.

Adverse Reactions: To minimize any adverse effect, the medication should be removed by irrigation at the first sign of irritation. In chronic stasis ulcers, it may be helpful to protect the easily irritated skin surrounding them with zinc oxide ointment, and to confine the drug to the lesion itself.

Dosage and Administration: *Topically,* in doses depending upon the site being treated and at the discretion of the physician. Package literature should be consulted for specific details applicable to each dosage form.

Availability:
FURACIN®: **(Norwich-Eaton)**
Soluble Dressing, 0.2% in tubes of 28 and 56 gm and in jars of 135 and 454 gm and 5 lb.
Soluble Powder, 0.2% dissolved in a water-soluble powder of polyethylene glycol in shaker-top vials of 14 gm.
Topical Cream, 0.2% in tubes of 14 and 28 gm and in jars of 368 gm.

NITROGLYCERIN

Chemical Name: Glyceryl trinitrate.

Description: Nitroglycerin occurs as a volatile liquid which has explosive potential. The addition of carbohydrates renders it nonexplosive. It is thought to produce vasodilation by relaxing the smooth muscles of the wall of the blood vessels thus increasing blood supply to the myocardium. When taken sublingually, vasodilator effects appear within 2 to 3 minutes and persist for about 10 to 20 minutes. Tolerance to the drug becomes noticeable within a few days and is of considerable magnitude within 2 to 3 weeks.

Nitroglycerin is hydrolyzed in the blood stream to glycerol and nitrite; the nitrite is oxidized in part to nitrate. Repeated administration of therapeutic doses does not induce toxic effects except in those individuals who are hypersensitive to it. A sublingual dose not exceeding 0.6 mg will cause a decrease in heart size, a slight lowering of blood pressure and a slight increase in cardiac output. However, it decreases the output and work of the heart in patients with angina pectoris.

Indications: Prophylactic management of angina pectoris.

Contraindications: Idiosyncrasy to nitroglycerin, early myocardial infarction, glaucoma, hypotension, increased intracranial pressure, and severe anemia.

Precautions: Dosage forms other than sublingual tablets are intended for prophylactic use only; the sublingual tablets should be used for relief of an acute anginal attack. Tolerance to the drug may develop when used for prolonged periods. The development of blurred vision or dry mouth warrants discontinuation of the drug. If given to patients with glaucoma, extreme caution should be exercised in order to avoid an increase in ocular pressure.

Adverse Reactions: As with other nitrites, transient headache, postural hypotension, nausea and vomiting may occur. Overdosage may cause flushing, dizziness, tachycardia, headache and syncope.

Dosage and Administration: Usually 0.4 to 0.6 mg *sublingually* every 2 to 3 hours as required. For acute attacks, 0.4 mg may be taken sublingually every 5 minutes until pain is relieved. Timed-release dosage forms may be taken *orally* before breakfast and at bedtime (intervals of 12 hours). *Topically,* usually 1 to 2 inches of ointment every 3 to 4 hours. Some patients may require 4 to 5 inches. The ointment is spread on the special dose-measuring applicator and applied in a thin, uniform layer to skin of chest, abdomen or anterior thighs without massaging or rubbing. *Do not use fingers.* To determine optimal dose, start with 1 inch, increase dose ½ inch at a time until headache occurs, then drop back to optimal dose that does not cause headache. If treatment is to be discontinued, gradually reduce dose and frequency of application over a period of 4 to 6 weeks to prevent characteristic nitroglycerin withdrawal reactions.

Availability:
NITRO-BID®: **(Marion)**
Ointment, 2% in tubes of 20 and 60 gm and in Uni-Rx Paks of 20 and 60 gm in cartons of 6.
Plateau Capsules (sustained-release), 2.5, 6.5 and 9 mg in bottles of 60 and 100 and in Uni-Rx Paks (unit-dose) packages of 60 and 100 in cartons of 10; 9 mg in bottles of 60.
NITROGLYCERIN Capsules (timed-disintegration), 2.5 and 6.5 mg in bottles of 60 and 100. **(Lederle)**
NITROGLYCERIN Sublingual Tablets, 0.15, 0.3, 0.4 and 0.6 mg in bottles of 100. **(Lilly)**
NITROGLYN Tablets, (sustained-action), 1.3, 2.6 and 6.5 mg in bottles of 100 and 1000. **(Key Pharm.)**
NITROL® Ointment, 2% in tubes of 30 and 60 gm. **(Kremers-Urban)**
NITROSPAN® Capsules (sustained-release, micro-dialysis cells), 2.5 mg in bottles of 100. **(USV)**
NITROSTAT® Sublingual Tablets, 0.15, 0.3, 0.4 and 0.6 mg in bottles of 100 and in convenience packages of 100 (4 x 25). **(Parke-Davis)**
NITROVAS® Tablets, 2.6 mg (timed-disintegration) in bottles of 100 and 1000. **(Amfre-Grant)**

NITROPRUSSIDE SODIUM

Chemical Name: Sodium nitrosylpentacyanoferrate.

Description: Nitroprusside sodium is a potent, rapid-acting antihypertensive agent. The commercial product occurs as a reddish-brown powder that is soluble in water. Solutions of the drug are photosensitive and should be protected from light.

Present evidence suggests that the hypotensive effects of nitroprusside sodium are caused by peripheral vasodilatation as a result of a direct action on the blood vessels, independent of autonomic innervation. Following intravenous infusion, the drug induces a rapid antihypertensive action, usually within 2 minutes which lasts about 15 minutes after infusion has been discontinued; therefore, continuous infusion is necessary to maintain the hypotensive effect. Concomitant use with ganglionic blocking agents augments this effect. Its brief duration of action is due to the drug's rapid conversion to thiocyanate.

Clinical studies with hypertensive and normotensive patients showed that the drug produces a marked lowering of the arterial blood pressure, a slight increase in heart rate, a mild decrease in cardiac output and a moderate diminution in total peripheral vascular resistance. In hypertensive patients, moderate doses induced renal vasodilatation approximately equivalent to the decrease in pressure without an appreciable increase in renal blood flow or a decrease in glomerular filtration. Renal response to reduction in pressure was more significant in renovascular hypertensive patients, with a marked increase in renin release occurring from the involved kidney at mean arterial pressures ranging from 90 to 137 mm Hg. Furthermore, the magnitude of renin release from the involved kidney was significantly greater when compared with that in normotensive patients, while in the contralateral, uninvolved kidney, no significant release of renin was detected during reduction of pressure. Animal studies revealed no relaxation in the smooth muscle of the uterus or duodenum.

Indications: Treatment of hypertensive crises. Oral antihypertensive agents should be given simultaneously while the hypertensive emergency is being brought under control. May also be used where hypotension is required to minimize bleeding during surgical procedures.

Contraindications: In the treatment of compensatory hypertension (e.g., arteriovenous shunt or coarctation of the aorta). There is no known contraindication to the use of nitroprusside with oral antihypertensive agents. Its use during surgery is contraindicated when the cerebral circulation is inadequate or when the patient is moribund.

Warnings: Since nitroprusside is a potent drug, it should be administered **only** as an intravenous infusion with 5% dextrose in water. **Important Note:** *Should not be given by direct injection.* Since the metabolite thiocyanate inhibits both the uptake and binding of iodine, cautious use of the drug is therefore essential in patients with hypothyroidism and severe renal impairment. Blood levels of the metabolite should be determined daily (should not exceed 10 mg/100 ml) if treatment is to be extended in these patients. Those who are receiving concomitant antihypertensive medications are more sensitive to the hypotensive effect of nitroprusside sodium; therefore, the dosage of this drug should be adjusted accordingly. When hypotensive anesthetic techniques are employed, tolerance to blood loss, anemia and hypovolemia may be diminished, and the pulmonary ventilation perfusion ratio may be altered. Considerable caution should be exercised in patients who are especially poor surgical risks. Until further clinical experience has been gained, the safe use of this drug in pregnant women and in children has not been confirmed.

Precautions: Because of its rapid antihypertensive action, adequate facilities, equipment, and personnel should be readily available for frequent and vigilant monitoring of blood pressure. When the infusion is slowed or discontinued, blood pressure usually begins to rise immediately and returns to pretreatment levels within 1 to 10 minutes. Elderly patients require special care and initial lower doses since they are more sensitive to the hypotensive effects of the drug. It is urgent that precise measurement of the flow rate be maintained and the use of an infusion pump, micro-drip regulator, or other such device be employed. If used continuously, a fresh solution should be prepared every 4 hours, and the solution should be protected from light. If the solution turns blue, green or dark red, it should be discarded.

Adverse Reactions: Too rapid administration of the solution may cause nausea, retching, diaphoresis, apprehension, headache, restlessness, muscle twitching, retrosternal discomfort, palpitations, dizziness, and abdominal pain. However, these reactions rapidly disappeared by either slowing the rate or temporarily discontinuing the infusion, and they did not reappear when the infusion was reinstated at a slower rate. One case of hypothyroidism following prolonged therapy has been reported. A patient with severe hypertension with uremia received 3.9 gm of the drug over a period of 21 days. There was no tachyphylaxis, but the patient developed signs of hypothyroidism together with retention of thiocyanate (9.5 mg/100 ml). The use of peritoneal dialysis reduced the thiocyanate level and the signs of hypothyroidism subsided.

Dosage and Administration: *Intravenously.* The contents of the vial should be dissolved in 5% dextrose in water; *no other diluent should be used.* Also, this solution should not be used as a vehicle for simultaneous administration of any other drug. In patients who are not receiving other antihypertensive drugs, the usual dose is 3 mcg/kg/minute (range of 0.5 to 10 mcg/kg/minute). Usually, an average of 200 mcg/minute (range of 20 to 400 mcg/minute) is sufficient to maintain the blood pressure at a level of 30 to 40% lower than that of the pretreatment diastolic pressure. For patients receiving concomitant antihypertensive medications, smaller doses are required. In order to avoid excessive levels of thiocyanate and to minimize the possibility of a precipitous drop in blood pressure, the maximum recommended dose is 800 mcg/minute. Care should be taken to avoid extravasation. After the blood pressure is controlled, oral therapy with other antihypertensive agents should be substituted.

Availability:
NIPRIDE® Powder for Injection in vials of 50 mg. **(Roche)**

NOLAMINE

Description: Each timed-release tablet contains chlorpheniramine maleate, 4 mg, phenindamine tartrate, 24 mg and phenylpropanolamine hydrochloride, 50 mg.

Indications: Relief of nasal congestion associated with the common cold, sinusitis, rhinitis, nasopharyngitis, rhinorrhea, and congestion associated with hay fever and other allergies.

Precautions: Use with caution in the presence of hypertension, hyperthyroidism or cardiovascular disease. Should drowsiness occur, patients should be advised not to engage in activities requiring alertness such as driving a car or operating dangerous machinery.

Adverse Reactions: Occasionally, drowsiness, tremors, dizziness and nervousness may occur.

Dosage and Administration: *Orally,* 1 tablet every 8 hours, in mild cases every 10 to 12 hours.

Availability:
NOLAMINE Tablets (pink) in bottles of 50 and 250. **(Carnrick)**

NORETHINDRONE

Chemical Name: 17-Hydroxy-19-nor-17α-pregn-4-en-20-yn-3-one.

Description: Norethindrone is a synthetic progestogen which differs structurally from norethynodrel only in the position of the double bond in the A ring of the steroid molecule. It occurs as a white, crystalline powder slightly soluble in water and freely soluble in alcohol.

On a weight basis, oral norethindrone is about twice as potent, and the acetate ester about 4 times as potent, as parenteral progesterone. Norethindrone and norethindrone acetate share the same onset and duration of action, and actions and uses of parenteral progesterone. Norethindrone, with or without estrogen, achieves its contraceptive effect by suppressing the secretion of gonadotropin.

Indications: Treatment of amenorrhea; in abnormal uterine bleeding due to hormonal imbalance in the absence of organic pathology, such as submucous fibroids or uterine cancer; and in endometriosis. It is employed either alone or formulated with ethinyl estradiol for the control of conception.

Contraindications: In patients with thrombophlebitis, thromboembolic disorders, cerebral apoplexy, or with a history of these conditions; in patients with markedly impaired liver function, known or suspected carcinoma of the breast, known or suspected estrogen-dependent neoplasia; and in undiagnosed abnormal genital bleeding.

For warnings, precautions, adverse reactions and dosage, see monograph on Mestranol + Ethynodiol Diacetate.

Availability:
MICRONOR® Tablets (green) 0.35 mg in Dialpak® dispensers of 35. **(Ortho)**
NORLUTATE® Tablets (as acetate), 5 mg in bottles of 50. **(Parke-Davis)**
NORLUTIN® Tablets, 5 mg in bottles of 50. **(Parke-Davis)**
NOR-Q.D.® Tablets (yellow), 0.35 mg in dispenser-packages of 42. **(Syntex)**

w/Ethinyl Estradiol

BREVICON® Tablets in Memorette® dispensers of 21 tablets in packages of 3 and in refill packages of 6. Each tablet contains norethindrone, 0.5 mg and ethinyl estradiol, 0.035 mg. The Memorette dispensers of 28 tablets contain in addition 7 orange, inert tablets. **(Syntex)**
LOESTRIN® 21 1/20 Tablets in Petipac® compact containers of 21 tablets in cartons of 5 and in refill packages of 5. Each white tablet contains norethindrone (as acetate), 1 mg and ethinyl estradiol, 0.02 mg. **(Parke-Davis)**
LOESTRIN® 21 1.5/30 Tablets in Petipac® compact containers of 21 tablets in cartons of 5 and in refill packages of 5. Each green tablet contains norethindrone (as acetate), 1.5 mg and ethinyl estradiol, 0.03 mg. **Parke-Davis)**
LOESTRIN® FE 1/20 Tablets in Petipac® compact containers of 28 tablets in cartons of 5. Each white tablet contains norethindrone (as acetate), 1 mg and ethinyl estradiol, 0.02 mg. Each brown tablet contains ferrous fumarate, 75 mg. Each compact or refill contains 21 white tablets and 7 brown tablets. **(Parke-Davis)**
LOESTRIN® FE 1.5/30 Tablets in Petipac® compact containers of 28 tablets in cartons of 5. Each green tablet contains norethindrone (as acetate), 1.5 mg and ethinyl estradiol, 0.03 mg. Each brown tablet contains ferrous fumarate, 75 mg. Each compact or refill contains 21 green tablets and 7 brown tablets. **(Parke-Davis)**
MODICON® Tablets in Dialpak™ dispensers of 21 and 28 tablets in packages of 3 and 6. Each tablet contains norethindrone, 0.5 mg and ethinyl estradiol, 0.035 mg. **(Ortho)**
NORLESTRIN® [21] Tablets in Petipac® compact containers of 21 tablets in cartons of 5 and in

packages of 5 compacts or refills of 21 tablets each. Each tablet contains norethindrone (as acetate), 1 mg and ethinyl estradiol, 0.05 mg. **(Parke-Davis)**
NORLESTRIN [28] 1 mg Tablets in packages of 5 compacts or refills of 28 tablets each. Each compack contains 21 yellow tablets Norlestrin-1 mg and 7 white, inert tablets. **(Parke-Davis)**
NORLESTRIN [Fe] 1 or 2.5 mg Tablets in Petipac® compact containers of 28 and in packages of 5 compacts or refills of 28 tablets each. Each yellow tablet contains norethindrone (as acetate), 1 mg and ethinyl estradiol, 0.05 mg. Each pink tablet contains norethindrone (as acetate), 2.5 mg and ethinyl estradiol, 0.05 mg. Each brown tablet contains ferrous fumarate, 75 mg. Each Petipac compact container contains 21 pink or yellow tablets and 7 brown tablets. **(Parke-Davis)**
OVCON®-35/OVCON-50 Tablets in packages of 28 tablets in cartons of 6. Each peach tablet [35] contains norethindrone, 0.4 mg and ethinyl estradiol, 0.035 mg. Each package contains 21 peach tablets and 7 green, inert tablets. Each yellow tablet [—50] contains norethindrone, 1 mg and ethinyl estradiol, 0.05 mg. Each package contains 21 yellow tablets and 7 green, inert tablets. **(Mead Johnson)**
ZORANE® 1/20, 1.5/30 and 1/50 Tablets in compact containers of 28 in cartons of 5. Each pink tablet contains norethindrone (as acetate), 1 mg and ethinyl estradiol, 0.02 mg. Each blue tablet contains norethindrone (as acetate), 1.5 mg and ethinyl estradiol, 0.03 mg. Each green tablet contains norethindrone (as acetate), 1 mg and ethinyl estradiol, 0.05 mg. Each compact contains 21 pink, blue or green tablets and 7 white, inert tablets. **(Lederle)**

NORGESTREL

Chemical Name: Norgestrel—*dl*-13-β-Ethyl-17-α-ethinyl-17-β-hydroxygon-4-en-3 - one.

Description: Norgestrel is a synthetic progestogen. Available data suggest that all of the biological activity of norgestrel resides in the *d*-enantiomer portion. Animal studies have shown that norgestrel possesses much more progestational activity than does progesterone or norethisterone, is devoid of androgenic activity at usual clinical doses, and is neither estrogenic nor converted in vivo to estrogen.

The contraceptive action of norgestrel alone has been reported to be less effective than those of the sequential or combination products containing both a progestogen and estrogen.

The combination of norgestrel and ethinyl estradiol acts primarily by suppressing the secretion of gonadotropin. Although the primary mechanism of action is inhibition of ovulation, the effectiveness of norgestrel and ethinyl estradiol may also result from other mechanisms of action such as hostility of the cervical mucus to sperm penetration and migration.

Indications: Oral contraception.

For contraindications, warnings, precautions and adverse reactions, see monograph on Mestranol + Ethynodiol Diacetate.

Dosage and Administration: *Orally. Norgestrel:* One tablet daily taken on a continuous dosage regimen starting on the 1st day of menstruation or in the immediate postpartum period. The tablets should be taken at the same time each day and continued, without interruption, throughout the whole course of the contraceptive program whether or not bleeding occurs. The physician should be consulted in the event of prolonged bleeding. The patient should be well informed that *strict adherence* to the regimen is important and that the risk of pregnancy increases with each tablet missed. For the first 2 weeks or until 14 tablets have been taken, a nonhormonal contraceptive agent should be employed in addition to norgestrel. *Norgestrel + Ethinyl Estradiol:* The dosage is 1 tablet daily from the 5th through the 24th or 25th day of the menstrual cycle or 21 days of treatment followed by 7 days of rest period during which no tablets are taken or an inert tablet is taken. If spotting or breakthrough bleeding occurs, the patient should be instructed to continue on the same regimen. The 5th day of the menstrual cycle is considered the 1st day medication is started.

Availability:

Norgestrel

OVRETTE® Tablets, 0.075 mg in Pilpak® dispensers of 28 tablets in packages of 6. **(Wyeth)**

Norgestrel + Ethinyl Estradiol

LO/OVRAL® Tablets, 0.3 mg of norgestrel and 0.03 mg of ethinyl estradiol in Pilpak® dispensers of 21 tablets in packages of 6 and in 3-Pak packages of 63 tablets. **(Wyeth)**

LO/OVRAL-28 Tablets, 0.3 mg of norgestrel and 0.03 mg of ethinyl estradiol (21 white tablets and 7 pink, inert tablets) in packages containing 6 Pilpak® dispensers of 28 tablets each. **(Wyeth)**

OVRAL® Tablets, 0.5 mg. of norgestrel and 0.05 mg of ethinyl estradiol in packages containing 3 or 6 Pilpak® dispensers of 21 tablets each. **(Wyeth)**

OVRAL-28 Tablets, 0.5 mg of norgestrel and 0.05 mg of ethinyl estradiol (21 white tablets and 7 pink, inert tablets) in packages containing 6 Pilpak® dispensers of 28 tablets each. **(Wyeth)**

NORTRIPTYLINE HYDROCHLORIDE

Chemical Name: 5-(3-Methylaminopropylidene)-10,11-dihydro-5*H*-dibenzo[a,d]cycloheptene hydrochloride.

Description: Nortriptyline hydrochloride is a tricyclic antidepressant drug structurally and pharmacologically related to amitriptyline. It is not an MAO (monoamine oxidase) inhibitor. In experimental animals, nortriptyline exhibits a disruptive action on the electroencephalogram and on operant behavior, an anticonvulsant action, a peripheral and central atropine-like action, antihistamine and antiserotonin effects, and some adrenergic blockade. As with amitriptyline, the manner in which it exerts its clinical antidepressant effect is uncertain.

Indications: Treatment of endogenous and, to a lesser extent, reactive depression, and associated symptoms such as anxiety, tension, insomnia, restlessness, disinterest and irritability.

Contraindications: Hypersensitivity to the drug. Administration of nortriptyline concomitantly with other tricyclic antidepressants or with MAO inhibitors is contraindicated. A medication-free period of at least 2 weeks should be observed when transferring patients from MAO inhibitors to nortriptyline. Also contraindicated during the acute recovery period following myocardial infarction. A potential cross-sensitivity between nortriptyline and other dibenzazepines should be considered.

Warnings: Patients with cardiovascular disease should be under close supervision because of the tendency of the drug to produce sinus tachycardia and to prolong the conduction time. Myocardial infarction, arrhythmia, and strokes have occurred. Because of its anticholinergic activity, the action of guanethidine and similar drugs may be blocked. Nortriptyline should be used with utmost caution in patients who have glaucoma, a history of urinary retention or hyperthyroidism. Also, patients with a history of seizures should be followed closely inasmuch as this drug is known to lower the convulsive threshold. Safe use in pregnant or lactating women or in children has not been established. Patients should be warned about the possibility of drowsiness if they must operate dangerous machinery or drive a motor vehicle.

Precautions: Leukocyte and differential counts and liver function studies should be performed prior to and during prolonged therapy. Alterations (both up and down) in blood sugar levels have been noted. Since the possibility of suicide exists in severe depression, seriously depressed patients should be carefully supervised during early therapy with nortriptyline. It is important that the least possible quantity of the drug be dispensed at any given time. The use of the drug alone in schizophrenic patients may result in an exacerbation of the psychosis or may activate latent schizophrenic symptoms which may require discontinuation of therapy. If the drug is given to overactive or agitated patients, increased anxiety and agitation may occur. In manic-depressive patients nortriptyline may cause symptoms of the manic phase to emerge. Close clinical surveillance and careful adjustment of the dosage are required when the drug is given in conjunction with sympathomimetic or anticholinergic agents as epileptiform seizures may occur. Concurrent ingestion with CNS depressants and alcohol may potentiate the adverse effects of this drug. Concomitant use of nortriptyline with electroconvulsive therapy (with or without atropine, short-acting barbiturates and muscle relaxants) has not been thoroughly studied; therefore, the physician should be aware that additional adverse reactions may occur. If possible, the drug should be discontinued for several days prior to elective surgery.

Adverse Reactions: Although not all of the following adverse effects have been reported with this drug, the pharmacologic similarities among the tricyclic antidepressant drugs require that each of the reactions be considered when nortriptyline is administered. *Cardiovascular*—Hypotension, hypertension, tachycardia, palpitation, myocardial infarction, arrhythmias, heart block, stroke. *Psychiatric*—Confusional states (especially in the elderly) with hallucinations, disorientation, delusions; anxiety, restlessness, agitation; insomnia, panic, nightmares, hypomania, exacerbation of psychosis. *Neurological*—Numbness, tingling, paresthesias of extremities, incoordination, ataxia, tremors; peripheral neuropathy, extrapyramidal symptoms; seizures, alteration in EEG patterns; tinnitus. *Anticholinergic*—Dry mouth and, rarely, associated sublingual adenitis, blurred vision, disturbance of accommodation, mydriasis; constipation, paralytic ileus; urinary retention, delayed micturition, dilation of the urinary tract. *Allergic*—Skin rash, petechiae, urticaria, itching, photosensitization (avoid excessive exposure to sunlight); edema (general or of face and tongue), drug fever, cross-sensitivity with other tricyclic drugs. *Hematologic*—Bone-marrow depression, including agranulocytosis; eosinophilia; purpura; thrombocytopenia. *Gastrointestinal*—Nausea and vomiting, anorexia, epigastric distress, diarrhea; peculiar taste, stomatitis, abdominal cramps, black-tongue. *Endocrine*—Gynecomastia in the male, breast enlargement and galactorrhea in the female; increased or decreased libido, impotence; testicular swelling; elevation or depression of blood sugar levels. *Other*—Jaundice (simulating obstructive); altered liver function; weight gain or loss; perspiration; flushing; urinary frequency, nocturia; drowsiness, dizziness, weakness, fatigue; headache, parotid swelling; alopecia. *Withdrawal Symptoms*—Though these are not indicative of addiction, abrupt cessation of treatment after prolonged therapy may produce nausea, headache, and malaise. Toxic overdosage may result in confusion, restlessness, agitation, vomiting, hyperpyrexia, muscle rigidity, hyperactive reflexes, tachycardia, ECG evidence of impaired conduction, shock, congestive heart failure, stupor, coma, and CNS stimulation with convulsions followed by respiratory depression. Deaths have occurred following overdosage with drugs of this class. No specific antidote is known. General supportive measures are indicated, with gastric lavage. Respiratory assistance is apparently the most effective measure when indicated. The use of CNS depressants may worsen the prognosis. Intramuscular paraldehyde or preferably diazepam provides anticonvulsant activity with less respiratory depression than do the barbiturates. The use of digitalis and/or pyridostigmine may be considered in case of serious cardiovascular abnormalities or cardiac failure. The value of dialysis has not been established.

Dosage and Administration: *Orally.* The usual adult dosage is 25 mg 3 or 4 times daily. Doses above 100 mg daily are not recommended. For elderly and adolescent patients, 30 to 50 mg daily in divided doses.

Availability:
AVENTYL®: **(Lilly)**
Liquid, 10 mg/5 ml in bottles of 1 pint.
Pulvules® (capsules), 10 and 25 mg in bottles of 100 and 500 and in 10 strips of 10 individually labeled blisters each containing 1 pulvule.
PAMELOR®: **(Sandoz)**
Capsules, 10 and 25 mg in bottles of 100 and 500 and in Sandopak®s (unit-dose) packages of 100.
Liquid, 10 mg/5 ml in bottles of 1 pint.

NOSCAPINE

Chemical Name. 2-Methyl-8-methoxy-6, 7-methylenedioxy-1-(6, 7-dimethoxy-3-phthalidyl)-1, 2, 3, 4-tetrahydroisoquinoline.

Description: Noscapine is a naturally occurring opium alkaloid of the benzylisoquinoline group and is structurally related to papaverine. It is chemically and pharmacologically distinct from morphine and produces no psychological or physical dependence. Next to morphine it is the most abundant of the alkaloids being present to the extent of 6% in the opium capsule. It resembles papaverine in its action on smooth muscle, and except for its antitussive action, it has no significant effect on the CNS in doses within therapeutic range. The use of noscapine is largely confined to treatment of cough due to respiratory tract infection. It is readily absorbed from the gastrointestinal tract but its metabolic fate has not been established.

Indications: Temporary relief of cough associated with the common cold.

Contraindications: Hypersensitivity to any of the components.

Precautions: Patients with high fever, persistent cough, or diabetes should take this medication only as directed by the physician. Patients should be cautioned not to exceed the recommended dosage.

Adverse Reactions: None reported.

Dosage and Administration: *Orally.* Adults and children over 12 years of age. 1 tablet or teaspoonful every 3 or 4 hours, or as directed by the physician.

Availability:
ACTOL EXPECTORANT®: **(Beecham)**
Syrup in bottles of 1 pint. Each 5 ml (teaspoonful) contains noscapine, 30 mg; guaifenesin, 200 mg and alcohol, 12.5%.
Tablets, 30 mg with guaifenesin, 200 mg in bottles of 100.

NOVACEBRIN w/FLUORIDE: see The Fluoride-Vitamins

NOVOBIOCIN

Description: Novobiocin is an antibiotic derived from cultures of *Streptomyces nivens (S. spheroides).* In vitro, novobiocin inhibits the growth of staphylococci, streptococci and diplococci. Gram-negative cocci are only moderately susceptible and there is little or no effect on gram-negative rods of the enteric group except for coliform bacteria and for strains of *Proteus vulgaris.* Novobiocin is primarily bacteriostatic rather than bactericidal in action. It is readily absorbed from the gastrointestinal tract; peak blood levels are attained within 2 to 4 hours and detectable amounts remain approximately 24 hours following a single oral dose. The drug diffuses well into the pleural, joint and ascitic fluids. It does not diffuse into the spinal fluid unless the meninges are inflamed. It is excreted in the bile, urine and feces.

Indications: Treatment of staphylococcal infections, particularly in patients sensitive to other antibiotics; in infections in which the causative organism is resistant to other antibiotics; and in urinary tract infections due to microorganisms resistant to other commonly employed antibacterial agents, notably certain strains of Proteus.

Contraindications: Hypersensitivity to novobiocin.

Warnings: The high incidence of adverse reactions including urticaria, maculopapular dermatitis, hepatic dysfunction and blood dyscrasias strongly suggests that this antibiotic should be reserved only for those serious infections in which less toxic antibiotics are either ineffective or contraindicated. Rapid and frequent emergence of resistant strains, especially staphylococci, readily occurs with novobiocin. Safe use in pregnant and lactating women has not been established. Jaundice due to hyperbilirubinemia has been reported to occur 3 times as frequently in newborn infants as in control infants. For this reason, administration of novobiocin to premature, newborn and young infants should be avoided unless indication is extremely urgent because of serious infections not susceptible to other antibacterial agents.

Precautions: Blood dyscrasias, including pancytopenia, leukopenia, agranulocytosis, anemia and thrombocytopenia, have been reported, and total and differential blood cell counts should be made routinely during therapy. If hyperbilirubinemia or BSP retention occurs, the drug should be discontinued. Intrahepatic biliary obstruction and hemolysis may occur. If continued therapy appears essential, liver function studies should be made periodically. If jaundice occurs or if a yellow pigment appears in the plasma, therapy should be discontinued, except in serious infections in which the infecting organisms are resistant to other antibacterial agents. Constant observation of the patient is essential and if a new infection appears, appropriate measures should be undertaken. Treatment should be discontinued if allergic reactions develop which are not readily controlled with antihistaminic agents.

Adverse Reactions: A relatively high incidence of hypersensitivity reactions has been noted usually characterized by skin eruptions. These include urticarial, erythematous, maculopapular or scarlatiniform rash; rarely, erythema multiforme (Stevens-Johnson syndrome). Hematopoietic reactions noted were blood dyscrasias such as leukopenia, eosinophilia with or without fever, anemia, pancytopenia, agranulocytosis, and thrombocytopenia. Hepatic dysfunction was manifested by jaundice, elevation of serum bilirubin concentration and impaired bromsulphalein excretion. Other reactions noted include alopecia, nausea and vomiting, loose stools and diarrhea, intestinal hemorrhage, and pain at the injection site.

Dosage and Administration: *Orally.* The usual adult dosage is 250 mg every 6 hours or 500 mg every 12 hours, with a maximum of 2 gm daily. Dosage for children ranges from 15 to 45 mg/kg of body weight daily in divided doses. *Intravenously* or *intramuscularly.* Adult dosage is 500 mg every 12 hours. Children with moderately severe infections may be given 15 mg/kg of body weight daily and for severe infections 30 mg/kg of body weight daily in 2 divided doses at intervals of 12 hours. Treatment should be continued for at least 48 hours after temperature has returned to normal and all evidence of infection has disappeared.

Availability:
ALBAMYCIN®: **(Upjohn)**
Capsules (as the sodium salt), 250 mg in bottles of 16 and 100.
Injection (as the sodium salt), 100 mg/ml in Mix-O-Vials® of 5 ml.
Syrup (as the calcium salt), 125 mg/5 ml in bottles of 60 ml.

NUCOFED Ⓒ III

Description: Each capsule and each 5 ml of syrup contains codeine phosphate, 20 mg and pseudoephedrine hydrochloride, 60 mg in a mint-flavored vehicle. Combines the salutary effects of a decongestant with that of an antitussive-analgesic agent.

Indications: Symptomatic relief of cough and congestion due to upper respiratory tract infections, the common cold, bronchitis, influenza and sinusitis.

Contraindications: Hypersensitivity to any of the components.

Warnings: Codeine phosphate may be habit-forming. This drug should not be taken by: individuals with persistent cough such as occurs with smoking, asthma, emphysema; or for cough that is accompanied by excessive secretions; those with chronic pulmonary disease, shortness of breath, high blood pressure, heart disease, diabetes or thyroid disease; and children taking other medication except under the recommendation and supervision of a physician. Patients should be informed: that constipation may occur or be aggravated; not to exceed the recommended dosage; and to consult the physician if symptoms do not improve within 7 days; tend to recur, or are accompanied by high fever, rash or persistent headache.

Adverse Reactions: Nervousness, dizziness, or sleeplessness may occur with overdosage.

Dosage and Administration: *Orally* every 4 to 6 hours. Adults, 1 capsule or 1 teaspoonful, not to exceed 6 capsules or teaspoonsful in a 24-hour period. Children 6 to 12 years of age, 1/2 teaspoonful, not to exceed 3 teaspoonsful in a 24-hour period; 2 to 6 years of age, 1/4 teaspoonful, not to exceed 1 1/2 teaspoonsful in a 24-hour period. The capsules are not recommended for children of any age and the syrup for those under 2 years of age.

Availability:
Ⓒ III NUCOFED®: **(Beecham)**
Capsules in bottles of 60.
Syrup (mint-flavored) in bottles of 1 pint.

NYLIDRIN

Chemical Name: *p*-Hydroxy-α-[1-[(1-methyl-3-phenylpropyl)amino]ethyl]benzyl alcohol hydrochloride.

Description: Nylidrin hydrochloride is a sympathomimetic amine and a beta-receptor stimulant with selective pharmacologic action on blood vessels of skeletal muscle similar to that of epinephrine. It produces a direct vasodilating action upon small arteries and arterioles. It has no significant effect on pulse rate or blood pressure. Nylidrin increases cardiac output but produces little or no change in heart rate or rhythm. It is rapidly absorbed from the gastrointestinal tract and has a prolonged action.

Indications: May be of use whenever an increase in blood supply is desirable, as in vasospastic disorders of the extremities, and inner ear: *peripheral vascular disease* (arteriosclerosis obliterans, thromboangiitis obliterans, diabetic vascular disease, night leg cramps, Raynaud's disease, ischemic ulcer, frostbite, acrocyanosis, acroparesthesia, thrombophlebitis, cold feet, legs and hands), *circulatory disturbances of the inner ear* (primary cochlear cell ischemia, cochlear stria vascular ischemia, macular or ampular ischemia and other disturbances due to labyrinthine artery spasm or obstruction).

Contraindications: Acute myocardial infarction, paroxysmal tachycardia, progressive angina pectoris and thyrotoxicosis.

Warnings: In patients with cardiac disease such as tachyarrhythmias and uncompensated congestive heart failure, the benefit-to-risk ratio should be weighed prior to therapy and reconsidered at intervals during treatment.

Adverse Reactions: Trembling, nervousness, weakness, dizziness (not associated with labyrinthine artery insufficiency), palpitations, nausea and vomiting may occur. Postural hypotension, while not reported, may also occur.

Dosage and Administration: *Orally.* The usual dosage is 3 to 12 mg 3 or 4 times daily.

Availability:
ARLIDIN® Tablets, 6 and 12 mg in bottles of 100 and 1000 and in single-dose strip dispenser cartons of 100 and 500. **(USV)**
NYLIDRIN HYDROCHLORIDE Tablets, 6 and 12 mg in bottles of 100 and 1000. **(Lederle)**

NYSTATIN

Description: Nystatin is an antifungal antibiotic derived from cultures of a strain of *Streptomyces noursei.* It is a polyene antibiotic of undertermined structural formula, and occurs as a hygroscopic, yellow or light-tan powder very slightly soluble in water and sparingly soluble in alcohol.

Nystatin has been found to inhibit the growth of yeast-like flora probably due to the drug's ability to bind to sterols present in the cell membrane of the organism. This action causes an increase in membrane permeability, thus allowing leakage of the intracellular components into the surrounding area. In concentrations of 2 units/ml or more, nystatin is fungistatic in vitro against a variety of fungi, including the principal fungi that are pathogenic to man. The antibiotic exhibits no appreciable activity against bacteria. Following oral administration, nystatin is poorly absorbed, no detectable blood levels are discernible at therapeutic doses, only traces are found in the plasma following considerably larger doses, and finally, most of the unabsorbed drug is excreted unchanged in the feces.

Indications: Topical nystatin, either alone or combined with other antifungal agents, is indicated for the treatment of cutaneous or vaginal mycotic infections caused by *Candida* (Monilia) *albicans.* Oral nystatin is intended for the prevention, as well as the treatment, of candidal infections. Specifically, oral nystatin is indicated for the treatment of candidal infections of the oral cavity, for intestinal candidiasis, and for protection against the possible overgrowth of monilia during antimicrobial or corticosteroid therapy.

Contraindications: In patients known to be hypersensitive to nystatin or to any other component, and in lesions due to nystatin-insensitive pathogens.

Precautions: At the first sign of a hypersensitivity reaction, the drug should be discontinued immediately and appropriate measures taken.

Adverse Reactions: Generally, nystatin has been found to be virtually nontoxic and nonsensitizing, and to be well tolerated by all age groups. In sensitive individuals irritation may occur following topical or intravaginal administration, in which case medication should be discontinued. Large oral doses have produced diarrhea and gastrointestinal distress, nausea and vomiting. For details on the component drugs, see their individual monographs.

Dosage and Administration: *Topical* preparations may be applied to affected area 2 or 3 times daily, or as indicated until healing is complete. Treatment should continue for 1 week after clinical cure is evident. *Intravaginally,* the usual dosage is 1 or 2 vaginal tablets (100,000 or 200,000 units) deposited high in the vagina (with applicator) once daily for about 2 weeks. To prevent thrush in the neonate, the pregnant woman may use 1 or 2 vaginal tablets for 3 to 6 weeks before term. *Orally,* the usual prophylactic and therapeutic dose is 1 tablet (500,000 units) 3 or 4 times daily. This dosage may be doubled if intestinal fungi are not adequately suppressed. Dosage for infants and children is generally 200,000 units 4 times daily.

Availability:

Nystatin

CANDEX® **(Dome)**
Creme, 100,000 units/gm in tubes of 15 gm.
Lotion, 100,000 units/ml in plastic bottles of 30 ml.
KOROSTATIN™ Vaginal Tablets, 100,000 units in packages of 14 and 28 with applicator. **(Holland-Rantos)**

MYCOSTATIN®: **(Squibb)**
Cream, 100,000 units/gm in a vanishing-cream aqueous base in tubes of 15 and 30 gm.
Ointment, 100,000 units/gm in tubes of 15 and 30 gm.
Oral Suspension (Dry Powder) in bottles of 24 doses with dropper calibrated at 1 ml. When reconstituted, each ml provides 100,000 units; also in a premixed cherry-mint flavored suspension in bottles of 60 ml with calibrated dropper.
Oral Tablets, 500,000 units in bottles of 100.
Powder for tissue culture, 500,000 units/gm in vials of 20 ml.
Topical Powder, 100,000 units/gm dispersed in talc in squeeze bottles of 15 gm.
Vaginal Tablets, 100,000 units dispersed in lactose with ethyl cellulose, stearic acid and starch in packages of 15 and 30 with applicator.

NILSTAT®: **(Lederle)**
Oral Suspension, 100,000 units/ml in bottles of 60 ml with dropper and 1 pint.
Oral Tablets, 500,000 units in bottles of 100 and in unit-dose packages of 100 (10 x 10).
Topical Cream, 100,000 units/gm in a vanishing-cream water base in tubes of 15 gm and in jars of 240 gm.
Topical Ointment, 100,000 units/gm in tubes of 15 gm.
Vaginal Tablets, 100,000 units in plastic units of blister-packed tablets of 15 and 30 with applicator.

O-V STATIN® Combination Package containing 21 Mycostatin Oral Tablets, 400,000 units each and 14 Mycostatin Vaginal Tablets, 100,000 units each with applicator. **(Squibb)**

Combinations

NYSTAFORM® Ointment, 100,000 units/gm with iodochlorhydroxyquin, 10 mg/gm in tubes of 15 gm. **(Dome)**

NYSTAFORM-HC Ointment, 100,000 units/gm with iodochlorhydroxyquin, 30 mg/gm and hydrocortisone (microdispersed), 10 mg/gm in tubes of 15 gm. **(Dome)**

OMNI-TUSS Ⓒ

Description: Each 5 ml (teaspoonful) contains:

Codeine phosphate	10 mg
Phenyltoloxamine*	5 mg
Chlorpheniramine*	3 mg
Ephedrine*	25 mg
Guaiacol carbonate	20 mg

*As cationic exchange resin complexes.

Indications: Relief of coughs associated with upper respiratory tract infections, bronchitis, bronchiectasis, bronchial asthma, emphysema, sinusitis, rhinitis, hay fever, or other allergic conditions.

Contraindications: Hypertension, cardiac disease, hyperthyroidism, prostatic hypertrophy, or sensitivity to any of the components.

Warnings: Codeine may be habit-forming, and should therefore be prescribed with the same degree of care as for other narcotic containing preparations.

Precautions: Patients should be cautioned against driving motor vehicles or operating machinery if drowsiness appears.

Adverse Reactions: Jitteriness, nausea, dry mouth, insomnia and constipation.

Dosage and Administration: *Orally.* Adults, 1 teaspoonful every 12 hours. Children 6 to 12 years of age, 1/2 teaspoonful every 12 hours.

Availability:
Ⓒ OMNI-TUSS® Suspension in bottles of 1 pint. **(Pennwalt)**

OPIUM ALKALOIDS Ⓒ

Description: Concentrated opium alkaloids consist of all the alkaloids of opium (as hydrochlorides) in highly purified form free from inert matter (waxes, gums, resins) and in approximately the same proportions in which they occur in nature.

Clinical evidence indicates that analgesic activity stems primarily from the morphine content which is about 50% anhydrous morphine. In addition, other alkaloids such as codeine, papaverine, etc. enhance the sedative and analgesic effects of morphine and tend to minimize its undesirable side effects. Thus, 20 mg of hydrochloride of opium alkaloids (morphine content, 10 mg) is therapeutically equivalent to 15 mg of morphine. One part of opium alkaloids (as hydrochlorides) is equivalent to 5 parts of opium.

Alleviates pain by its action on opiate receptors which function to inhibit ascending pain pathways. Onset of analgesia following parenteral administration occurs within 30 minutes, reaches a peak within 1 hour with continuing effect for up to 7 hours.

Indications: In all disorders in which the analgesic, sedative-hypnotic or narcotic effect of an opiate is needed: the relief of severe pain in place of morphine. Formulated with belladonna for antispasmodic action.

Contraindications: Bronchial asthma, narcotic idiosyncrasies and respiratory depression.

Warnings: May be habit-forming. Belladonna should not be used in patients with glaucoma or organic pyloric stenosis. It should be used with caution in prostatism, urinary retention, elderly patients and children under 6 years of age. If eye pain occurs, the drug should be discontinued. Patients should be cautioned not to exceed the prescribed dose if dryness of the mouth occurs and to discontinue use if rapid pulse, blurring of vision or dizziness results. Frequent and prolonged use of preparations containing belladonna should be avoided. In the event of rectal bleeding, proctologic examination is indicated.

Precautions: An addicting drug with an addiction liability equal to that of morphine. For this reason the same precautions should be taken in administering this drug as with morphine. Opium alkaloids require judicious use in infants, old and debilitated patients, and in patients with increased intracranial pressure, toxic psychosis, prostatic obstruction and myxedema.

Adverse Reactions: Adverse effects resemble those of morphine; most common are nausea, vomiting, constipation, dysuria, urinary retention, headache, miosis and respiratory depression. Overdosage is manifested by coma, pinpoint pupils, and depressed respiration. Nalorphine and levallorphan tartrate are effective antidotes in treating severe respiratory depression.

Dosage and Administration: *Intramuscularly or subcutaneously.* Adults, usually 5 to 20 mg. *Rectally,* 1 suppository 1 or 2 times daily.

Availability:
CII PANTOPON® Injection, 20 mg/ml in ampuls of 1 ml. **(Roche)**
CII OPIUM AND BELLADONNA (B&O) Suppositories, 60 mg of powdered opium and 16.2 mg of belladonna extract in cartons of 20. **(Wyeth)**

OPIUM TINCTURE, CAMPHORATED CIII

Synonym: Paregoric.

Description: Camphorated tincture of opium is a solution of powdered opium, anise oil, benzoic acid, camphor and alcohol which yields no less than 35 mg and no more than 45 mg of anhydrous morphine in each 100 ml. This preparation readily increases smooth muscle tone of the gastrointestinal tract, inhibits gastrointestinal motility and propulsion and diminishes digestive secretions. The upper portion of the small intestine, particularly the duodenum, is affected more than the ileum. Normal peristaltic movements are thus inhibited and the passage of intestinal contents delayed.

Indications: As a gastrointestinal sedative in the symptomatic treatment of uncomplicated diarrhea and for the relief of "colicky cramps" commonly associated with this condition. May be used alone or in combination with other antidiarrheal agents.

Contraindications: Hypersensitivity or idiosyncrasy to morphine or its derivatives or to any of the components, and in diarrheas caused by poisonous substances until the toxic material has been eliminated from the gastrointestinal tract.

Warnings: May be habit-forming. Generally, strict adherence to the recommended dosage will not produce euphoria or analgesia; however, prolonged use or excessive amounts have been found to cause psychic dependence and other untoward effects common to morphine.

Adverse Reactions: Although rarely noted, nausea and other gastrointestinal disturbances have occurred.

Dosage and Administration: *Orally.* Adults, the usual dosage is 5 to 10 ml every 2 hours up to, but not exceeding, 4 times daily until the diarrhea is controlled. Children, 0.25 to 0.5 ml/kg of body weight after each loose stool.

Availability:
CIII PAREGORIC:
Liquid, 2 mg/5 ml in bottles of 1 pint and 1 gallon. **(Lilly)**
Liquid, 2 mg/5 ml in bottles of 1 gallon. **(McKesson)**
Liquid, 2 mg/5 ml in bottles of 1 pint and 1 gallon and in unit-dose (individual cups) of 5 ml. **(Parke-Davis)**
Liquid, 2 mg/5 ml in unit-dose (patient's cups) of 5 ml. **(Philips Roxane)**

ORNADE

Description: Each sustained-release capsule contains:

Chlorpheniramine maleate	8 mg
Phenylpropanolamine hydrochloride	50 mg
Isopropamide iodide	2.5 mg

An antihistaminic agent is combined with decongestant and anticholinergic agents to provide symptomatic relief of sneezing, running nose, weeping and other symptoms of nasal congestion and upper respiratory tract distress. The isopropamide component generally provides antisecretory relief for up to 10 to 12 hours.

Indications: May be of use for prompt and prolonged relief of respiratory tract congestion and hypersecretion associated with vasomotor and allergic rhinitis. May also be considered for the relief of nasal congestion and hypersecretion associated with the common cold and sinusitis.

Contraindications: Hypersensitivity to any of the components; concurrent therapy with MAO inhibitors; severe hypertension; bronchial asthma; coronary artery disease; stenosing peptic ulcer; pyloroduodenal or bladder neck obstruction. Also contraindicated for use in children under 6 years of age.

Warnings: Patients should be advised of the potential hazard of activities requiring complete alertness or skill such as operating vehicles or machinery. Patients should also be cautioned about the possible additive effects of alcohol and other CNS depressants. Safe use of the drug during pregnancy has not been established and should be used in pregnant and nursing women or in women of childbearing potential only when the therapeutic benefits have been weighed against the possible hazards to the mother and child. The iodine in isopropamide iodide may alter PBI test results and will suppress I^{131} uptake; therefore, patients should be medication-free for 1 week before these tests are performed, or tests unaffected by exogenous iodides should be substituted.

Precautions: Use with caution in patients with cardiovascular disease, glaucoma, prostatic hypertrophy, or hyperthyroidism.

Adverse Reactions: Drowsiness; excessive dryness of nose, throat or mouth; nervousness or insomnia may occur on rare occasions, but are usually mild and transitory; nausea, vomiting, epigastric distress, diarrhea, rash, dizziness, weakness, tightness of chest, anginal pain, abdominal pain, irritability, palpitation, headache, incoordination, tremor, difficulty in urination, dysuria, thrombocytopenia, leukopenia, convulsions, hypertension, hypotension, anorexia, constipation, visual disturbances. Isopropamide may cause signs of iodine toxicity, manifested by acne and parotitis. Overdosage may be manifested by dryness of mouth, dysphagia, thirst, blurred vision, dilated pupils, photophobia, fever, rapid pulse and respiration, disorientation, and either excitation or depression of the CNS. Gastric lavage followed by saline cathartics should be administered to hasten evacuation of the drug from the gastrointestinal tract. Respiratory depression should be treated promptly by the use of oxygen and stimulants. If marked excitement is present, a short-acting barbiturate or chloral hydrate may be used.

Dosage and Administration: *Orally.* Adults and children over 6 years of age, 1 capsule every 12 hours. *Not to be administered to children under 6 years of age.*

Availability:
ORNADE® Spansule® (Capsule) in bottles of 50 and 500 and in single-unit packages of 100.

(Smith Kline & French)

ORPHENADRINE

Chemical Name: *N, N*-Dimethyl-2-(*o*-methyl-α-phenylbenzyloxy)ethylamine.

Description: Orphenadrine, a *tertiary* amine anticholinergic agent, is the *o*-methyl analog of diphenhydramine and is closely related to chlorphenoxamine. Available as the hydrochloride and citrate salts, they occur as bitter, white, crystalline powders; the former is very soluble in water and in alcohol, and the latter is sparingly soluble in water and slightly soluble in alcohol.

Orphenadrine reduces skeletal muscle spasm, primarily through an atropine-like central action on cerebral motor centers or on the medulla. The drug also exhibits postganglionic anticholinergic effects and some antihistaminic and local anesthetic action. Following oral administration, the drug is readily absorbed from the gastrointestinal tract, a peak effect is apparent in about 2 hours and persists for about 4 to 6 hours. Its metabolic fate is unknown.

Indications: Symptomatic treatment of Parkinson's syndrome, and acute spasm of voluntary muscles, regardless of location. With aspirin, phenacetin and caffeine, the combination may be used for the symptomatic relief of mild to moderate pain associated with acute musculoskeletal disorders.

Contraindications: In patients with glaucoma, pyloric or duodenal obstruction, stenosing peptic ulcers, prostatic hypertrophy, obstructions at the bladder neck, myasthenia gravis, achalasia of the esophagus, and cardiospasm. Since mental confusion, anxiety and tremors have been reported in patients taking orphenadrine and propoxyphene concurrently, it is recommended that the two drugs not be given simultaneously.

Warnings: Since safe use during pregnancy or lactation, or in women of childbearing potential has not been established, use of the drug in these patients should be governed by the potential benefits and the possible risks to the mother and child.

Precautions: Should be used with caution in patients with cardiac decompensation, coronary insufficiency, cardiac arrhythmias and tachycardia. Since prolonged, excessive use of phenacetin-containing preparations may result in nephrotoxicity, such compounds should be used with caution in patients with renal insufficiency. Periodic monitoring of blood, urine, and liver function values is advised.

Adverse Reactions: Reactions are due chiefly to the anticholinergic nature of the drug and may include dry mouth, tachycardia, palpitation, urinary hesitancy or retention, blurred vision, dilated pupils, increased ocular tension, weakness, nausea, vomiting, headache, dizziness, constipation, drowsiness, urticaria and other dermatoses, mental confusion in the elderly. Cases of aplastic anemia have been reported, although no causal relationship had been established. Some patients may experience transient episodes of lightheadedness or dizziness following injection of the citrate.

Dosage and Administration: *Intravenously* or *intramuscularly.* Adults, usually 60 mg (2 ml) every 12 hours. *Orally.* Adults, 1 tablet (100 mg) in the morning and 1 in the evening, or one 50-mg tablet 3 times daily. With APC, the dosage for adults is 1 or 2 tablets 3 or 4 times daily; children 6 to 12 years of age, 1 tablet 3 or 4 times daily. **Forte** tablets, ½ to 1 tablet 3 or 4 times daily. Safe use in children under 6 years of age has not been determined.

Availability:
DISIPAL® Tablets (hydrochloride), 50 mg in bottles of 100. **(Riker)**
NORFLEX®: **(Riker)**
Injection (citrate), 30 mg/ml in ampuls of 2 ml.
Tablets, 100 mg (citrate) in bottles of 100 and 500.
NORGESIC® Tablets, 25 mg (citrate) with phenacetin, 160 mg; aspirin, 225 mg and caffeine, 30 mg in bottles of 100 and 500. **Forte Tablets** contain twice these amounts and are available in bottles of 100 and 500. **(Riker)**

OS-CAL-MONE

Description: Each tablet contains:

Methyltestosterone	2.67 mg
Ethinyl estradiol	5.33 μg
Calcium carbonate (from oyster shell)	400 mg

Combined steroid and calcium therapy helps to stimulate osteoblastic activity, arrest the catabolic process in osteoporosis and promote positive calcium balance.

Indications: Prophylaxis and treatment of osteoporosis.

Contraindications: Patients with a history of established or suspected mammary or genital (including prostatic) malignancy, known or suspected estrogen-dependent neoplasia, undiagnosed abnormal genital bleeding, active thrombophlebitis or thromboembolic disorders or a past history of these conditions, and pregnant patients due to possible masculinization of the female fetus.

Precautions: Edema, which may occur in steroid-sensitive patients, can usually be alleviated by temporarily reducing the dosage or withholding the medication and/or by instituting a low-salt diet and a diuretic to the regimen. The development of jaundice indicates immediate discontinuation of therapy.

Adverse Reactions: Virilization, uterine bleeding and mastodynia may occur.

For complete details on the contraindications, warnings, precautions and adverse reactions, see the monograph on Testosterone and the Estrogens.

Dosage and Adminstration: *Orally,* 1 tablet 3 times daily after meals.

Availability:
OS-CAL-MONE® Tablets in bottles of 100, 500 and 1000. **(Marion)**

OTOCORT

Description: Each ml of solution contains:

Neomycin sulfate (equiv. to neomycin base)		3.5 mg
Polymyxin B sulfate	(2000 units)	0.2 mg
Hydrocortisone		0.1 %
Antipyrine		5 %
Dibucaine hydrochloride		0.25 %

with methylparaben, propylparaben, sodium bisulfite and glycerin in purified water.

The combination of antibacterial, antiinflammatory and anesthetic agents provides bactericidal activity against susceptible organisms.

Indications: Treatment of acute and chronic otitis externa.

Contraindications: Hypersensitivity to any of the components, and in individuals with tuberculous, fungal and viral conditions of the skin, especially herpes simplex, vaccinia and varicella. Also contraindicated in cases of perforated eardrum.

Precautions: As with all antibiotics, prolonged use may result in overgrowth of nonsusceptible organisms including fungi. If superinfection occurs, discontinue the medication and institute appropriate measures. Because of the hazard of ototoxicity, care should be exercised in patients with chronic otitis media.

Adverse Reactions: Sensitivity reactions of the skin due to neomycin. Also allergic cross-reactions with kanamycin, paromomycin, streptomycin, and possibly gentamicin may occur which might prevent their future use. The wide usage of topical neomycin has resulted in the emergence of bacterial strains resistant not only to neomycin but also to kanamycin, paromomycin and streptomycin as well.

Dosage and Administration: *Topically.* Before applying, the ear canal should be thoroughly cleansed and dried. Then instill 3 to 5 drops of solution 3 or 4 times daily, or if preferred, a gauze wick moistened with the medication may be used.

Availability:
OTOCORT® Solution in plastic squeeze drop bottles of 7 ml. **(Lemmon)**

OUABAIN

Description: Ouabain is a purified cardiac glycoside obtained from *Strophanthus gratus,* and is closely related chemically to digitalis glycosides. It is capable of producing all the pharmacodynamic actions of digitalis, e.g., primarily myocardial stimulation by a direct action on cardiac muscle. When given intravenously full digitalis effect is obtained within 2 hours. Ouabain is eliminated rapidly from the body, and the duration of its effect is short; therefore, cumulation is less likely to occur than with other substances possessing a digitalis-like action.

Indications: As an emergency measure in acute congestive heart failure. Also useful in the treatment of atrial or nodal paroxysmal tachycardia and atrial flutter.

Precautions: Since ouabain is a potent and rapidly acting drug, close observation of the patient is essential. This drug is not suitable for maintaining a digitalis effect, and the administration of a cardiac glycoside effective by the oral route should be instituted as soon as the emergency has passed. Extreme care must be exercised if ouabain is given to a patient who has frequent premature ventricular beats or who has received any preparation containing digitalis during the preceding 3 weeks. If nausea, vomiting, or extreme bradycardia occurs, or if cardiac arrhythmia develops, the drug should be discontinued.

Dosage and Administration: *Intravenously* (very slowly). Initially, 250 mcg; but in an emergency 500 mcg can be injected into the vein. After the initial injection, 100 mcg may be given hourly until the desired result is produced or until a total of 1 mg has been given within 24 hours.

Availability:
OUABAIN Injection, 250 mcg/ml in ampuls of 2 ml in cartons of 12. **(Lilly)**

OXACILLIN: see The Penicillins

OXANDROLONE

Chemical Name: 17β-Hydroxy-17α-methyl-2-oxa-5α-androstan-3-one.

Description: Oxandrolone is a steroid hormone chemically and physiologically related to methyltestosterone. Structurally, oxandrolone is unique in that ring A of the steroid nucleus is a lactone ring. In common with methyltestosterone and other androgenic anabolic hormones, oxandrolone increases retention of nitrogen, potassium and phosphorus and decreases amino acid catabolism. It has not been established whether or not this positive nitrogen balance indicates a primary benefit in the utilization of protein-building dietary substances. In experimental animals, oxandrolone appears to produce fewer androgenic effects than methyltestosterone when administered in doses producing an equivalent anabolic action. The functions of anabolic steroids are therefore similar to those of male sex hormones with the possibility that serious disturbances of growth and sexual development may develop if given to young children. The gonadotropic functions of the pituitary may be suppressed, and a direct effect on the testes may occur. The drug is generally regarded as a therapeutic adjuvant to enhance protein anabolism and to arrest the catabolic effects of various disease processes. An optimal balanced diet should be administered concomitantly with the drug to achieve full benefits of therapy.

Indications: Useful in promoting weight gain in patients who have lost weight after extensive surgery, chronic infections or severe trauma; to offset the protein catabolism associated with prolonged corticosteroid therapy, and to relieve bone pain accompanying osteoporosis.

Contraindications: In male patients with suspected or proved prostatic carcinoma, in those with benign prostatic hypertrophy with obstructive symptoms, in carcinoma of the male breast or in some women with breast cancer, in patients with nephroses or the nephrotic phase of nephritis, a history of hypersensitivity or toxic reaction to the drug, in patients with severe renal, cardiac or hepatic decompensation, hypercalcemia, prepubertal males, and patients easily stimulated. Also contraindicated in pregnant patients and in lactating women who are breast feeding their infants due to possible masculinization of the fetus or infant. Hypersensitivity to the drug is also a contraindication.

Warnings: Anabolic steroids do not enhance athletic ability.

Precautions: Routine caution is advocated when administering oxandrolone to patients with cardiac, renal or hepatic disease since edema may occur which may be further provoked by the concomitant administration of adrenal corticosteroids or ACTH. The occurrence of amenorrhea or menstrual irrgularities warrants discontinuation of therapy until the etiology has been established. Since anabolic steroids have been reported to increase prothrombin-time response in patients receiving anticoagulants and may thus precipitate hemorrhagic complications, the dosage of the anticoagulant may have to be decreased in order to maintain the prothrombin time at the desired therapeutic level. They have also been reported to alter glucose tolerance test. Diabetic patients should be followed carefully and their insulin or oral hypoglycemic dosage adjusted accordingly. Cautious use is advised in patients with benign prostatic hypertrophy and in those with a history of myocardial infarction or coronary artery disease. Serial determinations of serum cholesterol should be made at regular intervals and therapy adjusted if indicated in patients with cardiovascular complications. Additionally, serum and urinary calcium levels should be evaluated periodically in those patients suspected of hypercalcemia.

Adverse Reactions: Typical androgenic effects are rare, and are generally mild and usually reversible. In prepubertal males, phallic enlargement and increased frequency of erections have been noted. In postpubertal males, inhibition of testicular function, oligospermia and gynecomastia. In females, hirsutism, male-pattern baldness, deepening of the voice and clitoral enlargement have been reported. These changes are usually irreversible even after prompt discontinuance of therapy and are not prevented by concomitant use of estrogens. Also reported were menstrual irregularities and masculinization of the fetus. In both sexes, nausea, increased or decreased libido, acne (especially in females and prepubertal males), inhibition of gonadotropin secretion, bleeding in patients on concomitant anticoagulant therapy, premature closure of epiphyses in children, and alteration in the following clinical laboratory tests: The metyrapone test, glucose tolerance test, the thyroid function tests (a decrease in the PBI, in thyroxine-binding capacity and radioactive iodine uptake), the electrolyte retention of sodium, chlorides, water, potassium, phosphates and calcium, and liver function tests (increased serum cholesterol, and suppression of clotting factors II, V, VII, X). Decreased 17-ketosteroid excretion (with oral 17 α-alkyl substitution).

Dosage and Administration: *Orally.* Average adult dosage is 2.5 mg 2 to 4 times daily. Dosage may range from 2.5 to 20 mg daily, depending on individual need and response. Children, 0.25 mg/kg of body weight daily. Therapy for 2 to 4 weeks is usually adequate for both adults and children. Additional courses of therapy may be given on an intermittent schedule as indicated.

Availability:
ANAVAR® Tablets, 2.5 mg (white, scored) in bottles of 100. **(Searle)**

OXAZEPAM Ⓒ IV

Chemical Name: 7-Chloro-1,3-dihydro-3-hydroxy-5-phenyl-2*H*-1,4-benzodiazepin-2-one.

Description: Oxazepam is a psychotherapeutic agent structurally and pharmacologically related to chlordiazepoxide and diazepam but exhibits a shorter half-life. It appears to act at subcortical levels of the CNS through an effect on limbic structures. Oxazepam produces sedative, skeletal muscle relaxant and anticonvulsant activities. Therapeutic doses have little or no effect on the autonomic nervous system. Peak plasma levels are reached within 4 hours following an oral dose; excretion is primarily in the urine as the glucuronide conjugate.

Indications: Management and control of psychoneurotic states characterized by anxiety especially when associated with depression, tension, agitation, irritability and related symptoms; alcoholism characterized by acute tremulousness, inebriation or anxiety associated with alcohol withdrawal.

Contraindications: Hypersensitivity to oxazepam and in psychoses.

Warnings: Several studies have suggested an increased risk of congenital malformations associated with the use of minor tranquilizers during the first trimester of pregnancy; therefore, safe use during gestation or in women of childbearing potential has not been definitely established, and its use should be limited to those instances where the need justifies the potential hazards.

Precautions: Should be used with caution in patients, particularly elderly patients, in whom a drop in blood pressure may lead to cardiac complications. The possibility of psychic dependence or addiction should be borne in mind, particularly when it is administered to alcoholic patients or to those known to have been addicted to other drugs. Also tolerance to alcohol may be lowered. Abrupt withdrawal of oxazepam following prolonged administration of high dosage may result in epileptiform seizures or withdrawal symptoms similar to those produced by other sedative drugs. Because of possible drowsiness or dizziness, the drug should be administered with caution to patients performing hazardous tasks requiring alertness and physical coordination.

Adverse Reactions: The incidence of adverse effects is low. The expected side effects of drowsiness and ataxia are extensions of its pharmacologic actions. Other reports have included dizziness (mild and transient), vertigo, headache, syncope, mild paradoxical reactions such as excitement and stimulation of affect in psychiatric patients. Rarely noted were diffuse skin rashes (morbilliform, urticarial and maculopapular), nausea, lethargy, edema, slurred speech, tremor, altered libido, leukopenia, hepatic dysfunction including jaundice. The following may occur: paradoxical excitation with severe rage reactions, hallucinations, menstrual irregularities, change in EEG pattern, blood dyscrasias including agranulocytosis, blurred vision, diplopia, incontinence, stupor, disorientation, fever and euphoria.

Dosage and Administration: *Orally.* In mild to moderate psychoneurotic reactions, 10 to 15 mg 3 or 4 times daily. In severe psychoneurotic conditions and in alcoholism, 15 to 30 mg 3 or 4 times daily. The initial dosage for elderly or debilitated patients is 10 mg 3 times daily. If necessary, increase cautiously to 15 mg 3 or 4 times daily. Not indicated for use in children under 6 years of age; also dosage for children 6 to 12 years of age has not been established.

Availability:
Ⓒ SERAX®: **(Wyeth)**
Capsules, 10, 15 and 30 mg in bottles of 100 and 500 and in Redipak® (strip-pack) cartons of 25; 15 and 30 mg in Redipak cartons of 100.
Tablets, 15 mg in vials of 100.

OXETHAZAINE

Chemical Name: 2,2′-(2-Hydroxyethylimino)*bis*[*N*-(α,α-dimethylphenethyl)-*N*-methylacetamide].

Description: Oxethazaine is an active topical anesthetic. When a dilute solution is applied to mucous membranes, it produces a more potent anesthetic effect of longer duration than either cocaine or lidocaine. An 0.0005% solution of oxethazaine induces the same duration of anesthesia in rabbit cornea as does an 0.25% solution of cocaine, a 1% solution of lidocaine, or a 2% solution of procaine.

In vitro studies indicate that the drug produces an antispasmodic action on smooth muscle. It also antagonizes the action of histamine, serotonin, physostigmine and barium sulfate on smooth muscle. When given intravenously to dogs, it does not produce any effect on intestinal motility, nor does it inhibit the action of neostigmine bromide on intestinal motility.

A wide margin of safety appears to exist between the effective dose of oxethazaine in alumina gel and the oral toxic dose. In mice the oral LD_{50} of oxethazaine is approximately 400 mg of base/kg of body weight. Clinically, no toxic effects have been observed on continued ingestion of recommended therapeutic doses.

Indications: Adjunctive therapy for the treatment of esophagitis and peptic ulcer.

Contraindications: Hypersensitivity to any of the ingredients.

Warnings: Adequate diagnostic studies are recommended in all cases. The possibility of gastrointestinal carcinoma should be considered in patients with protracted or recurrent indigestion.

Precautions: Oxethazaine may produce or aggravate constipation unless dietary measures are followed.

Adverse Reactions: Rarely noted were glossitis, skin eruption, dizziness, faintness or drowsiness.

Dosage and Administration: *Orally.* 1 or 2 teaspoonsful 4 times daily, 15 minutes before meals and at bedtime. The recommended dosage should not be exceeded. It is preferably taken undiluted or may be followed by a sip of water. The drug is not recommended for children.

Availability:
OXAINE® M Suspension, 10 mg/5 ml in aluminum gel with magnesium hydroxide, in bottles of 360 ml. **(Wyeth)**

OXOIDS

Description: The combined action of the three components exerts an inhibitory influence on all divisions of the autonomic nervous system. Each tablet contains:

Phenobarbital	20 mg
Ergotamine tartrate	0.3 mg
Belladonna extract (equiv. to 0.1 mg of belladonna alkaloids)	8 mg

Indications: The management of disorders characterized by nervous tension and exaggerated autonomic response. Menopausal disorders with hot flushes, sweats, restlessness, and insomnia; cardiovascular disorders with palpitation, tachycardia, chest oppression, and vasomotor disturbances; gastrointestinal disorders with hypermotility, hypersecretion, and alternating diarrhea and constipation when due to autonomic upset; genitourinary disorders such as uterine cramps and premenstrual tension; and interval treatment of recurrent, throbbing headache.

Contraindications: Occlusive vascular disease (Raynauds, thromboangiitis obliterans, leutic arteritis, severe arteriosclerosis, coronary artery disease, thrombophlebitis), coronary heart disease, hypertension, impaired hepatic or renal function, sepsis, third trimester of pregnancy, glaucoma, severe pruritus, hypersensitivity to any of the components; porphyria.

Warnings: Phenobarbital may be habit-forming, and should therefore be administered with the same degree of care attendant with other barbiturate-containing preparations.

Precautions: Caution should be exercised if excessive or prolonged dosage is comtemplated, and consideration should be given to the possibility of peripheral vascular complications in patients highly sensitive to ergot.

Adverse Reactions: Blurred vision, dry mouth, flushing of skin and drowsiness occur rarely.

Dosage and Administration: *Orally.* Usually 4 tablets daily (1 in the morning, 1 at noon and 2 at bedtime). In more resistant cases, dosage may begin with 6 tablets daily, then reduce gradually at weekly intervals according to the response.

Availability:
OXOIDS® Tablets (blue) in bottles of 100 and 1000. **(Lemmon)**

OXOLINIC ACID

Chemical Name: 5-Ethyl-5,8-dihydro-8-oxo-1,3-dioxolo-(4,5-g)-quinoline-7-carboxylic acid.

Description: A quinolone derivative, oxolinic acid is a synthetic antibacterial agent for oral administration in the treatment of urinary tract infections. The therapeutic activity of the drug appears to be qualitatively similar to that of nalidixic acid but differs in that it offers a smaller (twice-a-day) dosage schedule, and also causes a higher incidence of CNS effects characterized by restlessness, insomnia, and dizziness. It occurs as a crystalline substances having properties of a weak organic acid. It has been found effective against many gram-negative organisms, including members of Escherichia, Proteus, Enterobacter and Klebsiella genera. It acts primarily by inhibiting DNA synthesis. The drug is readily absorbed from the gastrointestinal tract and is eliminated in the urine and feces as active and inactive metabolites. It does not appear to accumulate in serum on repeated dosage nor in the presence of moderately severe kidney impairment. An effective bactericidal concentration for most susceptible organisms (over 25 mcg/ml) is attained in the urine within 4 hours and therapeutic activity persists for about 12 hours. In vitro studies have indicated that bacterial resistance to the drug and cross resistance to nalidixic acid can develop. Disc susceptibility testing with the 2 mcg disc should be performed prior to administration of the drug, and if clinical response warrants it, periodically during treatment.

Indications: Treatment of initial or recurrent nonobstructive urinary tract infections caused by susceptible gram-negative organisms.

Contraindications: Patients with known hypersensitivity to the drug, those with a history of convulsive disorders, and infants and nursing mothers.

Warnings: Elderly patients require special care because the CNS-stimulant action of the drug is increased in this age group. Clinical experience has not established if the drug can be used safely (1) with other CNS stimulants, (2) for continuous treatment periods longer than 4 weeks, and (3) in pregnant women and in children.

Precautions: Oxolinic acid may enhance the effects of oral anticoagulants, warfarin, or bishydroxycoumarin by displacing significant amounts of these agents from serum albumin binding sites. It should be used cautiously in patients with severely impaired renal function, although patients with moderate or markedly impaired renal function showed no evidence of further impairment or damage to the kidneys or of interference with renal excretion of the drug. Should bacterial resistance develop, other specific agents should be instituted. Patients should be advised that in the event of dizziness they should use caution when performing activities requiring alertness or physical coordination.

Adverse Reactions: The most frequently reported reactions include insomnia, dizziness, nausea, nervousness, and headache. Those less frequently reported were abdominal pain or cramps, anorexia, vomiting, restlessness, weakness, diarrhea, constipation, itching, disturbances in liver function tests, and reductions in leukocyte counts. Rarely reported were swelling of the extremities, reduction in hematocrit/hemoglobin, eosinophilia, photophobia, palpitation, feelings of disorientation and/or agitation or acute anxiety, urticaria, rash, soreness of the mouth and gums, and metallic taste. A seizure occurred in one patient who had a known history of epilepsy, and hallucinations and hysteria were noted in a patient who received higher than the recommended dose. All of these reactions were usually reversible; nevertheless, treatment should be discontinued if side effects are unremitting. Overdosage is characterized by CNS stimulation and/or gastric irritation and require supportive treatment.

Dosage and Administration: *Orally.* The recommended treatment schedule is 1 tablet twice daily (may be given every 12 hours) for 2 weeks. Although susceptible organisms may be eradicated within a few days, the full 2-week course is recommended.

Availability:
UTIBID® Tablets, 0.75 gm in bottles of 50. **(Warner-Chilcott)**

OXTRIPHYLLINE

Description: Oxtriphylline is the choline salt of theophylline and yields 64.4% of anhydrous theophylline. It increases central respiratory stimulation, dilates the bronchioles and the pulmonary arterioles thus enhancing ventilation of the lungs. The arterial plasma carbon dioxide level is lowered and the amplitude, but not the rate, of respiration is intensified. Similar to other xanthines, oxtriphylline is known to increase cardiac output and vital capacity. Since tolerance to the drug rarely occurs, it is useful for long-term therapy of bronchospasm.

Indications: Relief of acute bronchial asthma and for reversible bronchospasm associated with chronic bronchitis and emphysema.

Warnings: Although results of studies with animals revealed no teratogenic effects on the fetus, the drug's safe use during pregnancy has not been established; therefore, its use in pregnant or lactating women or in women of childbearing potential requires that the expected therapeutic benefits be weighed against the possible hazards to the mother and child.

Precautions: Concurrent use of other xanthine containing preparations may lead to CNS stimulation, particularly in children.

Adverse Reactions: Gastric distress and, occasionally, palpitation, and CNS stimulation.

Dosage and Administration: *Orally.* Usual adult dosage, 200 mg 4 times daily, preferably after meals and at bedtime. Children 2 to 12 years of age, 100 mg/60 lbs of body weight 4 times daily.

Availability:
CHOLEDYL®: **(Warner-Chilcott)**
Elixir, 100 mg/5 ml in bottles of 1 pint. Alcohol, 20%.
Tablets, 100 mg (red) in bottles of 100; 200 mg (yellow) in bottles of 100 and 1000 and in unit-dose packages of 100 (10 x 10).

OXYBUTYNIN CHLORIDE

Chemical Name: 4-Diethylamino-2 butynyl phenylcyclohexylglycolate hydrochloride.

Description: Oxybutynin chloride, a synthetic anticholinergic agent, occurs as a white, crystalline solid that is readily soluble in water and acids, but relatively insoluble in alkalis. Its molecular weight is 393.9.

The pharmacological effects produced by this drug are due to its direct spasmolytic action on smooth muscle and to its antimuscarinic activity while exhibiting no blocking effect on autonomic ganglionic or skeletal neuromuscular transmission. It has been reported to provide symptomatic relief of the frequent urge to micturate notably in those patients with uninhibited neurogenic bladder by: (1) diminishing the frequency of bladder contractions; (2) delaying initial desire to void, and (3) increasing bladder capacity. Studies with rabbit detrusor muscle have shown that oxybutynin produces only 1/5 the anticholinergic activity of atropine, but 4 to 10 times the antispasmodic activity.

Following oral administration, the effects of the drug appear in approximately 30 minutes and are sustained for up to 6 hours. It is detoxified in the liver and excreted in the urine; distribution in body tissues has not been established.

Reproduction studies in hamsters, rabbits, rats and mice have not shown any definite evidence of impaired fertility or adverse effects on the animal fetus.

Indications: Relief of symptoms associated with voiding in patients with uninhibited neurogenic and reflex neurogenic bladder. Pretreatment examination should include cystometry and other appropriate diagnostic procedures. Cystometry should be repeated at appropriate intervals to evaluate response to therapy. The presence of infection requires treatment with an appropriate antimicrobial agent.

Contraindications: Glaucoma; obstructive disease of the gastrointestinal tract; paralytic ileus; intestinal atony of the elderly or debilitated patients; megacolon; toxic megacolon complicating ulcerative colitis; severe colitis; myasthenia gravis; obstructive uropathy; unstable cardiovascular status in acute hemorrhage, and hypersensitivity to the drug.

Warnings: In the presence of high environmental temperature, heat prostration can occur with the use of this drug, which may result in fever and heat stroke due to decreased perspiration. Diarrhea may be an early symptom of incomplete intestinal obstruction, especially in patients with ileostomy or colostomy. In this instance, treatment with oxybutynin would be inappropriate and possibly harmful. Since drowsiness or blurred vision may occur, patients should be cautioned not to engage in activities requiring alertness or skill. When prescribed for pregnant patients, the physician should carefully consider the benefits versus the risk to the fetus. Until further clinical studies assure its safe use, it is not recommended for children under 5 years of age.

Precautions: Administer with caution to patients with autonomic neuropathy; hepatic or renal disease; ulcerative colitis (large doses may suppress intestinal motility to the point of producing a paralytic ileus and the use of anticholinergics may precipitate or aggravate the serious complication of toxic megacolon); hyperthyroidism; coronary heart disease; congestive heart failure; cardiac arrhythmias; hypertension; prostatic hypertrophy; and hiatal hernia associated with reflux esophagitis which may be aggravated by anticholinergic drugs.

Adverse Reactions: Side effects of oxybutynin are typical of those produced by anticholinergic drugs and may include dry mouth, decreased sweating, urinary hesitance and retention, blurred vision, tachycardia, palpitations, mydriasis, cycloplegia, increased ocular tension, drowsiness, weakness, dizziness, insomnia, nausea, vomiting, constipation, bloated feeling, impotence, suppression of lactation, severe allergic reactions or drug idiosyncrasies including urticaria and other dermal manifestations. The symptoms of overdosage usually progress from an intensification of the side effect of CNS disturbances (from restlessness and excitement to psychotic behavior), circulatory changes (flushing, fall in blood pressure, circulatory failure), respiratory failure, paralysis and coma. Measures to be taken include immediate gastric lavage and intravenous injection of 0.5 to 2 mg of physostigmine, repeated as necessary up to a total of 5 mg. Fever may be treated symptomatically and extreme excitement with sodium thiopental 2% solution given slowly intravenously or chloral hydrate (100 to 200 ml of a 2% solution) by rectal infusion. In the event of progression of the curare-like effect to paralysis of the respiratory muscles, artificial respiration is required.

Dosage and Administration: *Orally.* The usual adult dosage is 1 tablet 2 or 3 times daily, and the maximal recommended dosage is 1 tablet 4 times daily. Children over 5 years of age, the usual dosage is 1 tablet twice daily, and the maximal recommended dosage is 1 tablet 3 times daily.

Availability:
DITROPAN® Tablets, 5 mg (blue) in bottles of 100 and 1000 and in Identification Paks (unit-dose) packages of 500. **(Marion)**

OXYCODONE Ⓒ II

Chemical Name: 14-Hydroxydihydrocodeinone.

Description: Oxycodone, a semisynthetic narcotic analgesic, is a codeine analogue and bears the same chemical relationship to codeine that oxymorphone does to morphine. Its analgesic potency, considered to be 5 to 6 times that of codeine, and addiction liability are closer to morphine, and should therefore be attended with the same considerations applied to other narcotic agents. Derived from the opium alkaloid thebaine, it occurs as a white, odorless, crystalline powder that is slightly soluble in water and soluble in alcohol and in chloroform. Oxycodone, generally used as the hydrochloride and terephthalate salts which are freely soluble in water and slightly soluble in alcohol, is available only as an ingredient in mixtures usually containing APC or acetaminophen. Its clinical value corresponds to that of methadone and codeine in that it retains at least ½ of its analgesic activity when administered orally. Readily absorbed from the gastrointestinal tract, onset of action is rapid and the initial effects are generally preceived within 10 to 15 minutes, reaching a peak within 30 to 60 minutes with relief of pain continuing for 4 to 5 hours. It is metabolized by the liver and excreted chiefly in the urine.

Indications: For the relief of moderate to moderately severe pain.

Contraindications: Unusual sensitivity to any of the components.

Warnings: Oxycodone may be habit-forming. Oxycodone can produce drug dependence of the morphine type and, therefore, has the potential for being abused. Psychic and physical dependence and tolerance may develop upon repeated use. The usual precautions associated with the administration of oral narcotic-containing preparations must be observed. Since mental and physical abilities may be impaired, patients should be cautioned not to engage in activities requiring alertness and skill. Concurrent use with other CNS depressants such as general anesthetics, phenothiazines, other tranquilizers, sedative-hypnotics, alcohol, and other narcotic analgesics may produce an addictive effect. When such combined therapy is contemplated, the dose of one or both agents should be reduced. The possible adverse effects on fetal development have not been established; therefore, it should be used in pregnant women only when the anticipated benefits outweigh the potential hazards to the fetus. Generally, drugs of this class are not recommended for use in pediatric patients. Preparations containing salicylates should be used with caution in the presence of peptic ulcer or abnormality of blood coagulation.

Precautions: The respiratory depressant effects of narcotics and their capacity to elevate cerebrospinal fluid pressure may be markedly exaggerated in the presence of head injury, other intracranial lesions or a preëxisting increase in intracranial pressure. Furthermore, narcotics produce adverse reactions which may obscure the clinical course of patients with head injuries. Narcotics may also obscure the diagnosis or clinical course in patients with acute abdominal conditions. Narcotic-containing preparations should be given with caution to elderly or debilitated patients, and to those with severe impairment of hepatic or renal function, hypothyroidism, Addison's disease, and prostatic hypertrophy or urethral stricture. Phenacetin has been reported to damage the kidneys when taken in excessive amounts for prolonged periods. Also, aspirin may enhance the effect of anticoagulants, and inhibit the uricosuric effect of uricosuric agents.

Adverse Reactions: Most frequently observed were lightheadedness, dizziness, sedation, nausea and vomiting. These effects appear to be more prominent in ambulatory than in nonambulatory patients, and some of these complications may be alleviated if the patient lies down. Other toxic reactions include euphoria, dysphoria, constipation, skin rash, and pruritus. Overdosage is characterized by respiratory depression, extreme somnolence which can progress to stupor or coma, skeletal muscle flaccidity, cold and clammy skin, and occasionally, bradycardia and hypotension. In severe overdosage, apnea, circulatory collapse, cardiac arrest and death may occur. Primary attention should be given to the reestablishment of adequate respiratory exchange through provision of a patent airway and the institution of assisted or controlled ventilation. Naloxone, nalorphine or levallorphan (specific antidotes) should be given to combat respiratory depression. Oxygen, intravenous fluids, vasopressors and other supportive measures should be employed as indicated. Gastric emptying may be useful in removing unabsorbed drug.

Dosage and Administration: *Orally,* every 6 hours. The usual adult dose is 1 tablet. *Demi-Tablets:* children 12 years of age or older, 1/2 tablet; 6 to 12 years of age, 1/4 tablet. Tablets should be taken preferably after meals or with milk. Not indicated for children under 6 years of age.

Availability:
CII PERCOCET®-5 Tablets contain oxycodone hydrochloride, 5 mg and acetaminophen, 325 mg in bottles of 100 and 500 and in blister-packs of 25 tablets in units of 250 tablets (10 cartons) and 1000 tablets (40 cartons). **(Endo)**
CII PERCODAN® Tablets contain oxycodone hydrochloride, 4.5 mg; oxycodone terephthalate, 0.38 mg; aspirin, 224 mg; phenacetin, 160 mg and caffeine, 32 mg in bottles of 100, 500 and 1000 and in blister-packs of 25 tablets in units of 250 tablets (10 cartons) and 1000 tablets (40 cartons). **(Endo)**
CII PERCODAN-DEMI Tablets contain 1/2 the amounts of oxycodone hydrochloride and terephthalate; the quantities of APC are identical in bottles of 100, 500 and 1000. **(Endo)**
CII TYLOX™ Capsules contain oxycodone hydrochloride, 4.5 mg; oxycodone terephthalate, 0.38 mg and acetaminophen, 500 mg in bottles of 100 and in unit-dose packages of 25. **(McNeil)**

OXYMETAZOLINE

Chemical Name: 6-*tert*-Butyl-3-(2-imidazolin-2-ylmethyl)-2,4-dimethylphenol monohydrate.

Description: Oxymetazoline is a sympathomimetic amine structurally and pharmacologically related to naphazoline, tetrahydrozoline and xylometazoline. When applied to the nasal mucous membranes, it reduces vasodilation and turgescence and restores the patency of sinus ostia and blocked air passages in a variety of infections and allergic disorders of the upper respiratory tract. It provides a longer-acting decongestant effect than that achieved with other imidazoline derivatives.

Indications: Symptomatic relief of nasal congestion of allergic or infectious origin, acute and chronic rhinitis, sinusitis and rhinosinusitis, and vasomotor rhinitis. It may also be useful as adjunctive aid in the treatment and prevention of middle ear infection. It is recommended for use on a nasal tampon to facilitate intranasal examination, or before nasal surgery.

Contraindications: Hypersensitivity to oxymetazoline and to any ingredient formulated with it.

Warnings: Extreme caution is advised in patients who are receiving MAO inhibitors since a severe hypertensive crisis may ensue. Overdosage may produce sedation in children. Safe use of oxymetazoline during pregnancy has not been established with respect to adverse effect upon fetal development. Therefore, the drug should not be used in women of childbearing potential and particularly during early pregnancy unless in the judgment of the physician the potential benefits outweigh the possible hazards.

Precautions: Oxymetazoline should be used with caution in patients with coronary artery disease, hypertension, hyperthyroidism, or diabetes. Only the pediatric preparation should be given to children under 6 years of age.

Adverse Reactions: These are usually mild and transitory and may include burning, stinging and dryness of nasal mucosa, sneezing, headache, lightheadedness, insomnia, and palpitations. Excessive and prolonged use may precipitate a rebound congestion, although this phenomenon has been infrequently noted.

Dosage and Administration: *Topically.* Adults and children over 6 years of age, 2 to 4 drops or 2 or 3 sprays of solution may be instilled into each nostril in the morning and at bedtime Children 2 to 5 years of age, 2 or 3 drops of the **pediatric** solution may be instilled into each nostril in the morning and at bedtime.

Availability:
AFRIN®: **(Schering)**
Nasal Spray (OTC), 0.5 mg/ml (0.05%) in plastic squeeze bottles of 15 and 30 ml.
Nose Drops, 0.5 mg/ml (0.05%) in dropper bottles of 20 ml.
Pediatric Nose Drops, 0.25 mg/ml (0.025%) in dropper bottles of 20 ml.

OXYMETHOLONE

Chemical Name: 17β-Hydroxy-2-(hydroxymethylene)-17-methyl-5α-androstan-3-one.

Description: Oxymetholone is a synthetic steroidal hormone chemically and physiologically related to methyltestosterone. Oxymetholone is primarily used for its protein anabolic effect and its catabolic inhibiting effect on tissue. Nitrogen balance is improved with anabolic agents, but only where there is sufficient intake of calories and protein. Whether this positive nitrogen balance is of primary benefit in the utilization of protein-building dietary substances has not been established. Oxymetholone has also been found to exert an erythopoietic action and has been advocated for use in anemias due to bone marrow failure or to deficient red cell production such as acquired aplastic anemia, congenital aplastic anemia, myelofibrosis and the hypoplastic anemias due to the administration of myelotoxic drugs. Its use however should not replace other supportive measures such as transfusion, correction of iron, folic acid, vitamin B-12 or pyridoxine deficiency, antibacterial therapy and the appropriate use of corticosteroids.

Certain clinical effects and adverse reactions demonstrate the androgenic properties of this class of drugs. Complete dissociation of anabolic and androgenic effects has not been achieved. The actions of anabolic steroids are therefore similar to those of male sex hormones with the possibility of causing serious disturbances of growth and sexual development if given to young children. They suppress the gonadotropic functions of the pituitary and may exert a direct effect upon the testes.

Human growth hormone appears to be the preferred treatment of pituitary dwarfism. If human growth hormone is not available, anabolic agents may be used to treat this condition.

Indications: Adjunctive therapy in senile and postmenopausal osteoporosis. Anabolic steroids are without value as primary therapy but may be of value in adjunctive therapy. Equal or greater consideration should be given to diet, calcium balance, physiotherapy and good general health-promoting measures. May be of benefit in the treatment of anemias caused by deficient red cell production that do not respond to the standard hematinic formulas. In pituitary dwarfism, anabolic agents may be used with care until growth hormone is more available. Also indicated for the treatment of aplastic anemia.

Contraindications: Carcinoma of the prostate or breast in male patients, carcinoma of the breast in some female patients, in pregnant women, in premature or newborn infants, in nephrosis or the nephrotic phase of nephrosis, hypersensitivity, and in hepatic dysfunction.

Warnings: Anabolic steroids do not enhance athletic ability.

Precautions: Hypercalcemia may develop both spontaneously and as a result of hormonal therapy in women with disseminated breast carcinoma. If it develops while on oxymetholone, the drug should be discontinued. Caution is required in administering these agents to patients with cardiac, renal, or hepatic disease. Edema may occur occasionally. Concomitant administration with adrenal steroids or ACTH may add to the edema. If amenorrhea or menstrual irregularities develop, the drug should be discontinued until the etiology is determined. Anabolic steroids may increase sensitivity to anticoagulants. Dosage of the anticoagulant may have to be decreased in order to maintain the prothrombin time at the desired therapeutic level. Anabolic steroids also have been shown to alter glucose tolerance tests. Diabetics should be followed carefully and the insulin or oral hypoglycemic dosage adjusted accordingly. Since oxymetholone contains a 17 alpha-alkly group, liver function should be checked at regular intervals in patients receiving this drug. Anabolic steroids should be used with caution in patients with benign prostatic hypertrophy. Serum cholesterol may increase or decrease during therapy; therefore, caution is required in administering these agents to patients with a history of myocardial infarction or coronary artery disease. Serial determinations of serum cholesterol should be made and therapy adjusted accordingly. Serum and urinary calcium levels should be determined periodically in those patients suspected of hypercalcemia. The drug may cause the retention of sodium and water and should therefore be given with caution to patients with cardiorenal disease. It may also impair liver function and should be administered with extreme caution to patients with a history of or suspected, hepatic dysfunction. Liver function should be evaluated periodically during therapy, especially in geriatric patients and in those taking the drug for prolonged periods; the drug should be discontinued at the first sign of toxicity.

Adverse Reactions: The following adverse reactions have been associated with anabolic therapy: *in males*—prepubertal such as phallic enlargement, increased frequency of erections. Postpubertal such as inhibition of testicular functions, testicular atrophy and oligospermia, impotence, chronic priapism, gynecomastia, epididymitis and bladder irritability. *In females*—hirsutism, male pattern baldness, deepening of the voice, clitoral enlargement and menstrual irregularities. These changes are usually irreversible even after prompt discontinuance of therapy and are not prevented by concomitant use of estrogens. *In both sexes*—nausea, increased or decreased libido, acne (especially in females and prepubertal males), habituation, excitation and sleeplessness, chills, bleeding in patients on concomitant anticoagulant therapy, premature closure of epiphyses in children, vomiting, diarrhea, jaundice with rarely hepatic necrosis and death. *Alterations in these clinical laboratory tests*—the metyrapone test, the FBS and glucose tolerance tests, the thyroid function tests: a decrease in the PBI, in thyroxine-binding capacity and radioactive iodine uptake and an increase in T^3 uptake by the rbc's or resin may occur. Free thyroxine is normal. Altered tests usually persist for 2 to 3 weeks after anabolic therapy has been discontinued. *The electrolytes*—retention of sodium, chlorides, water, potassium, phosphates and calcium. *Liver function tests*—increased BSP, increased or decreased serum cholesterol, increased SGOT, increased serum bilirubin, increased alkaline phosphatase, decrease in clotting factors II, V, VII and X. *Miscellaneous laboratory tests*—increased creatine and creatinine-excretion lasting up to two weeks after discontinuing therapy, decreased 17-ketosteroid excretion.

Dosage and Administration: *Orally.* Hormone therapy is adjunctive to and not a replacement for conventional therapy. Adequate amounts of calories and proteins must be given if a beneficial effect is to be attained. *Adults:* The usual dosage is 2.5 mg 3 times daily. The majority of patients show a favorable result at 7.5 mg/day. Doses up to 15 mg/day may be employed. Results have been seen in 10 days, but optimal results are usually obtained in 4 to 6 weeks. Duration of therapy will depend on the condition being treated and the appearance of adverse reactions. Therapy should be intermittent. *Children:* Adequate response has been observed in children up to the age of 12 years on dosage schedules of 2.5 mg/day and 5 mg/day. Four to 6 weeks of therapy should be followed by 1 month without anabolic steroids. Roentgenograms should then be taken to determine the amount of bone maturation. Therapy should be reinstituted as indicated. Since skeletal stimulation may continue for 6 months after therapy has been terminated, the drug should be discontinued well before bone maturation reaches the norm for the chronological age. Children over 12 years of age may be given adult doses. For aplastic anemia, the recommended daily dose for adults and children is 1 to 5 mg/kg/day; however, doses of 1 to 2 mg/kg/day have been found to be effective. Since response is usually delayed, a minimum trial of 3 to 6 months is recommended. Following remission, some patients may need to be maintained on a lower daily dosage regimen. A continued maintenance dose is usually necessary in patients with congenital aplastic anemia.

Availability:
ADROYD® Tablets, 5 mg in bottles of 50; 10 mg in bottles of 100. **(Parke-Davis)**
ANADROL®-50 Tablets, 50 mg in bottles of 100. **(Syntex)**

OXYMORPHONE CII

Chemical Name: 1-14-Hydroxydihydromorphinone hydrochloride.

Description: Oxymorphone hydrochloride, a potent analgesic, is a semisynthetic narcotic substitute for morphine. It occurs as a soluble salt that is soluble in water but sparingly soluble in alcohol.

When administered parenterally, 1 mg of oxymorphone is equivalent in analgesic activity to about 10 mg of morphine sulfate. The onset of action is rapid and the initial effects are usually perceived within 5 to 10 minutes, with relief of pain persisting for approximately 3 to 6 hours. Because the drug produces only mild sedation and causes little depression of the cough reflex, it may be particularly useful in postoperative patients.

Indications: Relief of moderate to severe pain, parenterally for preoperative medication, for support of anesthesia, for obstetrical analgesia, and for relief of anxiety in patients with dyspnea associated with acute left ventricular failure and pulmonary edema.

Contraindications: Hypersensitivity to morphine analogs. Safe use in children under 12 years of age has not been established.

Warnings: Oxymorphone may be habit-forming. Tolerance and addiction can develop; the addicting potential appears to be about the same as for morphine. Safe use of oxymorphone during pregnancy, in nursing mothers, or in women of childbearing potential requires that the possible benefits of the drug be weighed against the potential hazards to the mother and child.

Precautions: The usual precautions associated with the administration of all potent narcotic-analgesics must be observed. Some respiratory depression may occur particularly when other drugs with depressant action have been given previous to administration. The respiratory depressant effects of narcotics and their capacity to elevate cerebrospinal fluid pressure may be markedly exaggerated in the presence of head injury, other intracranial lesions, or a preexisting increase in intracranial pressure. Furthermore narcotics produce adverse reactions which may obscure the clinical course of patients with head injuries. Caution must be exercised when the drug is given to elderly or debilitated patients, and to patients who are known to be sensitive to CNS depressants, such as those with cardiovascular, pulmonary, or hepatic disease, hypothyroidism (myxedema), acute alcoholism, delirium tremens, convulsive disorders, bronchial asthma and kyphoscoliosis. Debilitated and elderly patients, and those with severe liver disease should receive smaller doses.

Adverse Reactions: The possible side effects that may occur include drowsiness, nausea, vomiting, miosis, itching, dysphoria, lightheadedness, headache and respiratory depression. Overdosage is characterized by respiratory depression, extreme somnolence which may progress to coma or stupor. In acute toxicity, apnea, circulatory collapse, cardiac arrest, and death may occur. Primary consideration should be given to the reestablishment of adequate respiratory exchange through provision of a patent airway and the institution of assisted or controlled ventilation. The narcotic antagonists naloxone, nalorphine or levallorphan are specific antidotes against respiratory depression. An appropriate dose should be administered preferably by the intravenous route. Oxygen, intravenous fluids, vasopressors, and other supportive measures should be employed as indicated.

Dosage and Administration: Initially, 1 to 1.5 mg *subcutaneously or intramuscularly,* repeated every 4 to 6 hours as needed; 0.5 mg *intravenously.* In nondebilitated patients., the dose can be cautiously increased until satisfactory pain relief is obtained. For analgesia during labor, 0.5 to 1 mg *intramuscularly* is recommended. *Rectally,* 1 suppository every 4 to 6 hours.

Availability:
Ⓒ NUMORPHAN® Hydrochloride: **(Endo)**
Injection, 1 mg/ml in ampuls of 1 and 1.5 ml and in vials of 15 ml; 1.5 mg/ml in ampuls of 1 ml and in vials of 10 ml.
Suppositories (rectal), 5 mg in cartons of 6.

OXYPHENBUTAZONE: see Phenylbutazone

OXYPHENCYCLIMINE HYDROCHLORIDE

Chemical Name: 1,4,5,6-Tetrahydro-1-methyl-2-pyrimidinylmethyl-α-phenylcyclohexaneglycolate monohydrochloride.

Description: Oxyphencyclimine is a synthetic *tertiary* amine anticholinergic, and occurs as a white, crystalline powder sparingly soluble in water.

The clinical effects exhibited by this drug are qualitatively similar to those of atropine. As with most *tertiary* amines, it has a direct spasmolytic action on smooth muscle but has little effect on skeletal neuromuscular or ganglionic transmission. The rationale for the use of anticholinergic agents in the treatment of peptic ulcer is based on the ability of these compounds to block acetylcholine at postganglionic, parasympathetic neuro-effector sites in smooth muscle and secretory glands. However, the drug cannot be relied upon to heal the ulcer, decrease the rate of or prevent recurrences or complications. Following oral administration, effects are apparent in 1 to 2 hours and persist for 8 to 12 hours.

Indications: Adjunctive therapy in selected cases of peptic ulcer. Combination with phenobarbital is desired to allay tension or apprehension which often complicates these disorders. The addition of hydroxyzine provides tranquilness when anxiety or emotional overtones are complicating factors.

Contraindications: Glaucoma; obstructive uropathy such as bladder neck obstruction due to prostatic hypertrophy; obstructive disease of the gastrointestinal tract as in achalasia, pyloroduodenal stenosis, etc.; paralytic ileus; intestinal atony of the elderly or debilitated patient; unstable cardiovascular status in acute hemorrhage, severe ulcerative colitis; toxic megacolon complicating ulcerative colitis; and myasthenia gravis. Hypersensitivity to the drug or to any of the components added to the formulation is also a contraindication.

Warnings: Use of the drug during pregnancy, lactation, or in women of childbearing potential requires that the potential benefits be weighed against the possible risks to mother and child. Elderly patients may react to even small doses of anticholinergics and sedatives with excitement, agitation, drowsiness and other untoward manifestations. In the presence of a high environmental temperature, heat prostration (fever and heatstroke due to decreased sweating) can occur with the use of this drug. Diarrhea may be an early symptom of incomplete intestinal obstruction, especially in patients with ileostomy or colostomy, in which case treatment with oxyphencyclimine would be inappropriate and possibly harmful. Phenobarbital should not be administered to individuals known to be addiction-prone or to those with a history of physical and/or psychological dependence to habit-forming drugs.

Precautions: Routine caution is advised when using anticholinergic drugs in patients with autonomic neuropathy; hepatic or renal disease; ulcerative colitis (large doses may suppress intestinal motility to the degree of precipitating a paralytic ileus which may lead to toxic megacolon); hyperthyroidism; coronary heart disease; congestive heart failure; cardiac tachyarrhythmias, tachycardia, hypertension, and nonobstructing prostatic hypertrophy; hiatal hernia associated with reflux esophagitis because drugs of this type have been found to aggravate this condition. It should be noted that oxyphencyclimine in the treatment of gastric ulcer may cause a delay in gastric emptying time and may complicate such therapy (antral stasis). The use of this drug in the presence of complications of bilary tract disease should not be relied upon. Extreme caution is indicated when prescribing this product in the presence of tachycardia, since heart rate may be increased. A curare-like action may develop with excessive dosages. Patients should be cautioned not to perform any hazardous operations requiring alertness of motor coordination. That hydroxyzine may potentiate the action of CNS depressants should be kept in mind, and their dosage should therefore be reduced.

Adverse Reactions: Reactions are typical of anticholinergic drugs: dry mouth (most common), less frequently occurring are xerostomia, urinary hesitancy or retention; blurred vision and tachycardia; palpitations; mydriasis; dilatation of the pupils; cycloplegia; increased ocular tension; loss of taste; headaches; nervousness; drowsiness; weakness; dizziness; insomnia; nausea; vomiting; impotence; suppression of lactation; constipation; bloated feeling; severe allergic reactions or drug idiosyncrasias including anaphylaxis; urticaria and other dermal manifestations; some degree of mental confusion and/or excitement especially in elderly patients; and decreased sweating. It should be noted that adrenergic innervation of the eccrine sweat glands on the palms of the hands and soles of the feet make complete control of sweating impossible. Reactions to hydroxyzine may include drowsiness, xerostomia and, with extremely large doses, involuntary motor activity.

Dosage and Administration: *Orally.* Adults, usually from 5 to 10 mg morning and night. With phenobarbital, 1 tablet morning, evening and at bedtime. With hydroxyzine, dosage is the same as for oxyphencyclimine alone. Proper diet and antacids should be used when indicated as concomitant therapy. Since safe use in pediatric patients has not been confirmed, it is not recommended for use in those of this age group.

Availability:
DARICON® Tablets, 10 mg in bottles of 60 and 500. **(Beecham)**
w/Phenobarbital (**Warning:** May be habit-forming.)
DARICON PB Tablets, 5 mg with phenobarbital, 15 mg in bottles of 100. **(Beecham)**
w/Hydroxyzine Hydrochloride
ENARAX® Tablets, 5 and 10 mg with hydroxyzine hydrochloride, 25 mg in bottles of 60. **(Beecham)**
VISTRAX® Tablets, 5 and 10 mg with hydroxyzine hydrochloride, 25 mg in bottles of 100. **(Pfizer)**

OXYPHENONIUM

Chemical Name: Diethyl(2-hydroxyethyl)methylammonium α-phenylcyclohexaneglycolate bromide.

Description: Oxyphenonium bromide, a synthetic anticholinergic, occurs as a crystalline substance that is freely soluble in water and sparingly soluble in alcohol. Aqueous solutions of oxyphenonium are neutral.

The antisecretory and antispasmodic effects of this drug result from the antimuscarinic and ganglionic blocking activity. The antimuscarinic activity of oxyphenonium is of longer duration than that of atropine. Recommended doses produce an inhibitory effect on gastric secretion and gastrointestinal motility through the antimuscarinic action, and by blocking the stimulating effect of acetylcholine at the parasympathetic nerve endings. CNS activity is generally lacking.

Indications: Treatment of peptic ulcer as adjunctive therapy.

Contraindications: Glaucoma, obstructive uropathy (bladder neck obstruction due to prostatic hypertrophy), obstructive disease of the gastrointestinal tract (achalasia, paralytic ileus, pyloroduodenal stenosis, etc.); intestinal atony in the elderly or debilitated patient, unstable cardiovascular status in acute hemorrhage, severe ulcerative colitis; toxic megacolon complicating ulcerative colitis; myasthenia gravis, and hypersensitivity to oxyphenonium.

Warnings: In the presence of a high environmental temperature, heat prostration can occur with the use of this drug, which may result in fever and heat stroke due to decreased sweating. Diarrhea may be an early symptom of incomplete intestinal obstruction, especially in patients with ileostomy or colostomy. In this instance, treatment with oxyphenonium would be inappropriate and possibly harmful. Since drowsiness and blurred vision may occur, patients should be cautioned not to engage in activities requiring alertness or skill. Safe use of this drug during pregnancy or in lactating women has not been established, therefore, the benefits to be gained must be weighed against the possible hazards to the mother and child.

Precautions: Administer with caution to patients with autonomic neuropathy, hepatic or renal disease; early evidence of ileus (as in peritonitis); ulcerative colitis (large doses may suppress intestinal motility to the point of producing a paralytic ileus and the use of anticholinergics may precipitate or aggravate the serious complication of toxic megacolon); hyperthyroidism, coronary heart disease, congestive heart failure; cardiac arrhythmias; hypertension; nonobstructing prostatic hypertrophy; hiatal hernia associated with reflux esophagitis, which may be aggravated by anticholinergic drugs. The use of oxyphenonium in the treatment of gastric ulcer may produce a delay in gastric emptying time and may complicate such therapy (antral stasis). It should not be employed in the presence of biliary tract disease and tachycardia. Cautious use is advised in debilitated patients with chronic lung disease, and in patients over 40 years of age because of the increased incidence of glaucoma in this age group. A curare-like action may occur with overdosage.

Adverse Reactions: Xerostomia; urinary hesitancy and retention; blurred vision; tachycardia; palpitations; mydriasis; dilation of the pupil; cycloplegia; increased ocular tension; loss of taste; headache; nervousness; drowsiness; weakness; dizziness, insomnia; nausea, vomiting; impotence; suppression of lactation; constipation; bloated feeling; severe allergic reactions or drug idiosyncrasies, including anaphylaxis, urticaria and other dermal manifestations; some degree of mental confusion or excitement or both, especially in elderly patients, and decreased sweating. Treatment of overdosage requires the same procedures as for atropine overdosage.

Dosage and Administration: *Orally.* 2 tablets 4 times daily for several days. **Note:** Not recommended for use in children.

Availability:
ANTRENYL® Tablets, 5 mg (white, scored) in bottles of 100. **(Ciba)**

OXYTETRACYCLINE HYDROCHLORIDE

Chemical Name: 4-Dimethylamino-1,4,4α,5,5α,6,11,12α-octahydro-3,5,6,10,12,12α-hexahydroxy-6-methyl-1,11-dioxo-2-naphthacenecarboxamide hydrochloride.

Description: Oxytetracycline is a salt of a yellow, amphoteric, crystalline antibiotic derived from the actinomycete, *Streptomyces rimosus*. It is closely related, chemically and pharmacologically, to other antibiotics of the tetracycline group. It is freely soluble in water forming solutions that are stable for at least 48 hours when stored at 4° C.

Oxytetracycline diffuses readily through the placenta into the fetal circulation, into the pleural fluid and, under some circumstances, into the cerebrospinal fluid. It appears to be concentrated in the hepatic system and excreted in the bile, so that it appears in the feces, as well as in the urine, in a biologically active form. Oxytetracycline is primarily bacteriostatic and is thought to exert its antimicrobial effect by the inhibition of protein synthesis. Oxytetracycline is active against a wide range of gram-negative and gram-positive organisms. The drugs in the tetracycline class have closely similar antimicrobial spectra, and cross resistance among them is common. Microorganisms may be considered susceptible if the M.I.C. (minimum inhibitory concentration) is not more than 4 mcg/ml and intermediate if the M.I.C. is 4 to 12.5 mcg/ml. Susceptibility plate testing: A tetracycline disc may be used to determine microbial susceptibility to drugs in the tetracycline class. If the Kirby-Bauer method of disc susceptibility testing is used, a 30 mcg tetracycline disc should give a zone of at least 19 mm when tested against an oxytetracycline-susceptible bacterial strain. Tetracyclines are readily absorbed and are bound to plasma proteins in varying degrees.

Indications: Oxytetracycline is indicted in infections caused by the following microorganisms: Rickettsiae (Rocky Mountain spotted fever, typhus fever and the typhus group, Q fever, rickettsialpox and tick fevers); *Mycoplasma pneumoniae* (PPLO, Eaton agent), agents of psittacosis and ornithosis, agents of lymphogranuloma venereum and granuloma inguinale, the spirochetal agent of relapsing fever *(Borrelia recurrentis).* The following gram-negative microorganisms: *Haemophilus ducreyi* (chancroid), *Pasteurella pestis* and *Pasteurella tularen-*

sis, Bartonella bacilliformis, Bacteroides species, *Vibrio comma* and *Vibrio fetus, Brucella species* (in conjunction with streptomycin). Oxytetracycline is indicated for treatment of infections caused by the following gram-negative microorganisms, when bacteriologic testing indicates appropriate susceptibility to the drug. *Escherichia coli, Enterobacter aerogenes* (formerly *Aerobacter aerogenes), Shigella* species, *Mimi* species and *Herellea* species, *Haemophilus influenzae* (respiratory infections), *Klebsiella* species (respiratory and urinary infections).

Oxytetracycline is indicated for treatment of infections caused by the following gram-positive microorganisms when bacteriologic testing indicates appropriate suceptibility to the drug: *Streptococcus pyogenes* (for upper respiratory infections due to Group A beta-hemolytic streptococci, penicillin is the usual drug of choice, including the prophylaxis of rheumatic fever), Alpha-hemolytic streptococci (viridans group), Enterococcus group (*Streptococcus faecalis), Diplococcus pneumoniae, Staphylococcus aureus,* skin and soft tissue infections.

Oxytetracycline is not the drug of choice in the treatment of any type of staphylococcal infections. When penicillin is contraindicated, tetracyclines are alternative drugs in the treatment of infections due to: *Neisseria gonorrhoeae, Treponema pallidum* and *Treponema pertenue* (syphilis and yaws), *Listeria monocytogenes, Clostridium* species, *Bacillus anthracis, Fusobacterium fusiforme* (Vincent's infection), *Actinomyces* species. In acute intestinal amebiasis or in severe acne, the tetracyclines may be a useful adjunct to therapy. Tetracyclines are indicated in the treatment of trachoma, although the infectious agent is not always eliminated, as judged by immunofluorescence. Inclusion conjunctivitis may be treated with oral oxytetracycline or with a combination of oral and topical agents.

Contraindications: This drug is contraindicated in patients who have shown hypersensitivity to any of the tetracyclines.

Warnings: The use of oxytetracycline during tooth development (last half of pregnancy, infancy, and childhood to the age of 8 years) may cause permanent discoloration of the teeth (yellow-gray-brown). This adverse reaction is more common during long-term use of the drugs but has been observed following repeated short-term courses. Enamel hypoplasia has also been reported. *Oxytetracycline, therefore, should not be used in this age group unless other drugs are not likely to be effective or are contraindicated.* If renal impairment exists, even usual oral or parenteral doses may lead to excessive systemic accumulation of the drug and possible liver toxicity. Under such conditions, lower than usual total doses are indicated and, if therapy is prolonged, serum level determinations of the drug are advisable. This hazard is of particular importance in the parenteral administration of tetracyclines to pregnant or postpartum patients with pyelonephritis. When used under these circumstances, the blood level should not exceed 15 mcg/ml and liver function tests should be undertaken at frequent intervals. Other potentially hepatotoxic drugs should not be prescribed concomitantly. In the presence of renal dysfunction, particularly during pregnancy, intravenous oxytetracycline therapy in daily doses exceeding 2 gm has been associated with deaths due to liver failure.

Photosensitivity manifested by an exaggerated sunburn reaction has been observed in some individuals taking tetracyclines. Patients apt to be exposed to direct sunlight or ultraviolet light should be advised that this reaction can occur with tetracycline drugs, and treatment should be discontinued at the first evidence of skin erythema. The antianabolic action of oxytetracycline may cause an increase in BUN. While this is not a problem in those with normal renal function, in patients with significantly impaired function, higher serum levels of this drug may lead to azotemia, hyperphosphatemia, and acidosis. Results of animal studies indicate that oxytetracycline crosses the placenta, is found in fetal tissues and can have toxic effects on the developing fetus (often related to retardation of skeletal development). Evidence of embryotoxicity has also been noted in animals treated early in pregnancy. All tetracyclines form a stable calcium complex in any bone-forming tissue. A decrease in the fibula growth rate has been observed in prematures given oral tetracycline in doses of 25 mg/kg every 6 hours. This reaction was shown to be reversible when the drug was discontinued. Oxytetracycline is present in the milk of lactating women who are taking a drug in this class.

Precautions: As with all intramuscular preparations, oxytetracycline intramuscular solution should be injected well within the body of a relatively large muscle. Adults: The preferred sites are the upper outer quadrant of the buttock, (i.e., gluteus maximus), and the mid-lateral thigh. Children: It is recommended that intramuscular injections be given preferably in the mid-lateral muscles of the thigh. In infants and small children the periphery of the upper outer quadrant of the gluteal region should be used only when necessary, such as in burn patients, in order to minimize the possibility of damage to the sciatic nerve. The deltoid area should be used only if well developed such as in certain adults and older children, and then only with caution to avoid radial nerve injury. Intramuscular injections should not be made into the lower and mid-thirds of the upper arm. As with all intramuscular injections, aspiration is necessary to help avoid inadvertent injection into a blood vessel. In common with other antibiotic preparations, use of this drug may result in overgrowth of nonsusceptible organisms, including fungi. If superinfection occurs, the antibiotic should be discontinued and appropriate therapy instituted. In venereal diseases when coexistent syphilis is suspected, a dark-field examination should be done before treatment is started and the blood serology repeated monthly for at least 4 months. Because oxytetracycline has been shown to depress plasma prothrombin activity, patients who are on anticoagulant therapy may require a downward adjustment of their anticoagulant dosage. In long-term therapy, periodic laboratory evaluation of organ systems, including hematopoietic, renal and hepatic studies should be performed. All infections due to group A beta-hemolytic streptococci should be treated for at least 10 days. Since bacteriostatic drugs may interfere with the bactericidal action of penicillin, it is advisable to avoid giving oxytetracycline in conjunction with penicillin.

Adverse Reactions: Local irritation may be present after intramuscular injection. The injection should be deep, with care taken not to injure the sciatic nerve nor inject intravascularly. *Gastrointestinal:* Anorexia, nausea, vomiting, diarrhea, glossitis, dysphagia, enterocolitis, and inflammatory lesions (with monilial overgrowth) in the anogenital region. These reactions have been caused by both the oral and parenteral administration of tetracyclines. *Skin:* Maculopapular and erythematous rashes. Exfoliative dermatitis has been reported but is uncommon. Photosensitivity is discussed above. *Renal toxicity:* Rise in BUN has been reported and is apparently dose-related. *Hypersensitivity reactions:* Urticaria, angioneurotic edema, anaphylaxis, anaphylactoid purpura, pericarditis, and exacerbation of systemic lupus erythematosus. Bulging fontanels have been reported in young infants following full therapeutic dosage. This sign disappeared rapidly when the drug was discontinued. *Blood:* Hemolytic anemia, thrombocytopenia, neutropenia, and eosinophilia have been reported. When given over prolonged periods, oxytetracycline has been reported to produce brown-black microscopic discoloration of thyroid glands. No abnormalities of thyroid function studies are known to occur.

Precautions, contraindications and adverse reactions associated with other components used in combination with oxytetracycline should be kept in mind, and may be found in their individual monographs.

Dosage and Administration: *Orally.* Adults, usually 250 mg 4 times daily; 500 mg 4 times daily may be required for severe infection. Children, the usual daily dose is 25 to 50 mg/kg of body weight divided into 4 equal doses. Therapy should be continued for at least 24 to 48 hours after symptoms and fever have subsided. For treatment of brucellosis, 500 mg of oxytetracycline 4 times daily for 3 weeks should be accompanied by streptomycin, 1 gm intramuscularly twice daily the 1st week and once daily the 2nd week. For the treatment of uncomplicated gonorrhea, 1.5 gm initially followed by 0.5 gm 4 times a day for a total of 9 gm. For the treatment of syphilis, a total of 30 to 40 gm in equally divided doses over a period of 10 to 15 days. Antacids containing aluminum, calcium, or magnesium impair absorption and should not be given to patients taking oral tetracyclines. Food and some dairy products also interfere with absorption; therefore, the drug should be given either 1 hour before or 2 hours after meals. Pediatric oral dosage forms should not be given with milk formulas and should be given at least 1 hour prior to feeding. In the treatment of streptococcal infections, therapy should be continued for at least 10 days. *Intramuscularly.* Adults, 250 mg administered once every 24 hours or 300 mg in divided doses at 8- to 12-hour intervals. Children, 15 to 25 mg/kg of body weight up to a maximum of 250 mg/single daily injection. Dosage may be divided and given at 8- to 12-hour intervals. *Intravenously.* Adults, usually 250 to 500 mg every 12 hours and should not exceed 500 mg every 6 hours. Children, usually 12 mg/kg/day divided into 2 doses; however, 10 to 20 mg/kg/day may be given depending upon the severity of the infection. Intravenous solutions should be injected directly into a vein; they should not be injected intramuscularly or subcutaneously. *Topically.* In treating superficial infections of the eye, ear, nose, throat and skin due to susceptible organisms, applications may be made locally from 1 to 3 times daily according to the needs and response of the patient. *Intravaginally.* Insert 1 tablet high into the vaginal vault twice daily (upon retiring and on arising) for 2 to 4 days.

Availability:

Oxytetracycline Hydrochloride

OXLOPAR® Capsules, 250 mg in bottles of 100 and in unit-dose packages of 100 (10 x 10). **(Parke-Davis)**

OXY-KESSO-TETRA® Capsules, 250 mg in bottles of 100 and 1000 and in unit-dose cartons of 100. **(McKesson)**

OXYTETRACYCLINE HYDROCHLORIDE Capsules, 250 mg in bottles of 100 and 1000. **(Lederle)**

TERRAMYCIN®: **(Pfizer)**

Capsules, 125 mg in bottles of 100; 250 mg in bottles of 16, 100 and 500 and in unit-dose packages of 100. Both contain glucosamine hydrochloride.

Intramuscular Injection, 50 mg/ml in multiple dose vials of 10 ml; 50 and 125 mg/ml in 2-ml ampuls (prescored) and in 2-ml disposable syringes (Isoject®).

Intravenous for Injection in vials of 250 mg buffered with 1 gm of ascorbic acid and in vials of 500 mg buffered with 2 gm of ascorbic acid.

Syrup, 125 mg/5 ml (calcium salt) with *N*-acetylglucosamine in bottles of 60 ml and 1 pint.

Tablets, 250 mg (film coated) in bottles of 100.

w/Hydrocortisone

TERRA-CORTRIL®: **(Pfizer)**

Ophthalmic Suspension, 5 mg with hydrocortisone, acetate, 15 mg/ml in dropper bottles of 5 ml.

Topical Aerosol Spray, 300 mg with hydrocortisone, 100 mg and polymyxin B sulfate, 100,000 units in aerosol cans of 85 gm.

Topical Ointment, 3% with hydrocortisone, 1% in tubes of 15 gm.

w/Nystatin

TERRASTATIN® Capsules, 250 mg with glucosamine, and nystatin, 250,000 units in bottles of 50.

w/Polymyxin B Sulfate

TERRAMYCIN®: **(Pfizer)**

Ophthalmic-Otic Ointment, 5 mg with polymyxin B sulfate, 10,000 units/gm in tubes of 3.5 gm.

Topical Powder, 30 mg with polymyxin B sulfate, 1000 units/gm in shaker-top cans of 30 gm.

Vaginal Tablets, 100 mg with polymyxin B sulfate, 100,000 units in cartons of 10.

TERRAMYCIN Topical Ointment, 30 mg with polymyxin B sulfate, 1000 units/gm in tubes of 15 and 30 gm. **(Pfipharmecs)**

OXYTOCIN

Description: Oxytocin is a synthetic, water-soluble polypeptide consisting of 8 amino acids. Pharmacologically and clinically, oxytocin is identical with the oxytocic principle of the posterior lobe of the pituitary body. Each ml of oxytocin injection represents the oxytocic activity of 10 U.S.P. or international posterior pituitary units.

Oxytocin acts directly on the smooth musculature of the uterus, particularly toward the end of pregnancy, during labor and immediately following delivery. It stimulates rhythmic contractions of the uterus, increases the frequency of existing contractions, and raises the tone of the uterine musculature. It also stimulates contraction of myoepithelial cells in the mammary gland postpartum and increases the flow of milk—but not the volume. These effects are discernible following parenteral, intranasal, buccal, or sublingual administration.

Following intramuscular injection, the effect on the uterus is manifest in 3 to 7 minutes and persists for 30 to 60 minutes; intravenously, within 1 minute and is of shorter duration; buccally, within 30 minutes and persisting for 30 to 60 minutes.

Indications: Induction or stimulation of labor at term; management of labor at appearance of anterior shoulder of infant; to expel the placenta; to control postpartum hemorrhage and atony; and to relieve breast engorgement associated with static lactation.

Contraindications: Cephalopelvic disproportion, fetal malpresentation, prematurity of unripe cervix, factors predisposing to uterine rupture (caesarean section, grand multiparity), factors predisposing to thromboplastin or amniotic fluid embolism (dead fetus, abruptio placentae), hypertonic patterns of uterine contractions, hypersensitivity, severe toxemia, and serious medical or obstetric conditions or fetal distress. Intranasal administration is not recommended for intrapartum use.

Warnings: Oxytocin and oxytocin citrate should always be used with caution and under constant medical supervision. Careful selection of patients is important when oxytocin is used for elective induction or for reinforcement of already existent labor. Pelvic adequacy must be considered and maternal and fetal conditions evaluated before administering this drug. The erroneous assumption of fetal maturity is a serious hazard in elective induction. The drug should not be used simultaneously, by more than one route, or with cyclopropane anesthesia. The buccal tablet should not be swallowed; it should remain in the buccal pouch undisturbed.

Precautions: Oxytocin should be administered only under complete obstetrical supervision. During the second stage of labor, the effects of this drug may be accentuated. The injudicious use of parenteral oxytocin has resulted in maternal deaths due to hypertensive episodes, water intoxication, subarachnoid hemorrhage, rupture of the uterus and fetal death due to various causes. In the multipara, oxytocin may be used safely after complete dilation of the cervix, when the drug is properly administered, and when other conditions are favorable. In the primipara, employment of a low forceps operation rather than employment of oxytocin may be advisable in some patients. Increased blood loss and afibrinogenemia can occur with this drug. Because of its antidiuretic effect, consideration should be given to the possibility of water intoxication, particularly when oxytocin is administered continuously by infusion and the patient is receiving fluids. Accidental swallowing of the buccal tablet is not harmful; however, the oxytocin action of the tablet is destroyed in the digestive tract.

Adverse Reactions: Anaphylactic reaction, fetal and neonatal bradycardia, cardiac arrhythmia, postpartum hemorrhage, and pelvic hematoma have been noted. Excessive dosage may result in uterine hypertonicity, spasm, tetanic contraction, or rupture. Occasionally noted were nausea, vomiting, and premature ventricular contractions. A fatality due to afibrinogenemia has been reported. Severe water intoxication with convulsions and coma has occurred following prolonged intravenous infusion.

Dosage and Administration: Induction or stimulation of labor, 10 units (1 ml) in 1 liter of 5% dextrose injection is *infused* initially at the rate of 0.5 ml/min, increased, if necessary, to 2 ml/min. When labor is initiated, infusion may be continued, the rate adjusted according to contractions of the uterus and the response of the fetus. Infusion should be discontinued if uterine motility interferes with the fetal heart tone at any time. Management of labor at appearance of anterior shoulder, 2 units *intravenously.* Postpartum hemorrhage or atony, *intravenous infusion* as outlined above, or 5 to 10 units *intramuscularly. Buccally,* 1 tablet initially, then 1 tablet every 1/2 hour until the desired response is obtained, then note the number of tablets in the cheeks and maintain that number until delivery or until a total of 15 tablets have been given. *Intranasally,* 1 short spray into 1 or both nostrils 2 to 3 minutes before nursing or pumping of the breast.

Availability:
OXYTOCIN Injection, 10 units/ml in Tubex® (disposable syringes) of 1 ml. **(Wyeth)**
PITOCIN®: **(Parke-Davis)**
Injection, 10 units/ml in ampuls of 0.5 and 1 ml and in Steri-Dose® (disposable syringes) of 1 ml.
Tablets, Buccal (as citrate), 200 units foil-wrapped in packages of 10.
SYNTOCINON®: **(Sandoz)**
Injection, 10 units/ml in ampuls of 0.5 and 1 ml.
Nasal Spray, 40 units/ml in squeeze bottles of 2 and 5 ml.

PABALATE

PABALATE-SF

Description: Each Pabalate tablet contains sodium salicylate, 300 mg and sodium aminobenzoate (PABA), 300 mg. Each Pabalate-SF (sodium free) tablet contains potassium salicylate, 300 mg and potassium aminobenzoate, 300 mg.

Paraaminobenzoic acid acts synergistically with the salicylates achieving greater efficacy on lower salicylate dosage.

Indications: Temporary relief of pain and inflammation associated with rheumatoid arthritis, and to supplant plain salicylate. Pabalate sodium free is useful in patients with rheumatic symptoms complicated by such conditions as congestive heart failure, essential hypertension, glomerulonephritis or pregnancy which make it necessary to restrict their sodium intake.

Contraindications: Hypersensitivity to any of the components, and in the presence of an active ulcer.

Warnings: A probable association exists between the use of enteric-coated tablets containing potassium salts with or without thiazide diuretics, and the incidence of serious small bowel ulceration. These small bowel lesions have caused obstruction, hemorrhage and perforation. Surgery was frequently required and deaths have occurred. Such preparations should be administered only when indicated, and should be discontinued immediately if abdominal pain, distention, nausea, vomiting or gastrointestinal bleeding occur. When prescribing Pabalate-SF for patients who are receiving concurrent potassium supplementation (e.g., to replace potassium excreted during thiazide therapy), it should be kept in mind that Pabalate-SF contains potassium. A decrease in supplemental potassium dosage should be considered in order to help avoid hyperkalemia.

Precautions: Concurrent administration of Pabalate with sulfonamides should be avoided, since the aminobenzoate component inhibits the bacteriostatic action of the sulfonamide. Hypoprothrombinemia has been observed during prolonged and intensive therapy with salicylates. If patients receiving such dosages are to undergo surgery, the prothrombin time should be evaluated. Pabalate is not recommended for individuals on a sodium restricted diet.

Adverse Reactions: Nausea and gastrointestinal upset, a fine rash with or without pruritus, urticaria have been noted. The occasional occurrence of mild salicylism may require adjustment in dosage.

Dosage and Administration: *Orally.* Average adult dosage is 2 tablets 4 times daily. In acute exacerbations, the dose may be increased as required. Tablets should not be taken within 1 hour of ingesting milk or antacids such as sodium bicarbonate. Suggested dosage plan for concurrent administration with steroid hormones, employ full doses of Pabalate-SF, adjust the dosage of cortisone or hydrocortisone gradually to the lowest level that suppresses symptoms.

Availability:
PABALATE® (OTC) in bottles of 100 and 500. **(Robins)**
PABALATE-SF (sodium free) in bottles of 100 and 500. **(Robins)**

PALAFLOR: see The Fluoride-Vitamins

PANAFIL
PANAFIL-WHITE

Description: Contains:

Papain powder	10%
Urea U.S.P.	10%
Water-soluble chlorophyll derivatives	0.5%

Panafil-White: Formulation is the same except for the deletion of chlorophyll—stabilized in a hydrophilic base.

The formulation provides effective enzymatic debridement of necrotic tissue and liquefaction of fibrinous, purulent exudates, thus promoting healthy granulation of tissues. Papain exerts its proteolytic activity over a wide pH (3 to 12) range. Chlorophyll derivatives add to the therapeutic effect by inhibiting the hemagglutinating and inflammatory properties of protein degradation products in the wound, as well as those of enzymatic digestion.

Indications: For continuous cleansing-healing action in the local treatment of indolent wounds and ulcers, as well as acute and chronic lesions complicated by sloughing or suppuration.

Precautions: Not for ophthalmic use.

Adverse Reactions: A small percentage of patients may experience a transient burning sensation. Occasionally, the profuse exudate resulting from enzymatic digestion may cause irritation. In such cases, more frequent changes of dressings will alleviate the discomfort.

Dosage and Administration: *Topically.* Apply directly to lesion and cover with gauze or linen dressing. Daily or twice daily changes of dressings preferred, but intervals of 2 to 3 days between redressings are satisfactory. May be applied under pressure dressings. At each redressing, the lesion should be irrigated with isotonic saline solution or other mild cleansing agent except hydrogen peroxide which may inactivate the enzymatic action of papain.

Availability:
PANAFIL® Ointment in tubes of 30 and 120 gm and in jars of 480 gm. **(Rystan)**
PANAFIL-WHITE Ointment in tubes of 30 gm. **(Rystan)**

PANCEBRIN

Description: Each ml contains:

Vitamin A (synthetic)	(5000 units)	1.5 mg
Vitamin D (synthetic)	(500 units)	12.5 μg
Thiamine hydrochloride		5 mg
Riboflavin (as riboflavin 5′ phosphate sodium)		1 mg
Pyridoxine hydrochloride		1.5 mg
Niacinamide		10 mg
Pantothenic acid (as sodium pantothenate)		1.5 mg
Ascorbic acid		30 mg
Alpha-tocopherol		1 mg

Indications: Prevention and treatment of multiple vitamin deficiencies when oral therapy is ineffective.

Contraindications: Hypersensitivity to thiamine. Subcutaneous injection is not recommended.

Precautions: The usual precautions pertaining to parenteral administration of any medication should be observed. This product may cause irritation at the injection site, or pain along the course of the vein.

Adverse Reactions: Flushing, dizziness, or faintness. Repeated injections may cause sensitization.

Dosage and Administration: The usual dosage is 2 ml *intramuscularly* 2 or 3 times weekly. In severe illnesses, 2 ml 1 to 3 times daily are recommended. When administered *intravenously,* the rate of injection should not exceed 1 ml/min.

Availability:
PANCEBRIN® Injection in multiple-dose vials of 10 ml. **(Lilly)**

PANCREATIN

Description: Pancreatin is an amorphous powdered substance containing enzymes, principally pancreatic, protease, amylase, trypsin, and pancreatic lipase, obtained from the pancreas of the hog. Official preparations must be capable of converting not less than 25 times its weight of U.S.P. Potato Starch Reference Standard into soluble carbohydrates in 5 minutes and 25 times its weight of casein into proteoses in 1 hour. Each mg of pancreatin contains 100 units of protease, 150 units of amylase and 20 units of lipase sufficient to digest in vitro 32 gm of dietary protein, 48 gm of dietary starch and 23 gm of dietary fat.

It is usually employed in the treatment of conditions, such as faulty digestion, in which the secretion of pancreatic juice is deficient. It also decreases the nitrogen and fat content of the stool.

Indications: For exocrine pancreatic insufficiency, usually due to chronic pancreatitis, pancreatectomy, cystic fibrosis or ductal obstruction caused by cancer of the pancreas, and for steatorrhea or malabsorption syndrome and postgastrectomy (Bilroth II and total).

Warnings: Pancreatic exocrine replacement therapy should not delay or supplant treatment of the primary disorder. Inhalation of the powder should be avoided.

Precautions: Use with caution in patients known to be sensitive to pork protein or enzymes. If sensitivity develops, the drug should be discontinued.

Adverse Reactions: Nausea or diarrhea may occur with high dosages.

Dosage and Administration: *Orally.* Adults, 4 to 8 gm daily in divided doses at intervals of 1 or 2 hours or taken before, during and within 1 hour after meals with an extra dose taken with food between meals. Children, initially, 300 to 600 mg with each meal. In severe deficiencies the dose may be increased if no nausea, vomiting or diarrhea occurs.

Availability:
PANCREATIN: **(Lilly)**
Enseals (3 x N.F.), 325 mg in bottles of 100 and 500.
Powder in packets of 120 gm in cartons of 6.
Tablets, 325 mg in bottles of 100 and 1000.
PANTERIC®: **(Parke-Davis)**
Capsules, 325 mg in bottles of 100.
Filmseals (enteric-coated, 3 x N.F.), 325 mg in bottles of 100.
Granules in bottles of 120 gm.
VIOKASE®: **(Viobin)**
Powder in bottles of 120 and 240 gm.
Tablets, 325 mg in bottles of 100 and 500.

PANCRELIPASE

Description: Pancrelipase is a concentrate of pancreatic enzymes of porcine origin with standardized lipase activity. On a weight basis, pancrelipase has 12 times the lipolytic activity of pancreatin N.F., and a trypsin and amylase content of at least 4 times that of pancreatin. In vitro studies demonstrate that 300 mg of the enzyme is capable of digesting 17 gm of fat, 34 gm of protein, and 40 gm of starch. In common with other pancreatic enzyme preparations, it is partially inactivated by gastric juice in vivo.

Indications: Replacement therapy in the symptomatic treatment of conditions in which pancreatic enzymes are absent from or present in insufficient amounts in the intestine (pancreatectomy, chronic pancreatitis), cystic fibrosis or obstruction caused by cancer of the pancreas, steatorrhea, and in conditions in which fat digestion is inadequate due to pancreatic-enzyme deficiency.

Precautions: The drug should be administered with caution to patients allergic to hog protein or enzymes. The proper balance between fat, protein and starch intake must be maintained to avoid indigestion.

Dosage and Administration: *Orally,* 1 to 3 capsules or tablets or 1 to 2 packets with each meal or "snack," or as directed. Children, 1 or 2 capsules or tablets with each meal. In severe deficiencies the frequency of dosage may be increased to hourly intervals if no nausea or diarrhea result.

Availability:
COTAZYM®: **(Organon)**
Capsules in bottles of 100 and 500. Each capsule contains 8000 units of lipase and 30,000 units each of protease and amylase plus other enzymes from whole hog pancreas with 25 mg of calcium carbonate precipitated.
-65B Capsules in bottles of 100. Each capsule contains in addition to the above 65 mg of mixed conjugated bile salts and 2 mg of cellulase.
Packets, 16,000 units in cartons of 250; 40,000 units (cherry-flavored) in cartons of 100.
ILOZYME® Tablets in bottles of 250. Each tablet contains 400 mg of pancrelipase (repre-

senting no less than 9600 units of lipase and 40,000 units each of protease and amylase). One tablet hydrolyzes no less than 40 gm each of casein and starch. **(Warren-Teed)**
PANCREASE™ Capsules (enteric-coated) in bottles of 100 and 250. Each capsule contains 4000 units of lipase, 20,000 units of amylase and 25,000 units of protease plus other enzymes from whole hog pancreas. **(Johnson & Johnson)**

PANCURONIUM BROMIDE

Chemical Name: 2 Beta, 16 beta-dipiperidine-5 alpha-androstane-3 alpha, 17-beta-diol diacetate dimethobromide.

Description: Pancuronium bromide is a nondepolarizing neuromuscular blocking agent—it blocks nervous impulses to skeletal muscles at the myoneural junctions and rapidly induces paralysis. It possesses all of the characteristic pharmacological actions of this class of drugs.

Pancuronium has been reported to be approximately 5 times as potent as *d*-tubocurarine. The onset and duration of action of the drug depend on the dose administered. Following an injection of 0.04 mg/kg of body weight, the curare effect occurs within 45 seconds, peak effect usually is attained within 4½ minutes, and almost complete recovery (90%) occurs within 1 hour. It is excreted unchanged in the urine.

Pancuronium appears to have little effect upon the circulatory system; the most frequently reported observation has been a slight rise in pulse rate. Laboratory tests and clinical observations have revealed that a histamine release rarely, if ever, occurs. Pancuronium is antagonized by acetylcholine, anticholinesterases, and potassium ion. Its action is increased by inhalation anesthetics such as halothane, diethyl ether, enflurane, and methoxyflurane, as well as quinine, magnesium salts, hypokalemia, some carcinomas, and certain antibiotics such as neomycin, streptomycin, kanamycin, gentamicin, and bacitracin. Its action may also be altered in the presence of dehydration, electrolyte imbalance, acid-base imbalance, renal disease, and by concomitant administration of other neuromuscular agents. No increase in the intensity and duration of action is noted from the use of thiobarbiturates, narcotic analgesics, nitrous oxide or droperidol.

Prior administration of succinylcholine, such as that used for endotrachael intubation, enhances the relaxant effect and duration of action of this drug. If succinylcholine is used prior to pancuronium, the administration of pancuronium should be delayed until the effects of succinycholine show signs of wearing off. Pancuronium has no known effect on consciousness, the pain threshold or cerebration.

Indications: Adjunct to anesthesia in order to induce skeletal muscle relaxation. It may also be employed to facilitate the management of patients undergoing mechanical ventilation.

Contraindications: In patients known to be hypersensitive to the drug or to the bromide ion.

Warnings: Pancuronium should be administered in carefully adjusted dosage by or under the supervision of experienced clinicians, who are familiar with its action and the possible complications that might occur following its use. The drug should not be administered unless facilities for intubation, artificial respiration, oxygen therapy and medication (reversal agents) are immediately available. The clinician must be prepared to assist or control respiration. Since small doses of pancuronium may produce serious and profound effects in patients with myasthenia gravis, the use of a peripheral nerve stimulator is especially valuable in assessing the effects of the drug in such patients. Safe use during pregnancy, in women of childbearing potential or in obstetrical patients has not been established. May be used in obstetrical anesthesia but the dosage should be reduced in patients receiving magnesium sulfate for toxemia of pregnancy because the magnesium ion enhances the neuromuscular blockade effect and reversal of pancuronium may therefore be unsatisfactory.

Precautions: Pancuronium should be used with caution in patients with preexisting pulmonary, hepatic or renal disease. Neostigmine, in conjunction with atropine, will usually antagonize the skeletal-muscle relaxant action of this agent, and therefore, should be readily on hand. Neostigmine should be accompanied by or preceded by an injection of atropine in order to minimize the incidence of cholinergic side effects, notably excessive secretions and bradycardia. Satisfactory reversal can be judged by adequacy of skeletal-muscle tone and respiration. A peripheral-nerve stimulator may also be used to monitor restoration of twitch height. Failure of prompt reversal (within 30 minutes) may occur in the presence of extreme debilitation, carcinomatosis, and with concomitant use of certain broad spectrum antibiotics or anesthetic and/or adjunctive agents which also enhance neuromuscular blockade or cause respiratory depression.

Adverse Reactions: *Neuromuscular:* the most frequently noted adverse reaction consists primarily of an extension of the drug's pharmacological actions beyond the time period needed for surgery and anesthesia. This reaction may vary from skeletal muscle weakness to profound and prolonged skeletal muscle relaxation, resulting in respiratory insufficiency or apnea. Inadequate reversal of the neuromuscular blockade by anticholinesterase agents has also been observed with pancuronium. These adverse reactions are managed by manual or mechanical ventilation until recovery is judged adequate. *Cardiovascular:* a slight increase in pulse rate is frequently noted. *Gastrointestinal:* salivation is sometimes noted during very light anesthesia, especially if no anticholinergic premedication is used. *Skin:* an occasional transient rash is noted. *Respiratory:* 1 case of wheezing, responding to deepening of the inhalational anesthetic, has been reported.

Dosage and Administration: *Intravenously.* In adults, the initial dose ranges from 0.04 to 0.1 mg/kg of body weight, followed by incremental doses starting at 0.01 mg/kg, if necessary. These increments slightly increase the magnitude of the blockade, and significantly increase the duration of this action. For endotrachael intubation, doses of 0.06 to 0.1 mg/kg of body weight are recommended. Conditions satisfactory for intubation are usually present within 2 to 3 minutes. Dosage-response studies in children under 10 years of age are insufficient; therefore, the drug is not recommended for use in this age group. The physician should be aware that infants during the first month of life are especially sensitive to nondepolarizing neuromuscular blocking agents.

Availability:
PAVULON® Injection, 1 mg/ml in multiple-dose vials of 10 ml; 2 mg/ml in ampuls of 2 and 5 ml. **(Organon)**

PAPAIN

Description: Papain is a combination of one or more proteolytic enzymes extracted from *Carica papaya.* The potency of the commercial preparation of papain is expressed in units established by the manufacturer. One W-C unit is that quantity of proteolytic enzymes extracted from *Carica papaya* which will clot 2.64 microliters of milk substrate in 2 minutes at 40° C. Its principal direct effect appears to be a proteolytic or depolymerizing action on soft fibrin deposits in acutely inflamed areas, with an increasing cell and tissue permeability. It thereby facilitates the reduction of inflammation, drainage of fluids and resolution of cellular debris, all of which enhance the body's normal physiologic and tissue-repair mechanisms. When administered in recommended doses, the proteolytic activity does not affect uninjured cells or tissues.

Indications: Relief of the combined symptoms related to episiotomy.

Contraindications: Concomitant use with anticoagulants. The drug is not recommended for patients with generalized or systemic infections or severe blood-clotting disorders, or for those patients with a prior allergic reaction to papain.

Warnings: Safe use during pregnancy has not been established.

Precautions: Should be used with caution in patients with severe renal or hepatic disease.

Adverse Reactions: Nausea, vomiting, diarrhea, dizziness, pruritus, rash, urticaria, and a mild local tingling at the site of buccal absorption.

Dosage and Administration: *Orally,* either chewed or swallowed with water, or administered buccally. Prophylactic dosage, 2 tablets 1 or 2 hours before episiotomy. Therapeutic dosage, 2 tablets 4 times daily for at least 5 days.

Availability:
PAPASE® Tablets, 100,000 units in bottles of 100 and 1000. **(Warner-Chilcott)**

PAPAVERINE HYDROCHLORIDE

Chemical Name: 6,7-Dimethoxy-1-veratrylisoquinoline hydrochloride.

Description: Papaverine hydrochloride is a benzylisoquinoline alkaloid prepared either synthetically or from opium. It does not contain a phenanthrene group as do morphine and codeine and does not evoke tolerance or addiction.

The main actions of papaverine are exerted on smooth surface muscle. It relaxes the smooth musculature of the large blood vessels, especially the coronary, peripheral, cerebral, and pulmonary arteries. This action is particularly evident when such vessels are in spasm. The muscle cell is not paralyzed by papaverine, and still responds to drugs and other stimuli causing contraction. The antispasmodic effect is a direct one and is unrelated to muscle contraction. The drug produces minimal actions on the CNS, although very large doses tend to produce some sedation and sleepiness in some individuals.

Perhaps by its direct vasodilating action on cerebral blood vessels, papaverine increases cerebral blood flow and decreases cerebral vascular resistance in normal individuals; oxygen consumption is unaltered. These effects may explain the benefit reported from the drug in cerebrovascular encephalopathy.

Like quinidine, papaverine acts directly on the myocardium to depress conduction and to prolong the refractory period. The drug raises the threshold for inducing ventricular fibrillation. The coronary vasodilator action could be an additional factor of therapeutic value when such rhythms are secondary to insufficiency or occlusion of the coronary arteries.

Papaverine undergoes complete destruction in the tissues. It is metabolized in the liver and about 90% of the drug is bound to plasma proteins.

Indications: Relief of cerebral and peripheral ischemia associated with arterial spasm and myocardial ischemia complicated by arrhythmias.

Contraindications: There are no known contraindications to oral administration. Intravenous injection is contraindicated in the presence of complete heart block since the drug may produce transient ectopic rhythms of ventricular origin, either premature beats or paroxysmal tachycardia.

Precautions: Use with caution in patients with glaucoma. Medication should be discontinued if hepatic hypersensitivity with gastrointestinal symptoms, jaundice, eosinophilia or altered liver function tests become evident.

Adverse Reactions: Rarely occurring were nausea, abdominal distress, anorexia, constipation or diarrhea, skin rash, malaise, drowsiness, vertigo, sweating, and headache. Patients given parenteral doses may experience a general feeling of discomfort, intensive flushing of the face, perspiration, an increase in the depth of respiration, increase in heart rate, a slight rise in blood pressure, or excessive sedation.

Dosage and Administration: *Orally, intramuscularly or intravenously.* Initially, 1 to 4 ml injected every 3 hours as indicated. In cardiac extrasystoles, 2 doses may be given 10 minutes apart. The usual oral dosage range for adults is from 100 to 300 mg 3 to 5 times daily. **Note:** The injection should not be added to Lactated Ringer's solution because precipitation occurs.

Availability:

Papaverine Hydrochloride

CERESPAN® Capsules, 150 mg (in sustained release, micro-dialysis cells) in bottles of 100 and 1000, in drums of 5000 and in single-dose blister packs in cartons of 100. **(USV)**

DIPAV Capsules (timed-release), 150 mg in bottles of 100 and 1000. **(Lemmon)**

DYLATE SR Capsules (sustained-release), 150 mg in bottles of 100 and 1000. **(Elder)**

PAPAVERINE HYDROCHLORIDE: **(Lederle)**

Capsules, (timed-release), 150 mg in bottles of 60, 100 and 1000.

Tablets, 60 and 100 mg in bottles of 100 and 1000.

PAPAVERINE HYDROCHLORIDE: **(Lilly)**

Injection, 30 mg/ml in ampuls of 1 and 2 ml and in vials of 10 ml.

Powder (synthetic, U.S.P.) in cans of 30 and 120 gm.

Tablets, 30 mg in bottles of 100; 60 and 100 mg in bottles of 100 and 1000; 200 mg in bottles of 100. All potencies are available in unit-dose (individually labeled blister units) cartons of 100.

PAPAVERINE HYDROCHLORIDE Tablets, 100 mg in bottles of 500. **(Merrell-National)**
PAPAVERINE HYDROCHLORIDE Capsules, 150 mg in bottles of 100 and 1000 and in unit-dose packages of 100. **(Philips Roxane)**
PAPAVERINE HYDROCHLORIDE Tablets, 100 mg in bottles of 100 and 1000. **(Rowell)**
PAVABID® Plateau Capsules (sustained-release), 150 mg in bottles of 100, 250, 1000 and 5000 in UDIP® (unit-dose) packages of 500 and in Un-Rx Paks (unit-dose) packages of 60 and 100 in cartons of 25. **(Marion)**
PAVABID HP Capsules, 300 mg in Uni-Rx Paks of 60. **(Marion)**
PAVAGRANT Capsules, 100 mg in bottles of 1000. **(Amfre-Grant)**
PAVAKEY® Capsules (sustained-release), 150 and 300 mg in bottles of 100 and 1000. **(Key Pharm.)**
SUSTAVERINE™ Capsules (sustained-release), 150 mg in bottles of 60. **(ICN)**
THERAPAV® Capsules (liquid-filled), 75 mg in bottles of 100; 150 mg in bottles of 100 and 500. **(Cooper)**

PARAMETHADIONE

Chemical Name: 3,5-Dimethyl-5-ethyloxazolidine-2,4-dione.

TRIMETHADIONE

Chemical Name: 3,5,5-Trimethyloxazoline-2,4-dione.

Description: Paramethadione is a synthetic anticonvulsant with low toxicity. A homolog of trimethadione, it differs only in the substitution of an ethyl for a methyl group on carbon 5. It occurs as an oily liquid which is only slightly soluble in water. Trimethadione occurs as a white crystalline powder, with a slight camphor-like odor which is soluble in water and freely soluble in alcohol.

Both drugs have been shown to prevent convulsions which would be expected from fatal doses of pentylenetetrazol and thujone in experimental animals. They display a less marked effect on convulsions induced by picrotoxin, procaine, cocaine and strychnine. Unlike the hydantoins and the antiepileptic barbiturates, neither drug has been demonstrated to modify the maximal seizure pattern in patients receiving electroconvulsive therapy. Paramethadione has a slightly greater sedative effect than trimethadione. With both drugs this sedative effect may increase to the point of ataxia when excessive doses are administered. Sleep, unconsciousness and respiratory depression were produced in animals given toxic doses of about 1 gm/kg for paramethadione, and 2 gm/kg for trimethadione. Paramethadione is less apt to cause photophobia than trimethadione, and has been found to be useful in some patients not controlled by trimethadione.

Both drugs are readily absorbed from the gastrointestinal tract. They are demethylated in the liver and slowly excreted in this form by the kidneys. Following a single large therapeutic dose, only about 3% of the unchanged drug can be detected in the urine. Their action is prolonged when they are administered in large hypnotic doses to animals with severe hepatic injury or with bilateral nephrectomy.

Indications: Control of petit mal seizures that are refractory to other drugs.

Contraindications: Hypersensitivity to paramethadione and trimethadione.

Warnings: Recent reports suggest that anticonvulsant drugs including para- and trimethadione are associated with an increased incidence of congenital malformation among the offspring of women receiving the drug at the time of conception and subsequent pregnancy. Therefore, the use of these drugs in pregnant women or in women of childbearing potential requires that the potential benefits be weighed against the possible hazards to the patient as well as to the fetus. However, these drugs should not be discontinued in those patients prone to major seizures because of the strong possibility of precipitating status epilepticus with its attendant hypoxia and risk to both the mother and fetus. Nonetheless, consideration should be given to discontinuing these agents prior to and during pregnancy when the nature, frequency and severity of the seizures do not constitute a serious threat to the patient. At the present time, it is not known whether or not even minor seizures pose some risk to the developing embryo or fetus.

Precautions: Skin eruptions indicate the need for prompt withdrawal of the drug, and any dermal manifestation should be allowed to heal completely before treatment is resumed, and then only with considerable caution. Patients should be under strict medical supervision during the initial period of treatment and complete blood and differential counts and urinalyses should be done every month. A moderate degree of neutropenia with or without a corresponding drop in the leukocyte count may occur, but this does not call for withdrawal of therapy unless the total number of neutrophils drops to 2500 or less; frequent blood examinations should be made when the count is less than 3000. More severe hematologic complications, including fatal aplastic anemia, have occurred. Patients should be advised to report immediately such complications as sore throat, fever, malaise, easy-bruising, petechiae, or epistaxis, or any other problem that may represent an infection or bleeding tendency. Ordinarily, these drugs should not be used in patients with severe blood dyscrasias or with severe impairment of the liver. Therapy should be discontinued on the appearance of persistent or increasing albuminuria, jaundice, or other signs of hepatitis, scotoma, a lupus erythematous-like or myasthenia gravis-like syndrome or enlargement of the lymph nodes. However, consideration should be given to the fact that abrupt discontinuation of treatment may precipitate petit mal status. A substitute anticonvulsant should be administered in order to protect the patient. Caution must be exercised in patients with disease of the retina or optic nerve. Concurrent administration of other drugs known to cause toxic effects should be avoided or used with extreme caution. Reports have suggested that anticonvulsant drugs may be associated with neonatal hemorrhage in infants born to mothers treated with these drugs during pregnancy. Such drug therapy appears to reduce the levels of vitamin K-dependent clotting factors in the infant, causing an increased tendency to hemorrhage in the neonatal period. It has been suggested that vitamin K be given prophylactically to such infants at birth. Safe use during lactation has not been established.

Adverse Reactions: Gastrointestinal effects reported are hiccups, nausea, vomiting, abdominal pain and gastric distress, anorexia and weight loss. Disturbances of the CNS have included photophobia, diplopia, hemeralopia, vertigo, increased irritability, insomnia, drowsiness, paresthesias, headaches, fatigue and malaise, and personality changes. Visual disturbances appear to be due to the retinal effect of these drugs and usually can be controlled by a reduction in dosage. Drowsiness tends to subside with continued therapy or can be controlled with decreased dosage. Skin rashes, bleeding gums, epistaxis, retinal and petechial hemorrhages, vaginal bleeding and certain blood dyscrasias including leukopenia, neutropenia, thrombocytopenia, pancytopenia, agranulocytosis and hypoplastic anemia have been noted. A lupus-erythematosus syndrome and a syndrome simulating malignant lymphoma have occurred. Lymphadenopathy with hepatosplenomegaly associated with pruritus in hypersensitive individuals has also occurred. If lupus-like manifestations or lymph node enlargement should appear, therapy is to be discontinued and the patient observed for improvement before specific treatment for lupus erythematosus or lymphoma is instituted. Other reactions observed were changes in blood pressure, albuminuria and nephrosis, hepatitis, and precipitation of grand mal seizures. A myasthenia gravis-like syndrome also has been associated with chronic administration of the drug and indicates a discontinuation of medication. Hair loss may occur in patients receiving paramethadione; rarely in those receiving trimethadione. Acute overdosage is manifested by nausea, drowsiness, dizziness, ataxia, and visual disturbances. Treatment is started by inducing emesis; gastric lavage may be considered as an alternative. General supportive measures will be necessary. A careful evaluation of liver and renal function and of the blood-forming organs should be made following recovery.

Dosage and Administration: *Orally.* The dosage of either drug is the same. The usual adult dosage ranges from 300 to 600 mg 3 to 4 times daily. It is advisable to start therapy at a dosage of 0.9 gm daily in divided doses with increments of 300 mg daily at weekly intervals until therapeutic results are achieved or until toxic symptoms appear. In children, the initial dosage should be in proportion to age and weight, usually 0.3 to 0.9 gm daily in 3 or 4 equally divided doses. Maintenance dosage depends on the least amount of drug necessary to achieve adequate control.

Availability:

Paramethadione

PARADIONE®: **(Abbott)**

Capsules, 150 and 300 mg in bottles of 100.

Oral Solution, 300 mg/ml in bottles of 50 ml with graduated dropper.

Trimethadione

TRIDIONE®: **(Abbott)**

Capsules, 300 mg in bottles of 100.

Dulcet® (Chewable Tablets), 150 mg in bottles of 100.

Oral Solution, 200 mg/5 ml in bottles of 1 pint.

PARAMETHASONE ACETATE: see The Adrenal Corticosteroids

PARATHYROID

Description: Parathyroid is a protein hormone obtained from beef glands. It is standardized to a potency of not less than 100 U.S.P. units/ml, each unit representing 1/100 of the amount required to raise the calcium content of 100 mg of the blood serum of normal dogs 1 mg within 16 to 18 hours after administration. When administered parenterally, it raises the serum calcium level (largely by mobilizing calcium from the bones) and decreases serum inorganic phosphorus with increased urinary excretion of both calcium and phosphorus. The rise in serum calcium begins in about 4 hours, reaches a maximum in 12 to 18 hours and returns to the previous level in 20 to 24 hours.

Indications: Treatment of acute hypoparathyroidism with tetany. Also used in various tests in order to establish the diagnosis of idiopathic and postoperative hypoparathyroidism.

Contraindications: Hypercalcemia.

Precautions: Use cautiously in the presence of renal or cardiac disease. The use of the drug should be accompanied by frequent blood calcium determinations. Preliminary skin tests should be undertaken before intravenous injection, and desensitization should be employed if the tests are positive. If parathyroid injection is to be added to other intravenous solutions, it is recommended that 2.5 to 5% dextrose be used since saline solutions often cause a precipitate to form.

Adverse Reactions: Symptoms of overdosage are anorexia, vomiting, diarrhea and weakness. Subcutaneous injection may cause a moderate inflammatory reaction.

Dosage and Administration: *Subcutaneously, intramuscularly* or *intravenously,* 20 to 40 units every 12 hours if necessary; usually given in conjunction with calcium salts and vitamin D. Dosage should be controlled so that the serum level does not exceed 12 mg/100 ml.

Availability:

PARATHYROID Solution, 100 units/ml in ampuls of 5 ml. **(Lilly)**

PAREGORIC: see Opium Tincture, Camphorated

PAREPECTOLIN Ⓒ

Description: Each 30 ml of suspension contains:

Paregoric (equiv. to 15 mg of opium)	3.7 ml
Pectin	162 mg
Kaolin	5.5 gm
Alcohol	0.69 %

Indications: Symptomatic relief of diarrhea.

Warnings: Opium may be habit-forming.

Precautions: Preparations containing opium should be used with caution in infants, aged or debilitated patients, those with increased intracranial pressure, toxic psychosis, myxedema, prostatic hypertrophy or obstruction.

Adverse Reactions: Excessive doses may produce side effects common to morphine and its derivatives.

Dosage and Administration: *Orally.* Usual adult dosage is 1 or 2 tablespoonsful. Usual children's dosage is 1 or 2 teaspoonsful. Children 1 year of age, 1/2 teaspoonful; 3 years of age, 1 1/2 teaspoonsful; 6 years of age, 2 teaspoonsful. Dosage should be taken after each loose bowel movement for no more than 4 doses in 12 hours.

Availability:
Ⓒ PAREPECTOLIN® Suspension in bottles of 120 and 240 ml. **(Rorer)**

PARGYLINE HYDROCHLORIDE

Chemical Name: *N*-Methyl-*N*-2-propynylbenzylamine hydrochloride.

Description: Pargyline hydrochloride is a nonhydrazine MAO inhibitor compound used in the treatment of hypertension. It lowers both the systolic and diastolic blood pressure without depressing the patient. The effect is primarily orthostatic and is similar to that produced by ganglionic blocking agents. The action of pargyline is cumulative; a latent period of a few days to several weeks may occur before the full effect is achieved, and the effects may persist for as long as 3 weeks after therapy is discontinued. It is rapidly excreted in the urine, largely in unchanged form.

Indications: Treatment of moderate to severe hypertension, especially severe diastolic hypertension. It is not recommended for mild or labile hypertension amenable to therapy with sedatives or thiazide diuretics. Combined with methyclothiazide for the treatment of congestive heart failure with coexisting edema. This combination is not indicated for initial therapy since the condition requires that treatment be titrated to the individual patient. However, if the fixed combination represents the dosage so determined, its use may be more convenient in patient management.

Contraindications: In patients with pheochromocytoma, paranoid schizophrenia, hyperthyroidism, or advanced renal failure. It is also contraindicated in patients with malignant hypertension, and in children under 12 years of age. In general, the following drugs or agents are contraindicated in patients receiving pargyline hydrochloride: Centrally acting sympathomimetic amines such as amphetamine and its derivatives (also found in anorectic preparations); peripherally acting sympathomimetic drugs such as ephedrine and its derivatives (also found in nasal decongestants, cold remedies and hay fever preparations); aged and natural cheese (e.g., Cheddar, Camembert, and Stilton), processed cheese and other foods (e.g., pickled herring, Chianti wine, chocolate, yeast extract, avocado, banana peels, pods of broad beans, and chicken livers) which require the action of bacteria or molds for their preparation or preservation, because of the presence of pressor substances such as tyramine. Cream cheese, ricotta cheese and cottage cheese can be allowed in the diet during therapy with pargyline, since their tyramine content is inconsequential. In some patients receiving this drug, tyramine may precipitate an abrupt rise in blood pressure accompanied by some or all of the following consequences: severe headache, chest pain, profuse sweating, palpitation, tachycardia or bradycardia, visual disturbances, stertorous breathing, coma, and intracranial bleeding (which could be fatal). A phenothiazine derivative or phentolamine may be administered parenterally for treatment of such an acute hypertensive reaction. *Parenteral* administration of reserpine or guanethidine may cause hypertensive reactions from sudden release of catecholamines. Parenteral use of these drugs is contraindicated during, and for at least one week following, treatment with pargyline. Imipramine, amitriptyline, desipramine, nortriptyline, or their analogues should not be used with pargyline. The use of these drugs with a monoamine oxidase inhibitor has been reported to cause vascular collapse and hyperthermia which may be fatal. A drug-free interval (about two weeks) should separate therapy with pargyline and use of these agents. Since MAO inhibitors have been reported to potentiate the pressor effects of L-Dopa, it is recommended that at least one month should elapse after the discontinuance of pargyline before L-Dopa is given. Methyldopa or dopamine, may cause hyperexcitability in patients receiving pargyline.

Warnings: Patients on therapy with pargyline should be cautioned not to take other drugs without the knowledge and consent of the physician. They should also be cautioned on the use of alcoholic beverages in any form. They should be made aware that orthostatic hypotension can occur, also to report promptly the occurrence of severe headaches or other unusual symptoms. Patients with angina should be carefully instructed not to increase their physical activities in response to a lessening of anginal symptoms or an increase in well-being which usually occurs during treatment with this drug. Diabetic patients present an additional risk in that severe drug-induced hypoglycemia may occur; consequently, an adjustment in the dosage of their antidiabetic medication may be required. Patients with impaired renal function may experience cumulative drug effects. Safe use of pargyline during pregnancy has not been established, and consideration should be given to the possible risks to the mother and fetus.

Precautions: Caffeine, alcohol, antihistamines, barbiturates, chloral hydrate and other hypnotics, sedatives, tranquilizers and narcotics (meperidine is contraindicated) should be used cautiously and at reduced dosage in patients taking this drug. Those with angina pectoris or other manifestations of coronary artery disease should be warned against an increase in physical activity or a belief that their coronary artery disease has been improved, and should be observed closely for the development of postural hypotension. Care should be taken to watch for increasing elevations of BUN or other signs of progressive renal failure and for evidence of accumulation of the drug. Complete blood counts, urinalyses and tests of liver function should be made periodically. Patients receiving the product for prolonged periods should be examined for any changes in color perception, visual fields, visual acuity and fundi. If symptoms of orthostatic hypotension develop, they usually can be prevented or minimized by careful adjustment of dosage. Weight gain and edema also have been observed, and pargyline therapy has been accompanied by congestive heart failure in some patients with reduced cardiac reserve. Use cautiously, if at all, in the presence of a febrile episode since the hypotensive effects of the drug may be increased. Patients should be warned against self-medication, particularly with cold tablets, nasal decongestants and reducing pills sold over the counter. Hypotension may be associated with the use of excess doses of pargyline. Give with caution, if at all, to patients with hyperactive or hyperexcitable personalities or to those on antiparkinsonian therapy (exacerbation of symptoms may occur). Hyperreflexia, hyperexcitement, schizophrenia and mania may occur when the drug is administered in high dosage. Since pargyline may augment the hypotensive effects of anesthetic agents and surgery, the drug should be discontinued at least 2 weeks prior to operation. The possibility of sensitivity reactions to methyclothiazide should be considered in patients with a history of allergy or bronchial asthma. All the precautions attendant on the use of the thiazide compounds should be observed.

Adverse Reactions: The most frequently occurring side effects are those associated with orthostatic hypotension (dizziness, weakness, palpitation, or fainting). These usually respond to a reduction of dosage. Patients should be warned against rising to a standing position too quickly, especially when getting out of bed. Severe and persistent orthostatic hypotension should be avoided by reduction in dosage and/or discontinuation of therapy. Mild constipation, fluid retention with or without edema, dry mouth, sweating, increased appetite, arthralgia, nausea and vomiting, headache, insomnia, difficulty in micturition, nightmares, impotence and delayed ejaculation, rash and purpura, have also been encountered. Hyperexcitability, increased neuromuscular activity (muscle twitching), and other extrapyramidal symptoms have been reported. Gain in weight may be due to either edema or increased appetite. Drug fever is extremely rare. In some patients reduction of blood sugar has been noted. Although the significance of this has not been elucidated, the possibility of hypoglycemic effects should be borne in mind. Congestive heart failure has been reported in patients with reduced cardiac reserve. Reported manifestations of overdosage include agitation, hallucinations, hyperreflexia, convulsions, and both hypotension and hypertension. Management must be attempted with extreme caution because of the potential for interaction with antidotal drugs. Conservative treatment aimed at the maintenance of normal temperature, respiration, blood pressure, and proper fluid and electrolyte balance has generally been successful.

For information on the contraindications, warnings, precautions, and adverse reactions associated with methyclothiazide, the general statement on the Thiazide Diuretics should be consulted.

Dosage and Administration: *Orally,* as a single daily dose. Initially, 25 mg daily but may be increased by 10 mg weekly until control is achieved. The initial dosage should range from 10 to 25 mg daily in elderly (over age 65) or sympathectomized patients. When the drug is added to an established antihypertensive regimen, the initial daily dosage should not exceed 25 mg, and should be less than 25 mg for elderly or sympathectomized patients. Maintenance dosage is established by increasing the initial dosage at weekly intervals, by increments of 10 mg. The average maintenance dosage is 50 to 75 mg daily. Pargyline with methyclothiazide, 1 or 2 tablets daily; however, therapy should be initiated with separate administration of the components, and dosage should be determined by individual titration of ingredients. The upper limits of daily dosage of the 2 components are 10 mg of methyclothiazide and 200 mg of pargyline hydrochloride. In general, dosage should be kept at the minimum level required to maintain a desirable reduction in blood pressure without encountering undue reactions.

Availability:
EUTONYL® Filmtab® (film-sealed tablets), 10, 25 and 50 mg in bottles of 100. **(Abbott)**
EUTRON® Filmtab (tablets), 25 mg with methyclothiazide, 5 mg in bottles of 100 and 500. **(Abbott)**

PAROMOMYCIN SULFATE

Description: Paromomycin sulfate is a broad spectrum antibiotic produced by *Streptomyces rimosus* var. *paromomycinus.* It occurs as a white, amorphous substance that is soluble in water. In vitro and in vivo antibacterial action of paromomycin closely parallels that of neomycin. Unlike other antibiotics used as amebicides, this drug is directly amebicidal, and since it is active in the intestinal lumen, it also suppresses enteric flora and subsequently the bacterial production of ammonia. It is poorly absorbed following oral administration, with almost 100% of the drug recoverable in the feces.

Indications: Treatment of acute and chronic intestinal amebiasis (*not effective in extraintestinal amebiasis*), and as adjunctive therapy in the management of hepatic coma.

Contraindications: In patients hypersensitive to paromomycin and in those with intestinal obstruction.

Precautions: Overgrowth of nonsusceptible organisms including fungi may occur; if new infections occur, appropriate measures should be instituted. This product should be used with caution in the presence of gastrointestinal ulceration because of possible absorption.

Adverse Reactions: Nausea, abdominal cramps, and diarrhea have been reported in patients on large doses.

Dosage and Administration: *Orally. Treatment of intestinal amebiasis,* the usual dose is 25 to 35 mg/kg of body weight daily, administered in 3 doses with meals, for 5 to 10 days. *Management of hepatic coma,* the usual adult dose is 4 gm daily in divided doses, given at regular intervals for 5 to 6 days.

Availability:
HUMATIN®: **(Parke-Davis)**
Kapseals® (Capsules), 250 mg in bottles of 16.
Syrup, 125 mg/5 ml in bottles of 60 ml.

PEDÍACOF Ⓥ

Description: Each 5 ml (teaspoonful) contains codeine phosphate, 5 mg; phenylephrine hydrochloride, 2.5 mg; chlorpheniramine maleate, 0.75 mg and potassium iodide, 75 mg with sodium benzoate, 0.2% as preservative and alcohol, 5%.

Indications: Relief of coughs due to colds, and coughs and congestive symptoms associated with infections of the upper respiratory tract, such as tracheobronchitis or laryngobronchitis, croup, pharyngitis, allergic bronchitis and infectious bronchitis.

Contraindications: Tuberculosis, hypersensitivity to iodides.

Warnings: Codeine phosphate may be habit-forming.

Precautions: Use with caution in patients with cardiac disorders, hypertension or hyperthyroidism. Pediacof may cause elevation of protein-bound iodine.

Adverse Reactions: Mild anorexia, constipation, and drowsiness.

Dosage and Administration: *Orally.* Children 6 to 12 years of age, 2 teaspoonsful; 3 to 6 years of age, 1 to 2 teaspoonsful; 1 to 3 years of age, ½ to 1 teaspoonful; 6 months to 1 year, ¼ teaspoonful. Suggested doses may be repeated every 4 to 6 hours as needed.

Availability:
Ⓒ PEDIACOF® Syrup in bottles of 1 pint and 1 gallon. **(Breon)**

PEMOLINE Ⓒ

Chemical Name: 2-Amino-5-phenyl-2-oxazolin-4-one.

Description: A mild CNS stimulant, pemoline has been found to be similar in pharmacologic activity to that of other known psychostimulants without producing any significant sympathomimetic activity. It is structurally different from the amphetamines and methylphenidate. The drug occurs as a white, tasteless, odorless powder that is practically insoluble in water and only slightly soluble in alcohol. Although clinical studies have not revealed its precise mode of action, studies with rats have shown that the drug is capable of increasing the rate of dopamine synthesis. Pemoline is well absorbed from the gastrointestinal tract with peak effects apparent within 2 to 4 hours. The serum half-life of the drug is approximately 12 hours. It is excreted by the kidneys as unchanged drug (43%) and as metabolites. Approximately 75% of an oral dose appears in the urine within a 24-hour period. Multiple-dose studies in adults at several dose levels indicate that serum levels stabilize in about 2 to 3 days. Clinical improvement appears to be gradual in children with minimal brain dysfunction. Employing the suggested schedule of dosage titration, significant benefit may not be evident until the third or fourth week of drug administration.

Indications: Treatment of minimal brain dysfunction as adjunctive therapy to other remedial measures (psychological, educational, social).

Contraindications: Known hypersensitivity or idiosyncrasy to the drug.

Warnings: Until further experience with regard to safe and effective use has been gained, it is not recommended for use in children under 6 years of age or for prolonged administration. Long-term use of stimulants has been reported to temporarily suppress the predicted growth pattern of children (i.e. weight and/or height); therefore, patients requiring prolonged treatment should be carefully monitored. Since pemoline is excreted chiefly by the kidneys, special care is required when administering the drug to children with impaired renal function. Due attention should be given to a potential interaction with other drugs especially those with CNS activity. It is generally recognized that during pregnancy, especially in the first trimester, all medications should be used with considerable caution. This recommendation also applies to lactating women until safe use has been assured. Excessive use of pemoline by unstable individuals may result in a psychological dependence; in these rare instances discontinuing the medication should be considered.

Precautions: In several patients, a delayed (several months) hypersensitivity reaction involving the liver has been recorded. This reaction is manifested by mild to moderate increases in transaminase (SGOT and SGPT) and in lactic dehydrogenase levels which appear to revert to pretreatment levels when therapy is discontinued. It is suggested that liver function be checked periodically when patients are receiving the drug in large doses or for prolonged periods. Another clinical finding was jaundice, but whether or not it was drug-induced has not been substantiated.

Adverse Reactions: The primary side effect attributable to pemoline was insomnia which, in the majority of cases, was transient in nature or responded to a reduction in dosage. Anorexia with weight loss occurred during the first few weeks of therapy; however, with continuing therapy, a return to normal weight usually occurred within 3 to 6 months. Other reported complaints were abdominal pain, skin rash, irritability, mild depression, nausea, dizziness, headache, drowsiness, hallucinations, dyskinetic movements of the lips, face, and extremities, and convulsions. Mild adverse effects appearing early in treatment often disappear with continuing use of the drug. Dosage reduction or drug withdrawal should be considered when reactions appear to be of a significant or protracted nature. Agitation, restlessness, hallucinations, and tachycardia generally indicate acute overdosage; treatment is essentially the same as that for an overdosage of any CNS stimulant. Management is primarily symptomatic and may include induction of emesis, or gastric lavage, sedation, and other appropriate supportive measures. Extracorporeal hemodialysis may be helpful, but forced diuresis or peritoneal dialysis appear to be of little value.

Dosage and Administration: *Orally* as a single dose each morning. The recommended initial dose is 37.5 mg; gradually increased using 18.75 mg at 1-week intervals until the desired clinical response is obtained. The mean daily effective dose ranges from 56.25 to 75 mg daily; the maximal recommended daily dose is 112.5 mg. Improvement is gradual and, while using the recommended schedule, significant benefit may not be evident until after 3 or 4 weeks of therapy. Drug administration should be interrupted occasionally to determine if behavioral symptoms sufficient to require continuing therapy recur.

Availability:
Ⓒ CYLERT®: **(Abbott)**
Chewable Tablets, 37.5 mg in bottles of 100.
Tablets, 18.75, 37.5 and 75 mg in bottles of 100.

PENICILLAMINE

Chemical Name: D-3-Mercaptovaline.

Description: Penicillamine is a thiol compound devoid of antibacterial activity. It occurs as a white or nearly white, crystalline powder that is soluble in water and in alcohol and insoluble in ether, acetone, benzene, and carbon tetrachloride. It chelates copper, iron, mercury, lead, and probably other heavy metals to form soluble complexes readily excreted by the kidneys. Copper is chelated by a combination of 2 molecules of penicillamine with 1 atom of the metal. In vitro, 1 gm of penicillamine combines with about 200 mg of copper; under in vivo conditions, this amount of penicillamine results in the excretion of about 2 mg of copper. The drug also combines with cystine to form a soluble disulfide complex that is readily excreted, and it disassociates some macroglobulins thus reducing the viscosity of plasma.

Indications: Treatment of Wilson's disease (hepatolenticular degeneration) and cystinuria.

Warnings: This drug should be used during pregnancy only when the considered benefits to the patient outweigh the possible risks to the fetus.

Precautions: The skin of the knees, elbows, shoulder blades and toes should be observed for extravasations of blood. Body temperature should be taken nightly for the first few months of therapy. Urinalyses, differential blood counts, direct platelet counts, and hemoglobin determinations should be performed every 3 days during the first month of therapy and every 10 days for 3 or 4 months thereafter. If a reaction occurs, penicillamine should be discontinued until the reaction subsides and then reinstituted at a lower dosage. Administration of an adrenocortical steroid may be helpful in patients who repeatedly develop a toxic reaction. The eyes, should be examined for cataracts before therapy is initiated, and at least twice yearly during therapy. Severe visual disturbances, probably due to drug-induced pyridoxine deficiency have been noted; therefore, supplemental administration of this vitamin is advisable. Since iron deficiency may develop in menstruating women and in children, the concomitant administration of an iron preparation without the sulfurated potash or resin is recommended. Patients with renal impairment should be under close observation and frequent liver and kidney function tests are advisable. Penicillamine is not recommended during pregnancy because of its affinity for metals.

Adverse Reactions: Penicillamine causes allergic reactions, the most common of which is a maculopapular or erythematous rash early in therapy, and occasionally accompanied by fever, arthralgia, or lymphadenopathy. Cross-sensitivity between penicillin and penicillamine may occur. Other adverse reactions that have been reported include the nephrotic syndrome, hepatic dysfunction, tinnitus, falling hair, urticaria, elevated sedimentation rate, eosinophilia, monocytosis, leukocytosis, thrombocytosis, thrombocytopenia, thrombotic thrombocytopenic purpura, bone marrow hyperplasia, leukopenia, agranulocytopenia with fatal outcome; nausea, vomiting, loss of appetite, and occasional diarrhea; rarely, thrombophlebitis, pancreatitis, cheilosis, glossitis, and gingivostomatitis, polymyositis, pemphigus, fever, mammary hyperplasia, peptic ulcer, myasthenia, elastosis perforans serpiginosa, elevated plasma levels of lactic dehydrogenase, hemolytic anemia and diffuse alveolitis. A disseminated lupus erythematosus-like syndrome has occurred. Impairment of taste (reversible) probably due to copper deficiency, and a syndrome closely resembling disseminated lupus erythematosus have been noted. Severe and ultimately fatal glomerulonephritis and intraalveolar hemorrhage (Goodpasture's syndrome) have occurred but are rare. Reversible optic neuritis, increased serum alkaline phosphatase and positive cephalin flocculation and thymol turbidity tests have been reported. Increased skin friability at sites especially subject to pressure or trauma with extravasations of blood may occur. These may be purpuric with external bleeding if the skin is broken or may appear as vesicles containing dark blood. Excessive wrinkling of the skin and the development of small, white papules at venipuncture and surgical sites probably result from drug-induced collagen defects. The chelating action of the drug may also cause increased excretion of other heavy metals such as zinc and mercury.

Dosage and Administration: *Orally. For Wilson's disease,* the initial dosage for adults and older children is 250 mg 4 times daily; subsequently based on the determination of the amount of copper in the urine, this may be increased to 4 to 5 gm daily in divided doses. For infants over 6 months of age and young children, 250 mg daily dissolved in fruit juice. Suggested doses are best taken on an empty stomach. *For cystinuria,* the dosage for adults and older children is 1 to 4 gm daily divided into 4 doses. Young children and infants, 30 mg/kg of body weight daily in 3 or 4 equally divided doses. If equal doses are not possible or if undue reactions necessitate a reduction in dosage, the largest amount should be given at bedtime with 2 glasses of water, and another 2 glasses during the night when the urine is more concentrated and more acidic than during the day. Effective therapy is indicated by the urinary excretion of 100 to 200 mg of cysteine a day in patients with no history of stone formation, and below 100 mg in those who have had stone formation and/or pain.

Availability:
CUPRIMINE® Capsules, 125 mg in bottles of 100; 250 mg in bottles of 50 and 100.

(Merck Sharp & Dohme)

THE PENICILLINS

Description: The penicillins are antibiotic substances derived from several species of *Penicillium;* and some are prepared by molecular manipulation of the basic penicillin nucleus, 6-aminopenicillanic acid. These antibiotics act by interfering with the synthesis and cross linkage of mucopeptides that are essential for the formation of the bacterial cell wall. Most are rapidly excreted in the urine, either unaltered or as metabolites, although some (ampicillin and nafcillin) appear in high concentrations in the bile and are reabsorbed from the intestine. Blood concentrations of the penicillins may be increased and prolonged by the use of probenecid, which reduces the rate of their renal tubular excretion.

Minimal effective concentrations in vitro vary considerably among species of bacteria and among the several penicillins. Some of the penicillins (amoxicillin, ampicillin, carbenicillin, hetacillin, penicillin G, penicillin V, phenethicillin and ticarcillin) are ineffective against penicillinase-secreting bacteria. Plasma protein binding, which may decrease the activity of these drugs, ranges from only 20% for ampicillin, amoxicillin and hetacillin, 40% for methicillin, 45% for ticarcillin, 50% for carbenicillin, 35 to 60% for penicillin G, 75 to 80% for phenoxymethyl penicillin and phenethicillin and 90% or more for cloxacillin, dicloxacillin, nafcillin and oxacillin. A loading dose of twice the normal average dose may be required for any penicillin with a protein binding capacity exceeding 70% so that a more prompt initial therapeutic blood level may be attained, especially in emergency situations. Drugs such as aspirin and phenylbutazone are capable of displacing penicillins from their plasma protein binding sites, thereby elevating the level of free penicillin in the serum. As with other antibacterial agents, it is not known whether a constant blood level of penicillin is more or less effective than a varying concentration.

The penicillins enter ascitic fluid and cross the placental barrier and are found in amniotic fluid, cord serum and human milk. Their diffusion into cerebrospinal fluid and brain is inadequate and occurs only with meningeal inflammation. However, they readily diffuse into most body tissues, including kidneys, liver, lungs, heart, spleen, skin, and intestines. The oral dose of penicillin G must be at least 5 times larger than the parenteral dose because of its susceptibility to hydrolysis by gastric acid, and it should be given when the stomach is empty to minimize gastric retention. For high but transient blood levels, penicillin G may be given intramuscularly or intravenously every 3 to 6 hours. When massive doses (e.g., 20 million units or more daily) are required, the drug must be given by intravenous infusion. For more sustained effects, a less soluble preparation (e.g., benzathine penicillin G or procaine penicillin G) is given intramuscularly at daily, weekly or monthly intervals depending upon the specific preparation; however, the low blood levels produced are effective only against very sensitive organisms.

Claims for the superiority of one penicillin over another on the basis of such characteristics as blood levels of effectiveness in vitro may be made invalid by the differences among the penicillins in their stability to acid, rates of absorption and excretion, minimal effective blood levels, and amount of protein binding.

Indications: Penicillin G remains the drug of choice for the treatment of infections caused by susceptible gram-positive cocci such as pneumococci, group A hemolytic streptococci, and sensitive staphylococci, except for patients who are allergic to the penicillins and when specific conditions make the use of one of the other penicillins preferable. Penicillin G is also preferred for infections caused by gonococci, clostridiae, *Bacillus anthracis, Corynebacterium diphtheriae,* and *Actinomyces* species. For infections caused by resistant penicillinase-producing staphylococci, a penicillinase-resistant penicillin such as oxacillin, cloxacillin, methicillin or nafcillin is indicated; they should not be used in infections caused by penicillin G-susceptible bacteria such as streptococci, except in mixed infections in which penicillinase-producing staphylococci also are present.

Ampicillin is the most effective penicillin in low concentrations against several gram-negative bacteria such as *E. coli, H. influenzae,* and species of *Proteus* and *Salmonella.* It is used orally for the treatment of less serious infections caused by these organisms, especially infections of the urinary and respiratory tracts.

Carbenicillin and ticarcillin are unique in their activity against Pseudomonas and some of the newly emerging pathogenic strains of such microorganisms as Herellea, Mima, Citrobacter and Serratia, which have shown susceptibility. Some strains of Pseudomonas have developed resistance fairly rapidly. However, in vitro synergism between carbenicillin or ticarcillin and gentamicin sulfate in certain strains of *Pseudomonas aeruginosa* has been demonstrated.

Reports indicate an increasing number of strains of staphylococci resistant to penicillin G, thus emphasizing the need for culture and sensitivity studies in treating suspected staphylococcal infections.

Penicillin is effective when given prophylactically to patients with rheumatic fever. It is also used in high dosage prior to tonsillectomy, tooth extraction, or other minor surgical procedures in patients with a history of rheumatic fever as well as rheumatic or congenital heart disease.

Oral penicillin is indicated in less serious infections, in those that have been brought under control by parenteral therapy, and for prolonged treatment; it should not be used initially for the treatment of meningitis, syphillis, or actinomycosis or as adjunctive prophylaxis for genitourinary instrumentation or surgery, lower intestinal tract surgery, sigmoidoscopy and childbirth. The penicillins may be used orally for the prophylaxis—but not the treatment—of streptococcal endocarditis. Parenteral therapy with the penicillins should be reserved for serious infections, and for patients who are not likely to follow instructions for oral therapy.

Contraindications: Penicillin is contraindicated in those patients who have shown hypersensitivity to penicillin or to the cephalosporins and other related allergens.

Warnings: Serious and occasionally fatal hypersensitivity (anaphylactoid) reactions have been reported in patients on penicillin therapy. Although anaphylaxis is more frequent following parenteral therapy, it has occurred in patients on oral therapy. These reactions are more likely to occur in individuals with a history of sensitivity to multiple allergens; therefore, a careful inquiry into the patient's clinical history should be made before initiating treatment with penicillin. If an allergic reaction occurs, the drug should be discontinued and the patient treated immediately with epinephrine. Oxygen, intravenous corticosteroids and airway management, including intubation should be administered as indicated. Mental disturbances including anxiety, confusion, agitation, depression, and hallucinations, generally lasting for

15 to 30 minutes, have been reported in individuals following single-dose schedules for gonorrhea. Safe use during pregnancy has not been established.

Precautions: It should be used with caution in patients having histories of allergies, asthma or both. Based on the results of skin-test studies, it is advisable to test patients for sensitivity before giving any penicillin, and it is essential to find out if the patient has a history of such sensitization. Additionally, an occasional individual may become sensitized to Procaine [Penicillin G Procaine] in which case the drug should be withdrawn and appropriate therapy instituted. Although the penicillins are relatively nonirritating to tissue, some produce pain on intramuscular injection, or local phlebitis on intravenous infusion. However, they are irritating to the CNS and should be injected intrathecally *only* when absolutely essential, and then only in small, well-diluted doses. In patients with inadequate renal function, there is danger that the intravenous administration of massive doses of penicillin G may cause hyperkalemia or convulsions due to irritation of the CNS; also those receiving high dosages of sodium penicillin G may experience congestive heart failure due to excessive sodium intake. Frequent evaluations of electrolyte balance, and of renal, cardiac and vascular status are recommended. Penicillin should not be administered orally to patients with severe illness, or with nausea, vomiting, gastric dilatation, cardiospasm, or intestinal hypermotility. Sensitivity of the organism to a particular penicillin should be determined by in vitro tests; resistance, especially by staphylococci, can develop during treatment. In streptococcal infections, therapy must be sufficient to eliminate the organism; otherwise, the sequelae of streptococcal disease may occur. Cultures should be taken following completion of treatment to determine whether or not the streptococci have been eradicated. As with other antibiotics, serious superinfections with resistant organisms, especially gram-negative bacteria such as *Pseudomonas species,* may occur. As with any potent drug, prolonged use should be accompanied by periodic assessment of hepatic, and hematopoietic functions as well as those of other organ systems. The possibility of mycotic or bacterial superinfection should be considered during therapy. If they occur, therapy with the drug should be discontinued and appropriate measures instituted.

Adverse Reactions: The most serious and common untoward effects produced by penicillin are allergic reactions. These reactions are more likely to occur in individuals with a history of allergy, asthma, hay fever, or urticaria. Numerous deaths have occurred from anaphylaxis after the injection of penicillin, some following its oral administration. The most common reactions to oral penicillin are glossitis, stomatitis, enterocolitis, pseudomembranous colitis, nausea, vomiting, epigastric distress, diarrhea, and black hairy tongue. Other allergic reactions include skin eruptions (maculopapular to exfoliative dermatitis), urticaria, reactions resembling serum-sickness, and laryngeal edema. Although fever and eosinophilia may frequently be the only reactions observed. Chills, edema, arthralgia, and prostration may also occur. Hemolytic anemia, thrombocytopenia, thrombocytopenic purpura, leukopenia, and agranulocytosis, neuropathy, and nephropathy are infrequent reactions, and are usually associated with high doses of parenteral penicillin. A moderate rise in serum glutamic oxaloacetic transaminase (SGOT) has also been noted. Other types of toxic reactions to the penicillins have been rare; however, methicillin has been associated with depression of the red bone marrow, as well as nephritis, in some patients.

The preceding discussed briefly the physiologic, clinical and therapeutic similarities of the penicillins as a group. In the discussions that follow, the individual monographs discuss specifically each of the following:

- Amoxicillin
- Ampicillin
- Carbenicillin
- Carbenicillin Indanyl Sodium
- Cloxacillin
- Dicloxacillin
- Hetacillin
- Methicillin
- Nafcillin
- Oxacillin
- Penicillin G
- Penicillin G, Benzathine
- Penicillin G, Procaine
- Phenoxymethyl Penicillin
- Ticarcillin

AMOXICILLIN

Chemical Name: D-(-)-alpha-amino-p-hydroxybenzyl penicillin trihydrate.

Description: Amoxicillin is a semisynthetic, acid-stable penicillin that is similar in bactericidal activity to ampicillin. It acts by interfering with the synthesis and cross-linkage of mucopeptides essential for the formation and integrity of the bacterial cell wall. Because it is not susceptible to destruction by gastric acid, it can be given without regard to meals. Plasma protein binding for amoxicillin, as well as for ampicillin, is 20% compared to 35 to 60% for penicillin G. Its serum half-life is 61.3 minutes.

The drug is well absorbed from the gastrointestinal tract, and diffuses readily into most body tissues and fluids; however, penetration into the cerebrospinal fluid and brain occurs only with meningeal inflammation. Most of the drug is excreted unchanged in the urine; its excretion can be delayed by the concurrent administration of probenecid. Probenecid inhibits the renal tubular secretion of penicillin thus increasing and prolonging the plasma concentration of the antibiotic.

Following a single 500-mg dose, approximate peak serum levels averaging 7.5 mcg/ml are generally attained in 1 hour and measurable serum levels are present for 8 hours or more. Amoxicillin is inactivated by penicillinase-producing organisms, particularly staphylococci. All strains of pseudomonas and most strains of Klebsiella and Enterobacter are also resistant to this antibiotic.

Indications: Treatment of susceptible strains of gram-negative organisms such as *H. influenzae, E. coli, P. mirabilis* and *N. gonorrhoeae* and gram-positive organisms such as streptococci (including *Streptococcus faecalis*), *D. pneumoniae* and nonpenicillinase-producing staphylococci.

For contraindications, warnings, precautions and adverse reactions, see general statement.

Dosage and Administration: *Orally.* For adults and children weighing 20 kg or more, 250 to 500 mg every 8 hours. For children, 20 to 40 mg/kg daily in divided doses every 8 hours. For infections due to *N. gonorrhoeae,* 3 gm as a single oral dose. *Pediatric drops:* children under 6 kg (13 lbs.) 0.5 to 1 ml; 6 to 8 kg (13 to 18 lbs), 1 to 2 ml. Dosage is repeated every 8 hours. Except for gonorrhea, treatment should be continued for a minimum of 48 to 72 hours beyond the time that the patient becomes asymptomatic or evidence of bacterial eradication has been obtained. It is recommended that there be at least 10 days' treatment for any infection caused by hemolytic streptococci in order to prevent the occurrence of acute rheumatic fever or glomerulonephritis.

Availability:

AMOXIL®: **(Beecham)**

Capsules, 250 mg in bottles of 15, 100 and 500 and in unit-dose cartons of 100; 500 mg in bottles of 15, 50 and 500 and in unit-dose cartons of 100.

Oral Suspension, 125 and 250 mg/5 ml in bottles of 80, 100 and 150 ml.

Pediatric Drops, 50 mg/ml in bottles of 15 ml with dropper.

LAROTID®: **(Roche)**

Capsules, 250 mg in bottles of 100 and 500; 500 mg in bottles of 50 and 500. Both strengths are also available in Tel-E-Dose® packages of 100 and in Prescription Paks of 18, either singly or in trays of 10.

Oral Suspension, 125 and 250 mg/5 ml in bottles of 80, 100 and 150 ml and in Tel-E-Dose (unit-dose) bottles of 5 ml.

Pediatric Drops, 50 mg/ml in bottles of 15 ml with dropper.

POLYMOX®: **(Bristol)**

Capsules, 250 mg in bottles of 100 and 500 and in Dosa-Trol® (unit-dose) cartons of 100; 500 mg in bottles of 50 and 100 and in Dosa-Trol cartons of 100.

Oral Suspension, 125 and 250 mg/5 ml in bottles of 80, 100 and 150 ml and in Dosa-Trol (unit-dose) bottles of 5 ml.

Pediatric Drops, 50 mg/ml in bottles of 15 ml with dropper.

ROBAMOX®: **(Robins)**

Powder for Oral Suspension, 125 and 250 mg/5 ml in bottles of 80 and 150 ml.

Robicaps® (Capsules), 250 mg in bottles of 100; 500 mg in bottles of 50.

TRIMOX®: **(Squibb)**

Capsules, 250 mg in bottles of 100 and 500; 500 mg in bottles of 50 and 500.

Powder for Oral Suspension, 125 and 250 mg/5 ml in bottles of 80, 100 and 150 ml and in Unimatic® (unit-dose) bottles of 5 ml in cartons of 100.

UTIMOX®: **(Parke-Davis)**

Capsules, 250 mg in bottles of 100 and 500 and in unit-dose cartons of 100; 500 mg in bottles of 100 and in unit-dose cartons of 100.
Powder for Oral Suspension, 125 and 250 mg/5 ml in bottles of 80, 100 and 150 ml.
WYMOX™: **(Wyeth)**
Capsules, 250 mg in bottles of 100; 500 mg in bottles of 50.
Powder for Oral Suspension, 125 and 250 mg/5 ml in bottles of 80, 100 and 150 ml.

AMPICILLIN

Description: Ampicillin is a semisynthetic penicillin produced by acylation of 6-aminopenicillanic acid with D-(-)-aα-aminophenylacetic acid. It is available as the trihydrate, a colorless or slightly buff-color crystalline solid soluble in water and as anhydrous ampicillin, a white, crystalline powder sparingly soluble in water. The sodium salt occurs as a white, crystalline powder soluble in water; after reconstitution for parenteral administration, solutions should be used within 1 hour.

The drug diffuses readily into most body tissues and fluids; however, penetration into cerebrospinal fluid occurs only with meningeal inflammation. Ampicillin is the least serum bound of all the penicillins, averaging 20% compared to 40 to 90% for the other penicillins.

Ampicillin is destroyed by penicillinase and is therefore inactivated by strains of penicillinase-producing staphylococci and gram-negative bacilli. Following oral administration, ampicillin is well-absorbed, more slowly than are other penicillins, reaching peak serum levels within 1 or 2 hours and decreasing slowly for about 8 hours. Following intramuscular injection, peak serum levels are generally attained more quickly and tend to be higher than those resulting from equal doses given orally; significant activity is present in serum 4 hours or more after intramuscular injection. Probenecid inhibits the renal tubular secretion of ampicillin thus producing an increased serum level of the antibiotic.

Indications: Treatment of infections due to susceptible strains of gram-negative bacteria (including *Shigellae, S. typhosa* and other salmonellae, *E. coli, H. influenzae, P. mirabilis, N. meningitidis* and *N. gonorrhoeae).* Other indications include infections due to such susceptible gram-positive organisms as pneumococci, and nonpenicillinase-producing staphylococci, alpha and beta hemolytic streptococci; and in infections of the urinary, respiratory and gastrointestinal tracts. However, clinical experience indicates that an increasing number of ampicillin-resistant Haemophilus, Shigella and Salmonella species are emerging. The drug is not recommended for the treatment of infections due to organisms susceptible to penicillin G. Formulated with probenecid for the treatment of uncomplicated gonorrhea (urethral, cervical, pharyngeal or rectal) due to *N. gonorrhoeae.*

Contraindications: In patients with a history of allergic reactions to penicillins or cephalosporins; and in infections caused by penicillinase-producing staphylococci or other penicillinase-producing agents. Probenecid is not recommended for patients with known blood dyscrasias, uric acid-kidney stones, or for those experiencing an acute attack of gout.

Warnings: See general statement; also the monograph on Probenecid.

Precautions: In the event of an allergic reaction, the drug should be discontinued and the patient treated with the usual agents: antihistamines, pressor amines, corticosteroids. The renal, hepatic and hematopoietic systems should be evaluated periodically when therapy is prolonged. Since experience is limited, the drug should be used with caution in premature and newborn infants. In the treatment of complications of gonorrheal urethritis, such as prostatitis and epididymitis, prolonged and intensive therapy is recommended. Cases of gonorrhea with a suspected primary lesion of syphilis should have darkfield examinations for *Treponema pallidum* before receiving treatment. In all other cases where concomitant syphilis is suspected, serologic studies should be done monthly for at least 4 months. Safe use during pregnancy has not been established. For other precautions, see general statement; also the monograph on Probenecid.

Adverse Reactions: Ampicillin is generally well tolerated. Complications that do occur are usually mild and consist most often of skin rashes (not related to a true penicillin allergy) and diarrhea. A few instances of moderate elevation of serum glutamic oxaloacetic transaminase

(SGOT) have been observed. Mild, transitory elevations of SGOT have been seen in individuals receiving larger doses (2 to 4 times) than usual and frequently repeated intramuscular injections. These observations do not necessarily mean that the liver is involved. For other possible adverse reactions, see general statement, also the monograph on Probenecid.

Dosage and Administration: *Orally:* Adults, 250 to 500 mg or more 4 times daily depending upon the condition being treated and its severity. Children, 50 to 100 mg/kg of body weight in equally divided doses at intervals of 6 to 8 hours. *Intramuscularly* or *intravenously:* Adults, 250 to 500 mg every 6 hours. Children, 50 mg/kg in divided doses every 6 to 8 hours. *Bacterial meningitis due to sensitive organisms:* adults and children 150 to 200 mg/kg/day in divided doses every 3 to 4 hours. Ampicillin and probenecid: For acute gonorrheal infections in adult males and females, 1 bottle contains the required amount of each drug for the single-dose treatment, and is taken at the direction of the physician. It is advised that cultures be obtained from the original site(s) of infection 7 to 14 days following the initial treatment. Package literature should be consulted for details.

Availability:

AMCILL®: **(Parke-Davis)**

Capsules (as trihydrate), 250 and 500 mg in bottles of 24, 100 and 500 and in unit-dose packages of 100.

Chewable Tablets (as trihydrate), 125 mg in bottles of 40.

Oral Suspension (as trihydrate), 125 and 250 mg/5 ml in bottles of 80, 100, 150 and 200 ml and in unit-dose packages of 5 and 10 ml.

Pediatric Drops (as trihydrate), 100 mg/ml in bottles of 20 ml with dropper.

AMCILL-S® for Injection (sodium ampicillin) in Steri-Vials® of 125, 250, 500 mg and 1 gm.

AMPICILLIN TRIHYDRATE: **(Lederle)**

Capsules (as trihydrate), 250 and 500 mg in bottles of 100 and 500.

Powder for Oral Solution (as trihydrate), 125 and 250 mg/5 ml in bottles of 100 and 200 ml.

AMPICILLIN TRIHYDRATE: **(McKesson)**

Capsules, 250 mg in bottles of 100 and 1000; 500 mg in bottles of 100 and 500.

Powder for Oral Suspension, 125 and 250 mg/5 ml in bottles of 100 and 200 ml.

OMNIPEN®: **(Wyeth)**

Capsules, 250 and 500 mg in bottles of 100 and 500 and in Redipak® (strip-pack) cartons of 100.

Pediatric Drops for Oral Solution, 100 mg/ml in bottles of 20 ml with dropper.

Powder for Oral Suspension, 125 and 250 mg/5 ml in bottles of 80, 100, 150 and 200 ml; 500 mg/5 ml in bottles of 100 ml. The 250 mg/5 ml is also available in Redipak® (individually wrapped pouches) in cartons of 20.

OMNIPEN®-N Injection in vials of 125, 250, 500 mg and 1, 2 and 10 gm; 500 mg in piggyback vials of 10.

PEN A®: **(Pfipharmecs)**

Capsules (as trihydrate), 250 mg in bottles of 100 and 500 and in unit-dose cartons of 100; 500 mg in bottles of 100 and in unit-dose cartons of 100.

Powder for Oral Suspension (as trihydrate), 125 and 250 mg/5 ml in bottles of 100 and 200 ml.

PEN A/N for Injection (sodium ampicillin) in vials of 250 and 500 mg and 1 gm. **(Pfizer)**

PENBRITIN®: **(Ayerst)**

Capsules, 250 mg in bottles of 100 and 500 and in unit-doses of 100; 500 mg in bottles of 50 and 500 and in unit-doses of 100.

Oral Suspension, 125 and 250 mg/5 ml in bottles of 100 and 200 ml.

Pediatric Drops, 100 mg/ml in bottles of 20 ml.

PENBRITIN®-S for Injection in vials of 125, 250, 500 mg and 1, 2 and 4 gm.

PENSYN®: **(Upjohn)**

Capsules (as trihydrate), 250 mg in bottles of 100 and 500; 500 mg in bottles of 100.

Powder for Oral Suspension (as trihydrate), 125 and 250 mg/5 ml in bottles of 80, 100, 150 and 200 ml.

POLYCILLIN®: **(Bristol)**

Capsules, 250 mg in bottles of 24, 100, 500 and 1000 and in Dosa-Trol® packs of 100; 500 mg in bottles of 16, 100 and 500 and in Dosa-Trol packs of 100.

Pediatric Drops, 100 mg/ml in bottles of 20 ml.

Powder for Oral Suspension, 125 mg/5 ml in bottles of 60, 80, 100, 150 and 200 ml and in

Dosa-Trol bottles of 5 ml; 250 mg/5 ml in bottles of 80, 100, 150 and 200 ml and in Dosa-Trol bottles of 5 ml; 500 mg/5 ml in bottles of 100 ml and in Dosa-Trol bottles of 5 ml.
POLYCILLIN®-N Injection (IM or IV) in vials of 125, 250 and 500 mg; in vials of 1, 2 and 2.5 gm and in piggyback vials of 500 mg and 1 and 2 gm.
PRINCIPEN®: **(Squibb)**
Capsules, 250 mg in bottles of 50, 100 and 500 and in Unimatic® cartons of 100 and 500; 500 mg in bottles of 16, 100 and 500 and in Unimatic cartons of 100 and 500.
Powder for Oral Suspension, 125 and 250 mg/5 ml in bottles of 80, 100, 150 and 200 ml and in Unimatic cartons of 100 unit-dose bottles of 5 ml.
PRINCIPEN-N Injection in vials of 125, 250, 500 mg and 1 and 2 gm.
SK-AMPICILLIN™: **(Smith Kline & French)**
Capsules, 250 and 500 mg in bottles of 24, 100 and 500.
Chewable Tablets, 125 mg in bottles of 40.
Pediatric Drops, 100 mg/ml in bottles of 20 ml.
Powder for Oral Suspension, 125 and 250 mg/5 ml in bottles of 100, 150 and 200 ml.
SK-AMPICILLIN-N™ Injection in vials of 500 mg.
TOTACILLIN®: **(Beecham)**
Capsules (as trihydrate), 250 mg in bottles of 100 and 500; 500 mg in bottles of 50 and 500. Both potencies are available in Dispensing packages of 20 and 40.
Oral Suspension (as trihydrate), 125 and 250 mg/5 ml in bottles of 80, 100, 150 and 200 ml.
TOTACILLIN-N Injectable (sodium ampicillin) in vials of 125, 250 and 500 mg and 1, 2 and 10 gm and in Piggyback units of 1 and 2 gm.

w/Probenecid

POLYCILLIN®-PRB Dry Powder, 0.5 and 3.5 gm (as trihydrate) with 1 gm of probenecid in single-dose bottles. **(Bristol)**
PRINCIPEN® with PROBENECID in single-dose packages containing 7 Principen capsules, 389 mg each and 2 probenecid tablets, 111 mg each. **(Squibb)**

CARBENICILLIN

Description: Carbenicillin is a benzylpenicillin derivative prepared synthetically by adding a carboxyl group to the basic penicillin nucleus, 6-aminopenicillanic acid. The disodium salt, available for parenteral use, occurs as an off-white, lyophilized powder freely soluble in water, and is compatible with most intravenous fluids. Each gram provides approximately 5.5 mEq Na^+.

Carbenicillin is acid-labile and is not effective when taken orally and must therefore be administered intramuscularly or intravenously. Following administration of 1 gm, serum levels reach a peak in 1 hour after intramuscular injection, in 15 minutes after intravenous injection, and persist in diminishing concentrations for 4 to 8 hours depending upon the route used. The plasma half-life in individuals with normal renal function is approximately 1 hour. Blood concentrations may be only slightly increased and prolonged by the concomitant administration of probenecid. Most of the drug (about 75%) is excreted unchanged in the urine.

Carbenicillin has demonstrated in vitro activity against a variety of susceptible gram-positive and gram-negative pathogens including *Pseudomonas aeruginosa* and *Proteus.* It is susceptible to inactivation by penicillinase-producing staphylococci.

Indications: Primarily for the treatment of the following infections due to susceptible *Ps. aeruginosa, Proteus* species (particularly indole-positive strains) and certain strains of *E. coli:* urinary tract, soft tissue, severe systemic infections and septicemia, and acute and chronic respiratory infections. Although improvement has been noted clinically, sterile microbial cultures cannot be expected in patients with chronic respiratory disease and cystic fibrosis. That the drug is also effective against gram-positive organisms should be kept in mind when mixed infections are present.

Contraindications: Known hypersensitivity to penicillins.

Warnings: Safe use during pregnancy has not been established. Before beginning therapy with a penicillin, careful inquiry should be made concerning previous hypersensitivity to penicillins, cephalosporins and other allergens. If an allergic reaction does occur, carbenicillin should be discontinued and antihistamines, pressor amines and corticosteroids should be readily available.

Precautions: The emergence of resistant organisms should be kept in mind. Special dosage recommendations should be strictly followed for patients with impaired renal function (creatinine clearance less than 30 ml/minute); if bleeding is evident, the antibiotic should be discontinued and appropriate measures instituted.

For other information, including additional warnings and precautions, see general statement.

Adverse Reactions: The following may occur: skin rash, pruritus, urticaria, drug fever, anaphylactic reactions, nausea, anemia, thrombocytopenia, leukopenia, neutropenia, eosinophilia, elevated SGOT and SGPT (particularly in children), convulsions or neuromuscular irritability (with excessively high doses), and pain at the injection site. Several uremic patients receiving as much as 24 gm of carbenicillin daily have developed hemorrhagic manifestations associated with abnormal clotting and prothrombin times. Bleeding stopped when the drug was withdrawn. Vein irritation and phlebitis have been reported on occasion, particularly when undiluted solution was injected directly into a vein.

Dosage and Administration: *Intramuscularly* or *intravenously.* For uncomplicated urinary tract infections: the usual adult dosage is 1 to 2 gm every 6 hours; children, 50 to 200 mg/kg of body weight daily in divided doses every 4 to 6 hours. For serious urinary tract infections: the usual adult dosage is 200 mg/kg of body weight daily given by intravenous drip; children, 50 to 200 mg/kg of body weight daily in divided doses every 4 to 6 hours. For septicemia and severe systemic, respiratory, or soft tissue infections: the usual adult dosage is 300 to 500 mg/kg of body weight daily (20 to 40 gm); children, 400 to 500 mg/kg daily administered intravenously in divided doses or by continuous drip. For infants, initially 100 mg/kg of body weight, followed by 75 mg/kg every 6 to 8 hours for 3 to 7 days, depending upon the weight of the infant, then 100 mg/kg every 6 hours, administered either intramuscularly or by intravenous infusion (15 min.). For infections complicated by renal insufficiency (creatinine clearance less than 5 ml/minute) adults, 2 gm every 8 hours; during peritoneal dialysis, 2 gm every 6 hours; during hemodialysis, 2 gm every 4 hours administered intravenously. Children, clinical data are insufficient to recommend an adequate dose. Package literature should be consulted for dosage details and for methods of preparing solutions.

Availability:
GEOPEN® Injection (IV/IM) in vials of 1, 2 and 5 gm and in piggyback vials of 2, 5 and 10 gm. **(Roerig)**

PYOPEN® in vials of 1, 2, 5 and 20 gm and in piggyback vials of 2, 5, 10 and 20 gm. **(Beecham)**

CARBENICILLIN INDANYL SODIUM

Description: Carbenicillin indanyl sodium is the sodium salt of the indanyl ester. It is an acid stable compound suitable for oral administration. The antibacterial activity is due to its rapid conversion to carbenicillin by hydrolysis. Although this antibiotic provides substantial in vitro activity against a variety of both gram-positive and gram-negative organisms, the most important aspect of its profile is in its antipseudomonal and antiproteus activity. Because of the high urine levels obtained following oral administration, the drug has demonstrated significant effectiveness in urinary tract infection due to susceptible strains of *E. coli, Pr. mirabilis* and *Pseudomonas.* In addition, in vitro data, not substantiated by clinical studies, suggest that the following pathogens are usually susceptible: *Pr. morganii, Pr. rettgeri, Pr. vulgaris, Aerobacter, Enterococci, Staphylococcus* (nonpenicillinase producing) and *Streptococci.* Most strains of *Klebsiella* species are often resistant to this antibiotic, and some strains of *Pseudomonas* have developed resistance to carbenicillin.

Indications: Treatment of acute and chronic infections of the upper and lower urinary tract and in asymptomatic bacteriuria due to susceptible strains of *Escherichia coli, Pr. mirabilis* and *Pseudomonas.* **Note:** Susceptibility testing should be performed prior to and during the course of treatment to detect the possible development of resistant organisms.

Warnings: Safe use in pregnant patients or in children has not been established.

Precautions: Periodic assessment of renal, hepatic and hematopoietic systems is recommended during therapy. Since carbenicillin is excreted by the kidneys, patients with severe renal impairment (creatinine levels below 10 ml/minute) will not achieve therapeutic urine levels of carbenicillin.

For other information, including contraindications, warnings, precautions, see general statement.

Adverse Reactions: The following may occur: nausea, vomiting, and diarrhea; skin rashes, urticaria, or pruritus; anemia, thrombocytopenia, leukopenia, neutropenia, and eosinophilia; mild SGOT elevations; flatulence, dry mouth, furry tongue, vaginitis, and abdominal cramps.

Dosage and Administration: *Orally.* The usual adult dosage is 1 to 2 tablets 4 times daily.

Availability:
GEOCILLIN® Tablets, 382 mg (equiv.) in bottles of 100. **(Roerig)**

CLOXACILLIN

Chemical Name: 6-[3-(*o*-Chlorophenyl)-5-methyl-4-isoxazolecarboxamido]-3,3-dimethyl-7-oxo-4-thia-1-azabicyclo[3,2,0]-heptane acid sodium salt.

Description: Sodium cloxacillin is the monohydrated sodium salt of a semisynthetic penicillin prepared by acylation of 6-aminopenicillanic acid. It occurs as a white, crystalline powder with a slight odor, very soluble in water.

Sodium cloxacillin is resistant to inactivation by penicillinase; it differs from methicillin in that it is slightly less resistant to staphylococcal penicillinase but is slightly more resistant to *B. cereus* penicillinase than the latter drug.

Peak plasma levels of sodium cloxacillin occur about 1 hour following oral administration. Although renal and biliary excretion is fairly rapid, effective plasma levels can be maintained for 4 to 6 hours after the drug is administered. The half-life of cloxacillin has been reported to be between 30 and 60 minutes.

Indications: Treatment of only those infections known to be due to penicillinase-producing staphylococci that are sensitive to the drug such as pneumococci, group A beta-hemolytic streptococci, and staphylococci resistant and sensitive to penicillin G. It may be used as initial therapy for any suspected staphylococcal infection until definitive cultures and sensitivity results are known. However, in serious, life-threatening infections, oral preparations of the penicillins should not be relied on for initial therapy.

Contraindications: Hypersensitivity to penicillins or cephalosporins.

Precautions: Should an allergic reaction occur, the drug should be discontinued and the patient treated with the usual agents: antihistamines, pressor amines and corticosteroids. Periodic assessment of the organ system function, including renal, hepatic and hematopoietic systems, should be made during prolonged therapy. For other precautions, see general statement.

Adverse Reactions: Gastrointestinal disturbances (nausea, epigastric discomfort, flatulence, and loose stools), elevated SGOT levels, wheezing and sneezing. For other adverse reactions, see general statement.

Dosage and Administration: *Orally.* Adults, 250 mg every 6 hours for mild-to-moderate infections, and 500 mg or more every 6 hours for more serious infections. Children, 50 mg/kg of body weight daily in divided doses at intervals of 6 hours. Larger doses may be required for severe infections. Children weighing more than 20 kg should receive the adult dosage schedule. The drug should be given 1 or 2 hours before meals. **Note:** Group A beta-hemolytic streptococcal infections should be treated for at least 10 days to help prevent the occurrence of acute rheumatic fever or acute glomerulonephritis.

Availability:
CLOXAPEN Capsules, 250 and 500 mg in bottles of 100. **(Beecham)**
TEGOPEN®: **(Bristol)**
Capsules, 250 and 500 mg in bottles of 100.
Granules for Oral Solution, 125 mg/5 ml in bottles of 100 and 200 ml.

DICLOXACILLIN

Description: Sodium dicloxacillin is the monohydrated sodium salt of a semisynthetic penicillin prepared by acylation of 6-aminopenicillanic acid with 3-(2,6-dichlorophenyl)-5-methyl-4-isoxazolyl carboxylic acid, and occurs as a white to nearly white powder freely soluble in water. The drug is relatively stable in acid media; the extent of inactivation by gastric acidity lies between that of penicillin G and phenoxymethyl penicillin.

Dicloxacillin is resistant to destruction by penicillinase. It is well-absorbed from the gastrointestinal tract; peak serum levels in fasting subjects usually are reached within 1 to 2 hours after an oral dose. Serum levels are somewhat more prolonged than those achieved with cloxacillin or oxacillin; average blood levels following oral or intramuscular administration are similar, although they may vary more from one patient to another with oral doses than with parenteral doses. Diffusion into the cerebrospinal fluid is poor unless the meninges are inflamed.

Indications: Treatment of infections known to be due to penicillinase-producing staphylococci sensitive to the drug. It may be used as initial therapy for any suspected staphylococcal infection until definitive cultures and sensitivity are known. However, the drug should not be relied upon for initial therapy in serious, life-threatening infections. Dicloxacillin is effective in the treatment of infections caused by pneumococci, group A beta-hemolytic streptococci, as well as staphylococci that are resistant or sensitive to penicillin G. Because of poor penetration into the cerebrospinal fluid, dicloxacillin is not indicated in the treatment of meningitis.

Contraindications: In patients with a history of allergic reactions to penicillins or cephalosporins.

Precautions: In the event of an allergic reaction, the drug should be discontinued and the patient treated with the usual agents: antihistamines, pressor amines, and corticosteroids. The renal, hepatic and hematopoietic systems should be evaluated periodically when therapy is prolonged. Since experience is limited, a dosage regimen for newborn infants has not been established. For other precautions, see general statement.

Adverse Reactions: Mildly elevated SGOT levels, minor changes in the results of cephalin flocculation tests without other evidence of hepatic dysfunction, and eosinophilia with or without overt allergic manifestations. For other adverse reactions, see general statement.

Dosage and Administration: *Orally* or *intramuscularly.* For mild to moderate upper respiratory and localized skin and soft tissue infections due to sensitive organisms: adults and children weighing 40 kg or more, 125 mg every 6 hours; children weighing less than 40 kg, 12.5 mg/kg/day in divided doses every 6 hours. For more severe infections such as those of the lower respiratory tract or disseminated infections: above dosages should be doubled. **Note:** Infections caused by group A beta-hemolytic streptococci should be treated for at least 10 days to help prevent the occurrence of acute rheumatic fever or acute glomerulonephritis.

Availability:
DYCILL® Capsules, 250 and 500 mg in bottles of 100. **(Beecham)**
DYNAPEN®: **(Bristol)**
Capsules, 125 and 250 mg in bottles of 24 and 100 and in Dosa-Trol® (unit-dose) bottles in packages of 100.
Powder for Oral Suspension, 62.5 mg/5 ml in bottles of 80 and 100 ml.
PATHOCIL®: **(Wyeth)**
Capsules, 250 mg in bottles of 25 and 100.
Powder for Oral Suspension, 62.5 mg/5 ml in bottles of 80 ml.
VERACILLIN® Capsules, 250 mg in bottles of 100; 500 mg in bottles of 50. **(Ayerst)**

HETACILLIN

Description: Hetacillin is a semisynthetic antibiotic derived from the penicillin nucleus 6-aminopenicillanic acid. Its antibiotic activity results from the rapid conversion of the hetacillin moiety to ampicillin. Oral preparations of hetacillin are acid stable and apparently well-absorbed, but food appears to retard the absorption. In the conversion of hetacillin to ampicillin at a pH of 7.1, the half-life of hetacillin is 20 minutes. Oral formulations of hetacillin and potassium hetacillin equivalent to 225 and 450 mg of ampicillin activity provide peak blood levels of 1.7 to 2.1 mcg/ml and 2.5 to 2.7 mcg/ml, respectively.

Hetacillin itself has not shown antibacterial action but upon conversion to ampicillin its bactericidal action is similar to that of benzyl penicillin. It appears to act by inhibiting biosynthesis of cell-wall mucopeptides. Ampicillin Susceptibility Test Disk, 10 mcg, should be used to estimate the in vitro susceptibility of bacteria to hetacillin.

For Indications, Contraindications, Warnings, Precautions and Adverse Reactions see monograph on Ampicillin.

Dosage and Administration: *Orally* in a fasting state. For mild-to-moderate infections, 225 mg and severe infections, 450 mg 4 times daily for patients weighing 90 lbs (40 kg) or more, and 2.5 or 5 mg/lb 4 times daily for patients weighing less than 90 lbs (40 kg). Treatment should be continued for 48 to 72 hours beyond the time the patient becomes asymptomatic or evidence of bacterial eradication has been obtained. Infections due to group A beta-hemolytic streptococci should be treated for a minimum of 10 days to help prevent the development of acute rheumatic fever or acute glomerulonephritis. Chronic urinary and gastrointestinal tract infections may require prolonged and intensive therapy at doses in excess of those recommended above. It may be necessary to maintain therapy for several weeks and to continue bacteriologic or clinical follow-up or both for several months after cessation of therapy.

Availability:
VERSAPEN®: **(Bristol)**
Pediatric Drops, 112.5 mg/ml (ampicillin activity) in bottles of 15 ml.
Powder for Oral Suspension, 112.5 and 225 mg/5 ml (ampicillin activity) in bottles of 100 and 200 ml.
VERSAPEN-K (potassium salt): **(Bristol)**
Capsules, 225 and 450 mg (ampicillin activity) in bottles of 100.

METHICILLIN

Description: Sodium methicillin is the monohydrate of the sodium salt of a penicillin produced synthetically by linking 6-aminopenicillanic acid with 2,6-dimethoxybenzoic acid. It occurs as a white or cream-color, crystalline powder freely soluble in water. Each gm of the commercial product is equivalent to 900 mg of sodium methicillin activity and is buffered with 50 mg of sodium citrate. Because it is not acid-resistant, it must be given parenterally.

Sodium methicillin resists inactivation by staphylococcal penicillinase and also resists degradation by *B. cereus* penicillinase. In comparable concentrations, methicillin is less effective than penicillin G against other gram-positive cocci, both in vitro and in vivo.

Following intramuscular injection, the drug is rapidly absorbed; peak blood concentrations are attained within 1 hour and therapeutic concentrations last from 4 to 6 hours. Approximately 40% of the drug is protein bound. Methicillin is rapidly excreted, chiefly intact, in the urine and bile and requires frequent injections to maintain adequate blood levels. It is well distributed in various body fluids and tissues, but penetration into the cerebrospinal fluid is not readily accomplished unless the tissues are inflamed.

Indications: Treatment of infections due to penicillinase-producing staphylococci sensitive to the drug. It may be used as initial therapy for any suspected staphylococcal infection until definitive culture and sensitivity results are known. Methicillin is effective only in the treatment of infections caused by pneumococci, group A beta-hemolytic streptococci and staphylococci that are both resistant and sensitive to penicillin G. The drug is not recommended for the treatment of infections due to organisms sensitive to penicillin G, penicillin V or phenethicillin. The number of strains of staphylococci resistent to methicillin has been reported to be increasing.

Contraindications: Hypersensitivity to penicillins or cephalosporins.

Precautions: In the event of an allergic reaction, the drug should be discontinued and the patient treated with the usual agents: antihistamines, pressor amines, and corticosteroids. The renal, hepatic and hematopoietic systems should be evaluated periodically when therapy is prolonged. For other precautions, see general statement.

Adverse Reactions: Abnormal renal function including hematuria, casts and azotemia (nephritis), and neutropenia with evidence of bone marrow depression. For other possible adverse reactions, see general statement.

Dosage and Administration: *Intramuscularly.* Adults, 1 gm every 4 or 6 hours. Infants and children, 25 mg/kg of body weight every 6 hours. *Intravenously.* Adults, 1 gm every 6 hours using 50 ml of isotonic solution at the rate of 10 ml/minute. Infants and children, specific dosage recommendations have not been established. Therapy should be continued for 48 hours after the patient has become afebrile. **Note:** Higher doses should be administered in very severe infections and therapy should be continued for at least 1 to 2 weeks after the patient has become asymptomatic and cultures are sterile. Treatment of osteomyelitis may require several months of intensive therapy.

Availability:
AZAPEN® Injection (buffered) in vials of 1, 4 and 6 gm. **(Pfizer)**
CELBENIN® Injection (buffered) in vials of 1, 4, 6 and 10 gm and in piggyback vials of 1, 2 and 6 gm. **(Beecham)**
STAPHCILLIN® Injection (buffered) in dry-filled vials of 1, 4 and 6 gm and in piggyback vials of 1 and 4 gm. **(Bristol)**

NAFCILLIN

Description: Sodium nafcillin is the sodium salt of a semisynthetic penicillin produced by linking 6-aminopenicillanic acid with 2-ethoxy-1-naphthoic acid. It occurs as white to off-white crystals freely soluble in water. The drug is inactivated in acid media.

Nafcillin is resistant to destruction by staphylococcal penicillinase. It is well-absorbed following intramuscular injection; peak serum concentrations are reached within 1/2 to 1 hour, but only a negligible concentration remains after 4 to 6 hours. When given orally, peak blood concentrations occur within 1 to 2 hours, and by the 4th hour therapeutic concentrations are generally very low. Approximately 90% of a single intravenous dose is excreted in the bile; some reabsorption from the small intestine occurs. Clinical studies indicate that the drug is distributed to virtually all body tissues; however, it does not penetrate well into cerebrospinal fluid.

Indications: Treatment of infections caused by staphylococci that are resistant to penicillin G and those infections caused by staphylococci, pneumococci, and streptococci that are sensitive to penicillin G but primarily for therapy of penicillin G-resistant staphylococcal infections.

Contraindications: Hypersensitivity to penicillins or cephalosporins.

Precautions: In the event of an allergic reaction, the drug should be discontinued and the patient treated with the usual agents: antihistamines, pressor amines, and corticosteroids. For other precautions, see general statement.

Adverse Reactions: Hay fever, asthma, drug fever, nausea, vomiting, diarrhea, and thrombophlebitis.

Dosage and Administration: *Intravenously.* Adults, 0.5 to 1 gm every 4 hours. The dose should be dissolved in sodium chloride solution either in 15 to 30 ml and injected over a period of 10 minutes or in 100 to 150 ml and given by slow intravenous drip. *Intramuscularly.* Adults, 500 mg every 4 to 6 hours. Infants and children, 25 mg/kg of body weight twice daily. *Orally.* Adults, 250 mg to 1 gm every 4 to 6 hours, depending on the severity of the infection. Children, 250 mg 3 times daily or 25 to 50 mg/kg of body weight daily in 4 divided doses. Oral dosage should be taken 1 or 2 hours before meals.

Availability:
NAFCIL™ Injection (as sodium salt) in vials of 0.5, 1 and 2 gm and in piggyback vials of 1 and 2 gm. **(Bristol)**
UNIPEN®: **(Wyeth)**
Capsules (as monohydrate), 250 mg in bottles of 100 and in Redipak® (unit-dose) cartons of 100.
Injection (as monohydrate) in vials of 0.5, 1 and 2 gm and in piggyback vials of 1, 2 and 4 gm.

Oral Solution (as monohydrate), 250 mg/5 ml in bottles of 100 ml with 1 vial of diluent.
Tablets (as monohydrate), 500 mg in bottles of 50.

OXACILLIN

Description: Sodium oxacillin is the monohydrate of the sodium salt of a semisynthetic penicillin prepared by acylation of 6-aminopenicillanic acid with 5-methyl-3-phenyl-4-isoxazolecarboxylic acid. It occurs as a colorless, crystalline solid freely soluble in water.

Oxacillin is similar to dicloxacillin with regard to stability in acid media and to resistance to inactivation by penicillinase. In vitro studies, using comparable concentrations, show it to be less effective than penicillin G against streptococci, pneumococci, and penicillin G-sensitive staphylococci, but more effective than methicillin when used against penicillin G-resistant strains of *Staphylococcus aureus.* The drug is rapidly but incompletely (approximately 60%) absorbed from the gastrointestinal tract; absorption is more efficient when taken on an empty stomach. Doses of 0.5 to 1 gm produce average maximal serum concentrations of 4 to 8 mcg/ml in 1 hour. The drug is well absorbed following intramuscular administration, average peak serum levels are usually reached in ½ hour, diminishing over a period of about 4 hours. The drug diffuses into synovial fluid and, in small amounts, into pleural fluid and bronchial secretions; examination of peritoneal or pericardial fluid 1 hour after oral administration showed no detectable concentrations of the antibiotic. It has been found to be present in bile, amniotic fluid, cord serum, in the milk of lactating women, and in trace amounts in normal cerebrospinal fluid.

Indications: Treatment of infections known to be due to penicillinase-producing staphylococci sensitive to the drug. It may be used as initial therapy for any suspected staphylococcal infection until definitive cultures and sensitivity results are known. The drug should not be relied on *orally* for initial therapy in serious, life-threatening situations. Oxacillin is effective in the treatment of infections caused by pneumococci, group A beta-hemolytic streptococci, and staphylococci that are resistant and sensitive to penicillin G.

Contraindications: In patients with a history of allergic reactions to penicillins or cephalosporins.

Warnings: See general statement.

Precautions: In the event of an allergic reaction, the drug should be discontinued and the patient treated with the usual agents: antihistamines, pressor amines, and corticosteroids. The renal, hepatic and hematopoietic systems should be evaluated periodically when therapy is prolonged. For other precautions, see general statement.

Adverse Reactions: Moderately elevated SGOT and SGPT levels and a rare case of reversible hepatocellular dysfunction have been reported. Transient hematuria, albuminuria and azotemia have been noted in some neonates and infants receiving high doses of the drug (150 to 175 mg/kg/day). Other reactions reported were granulocytopenia, leukopenia and thrombophlebitis. For other possible adverse reactions, see general statement.

Dosage and Administration: *Orally.* For mild to moderate upper respiratory and localized skin and soft tissue infections due to sensitive organisms: adults, 500 mg every 4 to 6 hours for at least 5 days; children, 50 mg/kg/day in divided doses every 6 hours for at least 5 days. For more severe infections, the above dosages may be doubled. Children weighing more than 40 kg may be given adult dosages. *Intramuscularly* or *intravenously:* mild to moderate infections, 250 to 500 mg for adults every 4 to 6 hours; children, 50 mg/kg/day in divided doses 4 times daily. For more severe or serious infections, 500 mg to 1 gm for adults every 4 to 6 hours; children, 50 to 100 mg/kg/day in 4 equally divided doses. Very severe infections usually require very high doses and prolonged therapy. **Note:** Infections caused by group A beta-hemolytic streptococci should be treated for at least 10 days to help prevent the occurrence of acute rheumatic fever or acute glomerulonephritis.

Availability:
BACTOCILL®: **(Beecham)**
Capsules, 250 and 500 mg in bottles of 100 and in unit-dose cartons of 100 (10 × 10).

For injection in vials of 500 mg and 1, 2, 4 and 10 gm and in piggyback vials of 1 and 2 gm.
PROSTAPHLIN®: **(Bristol)**
Capsules, 250 and 500 mg in bottles of 48 and 100 and in Dosa-Trol® (unit-dose) bottles in packages of 100.
For injection in vials of 250 and 500 mg and 1, 2 and 4 gm and in piggyback vials of 1, 2 and 4 gm.
Powder for Oral Suspension, 250 mg/5 ml in bottles of 100 ml.

PENICILLIN G

Description: Penicillin G (benzyl penicillin) is a natural penicillin, extracted from the mycelial phase of certain species of the mold *Penicillium* grown in submerged fermenter cultures. It appears to be the most active of all the penicillins against staphylococci, streptococci, and pneumococci, and gram-negative bacilli, with the exception of penicillinase-producing staphylococci. Potassium penicillin G is a white, crystalline powder which is moderately hygroscopic. In aqueous solution, it retains substantially full potency for several days at temperatures below 15° C, but it is rapidly inactivated by acids, alkalies, and oxidizing agents.

Oral preparations of penicillin G are only slightly affected by normal gastric acidity (pH of 2 to 3.5); however, a pH of 2 rapidly destroys the antibiotic. Oral penicillin G is absorbed in the upper small intestine, chiefly the duodenum; maximal blood concentrations are attained within 30 to 60 minutes. Based on serum level and urinary excretion data, approximately 30% of the dose is absorbed, the rest passes into the colon where it is largely inactivated by bacteria; only a small amount is excreted by the feces. For this reason about 4 to 5 times the dose of oral penicillin G must be given to obtain a blood level comparable to that obtained with parenteral penicillin G. Since gastric acidity, stomach emptying time and other factors affecting absorption may vary considerably, serum levels may be appreciably reduced to nontherapeutic levels in certain individuals.

Aqueous penicillin G is rapidly absorbed following both intramuscular and subcutaneous injection, and peak blood levels are attained within 15 to 30 minutes. Approximately 60% of the total dose of 300,000 units is excreted in the urine within a 5-hour period. For this reason, high and frequent doses are required to maintain the elevated serum levels desirable in treating certain severe infections in individuals with normal kidney function. In neonates and young infants and in individuals with impaired kidney function, excretion is considerably delayed.

Indications: Oral penicillin G is intended for the treatment of mild to moderately severe infections due to organisms sensitive to low serum levels of penicillin G. Parenteral penicillin G is indicated in the therapy of severe infections when rapid and high blood levels are required. **Note:** Recent reports have indicated a rise in penicillin G-resistant staphylococcal strains.

For further information regarding contraindications, warnings, precautions and adverse reactions, see general statement.

Dosage and Administration: *Orally, intramuscularly* or *subcutaneously.* The oral dose should be given at least 1 hour before or 2 hours after meals. The usual dosage recommendations for adults and children 12 years of age and over are as follows: *Streptococcal infections,* mild to moderately severe, of the upper respiratory tract and including scarlet fever and mild erysipelas—200,000 to 250,000 units every 6 to 8 hours for mild infections; 400,000 to 500,000 units every 8 hours for moderately severe infections. Treatment should be continued for 10 days. Pneumococcal infections, mild to moderately severe, of the respiratory tract, including otitis media—400,000 to 500,000 units every 6 hours until the patient has been afebrile for at least 2 days. Staphylococcal infections, mild infections of the skin and soft tissue (culture and sensitivity tests should be performed)—200,000 to 500,000 units every 6 to 8 hours until infection is cured. Fusospirochetosis (Vincent's infection) of the oropharynx, mild to moderately severe infections—400,000 to 500,000 units every 6 to 8 hours. For the prevention or recurrence following rheumatic fever and/or chorea—200,000 to 250,000 units twice daily on a continuous basis. To prevent bacterial endocarditis in patients with rheumatic or congenital heart lesions who are to undergo dental or minor upper respiratory tract surgery or instrumentation—600,000 units of aqueous procaine penicillin G mixed with 200,000 units of aqueous penicillin G *intramuscularly* 1 hour before the procedure and once daily for the 2 days following the procedure. **Note:** Therapy for children under 12 years of age is calculated on the basis of body weight. For infants and small children, the suggested dose is 25,000 to 90,000 units/kg/day in 3 to 6 divided doses.

Availability:

Potassium Penicillin G

For Injection (buffered, dry) in vials of 200,000, 500,000, 1 and 5 million units. **(Lilly)**
For Injection (buffered, dry) in vials of 1 and 5 million units. **(Parke-Davis)**
For Injection (buffered, dry) in vials of 1, 5, 10, and 20 million units. **(Squibb)**
For Injection (crystalline, dry), 20 million units in vials of 100 ml. **(Lilly)**
Powder for Oral Solution, 200,000 and 400,000 units/5 ml in vials of 100 and 200 ml. **(Lederle)**
Tablets (buffered), 250,000 and 400,000 units in bottles of 100 and 1000. **(Lederle)**
Tablets (buffered), 100,000 and 250,000 units in bottles of 12 and 100. **(Lilly)**
Tablets (buffered), 400,000 units in unit-dose bottles of 100 (10 × 10). **(Parke-Davis)**
Tablets (buffered), 200,000 and 250,000 units in bottles of 100 and 1000; 400,000 units in bottles of 100 and 1000 and in Redipak® (unit-dose) cartons of 100. **(Wyeth)**
KESSO-PEN®: **(McKesson)**
Powder for Syrup, 200,000 and 400,000 units/5 ml in bottles of 100 and 200 ml.
Tablets, 200,000, 250,000 and 400,000 units in bottles of 100 and 1000.
PENTIDS®: **(Squibb)**
Powder for Syrup (buffered), 200,000 and 400,000 units/5 ml in bottles of 100 and 200 ml and in Unimatic® cartons of 5 ml.
Tablets (buffered), 200,000 units in bottles of 100; 400,000 units in bottles of 16 and 100; 800,000 units in bottles of 30 and 100. All strengths are available in Unimatic® (unit-dose) cartons of 100.
PFIZERPEN® Injection (buffered, dry) in vials of 1, 5 and 20 million units. **(Pfizer)**
PFIZERPEN G: **(Pfipharmecs)**
Powder for Oral Suspension, 400,000 units/5 ml in bottles of 100 and 200 ml.
Tablets, 200,000 units in bottles of 100 and 500; 250,000 units in bottles of 100; 400,000 units in bottles of 100 and 1000 and in unit-dose packs of 100; 800,000 units in bottles of 100.
SK-PENICILLIN G™: **(Smith Kline & French)**
Powder for Oral Suspension, 200,000 and 400,000 units/5 ml in bottles of 100 and 200 ml.
Tablets, 400,000 units in bottles of 100 and 1000; 800,000 units in bottles of 100.
SUGRACILLIN® Granules, 125,000 units/5 ml in bottles of 60 ml; 250,000 units/5 ml in bottles of 80 and 150 ml. **(Upjohn)**

Sodium Penicillin G

For Injection (buffered, dry) in vials of 5 million units. **(Squibb)**
For Injection (crystalline, dry) in vials of 1 million units. **(Upjohn)**

PENICILLIN G, BENZATHINE

Description: Benzathine penicillin G is a repository penicillin compound which provides blood levels for long periods following intramuscular administration. This property is the result of its extremely low solubility in water. It is known chemically as dibenzylethylenediamine dipenicillin G.

Following intramuscular administration, benzathine penicillin G is absorbed very slowly into the blood stream from the site of injection and converted by hydrolysis to penicillin G. This combination of hydrolysis and slow absorption results in much lower serum levels than other parenteral penicillins. Approximately 60% of penicillin G is bound to serum protein. The drug is distributed throughout the body tissues in widely varying amounts. Highest levels are found in the kidneys with lesser amounts in the liver, skin and intestines. Penicillin G penetrates, to a lesser degree, into all other tissues and the spinal fluid. With normal kidney function, the drug is excreted rapidly by tubular excretion. In neonates and young infants and in individuals with impaired kidney function, excretion of penicillin G is considerably delayed.

Indications: Treatment and prevention of infections caused by penicillin-sensitive organisms including syphilis.

For information regarding contraindications, warnings, precautions and adverse reactions, see general statement.

Dosage and Administration: *Intramuscularly.* Injection should be made deep into the upper outer quadrant of the buttock. *For streptococcal (group A) upper respiratory infections such as pharyngitis,* a single injection of 1,200,000 units for adults; 900,000 units for older children, and 300,000 to 600,000 units for infants and children under 60 pounds. *For venereal infections (syphilis, primary, secondary* and *latent),* 2.4 million units (1 dose). *Late tertiary and neurosyphilis,* 2.4 million units at intervals of 1 week for 3 doses. *For congenital syphilis,* children under 2 years of age, 50,000 mg/kg of body weight; 2 to 12 years of age, dosage should be adjusted based on the adult dosage schedule. *For yaws, bejel and pinta,* 1.2 million units (1 injection). *For prophylaxis of rheumatic fever and glomerulonephritis,* 1,200,000 units once a month or 600,000 units twice a month. *Orally. For streptococcal and pneumococcal (upper respiratory tract) infections and staphylococcal (skin and soft tissue) infections,* 400,000 to 600,000 units every 4 to 6 hours. Treatment for streptococcal infections should be continued for 10 days, and for pneumococcal infections until the patient has been afebrile for 2 days. *For the prophylaxis of rheumatic fever and/or chorea,* 200,000 units twice daily on a continuing schedule. Dosage for children under 12 years of age is calculated according to body weight. The suggested dose for infants and small children is 25,000 to 90,000 units/Kg daily in 3 to 6 divided doses.

Availability:

Benzathine Penicillin G

BICILLIN®: **(Wyeth)**

Long-Acting Injection, 300,000 units/ml in vials of 10 ml; 600,000 units/ml in 1-, 1.5-, 2- and 4-ml disposable syringes with needle (Tubex®).

Oral Suspension, 150,000 and 300,000 units/5 ml in bottles of 60 ml.

Tablets, 200,000 units in bottles of 36.

PERMAPEN® Aqueous Suspension, 600,000 units/ml in Isoject®s (disposable prefilled syringe and needle unit) of 1 and 2 ml. **(Pfizer)**

w/Procaine Penicillin G

BICILLIN® C-R *Injection* (aqueous suspension), 150,000 units with procaine penicillin G, 150,000 units/ml in vials of 10 ml; 300,000 units of each in 1-ml disposable syringe with needle; 600,000 units/ml of each in 2- and 4-ml disposable syringe with needle; 900,000 units with procaine penicillin G, 300,000 units in Tubex® (disposable syringes) of 2 ml. **(Wyeth)**

PENICILLIN G, PROCAINE

Description: Procaine penicillin G, a slightly soluble salt produced by incorporation of procaine into the penicillin molecule, is a white, microcrystalline powder with a potency of 1009 penicillin units/mg.

Following intramuscular injection, procaine penicillin G has a more prolonged duration of action than injectable solutions of the sodium or potassium salts of penicillin. Because of the slow release of penicillin G from procaine penicillin, continuous and prolonged therapeutic blood levels are maintained. In most patients, an intramuscular dose will retain a blood level of at least 0.03 units/ml for 24 hours.

See general statement for indications, contraindications, warnings, precautions and adverse reactions.

Dosage and Administration: *Intramuscularly,* 600,000 to 1,000,000 units daily for 5 to 10 days or as directed by the physician.

Availability:

Procaine Penicillin G

CRYSTICILLIN® A.S. Suspension for Injection, 300,000 units/ml in vials of 10 ml; 600,000 units/1.2 ml in vials of 1.2 and 12 ml. **(Squibb)**

DURACILLIN® A.S. Aqueous Suspension for Injection, 300,000 units/ml in Hyporets® (1-ml disposable syringes) and ampuls of 1 and 10 ml; 300,000/0.6 ml in 1.2 ml disposable syringe with needle. **(Lilly)**

PFIZERPEN®-AS Aqueous Suspension for Injection, 300,000 units/ml in vials of 10 ml; 600,000 units/ml in prefilled disposable syringes (Isoject®) of 1, 2 and 5 ml. **(Pfizer)**

WYCILLIN® Suspension for Injection, 300,000 units/ml in vials of 10 ml and 1-ml Tubex® (disposable syringes) with needle; 600,000 units/ml in 1-, 2- and 4-ml disposable syringe with needle. **(Wyeth)**

w/Probenecid

WYCILLIN® with PROBENECID in a combination package containing two 4-ml disposable syringes each containing 2,400,000 units of penicillin G procaine and 2 tablets each containing 0.5 gm of probenecid. **(Wyeth)**

PHENOXYMETHYL PENICILLIN

Description: Phenoxymethyl penicillin (penicillin V) is a phenoxymethyl analog of penicillin G. It occurs as a white, odorless, crystalline powder that is very slightly soluble in water. The potassium salt is very soluble in water.

Phenoxymethyl penicillin, unlike penicillin G, is quite stable in gastric juice and is readily absorbed from the gastrointestinal tract. It may be given with meals; however, blood levels are slightly higher when the drug is given on an empty stomach. Average blood levels are 2 to 5 times higher than the levels following the same dose of oral penicillin G, and also shows much less individual variation.

Once absorbed, about 80% of the compound is bound to serum protein. Tissue levels are highest in the kidneys, with lesser amounts in the liver, skin, and the intestines. Small amounts are found in other body tissues and in the cerebrospinal fluid. The drug is excreted as rapidly as it is absorbed in individuals with normal kidney function; however, recovery of the drug from the urine indicates that only about 25% of the dose given is assimilated. In neonates, young infants, and in individuals with impaired kidney function, excretion is considerably delayed.

Indications: Treatment of mild to moderately severe infections due to penicillin-susceptible organisms including streptococcal infections without bacteremia, pneumococcal infections, staphylococcal infections, and fusospirochetosis (Vincent's gingivitis and pharyngitis), and for the prevention of rheumatic fever and bacterial endocarditis. **Note:** An increasing number of strains of staphylococcal organisms resistant to penicillin G have been reported. Therefore, culture and sensitivity studies are indicated when treating suspected staphylococcal infections.

For complete details on contraindications, warnings, precautions and adverse reactions, see general statement.

Dosage and Administration: *Orally.* The recommended dosages for adults and children over 12 years of age are as follows: *For streptococcal infections,* 200,000 to 400,000 units every 6 to 8 hours for 10 days; for mild to moderately severe streptococcal pharyngitis, 800,000 units every 12 hours may be used as an alternate regimen. *For pneumococcal infections,* 400,000 to 800,000 units every 6 hours until the patient has been afebrile for at least 2 days. *For staphylococcal infections and fusospirochetosis,* 400,000 to 800,000 units every 6 to 8 hours. For the prevention of recurrence following rheumatic fever and chorea, or both, 200,000 to 250,000 units twice daily on a continuous basis. To prevent bacterial endocarditis in patients with rheumatic or congenital heart lesions who are to undergo dental or upper respiratory tract surgery or instrumentation, 800,000 units 1 hour before the procedure and 400,000 units every 6 hours for the remainder of that day and for 2 days or longer following the procedure. **Note:** Therapy for children under 12 years of age is calculated on the basis of body weight. For infants and small children, the suggested dose is 25,000 to 90,000 units/kg of body weight daily in 3 to 6 divided doses. To avoid any after effects due to streptococcal infection, therapy must be sufficient (10 days minimum) to eliminate the organisms, and upon completion of treatment, culture studies should be performed to determine whether or not the streptococci have been completely eradicated.

Availability:

Phenoxymethyl Penicillin

V-CILLIN® Drops, 125 mg/0.6 ml in 12-dose bottles. **(Lilly)**

Potassium Phenoxymethyl Penicillin

BETAPEN®-VK: **(Bristol)**

Powder for Oral Solution, 125 and 250 mg/5 ml in bottles of 100 and 200 ml.

Tablets, 250 mg (400,000 units) in bottles of 100 and 1000; 500 mg (800,000 units) in bottles of 100.

COMPOCILLIN®-VK: **(Ross)**
Filmtab® (tablets), 250 and 500 mg in bottles of 100 and 500.
Granules for Oral Solution, 125 and 250 mg/5 ml in bottles of 100 and 200 ml.
LEDERCILLIN® VK: **(Lederle)**
Powder for Oral Solution, 125 and 250 mg/5 ml in bottles of 100, 150 and 200 ml.
Tablets, 250 and 500 mg in bottles of 100 and in Clinipaks® (unit-dose) packages of 100 (10 × 10) and 1000 (50 × 20); the 250 mg are also available in bottles of 1000.
PENAPAR VK® Tablets, 250 mg (400,000 units) in bottles of 100 and 1000 and in unit-dose packages of 100; 500 mg (800,000 units) in bottles of 100. **(Parke-Davis)**
PEN•VEE® K: **(Wyeth)**
Powder for Oral Solution, 125 and 250 mg/5 ml in bottles of 100, 150 and 200 ml; 250 mg/5 ml is also available in Redipak® (individually wrapped pouches) in cartons of 20.
Tablets, 125 mg in bottles of 36; 250 and 500 mg in bottles of 100 and 500 and in Redipak®s of 100 (cartons of 5 × 20 strips); the 500 mg tablets are also available in bottles of 25.
PFIZERPEN VK®: **(Pfipharmecs)**
Powder for Oral Solution, 125 and 250 mg/5 ml in bottles of 100 and 200 ml.
Tablets, 250 mg in bottles of 100 and 1000 and in unit-dose cartons of 100; 500 mg in bottles of 100.
ROBICILLIN VK®: **(Robins)**
Powder for Oral Solution, 125 and 250 mg/5 ml in bottles of 100 and 200 ml.
Tablets, 250 mg (400,000 units) in bottles of 100 and 1000; 500 mg (800,000 units) in bottles of 100 and 500.
SK-PENICILLIN VK®: **(Smith Kline & French)**
Powder for Oral Solution, 125 and 250 mg/5 ml in bottles of 100 and 200 ml.
Tablets, 250 mg in bottles of 100 and 500; 500 mg in bottles of 100.
UTICILLIN® VK: **(Upjohn)**
Granules for Oral Solution, 125 and 250 mg/5 ml in bottles of 100 and 200 ml.
Tablets, 250 mg in bottles of 100 and 1000; 500 mg in bottles of 100.
V-CILLIN K®: **(Lilly)**
Powder for Oral Solution, 125 mg/5 ml in bottles of 40, 100, 150 and 200 ml and in Identi-Dose® of 5 ml (each package consists of 100 individually labeled bottles of 1 dose each); 250 mg/5 ml in bottles of 100, 150 and 200 ml and in Identi-Dose of 100.
Tablets, 125 mg in bottles of 50 and 100 and in unit-dose packages of 100; 250 and 500 mg in bottles of 24, 100 and 500 and in unit-dose packages of 100.
VEETIDS®: **(Squibb)**
Powder for Oral Solution, 125 and 250 mg/5 ml in bottles of 100 and 200 ml.
Tablets, 250 and 500 mg in bottles of 100 and in Unimatic® cartons of 100.

TICARCILLIN

Chemical Name: 6-[(Carboxy-3-thienylacetyl)amino]-3,3-dimethyl-7-oxo-4-thia-l-azabicyclo [3.2.0]-heptane-2-carboxylic acid disodium.

Description: Ticarcillin is a semisynthetic antibiotic derived from the penicillin nucleus 6-aminopenicillanic acid. It is available as the disodium salt, a white or pale yellow powder that is very soluble in water; after reconstitution for parenteral administration, the solution is clear, colorless or pale yellow, having a pH of 6 to 8.

Ticarcillin has demonstrated in vitro activity against a variety of gram-positive and gram-negative organisms including *Pseudomonas aeruginosa* and *Proteus,* although some strains of *Pseudomonas* usually develop resistance fairly rapidly. Some pathogenic strains of microorganisms such as *Mima, Herellea, Citrobacter* and *Serratia* also have been shown to be susceptible. Since it is not absorbed when taken orally, the drug must therefore be administered intramuscularly or intravenously. It readily diffuses into tissues and interstitial fluid, and can be detected in the bile, and in the cerebrospinal and pleural fluids. Following administration of 1 gm intramuscularly, peak serum levels of 31 mcg/ml are reached in ½ hour and persists in diminishing concentrations for approximately 6 hours. Somewhat higher and more prolonged serum levels can be achieved with the concurrent administration of probenecid. Serum levels of 10 to 25 mcg/ml usually are effective against most susceptible organisms; however, 60 mcg/ml or greater are needed for *Pseudomonas.* Ticarcillin should be used preferably with gentamicin in the treatment of infections caused by *Pseudomonas,* since this combination has synergistic effects against these pathogens.

As with other penicillins, the drug is eliminated by glomerular filtration and tubular secretion. It is not highly bound to serum protein (approximately 45%) and is excreted unchanged in high concentrations in the urine. Following administration of a 1- to 2-gm dose intramuscularly, urine concentrations of 2 to 4 mg/ml may be obtained in patients with normal renal function; also, the serum half-life is about 70 minutes. Ticarcillin is susceptible to destruction by penicillinase-producing staphylococci.

Indications: Primarily for infections due to sensitive strains of *Pseudomonas aeruginosa, Proteus* (both indole-positive and indole-negative), *Escherichia coli, Enterobacter* and *Streptococcus faecalis:* urinary tract, skin and soft tissue, severe systemic infections and septicemia and acute and chronic respiratory tract infections. Although improvement has been noted clinically, sterile microbial cultures cannot be expected in patients with chronic respiratory disease or cystic fibrosis. That the drug is also effective against gram-positive organisms should be kept in mind when mixed infections are present.

Contraindications: Patients with a history of allergic reactions to other penicillins.

Warnings: Patients, especially those with poor renal function, who are receiving high doses of ticarcillin may develop hemorrhagic conditions associated with abnormal clotting and prothrombin times; however, these usually revert to normal upon withdrawal of the medication.

Precautions: Because 1 gm of ticarcillin contains approximately 6.5 mEq of sodium ion, the electrolyte and cardiac status of the patient should be carefully monitored. In addition, the serum potassium levels should be measured periodically, since hypokalemia has been reported to have occurred in a few patients.

For other information, including warnings and precautions, see general statement.

Adverse Reactions: The following may occur: skin rashes, pruritus, urticaria, drug fever, nausea and vomiting, anemia, thrombocytopenia, leukopenia, neutropenia, eosinophilia, elevated SGOT and SGPT, convulsions or neuromuscular irritability (with excessively high doses), and pain at the injection site. Vein irritation and phlebitis have been reported on occasion, particularly when undiluted solution was injected directly into a vein. Hypokalemia may be corrected by the addition of potassium salts.

Dosage and Administration: *Intravenous infusion.* For bacterial septicemia, respiratory tract and soft tissue infections: Adults and children, 200 to 300 mg/kg of body weight daily in divided doses every 3, 4 or 6 hours. Generally, dosages depend upon the weight of the patient and the severity of the infection, but the usual recommended dosage is 3 gm daily in divided doses. For complicated urinary tract infections: Adults and children, 150 to 200 mg/kg daily in divided doses every 4 or 6 hours. *Intramuscularly* or *intravenously* (direct). For uncomplicated urinary tract infections: Adults, 1 gm every 6 hours; children, 50 to 100 mg/kg daily in divided doses every 6 or 8 hours. For infections complicated by renal insufficiency: The initial loading dose is 3 gm *intravenously,* followed by intravenous doses based on creatinine clearance or type of dialysis (creatinine clearance less than 10 ml/minute, 2 gm every 12 hours; with hepatic dysfunction, 2 gm every 24 hours; during peritoneal dialysis, 3 gm every 12 hours; and patients on hemodialysis, 3 gm after each dialysis). For infants, the usual initial dose is 100 mg/kg of body weight, followed by 75 mg/kg every 4, 6 or 8 hours for 1 or 2 weeks, depending upon the age and weight of the child. Package literature should be consulted for dosage details and for methods of preparing solutions.

Availability:
TICAR® Injection (as disodium salt) in vials of 1, 3 and 6 gm and in piggyback bottles of 3 gm.
(Beecham)

PENTAERYTHRITOL TETRANITRATE

Description: Pentaerythritol tetranitrate, the nitric acid ester of the tetrahydric alcohol, occurs as a white, crystalline powder sparingly soluble in water and in alcohol.

The coronary vasodilation produced by pentaerythritol tetranitrate is believed to be due to the release of its nitrite ions. Because of its antispasmodic action on the smooth muscle of the coronary vessels, the drug increases myocardial blood flow and oxygen supply without significantly changing pulse rate, blood pressure and cardiac output.

Following oral administration, the effect of the drug occurs within 1 hour and persists for 4 to 5 hours.

Indications: May be of use in the management, prophylaxis or treatment of anginal attacks; intended to reduce the number of episodes and the severity of anginal pain, but not to abort the acute anginal episode. Pentaerythritol tetranitrate with nitroglycerin is indicated for the rapid relief of acute episodes. Combined with a barbiturate or meprobamate, to provide sedative action, thus decreasing anxiety, tension and physical agitation.

Contraindications: Hypersensitivity to any of the components.

Warnings: Data supporting the use of pentaerythritol tetranitrate during the early days of the acute phase of myocardial infarction are insufficient to establish safety. This drug can act as a physiological antagonist to norepinephrine, acetylcholine, histamine and many other agents.

Precautions: Should be used with caution in patients with glaucoma. Tolerance to this drug, and cross-tolerance to other nitrites and nitrates may occur.

Adverse Reactions: Predominantly rash and/or exfoliative dermatitis (which requires withdrawal of medication), headache, and gastrointestinal distress (usually mild and transient with continuation of medication); however, in some instances severe, persistent headaches may occur. Also reported were cutaneous vasodilatation with flushing; transient episodes of dizziness and weakness, as well as other signs of cerebral ischemia associated with postural hypotension. Marked sensitivity to the hypotensive effects of pentaerythritol tetranitrate and severe responses such as nausea, vomiting, weakness, restlessness, pallor, perspiration and collapse can occur, even with the usual therapeutic doses; alcohol may enhance this effect.

For complete data on any of the components formulated with pentaerythritol tetranitrate, see their respective monographs.

Dosage and Administration: *Orally,* 1 to 2 tablets 4 times daily, taken at least 1/2 hour before meals or 1 hour after meals and at bedtime, or 1 capsule every 12 hours on an empty stomach. May be administered in individualized doses up to 160 mg daily. Peritrate with nitroglycerin, 1 tablet *sublingually* as needed, but not to exceed 8 tablets in 24 hours.

Availability:

Pentaerythritol Tetranitrate

Tablets, 10 and 20 mg in bottles of 1000. **(Lederle)**

Tablets, 10 and 20 mg in bottles of 1000. **(Philips Roxane)**

DUOTRATE® Plateau Caps® (sustained-release capsules), 30 and 45 mg in bottles of 100, 500 and 1000. **(Marion)**

METRANIL™ Duracap® (capsules), 80 mg in bottles of 60 and 500. **(Meyer)**

NEO-COROVAS Tymcaps (timed-disintegrating capsules), 30 mg in bottles of 60, 100, 120, 500 and 1000; 80 mg in bottles of 100 and 1000. **(Amfre-Grant)**

PENTRITOL® Tempules® (timed-release), 30 mg in bottles of 100 and 250; 60 mg in bottles of 60 and 250. **(Armour)**

PERITRATE®: **(Warner-Chilcott)**

Tablets, 10 and 20 mg in bottles of 100 and 1000; 20 mg in punch-out blisterpack strips of 10 tablets in cartons of 10 strips (10 x 10); 40 mg in bottles of 100.

SA Tablets (sustained-action), 80 mg in bottles of 100 and 1000 and in unit-dose packages of 100.

SK-PETN™ Tablets, 10 and 20 mg in bottles of 100. **(Smith Kline & French)**

w/Barbiturate (**Warning:** May be habit-forming.)

COROVAS Tymcaps (timed-disintegrating capsule), 30 mg with secobarbital, 50 mg in bottles of 60, 120, 500 and 1000. **(Amfre-Grant)**

PERITRATE® with PHENOBARBITAL: **(Warner-Chilcott)**

Sustained-Action Tablets, 80 mg with phenobarbital, 45 mg in bottles of 100 and 1000.

Tablets, 10 and 20 mg with phenobarbital, 15 mg in bottles of 100 and 1000.

w/Meprobamate

EQUANITRATE® Tablets, 10 and 20 mg with meprobamate, 200 mg in bottles of 50. **(Wyeth)**

MILTRATE® Tablets, 10 and 20 mg with meprobamate, 200 mg in bottles of 100. **(Wallace)**

Miscellaneous

CARTRAX® Tablets, 10 and 20 mg with hydroxyzine hydrochloride, 10 mg in bottles of 100. **(Roerig)**

PERITRATE® with NITROGLYCERIN Sublingual Tablets, 10 mg with nitroglycerin, 0.3 mg in bottles of 50. **(Warner-Chilcott)**

PENTAGASTRIN

Chemical Name: N-t-Butyloxycarbonyl-B-alanyl-L-tryptophyl-L-methionyl-L-aspartyl-L-phenylalanyl amide.

Description: Pentagastrin is a synthetic pentapeptide containing the carboxyl terminal tetrapeptide amide fraction found in all natural gastrins. It has been noted to possess all the physiologic and phamacologic effects of the natural hormones. It occurs as a colorless, crystalline solid that is soluble in dimethylformamide and dimethylsulfoxide and is almost insoluble in water, alcohol, ether, benezene, chloroform, and ethyl acetate. The commercial product contains the ammonium salt of the peptide that is soluble in water in concentrations of 1 mg/ml.

The recommended subcutaneous dose of 6 mcg/kg of body weight will produce peak acid output equivalent to that produced by 40 mcg/kg of histamine acid phosphate or 1500 mcg/kg of betazole hydrochloride, an analog of histamine. This response is repeated when equal doses are given to the same individual. However, if the dose exceeds this amount, pentagastrin may inhibit gastric acid secretion. The drug exerts its effect in approximately 10 minutes with maximal response occurring in most patients 20 to 30 minutes after administration. Duration of activity usually ranges from 60 to 80 minutes. The plasma half-life is thought to be less than 10 minutes. Current reports indicate that the drug is inactivated in the liver, kidney and upper intestinal tract. Pentagastrin has been found to interact with other peptide hormones such as cholecystokinin-pancreozymin, secretin, and glucagon. No biochemical abnormality which might indicate specific organ toxicity has been encountered.

Indications: A diagnostic agent for evaluating gastric acid secretory function. It is useful in testing anacidity in patients with suspected pernicious anemia, atrophic gastritis or gastric carcinoma; for hypersecretion in patients with suspected duodenal ulcer or postoperative stomal ulcer, and for the diagnosis of Zollinger-Ellison tumor; also for determining the adequacy of acid-reducing operations for peptic ulcer.

Contraindications: Previous hypersensitivity or an allergic response to the drug.

Warnings: The use of pentagastrin in pregnant patients has not been evaluated; therefore, the benefits to be derived from the drug must be weighed against the possible harm to the mother and/or fetus. Clinical reports are insufficient to recommend the use of, or to establish a proper dose, in children.

Precautions: Cautious use is advised in patients with pancreatic, hepatic, or biliary disorders. As with gastrin, the drug could, in some instances, stimulate secretion of pancreatic enzyme and bicarbonate output, as well as biliary flow.

Adverse Reactions: The drug has been reported to cause fewer and less severe cardiovascular and other complications than does histamine or betazole hydrochloride. Those usually associated with the use of pentagastrin include gastrointestinal reactions characterized by abdominal pain, desire to defecate, nausea, vomiting, borborygmi, and blood-tinged mucus; cardiovascular reactions manifested by flushing, and tachycardia; CNS reactions manifested by dizziness, faintness or lightheadedness, drowsiness, sinking feeling, transient blurring of vision, tiredness, and headache. Other reactions reported include shortness of breath, heavy sensation in arms and legs, tingling sensation in the fingers, chills, sweating, generalized burning sensation, warmth, pain at the site of injection and bile in collected specimens. Allergic and hypersensitivity reactions may occur in some patients.

Dosage and Administration: *Subcutaneously.* Adults, 6 mcg/kg of body weight.

Availability:

PEPTAVLON® Injection, 0.25 mg/ml (250 mcg) in ampuls of 2 ml in cartons of 10. **(Ayerst)**

PENTAZOCINE

Chemical Name: 1,2,3,4,5,6-Hexahydro-*cis*-6,11-dimethyl-3-(3-methyl-2-butenyl)-2,6-methano-3-benzazocin-8-ol.

Description: Pentazocine is a non-narcotic, synthetic analgesic of the benzazocine series and occurs as a white, crystalline substance soluble in acidic aqueous solution.

The parenteral administration of a 30-mg dose has been found to be as effective as 10 mg of morphine or 75 to 100 mg of meperidine. Oral administration of a 50-mg dose appears to be equivalent in analgesic effect to 60 mg of codeine. As with opiate analgesics, pentazocine possesses hypnotic effects and decreases gastrointestinal motility. It antagonizes, to some extent, the analgesic effects of morphine, meperidine, and phenazocine; its antagonistic activity is 1/50 that of nalorphine. In addition, it reverses, incompletely, the cardiovascular, respiratory, and behavioral depression induced by narcotic agents. Onset of significant analgesia usually occurs within 15 to 30 minutes following oral administration; 15 to 20 minutes following intramuscular or subcutaneous administration, and 2 to 3 minutes following intravenous administration.

Pentazocine is extensively metabolized with less than 13% appearing in the urine as unchanged drug and up to 30% as a glucuronide conjugate.

Indications: *Orally,* for the relief of moderate to severe pain. *Parenterally,* for preoperative analgesia and sedation, control of postoperative pain, relief of pain during labor, and for other types of pain requiring a potent analgesic.

Contraindications: Hypersensitivity to pentazocine.

Warnings: Use with extreme caution, and only if the drug is deemed essential, in patients with head injury and other intracranial lesions or with a preexisting increase in intracranial pressure; pregnant patients (except those in labor), women delivering premature infants; emotionally unstable patients; those with a history of drug dependence or abuse (withdrawal symptoms may follow abrupt discontinuance of the drug), and patients who have had acute CNS manifestations (hallucinations, disorientation, and confusion) while receiving pentazocine. The drug is not recommended for children under 12 years of age because of limited clinical experience in this age group. Since sedation, dizziness, and occasional euphoria have been noted, ambulatory patients should be cautioned not to engage in hazardous tasks that require alertness or physical coordination. The compound containing aspirin should be used with special care in the presence of peptic ulcer, in conjunction with anticoagulant therapy, or in any situation in which the effects of aspirin may be deleterious. Constant rotation of the injection site is essential in order to reduce tissue damage characterized by severe sclerosis of the skin, subcutaneous tissue, and underlying muscle.

Precautions: Use cautiously and in low dosage in patients with respiratory depression, obstructive respiratory condition or cyanosis. Administer with utmost caution to patients dependent on narcotics since mild withdrawal symptoms have been noted. Periodic renal or hepatic function tests should be performed when the drug is given to patients with impaired kidney or liver function. Pentazocine is additive to, or may potentiate the effects of, other CNS depressants; therefore, caution should be observed when the drug is used concomitantly with these agents to avoid overdosage. It should be administered with care in patients with myocardial infarction who exhibit nausea and vomiting, or in those who are prone to seizures, and in patients about to undergo biliary surgery since spasm of the sphincter of Oddi may occur.

Adverse Reactions: Reports have included nausea, vomiting, dizziness, lightheadedness, sedation, euphoria, headache. Infrequently noted were constipation, weakness, disturbed dreams, insomnia, syncope, visual blurring and focusing difficulty, depression, hallucinations, flushing, rash, hypotension, tachycardia. Rarely noted were abdominal distress, anorexia, diarrhea, confusion, tremor, irritability, excitement, tinnitus, chills, urticaria, depression of white blood cells especially granulocytes which is usually reversible, moderate transient eosinophilia, respiratory depression, urinary retention, toxic epidermal necrolysis, allergic reactions including edema of the face. *There have been rare reports of possible abstinence syndromes in newborns after prolonged use during pregnancy.* Clinical experience with pentazocine overdosage has been insufficient to define the signs and symptoms of this condition. Signs of salicylate overdosage include headache, dizziness, confusion, tinnitus, diaphoresis, thirst, nausea, vomiting, diarrhea, tachycardia, tachypnea, Kussmal breathing, convulsions and coma. Death is usually caused by respiratory failure.

Dosage and Administration: The parenteral dosage for general pain states, except obstetrics, is 30 mg every 3 to 4 hours as needed. Doses up to 60 mg may be given with caution. Obstetric, 30 mg *intramuscularly* during labor, or 20 mg *intravenously* when contractions become regular; may be repeated once or twice every 2 or 3 hours. The usual oral dosage is 1 or 2 tablets every 3 or 4 hours. **Caution:** Because precipitation will occur, the parenteral solutions should not be mixed in the same syringe with soluble barbiturates.

Availability:

Pentazocine

TALWIN® Injection (as lactate), 30 mg/ml in Uni-Amp® (individual unit-dose ampuls) of 1, 1.5 and 2 ml, in ampuls of 1, 1.5 and 2 ml and in multiple dose vials of 10 ml; 30, 45 and 60 mg in Carpuject®s (half-filled syringes) of 2 ml. **(Winthrop)**

TALWIN 50 Tablets (as hydrochloride), 50 mg (peach, scored) in bottles of 100 and in unit-dose packages of 100. **(Winthrop)**

Combinations

TALWIN® COMPOUND Caplets® (tablets) 12.5 mg (equiv. to base) with acetylsalicylic acid (aspirin), 325 mg in bottles of 100. **(Winthrop)**

PENTOBARBITAL SODIUM (C-II)

Chemical Name: 5-Ethyl-5-(1-methylbutyl)barbiturate sodium.

Description: Pentobarbital sodium, a short-acting barbiturate which produces a sedative-hypnotic effect and some degree of analgesia, occurs as a white, odorless, slightly bitter, crystalline powder very soluble in water and freely soluble in alcohol. Aqueous solutions decompose slowly on standing and rapidly on boiling.

Following oral administration, onset of action occurs within 15 to 30 minutes, lasts for 3 to 6 hours and has a half-life of 21 to 42 hours. Pentobarbital sodium is metabolized primarily in the liver to an inactive metabolite; only a negligible amount of the drug appears in the urine in unchanged form.

Indications: *Orally* as a sedative or hypnotic for insomnia. *Parenterally* for rapid onset of action or precise control of hypnotic level. It may be used as a preanesthetic medication, for the induction of general anesthesia, or as an adjunct during labor. It may also be employed to provide hypnosis or sedation during diagnostic or manipulative procedures, as a diagnostic or therapeutic aid in psychiatry (narcoanalysis and narcotherapy), or for producing rapid sedation in acutely disturbed psychiatric patients; also for emergency control of convulsive states, particularly those associated with tetanus, status epilepticus, and toxic reactions to strychnine and local anesthetics.

Contraindications: Hypersensitivity, latent or manifest porphyria or a familial history of intermittent porphyria, uncontrolled pain, history of confusion, restlessness or abnormal reaction to hypnotics, impaired liver function, addiction-prone individuals or those with severe respiratory depression.

Warnings: Pentobarbital may be habit-forming. Intravenous administration should not be attempted without adequate provisions for supporting respiration and circulation; too rapid administration may result in adverse respiratory and circulatory reactions, and should be avoided. Intramuscular injection should not exceed 5 ml at any one site because of possible tissue irritation. Pentobarbital may increase the rate of hepatic metabolism of coumarin anticoagulants; therefore, the dosage of the anticoagulant should be adjusted accordingly when used concomitantly with this drug. Furthermore, the respiratory-depressant effects of pentobarbital may be increased when used concomitantly with such drugs as antihistamines, tranquilizers, other sedatives or hypnotics, ether, alcohol, or curare-like drugs. Safe use during pregnancy has not been established with respect to adverse effects upon fetal development. Therefore, when intended for use in pregnant patients, the physician should weigh carefully the benefits to the mother versus the hazards to the fetus. Excessive doses during labor may result in depression of the newborn, and the clinician should be aware that premature infants are particularly susceptible to the depressant effects of the drug; thus due caution should be exercised when delivery of a premature infant is anticipated. Prolonged use of barbiturates, even in therapeutic dosages, can result in psychic dependence. Withdrawal symptoms may occur after chronic use of large doses, resulting in delirium, convulsions, or death. It is advised to use utmost care when administering barbiturates to individuals in anxiety states involving impending depression or suicidal tendencies.

Precautions: Caution is essential when the drug is administered in the presence of any respiratory difficulty. Special care should be taken when pentobarbital is administered to patients in whom the hypnotic effect may be prolonged or intensified, as in those suffering from shock, severe liver disease, uremia, or after recent administration of other respiratory depressants. Considerable caution is essential in patients with severe anemia or congestive heart failure, in debilitated patients, in the presence of status asthmaticus, impaired respiratory or circulatory function. Since pentobarbital is detoxified primarily in the liver, it should be used with caution in patients with hepatic impairment. Solutions of the drug are highly alkaline; therefore, extreme care should be exercised to avoid perivascular extravasation or intraarterial injection. Extravascular injection may cause local tissue damage with subsequent necrosis. The consequences of intraarterial injection may vary from transient pain along the course of the artery to gangrene of the limb. Signs of accidental injection by this route include, in addition to pain, delayed onset of hypnosis, pallor and cyanosis of the extremity, and patchy discoloration of the skin. Any complaint of pain in the limb warrants discontinuing the injection. Hypotension may result from intravenous administration, particularly in patients with hypertension. Following the use of pentobarbital in office procedures, the patient should be cautioned not to engage in hazardous occupations requiring coordination or skill such as driving a motor vehicle for the remainder of the day.

Adverse Reactions: Idiosyncratic reactions such as excitement, pain or hangover; coughing, hiccoughing, laryngospasm, and chest-wall spasm have followed intravenous use of pentobarbital. Bronchospasm may occur in individuals with bronchial asthma. Allergic reactions including localized swellings and erythematous dermatitis have been observed particularly in patients subject to asthma, urticaria, angioedema and similar conditions. Psychological dependence on the drug can occur. Other possible reactions that may occur include respiratory depression, apnea, circulatory collapse, drowsiness, lethargy, nausea and vomiting. Overdosage is manifested by coma, hypothermia followed by fever, sluggish or absent reflexes, respiratory depression, and gradual appearance of circulatory collapse and pulmonary edema. Maintaining adequate ventilation and blood pressure and employing the usual supportive measures are recommended. Dialysis may be helpful. Analeptic drugs have been used with varying success.

Dosage and Administration: *Orally.* Adults, 20 to 30 mg 3 or 4 times daily for daytime sedation, or 100 mg at bedtime. Children, 8 to 30 mg for daytime sedation, depending upon age. The hypnotic dose should be adjusted according to age and weight. *Rectally:* adults, 1 suppository (200 mg). Children, 15 to 150 mg depending upon age and weight. *Intramuscularly:* adults, usually, 150 to 200 mg; children, 25 to 80 mg. *Intravenously:* adults, initially 100 mg, increased if necessary to a total of 200 to 500 mg. Dosage should be reduced proportionately for children. **Note:** The injection should not be administered if precipitation has occurred.

Availability:

Ⓒ II NEBRALIN® Tablets (timed-release), 90 mg in bottles of 50. **(Dorsey)**

Ⓒ II NEMBUTAL®: **(Abbott)**

Capsules, 30 mg in bottles of 100; 50 and 100 mg in bottles of 100, 500 and 1000 and in Abbo-Pac® (unit-dose) packages of 100.

Elixir, 20 mg/5 ml in bottles of 1 pint and 1 gallon and in Abbo-Pac (unit-dose) bottles of 5 ml in cartons of 25.

Gradumet® (long-release), 100 mg in bottles of 100, 500 and 5000, in strip-packages of 25 and in Abbo-Pac of 100.

Injection, 50 mg/ml in ampuls of 2 and 5 ml and in mutiple-dose vials of 20 and 50 ml.

Ⓒ III *Suppositories,* 30, 60, 120, and 200 mg in cartons of 12.

Ⓒ II PENTOBARBITAL SODIUM Capsules, 100 mg in bottles of 100 and 1000. **(ICN)**

Ⓒ II PENTOBARBITAL SODIUM Capsules (Pulvules®), 100 mg in bottles of 100. **(Lilly)**

Ⓒ-II PENTOBARBITAL SODIUM Capsules, 100 mg in bottles of 1000 and in unit-dose packages of 100 (10 strips × 10). **(Parke-Davis)**

Ⓒ-II PENTOBARBITAL SODIUM: **(Wyeth)**

Capsules, 100 mg in Redipak® (strip-pack) cartons of 25.

Injection, 50 mg/ml in disposable syringes (Tubex®) of 1 and 2 ml in Tamp-R-Tel® (tamper-resistant) packages of 10.

Combinations

Ⓒ-III CARBRITAL® Capsules (Kapseals®) 50 mg with carbromal, 120 mg in bottles of 100; 100 mg with carbromal, 240 mg in bottles of 100 and 1000 and in unit-dose packages of 100 (10 strips x 10). **(Parke-Davis)**

Ⓒ-III NIPIRIN Capsules, 32 mg (as base) with aspirin, 325 mg in bottles of 1000. **(Elder)**

PENTYLENETETRAZOL

Chemical Name: 6,7,8,9-Tetrahydro-5*H*-tetrazoloazepine.

Description: Pentylenetetrazol stimulates all parts of the CNS but its action on motor function and the respiratory and vasomotor centers is most pronounced. It has also been shown to enhance synaptic transmission. Readily absorbed, it is rapidly metabolized in the liver, and approximately 75% of the drug is excreted through the kidneys. It occurs as white crystals that are freely soluble in water.

Indications: *Orally* to enhance mental and physical activity of geriatric patients. When niacin is combined with the drug, it helps to increase cerebral blood flow; vitamins are added to help combat the nutritional deficiencies resulting from poor food assimilation as well as irregular eating habits. *Parenterally* as an antidote in respiratory depression and failure due to intoxication with barbiturates, alcohol, chloral hydrate, and other CNS depressants that are antagonized by this drug.

Contraindications: None known.

Warnings: Safe use during pregnancy has not been established.

Precautions: Care should be exercised in patients with a low convulsive threshold or with a focal brain lesion, or severely impaired liver function. Cautious use is advised in patients with peptic ulcer, gallbladder or liver diseases. Caution should also be exercised when administering high doses to patients with heart disease. Bradycardia, splanchnic vasodilation and conduction disturbances may occur with a resultant fall in blood pressure. Niacin may potentiate hypotensive drugs and phenothiazine derivatives and may inactivate fibrinolysin. Since decreased glucose tolerance and mild diabetes have been reported with average or excessive doses of niacin, the drug should be used with caution in diabetic patients.

Adverse Reactions: Occasionally, pruritus due to niacin. Parenteral high doses may precipitate clonic convulsions.

Dosage and Administration: *Orally,* initial dosage is 200 mg 3 or 4 times daily; maintenance, 100 mg 3 or 4 times daily. In depression from barbiturates, 5 ml of a 10% solution can be injected *intravenously* within 3 to 5 seconds; subsequent *intramuscular* injections of 1 to 2 ml of a 10% solution may be given. The interval and frequency of the medication must be governed solely by the clinical response.

Availability:

Pentylenetetrazol

METRAZOL®: **(Knoll)**

Liquid, 100 mg/5 ml in bottles of 1 pint.

Sterile Solution, 100 mg/ml (10%) in vials of 1 ml in cartons of 10.

Tablets, 100 mg in bottles of 100 and 1000.

w/Niacin

GERONIAZOL®: **(Philips Roxane)**

Elixir, 200 mg with niacin, 100 mg/5 ml in bottles of 1 pint. Alcohol, 12%.

TT Tablets (Temporol), 300 mg with niacin, 150 mg in bottles of 100 and 500.

NICO-METRAZOL®: **(Knoll)**
Elixir, 100 mg with niacin, 50 mg/5 ml in bottles of 1 pint and 1 gallon. Alcohol, 15%.
Tablets, 100 mg with niacin, 50 mg in bottles of 100 and 1000.

w/Vitamin B Complex

VITA-METRAZOL®: **(Knoll)**
Elixir in bottles of 1 pint. Each 5 ml contains pentylenetetrazol, 100 mg with niacinamide, 10 mg and 1 mg each of thiamine and pyridoxine; 1.4 mg of riboflavin-5 phosphate sodium and 2 mg of *d*-panthenol in a 15% alcoholic solution.
Tablets in bottles of 100. Each tablet contains, pentylenetetrazol, 100 mg with niacinamide, 10 mg and 1 mg each of thiamine, riboflavin, and pyridoxine and 25 mg of ascorbic acid.

PERCOBARB Ⓒ II

Description: Each capsule contains:

Oxycodone hydrochloride	4.5 mg
Oxycodone terephthalate	0.38 mg
Hexobarbital	100 mg
Aspirin	224 mg
Phenacetin	160 mg
Caffeine	32 mg

Oxycodone is a semisynthetic narcotic analgesic with CNS actions similar to those of morphine. Its therapeutic value corresponds to that of codeine and methadone in that it retains at least 1/2 of its analgesic activity when administered orally.

Indications: Relief of mild to moderately severe pain.

Contraindications: In patients hypersensitive to any of the components, and in the presence of intermittent porphyria.

Warnings: Oxycodone and hexobarbital may be habit-forming. Oxycodone can produce drug dependence of the morphine type and, therefore, has the potential for being abused. Psychic and physical dependence and tolerance may develop upon repeated use. The usual precautions associated with the administration of oral narcotic-containing preparations must be observed. Since mental and physical abilities may be impaired, patients should be cautioned not to engage in activities requiring alertness or skill. Concurrent use with other CNS depressants such as general anesthetics, phenothiazines, other tranquilizers, sedative-hypnotics, alcohol, and other narcotic analgesics may produce an additive effect. When such combined therapy is contemplated, the dose of one or both agents should be reduced. The possible adverse effects on fetal development has not been established; therefore, it should be used in pregnant women only when the anticipated benefits outweigh the potential hazards to the fetus. This product is not recommended for use in children under 12 years of age. Preparations containing salicylates should be used with caution in the presence of peptic ulcer or abnormality of blood coagulation.

Precautions: The respiratory depressant effects of narcotics and their capacity to elevate cerebrospinal fluid pressure may be markedly exaggerated in the presence of head injury, other intracranial lesions or a preexisting increase in intracranial pressure. Furthermore, narcotics and barbiturates produce adverse reactions which may obscure the clinical course of patients with head injuries. Narcotics may also obscure the diagnosis or clinical course in patients with acute abdominal conditions. Narcotic-containing preparations should be given with caution to elderly or debilitated patients, and to those with severe impairment of hepatic or renal function, hypothyroidism, Addison's disease, and prostatic hypertrophy or urethral stricture. Phenacetin has been reported to damage the kidneys when taken in excessive amounts for prolonged periods. Also, aspirin may enhance the effect of anticoagulants, and inhibit the uricosuric effect of uricosuric agents.

Adverse Reactions: Most frequently observed were lightheadedness, dizziness, sedation, nausea and vomiting. Others which may occur include euphoria, dysphoria, constipation, and pruritus. Idiosyncrasy to barbiturates is usually manifested in the form of "hangover," excitement, or pain. Overdosage is characterized by respiratory depression, extreme somnolence which can progress to stupor or coma, skeletal muscle flaccidity, cold and clammy skin, and occasionally bradycardia and hypotension. In severe overdosage, apnea, circulatory collapse, cardiac arrest and death may occur. The ingestion of very large amounts of this product may, in addition, result in barbiturate poisoning and in acute salicylate intoxication. Primary attention should be given to the reestablishment of adequate respiratory exchange through provision of a patent airway and the institution of assisted or controlled ventilation. Naloxone, nalorphine or levallorphan (specific antidotes) should be given to combat respiratory depression. Oxygen, intravenous fluids, vasopressors and other supportive measures should be employed as indicated. Hemodialysis may be necessary to remove the barbiturate.

Dosage and Administration: *Orally.* Usual adult dosage is 1 capsule every 6 hours, preferably after meals or with milk.

Availability:
Ⓒ PERCOBARB® Capsules in bottles of 100 and 500. **(Endo)**

PERCOGESIC with CODEINE Ⓒ

Description: Each tablet contains codeine phosphate, 32.4 mg; acetaminophen, 325 mg and phenyltoloxamine citrate, 30 mg.

Indications: Treatment of moderate acute pain that usually accompanies bursitis, sinusitis, neuralgias, dysmenorrhea, myalgias, arthritides, rheumatoid conditions, headache, tension headache, toothaches, and pain due to dental procedures, and for the relief of symptoms of the common cold, fever, and other discomforts associated with systemic viral infections.

Contraindications: Hypersensitivity to any of the components.

Warnings: Codeine phosphate may be habit-forming; therefore, the general precautions for the use of narcotics should be considered when prescribing this preparation. Administration is not recommended for more than 7 days.

Precautions: Because of its drying action on the respiratory mucosa, the indiscriminate use of codeine may precipitate severe respiratory insufficiency resulting from increased viscosity of the bronchial secretions and suppression of the productive cough. The CNS-depressant effects of codeine may be enhanced by such drugs as the phenothiazines, the MAO inhibitors, and the tricyclic antidepressants, and may be additive when used with other CNS depressants. Since drowsiness may occur, patients should be cautioned not to engage in activities requiring alertness or physical coordination.

Adverse Reactions: Nausea, vomiting, constipation, drowsiness and miosis.

Dosage and Administration: *Orally.* Adults, 1 or 2 tablets every 4 hours. Children 5 to 12 years of age, 1/2 the adult dosage.

Availability:
Ⓒ PERCOGESIC® with CODEINE Tablets in bottles of 100 and 1000. **(Endo)**

PERIHEMIN

Description: Each capsule contains:

Cyanocobalamin (vitamin B-12)	5 μg
Intrinsic factor concentrate	25 mg
Ferrous fumarate (elemental iron, 66 mg)	160 mg
Folic acid	0.33 mg
Ascorbic acid	50 mg

Indications: Treatment of hypochromic, microcytic and macrocytic hyperchromic anemias.

Warnings: Folic acid is improper therapy in the treatment of pernicious anemia and other megaloblastic anemias where vitamin B-12 is required.

Precautions: Not all patients with pernicious anemia show satisfactory therapeutic responses to oral vitamin B-12-intrinsic factor preparations. In addition, some patients with an initial good response appear to become refractory to intrinsic factor after varying periods of oral therapy. Periodic examinations and laboratory studies of pernicious anemia patients are essential and recommended. Failure of response, or inadequate response, is an indication for parenteral vitamin B-12 generally recognized as the preferred treatment of this condition. This preparation should not be relied upon to correct the folic acid deficiency characterizing sprue or the malabsorption syndromes, as therapeutic amounts of folic acid should be administered in these conditions.

Adverse Reactions: Allergic sensitization has been reported following both the oral and parenteral administration of folic acid. Excessive ingestion of iron-containing preparations may lead to gastrointestinal hemorrhage in children.

Dosage and Administration: *Orally.* Children over 12 years of age and adults, 1 capsule 3 times daily with or after meals.

Availability:
PERIHEMIN® Capsules in bottles of 100 and 500. **(Lederle)**

PERPHENAZINE: see The Phenothiazines

PERTUSSIS IMMUNE GLOBULIN, HUMAN

Description: A solution (16.5%) of the gamma globulin fraction of blood from adult human donors who have been hyperimmunized with phase I pertussis vaccine. The antibody content, as determined by agglutination tests, is about 16 times that of unconcentrated human immune serum.

Indications: Passive prevention and treatment of whooping cough.

Precautions: Should not be administered intravenously.

Adverse Reactions: Soreness at the injection site and, rarely, a systemic reaction.

Dosage and Administration: *Intramuscularly.* Prophylactically, 1.25 ml as soon as possible after exposure and another dose 1 week later. If exposure continues, dosage may be repeated every 1 or 2 weeks. Therapeutically, 1.25 ml initially and 1.25 ml every day or 2 until signs of recovery are apparent. For critically ill children, the initial dosage may be doubled. In pertussis pneumonitis, therapy may be combined with antibiotics.

Availability:
HYPERTUSSIS® in vials of 1.25 ml. **(Cutter)**

PHAZYME-PB Ⓒ IV

Description: Each two-phase release tablet contains in the outer layer for prompt release in the stomach 20 mg of activated simethicone. The enteric-coated core releases in the small intestine 240 mg of pancreatin, 40 mg of activated simethicone and 15 mg of phenobarbital.

Indications: Relief of discomfort due to gastrointestinal gas resulting from aerophagia, dyspepsia, faulty digestion and food intolerance. Also for relief of gas distress associated with other functional or organic conditions such as diverticulitis, spastic colitis, hyperacidity, postcholecystectomy syndrome and chronic cholecystitis.

Contraindications: Hypersensitivity to any of the ingredients.

Warnings: Phenobarbital may be habit-forming.

Precautions: Since drowsiness may occur, patients should be cautioned not to engage in activities requiring alertness and physical coordination.

Adverse Reactions: Those associated with phenobarbital are dry mouth, blurred vision, dizziness, palpitation, nausea, and constipation. For additional contraindications, warnings, precautions and adverse reactions pertaining to phenobarbital, see specific monograph.

Dosage and Administration: *Orally,* 1 or 2 tablets with meals and upon retiring, or as required.

Availability:
(C-IV) PHAZYME®-PB Tablets (yellow) in bottles of 100 and 1000. **(Reed & Carnrick)**

PHELANTIN (C-III)

Description: Each Kapseal contains phenytoin, 100 mg; phenobarbital, 30 mg and methamphetamine hydrochloride, 2.5 mg.

Indications: Control of grand mal and psychomotor seizures.

Contraindications: Methamphetamine hydrochloride is contraindicated in patients with moderate to severe hypertension, advanced symptomatic cardiovascular disease, arteriosclerosis, hyperthyroidism, during pregnancy and in patients receiving MAO inhibitors during or within 14 days of treatment, in patients hypersensitive to any of the components. For other contraindications, see monograph on Phenytoin and Phenobarbital.

Warnings: Phenobarbital may be habit-forming. Clinical reports suggest that the use of anticonvulsant drugs in pregnant women may have a teratogenic effect on the unborn child. While a definite cause and effect relationship has not been firmly established, it is recommended that the medication be discontinued prior to and during gestation, primarily in patients in whom withdrawal would not constitute a serious threat. However, these drugs should not be suspended in patients inclined to major seizures because of the strong possibility of precipitating status epilepticus with its attendant hypoxia and risk to both the mother and fetus. At present, it is not known whether or not even minor seizures incur some hazard to the developing embryo or fetus.

Precautions: If drowsiness develops, patients should be warned not to engage in activities requiring alertness such as driving or operating machinery. Methamphetamine should be administered with caution, if at all, to patients with hyperexcitability states or to those receiving CNS stimulants. It should also be used with caution in elderly, debilitated or asthenic patients or in those with psychopathic personalities or a history of suicidal or homicidal tendencies. Psychic dependence or addiction may occur, particularly when administered to alcoholic patients or to those with a history of drug addiction. Hyperglycemia, resulting from the drug's inhibitory effect on insulin release, has been reported. Phenytoin may also raise the blood sugar level in patients already suffering from hyperglycemia. Osteomalacia has been associated with anticonvulsant therapy including phenytoin and/or phenobarbital. For additional precautions, see monograph on Phenytoin and Phenobarbital.

Adverse Reactions: Methamphetamine may induce nervousness, insomnia, irritability, talkativeness, dizziness, headache, blurred vision, mydriasis, hyperexcitability, hypertension, hypotension, tachycardia, palpitation, nausea, vomiting, abdominal cramps, diarrhea or constipation, dry mouth, anorexia, metallic taste, and paradoxical increased depression or agitation in depressed patients. For additional adverse reactions, see monograph on Phenytoin and Phenobarbital.

Dosage and Administration: *Orally.* The recommended initial dosage for children over 6 years of age and adults is 1 capsule 2 or 3 times daily. Dosage can be adjusted gradually until the desired effect is reached. Maintenance dosage for adults is 3 to 4 capsules daily; children 2 or 3 capsules daily.

Availability:
(C-III) PHELANTIN® Kapseals® (capsules) in bottles of 100. **(Parke-Davis)**

PHENACEMIDE

Chemical Name: Phenylacetylurea.

Description: Phenacemide is a synthetic anticonvulsant that produces only minor sedative action. In preclinical studies, the drug has been found to elevate the threshold for minimal electroshock convulsions and to abolish the tonic phase of maximal electroshock seizures when given in doses well below those causing neurological signs. The drug prevents or modifies seizures induced by pentylenetetrazol or other convulsant agents. In comparative tests, it was found to be equal to or more effective than other commonly used anticonvulsants against focal seizures of a psychomotor type which were induced in mice by low frequency stimulation of the cerebral cortex. Studies in mice also suggest that when phenacemide is added to a mephenytoin, phenobarbital or trimethadione regimen, it exerts a synergistic anticonvulsant effect.

Following oral administration, phenacemide is readily absorbed from the intestine and following a single dose its duration of action is approximately 5 hours. It is metabolized in the liver into inactive metabolites which are excreted by the kidney.

Indications: Control of severe epilepsy, particularly mixed forms of psychomotor seizures that are refractory to other drugs.

Contraindications: Hypersensitivity to phenacemide.

Warnings: There is strongly suggestive evidence that the incidence of birth defects is increased with the use of anticonvulsant drugs during pregnancy. Therefore, use in pregnant or lactating women or in women of childbearing potential requires that the expected benefits be weighed against the possible hazards. However, these drugs should not be discontinued in those patients prone to major seizures because of the strong possibility of precipitating status epilepticus with its attendant hypoxia and risk to both the mother and fetus. Nonetheless, consideration should be given to discontinuing these agents prior to and during pregnancy when the nature, frequency and severity of the seizures do not constitute a serious threat to the patient. At the present time, it is not known whether or not even minor seizures pose some risk to the developing embryo or fetus.

Precautions: Phenacemide should be administered only to those patients found refractory to other anticonvulsants. Since the drug can produce serious side effects as well as direct organ toxicity, it is advisable to hospitalize the patient during the first week of treatment. Particular care is essential if treatment warrants the concurrent use of other anticonvulsants known to produce similar toxic effects. Phenacemide is particularly prone to cause serious personality changes, including psychosis and suicidal depression. Accordingly, patients or their families should be made aware that if the patient experiences a decreased interest in surroundings, depression, or aggressiveness that these are early manifestations of a developing psychosis. Severe or exaggerated personality changes, signs of liver damage, urinary dysfunction, rash or marked depression of the blood count are indications for immediate withdrawal of the drug. Blood counts, kidney and liver function tests should be made prior to treatment and regularly during treatment. Deaths attributable to liver damage and aplastic anemia during therapy with this product have been reported. Patients with a history of allergy require special care, and the drug should be immediately withdrawn at the first sign of a skin rash or other allergic manifestation. When given to mothers during pregnancy, phenacemide may cause neonatal hemorrhage; it has been suggested that vitamin K be administered prophylactically to such infants at birth.

Adverse Reactions: Personality changes which may lead to attempted suicide, and toxic psychoses; gastrointestinal disturbances, anorexia and weight loss, headaches, drowsiness, dizziness, insomnia, paresthesia, hepatitis, blood dyscrasias, skin rash, and nephritis. Symptoms of acute overdosage include excitement or mania, followed by drowsiness, ataxia and coma. In one instance of acute overdosage, dizziness was followed by coma which lasted approximately 24 hours. Patients should be advised to report all such signs immediately, especially during the first 6 months of therapy. A careful evaluation of liver and kidney function, mental state, and the blood-forming organs should be made following recovery.

Dosage and Administration: *Orally.* Dosage must be based on the response of the patient. Adults: Suggested initial dosage is 500 mg 3 times daily with meals, gradually increasing with additional 500 mg daily at weekly intervals to an average dosage of 2 to 3 gm/day; although some patients may require as much as 5 gm daily. Children 5 to 10 years of age, 1/2 adult dosage.

Availability:
PHENURONE® Tablets, 500 mg in bottles of 100. **(Abbott)**

PHENAZOPYRIDINE

Chemical Name: 2,6-Diamino-3-phenylazopyridine.

Description: Phenazopyridine hydrochloride, an azo dye, occurs as a red, crystalline powder with a violet luster.

Phenazopyridine is excreted in the urine where it exerts a topical analgesic effect on the mucosa of the urinary tract. This action helps to relieve pain, burning, urgency and frequency. Since this agent is an analgesic, it should be employed only for the relief of symptoms. Because it is compatible with antibacterial therapy, the drug can therefore help to relieve pain and discomfort while antibacterial therapy controls the infection.

Indications: Symptomatic relief of pain and discomfort resulting from irritation of the lower urinary tract mucosa due to infection, trauma, surgery, endoscopic procedures, or to the passage of sounds or catheters.

Contraindications: Renal insufficiency.

Precautions: A yellowish tinge of the skin or sclerae may indicate accumulation due to impaired renal excretion and the need to discontinue therapy.

Adverse Reactions: Occasional gastrointestinal disturbances.

Dosage and Administration: *Orally.* Average adult dosage is 200 mg 3 times daily after meals. Patients should be told that the drug may produce a reddish-orange discoloration of the urine.

Availability:
PYRIDIUM® Tablets, 100 and 200 mg in bottles of 100 and 1000 and in unit-dose packages of 100. **(Warner-Chilcott)**

PHENDIMETRAZINE TARTRATE (C-III)

Chemical Name: 3,4-Dimethyl-2-phenylmorpholine tartrate.

Description: Phendimetrazine tartrate is an anorexigenic agent with properties and functions similar to those of the amphetamines. It occurs as a white, odorless powder that is bitter to the taste; it is soluble in water, methanol and alcohol.

Pharmacologic actions include stimulation of the CNS and elevation of blood pressure. Tachyphylaxis and tolerance have also been demonstrated. The limited usefulness of this agent should be measured against the possible risk factors inherent in its use. Available clinical data are insufficient to establish that this drug acts primarily on the appetite-control centers of the hypothalamus. Other CNS action or metabolic effects may also be involved.

Following oral administration, phendimetrazine provides peak blood levels in 1 hour after a single dose; continuing anorexigenic activity persists for approximately 4 to 5 hours. To obtain maximal results, the drug should be used in conjunction with dietary discretion, moderate exercise, and psychologic support.

Indications: Recommended for short-term use (a few weeks) as an adjunct to a program of caloric restriction and other measures in the management of exogenous obesity.

Contraindications: Advanced arteriosclerosis, major coronary artery disease, cardiac decompensation, moderate to severe hypertension, hyperthyroidism, in agitated or emotionally unstable patients, concomitant use with other CNS stimulants, patients with a history of drug abuse, and in those with known hypersensitivity or idiosyncrasy to sympathomimetic amines. It is also contraindicated during or within 14 days after receiving MAO inhibitors.

Warnings: Since tolerance to the drug usually develops within a few weeks, the recommended dose should not be exceeded in an attempt to increase the anorectic effect. Although abuse of phendimetrazine is rare when it is used under strict medical supervision, the physician should keep in mind the possibility of its occurrence in susceptible individuals. There are reports of patients who have increased the dosage to many times that recommended. Abrupt cessation following prolonged high dosage administration results in extreme fatigue, mental depression as well as changes on the sleep EEG. Chronic intoxication is manifested by severe dermatoses, marked insomnia, irritability, hyperactivity, personality changes, and psychosis —often clinically indistinguishable from schizophrenia. Patients should be cautioned not to engage in hazardous activities such as driving a motor vehicle. This drug is not recommended for use in pregnant women or in children under 12 years of age.

Precautions: Phendimetrazine may be used with caution in patients with mild hypertension. Patients with diabetes mellitus should be followed closely since dosage requirements of the antidiabetic drugs may be altered with the use of anorectic agents and concomitant dietary restriction.

Adverse Reactions: The incidence and frequency of adverse effects produced by this drug are not significantly different from those of other amphetamine-like compounds. Those noted include overstimulation, restlessness, insomnia, agitation, flushing, tremor, sweating, dizziness, headache, psychotic states, blurring of vision; palpitation, tachycardia, elevated blood pressure; mouth dryness, nausea, diarrhea, constipation, stomach pain; urinary frequency, dysuria, and changes in libido. Abuse of the drug may be associated with intense psychological dependence and severe social dysfunction. Severe overdosage may result in convulsions, coma, and death. The management of overdose is primarily symptomatic and includes sedation with a barbiturate. If hypertension is marked, the use of a nitrate or rapid-acting alpha receptor-blocking agent should be considered. Experience with hemodialysis or peritoneal dialysis is inadequate to permit recommendations for its use.

Dosage and Administration: *Orally.* The usual dosage is 1 tablet 2 or 3 times daily, 1 hour before meals. Dosage should be adjusted to the needs of the patient and may range from 1/2 tablet daily to 2 tablets 2 or 3 times daily.

Availability:

CIII BONTRIL PDM Tablets, 35 mg in bottles of 100 and 1000.	**(Carnrick)**
CIII MINUS Tablets, 35 mg in bottles of 100 and 1000.	**(Amfre-Grant)**
CIII PHENDIMETRAZINE TARTRATE Tablets, 35 mg in bottles of 1000.	**(Elder)**
CIII PLEGINE® Tablets, 35 mg in bottles of 100 and 1000.	**(Ayerst)**
CIII STATOBEX® Capsules, 35 mg in bottles of 100 and 1000.	**(Lemmon)**
CIII STATOBEX-G Tablets, 35 mg in bottles of 100 and 1000.	**(Lemmon)**

PHENELZINE SULFATE

Chemical Name: 2-Phenylethylhydrazine dihydrogen sulfate.

Description: Phenelzine sulfate, a monoamine oxidase inhibitor of the hydrazine group, occurs as a white, crystalline solid freely soluble in water.

Clinical evidence indicates that phenelzine sulfate is useful in the treatment of depressive illnesses, and appears to be most effective in endogenous depressions. In responsive patients, there is a latent period before onset of action; the maximal effect usually occurs within 1 to 2 weeks.

Indications: May be of use in the treatment of moderate to severe depressive states in adults. It is generally indicated for the treatment of endogenous depression, the depressive phase of manic depressive psychosis and exogenous (reactive) depression. It should not be used in the treatment of mild depression or that due to an appropriate response to temporary stress.

Contraindications: Known hypersensitivity to the drug, elderly or debilitated patients, patients with a cerebrovascular defect, cardiovascular disease, hypertension, a history of headache, pheochromocytoma, a history of liver disease or abnormal liver function tests, congestive heart failure, concomitant use of CNS depressants or stimulants, sympathomimetic drugs, guanethidine, other MAO inhibitors or foods containing a high tyramine content such as aged cheese and wines.

Warnings: Because the most serious reactions involve changes in blood pressure, phenelzine should not be given to elderly or debilitated patients, or to those who have hypertension, cardiovascular or cerebrovascular disease. Also it is not recommended in patients who have frequent or severe headaches, because the manifestation of headache during therapy may be the first symptom of a hypertensive reaction to the drug. Intracranial bleeding has been reported in association with increased blood pressure. Blood pressure should be observed frequently to detect evidence of any pressor response. Phenelzine should be discontinued at least 10 days prior to elective surgery requiring anesthesia. Long-term studies with mice have shown a potential for drug-induced pulmonary and vascular tumors.

Precautions: If a hypertensive crisis occurs, medication should be discontinued and therapy to lower blood pressure should be instituted immediately. The drug should be used cautiously in seriously depressed patients in whom the possibility of suicide is a problem. Schizophrenic patients may present with excessive stimulation; and in manic-depressive states, it may result in a swing from a depressive to a manic phase. Imipramine, desipramine, MAO inhibitors, nortriptyline, or amitriptyline should not be given with or for at least 2 weeks after discontinuation of phenelzine in order to avoid a hypertensive crisis. Also caution is advised when this agent is used in combination with antihypertensive drugs, including thiazide diuretics since a hypotensive episode may occur. Because it may produce excessive stimulation, the drug should be used cautiously in overactive, overstimulated, or agitated patients. Patients should be warned not to eat cheese or to take proprietary drugs that contain pressor agents (e.g., certain cold remedies, hay fever preparations, or anorexiants), or CNS depressants such as alcohol and narcotic drugs while undergoing therapy with this drug. They should be instructed to report promptly the occurrence of headache or other unusual symptoms. Those undergoing treatment with phenelzine should be closely followed for symptoms of postural hypotension; also adequate precautions should be taken when treating epileptic patients. Diabetic patients should be closely observed for any alterations in glucose metabolism or potentiation of their hypoglycemic drug. Caution should also be observed when used concomitantly with barbiturates or rauwolfia alkaloids. Safe use during pregnancy or lactation or in women of childbearing potential, and in children under 16 years of age has not been established.

Adverse Reactions: The most important reaction associated with the use of phenelzine is the occurrence of a hypertensive crisis which has in some instances been fatal. Other undesirable effects have included dizziness, constipation, dry mouth, postural hypotension, drowsiness, weakness and fatigue, edema, gastrointestinal disturbances, blurred vision, glaucoma, sweating, skin rash, jitteriness, palilalia, urinary retention, euphoria, nystagmus, sexual disturbances, hypernatremia, hypomania, agitation, ataxia, shock-like coma, edema of the glottis, transient respiratory and cardiovascular depression, leukopenia, toxic delirium, reversible jaundice, manic reaction, convulsions, acute anxiety reaction and precipitation of schizophrenia, and fatal progressive necrotizing hepatocellular damage. In severe overdosage, the initial manifestation is faintness, with hypotension and, occasionally precordial pain and intense headache. Hyperactivity and marked agitation may also occur. Cool and clammy skin with profuse perspiration, coma, seizures, and signs of peripheral circulatory collapse have been known to occur. In some cases trismus and opisthotonos may be observed, the pulse may become fast and irregular, and respiration may become shallow. Measures generally found helpful include bed rest, maintenance of hydration and electrolyte balance, avoidance of CNS stimulants and, when indicated, the use of an intravenous phenothiazine.

Dosage and Administration: *Orally.* Recommended initial dosage for adults is 15 mg 3 times daily. Dosage should then be increased to at least 60 mg daily at a fairly rapid pace consistent with patient tolerance, but 90 mg daily may be necessary to obtain a satisfactory response. Many patients do not show a clinical response until treatment at 60 mg has been continued for at least 4 weeks. After maximum benefit is obtained, usually in 2 to 6 weeks, dosage should be reduced over a period of several weeks to a maintenance level; this may be as low as 15 mg daily or every other day. The maximum recommended daily dose is 90 mg.

Availability:
NARDIL® Tablets, 15 mg in bottles of 100. **(Warner-Chilcott)**

PHENINDIONE

Chemical Name: 2-Phenyl-1,3-indandione.

Description: Phenindione, a short-acting indandione, is a synthetic anticoagulant with action and uses similar to those of bishydroxycoumarin and its derivatives, although it is unrelated chemically. It inhibits hepatic synthesis of factors II, VII and X, thereby producing an anticoagulant effect through reduction of prothrombin concentration of the blood. Following oral administration, therapeutic levels are reached within 18 to 24 hours; when the drug is discontinued the prothrombin time of the blood usually returns to normal within 24 to 48 hours.

Indications: Prophylaxis and treatment of venous thrombosis and its extension, treatment of atrial fibrillation with embolization, prophylaxis and treatment of pulmonary embolism, and as an adjunct in the treatment of coronary occlusion.

Contraindications: Patients who are bleeding or who have hemorrhagic tendencies, those with open wounds, ulcerating or granulomatous lesions or extensive denudation of skin, visceral carcinoma, ulcerations of the gastrointestinal tract, subacute bacterial endocarditis, severe liver or kidney disease, severe uncontrolled hypertension, recent or contemplated surgery of the eye, brain, or spinal cord, continuous tube drainage of the stomach or small intestine, and initial elevated prothrombin time, or deficiency of vitamin K or ascorbic acid.

Warnings: The effects of the drug tend to be cumulative and prolonged; therefore, caution should be exercised when administered in any condition where added risk of hemorrhage is present. At the earliest sign of bleeding the drug should be withdrawn. Dosage should be controlled by periodic determination of prothrombin time, since determinations of clotting and bleeding times are not effective measures for control of therapy. Agranulocytosis and hepatitis have been associated with the use of oral anticoagulants; patients should be instructed to report promptly any prodromal symptoms such as marked fatigue, chills, fever, or sore throat. Periodic blood studies and liver function tests are required, and therapy should be terminated if leukopenia or symptoms of hypersensitivity (dermatitis or fever) occur. Rash, persistent albuminuria, or fever of undetermined origin are signs of impending toxicity. Because of the possibility of renal damage, urine should be tested periodically. Oral anticoagulants pass through the placental barrier, and have been reported to cause fetal hemorrhage and intrauterine death. Also, it has been strongly suggested that they may be responsible for the congenital malformations (nasal hypoplasia and other abnormalities consistent with a diagnosis of chondrodysplasia punctate) appearing in children born to mothers who received oral anticoagulants during pregnancy. Consequently, if these drugs must be used in pregnant patients, such patients should then be made well aware of the potential risk.

Precautions: Use with caution in patients with active tuberculosis, moderate hypertension, mild liver or kidney disease, severe diabetes, in patients with indwelling catheters, during menstruation, and the postpartum period, or in patients with a past history of ulcerative disease of the gastrointestinal tract, or any occupation which carries a hazard of significant physical injury, or exposure to DDT and chlordane. Special care is needed in the presence of hepatic disorders, vitamin K deficiency, congestive heart failure, diarrhea, poor nutritional state, collagen disease, disorders of the pancreas, fever, cachexia, renal insufficiency, x-ray therapy, scurvy, and alcoholism since these conditions increase the response to these agents. Conversely, edema, hyperlipidemia, diabetes mellitus, hypercholesterolemia, visceral carcinoma, myxedema, and hereditary resistance to the oral anticoagulants decrease the response.

It is of utmost importance that no other drug be administered with phenindione without full appreciation of its potential for interacting with it, thereby increasing or decreasing its anticoagulant effect. Fatalities have been reported from interactions affecting the metabolism of oral anticoagulants or their binding to plasma proteins. Drugs which may stimulate metabolic degradation of this anticoagulant include phenobarbital as well as other barbiturates, glutethimide, meprobamate, rifampin, ethchlorvynol, and griseofulvin. In addition, oral contraceptives, ACTH, and adrenocorticosteroids have been reported to reduce the response to oral anticoagulants. Patients receiving these drugs may require larger doses of phenindione to achieve an optimal anticoagulant effect. When these drugs are discontinued, it may be necessary to reduce the dose of phenindione. Such drugs as phenylbutazone, oxyphenbutazone, diazoxide, chloral hydrate, and mefenamic, ethacrynic, and nalidixic acids may increase the quantity of free drug available by displacing phenindione from protein binding sites. Quinine, quinidine, and salicylates in large doses depress prothrombin formation in the liver, and thus may increase the patient's sensitivity to phenindione and cause hemorrhage. Broad-spectrum antibiotics, which suppress the organisms comprising the normal bacterial flora of the intestine and reduce the production of vitamin K, may increase anticoagulant activity, but this is not usually observed unless there is a dietary deficiency of vitamin K. Other drugs which have been reported to cause an exaggerated response and a prolonged prothrombin time include methylthiouracil, propylthiouracil, phenyramidol, disulfiram, dextrothyroxine, clofibrate, glucagon, chloramphenicol, nortriptyline, and various anabolic steroids.

Oral anticoagulants have been reported to inhibit the enzymatic degradation of phenytoin in the liver thus leading to increased serum levels and prolonged half-life of phenytoin which could result in drug intoxication. Conversely, phenytoin stimulates the metabolism of oral anticoagulants, thereby decreasing their serum levels and thus increasing the plasma prothrombin-proconvertin concentrations. Oral anticoagulants also are known to potentiate the hypoglycemic effect of tolbutamide by inhibiting its degradation in the liver. They have also been known to elevate the serum levels of chlorpropamide and phenobarbital. Therefore, with the addition or withdrawal of any of these drugs, there is the danger of either inadequate anticoagulant response to phenindione or bleeding. In such cases, the dosage of this drug should be carefully regulated, or its use discontinued.

Adverse Reactions: The principal toxic effect is hemorrhage and this may occur even with therapeutic doses and with a prothrombin time within the usual therapeutic range. The occurrence of significant gastrointestinal or urinary tract bleeding may indicate the presence of an underlying occult lesion. Following are some of the adverse reactions which have been reported with oral anticoagulants and which may occur with phenindione. These include bleeding from peptic ulcer or carcinoma, nausea, vomiting, diarrhea, steatorrhea; hematuria, nephropathy; anemia, leukopenia, failure of myeloid maturation, atypical mononuclear cells, eosinophilia, leukemoid reaction, agranulocytosis, aplastic anemia, thrombocytopenia, Factor IX deficiency, leukocyte agglutinins; hepatitis, jaundice; rash; pruritus, alopecia, dermatitis, urticaria; paralysis of accommodation, sore throat and mouth, and fever. Overdosage may result in hematuria, hemorrhage from wounds and ulcerative lesions, bleeding from the mucous membranes, and widespread petechiae and ecchymotic hemorrhages. Paralytic ileus and intestinal obstruction from submucosal or intramural hemorrhage may also occur. Hemorrhagic necrosis (bleeding into the skin and subcutaneous tissue with necrosis, vasculitis and thrombosis) of the female breast, and other areas has been reported. Rarely reported was priapism. Uterine bleeding may be excessive, but menstrual flow is usually normal.

Dosage and Administration: *Orally.* The prothrombin clotting time should be determined during the first 3 days of therapy and thereafter as indicated by the patient's response. Initial daily dose is 100 to 150 mg twice daily, in the morning and at bedtime. Patients weighing less than 70 kg should be given 200 mg daily while those weighing more should receive 300 mg. Maintenance dosage may vary from 50 to 100 mg daily in divided doses with an average of 75 mg daily. Dosage should be adjusted as necessary, in accordance with prothrombin time determinations.

Availability:
HEDULIN® Tablets, 50 mg in bottles of 100 and 1000. **(Merrell-National)**

PHENMETRAZINE Ⓒ-II

Chemical Name: 2-Phenyl-3-methyltetrahydro-1, 4-oxazine hydrochloride.

Description: Phenmetrazine, an amphetamine congener, occurs as a white to off-white, crystalline powder very soluble in water and freely soluble in alcohol. It is a sympathomimetic amine chemically related to the oxine group of compounds. It is readily absorbed from the gastrointestinal tract, and its effects persist for about 4 hours following oral administration.

Pharmacologic actions include stimulation of the CNS and elevation of blood pressure. Tachyphylaxis and tolerance have also been demonstrated. The limited usefulness of this agent should be measured against the possible risk factors inherent in its use. Available clinical data are insufficient to establish that this drug acts primarily on the appetite-control centers of the hypothalamus. Other CNS actions, or metabolic effects may also be involved.

Indications: Exogenous obesity as a short-term (a few weeks) adjunct in a regimen of weight reduction based on caloric restriction.

Contraindications: Advanced arteriosclerosis, symptomatic cardiovascular disease, moderate to severe hypertension, hyperthyroidism, glaucoma, known hypersensitivity or idiosyncrasy to sympathomimetic amines, and agitated states; in patients with a history of drug abuse; concomitant use of MAO inhibitors or CNS stimulants. The use of phenmetrazine within 14 days following the administration of monoamine oxidase inhibitors may result in hypertensive crises.

Warnings: Since tolerance to the drug usually develops within a few weeks, the recommended dose should not be exceeded in an attempt to increase the anorectic effect. Instances involving abuse and addiction to the drug have been reported. Abrupt cessation following prolonged high dosage administration results in extreme fatigue and mental depression as well as reversible changes noted on the sleep EEG. Manifestations of chronic intoxication include severe dermatoses, marked insomnia, irritability, hyperactivity and personality changes. The most severe manifestation of chronic intoxication is psychosis often clinically indistinguishable from schizophrenia. Patients should be cautioned that phenmetrazine may impair their ability to engage in potentially hazardous activities such as operating machinery or driving a motor vehicle. Safe use during pregnancy has not been established; therefore, it should not be given to women who are or who may become pregnant, particularly to women in the first trimester of pregnancy, unless in the opinion of the physician the potential benefits outweigh the possible risks. The drug is not recommended for use in children under 12 years of age.

Precautions: Caution should be exercised in patients with mild hypertension. Insulin requirements in diabetes mellitus may be altered; also psychological disturbances have been reported in female patients who were on a restrictive diet with or without the concomitant use of an anorectic agent. The hypotensive effect of guanethidine may be decreased in patients taking this drug. The least amount feasible should be prescribed or dispensed at one time in order to minimize the possibility of overdosage.

Adverse Reactions: Complications noted were palpitation, tachycardia, elevation of blood pressure; overstimulation, restlessness, dizziness, insomnia, euphoria, dysphoria, tremor, headache, rarely psychotic episodes at recommended doses; dryness of mouth, unpleasant taste, diarrhea, constipation, and other gastrointestinal disturbances; urticaria; impotence and changes in libido. Manifestations of acute overdosage include restlessness, tremor, hyperreflexia, rapid breathing, confusion, assaultiveness, hallucinations, and panic states. Fatigue and depression usually follow CNS stimulation. Cardiovascular effects are manifested by arrhythmias, hypertension, or hypotension and circulatory collapse. Gastrointestinal symptoms include nausea, vomiting, diarrhea and abdominal cramps. Severe intoxication may result in convulsions, coma, and death. Management of acute intoxication is largely symptomatic and includes lavage and sedation with a barbiturate. Hemodialysis or peritoneal dialysis is not recommended. Acidification of the urine should increase excretion of this drug. Intravenous phentolamine has been suggested for possible acute, severe hypertension if this complicates phenmetrazine overdosage.

Dosage and Administration: *Orally.* Usual adult dosage is 25 mg 2 or 3 times daily, taken 1 hour before meals. Dosage should be adjusted to individual response and tolerance and may range from 12.5 mg twice daily to a maximum of 25 mg 3 times daily. Since the prolonged-action tablets provide appetite suppression of approximately 12 hours, the time of administration should be determined by the period of the day over which the anorectic effect is desired.

Availability:
Ⓒ(II) PRELUDIN®: **(Boehringer Ingelheim)**
Endurets® (prolonged-action tablets), 50 and 75 mg in bottles of 100.
Tablets, 25 mg in bottles of 100.

PHENOBARBITAL Ⓒ(IV)

Chemical Name: 5-Ethyl-5-phenylbarbituric acid.

Description: Phenobarbital, a long-acting barbiturate, occurs as a white, crystalline powder very slightly soluble in water and freely soluble in alcohol. Phenobarbital sodium occurs as a bitter, white, crystalline powder, or as granules or flakes very slightly soluble in water, but soluble in alcohol.

Phenobarbital is useful as a long-acting sedative and hypnotic in the treatment of conditions in which mild, relatively prolonged sedation is desirable. Its action appears to be more potent and persistant than barbital but slower in effect. The cerebral cortex and the reticular activating system are the most sensitive to barbiturate effects; the cerebellar, vestibular and spinal systems are less sensitive; and the vital medullary systems concerned with respiration and circulation are least sensitive. The barbiturates produce sleep which closely resembles physiologic sleep, subjectively and on EEG record.

Phenobarbital is a respiratory depressant by virtue of its direct effect on the medullary respiratory center. It diminishes and, in high doses, may abolish the sensitivity of the respiratory center to its normal stimulus, carbon dioxide.

Ordinary hypnotic doses have no significant effect on the cardiovascular system. Phenobarbital tends to decrease the tonus of the gastrointestinal musculature. It has no direct injurious effect on the normal kidney. Severe oliguria or anuria may occur in acute barbiturate poisoning largely as a result of the marked hypotension.

Small doses usually produce pronounced sedative and antispasmodic action, larger doses hypnotic and anticonvulsant action. Following administration, sedative action appears in about 1 hour and continues for 10 to 16 hours.

Indications: When a general sedative, antispasmodic, or a long-acting hypnotic is indicated; as an adjunct to analgesics and antispasmotics, and as an anticonvulsant in epilepsy used either alone, or in some cases, combined with other anticonvulsant drugs.

Contraindications: Hypersensitivity to barbiturates, uncontrolled pain, known addiction to sedative-hypnotics, latent or manifest porphyria or a familial history of intermittent porphyria, history of confusion or restlessness from hypnotics, history of abnormal reaction to barbiturates, severe pulmonary insufficiency, premonitory signs or symptoms of hepatic coma, and nephritis.

Warnings: Phenobarbital may be habit-forming. Tolerance, psychological and/or physical dependence may occur; therefore, special care should be exercised in the treatment of emotionally unstable patients and those with a history of alcoholism or other drug dependence because of the possibility of such patients increasing the dosage on their own initiative. Manifestations of chronic intoxication include ataxia, slurred speech, and vertigo. Abrupt cessation after prolonged ingestion of large doses may result in withdrawal symptoms, which may include tremulousness, weakness, insomnia, convulsions, and delirium. Such withdrawal symptoms have also been observed in newborn infants whose mothers required anticonvulsant therapy. Appropriate management includes hospitalization and gradual withdrawal over a period of several days. Safe use of barbiturates during pregnancy has not been established; therefore, they should be used only when the expected therapeutic benefits outweigh the possible hazards. Barbiturates readily cross the placental barrier and if administered during labor they may have a depressant effect on the fetus; infants born to the mothers receiving these drugs may have difficulty in breathing spontaneously. Small amounts have been detected in the milk of nursing mothers who have been receiving large doses. Status epilepticus may result from the abrupt discontinuation of phenobarbital even when administered in small daily doses in the treatment of epilepsy. Since barbiturates stimulate the activity of hepatic enzymes responsible for drug metabolism, they may decrease the blood concentration and clinical effectiveness of such drugs as antihistamines, steroids, vitamin D, etc., when given concurrently. Also, they may lower the blood level of coumarin anticoagulants and thus shorten prothrombin time. The sedative effect represents a hazard in ambulatory patients whose activities require alertness and motor coordination.

Precautions: Use with caution in patients with renal or hepatic impairment when excretion may be delayed; in debilitated or elderly patients, particularly those with cerebral arteriosclerosis, who may experience accentuated nocturnal confusion, excitement or depression under barbiturate therapy; in patients previously addicted to barbiturates; and in patients with fever, hyperthyroidism, diabetes mellitus, severe anemia, congestive heart failure and any condition in which respiratory depression may occur. Occasional "hangover" may occur. Hypersensitive patients may develop restlessness, excitement, skin rashes, fever, and collapse. Continued uncontrolled use may cause habituation. Overdosage may result in stupor, lowered body temperature, feeble heart action, depression or paralysis of the respiratory centers.

Extreme caution should be exercised to avoid perivascular extravasation or intraarterial injection. Extravascular injection may cause local tissue damage with subsequent necrosis. The consequences of intraarterial injection may vary from transient pain along the course of the artery to gangrene of the limb. Signs of accidental injection by this route include, in addition to pain, delayed onset of hypnosis, pallor and cyanosis of the extremity, and patchy discoloration of the skin. Any complaint of pain in the limb warrants discontinuation of the injection.

In cases of great debility or pulmonary disease, shock, or uremia, phenobarbital should be used with extreme caution. Special care is needed when the drug is given to patients also receiving ether or curare-like drugs because a synergistic respiratory depressant effect may ensue. Phenobarbital may have an additive effect with other barbiturates, tranquilizers, alcohol, centrally acting analgesics, hypnotics, and anesthetics which can result in excessive depression when administered concurrently with any of these drugs.

Adverse Reactions: Dizziness, headache, "hangover", confusion (particularly in the elderly), paradoxical excitation, exacerbation of preexisting pain; nausea, vomiting, epigastric pain; hypotension, megaloblastic anemia, agranulocytosis, thrombocytopenia; facial edema, skin rash, bullae and vesicles, purpura, erthema multiforme, and rarely, exfoliative dermatitis. Rickets and osteomalacia may develop due to increased vitamin D metabolism. Severe allergic reactions may result in degenerative changes in the liver. Acute overdosage primarily involves the central nervous and cardiovascular systems and includes shock, coma and death. Respiratory depression and renal failure may occur. Mild overdosage usually resembles alcohol intoxication. In acute barbiturate toxicity, general physiologic supportive measures should be undertaken immediately. Most important of these is correction of anoxia, which may be accomplished by removal of airway obstruction, oxygen administration, artificial respiration or analeptic therapy, or a combination of these procedures. However analeptic therapy should be avoided unless a definite need exists. Absorption of the drug should be minimized by emesis, gastric lavage, or gastric aspiration. Peritoneal dialysis or hemodialysis may be life-saving in severe poisoning. If renal function is satisfactory, forced diuresis and alkalization of the urine will hasten the excretion of the barbiturate.

Dosage and Administration: *Orally.* The sodium salt may also be administered *rectally, subcutaneously, intramuscularly* or *intravenously.* Recommended adult sedative dosage is 16 to 32 mg 2 to 4 times daily; the hypnotic dose is 100 to 320 mg. Total daily dosage should not exceed 600 mg. The intravenous dose should not exceed 300 mg and should be given at a maximum rate of 50 mg/minute. The sedative dosage for children is 8 to 16 mg 2 or 3 times daily. *For epilepsy,* single doses of 30 to 120 mg, repeated at intervals; their frequency will be determined by the patient's response. More than 300 mg is seldom required, and the dose should rarely, if ever, exceed 600 mg. *In status epilepticus, maniacal conditions, or delirium tremens,* intramuscular or intravenous injection of doses up to 600 mg may be required. When intravenous administration of large doses is indicated, the drug should be injected slowly at a rate not in excess of 30 to 60 mg/minute. *Nervous vomiting* may be controlled by intramuscular injection of 60 to 120 mg every 4 hours.

Availability:

Phenobarbital

Ⓒ IV ESKABARB® Spansule® (sustained-release capsules), 65 and 100 mg in bottles of 50. **(Smith Kline & French)**

Ⓒ IV LUMINAL® Ovoids (sugar-coated, oval-shaped tablets), 16 and 32 mg in bottles of 250. **(Winthrop)**

Ⓒ IV PHENOBARBITAL Elixir, 15 mg/3.75 ml in Abbo-Pac® (single-dose) bottles of 3.75 ml; 20 mg/5 ml in Abbo-Pacs of 5 ml in cartons of 100. **(Abbott)**

Ⓒ IV PHENOBARBITAL Tablets, 15 and 30 mg in bottles of 1000 and in single-units of 90. **(ICN)**

Ⓒ IV PHENOBARBITAL: **(Lederle)**

Elixir, 20 mg/5 ml in bottles of 1 pint.

Tablets, 15 and 30 mg in bottles of 1000 and 5000.

Ⓒ PHENOBARBITAL: **(Lilly)**
Elixir, 20 mg/5 ml in bottles of 1 pint and 1 gallon.
Tablets, 15 and 30 mg in bottles of 100, 1000 and 5000 and in blister strips of 100 (10 x 10); 60 and 100 mg in bottles of 100 and 1000 and in blister strips of 100 (10 x 10).
Ⓒ PHENOBARBITAL: **(McKesson)**
Elixir, 20 mg/5 ml in bottles of 1 pint and 1 gallon.
Tablets, 16 and 32 mg in bottles of 1000 and 5000; 65 mg in bottles of 1000.
Ⓒ PHENOBARBITAL Elixir, 20 mg/5 ml in bottles of 1 gallon. **(Merrell-National)**
Ⓒ PHENOBARBITAL: **(Parke-Davis)**
Elixir, 20 mg/5 ml in bottles of 1 pint and 1 gallon and in unit-doses of 5 ml in cartons of 100.
Liquid, 100 mg/5 ml in unit-dose patient cups of 5 ml in cartons of 100.
Tablets, 15, 30, 60 and 100 mg in bottles of 1000 and in unit-dose packages of 100 (10 x 10).
Ⓒ PHENOBARBITAL: **(Philips Roxane)**
Elixir, 20 mg/5 ml in bottles of 1 gallon and in unit-dose patient cups of 5 ml in cartons of 100 (10 x 10).
Tablets, 15, 30, 60 and 100 mg in bottles of 1000 and in unit-dose blister packs of 100.
Ⓒ PHENOBARBITAL Elixir, 20 mg/5 ml in bottles of 1 gallon. **(Upjohn)**
Ⓒ PHENOBARBITAL: **(Wyeth)**
Elixir, 20 mg/5 ml in bottles of 1 gallon and in Redipak® (unit-dose) of 5 ml in cartons of 25.
Tablets, 15, 30, and 100 mg in Redipak® (unit-dose) of 25 and 100; 60 mg in Redipak (unit-dose) of 25.
Ⓒ SEDADROPS® Liquid, 16 mg/ml in bottles of 30 ml with dropper. **(Merrell-National)**
Ⓒ SK-PHENOBARBITAL™ Tablets, 15 and 30 mg in bottles of 1000. **(Smith Kline & French)**

Phenobarbital Sodium

Ⓒ LUMINAL® SODIUM Injection, 130 mg/ml in ampuls of 1 ml. **(Winthrop)**
Ⓒ PHENOBARBITAL SODIUM Powder for Injection in ampuls containing 120 mg. **(Lilly)**
Ⓒ PHENOBARBITAL SODIUM Injection, 60 and 130 mg/ml in Tubex® (disposable syringes) of 1 ml in Temp-R-Tel® (tamper-resistant) packages of 10. **(Wyeth)**

PHENOLSULFONPHTHALEIN

Chemical Name: α-Hydroxy-α,α-*bis*(*p*-hydroxyphenyl)-*o*-toluenesulfonic acid γ-sultone.

Description: Phenolsulfonphthalein is a nonirritating dye, rapidly absorbed after intramuscular injection and excreted unchanged chiefly in the urine. Following intramuscular injection, 40 to 50% of the dye is eliminated in the urine in the first hour and 60 to 75% at the end of 2 hours. After intravenous injection, 25 to 45% is eliminated in 15 minutes, 50 to 65% in 30 minutes and 65 to 80% after 1 hour. Excretion of the dye is diminished in the presence of cardiac failure, particularly after intramuscular injection.

The sensitivity test requires that 0.1 ml of a 1:100 dilution of dye be injected intradermally. Patients who are sensitive will show a clear-cut pseudopodia within 15 to 20 minutes, and at 30 minutes; these will have blended into a more general edema without pseudopodia.

Indications: Diagnostic agent for determining kidney function.

Precautions: A lapse of at least 24 hours should be allowed between the PSP test and a prior BSP test. Patients with a history of allergy should be tested for sensitivity. It should be borne in mind that patients with gout or those receiving acidic drugs may show false impairment of renal function. An occasional idiosyncrasy may occur in some patients which may readily respond to treatment with antihistamines or epinephrine.

Dosage and Administration: The patient is first given a glass of water, preferably 1 to 1½ hours before injecting the dye. Just before injection, the patient's bladder should be completely emptied and 1 ml of the solution injected into the gluteal muscles, or intravenously. If given intramuscularly, collect the urine secreted during 1 hour and 10 minutes, also during a second hour, and estimate the amount of dye excreted, colorimetrically. If given intravenously, collections and estimations may be made at the end of 15 or 30 minutes or 1 hour.

Availability:
PHENOLSULFONPHTHALEIN Injection, 6 mg/ml in ampuls of 1 ml and in 1-ml disposable units. **(Hynson, Westcott & Dunning)**

THE PHENOTHIAZINES

Description: The phenothiazines are derived from a 3-ringed molecule in which 2 benzene rings are linked by a sulfur atom and a nitrogen atom. The members of the group differ according to the nature of the substituents at C_2 and C_{10} which influences not only their potency but also their pharmacologic activity respectively. Modification of the molecule alters the tranquilizing activity and toxicity to some extent, but in some instances has led to the synthesis of compounds that exhibited primarily antipruritic, antiemetic, antidepressant and, in the case of methotrimeprazine, analgesic activity.

The phenothiazines consist of 3 main groups: the aliphatic, piperidine and piperazinyl groups at C_{10}. Halogen, methoxy or thiomethyl groups are the substituents at C_2. All of the phenothiazines used in psychiatry contain a 3-carbon bridge between the ring and side chain nitrogen atoms. This is in contrast to the anticholinergic phenothiazines used in the treatment of parkinsonism and to the antihistaminic phenothiazines which have only 2 carbons separating the nitrogens.

The relation of their biochemical activity to their pharmacologic activity is not clear. The phenothiazines appear to inhibit the succinoxidase system, oxidative metabolism, phospholipid synthesis and cholinesterase activity; to depress glycolysis, the synthesis of glutamine and the incorporation of glycine into protein. Unlike the barbiturates and other sedative preparations used for the treatment of anxiety, the phenothiazines not only act upon the CNS but also exert significant effects upon organ systems throughout the body. Experimental and clinical studies suggest that they act on the hypothalamus and are believed to depress various components of the mesodiencephalic activating system (reticular formation) which controls basal metabolism and body temperatures, wakefulness, vasomotor tone, emesis, and hormonal balance, in addition to exerting a peripheral autonomic effect of varying degrees.

Reproduction studies in rodents have demonstrated a potential for embryotoxicity, increased neonatal mortality, and transfer of the drug in the mother's milk during lactation. Tests in offspring of drug-treated rodents showed decreased performance. The possibility of permanent neurological damage cannot be excluded. There is no adequate data regarding the significance of this in clinical reports.

Indications: The phenothiazines are used for the treatment of symptoms commonly associated with such neuropsychiatric conditions as psychomotor agitation, senile and arteriosclerotic psychoses, obsessive and phobic reactions, schizophrenia, manic-depressive states, neurodermatitis, melancholia, paranoid psychoses, and hysteria. They are useful in controlling emotional and anxiety-tension states, in mitigating the acute and chronic withdrawal symptoms of drug addiction and alcoholism, in treating various conditions of nausea and vomiting, in treating refractory hiccups, and for their potentiating effect on other drugs such as analgesics, general anesthetics, and muscle relaxants. It is well to bear in mind that the individual phenothiazines vary in their capabilities in different neuropsychiatric and other conditions.

Contraindications: The presence of bone marrow depression, blood dyscrasias, liver damage, or renal insufficiency precludes the use of phenothiazines. In circulatory collapse, comatose or greatly depressed states caused by CNS depressants, in patients taking large amounts of antihistamines, barbiturates, alcohol, narcotics, or analgesics, and in those with suspected or established subcortical brain damage with or without hypothalmic damage, since a severe hyperthermic reaction may occur. Patients with special medical disorders such as Parkinsons' disease, cerebral arteriosclerosis, coronary heart disease, mitral insufficiency or pheochromocytoma and those who have exhibited idiosyncrasy to other centrally acting drugs may experience severe reactions to these compounds. Also in those patients who previously had experienced phenothiazine-induced blood dyscrasias or severe allergic reactions, such as anaphylactoid reactions, asthma, or laryngeal edema. It should also be noted that severe hypertensive heart disease or hypotension is a contraindication to phenothiazine administration. Cross-sensitivity between the phenothiazines may occur.

Warnings: Patients in whom phenothiazine-induced jaundice has occurred should be given these compounds only when, in the judgment of the physician, they are considered essential to the welfare of the patient. Since drowsiness may occur, patients should be cautioned not to engage in activities requiring alertness or mechanical skill. They should also be warned that the effects of alcohol and other CNS depressants may be potentiated, and that these compounds may also counteract the antihypertensive effect of guanethidine and related compounds. Because of their anticholinergic action, the phenothiazines should be employed with considerable care in patients with a history of glaucoma or prostatic hypertrophy. Since potential adverse effects upon fetal development have not been confirmed, these drugs should not be used in women of childbearing potential, particularly during the first trimester of pregnancy, or in lactating women, unless in the judgment of the physician, the potential benefits outweigh the possible risks.

Precautions: The phenothiazines should be used cautiously, if at all, in patients with arteriosclerosis, cardiovascular disease or similar conditions, in those patients in whom any sudden change in blood pressure might lead to serious complications of the cardiovascular system, and in patients who have reacted unfavorably to other phenothiazine derivatives or to insulin or electroconvulsive therapy. Use with caution in instances where CNS depressants (opiates, analgesics, anesthetics, antihistamines, barbiturates, and alcohol) may be potentiated—the dose of a narcotic or barbiturate should be reduced 1/4 or 1/2 the usual amount when used together with phenothiazine derivatives; in patients with a history of convulsive disorders, and in patients with jaundice. Since the phenothiazines lower the convulsive threshold, routine caution is essential in patients with a history of epilepsy. However, they do not potentiate the anticonvulsant action of barbiturates; therefore, adequate dosage of the appropriate anticonvulsant (including barbiturates) must be maintained. If hypotension occurs, epinephrine is not recommended, since phenothiazines may reverse the epinephrine-pressor effects which may result in a paradoxical further lowering of blood pressure.

Cautious use is required in patients receiving atropine or related compounds because of additive anticholinergic effects; and in those exposed to extreme heat or organophosphate insecticides. Patients with acute or chronic respiratory impairment, particularly children, should receive special care because the cough reflex can be suppressed. Those phenothiazines with antiemetic effects may mask the signs and symptoms of overdosage of toxic drugs or may obscure conditions such as brain tumor or intestinal obstruction. The phenothiazines may produce some degree of physical dependence and abrupt withdrawal, particularly after high-dose therapy; also may cause gastritis, nausea and vomiting, dizziness and tremulousness. However, the incidence of these effects can usually be reduced by decreasing the dosage gradually. Patients on long-term therapy, especially those who are on high doses, should be evaluated periodically to decide whether the maintenance dosage could be lowered or drug therapy could be discontinued. Phenothiazines should be used with extreme care in patients with liver dysfunction, and in those with a history of ulcer disease; aggravation of preexisting peptic ulcer has been noted.

Close supervision of children with an acute illness or dehydration is advised, because of their greater susceptibility to dystonias associated with phenothiazine therapy. Overdosage should be avoided when phenothiazine derivatives are used concomitantly with other depressant drugs. Therapy with phenothiazine derivatives should be discontinued at least 5 days before elective surgical procedures on psychotic patients. Prolonged therapy with these compounds may produce white and yellowish granulations in the anterior capsule and adjoining subcapsular part of the lens and in the cornea. These changes do not appear to affect visual function but may terminate as lenticular opacities. Lactation, gynecomastia and other alterations in reproductive function may also occur with extended therapy.

Adverse Reactions: While certain of the side effects listed below are unquestionably due to the phenothiazines, others may possibly represent manifestations of the underlying psychiatric condition, concurrent disease, or joint action of the drug with other therapeutic agents. Side effects which may occur can be classified as follows: *Blood dyscrasias and liver disorders:* leukopenia, hemolytic anemia, agranulocytosis, purpura, pancytopenia, eosinophilia, cholestatic jaundice, and xanthomatous biliary cirrhosis. *Cardiovascular:* severe acute hypotension (particularly in patients with pheochromocytoma or mitral insufficiency), cardiac arrhythmias (including various degrees of A-V block, T-wave changes and paroxysmal tachycardias). *Extrapyramidal syndromes:* Parkinson-like syndrome manifested as tremors, rigidity, akinesia, shuffling gait, postural abnormalities, pill-rolling movements, mask-like facies, and excessive salivation. Dyskinesias, commonly involving muscles about the face and neck, such as protrusion of tongue, mandibular tics, difficulty in speaking and swallowing, oculogyric crisis, perioral spasm, torticollis, hyperextension of neck and trunk, clonic and tonic contraction of other muscle groups. Profuse sweating, pallor and fever may accompany these symptoms. Akathisia, as manifested by motor restlessness varying in intensity from a feeling of inner disquiet to inability to sit still or sleep; complete intolerance to inactivity.

Two of the 4 initial controlled studies suggested that side effects may occur with butaperazine somewhat more frequently than with other phenothiazines. The extrapyramidal side effects, as with all phenothiazines, generally appear to increase in frequency and sometimes in severity as the dose is increased. Such reactions are seldom serious and usually disappear within 1 or 2 days or less after the dose is reduced or the drug temporarily discontinued. However, irreversible dyskinesias have been reported with this class of drugs. An antiparkinsonian drug may be administered for more prompt control of extrapyramidal reactions. *Skin disorders:* erythema, eczema, exfoliative dermatitis, melanin pigmentation, and photosensitivity. *Endocrine imbalance:* delayed ovulation and menstruation, false pregnancy tests, amenorrhea, lactation, and increased libido in women; inhibition of ejaculation, gynecomastia and impotence in men. *Autonomic reactions:* dry mouth, nausea and vomiting, constipation, fecal impaction, paralytic ileus, blurred vision, miosis, mydriasis, increase in appetite (weight gain), peripheral edema, nasal congestion, tachycardia, change in body temperature (up or down), bladder paralysis, hyperglycemia, hypoglycemia and glycosuria. *Ocular reactions:* aggravation of glaucoma, mydriasis, pigmentary retinopathy, corneal and lens deposits and photophobia. *Allergic reactions:* urticaria, asthma, laryngeal edema, and anaphylaxis. *Miscellaneous:* weight gain, fainting, dizziness, drowsiness, convulsive seizures, depression, insomnia, fatigue, edema, paradoxical exacerbation of psychosis, and possibly teratogenic effects. Hyperreflexia has been reported in the newborn when a phenothiazine was used during pregnancy. Grand mal seizures, catatonic-like states, psychotic symptoms, cerebral edema, and abnormalities of cerebrospinal fluid proteins have been observed. **Note:** Occasionally, sudden death has been reported in patients who have been taking phenothiazines. In some patients death appeared to be due to cardiac arrest or to asphyxia due to failure of the cough reflex. In some the cause could not be determined nor could it be established that death was due to phenothiazine therapy. Available evidence indicates a relationship between phenothiazine therapy and the occurrence of systemic lupus erythematosus-like syndrome.

Tardive dyskinesia may appear in some patients on long-term therapy or may occur after therapy with these compounds has been discontinued. The risk appears to be greater in elderly patients on high-dose therapy, especially female patients. The symptoms are persistent and in some patients appear to be irreversible. The syndrome is characterized by rhythmical involuntary movements of the tongue, face, mouth or jaw (e.g., protrusion of the tongue, puffing of cheeks, puckering of mouth, chewing movements). These may be accompanied by involuntary movements of the extremities. There is no known treatment for this condition; antiparkinsonian agents usually do not alleviate the symptoms. It is advised that the phenothiazine agent be discontinued if the above phenomena appear. If treatment is reinstituted, or dosage of the particular drug increased, or another drug substituted, the syndrome may be masked. It has been reported that fine vermicular movements of the tongue may be an early sign of the syndrome, and that the full-blown syndrome may not develop if medication is withdrawn when lingual vermiculation appears. Elderly patients, especially female patients, and probably all patients over 50 years of age should be carefully observed.

Dosage and Administration: The dose of the phenothiazine derivatives varies with the preparation, potency, administration and the clinical use (i.e., psychosis versus neurosis). They may be given *orally, rectally, intramuscularly, intravenously* and occasionally *subcutaneously.* Dosage will also depend upon the severity of the condition and the response to treatment. Initial doses should be small and then gradually increased until the desired therapeutic response is obtained. When response is satisfactory, dosage should be reduced to the smallest amount necessary to maintain relief of symptoms. In general, dosages in the lower range are usually sufficient for most elderly patients. Since they appear to be more susceptible to hypotension and neuromuscular reactions, such patients should be observed closely, and any increase in their dosage schedule should be made with utmost care. These recommendations also apply to individuals who are debilitated or emaciated, or who are considered to be poor-risk patients. Oral treatment should replace parenteral as soon as possible. Abrupt withdrawal of the drug is not advocated especially in patients who have been receiving large doses for extended periods. Intramuscular injection should be made deep into a large muscle mass and the patient should be lying down and should remain in this position for at least 1 hour after the injection. Since parenteral administration of phenothiazines may cause postural hypotension, this mode of administration should be reserved for hospitalized patients. Some clinicians recommend simultaneous administration of antiparkinsonian agents in order to avoid extrapyramidal reaction.

The preceding discussed briefly the physiologic, clinical and therapeutic similarities of the phenothiazines as a group. In the discussions that follow, each individual monograph deals specifically with each of the following:

- Acetophenazine Maleate
- Butaperazine Maleate
- Carphenazine Maleate
- Chlorpromazine Hydrochloride
- Ethopropazine Hydrochloride
- Fluphenazine
- Mesoridazine
- Methdilazine Hydrochloride
- Methotrimeprazine Hydrochloride
- Perphenazine
- Piperacetazine
- Prochlorperazine
- Promazine Hydrochloride
- Promethazine Hydrochloride
- Propiomazine Hydrochloride
- Thiethylperazine Maleate
- Thioridazine Hydrochloride
- Trifluoperazine
- Triflupromazine Hydrochloride
- Trimeprazine Tartrate

ACETOPHENAZINE MALEATE

Chemical Name: 10-[3-[4-(2-Hydroxyethyl)-1-piperazinyl]propyl]phenothiazin-2-yl methyl ketone dimaleate.

Description: Acetophenazine maleate is a phenothiazine of the piperazine group. Although its precise mechanism of action has not been established, it appears to act at all levels of the CNS as well as on other organ systems.

Indications: Management of manifestations of psychotic disorders. It has been shown to be ineffective in the management of behavioral disorders in patients with mental retardation.

Contraindications: In comatose or severely depressed states due to CNS depressants, bone marrow depression, hypersensitivity, and cross sensitivity to other phenothiazines.

Warnings: Acetophenazine may impair the mental and/or physical abilities required for the performance of hazardous tasks that require alertness or skill; the patient should be cautioned accordingly. The use of alcohol should be avoided since additive effects and hypotension may occur. The possible benefits must be weighed against the potential hazards when this drug is administered to pregnant or lactating women or to women of childbearing potential. Safety and effectiveness in children have not been established; therefore, the drug is not recommended for the pediatric age group.

Adverse Reactions: Extrapyramidal symptoms are more commonly noted, but sedative effects, jaundice, and blood dyscrasias are less frequently seen with acetophenazine maleate.

For other indications, contraindications, warnings, precautions and adverse reactions, see general statement.

Dosage and Administration: *Orally.* The usual adult dosage is 20 mg 3 times daily. Dosage ranges between 40 and 80 mg daily in divided doses. For hospitalized patients, the optimum total daily dosage ranges from 80 to 120 mg administered in divided doses. Certain hospitalized patients with severe schizophrenia have received doses as high as 400 to 600 mg daily.

Availability:
TINDAL® Tablets, 20 mg in bottles of 100. **(Schering)**

BUTAPERAZINE MALEATE

Chemical Name: 1-[10-[3-(4-Methyl-1-piperazinyl)-propyl]phenothiazin-2-yl]-1-butanone dimaleate.

Description: Butaperazine maleate, a member of the piperazine group of phenothiazine tranquilizers, is closely related structurally to prochlorperazine, differing only in the substitution of a butyryl group for the chloro group at the 2 position of the latter compound. Butaperazine maleate occurs as a yellow, crystalline powder slightly soluble in water and in alcohol.

Indications: Butaperazine is a potent psychotherapeutic agent indicated only in the management of chronic schizophrenic patients who are under close psychiatric supervision. The following target symptoms have been shown to respond to butaperazine therapy: hallucinations, delusions, hyperactivity, agitation, aggression, hostility, assaultiveness, excitement, destructiveness, anxiety, tension and confusion. The drug currently is not recommended for the management of psychoneurosis, ordinary nervous disorders, or for children under 12 years of age.

Contraindications: Comatose patients, especially those whose depression is due to barbiturates, narcotics, alcohol, analgesics, antihistamines, or other drugs. The drug should not be used in the presence of circulatory collapse, bone-marrow depression, or in patients with a history of jaundice, blood dyscrasias or hypersensitivity related to other phenothiazines.

Warnings: Those taking this drug should not operate a motor vehicle or hazardous machinery or engage in operations which require alertness. Patients should be advised against the use of alcohol during treatment with this or any phenothiazine derivative. When butaperazine is combined with barbiturates, analgesics, narcotics, antihistamines, or other CNS-acting drugs, the dosage of both should be reduced to 1/2 the conventional dosage. Since safe use of this drug during pregnancy has not been established, its use in women who are or who may become pregnant is not recommended currently unless, in the opinion of the physician, potential therapeutic benefits clearly outweigh the possible risks.

Precautions: Butaperazine should be used with caution in patients who are about to receive general anesthesia. As with other phenothiazines, it should be used with caution in patients with glaucoma, cardiovascular disease, hypotension, or epilepsy. Therapy in elderly and debilitated patients should be initiated with a low dose. If hypotension occurs, the patient should be placed in a recumbent position and, if a vasopressor is indicated, levoarterenol or phenylephrine should be used. Epinephrine is contraindicated because of its tendency to decrease blood pressure in the presence of phenothiazines. Blood counts and reliable liver function studies are generally advisable at periodic intervals. Because of its antiemetic effect, butaperazine may mask the symptoms of drug overdosage, intestinal obstruction or brain tumor. If extrapyramidal manifestations appear, they may be relieved by dosage reduction, an antiparkinsonian drug, or sedation. When resuming butaperazine therapy after an interval without the drug, a lower starting dose should be employed. Exaggerated response to atropine, environmental heat and phosphorus insecticides have been reported in association with phenothiazine therapy.

Adverse Reactions: Studies have shown that side effects occur more frequently with butaperazine than with the other phenothiazines. The extrapyramidal side effects generally appear to increase in frequency and sometimes in severity as the dose is increased.

For other indications, contraindications, warnings, precautions, and adverse reactions, see general statement.

Dosage and Administration: *Orally.* For the average adult, 5 to 10 mg 3 times daily initially and increased by increments of 5 to 10 mg every few days until the maximal response is achieved. Dosage schedules should be adjusted to the needs of the individual patient. Dosage in excess of 100 mg/day is not recommended, nor should the drug be used at any dosage in children under 12 years of age until the drug's safety in this age group has been established. Dosages should be adjusted weekly in the early stages of therapy. If mild or moderate side effects occur, dosage should be decreased gradually to a maintenance level and/or an antiparkinsonian agent added in appropriate doses. After discharge from the hospital or after acute symptoms have subsided, patients may be kept on a maintenance dosage of 1/4 to 1/2 the dose required during the acute phase. The effective dosage will vary with the severity and duration of the patient's illness. Patients maintained on butaperazine should be seen at regular intervals to minimize the occurrence of a relapse. Best results are obtained when patients are carefully supervised and drug therapy is continued for extended periods.

Availability:
REPOISE® Film-coated Tablets (as maleate), 5 mg (yellow), 10 mg (green) and 25 mg (orange) in bottles of 100 and 500. **(Robins)**

CARPHENAZINE MALEATE

Chemical Name: 1-[10-[3-[4-(2-Hydroxyethyl)-1-piperazinyl]propyl]phenothiazine-2-yl]-1-pro-panone dimaleate.

Description: Carphenazine maleate, a relatively short-acting, psychopharmacologic agent, is a piperazine-type phenothiazine compound. Its spectrum of activity is similar to that of perphenazine, trifluoperazine and fluphenazine. Carphenazine maleate occurs as a yellow powder that is slightly soluble both in water and in alcohol.

Although its exact mode of action has not been determined, it appears to act at all levels of the CNS and on multiple organ systems. Teratogenic effects were not observed in rats and rabbits given 7.5 and 20 times the clinical therapeutic dose.

Indications: Relief of symptoms of schizophrenia such as agitation, anxiety, and tension.

Contraindications: In comatose or greatly depressed states due to CNS depressants including excessive psychomotor agitation; prior hypersensitivity reaction including jaundice and blood dyscrasias, cross sensitivity to other phenothiazines, and bone marrow depression.

Warnings: Since carphenazine may impair mental and/or physical abilities, patients should be cautioned not to engage in any activities that require alertness or skill. The therapeutic benefits must be weighed against the potential hazards when carphenazine is administered to pregnant or lactating women or to women of childbearing potential. This drug is not recommended for use in the pediatric age group since safety and effectiveness have not been established. The use of alcohol should be avoided since additive effects and hypotension may occur.

Precautions: Because of carphenazine's anticholinergic properties, it should be used with caution in patients who might be exposed to extreme heat or who are receiving atropine or related drugs; also in those who might be exposed to phosphorus insecticides. Carphenazine's antiemetic effect noted in animal studies may mask signs of overdosage of toxic drugs and obscure conditions such as intestinal obstruction and brain tumor.

Adverse Reactions: Extrapyramidal symptoms are more commonly noted, but sedative effects, jaundice, and blood dyscrasias are less frequently seen with carphenazine maleate.

For the mode of action, other indications, contraindications, precautions and adverse reactions associated with phenothiazine therapy, see general statement.

Dosage and Administration: *Orally.* The usual adult dosage is 12.5 to 25 mg (or 50 mg in chronic patients) 2 or 3 times daily, increasing gradually at weekly intervals until maximum response is obtained. Dosage may then be reduced to the lowest effective maintenance level. Patients with acute symptomatology may respond to a dose of 100 mg daily; doses above 400 mg daily are not recommended.

Availability:
PROKETAZINE® Tablets, 12.5 mg (yellow), 25 mg (orange) and 50 mg (pink) in bottles of 50.
(Wyeth)

CHLORPROMAZINE HYDROCHLORIDE

Chemical Name: 2-Chloro-10-(3-dimethylaminopropyl)phenothiazine hydrochloride.

Description: Chlorpromazine hydrochloride is a dimethylamine derivative of phenothiazine. It occurs as a grayish-white, water-soluble powder; a 5% solution has a pH of approximately 4.5. Unlike promethazine, to which it is closely related chemically, chlorpromazine produces inadequate antihistaminic action.

The drug is readily absorbed from the gastrointestinal tract and is distributed throughout the tissues with highest concentration appearing in the lungs, liver and spleen. It undergoes sulfoxidation and partial or complete demethylation to form nonpolar metabolites which are excreted in the urine. It also undergoes oxidation at the 3 and 7 position of the 3-ring molecule and conjugation with glucuronic acid. Following its ingestion, trace amounts of the free drug and its metabolites may be detected in the body for as long as 6 to 12 months.

Indications: Chlorpromazine is used in general medical practice in the management of symptoms of psychotic disorders and those of manic-depressive states; for the control of nausea and vomiting, acute intermittent porphyria, restlessness and apprehension prior to surgery, and excessive anxiety, tension and agitation as seen in neurosis; for the relief of intractable hiccups, and as an adjunct in the treatment of tetanus. May also be useful in mild alcoholic states to control agitation, tension, nausea and vomiting; in children with moderate to severe agitation, hyperactivity or aggressiveness, in patients with cancer as an adjuvant to control apprehension and suffering, as a means of reducing (by potentiation) the amounts of narcotic, sedatives and anesthetics required.

Contraindications: Comatose states, presence of large amounts of CNS depressants, and bone marrow depression.

Warnings: Caution should be exercised when chlorpromazine is administered to children for the treatment of vomiting. Generally, antiemetics are not recommended for use in treating uncomplicated short-term vomiting in children or vomiting of unknown etiology, but only for those cases in which the vomiting is prolonged and of known etiology. The possible development of drug-induced extrapyramidal symptoms may confuse the diagnosis of Reye's syndrome or other encephalopathy. Although unconfirmed, some suspicion exists that because chlorpromazine is potentially hepatotoxic, it may contribute to or adversely affect the course of Reye's syndrome, and its use should be avoided in suspected cases.

Precautions: Chlorpromazine does *not* intensify the anticonvulsant action of barbiturates or other such drugs. Therefore, when used together with this phenothiazine, the dosage of the anticonvulsant agent should not be reduced, instead the initial dose of chlorpromazine should be lower, and should then be increased as needed.

Adverse Reactions: Those which may be experienced with chlorpromazine include mild to moderate drowsiness; jaundice (the clinical characteristic resembles infectious hepatitis, with laboratory features of obstructive jaundice, rather than those of parenchymal damage); agranulocytosis, eosinophilia, leukopenia, hemolytic anemia, thrombocytopenic purpura, and, rarely, pancytopenia; postural hypotension, simple tachycardia, syncope and dizziness, and EKG changes. Sudden death, apparently due to cardiac arrest, has been reported, but whether or not it was drug-induced has not been established. Also noted were such reactions as neuromuscular (extrapyramidal) reactions, closely resembling parkinsonism, hyperreflexia in the newborn, persistent tardive dyskinesia; psychotic symptoms and catatonic-like states, convulsive seizures (petit mal and grand mal), abnormality of the cerebrospinal fluid proteins; allergic reactions of a mild urticarial type or photosensitivity, contact dermatitis; endocrine disorders manifested by lactation and moderate breast engorgement, false-positive pregnancy tests, amenorrhea and gynecomastia, hyperglycemia, hypoglycemia and glycosuria; occasional dry mouth, nasal congestion; constipation; adynamic ileus; urinary retention; miosis and mydriasis; skin pigmentation and ocular changes may occur on long-term therapy. Other complications that may occur include mild fever usually after large intramuscular doses; hyperpyrexia; increases in appetite and weight; peripheral edema; and a systemic lupus erythematosus-like syndrome.

For other contraindications, warnings, precautions and adverse reactions, see general statement.

Dosage and Administration: *Orally, intramuscularly, intravenously* or *rectally,* in doses according to the condition being treated and the response of the patient. While 100 mg to 1 gm may be necessary to treat severe emotional disorders, 25 mg may control vomiting. For *agitated psychotics,* the initial dosage is 25 to 50 mg orally 3 times daily, gradually increased until the desired effect is achieved. Daily dosage of 200 mg is not unusual, and some patients may require 800 mg daily. The rectal dose is usually twice the oral dose. The usual intramuscular dose is 25 to 50 mg 1 to 3 times daily. Intramuscular injections should be administered by deep slow injection into the upper outer quadrant of the buttock. Intravenous injection is recommended only for severe hiccups and surgery. Subcutaneous injection should be avoided. Children's dosage is 0.5 mg/kg of body weight every 4 to 6 hours. The maximal daily dose is 50 mg for children under 5 years of age, 75 mg for children 5 to 12 years of age. Higher doses may be necessary for psychiatric cases.

Availability:

Chlorpromazine Hydrochloride

Concentrate, 30 and 100 mg/ml in bottles of 240 ml. **(Lederle)**

Injection, 25 mg/ml in disposable syringes (Tubex®) of 1 and 2 ml with needle. **(Wyeth)**
Syrup, 10 mg/ml in bottles of 120 ml. **(Lederle)**
Tablets, 50 mg in bottles of 1000. **(Elder)**
Tablets, 10, 25, 50, 100 and 200 in bottles of 100 and 1000; 50 and 100 mg in bottles of 120; 200 mg in unit-dose packages of 100. **(Lederle)**
Tablets, 10, 25, 50, 100 and 200 mg in bottles of 100 and 1000 and in unit-dose packages of 100. **(Philips Roxane)**
CHLOR-PZ® Tablets, 10, 25, 50, 100 and 200 mg in bottles of 100 and 1000. **(USV)**
PROMAPAR® Tablets, 10, 25, 50, 100 and 200 mg in bottles of 100 and 1000 and in unit-dose packages of 100. **(Parke-Davis)**
THORAZINE®: **(Smith Kline & French)**
Injection, 25 mg/ml in ampuls of 1 and 2 ml and in multiple-dose vials of 10 ml.
Liquid Concentrate, 30 mg/ml in bottles of 120 ml and 1 gallon; 100 mg/ml in bottles of 240 ml.
Spansule® Capsules (timed-disintegration), 30, 75, 150 and 200 mg in bottles of 50 and 500; 300 mg in bottles of 50. All potencies in single-unit packages of 100.
Suppositories, 25 and 100 mg in cartons of 12.
Syrup, 10 mg/5 ml in bottles of 120 ml.
Tablets, 10, 25, 50, 100 and 200 mg in bottles of 100 and 1000 and in blister strips of 10 tablets in cartons of 10.

ETHOPROPAZINE HYDROCHLORIDE

Chemical Name: 10-[2-(Diethylamino)propyl]phenothiazine hydrochloride.

Description: Ethopropazine hydrochloride is a phenothiazine derivative possessing both atropine-like and antihistaminic activity. It exhibits ganglionic blocking action with depression of the CNS system. Ethopropazine hydrochloride occurs as white to off-white, water-soluble crystals that are only slightly soluble in alcohol.

The drug exerts significant parasympatholytic actions among a wide variety of pharmacologic effects. Although its precise mode of action has not been determined, it appears to exert a marked influence upon the neuromuscular symptoms of Parkinson's disease.

It differs from other phenothiazine compounds in that it does not potentiate CNS depressants nor does it have antiemetic action. Ethopropazine may be used either alone or in combination with such drugs as atropine, stramonium, dextroamphetamine and the antihistamines.

Oral administration of a single dose produces significant blood levels within ½ to 1 hour; therapeutic action continues for about 4 hours.

Indications: In parkinsonism and drug-induced extrapyramidal symptoms.

Contraindications: In patients with glaucoma or prostatic hypertrophy.

Warnings: Safe use during pregnancy has not been established; therefore, it is not recommended unless the expected benefits outweigh the possible risks. Patients receiving this drug should be cautioned not to engage in hazardous occupations that require alertness or skill.

Precautions: Cautious use is required in patients for whom parasympatholytic action would be undesirable. Antiparkinsonian agents, when used to treat phenothiazine- or reserpine-induced extrapyramidal reactions in patients with mental disorders, may exacerbate the mental symptoms and precipitate a toxic psychosis. Permanent extrapyramidal symptoms have been noted with prolonged phenothiazine therapy, and the possibility that ethopropazine may mask the development of these symptoms has not been established.

Adverse Reactions: The most common effects reported are drowsiness, dizziness, and a cerebral reaction consisting of fogginess, inability to think, lassitude, forgetfulness and confusion. Parasympatholytic effects such as dry mouth, nausea, vomiting, blurred vision, diplopia, constipation and urinary retention are rarely severe and either disappear as therapy is continued or diminish as the dosage is reduced. Less commonly observed effects include epigastric discomfort, muscular cramping, paresthesia, a sensation of heaviness of limbs, skin rash and, with high doses, transient hypotension. The following are possible on theoretical grounds: electroencephalographic slowing, electrocardiographic abnormalities (e.g., tachycardia), rarely hematologic reactions (agranulocytosis, pancytopenia, purpura), certain endocrinologic disturbances, jaundice, pigmentation of the cornea, lens, retina and skin.

Dosage and Administration: *Orally.* Initially, dosage is usually 50 mg once or twice daily, increased gradually if necessary. Patients with mild to moderate symptoms are frequently controlled with 100 to 400 mg daily. Severe cases may require further gradual increases to 500 or 600 mg or more daily.

Availability:
PARSIDOL® Tablets, 10, 50 and 100 mg in bottles of 100. **(Warner-Chilcott)**

FLUPHENAZINE

Chemical Name: 4-[3-[2-(Trifluoromethyl)phenothiazin-10-yl]propyl]-1-piperazine ethanol.

Description: Fluphenazine is a trifluoromethyl phenothiazine derivative intended for the management of schizophrenia. It is closely related chemically to trifluoperazine. On a weight basis, it is considered the most potent of all the phenothiazines.

Although the mechanism of action of fluphenazine is not known, it appears to be active at all levels of the CNS as well as on organ systems. Experimental and clinical studies suggest that fluphenazine has a more potent and more prolonged duration of action than either triflupromazine or chlorpromazine. Because of its chemical structure, hypotension is less likely to occur, and it appears to have less sedative effects; also it does not potentiate CNS depressants and anesthetics to the same degree as do some of the other phenothiazines.

The esterification of fluphenazine markedly prolongs the drug's duration of effect without unduly attenuating its beneficial action. The onset of action generally appears between 24 and 72 hours after injection, and the effects of the drug on psychotic symptoms become significant within 48 to 96 hours. Amelioration of symptoms then continues for 1 to 3 weeks or longer, with an average duration of effect of about 2 weeks.

Indications: Management of manifestations of schizophrenia. The drug is of no value in the management of behavioral problems in patients who are mentally retarded.

Contraindications: In patients with suspected or established subcortical brain damage, with or without hypothalamic damage, since a hyperthermic reaction with temperatures in excess of 104° F may occur. This reaction may be delayed up to 14 to 16 hours after the drug has been administered. It is recommended that the body be totally covered with ice; the use of antipyretics may be helpful. Parenteral use is contraindicated in patients who are comatose or who are in severely depressed states. The presence of blood dyscrasias, liver damage or renal insufficiency precludes the use of this drug.

Precautions: The effects of atropine may be potentiated in some patients receiving fluphenazine because of added anticholinergic effects. Special caution is advised in patients with mitral insufficiency or other cardiovascular diseases and pheochromocytoma. The possibility of liver damage, pigmentary retinopathy, lenticular and corneal deposits, and development of irreversible dyskinesia should be considered when patients are on prolonged therapy. Parenteral administration should be undertaken at the direction of a physician experienced in the clinical use of psychotropic drugs, particularly phenothiazine derivatives. Furthermore, facilities should be readily available for periodic checking of hepatic function, renal function, and the hematopoietic system. The physician should be alert for the possible development of "silent pneumonias."

For other contraindications, warnings, precautions and adverse reactions, see general statement.

Dosage and Administration: *Orally, intramuscularly* or *subcutaneously.* Depending on the severity and duration of symptoms, the total oral or parenteral daily dosage for *adult* psychotic patients may range from 2.5 to 10 mg and should be divided and administered at intervals of 6 to 8 hours. The smallest amount that will produce the desired results must be carefully determined for each patient. The *oral* dose is usually 2 to 3 times the *parenteral* dose. Daily maintenance *oral* doses of 1 to 5 mg are often given as a single daily dose. For geriatric patients, the suggested initial *oral* dose is 1 to 2.5 mg daily, adjusted according to the response of the patient. *Parenterally,* a dose of 12.5 to 25 mg every 4 weeks of the *decanoate* ester or 25 mg every 2 weeks of the *enanthate* ester is recommended for most patients.

Availability:

Fluphenazine Decanoate

PROLIXIN DECANOATE Injection, 25 mg/ml (in sesame oil) in Unimatic® syringes (single-dose) of 1 ml and in vials of 5 ml. **(Squibb)**

Fluphenazine Enanthate

PROLIXIN® Injection, 25 mg/ml in Unimatic® syringes (single-dose) of 1 ml and in vials of 5 ml. **(Squibb)**

Fluphenazine Hydrochloride

PERMITIL®: **(Schering)**

Chronotab® Tablets (repeat-action), 1 mg in bottles of 60 and 250.

Oral Concentrate, 5 mg/ml in bottles of 120 ml with calibrated dropper.

Tablets, 0.25, 2.5 and 5 mg in bottles of 50; 10 mg in bottles of 1000.

PROLIXIN®: **(Squibb)**

Elixir, 0.5 mg/ml in bottles of 60 ml (with dropper) and 1 pint.

Injection (IM only), 2.5 mg/ml in multiple-dose vials of 10 ml.

Tablets, 1, 2.5, 5, and 10 mg in bottles of 50 and 500; 2.5 and 5 mg in Unimatic® (single-dose) cartons of 100.

MESORIDAZINE

Chemical Name: 10-[2(1-Methyl-2-piperidyl)ethyl]-2-methylsulfinyl)-phenothiazine [as the besylate].

Description: Mesoridazine is the besylate salt of an intermediate oxidation product of thioridazine metabolism. It differs structurally from thioridazine in that a sulfoxide group is attached to the thiomethyl group at position 2 in the side chain of the phenothiazine nucleus. Mesoridazine besylate occurs as a pale-yellow, crystalline powder freely soluble in water, chloroform or methanol, and sparingly soluble in alcohol. The parenteral solution is adjusted to pH 4 to 5, is photosensitive and should therefore be protected from light.

The drug is well absorbed from muscle or the gastrointestinal tract. Following oral administration, a peak blood level is reached in about 2 hours which persists for 4 to 6 hours. Following intramuscular injection, a peak blood level is reached in 30 minutes and is maintained for 6 to 8 hours. The drug is excreted in the bile, urine and feces. Urinary and fecal excretion is slow and still incomplete 5 days after administration.

The pharmacodynamic spectrum of mesoridazine is similar to that of other phenothiazines, particularly that of chlorpromazine and thioridazine.

Indications: Treatment of schizophrenia, behavioral problems in mental deficiency and chronic brain syndrome, acute and chronic alcoholism, and psychoneurotic manifestations.

Contraindications: Hypersensitivity to the drug, severe depression of the CNS or comatose states from any cause.

Warnings: Phenothiazines should be used with caution in those patients whose activities require complete alertness; dosage should be increased gradually. Mesoridazine may be used during pregnancy only when the anticipated benefits outweigh the potential risks to mother and fetus. Use of the drug in children under 12 years of age is *not* recommended. It is well to bear in mind that phenothiazines may potentiate CNS depressants as well as atropine and insecticides containing phosphorus.

Precautions: While not presently attributable to mesoridazine, ocular changes have been observed with other phenothiazines. To avoid the possible hypotensive effects, parenteral administration should be reserved for bedfast patients or for acute ambulatory cases, and patients should be kept in a supine position for at least 30 minutes after injection. Leukopenia and/or agranulocytosis have been associated with phenothiazine therapy. A single case of transient granulocytopenia has been reported with this drug. Since convulsive seizures have been known to occur, patients receiving anticonvulsant medication should be maintained on that regimen while receiving mesoridazine.

For additional contraindications, warnings and precautions associated with phenothiazines, see general statement.

Adverse Reactions: Compared with other phenothiazines, mesoridazine exhibits a low incidence of reactions. Except for tremor and rigidity, reactions in general were the result of relatively high doses taken early in therapy. The following have been reported: *CNS*—drowsiness, Parkinson's syndrome, dizziness, weakness, tremor, restlessness, ataxia, dystonia, rigidity, slurred speech, akathisia, and motor reactions (opisthotonos). *Autonomic*—dry mouth, nausea and vomiting, fainting, nasal congestion, photophobia, constipation and blurred vision. *Endocrine*—inhibited ejaculation and lactation. *Dermatologic*—rash, pruritus, hypertrophied papillae of tongue, and angioneurotic edema. *Cardiovascular*—hypotension, cardiac arrhythmia. Changes in the electrocardiogram apparently due to altered myocardial polarization have been observed in some patients. These include prolonged Q-T interval, lowered and inverted T wave and the appearance of a change tentatively identified as a bifid T or U wave. They are noticed in patients receiving other phenothiazines, but do not appear to be related to actual myocardial damage.

For other reactions associated with phenothiazines generally, see general statement.

Dosage and Administration: *Orally. Schizophrenia:* initially, 50 mg 3 times daily; optimal dosage range is 100 to 400 mg daily. *Organic Brain Disorders:* initially, 25 mg 3 times daily; optimal dosage range is 75 to 300 mg daily. *Alcoholism:* initially, 25 mg twice daily; optimal dosage range is 50 to 200 mg daily. *Psychoneuroses:* initially, 10 mg 3 times daily; optimal dosage range is 30 to 150 mg daily. *Intramuscularly,* 25 mg initially, repeated in 1/2 to 1 hour if necessary; optimal dosage range is 25 to 200 mg daily.

Availability:
SERENTIL®: **(Boehringer Ingelheim)**
Concentrate, 25 mg/ml in bottles of 120 ml with graduated dropper.
Injection, 25 mg/ml in ampuls of 1 ml.
Tablets, 10, 25, 50 and 100 mg in bottles of 100.

METHDILAZINE HYDROCHLORIDE

Chemical Name: 10-[(1-Methyl-3-pyrrolidinyl)methyl] phenothiazine hydrochloride.

Description: Methdilazine hydrochloride is a phenothiazine derivative possessing antihistaminic and antipruritic activity. It has been postulated that the antipruritic action may be due to the analgesic action of the phenothiazine drugs.

Indications: Symptomatic relief of pruritic symptoms in urticaria.

Contraindications: Idiosyncrasy or hypersensitivity to phenothiazine drugs; jaundice or a history of jaundice; CNS depression due to barbiturates, alcohol, narcotics, and analgesics; asthma; narrow-angle glaucoma; prostatic hypertrophy; stenosing peptic ulcer; pyloroduodenal obstruction; bladder neck obstruction; premature or newborn infants; acutely ill or dehydrated children, and concomitant use with other phenothiazines, antihistaminics, or MAO inhibitors.

Warnings: Patients should be warned not to engage in any activity requiring alertness or skill since drowsiness may occur. Safe use of methdilazine during pregnancy has not been established; therefore, the therapeutic benefits must be weighed against the potential hazards to the fetus. Overdosage or accidental ingestion of large quantities in children may result in convulsions or death. Special care is required when methdilazine is given to elderly patients who generally are more prone to untoward reactions. If neuromuscular reactions occur, the drug should be withdrawn and not reinstated.

Precautions: The potential atropine-like effects of this drug should be considered before prescribing for each patient, especially for those with inactive asthma. Cautious use is required in patients receiving CNS depressants, opiates, analgesics, barbiturates and sedatives, as potentiation of their effects may occur.

Adverse Reactions: Drowsiness, dizziness, gastrointestinal disturbances, jitteriness, dryness of the mucous membranes, headache, and skin rash have been reported. Rarely observed were extrapyramidal symptoms such as tremors, spasticity, painful constriction of skeletal muscles, and dystonias.

Dosage and Administration: *Orally,* 2 to 4 times daily; adults, 8 mg and children over 3 years of age, 4 mg. Chewable tablets should be chewed and swallowed promptly.

Availability:
TACARYL®: **(Westwood)**
Chewable Tablets, 3.6 mg in bottles of 100.
Syrup, 4 mg/5 ml in bottles of 1 pint.
Tablets, 8 mg in bottles of 100.

METHOTRIMEPRAZINE HYDROCHLORIDE

Chemical Name: 2-Methoxy-10 (2-methyl-3-dimethylaminopropyl)-phenothiazine hydrochloride.

Description: Methotrimeprazine is a phenothiazine derivative structurally related to trimeprazine. It differs structurally from the latter only in the presence of a methoxy group at the 2 position on the phenothiazine nucleus. It occurs as a white, crystalline powder freely soluble in water and in alcohol.

Methotrimeprazine, when administered parenterally, exerts analgesic and sedative effects. Its analgesic effect in chronic pain is comparable to that of morphine and meperidine, without any evidence of habituation, addiction or dependence with large doses and with long-term administration. In addition, it also exhibits antihistaminic, anticholinergic and antiadrenalin activity. The drug is actively metabolized into sulfoxides and glucuronic conjuates and largely excreted into the urine as such. Only small amounts of the unchanged drug is excreted in the feces and in the urine (1%). Following injection, the drug exerts its analgesic effect in about ½ hour and is maintained for about 4 hours. There have been no reports of toxicity to the fetus when used during labor. Studies have shown that the drug, in recommended doses, usually does not depress respiration, or the cough reflex.

Indications: Relief of pain of various types and degrees of severity and for sedation. It is recommended for obstetrical analgesia and sedation, and as a preanesthetic and postoperative medication. The phenothiazine-type action of the drug may also allay accompanying anxiety and apprehension, thereby reducing the need for other drugs which may have depressant effects.

Contraindications: Concurrent use with antihypertensive drugs including MAO inhibitors; in patients with a history of sensitivity to phenothiazines; in the presence of overdosage of CNS depressants or comatose states, severe myocardial, renal or hepatic disease, and clinically significant hypotension; and in patients under 12 years of age, until more experience has been obtained in this age group.

Warnings: Following administration of the drug, orthostatic hypotension, fainting, or dizziness may occur. Ambulation should be avoided or carefully supervised for at least 6 hours following the initial dose. Tolerance to this effect usually develops with continual administration. The drug should be used with caution in women of childbearing potential and during early pregnancy; there is no evidence of adverse developmental effect when used during late pregnancy or labor. Animal studies have shown that the drug may affect fertility adversely and that it may depress spermatogenesis (with large doses). Because of its additive effect when used with other analgesic and sedative drugs, methotrimeprazine dosage and that of other CNS depressants should be reduced and critically adjusted when used concomitantly or when sequence of use results in overlapping of drug effects.

Precautions: Should be used cautiously when combined with atropine, scopolamine or succinylcholine to avoid tachycardia, a fall in blood pressure and undesirable CNS effects. Geriatric and debilitated patients and those with heart disease are more sensitive to the effects of phenothiazines. A low initial dose is recommended for these patients, and subsequent doses adjusted according to response and tolerance. The pulse rate, blood pressure and general circulatory status should be evaluated frequently until dosage requirements and response have been stabilized. When long-term use is anticipated, periodic blood counts and liver function studies are recommended. Epinephrine should *not* be used to treat hypotensive episodes, since a paradoxical fall in blood pressure may result. Levarterenol should be reserved for hypotension unresponsive to other vasopressors.

Adverse Reactions: The most important effects have been those associated with orthostatic hypotension including fainting or syncope and weakness. Other reactions include disorientation, dizziness, drowsiness, excessive sedation, weakness, slurred speech, abdominal discomfort, nausea, vomiting, dry mouth, nasal congestion, difficult urination, chills, uterine inertia, pain at the injection site, local inflammation and swelling, agranulocytosis, jaundice, and other effects usually associated with phenothiazines (see general statement).

Dosage and Administration: *Intramuscularly* into a large muscle mass. The drug may be mixed in the same syringe *only* with atropine or scopolamine. The usual adult dosage *for analgesia* is 10 to 20 mg every 4 to 6 hours as required, with adjustment of subsequent doses for acute or intractable pain. Dosage may vary from 5 to 40 mg at intervals of 1 to 24 hours. *For obstetrical analgesia,* an initial dose of 15 to 20 mg during labor is usually sufficient; may be repeated at intervals as the clinical situation warrants. *For preanesthetic medication,* the dose varies from 2 to 20 mg administered 45 minutes to 3 hours before surgery. A dose of 10 mg is often satisfactory. Atropine sulfate, or scopolamine hydrobromide may be used concurrently but in lower than usual doses. *For postoperative analgesia,* a dose of 2.5 to 7.5 mg immediately following surgery is suggested. Subsequent doses should be adjusted and administered at intervals of 4 to 6 hours as needed.

Availability:
LEVOPROME® Injection, 20 mg/ml in ampuls of 1 ml and in vials of 10 ml. **(Lederle)**

PERPHENAZINE

Chemical Name: 4-[3-(2-Chlorophenothiazin-10-yl)propyl]-1-piperazineethanol.

Description: Perphenazine is a phenothiazine derivative that possesses strong antiemetic effects and little hypotensive or sedative effects. It is structurally related to fluphenazine and differs only in the replacement of a trifluoromethyl group with a chlorine atom at the 2 position on the phenothiazine nucleus. It is a light-sensitive, crystalline compound that is practically insoluble in water, soluble in acetone and freely soluble in alcohol.

Indications: Management of the manifestations of psychotic disorders; and the control of severe nausea and vomiting in adults. May also be effective in the management of neurosis.

Warnings: Not recommended for use in children under 12 years of age.

For contraindications, other warnings, precautions and adverse reactions, see general statement.

Dosage and Administration: *Orally:* **Tablets:** Dosage must be adjusted to the individual requirements of each patient, the severity of the condition and the response obtained. Adult dosage—Anxiety and tension states, 2 or 4 mg 3 times daily (total daily dose larger than 16 mg seldom required). Moderately disturbed outpatients, 4 to 8 mg 3 times daily (use of dosage greater than 24 mg daily should be avoided in ambulatory outpatients). Hospitalized psychiatric patients, 8 to 16 mg 2 to 4 times daily (total daily dosage should not exceed 64 mg). Nausea and vomiting, average dosage range is 8 to 16 mg daily in divided dosage (occasionally 24 mg may be necessary). Dosage in children over 12 years of age—lowest range of adult dosage. **Repetabs:** Adult dosage—Anxiety and tension states, 1 Repetab once or twice daily; moderately disturbed outpatients, 1 or 2 Repetabs morning and night; hospitalized psychiatric patients, 1 to 4 Repetabs morning and night; do not exceed 64 mg daily; nausea and vomiting, 2 Repetabs may be given initially in acute cases, average dose is 1 Repetab night and morning. Dosage in children over 12 years—1 Repetab night and morning. **Concentrate:** 8 to 16 mg diluted in 1 or 2 fl oz of fruit juice, milk, coffee or other palatable beverage 2 to 4 times daily depending on severity of symptoms and individual response. **Injection:** *Intramuscularly* or, in selected patients, *intravenously.* Dosage should be individualized as needed. Usual initial dose is 5 mg and may be repeated every 6 hours. Total daily *intramuscular* dosage should not exceed 15 mg in ambulatory patients or 30 mg in hospitalized patients. *Intravenous* dosage should be given as a diluted solution via either fractional injection or slow drip infusion. Discontinue as soon as symptoms subside; dosage should not exceed 5 mg.

Availability:
TRILAFON®: **(Schering)**
Concentrate, 16 mg/5 ml in bottles of 120 ml with graduated dropper.
Injection, 5 mg/ml in ampuls of 1 ml.
Repetabs® (repeat-action tablets), 8 mg in bottles of 100.
Tablets, 2, 4, 8 and 16 mg in bottles of 50 and 500.

PIPERACETAZINE

Chemical Name: 10- 3-[4-(2-Hydroxymethyl)piperidino]-propyl phenothiazin-2-yl methyl ketone.

Description: Piperacetazine, a piperidine derivative of phenothiazine, possesses not only tranquilizing and sedative properties but also antiemetic properties. It is considered to be one of the more potent members of this group of tranquilizing agents, and can be employed for both long and short term therapy.

In animals the pharmacologic action of piperacetazine was found to be similar to that of other phenothiazines. A study with 153 psychotic male patients showed that the therapeutic effect of piperacetazine differed little from that of chlorpromazine but that the incidence of toxic responses was less. It was noted that orthostatic hypotension could usually be avoided by administering the initial doses at low levels. When the drug was abruptly withdrawn, there was no evidence of habituation, addiction, or withdrawal reaction of any degree. Also funduscopic examination of 87 of the patients who had received piperacetazine for almost 2 years showed no evidence of drug-associated ocular changes.

Indications: Used primarily for the control of hyperactivity, agitation, and anxiety states associated with acute and chronic schizophrenic reactions. These include chronic undifferentiated, paranoid, catatonic, hebephrenic, simple schizoaffective and acute undifferentiated schizophrenias.

Contraindications: In patients with known hypersensitivity to phenothiazines; in the presence of thrombocytopenia or other blood dyscrasias, bone marrow depression, or significant liver disease. Cross-sensitivity between the phenothiazines may occur. See general statement.

Warnings: Since mental and physical abilities may be impaired, it is advised that patients be cautioned not to engage in hazardous tasks requiring alertness or skill. Concomitant use with alcohol should be avoided due to a potential additive effect. Patients with known suicidal tendencies should not be given this drug except under strict medical supervision. If the drug is considered for administration to pregnant women, the possibility of risk to the fetus must be weighed against the expected therapeutic benefits. Until further clinical studies assure its safe use, it is not recommended for children under 12 years of age. See general statement.

Precautions: The antiemetic effect of piperacetazine may mask the toxicity of other drugs or obscure the development of a serious organic condition. Caution is required when the drug is administered to patients who are taking atropine or related drugs, barbiturates or narcotics; to those who have been exposed to extreme heat or to phosphorus insecticides, and to those with a history of epilepsy or peptic ulcer. Caution also is necessary in patients who may have respiratory impairment due to acute pulmonary infection or chronic respiratory disorders such as severe asthma or emphysema. Because of possible drug-associated photosensitivity, patients should be warned against undue exposure to sunlight. Any sign of blood dyscrasias requires immediate discontinuance of the drug and the institution of appropriate measures. The possible occurrence of liver damage, pigmentary retinopathy, lenticular or corneal deposits, and the development of irreversible dyskinesias must be considered when therapy is prolonged. See general statement.

Adverse Reactions: Drowsiness, sedation, dizziness, orthostatic hypotension, gastritis, syncope, edema, erythematous dermatitis, and extrapyramidal reactions were the most commonly noted but were reversible when the dosage was modified or the drug discontinued. Rarely observed were urinary retention, pedal edema, convulsions, nausea, emesis and bradycardia. See general statement.

Dosage and Administration: *Orally.* Dosage should be individualized throughout the entire course of treatment. Initially 20 to 40 mg daily in divided doses. For maintenance therapy, up to 160 mg daily in divided doses has been satisfactorily tolerated by many patients.

Availability:
QUIDE® Tablets, 10 mg (orange) and 25 mg (yellow) in bottles of 100. **(Dow)**

PROCHLORPERAZINE

Chemical Name: 3-Chloro-10-[3-(4-methyl-1-piperazinyl)propyl]phenothiazine.

Description: Prochlorperazine is a phenothiazine of the piperazine subgroup. The dimaleate salt occurs as minute crystals that are very slightly soluble in water, slightly soluble in alcohol and practically insoluble in ether, benzene, and chloroform. It differs structurally from trifluoperazine only in the replacement of a trifluoromethyl group with a chlorine atom at the 2 position on the phenothiazine nucleus.

Prochlorperazine is an effective antiemetic and a tranquilizer with specific action in psychic and psychosomatic conditions. Extrapyramidal symptoms are relatively common, particularly at higher doses, but may appear in patients taking moderate doses; also motor restlessness and dystonias occur as well. On a weight basis, it is more potent than chlorpromazine but produces less hypotension.

Indications: Control of severe nausea and vomiting and the management of manifestations of psychotic disorders. May be useful in the control of excessive anxiety, tension and agitated states usually seen in neurosis or associated with somatic conditions.

Contraindications: In comatose or severely depressed states due to CNS depressant drugs, and in the presence of bone marrow depression. It is also contraindicated in pediatric surgery.

Warnings: A previous hypersensitivity reaction (blood dyscrasias, jaundice) to a phenothiazine precludes its use unless in the judgment of the physician the potential benefits outweigh the possible hazards. Caution should be exercised when prochlorperazine is administered to children for the treatment of vomiting. Generally, antiemetics are not recommended for use in treating uncomplicated short-term vomiting in children or vomiting of unknown etiology, but only for those cases in which the vomiting is prolonged and of known etiology. The possible development of drug-induced extrapyramidal symptoms may confuse the diagnosis of Reye's syndrome or other encephalopathy. Although unconfirmed, some suspicion exists that because prochlorperazine is potentially hepatotoxic, it may contribute to or adversely affect the course of Reye's syndrome, and its use should be avoided in suspected cases.

Precautions: The antiemetic effect may mask signs of overdosage of toxic drugs or may obscure the diagnosis of such conditions as intestinal obstruction and brain tumor. Aspiration of vomitus has occurred in a few post-surgical patients who have received prochlorperazine as an antiemetic. Although no causal relationship has been established, this possibility should be considered during post-surgical care. Most elderly patients, and children with acute illnesses (e.g., chickenpox, CNS infections, measles, gastroenteritis) or dehydration appear to be much more susceptible to neuromuscular reactions, particularly dystonias, than adults; therefore, the drug should be used only under close supervision in such patients.

Adverse Reactions: Those usually noted with prochlorperazine include drowsiness, dizziness, amenorrhea, skin reaction, hypotension, cholestatic jaundice, leukopenia, agranulocytosis, neuromuscular (extrapyramidal) reactions characterized by motor restlessness resembling parkinsonism or of the dystonic type (spasm of the neck muscles which may progress to torticollis, extensor rigidity of back muscles which may progress to opisthotonos, carpopedal spasm, trismus, difficulty in swallowing, oculogyric crisis and protrusion of the tongue), pseudo-parkinsonism, persistent tardive dyskinesia, and contact dermatitis.

For other contraindications, warnings, precautions and adverse reactions, see the general statement.

Dosage and Administration: *Orally.* **Tablets:** 5 to 10 mg 3 or 4 times daily. In resistant cases, dosage may be increased gradually until symptoms are controlled or side effects become bothersome. The 25-mg tablet is primarily for use in hospitalized psychiatric patients. **Con-**

centrate: To insure palatability and stability, add the desired dose to 60 ml or more of diluent *just prior to administration.* The vehicles suggested for dilution include tomato or fruit juice, milk, simple syrup, orange syrup, carbonated beverages, coffee, tea, or water, as well as soups, puddings, etc. The concentrate is intended for institutional use *only,* and should not be given to children. **Spansule (capsules):** Most patients respond well to one 15-mg capsule taken upon arising or one 10-mg Spansule every 12 hours. *Intramuscularly.* **Ampuls:** Initial dose, 5 to 10 mg (1 to 2 ml), should be injected deeply into the upper outer quadrant of the buttock. Repeat, if necessary, at intervals of 3 to 4 hours. Total parenteral dosage in 24 hours should not exceed 40 mg. May also be injected *intravenously. Intravenous infusion:* 20 mg (4 ml)/liter of isotonic solution. *Rectally.* **Suppositories:** 25 mg 2 times daily; children 20 to 29 lbs of body weight, 2.5 mg 1 or 2 times daily, not to exceed 7.5 mg daily; 30 to 39 lbs, 2.5 mg 2 or 3 times daily, not to exceed 10 mg daily; 40 to 80 lbs, 2.5 mg 3 times daily or 5 mg 2 times daily, not to exceed 15 mg daily. It is not recommended for children under 20 lbs in weight or 2 years of age, except where potentially lifesaving. For complete dosage schedule, see package literature.

Availability:
COMPAZINE®: **(Smith Kline & French)**
Concentrate, 10 mg/ml in bottles of 120 ml.
Injection, 5 mg/ml in ampuls of 2 ml, in disposable syringes of 2 ml and in multiple-dose vials of 10 ml.
Spansule® (capsules), 10, 15 and 30 mg in bottles of 50 and 500 and in single-dose packages of 100; 75 mg in bottles of 50.
Suppositories, 2.5, 5 and 25 mg in cartons of 12.
Syrup, 5 mg/5 ml in bottles of 120 ml.
Tablets, 5 and 10 mg in bottles of 100 and 1000 and in blister-strips of 10 in cartons of 10; 25 mg in bottles of 100 and 1000.

PROMAZINE HYDROCHLORIDE

Chemical Name: 10-(3-Dimethylaminopropyl)phenothiazine hydrochloride.

Description: Promazine hydrochloride is a member of the group of phenothiazines containing an acyclic aliphatic moiety at the 10 position. Its chemical structure differs from that of triflupromazine only in the replacement of the trifluoromethyl group with a hydrogen atom at the 2 position on the phenothiazine ring. Promazine hydrochloride occurs as a hygroscopic, white, crystalline salt that is freely soluble in water, soluble in alcohol and practically insoluble in ether and benzene. Aqueous solutions of the drug are slightly acid. The mechanism whereby its therapeutic action takes place has not been fully understood; however, it appears to be in the hypothalmic region of the mesodiencephalon; exerts primary depressant action on the activity of the brain stem reticular formation. It possesses both antiemetic and antipsychotic activity.

Peak blood levels of promazine are observed in dogs 20 minutes following intraabdominal injection. These levels decline gradually throughout the following 48 hours. About 60% of the dose is excreted in the urine and the remainder in the feces. By means of paper chromatography, 6 metabolites of promazine have been distinguished. The drug differs in producing minimal sedation with a more marked taming effect than other phenothiazines of similar chemical structure. The preferred parenteral route of administration is by intramuscular injection; routine use of the intravenous route is not recommended.

Indications: Management of the manifestations of psychotic disorders. May also be effective in the control of nausea and vomiting, for the relief of apprehension prior to surgery, and for reducing agitation and tension associated with mild alcoholic withdrawal.

Contraindications: Intraarterial injection, in patients hypersensitive to promazine, and in the presence of bone marrow depression.

Adverse Reactions: The most common are drowsiness and orthostatic hypotension which will usually disappear on continued therapy or can be controlled by decreasing the dose. Rarely occurring are leukopenia or agranulocytosis.

For complete data, refer to the general statement.

Dosage and Administration: *Orally, intramuscularly* or *intravenously.* The amount, route and frequency of administration should be governed by the severity of the condition treated and the response of the patient. The oral route should be used whenever possible; when the effect produced by oral dosage will not produce a sufficient response, it may be given parenterally. In the management of severely agitated patients, it is recommended that promazine be given intramuscularly in initial doses of 50 to 150 mg depending on the degree of excitation. In general, these doses are sufficient but, if the desired calming effect is not apparent within 30 minutes, additional doses up to a total of 300 mg may be given. Once the desired control is obtained, the drug may then be given orally. The oral or intramuscular dose is 10 to 200 mg at 4 to 6 hour intervals depending upon the response of the patient. In less severe disturbances, dosage should be adjusted downward. Maintenance dosage may range from 10 to 200 mg given at 4 to 6 hour intervals. When tablet medication is unsuitable or refused, the syrup or liquid concentrate may be used by diluting in appropriate citrus or chocolate-flavored drinks. The degree of CNS depression induced by promazine has not been great; however, in the acutely inebriated patient the initial dose should not exceed 50 mg to be sure that the depressant effect of alcohol is not enhanced. *Antiemetic*—The usual dose is 25 to 50 mg repeated at 4 to 6 hour intervals. When active vomiting or severe nausea precludes oral medication, intramuscular administration in 50 mg doses will usually control the symptom. Oral medication should be resumed as soon as feasible. *Potentiation of Analgesics*—In presurgical sedation, the drug is administered intramuscularly usually in 50 mg doses and in conjunction with reduced doses of analgesics such as meperidine. In general, doses of analgesics and sedatives may be reduced by 1/3 to 1/2 when promazine is used as an adjunct. Promazine may also be used intravenously in 50 mg doses but careful supervision of the patient must be maintained to avoid the development of hypotension. In acute episodes of chronic psychotic disease in children over 12 years of age, 10 to 25 mg every 4 to 6 hours.

Availability:
SPARINE®: **(Wyeth)**
Concentrate, 30 mg/ml in bottles of 120 ml with dropper; 100 mg/ml in bottles of 30 ml with dropper.
Injection, 25 mg/ml in vials of 10 ml and in 1- and 2-ml disposable syringes with needles. (Tubex®); 50 mg/ml in vials of 2 and 10 ml and in 1- and 2-ml disposable syringes with needle (Tubex®).
Syrup, 10 mg/5 ml in bottles of 120 ml.
Tablets, 10 and 200 mg in bottles of 50; 25, 50 and 100 mg in bottles of 50 and 500.

PROMETHAZINE HYDROCHLORIDE

Chemical Name: 10-(2-Dimethylaminopropyl)phenothiazine hydrochloride.

Description: Promethazine hydrochloride, a dimethylamino-isopropyl derivative of phenothiazine, occurs as a crystalline substance that is freely soluble in water, soluble in alcohol and chloroform and practically insoluble in acetone and ether. In addition to its antihistaminic action, which is of marked potency and prolonged duration, it also provides antiemetic as well as anticholinergic actions so that it is useful in a variety of clinical situations. It is relatively free of extrapyramidal stimulation that is associated with other phenothiazine derivatives. Although it does not block the release of histamine, its antihistaminic effect is due to its antagonizing action on most, but not all, of the pharmacological effects of histamine. The duration of action is usually from 4 to 6 hours.

Indications: Preoperatively to relieve apprehension, relax the patient and produce light sleep. Reduces the amount of sedatives and analgesics required; prevents or controls nausea and vomiting. During surgery, permits reduced amounts of anesthetics and controls nausea, vomiting and hiccups. Postoperatively, reduces requirements for analgesics, controls nausea and vomiting and provides patient with continued sedation. Useful in all surgical procedures, especially in those complicated by age (pediatric or geriatric patients); when vomiting, apprehension or anxiety is particularly troublesome; and in obstetric patients. Produces a state of quiescence in which patient is relieved of apprehension and is indifferent to environment. Although light sleep is induced, patient can readily be aroused to clear consciousness, to answer questions, and can cooperate with surgeon and anesthesiologist. In obstetric management, therapeutic benefits are accomplished with no maternal or fetal depression. Potent antihistaminic in the management of all allergic conditions known to respond to antihistaminic therapy; will ameliorate and control minor blood transfusion reactions of allergic origin. Useful as a nighttime sedative; useful in the prophylaxis of swelling, pain and trismus in dental surgery; actively controls motion sickness; also helpful as therapy for anaphylactic reactions adjunctive to epinephrine and other standard measures after the acute manifestations have been controlled.

Contraindications: Comatose states, bone marrow depression, idiosyncrasy or hypersensitivity to promethazine, asthmatic attack, narrow-angle glaucoma, prostatic hypertrophy, stenosing peptic ulcer, pyloroduodenal obstruction, bladder neck obstruction, patients receiving MAO inhibitors, or those who have received large amounts of CNS depressants (alcohol, barbiturates, narcotics), disorders of the lower respiratory tract, newborn or premature infants, and acutely ill or dehydrated children (increases susceptibility to dystonias). **Important note:** *Promethazine should not be injected intraarterially.* Inadvertant intraarterial injection, or periarterial injection, may result in serious vascular damage and gangrene.

Warnings: Care should be exercised not to allow perivascular extravasation since under such circumstances chemical irritation may occur. Promethazine is not recommended for treatment of uncomplicated vomiting in children and its use should be limited to prolonged vomiting of known etiology. The possible development of drug-induced extrapyramidal symptoms may confuse the diagnosis of Reye's syndrome or other encephalopathy. Although unconfirmed, some suspicion exists because promethazine is potentially hepatotoxic, it may contribute to or adversely affect the course of Reye's syndrome, and its use should be avoided in such cases.

Precautions: Antiemetics may mask the symptoms of an unrecognized disease or drug overdosage and thereby interfere with diagnosis. Patients in pain who have received inadequate or no analgesia have been noted to develop "athetoid-like" movements of the upper extremities following the parenteral administration of promethazine; however, these symptoms usually disappear upon adequate control of the pain.

Adverse Reactions: Rarely leukopenia or agranulocytosis. Signs of overdosage include excitation, ataxia, incoordination, athetosis, convulsion and coma. Common signs in children are fixed, dilated pupils; fever and a flushed face. Treatment is symptomatic and supportive.

For complete data, see general statement.

Dosage and Administration: *Orally, intramuscularly, intravenously* and *rectally.* Intravenous administration should not exceed 25 mg/ml/minute. Barbiturates should be eliminated or reduced by at least 1/2 with promethazine HCl; meperidine, morphine, other analgesic depressants should be reduced by 1/4 to 1/2. *Sedation:* Children—12.5 to 25 mg orally or by rectal suppository at bedtime. Adults usually require 25 to 50 mg for nighttime, presurgical or obstetric sedation. *Presurgical care:* 12.5 to 25 mg doses for children and 50 mg for adults the night before surgery; relieves apprehension and produces a quiet sleep. Preoperative medication in children, 0.5 mg/lb of body weight, in combination with an equal dose of meperidine and an appropriate dose of an atropine-like drug. Suppositories: 25 mg in children up to 3 years and 50 mg in older children may be used instead of oral or parenteral medication. Usual adult dosage is 50 mg with equal amount of meperidine and required amount of a belladonna alkaloid. Postoperative sedation and potentiation of analgesics may be obtained by administration of 12.5 to 25 mg in children and 25 to 50 mg in adults. *Obstetric sedation:* Early stages of labor, 50 mg. When labor is definitely established administer from 25 to 75 mg average dose, 50 mg intramuscularly or intravenously with an equal dose of meperidine and amnesic agents as indicated. If average doses are used, it is rarely necessary to repeat medication during course of normal labor. If required, 25 to 50 mg doses, with or without a reduced dose of analgesic, may be repeated once or twice at 3- to 4-hour intervals. *Nausea and vomiting:* For active therapy of nausea and vomiting, average dose is 25 mg. When oral medication cannot be tolerated, give intravenously, intramuscularly or by suppository. From 12.5 to 25 mg doses may be repeated as necessary at 4- to 6-hour intervals. For prophylaxis of nausea and vomiting, as during surgery and in the postoperative period, average dose is 25 mg repeated at 4- to 6-hour intervals as necessary. In pregnancy, it is suggested that 25 mg be given orally or by suppository on retiring; 12.5 to 25 mg in the morning, if necessary. *Motion sickness:* Adults—average dose is 25 mg twice daily. Initial dose 1/2 to 1 hour before travel, repeated 8 to 12 hours later if needed. Children—12.5 to 25 mg twice daily. *Allergy:* Average oral dose is 25 mg before retiring; 6.25 to 12.5 mg may be taken before meals and on retiring. After initiation of treatment, dosage should be adjusted to smallest amount adequate to relieve symptoms. When oral route is not feasible, suppositories, 25 mg, or injection, 25 mg intravenously or intramuscularly, may be used. Dose may be repeated within 2 hours if necessary, but oral therapy should be initiated if indicated. Children tolerate promethazine HCl well and may be given dosage in same range as adults. As preoperative medication, postoperative sedative, or in 25-mg doses prior to or during blood transfusion, minor transfusion reactions of an allergic nature will be prevented or controlled. *Dentistry:* For sedation and prophylaxis of swelling, pain and trismus following extractions or other oral surgical procedures, 25 mg 12 to 24 hours prior to procedure, repeated 1 to 1½ hours preoperatively. Postoperatively, 12.5 to 25 mg at 6-hour intervals provides for more consistent reduction of edema.

Availability:

Promethazine Hydrochloride

Expectorant, 5 mg/5 ml in bottles of 120 ml, 1 pint and 1 gallon. **(Lederle)**
Injection, 25 and 50 mg/ml in ampuls of 1 ml. **(Knoll)**
Injection, 25 mg/ml (IM & IV) and 50 mg/ml (IM only) in Uni-Amp® and in ampuls of 1 ml and in multiple-dose vials of 10 ml. **(Winthrop)**
Tablets, 25 and 50 mg in bottles of 100 and 1000. **(Lederle)**
PHENERGAN®: **(Wyeth)**
Injection, 25 and 50 mg/ml in ampuls of 1 ml and in 1-ml Tubex® (cartridge-needle unit).
Rectal Suppositories, 12.5, 25 and 50 mg in cartons of 12 and in Redipak® cartons of 25.
Syrup, 6.25 and 25 mg/5 ml in bottles of 1 pint.
Tablets, 12.5 mg in bottles of 100 and 1000 and in Redipak® cartons of 100; 25 mg in bottles of 100, 1000 and in Redipak® cartons of 25 and 100; 50 mg in bottles of 100.
REMSED Tablets, 50 mg in bottles of 100. **(Endo)**

Combinations

PHENERGAN®: **(Wyeth)**
Compound Tablets in bottles of 50. Each tablet contains promethazine hydrochloride, 6.25 mg; pseudoephedrine hydrochloride, 60 mg and acetylsalicylic acid, 600 mg.
Expectorant, Pediatric, with Dextromethorphan in bottles of 120 and 180 ml, 1 pint and 1 gallon. Each 5 ml (teaspoonful) contains promethazine hydrochloride, 5 mg; dextromethorphan hydrobromide, 7.5 mg; fluidextract ipecac, 0.17 minims and potassium guaiacolsulfonate, 44 mg; with citric acid and sodium citrate and alcohol, 7%.
Expectorant Plain in bottles of 120 and 180 ml, 1 pint and 1 gallon. Each 5 ml is identical in composition to the Pediatric Expectorant with Dextromethorphan, minus the dextromethorphan.
Ⓒ *Expectorant with Codeine* in bottles of 120 and 180 ml, 1 pint and 1 gallon. Each 5 ml is identical in composition to the Plain Expectorant plus the addition of 10 mg of codeine phosphate.
PHENERGAN®-D Tablets in bottles of 100. Each tablet contains promethazine hydrochloride, 6.25 mg and pseudoephedrine hydrochloride, 60 mg.
PHENERGAN® VC:
Expectorant, Plain in bottles of 120 and 180 ml, 1 pint and 1 gallon. Each 5 ml is identical in composition to Phenergan Expectorant Plain plus the addition of phenylephrine hydrochloride, 5 mg.
Ⓒ *Expectorant with Codeine* in bottles of 120 ml, 1 pint and 1 gallon. Each 5 ml is identical in composition to the Plain Expectorant plus the addition of codeine phosphate, 10 mg and phenylephrine hydrochloride, 5 mg.
PROMETHAZINE HYDROCHLORIDE: **(Lederle)**
Ⓒ *Expectorant with Codeine* in bottles of 120 ml, 1 pint and 1 gallon. Each 5 ml contains promethazine hydrochloride, 5 mg and codeine phosphate, 10 mg.
Ⓒ *VC Expectorant* in bottles of 120 ml, 1 pint and 1 gallon. Each 5 ml contains promethazine hydrochloride, 5 mg; phenylephrine hydrochloride, 5 mg and codeine phosphate, 10 mg.
PROMEX Expectorant in bottles of 120 ml, 1 pint and 1 gallon. Each 5 ml contains promethazine hydrochloride, 5 mg; fluidextract ipecac, 17 minims; potassium guaiacolsulfonate, 44 mg and alcohol, 7%. **(Lemmon)**

PROPIOMAZINE HYDROCHLORIDE

Chemical Name: 1-[10-(2-Dimethylaminopropyl)phenothiazin-2-yl]-1-propane.

Description: Propiomazine hydrochloride is a phenothiazine derivative structurally and pharmacologically related to promethazine. It differs structurally from promethazine only in the presence of a propionyl group at the 2 position on the phenothiazine nucleus. Propiomazine occurs as a yellowish, crystalline powder soluble in water and slightly soluble in alcohol. Aqueous solutions of the drug are slightly acidic and are incompatible with barbiturate salts and other alkaline substances.

Indications: Used as a sedative and antiemetic in surgical and obstetrical procedures; as an adjunct to anesthesia.

Contraindications: Intraarterial injection because of the possible occurrence of arterial or arteriolar spasm with resultant impairment of local circulation.

Precautions: When used concurrently, the dose of barbiturates should be reduced by at least 1/2; the dose of meperidine, morphine, and other analgesic depressants should be reduced by 1/4 to 1/2. Intravenous injection should be made only into vessels previously undamaged by multiple injections or trauma; perivascular extravasation should be avoided. In the event of dizziness or drowsiness, patients should be cautioned not to engage in activities requiring alertness such as driving a car or engaging in a hazardous occupation. Safe use during pregnancy has not been established.

Adverse Reactions: Dry mouth, elevated blood pressure, hypotension and tachycardia.

For complete data, see general statement.

Dosage and Administration: *Intravenously* or *intramuscularly* in doses of 10 to 40 mg. Propiomazine relieves apprehension and induces a quiet sleep from which the patient can be easily aroused. Adults usually require 20 mg for nighttime sedation; presurgical or obstetrical sedation may be obtained. *Presurgical care:* 20 mg intramuscularly the night before surgery relieves apprehension and produces a quiet sleep in adults. The usual adult dosage for preoperative medication is 20 mg of propiomazine with 50 mg of meperidine both intravenously or intramuscularly. Although 20 mg of propiomazine is sufficient for most patients, for adequate sedation some will require as much as 40 mg intravenously or intramuscularly at the discretion of the physician. The desired amount of belladonna alkaloids may be added as required. Sedation during surgery with local, nerveblock or spinal anesthesia may be obtained by the intravenous or intramuscular administration of 10 to 20 mg. Postoperative sedation and enhancement of analgesic effects may be obtained in adults by the intravenous or intramuscular administration of 10 to 20 mg. *Obstetrics:* the intravenous or intramuscular administration in doses of 20 mg will provide sedation and relieve apprehension in the early stages of labor. Some patients may require up to 40 mg. When labor is definitely established, administer 20 to 40 mg of propiomazine intramuscularly or intravenously with 25 to 75 mg of meperidine (average dose 50 mg). Amnesic agents may be administered as necessary. If the average doses of propiomazine and meperidine are used, it is seldom necessary to repeat the medication during normal labor. If necessary, additional doses may be repeated at 3-hour intervals. Neither prolongation of labor nor significant maternal or fetal depression has been observed. *Dentistry:* For sedation during dental surgery under local or general anesthesia, propiomazine should be administered intravenously or intramuscularly in doses of 10 to 30 mg. The usual dose will be 20 mg, but some patients may require the full amount. *Pediatrics:* Propiomazine hydrochloride has been used in children as a sedative the night before surgery and for preanesthetic and postoperative medication. In children under 60 pounds of body weight, dosage of propiomazine should be calculated on a basis of 0.25 to 0.5 mg/pound of body weight. The higher dosage recommendation should be necessary only in the extremely nervous excitable child.

Availability:
LARGON® Injection, 20 mg/ml in ampuls of 1 and 2 ml and in 1- and 2-ml Tubex® (disposable syringes) with needle. **(Wyeth)**

THIETHYLPERAZINE MALEATE

Chemical Name: 2-(Ethylthio)-10-[3-(4-methyl-1-piperazinyl)propyl]phenothiazine dimaleate.

Description: Thiethylperazine is a phenothiazine derivative that exerts a pronounced anti-emetic-antinauseant activity and effectively controls vertigo associated with pathology of the inner ear. Its specificity of action provides a favorable therapeutic index for control of vomiting and vertigo with relative freedom from psychotropic effects.

Indications: Control of vertigo and accompanying nausea and vomiting due to various etiologies.

Contraindications: Pregnancy; children under 12 years of age; severe CNS depression; comatose states due to any cause; intravenous administration.

Precautions: It is obvious that sound clinical judgment must be exercised in determining whether vomiting represents a warning of organic abnormality, and that this must first be recognized before employing this drug. In excessive doses thiethylperazine may produce extrapyramidal stimulation with the varied symptom complex characteristic of this complication. While no hepatic, hematopoietic or renal toxicity has been reported at recommended dose levels, it should be remembered that these reactions may occur with phenothiazine drugs.

Adverse Reactions: Drowsiness and dryness of the mouth may occur. Orthostatic hypotension may be manifested at higher dose levels.

For complete data, see general statement.

Dosage and Administration: *Orally, rectally* or *intramuscularly (deep).* The usual dosage is from 10 to 30 mg daily. Usually the initial dose is given by intramuscular injection or rectally; subsequent doses may be given by the same route or orally.

Availability:
TORECAN®: **(Boehringer Ingelheim)**
Injection, 5 mg/ml in ampuls of 2 ml.
Suppositories, 10 mg in cartons of 12.
Tablets, 10 mg in bottles of 100.

THIORIDAZINE HYDROCHLORIDE

Chemical Name: 2-Methylmercapto-10-[2-(N-methyl-2-piperidyl)ethyl] phenothiazine.

Description: Thioridazine, a phenothiazine derivative, differs structurally from other phenothiazines in that a thiomethyl group replaces a halogen in position 2 on the phenothiazine nucleus. Thioridazine's basic pharmacological activity is similar to that of other phenothiazines. It occurs as a white to slightly yellow, granular powder, having a faint odor and a very bitter taste. It is soluble in both water and alcohol.

Thioridazine shows greater specificity of psychotherapeutic action, less frequent extrapyramidal stimulation, and is without appreciable antiemetic action.

Indications: Management of the manifestations of psychotic disorders. May be effective in the relief of symptoms of neurotic depressive reactions, alcohol withdrawal syndrome, intractable pain, senility; psychoses, agitated states such as schizophrenia, manic psychoses and toxic psychoses and agitated depression, and in the control of moderate to severe agitation, hyperactivity, or aggressiveness in disturbed children.

Contraindications: Hypersensitivity to the drug, severe CNS depression or comatose states, and in children under 2 years of age.

Precautions: Leukopenia and/or agranulocytosis and convulsive seizures have been reported but are infrequent. Thioridazine has been shown to be helpful in the treatment of behavioral disorders in epileptic patients, but anticonvulsant medication should also be maintained. Pigmentary retinopathy, which has been observed primarily in patients taking larger than recommended doses, is characterized by diminution of visual acuity, brownish coloring of vision, and impairment of night vision; examination of the fundus discloses deposits of pigment. Female patients appear to have a greater tendency to orthostatic hypotension than male patients. The administration of epinephrine should be avoided in the treatment of drug-induced hypotension in view of the fact that phenothiazine may induced a reversed epinephrine effect. Should a vasoconstrictor be required, the most suitable are levarterenol and phenylephrine.

Adverse Reactions: Most side effects are mild and transient. These usually include drowsiness (occasional) and pseudoparkinsonism and other extrapyramidal symptoms (infrequent). Nocturnal confusion, hyperactivity, lethargy, psychotic reactions, restlessness, and headache have been reported but are extremely rare. Other reactions noted include dryness of mouth, blurred vision, constipation, nausea, vomiting, diarrhea, nasal stuffiness, pallor, galactorrhea, breast engorgement, amenorrhea, inhibition of ejaculation, peripheral edema, dermatitis and skin eruptions of the urticarial type, photosensitivity (very rare), ECG changes, and rare cases described as parotid swelling.

For complete data, see general statement.

Dosage and Administration: *Orally.* Dosage must be individualized according to condition and degree of psychomotor agitation and response. The smallest effective dosage should be determined for each patient. Adults: the usual initial dose is 10 mg 2 to 4 times daily for mild emotional disturbances, 25 mg 3 times daily for moderately disturbed patients, and 50 to 100 mg 3 times daily in ambulatory psychotic patients; for hospitalized patients, 200 mg 3 or 4 times daily. Children's dosage ranges from 0.5 to a maximum of 3 mg/kg of body weight. For children with moderate disorders, 10 mg 2 or 3 times daily is the usual starting dose. For hospitalized, severely disturbed or psychotic children, 25 mg 2 or 3 times daily. Dosage may be increased gradually until optimum therapeutic effect is obtained or the maximum has been reached. **Note:** Not recommended for use in children under 2 years of age.

Availability:

MELLARIL®: **(Sandoz)**

Concentrate, 30 and 100 mg/ml in bottles of 120 ml with measured dropper; 30 mg/ml also available in bottles of 1 pint.

Tablets, 10, 15, 25, 50, 100, 150 and 200 mg in bottles of 100 and 1000.

MELLARIL-S™ Suspension (as base), 25 and 100 mg/5 ml in bottles of 1 pint. **(Sandoz)**

TRIFLUOPERAZINE

Chemical Name: 10-[3-(4-Methylpiperazin-1-yl)propyl]-2-trifluoromethylphenothiazine.

Description: Trifluoperazine, a member of the piperazine subgroup of phenothiazines, occurs as a hygroscopic, cream-color, fine powder that is freely soluble in water. Aqueous solutions of 5% concentration have a pH of 2.2. Trifluoperazine is closely related structurally to prochlorperazine, differing only in that it replaces the chlorine atom with a trifluoromethyl group at the 2 position on the phenothiazine nucleus. It relieves anxiety, agitation and tension without sedative or euphoric effects.

For the mode of action, indications, contraindications, precautions, and other adverse reactions, see general statement.

Indications: Management of the manifestations of psychotic disorders. May also be of use in controlling excessive anxiety, tension and agitation as seen in neuroses or associated with somatic conditions.

Adverse Reactions: Extrapyramidal symptoms, akathisia, and drowsiness.

Dosage and Administration: *Orally.* Adults—in general or psychiatric office practice, 1 to 2 mg twice daily; in hospitalized or adequately supervised patients, 2 to 5 mg twice daily; in acutely ill, hospitalized patients, as much as 40 mg daily or more may be given. Optimum dosage levels should be reached within 2 or 3 weeks. Children, 6 to 12 years of age—1 mg once or twice daily depending upon size of child and only when child is adequately supervised or hospitalized. *Intramuscularly,* injected deeply, for prompt control of severe symptoms: Adults—1 to 2 mg (1/2 to 1 ml) every 4 to 6 hours as needed, with oral therapy resumed as soon as feasible; children, 6 to 12 years of age—1 mg (1/2 ml) once or twice daily until symptoms subside, usually within 24 hours, after which oral therapy should be resumed. Intramuscular dosage should not exceed 10 mg daily for adults except in patients with exceptionally severe symptoms.

Availability:
STELAZINE®: **(Smith Kline & French)**
Injection, 2 mg/ml in multiple-dose vials of 10 ml.
Solution (Concentrate), 10 mg/ml in bottles of 60 ml in cartons of 12.
Tablets, 1, 2, 5 and 10 mg in bottles of 100 and 1000 and in single-unit packages of 100.

TRIFLUPROMAZINE HYDROCHLORIDE

Chemical Name: 10-[3-(Dimethylamino)propyl]-2-trifluoromethylphenothiazine.

Description: Triflupromazine, a derivative of dimethylaminopropyl subgroup of phenothiazines, occurs as a crystalline substance that is soluble in water, alcohol, and acetone. The pH of a 2% aqueous solution is 4.1; if the pH is raised to 6.4, precipitation of the free base occurs. It is closely related structurally to chlorpromazine and promazine, differing only in the nature of the substituted group at the 2 position of the phenothiazine nucleus. Adverse effects are similar to those observed with chlorpromazine, but there is a higher incidence of extrapyramidal symptoms. It is employed in treating disturbed psychotic patients by decreasing excessive psychomotor behavior, modifying the disturbing effects of delusions and rendering the patient more amenable to psychotherapy and in the prevention and control of nausea and vomiting from various commonly encountered causes; and for pre- and postoperative tranquilization.

Indications: Management of the manifestations of psychotic disorders with the exception of depressive reactions, for the control of severe nausea and vomiting.

Contraindications: In suspected or established subcortical brain damage with or without hypothalamic damage.

Precautions: Cautious use is advised in patients with a history of convulsive disorders; mitral insufficiency or pheochromocytoma, and idiosyncrasy to phenothiazines.

For complete data, see general statement.

Dosage and Administration: For psychotic disorders: *Orally,* the recommended initial dose is 100 to 150 mg daily and the maintenance dose is 30 to 150 mg daily. The recommended dosage for children is 2 mg/kg of body weight up to a maximum total daily dose of 150 mg in divided doses. *Intramuscularly,* the recommended dose for adults is 60 to 150 mg and for children is 0.2 to 0.25 mg/kg up to a maximum total daily dose of 10 mg. The drug should not be administered to children under 2½ years of age. **For nausea and vomiting:** *Orally,* the recommended dose for adults is 20 to 30 mg daily and for children is 0.2 mg/kg up to a maximum total daily dose of 10 mg divided into 3 doses. *Intramuscularly,* the recommended dose for adults is 5 to 15 mg as a single dose which may be repeated every 4 hours up to a maximum total daily dose of 60 mg; for elderly or debilitated patients is 2.5 mg up to a maximum total daily dose of 15 mg, and for children is 0.2 to 0.25 mg/kg up to a maximum total daily dose of 10 mg. *Intravenously,* the recommended adult dose is 1 to 3 mg daily; this route of administration is not intended for use in children.

Availability:
VESPRIN®: **(Squibb)**
Injection, 10 mg/ml in vials of 10 ml and in Unimatic® syringes (single-dose) of 1 ml; 20 mg/ml in vials of 1 ml.
Suspension (High Potency), 50 mg/5 ml in bottles of 120 ml.
Tablets, 10, 25 and 50 mg in bottles of 50 and 500; the 10 and 25 mg tablets are also available in Unimatic® (single-dose) containers of 100.

TRIMEPRAZINE TARTRATE

Chemical Name: 10-[3-(Dimethylamino)-2-methylpropyl]phenothiazine tartrate.

Description: Trimeprazine, a member of the dimethylamine subgroup of phenothiazines, occurs as a crystalline substance that is soluble in water and only slightly soluble in alcohol. The drug has a potent and rapid antipruritic action in a variety of conditions, both dermatologic and nondermatologic. Also, it has demonstrated an antagonistic action to serotonin and to histamine and a blocking effect in conditioned-response tests, a property apparently correlated with tranquilizing effects in clinical use.

Indications: For the symptomatic relief of pruritic symptoms in urticaria. May also be useful in the relief of pruritic symptoms in neurodermatitis, allergic, contact and atopic dermatitis, chickenpox, and in pruritus ani et vulvae.

Precautions: Since trimeprazine has slight antiemetic action, it may obscure signs of intestinal obstruction, brain tumor, or overdosage of toxic drugs.

Adverse Reactions: Drowsiness, dizziness, dryness of mucous membranes, gastrointestinal upset, cholestatic jaundice, extrapyramidal reactions, and blood dyscrasias including leukopenia and agranulocytosis have been observed.

For the mode of action, other indications, contraindications, precautions and adverse reactions, see general statement.

Dosage and Administration: *Orally.* Dosage should always be adjusted according to the severity of symptoms and the response of the patient. Starting dosage: Adults—1 tablet (2.5 mg) 4 times daily or 1 Spansule (5 mg) twice daily; children 7 to 12—1 tablet 3 times daily or 1 Spansule at night; 3 to 6—1 tablet or 1 teaspoonful (2.5 mg) of syrup 3 times daily; 2 and younger—½ teaspoonful (1.25 mg) 3 times daily. In patients with severe or refractory symptoms, a higher dosage schedule is indicated: Adults—2 tablets 4 times daily or 2 Spansules every 12 hours; children 7 to 12—1 tablet 4 times daily or 1 Spansule every 12 hours; 3 to 6—1 tablet or teaspoonful of syrup 4 times daily; 2 and younger—½ teaspoonful of syrup 4 times daily. Total daily dosages should not exceed 5 mg for children 2 years old or younger or 10 mg for children 3 to 12. **Note:** Trimeprazine tartrate is not recommended for use in infants under 6 months of age, and the extended-release product is not recommended for children younger than 6 years of age.

Availability:

TEMARIL®: **(Smith Kline & French)**

Spansule® (extended-release capsules), 5 mg in bottles of 50 and in single-unit packages of 100.

Syrup, 2.5 mg/5 ml in bottles of 120 ml. Alcohol, 7.5%.

Tablets, 2.5 mg in bottles of 100 and 1000 and in single-unit packages of 100.

PHENOXYBENZAMINE

Chemical Name: *N*-(2-Chloroethyl)-*N*-(1-methyl-2-phenoxyethyl)benzylamine.

Description: Phenoxybenzamine hydrochloride is a long-acting adrenergic blocking agent structurally related to dibenamine and azapetine. It occurs as colorless crystals slightly soluble in water and soluble in alcohol.

Phenoxybenzamine apparently blocks the *alpha* receptor sites at the postganglionic synapse of sympathetic nerves. These receptor sites are then unable to react to endogenous or exogenous sympathomimetic agents. With the exception of the cardiac action of epinephrine, the drug blocks the excitatory effects of epinephrine, including vasoconstriction and contraction of exocrine gland smooth muscle, and reverses the pressor effects. Muscular, cutaneous, and pulmonary vascular systems are dilated but renal, hepatic, and cerebral blood flow, and cardiac output are not affected. Phenoxybenzamine appears to produce a variable reduction in blood pressure and, in high doses, it appears to prevent epinephrine-induced cardiac arrhythmias.

Following oral administration, about 30% of the drug is absorbed, and therapeutic action occurs in about 2 hours. When sufficient phenoxybenzamine is given to produce complete blockade, the duration of action is 24 to 36 hours. Its exact metabolic fate is unknown; however, it is excreted in the urine and bile.

Indications: Treatment of pheochromocytoma and control of episodes of hypertension and sweating. If severe tachycardia is present, concomitant use of a beta-adrenergic blocking agent is recommended. May also be useful in peripheral vasospastic disorders such as Raynaud's syndrome, acrocyanosis and frostbite sequelae.

Contraindications: When a fall in blood pressure may be undesirable.

Warnings: Concomitant administration with drugs having prominent alpha adrenergic blocking effects may result in an exaggerated hypotensive response and tachycardia. Also, phenoxybenzamine should not be used in patients with compensated congestive heart failure because the tachycardia which sometimes accompanies high doses may precipitate frank cardiac failure.

Precautions: Use with caution in patients with marked cerebral or coronary arteriosclerosis or renal damage. May aggravate symptoms of respiratory infections. It is not recommended for disorders involving the larger blood vessels in which direct-acting vasodilators are the preferred therapy.

Adverse Reactions: Nasal congestion, miosis, and inhibition of ejaculation may occur; these symptoms tend to decrease as therapy is continued. Gastrointestinal irritation has also been noted. Overdosage may be manifested by postural hypotension resulting in dizziness or fainting; tachycardia, particularly postural; vomiting; lethargy, or shock.

Dosage and Administration: *Orally.* Recommended initial dosage is 10 mg daily in a single dose. Dosage may be increased in increments of 10 mg daily at intervals of 4 days. Maintenance dosage usually ranges from 20 to 60 mg daily, given in single or divided doses. Two to 4 weeks of therapy may be required before maximal.response is obtained.

Availability:
DIBENZYLINE® Capsules, 10 mg in bottles of 100. **(Smith Kline & French)**

PHENOXYMETHYL PENICILLIN: see The Penicillins

PHENPROCOUMON

Chemical Name: 3-(α-Ethylbenzyl)-4-hydroxycoumarin.

Description: Phenprocoumon, one of the longer-acting of the oral anticoagulant agents, is a coumarin derivative. It depresses the plasma prothrombin activity of the blood by interfering with the hepatic synthesis of several coagulation factors [factor II (prothrombin), factor VII (proconvertin), factor IX (Christmas factor, plasma thromboplastin component) and factor X (Stuart-Prower)].

Phenprocoumon is readily absorbed from the gastrointestinal tract. Depending upon the loading dose a therapeutic degree of hypothrombinemia may be achieved within 24 to 36 hours, with peak effect occurring within 48 to 72 hours; the duration of action is from 7 to 14 days.

Indications: Prophylaxis and treatment of thromboembolic diseases.

Contraindications: In active ulcerative disease or overt bleeding within the gastrointestinal, genitourinary or respiratory tracts; cerebrovascular system: aneurysms (cerebral, dissecting aortic), pericardial effusions, subacute bacterial endocarditis; in hemorrhagic blood dyscrasias such as hemophilia, thrombocytopenic purpura, or those associated with coagulation defects; in surgery of the CNS or eye or in traumatic surgery that results in large open surfaces; where laboratory facilities are inadequate or patient cooperation is lacking; previous anaphylactic or hypersensitivity reaction to phenprocoumon.

Warnings: The use of phenprocoumon represents a risk to the fetus since the drug crosses the placental barrier. Congenital malformations, including nasal hypoplasia and other abnormalities consistent with a diagnosis of chondrodysplasia punctata as well as fetal hemorrhage and intrauterine deaths have been reported. Therefore, extreme caution must be exercised when administering the drug to pregnant patients. Caution is also required when giving the drug to nursing mothers, in the presence of cachexia or a prolonged dietary deficiency of vitamin K, in moderate or severe hepatic or renal insufficiency, in the presence of infectious diseases, or a disturbance of the intestinal flora, in patients with indwelling catheter or in those with moderate to severe hypertension. When hemorrhage occurs during oral anticoagulant therapy, the possibility of organic lesions such as a neoplasm should be considered.

Precautions: Response to phenprocoumon may be altered by changes in the patient's diet, environment, physical state, and by the concomitant administration of other drugs such as salicylates which accentuate the anticoagulant effect and of phenobarbital which is antagonistic. Periodic determination of the prothrombin time is essential.

Adverse Reactions: Excessive prothrombinopenia (with or without bleeding), alopecia, anorexia, nausea, vomiting, diarrhea, urticaria, erythema, dermatitis, hemorrhagic infarction, necrosis of the skin and cyanosis of the toes have been noted.

For complete information on potential drug interactions, see monograph on Bishydroxycoumarin.

Dosage and Administration: *Orally.* To initiate therapy, the usual dose is 24 mg. Dosage should be gauged according to prothrombin activity, and the blood prothrombin time should be determined prior to and 24 hours after the administration of the initial dose. Thereafter, the prothrombin time should be measured every 24 to 48 hours for the first week, once or twice weekly for the next 3 or 4 weeks and once semimonthly or monthly for patients on long-term treatment. The maintenance dose is variable, the average daily dose being 0.75 to 6 mg. The exact amount should be adjusted according to the response of the patient as determined by prothrombin activity.

Availability:
LIQUAMAR® Tablets, 3 mg in bottles of 100 and 1000. **(Organon)**

PHENSUXIMIDE

Chemical Name: *N*-Methyl-2-phenylsuccinimide.

Description: Phensuximide, an anticonvulsant drug, is prepared by the chemical reaction of methylamine on phenylsuccinic acid. It occurs as fine crystals slightly soluble in water and readily soluble in alcohol. Aqueous solutions are fairly stable at pH 2 to 8, but hydrolysis occurs under more alkaline conditions.

Phensuximide suppresses the paroxysmal spike and wave pattern which is common in petit mal seizures. The frequency of epileptiform attacks is reduced, apparently by depression of the motor cortex and elevation of the threshold of the CNS to convulsive stimuli.

The drug is readily and promptly absorbed following oral ingestion, and is not bound to plasma proteins. It is rapidly metabolized by the hepatic microsomal and other enzymes to the N-demethyl and parahydroxyphenyl derivatives and other metabolites; renal excretion of unchanged drug is negligible.

Indications: Control of petit mal epilepsy.

Contraindications: Phensuximide should not be used in patients with a history of hypersensitivity to succinimides.

Warnings: Blood dyscrasias, including some with fatal outcome, have been reported to be associated with the use of succinimides; therefore, periodic blood counts should be performed. It has been reported that succinimides have produced morphological and functional changes in animal liver. Also, clinical reports have indicated abnormalities in liver and renal function. For these reasons, phensuximide should be administered with extreme caution to patients with known liver or renal disease. Periodic urinalysis and liver function studies are advised for all patients receiving this drug.

Systemic lupus erythematosus has been reported with the use of succinimides; the physician should consider this possibility. Animal reproduction studies for related succinimides have shown an increase in the number of stillbirths and ossification defects in neonatal rats. While a number of reports suggest that the use of anticoagulant drugs in pregnant women may have a teratogenic effect on the unborn infant, a definite cause and effect relationship has not been firmly established. It is recommended that the medication be discontinued prior to or during pregnancy, primarily in patients in whom withdrawal would not pose a serious threat. However, these drugs should not be withheld in patients prone to major seizures because of the strong possibility of precipitating status epilepticus with its attendant hypoxia and risk to both the mother and fetus. It is not known whether or not even minor seizures constitute some risk to the developing embryo or fetus. Phensuximide may impair the mental and/or physical abilities required for the performance of potentially hazardous tasks, such as driving a motor vehicle or other such activity requiring alertness and physical coordination; the patient should be cautioned accordingly.

Precautions: Phensuximide, when used alone in mixed types of epilepsy, may increase the frequency of grand mal seizures in some patients. As with other anticonvulsants, it is important to proceed slowly when increasing or decreasing dosage, as well as when adding or eliminating other medication. Abrupt withdrawal of this drug may precipitate petit mal status.

Adverse Reactions: Those generally associated with the use of succinimides include the following: *Gastrointestinal reactions*—nausea or vomiting, vague gastric upset, cramps, anorexia, diarrhea, weight loss, epigastric and abdominal pain, and constipation. *Hemopoietic reactions*—eosinophilia, granulocytopenia, transient leukopenia, agranulocytosis, aplastic anemia, monocytosis, and pancytopenia. *CNS reactions*—drowsiness, ataxia or dizziness, irritability and nervousness, headache, blurred vision, photophobia, hiccups, dreamlike state, lethargy, hyperactivity, fatigue, and insomnia. Drowsiness, ataxia, and dizziness have been the most frequent side effects noted. Psychologic abnormalities may be manifested by confusion, instability, mental slowness, depression, hypochondriacal behavior, disturbances of sleep, night terrors, inability to concentrate, and aggressiveness. These effects may be noted particularly in patients who have previously exhibited psychological abnormalities. There have been rare reports of psychosis, suicidal behavior, auditory hallucinations, increased libido and increased state of depression. *Reactions to the integumentary system*—urticaria, Stevens-Johnson syndrome, pruritic erythematous rashes, skin eruptions, erythema multiforme, and systemic lupus erythematosus. *Genitourinary reactions*—urinary frequency, renal damage, and hematuria. *Miscellaneous reactions*—periorbital edema, hyperemia, alopecia, muscular weakness, myopia, vaginal bleeding, swelling of the tongue, gum hypertrophy and hirsutism.

Dosage and Administration: *Orally*, 0.5 to 1 gm 2 or 3 times daily. The total dosage for adults, regardless of age, may vary between 1 and 3 gm/day, the average being 1.5 gm. For pediatric administration, the usual dose may vary from 0.6 to 1.2 gm 2 or 3 times daily. May be administered in combination with other anticonvulsants when other forms of epilepsy coexist with petit mal.

Availability:
MILONTIN®: **(Parke-Davis)**
Kapseals® (Capsules), 250 and 500 mg in bottles of 100.
Suspension, 300 mg/5 ml in bottles of 1 pint.

PHENTERMINE Ⓒ IV

Chemical Name: α,α-Dimethylphenethylamine (phenyl-tertiary-butylamine).

Description: Phentermine, a highly complex molecule, is available as a cation exchange resin complex of sulfonated polystyrene or as the hydrochloride salt. Phentermine resin is a coarse, granular substance practically insoluble in water. The hydrochloride salt occurs as a bitter, white, crystalline powder soluble in water and in alcohol.

This compound produces an anorexigenic effect and loss of weight. The resin complex of phentermine appears to have no physiologic or pharmacologic effects until it reacts with cations (H^+, K^+, Na^+, etc.) in the gastrointestinal tract. It is released from the resin complex at a rate depending upon the total concentration of these cations. Since the concentration is fairly constant throughout the entire gastrointestinal tract, predictable, continuous, and controlled ionic release occurs over a period of 10 to 14 hours. Phentermine is a sympathomimetic amine with pharmacologic activity similar to the prototype [amphetamines] of this class. It exerts relatively weak peripheral and central excitatory effects but produces significant anorectic activity. The resin-complex form appears to be less than one-half as toxic as the free drug.

Indications: Treatment of exogenous obesity as a short-term adjunct (a few weeks) in a regimen of weight reduction based on caloric restriction.

Contraindications: Advanced arteriosclerosis, symptomatic cardiovascular disease, moderate to severe hypertension, hyperthyroidism, known hypersensitivity or idiosyncrasy to the sympathomimetic amines, glaucoma, agitated states, patients with a history of drug abuse, and during or within 14 days following the administration of monoamine oxidase inhibitors (a hypertensive crisis may result).

Warnings: Tolerance to the anorectic effect usually develops within a few weeks. When this occurs, the recommended dose should not be exceeded in an attempt to increase the effect; rather the drug should be discontinued. Sympathomimetic drugs may mask extreme fatigue which can impair the ability to perform potentially hazardous activities (e.g., operating machinery or vehicles); therefore, patients should be cautioned accordingly. Phentermine has a significant potential for abuse. Tolerance and extreme psychological dependence have occurred; there are reports of patients who have increased the dosage to many times that recommended. Abrupt cessation following prolonged high dosage administration results in extreme fatigue and mental depression; changes have also been noted on the sleep EEG.

Manifestations of chronic intoxication include severe dermatoses, marked insomnia, irritability, hyperactivity, and personality changes. The most severe manifestation of chronic intoxication is psychosis, often clinically indistinguishable from schizophrenia. Safe use during pregnancy has not been established; therefore, use of this drug by women who are or who may become pregnant requires that the potential benefit be weighed against the possible hazard to the mother and infant. Phentermine is not recommended for use in children under 12 years of age.

Precautions: Use cautiously in patients with mild hypertension. It should be considered that the insulin requirements in diabetes mellitus may be altered in association with the use of phentermine and the concomitant dietary regimen. It may also decrease the hypotensive effect of guanethidine. The smallest quantity feasible should be prescribed or dispensed at one time in order to minimize the possibility of overdosage.

Adverse Reactions: *Cardiovascular:* Palpitation, tachycardia, elevation of blood pressure. *CNS:* Overstimulation, restlessness, dizziness, insomnia, euphoria, dysphoria, tremor, headache; rarely, psychotic episodes at recommended doses. *Gastrointestinal:* Dryness of the mouth, unpleasant taste, diarrhea, constipation, other gastrointestinal disturbances. *Allergic:* Urticaria. *Endocrine:* Impotence, changes in libido. Manifestations of acute overdosage may include restlessness, tremor, hyperreflexia, rapid respiration, confusion, assaultiveness, hallucinations, and panic states. Fatigue and depression usually follow the central stimulation. Cardiovascular effects include arrhythmias, hypertension or hypotension and circulatory collapse. Gastrointestinal symptoms may be manifested by nausea, vomiting, diarrhea, and abdominal cramps. Fatal poisoning usually terminates in convulsions and coma. Management of acute intoxication is largely symptomatic and includes gastric lavage and sedation with a barbiturate. Experience with hemodialysis or peritoneal dialysis is inadequate to permit recommendation in this regard. Acidification of the urine increases excretion of phentermine. If severe hypertension complicates overdosage, intravenous phentolamine has been suggested.

Dosage and Administration: *Orally,* 1 capsule daily before breakfast or 10 to 14 hours before retiring or 1 tablet 3 times daily before meals. For highly responsive individuals, 15 mg may be sufficient; for others 30 mg may be required.

Availability:

Ⓒ ADIPEX 8™: **(Lemmon)**

Capsules (as hydrochloride), 8 mg in bottles of 100 and 1000.

Tablets (as hydrochloride), 8 mg in bottles of 100 and 1000.

Ⓒ ADIPEX-P™. **(Lemmon)**
Capsules (as hydrochloride), 30 mg (equiv. to 24 mg phentermine) in bottles of 100 and 1000.
Tablets (as hydrochloride), 37.5 mg (equiv. to 30 mg of phentermine) in bottles of 100 and 1000.
Ⓒ IONAMIN® (as cationic exchange resin complex), 15 and 30 mg in bottles of 100 and 400. **(Pennwalt)**
Ⓒ FASTIN® Capsules (as hydrochloride), 30 mg (equiv. to 24 mg of phentermine) in bottles of 100. **(Beecham)**

PHENTOLAMINE

Chemical Name: 2-[*N*-(m-Hydroxyphenyl)-*p*-toluidinomethyl]imidazoline.

Description: Phentolamine mesylate is an *alpha* adrenergic blocking agent chemically and pharmacologically related to tolazoline. It occurs as a white, odorless, crystalline powder freely soluble in water and in alcohol.

Phentolamine selectively inhibits responses to adrenergic stimuli that are mediated by *alpha* receptors (primarily excitatory responses of smooth muscles and exocrine glands). It produces a fall in blood pressure by means of its vasodilating effect due primarily to a direct action on vascular smooth muscle and its cardiac stimulating effect; it produces a direct stimulant action on cardiac muscle.

Phentolamine appears to be only about 20% as active when given orally as when administered parenterally. About 10% of an injected dose is recovered in the urine as active drug; the fate of the remainder is unknown.

Indications: *Orally* and *parenterally* for use in the medical management of patients with pheochromocytoma to prevent paroxysmal attacks prior to surgical treatment; preoperatively and during actual removal of the tumor; and to prevent or control hypertensive episodes that may occur as the result of stress and manipulation of the tumor. *Parenterally,* the drug is also useful in preventing or counteracting dermal necrosis and sloughing caused by intravenous administration or extravasation of norepinephrine and as a diagnostic test for pheochromocytoma.

Contraindications: Myocardial infarction, a history of myocardial infarction, coronary insufficiency, angina or other evidence suggestive of coronary artery disease, and hypersensitivity to phentolamine or to related compounds.

Warnings: Myocardial infarction, cerebrovascular spasm, and cerebrovascular occlusion have been reported to occur following the administration of phentolamine, usually in association with marked hypotensive episodes with shock-like states which occasionally follow parenteral administration. For screening tests in patients with hypertension, the generally available urinary assay of catecholamines or other biochemical assays have largely supplanted the phentolamine and other pharmacological tests for reasons of accuracy and safety. The phentolamine test is not the procedure of choice and should be reserved for cases in which additional confirmatory evidence is necessary, and the relative risks involved in conducting the test have been considered. Safe use of this drug in pregnant or lactating women has not been established; therefore, the benefits to be derived must be weighed against the potential hazards to the mother and child.

Precautions: Tachycardia and cardiac arrhythmias may occur; therefore, whenever possible, administration of this drug should be deferred until cardiac rhythm returns to normal.

Adverse Reactions: Acute and prolonged hypotensive episodes, tachycardia, and cardiac arrhythmias have been reported, most frequently after parenteral administration. In addition, weakness, dizziness, flushing, orthostatic hypotension, nasal stuffiness, nausea, vomiting, and diarrhea may occur.

Dosage and Administration: *Intramuscularly* or *intravenously* for diagnosis and therapy of pheochromocytoma. It is essential that certain precautions be taken to eliminate the possibility of false positive or false negative responses. These involve withholding all but most essential medication for 24 to 72 hours prior to test, obtaining accurate basal blood pressure, correct positioning of the patient, and double checking by means of a histamine test. For complete information regarding the phentolamine test for pheochromocytoma and on its use in counteracting ischemic necrosis, consult the package literature. *Orally.* To control and prevent paroxysmal attacks prior to surgery, 1 tablet 4 to 6 times daily. In severe cases, higher dosages may be required. Children, 1/2 tablet 4 to 6 times daily.

Availability:
REGITINE®: **(Ciba)**
Injection (lyophilized, as mesylate) in vials of 5 mg with 1-ml ampul of Sterile Water for Injection.
Tablets (as hydrochloride), 50 mg in bottles of 100.

PHENYLBUTAZONE

Chemical Name: 4-Butyl-1,2-diphenyl-3,5-pyrazolidinedione.

OXYPHENBUTAZONE

Chemical Name: 4-Butyl-1-(*p*-hydroxyphenyl) 2-phenyl-3,5-pyrazolidinedione.

Description: Phenylbutazone, and oxyphenbutazone, the monohydrate of the *para*-hydroxy analog and a major metabolite of phenylbutazone, are closely related chemically and pharmacologically, including toxic effects, to the pyrazolines (pyrazole compounds amidopyrine and antipyrine). Phenylbutazone occurs as a white or yellowish, bitter powder very slightly soluble in water and in alcohol.

On a weight basis, phenylbutazone and oxyphenbutazone are about equal as antiinflammatory agents, but the analgesic effect of the latter is about 1/3 that of the former. Both retain sodium, chloride and water, presumably by enhancing renal tubular reabsorption, but they do not affect the excretion of potassium. With usual dosages, neither drug has clinically significant uricosuric activity. In experimental animals, oxyphenbutazone has been shown to be less ulcerogenic; in clinical use it may cause less gastric irritation than does phenylbutazone.

Indications: Gout, rheumatoid arthritis, rheumatoid spondylitis, osteoarthritis, psoriatic arthritis, acute superficial thrombophlebitis, painful shoulder (peritendinitis, capsulitis, bursitis, and acute arthritis of the shoulder), and a variety of local inflammatory conditions.

Important Note: Neither phenylbutazone nor oxyphenbutazone should ever be given casually. Each patient should be carefully evaluated before treatment is started and should remain constantly under the close supervision of the physician. Therapy should not be initiated until a careful detailed history and a complete physical and laboratory examination including blood count, urinalysis, etc., of the patient has been performed. See Warnings and Precautions.

Contraindications: In children 14 years of age or less, and in senile patients, in individuals with a history of, or symptoms of gastrointestinal inflammation or ulceration, including severe or recurrent or persistent dyspepsia, in those with a history of, or presence of drug allergy; blood dyscrasias, renal, hepatic or cardiac dysfunction; hypertension; thyroid disease; systemic edema; salivary gland enlargement or stomatitis due to the drug; polymyalgia rheumatica, and temporal arteritis. Phenylbutazone and oxyphenbutazone are contraindicated when the patient is receiving other potent chemotherapeutic agents, and also in patients who are on long-term anticoagulant therapy.

Warnings: The known factors affecting the incidence of toxic reactions are age, weight, dosage, duration of therapy, existence of concomitant diseases, and concurrent potent chemotherapy. Careful instructions to, and observations of, the individual patient are essential to the prevention of serious, life-threatening adverse reactions. This is especially true in the elderly patient (60 years and over) who have an increased susceptibility to the toxicity of the drug. The lowest effective dose for the specific individual should be the continuous goal of therapy with this drug. In each patient, the risk of severe, and even fatal drug reactions must be weighed against the possible drug benefits initially unpredictable for the individual. Phenylbutazone should be restricted to treatment periods of *1-week* duration. The appearance of clinical edema is an indication to discontinue treatment with the drug. Animal reproduction studies thus far, though inconclusive, exhibit evidences of embryotoxicity. Therefore, it is recommended that the drug be used with caution in the first trimester of pregnancy, weighing the potential risks against the benefits. Pregnant women and nursing mothers should receive phenylbutazone or oxyphenbutazone with caution since either drug may appear in cord blood and breast milk. Serious, even fatal blood dyscrasias, including aplastic anemia may occur suddenly despite regular repeated hemograms, and may become manifest many days or weeks after withdrawal of the drug. Any significant change in the total white count, relative decrease in granulocytes, appearance of immature forms, or fall in hematocrit should be a signal for immediate cessation of therapy and a complete hematologic investigation. Unexplained bleeding involving the CNS, adrenal glands, and gastrointestinal tract has occurred due to therapy with these drugs. They may potentiate the pharmacologic action of insulin, sulfonylurea, and sulfonamide-type agents. Patients receiving such concomitant therapy should be carefully observed for this effect. Both drugs reduce the iodine uptake by the thyroid. Both nontoxic and toxic goiters and myxedema due to therapy with either drug have been reported. The development of blurred vision while on one of these drugs can be a significant toxic symptom worthy of a complete ophthalmological examination. In patients *under sixty years of age* swelling of the ankles or face alone may be prevented by reducing the dosage. Otherwise, the appearance of clinical edema is an indication to discontinue the drug.

Precautions: Patients taking phenylbutazone or oxyphenbutazone should remain under close supervision of the physician and should be warned to report immediately the occurrence of fever, sore throat, lesions in the mouth, salivary gland enlargement, weight gain, edema, and black or tarry stools, or any other sign or symptom pertinent to the individual case. Periodic visits with the patient should include verbal evaluation and physical examination for signs of toxic reactions, check of patient's weight to detect significant water retention, and complete blood counts at weekly intervals during the early phase of therapy and at intervals of 2 weeks thereafter to guard against the possibility of blood dyscrasia. While on either drug, patients should be cautioned about participation in activity necessitating alertness and coordination, as driving a car, etc. Although a definite causal relationship to drug therapy has not been firmly established, cases of leukemia have been reported in patients with a history of short- and long-term therapy. The overwhelming majority of these patients were over 40 years of age. It should also be recognized that arthritic-type pains can be the presenting symptom of leukemia.

Adverse Reactions: Phenylbutazone or oxyphenbutazone is a potent drug; its misuse can lead to serious results. Detailed information on their use should be thoroughly reviewed before undertaking therapy. *Gastrointestinal:* Ulcerative esophagitis; acute and reactivated gastric and duodenal ulcer with perforation and hemorrhage; ulceration and perforation of large bowel; occult gastrointestinal bleeding with anemia; gastritis; epigastric pain; hematemesis; dyspepsia; nausea, vomiting and diarrhea; abdominal distention. *Hematologic:* Agranulocytosis, aplastic anemia, hemolytic anemia, anemia due to blood loss including occult gastrointestinal bleeding, thrombocytopenia, pancytopenia, leukemia, leukopenia, bone marrow depression. *Fluid, electrolyte disturbances:* Sodium and chloride retention, water retention and edema, plasma dilution, respiratory alkalosis, metabolic acidosis. *Hepatic:* Fatal and nonfatal hepatitis (cholestasis may or may not be prominent). *Dermatologic:* Petechiae, purpura without thrombocytopenia, toxic pruritus, erythema nodosum. *Allergic reactions:* All allergic reactions require *prompt* and *permanent withdrawal* of phenylbutazone or oxyphenbutazone. Erythema multiforme; Stevens-Johnson syndrome, Lyell's syndrome, toxic necrotizing epidermolysis; exfoliative dermatitis; serum sickness; hypersensitivity angiitis (polyarteritis); anaphylactic shock; urticaria; arthralgia; fever; rashes. *Renal:* Proteinuria, hematuria, oliguria, anuria, renal failure with azotemia, glomerulonephritis, acute tubular necrosis, nephrotic syndrome, bilateral renal cortical necrosis, renal stones, ureteral obstruction with uric acid crystals due to the uricosuric action of this drug, impaired renal function. *Cardiovascular:* Cardiac decompensation, hypertension, pericarditis, diffuse interstitial myocarditis with muscle necrosis, perivascular granulomata, aggravation of temporal arteritis in patients with polymyalgia rheumatica. *Ocular:* Optic neuritis, blurred vision, retinal hemorrhage, toxic amblyopia, retinal detachment. *Otic:* Hearing loss. *Metabolic-endocrine:* Hyperglycemia, thyroid hyperplasia, toxic goiter, association of hypothyroidism and hyperthyroidism (causal relationship not established). *CNS:* Agitation, confusional states, lethargy. *CNS reactions associated with overdosage:* Convulsions, euphoria, psychosis, depression, headaches, hallucinations, giddiness, vertigo, coma, hyperventilation, insomnia. *Miscellaneous:* Ulcerative stomatitis, salivary gland enlargement.

Dosage and Administration: *Orally. Rheumatoid arthritis, rheumatoid spondylitis, osteoarthritis, psoriatic arthritis* and *painful shoulder:* adults, 100 to 200 mg 3 times daily for 1 week initially, followed by 100 to 200 mg daily as maintenance (not to exceed 400 mg daily). *Acute gouty arthritis:* 400 mg initially, followed by 100 mg every 4 hours for not more than 1 week. *Acute superficial thrombophlebitis:* 200 mg 3 times daily for the first 2 or 3 days, followed by 100 mg 3 times daily for not more than 10 days.

To minimize gastric upset, phenylbutazone or oxyphenbutazone should always be taken immediately before or after meals or with a full glass of milk. The capsules containing antacids should be substituted if dyspeptic symptoms occur.

Availability:

Phenylbutazone

AZOLID® Tablets, 100 mg in bottles of 100 and 1000. **(USV)**

AZOLID®-A Capsules, 100 mg with dried aluminum hydroxide gel, 100 mg and magnesium trisilicate, 150 mg in bottles of 100 and 1000. **(USV)**

BUTAZOLIDIN® Tablets, 100 mg in bottles of 100 and 1000. **(Geigy)**

BUTAZOLIDIN® ALKA Capsules, 100 mg with dried aluminum hydroxide gel, 100 mg, and magnesium trisilicate, 150 mg in bottles of 100 and 1000, in unit-dose blister packages of 100 and 1000. **(Geigy)**

STERAZOLIDIN® Capsules, 50 mg with prednisone, 1.25 mg: dried aluminum hydroxide gel, 100 mg and magnesium trisilicate, 150 mg in bottles of 100. **(Geigy)**

Oxyphenbutazone

OXALID® Tablets, 100 mg in bottles of 100 and 1000. **(USV)**

TANDEARIL® Tablets, 100 mg in bottles of 100 and 1000. **(Geigy)**

PHENYLEPHRINE HYDROCHLORIDE

Chemical Name: 1-*m*-Hydroxy-α-[(methylamino) methyl]benzyl alcohol hydrochloride.

Description: Phenylephrine hydrochloride is a synthetic sympathomimetic compound structurally similar to epinephrine and ephedrine.

Phenylephrine is a potent sympathomimetic agent of relatively low toxicity. It is as effective a vasoconstrictor and pressor substance as epinephrine or ephedrine; causes little or no tachycardia, irregularity in pulse rate, or CNS stimulation. Phenylephrine is stable and effective orally, more lasting in action than epinephrine, and does not lose its effectiveness upon repeated administration. A prompt, short-acting mydriatic, it causes little or no cycloplegia or irritation.

Indications: Temporary relief of nasal congestion, hay fever, sinusitis, and head colds; as an ophthalmic decongestant and vasoconstrictor and for pupil dilatation in uveitis (posterior synechiae), wide-angle glaucoma, surgery, refraction, ophthalmoscopic examination, and diagnostic procedures; for the treatment of orthostatic hypotension; to maintain adequate blood pressure during severe hypotensive states and shock; in the treatment of paroxysmal supraventricular tachycardia; for the prevention and treatment of hypotension associated with spinal anesthesia; for the prolongation of spinal anesthesia; and as a vasoconstrictor for regional anesthesia. Zinc is added for its astringent properties.

Contraindications: Narrow-angle glaucoma, hypertension, ventricular tachycardia. The 10% solution should not be used in infants.

Precautions: Should be used cautiously, if at all, in patients with hypertension or ventricular tachycardia and should be employed only with considerable caution in elderly patients or in patients with hyperthyroidism, bradycardia, partial heart block, or myocardial disease. Vasopressors have been found to cause serious cardiac arrhythmias in patients undergoing halothane anesthesia and therefore should be used only with extreme caution, or not at all. The 10% ophthalmic solution should be used with caution in patients with advanced arteriosclerotic conditions or severe hypertension. Phenylephrine may be used in patients with glaucoma when temporary dilatation of the pupil may free adhesions or when vasoconstriction of intrinsic vessels may lower intraocular tension; these advantages may temporarily outweigh the danger from coincident dilatation of the pupil. It should be used cautiously and in small doses in patients receiving MAO inhibitors, adrenergic and ganglionic blocking agents, rauwolfia and veratrum alkaloids, phenothiazines tranquilizers, and tricyclic antidepressants. If combined with oxytocics during obstetrical procedures, a severe persistent hypertension may occur and may result in the rupture of a cerebral blood vessel in the postpartum period.

Adverse Reactions: It is well to bear in mind that phenylephrine is, in fact, a sympathomimetic drug related to epinephrine and ephedrine, and that although the incidence is rare, it may produce such reactions as tremor, pallor, perspiration, palpitation or collapse. Administered intravenously to patients with paroxysmal tachycardia, overdosage may induce ventricular extrasystoles and short paroxysms of ventricular tachycardia, a sensation of fullness in the head, and tingling of the extremities.

Dosage and Administration: *Orally.* Adults, 2 tablets 3 or 4 times daily, or 1 timed-release tablet 3 times daily. *Subcutaneously or intramuscularly*, the usual dose is from 2 to 5 mg with a range of 1 to 10 mg. The initial dose should not exceed 5 mg. *Intravenously*, 10 to 20 mg in 500 ml of an isotonic infusion solution at a rate adjusted to maintain blood pressure. *Topically*, 1 or 2 drops of the 2.5% ophthalmic solution or 1 drop of the 10% solution into the conjunctiva. For complete details, consult package literature. *Spray or drops*, adults—instill 3 sprays or drops into each nostril; children over 3 years of age—1 or 2 sprays into each nostril. Administer when necessary but not more than 5 times daily.

Availability:

BIOMYDRIN®: **(Warner-Chilcott)**

Nasal Drops (OTC), 0.25% in bottles of 15 ml with dropper.

Nasal Spray (OTC), 0.25% in bottles of 15 ml with atomizer.

MYDFRIN™ Ophthalmic Solution, 2.5% in plastic dropper bottles of 5 ml. **(Alcon)**

NEO-SYNEPHRINE®: **(Winthrop)**

Injection, 10 mg/ml in ampuls of 1 ml.

Nasal Spray (OTC), 0.25 and 5% in squeeze bottles of 22.5 ml.

Ophthalmic Solution (low surface tension), 2.5% in Mono-Drop® (plastic dropper) bottles of 15 ml; 10% in Mono-Drop® (plastic dropper) bottles of 5 ml.

Ophthalmic Solution (viscous), 10% in Mono-Drop® (plastic dropper) bottles of 5 ml.

PYRACORT®-D Nasal spray (OTC), 0.5% in plastic spray bottles of 22.5 ml. **(Lemmon)**

Combinations

RHINEX® D-Lay Tablets, 2.5 mg with chlorpheniramine maleate, 1.25 mg and aspirin, 150 mg in bottles of 100 and 1000. **(Lemmon)**

RHINEX DM Tablets, 5 mg with chlorpheniramine maleate, 2 mg and dextromethorphan hydrochloride, 10 mg in bottles of 100 and 1000. **(Lemmon)**

SINGLET® Tablets (timed-release), 40 mg with chlorpheniramine maleate, 8 mg and acetaminophen, 500 mg in bottles of 100. **(Dow)**

PHENYLMERCURIC ACETATE

Description: Phenylmercuric acetate occurs as small, lustrous crystals slightly soluble in water and soluble in alcohol. The concentrated solution contains 0.2% phenylmercuric acetate in a buffered solvent of 50% alcohol, de-ionized water, sodium acetate, acetic acid and boric acid to attain an acid pH of 4.1. The jelly contains 0.02% phenylmercuric acid in a special base containing boric acid, with acetic acid added to attain a pH of 4.

Indications: Adjunctive therapy in trichomoniasis, bacterial infections, moniliasis, mixed infections, nonspecific leukorrhea, post-cauterization therapy in the treatment of cervical pathology.

Adverse Reactions: Erythematous or vesicular eruptions may occur; if these appear, treatment should be discontinued.

Dosage and Administration: *Intravaginally* as a douche, add from 1 to 3 tablespoonsful to 1 quart of water, depending upon the potency of the solution desired. May be used concomitantly with gentian violet. After douching, insert 1 applicatorful of jelly daily and continue through the menstrual period (douches are omitted during the menstrual period); this procedure should be continued for 6 to 8 weeks or longer if necessary. As a prophylactic, the jelly should be inserted during the 2 menstrual periods following cessation of daily use. Following cervical cauterization, the jelly should be instilled only upon retiring; no douches are required except prior to gynecological examination.

Availability:
NYLMERATE: **(Holland-Rantos)**
Jelly, 0.02% in tubes of 80 and 136 gm with or without applicator.
Solution Concentrate, 0.2% in bottles of 1 pint with measuring cup.

PHENYLPROPANOLAMINE HYDROCHLORIDE

Chemical Name: α-(l-Aminoethyl)benzyl alcohol hydrochloride.

Description: Phenylpropanolamine is a sympathomimetic agent closely related pharmacologically to ephedrine and epinephrine. It is approximately equal in potency to ephedrine but usually causes less CNS stimulation. In common with other sympathomimetic amines, the drug causes vasoconstriction and blanching of the nasal mucosa. It occurs as a white, crystalline powder freely soluble in water and in alcohol.

Indications: Symptomatic relief of nasal congestion associated with the common cold, rhinitis, sinusitis, nasopharyngitis, or allergic conditions such as hay fever and allergic rhinitis. Combined with dextromethorphan for temporary relief from coughing and nasal congestion associated with the common cold. Parenterally, as a vasopressor during surgery, particularly during spinal anesthesia.

Precautions: Use with caution in patients with hypertension, cardiovascular disease, hyperthyroidism or diabetes. Large doses may cause hypertension, tachycardia, nervousness, restlessness or insomnia. Should not be administered to patients receiving MAO inhibitors. Close supervision and careful adjustment of dosages are required if given with tricyclic antidepressants. Symptoms of overdosage may include rapid pulse and respiration, disorientation, elevated blood pressure, tachycardia, dilated pupils, headache, CNS stimulation, nausea and vomiting, gastrointestinal upset, and anorexia.

Dosage and Administration: *Orally.* Adults, 25 mg at intervals of 3 or 4 hours to 50 mg at intervals of 6 to 8 hours as indicated. Children 8 to 12 years of age, 25 mg 3 times daily. *Elixir,* for adults 2 teaspoonsful and children 1 teaspoonful 3 times daily. *Liquid,* for adults and children over 12 years of age 2 teaspoonsful; children 4 to 12 years, 1 teaspoonful, and those 2 to 4 years, ½ teaspoonful taken 4 times daily. *Intramuscularly,* 0.5 to 1 ml to initiate symptomatic therapy.

Availability:
Phenylpropanolamine Hydrochloride
Injection, 75 mg/ml in ampuls of 30 ml. **(Various Mfrs.)**
PROPADRINE®: **(Merck Sharp & Dohme)**
Capsules (OTC), 25 mg in bottles of 100 and 500; 50 mg in bottles of 100.
Elixir (OTC), 20 mg/5 ml in bottles of 1 pint.
Combinations
ORNACOL®: **(Smith Kline & French)**
Capsules (OTC), 25 mg with dextromethorphan hydrobromide, 30 mg in bottles of 20 and 100.
Liquid (OTC), 12.5 mg/5 ml with dextromethorphan hydrobromide, 15 mg/5 ml in bottles of 120 ml.

PHENYTOIN

Chemical Name: 5,5-Diphenyl-2,4-imidazolidinedione.

Description: An anticonvulsant agent which is structurally and pharmacologically related to mephenytoin and ethotoin. It occurs as a white powder practically insoluble in water and slightly soluble in alcohol. The sodium salt of phenytoin occurs as a white, hygroscopic powder freely soluble in water and soluble in alcohol.

Its precise mechanism of action is not known but the drug apparently prevents or reduces the severity and frequency of epileptiform attacks by causing a reduction in the voltage, frequency and spread of electrical discharges within the motor cortex, with relatively little hypnotic and narcotizing effects. Possibly by promoting sodium efflux from neurons, phenytoin tends to stabilize the threshold against hyperexcitability caused by excessive stimulation or environmental changes capable of reducing membrane sodium gradient. This includes the reduction of post-tetanic potentiation at synapses. Loss of post-tetanic potentiation prevents cortical seizure foci from detonating adjacent cortical areas. The sodium salt [phenytoin sodium] reduces the maximal activity of brain stem centers responsible for the tonic phase of grand mal seizure.

Because phenytoin sodium is slowly absorbed following intramuscular injection, patients stabilized on a daily oral regimen of the drug may experience a drop in peak blood levels to 50 to 60% of stable levels if crossed over to an equal intramuscular dose. In order to achieve rapid therapeutic levels, the drug should be given intravenously. Approximately 70 to 90% is bound to plasma proteins, mainly albumin, and the plasma half-life following oral ingestion averages 22 hours, with a range of 7 to 10 days after initiation of therapy with a recommended daily dose of 300 mg. The clinically effective serum level is usually 10 to 20 mcg/ml. The major portion of phenytoin is excreted in the bile as inactive metabolites which are then reabsorbed from the intestinal tract and excreted in the urine. The parahydroxyphenyl derivative is the principal metabolite and accounts for about 60 to 70% of a single dose of the drug.

Indications: Grand mal epilepsy, psychomotor seizures. Parenterally for use in the treatment of status epilepticus and control of seizures in neurosurgery.

Contraindications: Phenytoin is contraindicated in those patients with a known hypersensitivity to hydantoin products; in the presence of sinus bradycardia, sino-atrial block, second and third degree A-V block, and in patients with Adams-Stokes syndrome.

Warnings: Since blood dyscrasias have occurred after phenytoin therapy, hemoglobin level and the white-cell count should be checked at appropriate intervals. Certain drugs which may be given concurrently with this product seem to enhance the action of phenytoin, possibly by inhibiting its metabolism in the liver. These include bishydroxycoumarin, phenylbutazone, sulfaphenazole, disulfiram, and isoniazid. Tricyclic antidepressants in high doses may precipitate seizures and the dosage of phenytoin may have to be adjusted. Phenobarbital and other barbiturates may enhance the speed of metabolism. This effect, however, is variable and unpredictable. Other drugs, in addition to those listed above, when given concurrently with phenytoin, may influence its metabolic rate. The results of certain clinical laboratory tests, e.g., metyrapone, 1-mg dexamethasone, and protein-bound iodine, may be altered if the patient has been receiving this drug. *Subcutaneous or perivascular injection should be avoided because of the highly alkaline nature of the solution.* Intravenous injection should be *very slow* (at a rate not exceeding 1 ml of solution (50 mg) phenytoin/minute). The addition of phenytoin solutions to intravenous infusions is not recommended due to its instability and resultant precipitation. The solution should not be used if haziness or precipitate develops. The possibility of a severe convulsive seizure caused by a marked hypoglycemic state such as that resulting from an adenoma of the pancreas has been stressed. A blood sugar test should be made whenever this possibility is suspected. Patients should be observed for signs of anoxia, respiratory depression, or circulatory involvement. Recent reports strongly suggest an association between the use of anticonvulsant drugs and an increased incidence of birth defects in the offspring. Therefore, use during pregnancy, lactation or in women of childbearing age requires that the potential benefits be weighed against possible hazards to the patient and fetus. It is strongly advised that anticonvulsant therapy not be discontinued in patients in whom the drug is administered to prevent major seizures because of the potential of precipitating status epilepticus with attendant hypoxia, and risk to both the mother and the unborn child. Consideration should, nevertheless, be given to discontinuation of anticonvulsants prior to and during gestation when the nature, frequency and severity of the seizures do not constitute a serious threat to the patient. At present, it is not known whether even minor seizures pose some risk to the developing embryo or fetus.

Precautions: Ingestion of alcohol may interfere with the action of anticonvulsants. It is important to proceed slowly when increasing or decreasing dosage, as well as when adding or eliminating other medication. Abrupt withdrawal of anticonvulsant medication can precipitate status epilepticus. Because blood levels are substantially affected by the differences in dissolution and absorption rates, the physician is advised to keep the patient on the same product and dosage form, and if these must be changed, to check blood levels regularly. Phenytoin has been associated with reversible lymph node hyperplasia, osteomalacia, and hyperglycemia (resulting from the drug's inhibitory effect on insulin release), and may further raise the blood sugar level in hyperglycemic patients. The drug should be discontinued if a skin rash appears. If the rash is exfoliative, purpuric, or bullous, use of the drug should not be resumed. If the rash is a milder type (measles-like or scarlatiniform), therapy may be resumed after the rash has completely disappeared. If the rash recurs upon reinstitution of therapy, further medication with this drug is contraindicated. Phenytoin should be used with care in patients with hypotension and severe myocardial insufficiency. Also, patients with impaired liver function, elderly patients, or those who are gravely ill, may show early signs of toxicity.

Adverse Reactions: *CNS:* The most common manifestations encountered with phenytoin therapy are referable to this system. These include nystagmus, ataxia, slurred speech, and mental confusion. Dizziness, insomnia, transient nervousness, motor twitchings, and headache have also been observed. These side effects may disappear with continuing therapy at a reduced dosage level. *Gastrointestinal System:* Phenytoin may cause nausea, vomiting, and constipation. Administration of the drug with or immediately after meals may help prevent gastrointestinal discomfort. *Integumentary System:* Dermatological manifestations sometimes accompanied by fever have included scarlatiniform or morbilliform rashes. Other more serious forms which may be fatal have included bullous, exfoliative, or purpuric dermatitis, lupus erythematosus, and Stevens-Johnson syndrome. *Hemopoietic System:* Hemopoietic complications, some fatal, have occasionally been reported in association with administration of phenytoin. These have included thrombocytopenia, leukopenia, granulocytopenia, agranulocytosis, and pantocytopenia. While macrocytosis and megaloblastic anemia have occurred, these conditions usually respond to folic acid therapy. The occasional occurrence of lymphadenopathy indicates the need to differentiate such a condition from other lymph gland pathology. *Other:* Gingival hyperplasia occurs frequently, while polyarthropathy and hirsutism occur occasionally. Toxic hepatitis, liver damage, and periarteritis nodosa may occur and can be fatal. Fatalities due to cardiac arrest, ventricular fibrillation, ventricular standstill, tonic seizures, and respiratory arrest have been reported following intravenous administration of phenytoin. Alterations of cardiac and respiratory function can be produced by too rapid administration of the drug intravenously. Complications may occur more readily in elderly patients and in gravely ill patients.

Dosage and Administration: *Orally.* Initial dosage is 100 mg 3 times daily, optimum dosage to be determined for each patient individually. For most adults, 300 or 400 mg is a satisfactory maintenance dosage, increased to 0.6 gm if necessary. The recommended initial dosage for children is 5 mg/kg/day in 2 or 3 equally divided doses, with subsequent dosage individualized to a maximum of 300 mg daily. For most children, 4 to 8 mg/kg/day is a satisfactory maintenance dosage, but children over 6 years of age may require the minimal adult dosage of 300 mg/day. An alternative procedure is to give the drug on a once-a-day schedule because of the long half-life of phenytoin, a single daily dose is as effective as divided doses. All doses should be taken with at least a half glass of water to reduce gastric irritation. Phenobarbital or bromides, if previously administered, should be withdrawn gradually, by overlapping therapy. *Intravenously.* Status epilepticus, 150 to 250 mg of sodium solution at a rate not to exceed 1 ml (50 mg)/minute followed by 100 to 150 mg 30 minutes later if necessary. Children's dose is proportionately less. *Intramuscularly.* Neurosurgical prophylaxis, 2 to 4 ml (100 to 200 mg) 3 or 4 times during the 24 hours before surgery, or during surgery at 4-hour intervals and continuing into the postoperative period. When oral administration is to be resumed following intramuscular usage, the oral dosage should be properly adjusted (usually reduced by 50% the previous oral dosage) for 1 week to prevent excessive plasma levels due to the sustained release from intramuscular tissue sites.

Availability:

Phenytoin

DILANTIN®: **(Parke-Davis)**

Infatabs® (flavored tablets), 50 mg in bottles of 100 and in unit-dose packages of 100 (10 x 10).
Oral Suspension, 30 and 125 mg/5 ml in bottles of 240 ml.

Phenytoin Sodium

DILANTIN®: **(Parke-Davis)**
Capsules (Kapseals®), 30 and 100 mg in bottles of 100 and 1000 and in unit-dose packages of 100.
Injection, 50 mg/ml in ampuls (ready mixed) of 2 and 5 ml with disposable syringe in packages of 10 and in Steri-Dose® disposable syringes of 2 ml.
Powder in bottles of 30 gm.
w/Phenobarbital Capsules (Kapseals®), 100 mg with either 16 mg or 32 mg of phenobarbital (**Warning:** may be habit-forming) in bottles of 100 and 1000 and in unit-dose packages of 100.
PHENYTOIN SODIUM Capsules, 100 mg in bottles of 1000 and in unit-dose packages of 100. **(Lederle)**

PHTHALYLSULFATHIAZOLE: see The Sulfonamides

PHYSOSTIGMINE

Description: Physostigmine, an alkaloid obtained from *Physostigma venenosum*, produces pupillary constriction and spasm of accommodation through inactivation of cholinesterase. This effect permits intensive action of acetylcholine on the effector cells of the ciliary muscle and the sphincter muscle of the iris. It induces prompt action which occurs within 2 minutes after instillation, reaches a maximum within 1 to 2 hours, and persists for 12 to 36 hours.

Indications: Management of glaucoma.

Contraindications: In inflammatory disease of the iris or ciliary body.

Warnings: Overdosage may produce symptoms of systemic cholinesterase inhibitor toxicity.

Precautions: Use with caution in vagotonic states. Sensitivity to the drug may develop.

Adverse Reactions: Physostigmine may induce hyperreactivity of the pupillary and accommodative reflexes with resultant temporary decrease of visual acuity. Increased tonus of skeletal muscle or twitching of the lid may result following topical instillation into the conjunctival sac. Long-term use may produce changes in the pigmented epithelium of the iris. Chronic conjunctival irritation often occurs. Contact allergic dermatitis may also develop after prolonged use.

Dosage and Administration: *Topically,* instill 1 or 2 drops into eye; repeat as necessary to obtain miosis; or as directed by the physician.

Availability:
ISOPTO® ESERINE Ophthalmic Solution (as salicylate), 0.25 and 0.5% in Drop-Tainer® (dropper bottles) of 15 ml. **(Alcon)**
ISOPTO® P-ES Ophthalmic Solution, 0.25% (as salicylate) with pilocarpine hydrochloride, 2% in Drop-Tainer® (dropper bottles) of 15 ml. **(Alcon)**

PHYTONADIONE

Synonym: Vitamin K_1.

Chemical Name: 2-Methyl-3-phytyl-1,4-naphthoquinone.

Description: Phytonadione is a prothrombogenic vitamin that possesses the physiological activity of natural vitamin K. It occurs as a clear, yellow, very viscous, odorless or nearly odorless liquid.

Phytonadione has been reported to produce a more prompt, potent, and prolonged action than do the vitamin K analogues. The prothrombogenic effect usually occurs within 6 to 10 hours following oral administration and within 1 to 2 hours following intravenous administration. A normal prothrombin level may often be obtained within 12 to 14 hours.

Indications: To reverse anticoagulant-induced hypoprothrombinemia, and for the prophylaxis and therapy of hemorrhagic disease of the newborn. Also useful in hypoprothrombinemia due to (1) antibacterial therapy, (2) factors limiting absorption or synthesis of vitamin K (e.g., obstructive jaundice, biliary fistula, sprue, ulcerative colitis, celiac disease, intestinal resection, cystic fibrosis of the pancreas, and regional enteritis, or (3) to the toxic action of certain drugs (e.g., salicylates).

Contraindications: Hypersensitivity to phytonadione or to any component formulated with it.

Warnings: Occasionally, pain, swelling and tenderness at the injection site may occur. Severe reactions, including fatalities, have occurred during and immediately after intravenous injection, even when precautions have been taken to dilute the solution and to avoid rapid infusion. These reactions were reported to resemble hypersensitivity or anaphylaxis, including shock and cardiac and/or respiratory arrest, and to have occurred in some patients who had received the drug for the first time. Therefore, the intravenous route should be restricted to those situations where other routes are not feasible and the serious risk involved is considered justified. Attention must be paid to the fact that when hypoprothrombinemia due to anticoagulant therapy results in severe hemorrhage, no vitamin K preparation is a substitute for the use of whole blood transfusion, but should be considered as adjunctive therapy. To avoid overzealous correction of anticoagulant-induced hypoprothrombinemia, the minimum effective dose should be used, and the prothrombin time should be checked regularly. Phytonadione will not counteract the anticoagulant action of heparin.

Precautions: To minimize the occurrence of reactions, rapid intravenous administration of the colloidal solution should be avoided—the rate must not exceed 5 mg/minute. Excessive doses of phytonadione may cause temporary refractoriness to anticoagulants of the coumarin type, and larger doses may be necessary when reinstituting anticoagulant therapy. No adequate information is available as to whether or not this drug may affect fertility in male or female patients or have a teratogenic potential or other adverse effect on the fetus.

Adverse Reactions: Transient "flushing sensations" and "pecular" sensations of taste have been observed, as well as instances of dizziness, rapid and weak pulse, profuse sweating, brief hypotension, dyspnea and cyanosis. The possibility of allergic sensitivity, including an anaphylactoid reaction, should be kept in mind, especially since deaths have been reported following intravenous administration. Hyperbilirubinemia in the newborn has been reported with large doses. Kernicterus has not been noted following parenteral administration at therapeutic dose levels.

Dosage and Administration: *Orally*. To modify anticoagulant effects, 2.5 to 10 mg up to 25 mg (rarely 50 mg) initially. If prothrombin time has not been satisfactorily shortened in 12 to 48 hours, repeat the dose. For surgery, up to 50 mg given at least 24 hours preoperatively, along with temporary discontinuance of anticoagulant, is recommended to restore prothrombin to a safer limit for the operative period. For hypoprothrombinemia due to obstructive jaundice and biliary fistula, a range of 2 to 20 mg or more daily may be required with concomitant administration of bile salts; gastrointestinal disorders interfering with vitamin absorption, 5 to 15 mg or more daily; salicylates, 25 to 50 mg or more; antibiotics or sulfonamides, up to 15 mg. *Parenterally*. For actual or imminent hemorrhage, 5 to 25 mg *intravenously*. For potential but remote threat of hemorrhage, 1 to 25 mg *intramuscularly* or *intravenously*.

Availability:
AquaMEPHYTON® Injection, 2 mg/ml in ampuls of 0.5 ml; 10 mg/ml in ampuls of 1 ml and in vials of 2.5 and 5 ml. **(Merck Sharp & Dohme)**
KONAKION® Injection (IM only), 2 mg/ml in ampuls of 0.5 ml; 10 mg/ml in ampuls of 1 and 2.5 ml. **(Roche)**
MEPHYTON Tablets, 5 mg in bottles of 100. **(Merck Sharp & Dohme)**

PILOCARPINE

Description: Pilocarpine is an alkaloid obtained from *Pilocarpus jaborandi*. It contracts the pupil by acting directly on the myoneural junction of the sphincter muscle in the iris. Onset of action begins within 15 to 30 minutes, reaches a maximum in approximately 75 minutes and persists for 4 to 8 hours. Spasm of accommodation also begins in about 15 minutes and persists for 2 or 3 hours.

Indications: Treatment of primary simple (open-angle) glaucoma, acute narrow-angle and secondary glaucomas, in congenital glaucoma, in the reduction of intraocular tension pre- and postoperatively, as an antidote for mydriasis. Compounded with epinephrine for synergistic action, thus producing greater reduction in intraocular pressure; it is also used to improve the appearance of the eye through its rapid blanching properties, and to help offset the tissue irritation which usually accompanies the use of pilocarpine.

Contraindications: In cases where constriction is undesirable such as acute iritis, secondary glaucoma, and acute inflammatory disease of the anterior segment, and in patients sensitive to any of the ingredients.

Warnings: For topical ophthalmic use only.

Precautions: Should be used with caution in closed-angle glaucoma, vascular hypertension or both, and in patients with bronchial asthma. Discontinue medication if irritation or sensitization occur.

Adverse Reactions: Prolonged use may produce innocuous extra-cellular pigmentation in the palpebral conjunctiva. Conjunctival irritation may occur frequently. Occipital headaches, palpitation, paleness, acceleration of heart beat, trembling and perspiration have been observed on rare occasions.

Dosage and Administration: *Topically* by instillation into the conjunctival sac. In simple open-angle glaucoma, initially 1 or 2 drops of a 1 or 2% solution every 6 to 8 hours; if not well tolerated an 0.25 or 0.5% solution may be used. Concentration and frequency may be increased as required. In acute narrow-angle and secondary glaucomas prior to surgery, 1 or 2 drops of a 2% solution every minute for 5 minutes, then 1 or 2 drops every 5 minutes for 25 minutes followed by 1 or 2 drops 3 or 4 times each hour until a satisfactory response is attained. To avoid a bilateral attack 3 drops of a 1% solution every 8 hours may be instilled into the unaffected eye. In congenital glaucoma, 1 or 2 drops of a 2% solution every 6 hours, then every 10 minutes for 30 minutes immediately prior to surgery. To counteract cycloplegics, 1 or 2 drops of a 1 or 2% solution as needed. Pilocarpine and phenylephrine, 1 or 2 drops 2 to 4 times daily. The ocusert unit is placed in the eye by the patient according to the physician's instructions.

Availability:

Pilocarpine Hydrochloride

ALMOCARPINE® Ophthalmic Solution, 1, 2 and 4% in Steri-Tainer® dropper bottles of 15 ml. **(Ayerst)**

ISOPTO® CARPINE Ophthalmic Solution, 0.5, 1, 2, 3, 4 and 6% in Drop-Tainer® (dropper bottles) of 15 and 30 ml; 0.25, 1.5, 5, 8 and 10% in Drop-Tainer® bottles of 15 ml. **(Alcon)**

MI-PILO® Ophthalmic Solution, 1, 2 and 4% in dropper bottles of 15 ml. **(Barnes-Hind)**

OCUSERT PILO-20/-40 Sterile System releases 20 or 40 mcg/hour for 1 week in packages of 8 individual units. **(Ciba)**

PILOCAR® Ophthalmic Solution, 0.5, 1, 2, 3 and 6% in dropper-tip bottles of 15 ml; 1, 2 and 4% in dropperette applicators of 1 ml. **(Smith, Miller & Patch)**

PILOMIOTIN® Ophthalmic Solution, 1, 2 and 4% in dropper bottles of 15 ml. **(Smith, Miller & Patch)**

Combinations

E-CARPINE® Ophthalmic Solution, 1, 2, 3, 4 and 6% with epinephrine bitartrate equivalent to 0.5% epinephrine in Drop-Tainer® bottles of 15 ml. **(Alcon)**

Pilocarpine Nitrate

P. V. CARPINE® Liquifilm® Ophthalmic Solution, 0.5, 1, 2, 3, 4 and 6% in dropper bottles of 15 ml. **(Allergan)**

PIPERACETAZINE: see The Phenothiazines

PIPERAZINE

Description: Piperazine, an anthelmintic, is available as the citrate. Piperazine citrate occurs as a white, crystalline powder soluble in water and insoluble in alcohol. The drug produces a paralysis of ascaris muscle with resultant expulsion of the worm through intestinal peristalsis. Systemic absorbtion of piperazine is variable and the drug is excreted essentially unchanged.

Indications: Treatment of infections due to pinworms (*Enterobius vermicularis*), and roundworms (*Ascaris lumbricoides*).

Contraindications: In patients with impaired renal or hepatic function, convulsive disorders, or a history of hypersensitivity reactions to the drug and its salts.

Warnings: Because of potential neurotoxicity of this drug, especially in children, prolonged or repeated treatment in excess of that recommended should be avoided. Safe use during pregnancy has not been established.

Precautions: Supportive therapy and special care is indicated in patients with severe malnutrition, or anemia. If CNS, gastrointestinal, or hypersensitivity reactions occur, the drug should be discontinued.

Adverse Reactions: *Orally.* Those reported have been usually due to excessive dosage. These include: *Gastrointestinal*—nausea, vomiting, abdominal cramps, and diarrhea. *CNS*—headache, vertigo, ataxia, tremors, choreiform movements, muscular weakness, hyporeflexia, paresthesia, blurring of vision, paralytic strabismus, convulsion, EEG abnormalities, sense of detachment, and memory defect. *Hypersensitivity*—urticaria, erythema multiforme, purpura, fever, and arthralgia.

Dosage and Administration: *Orally. For pinworm infection:* Adults and children, a single daily dose of 65 mg/kg of body weight with a maximum daily dose of 2.5 gm for 7 consecutive days. *For roundworm infections*, once daily for 2 consecutive days. For adults, 3.5 gm and for children, 75 mg/kg of body weight with a maximum daily dose of 3.5 gm. In severe infections, the course may be repeated after a 1-week rest period. In instances where repeated therapy is not practicable, a single dose of 70 mg/lb of body weight, up to a maximum of 3 gm, may be given.

Availability:
ANTEPAR®: **(Burroughs Wellcome)**
Syrup, 550 mg/5 ml (as citrate) equiv. to 500 mg of piperazine hexahydrate in bottles of 1 pint.
Tablets, 550 mg (as citrate) equiv. to 500 mg of piperazine hexahydrate in bottles of 100 and 1000.

PIPEROCAINE HYDROCHLORIDE

Chemical Name: y-(2-Methylpiperidyl) propyl benzoate hydrochloride.

Description: Piperocaine hydrochloride, a benzoic acid ester, occurs as a white, odorless, crystalline powder freely soluble in water and soluble in alcohol. Aqueous solutions are acid to litmus; they are stable and retain their potency after sterilization by boiling or autoclaving.

Piperocaine is an effective topical anesthetic for surface anesthesia of the mucous membranes, and for infiltration, regional and caudal anesthesia. Compared with procaine, its effect is more potent and more toxic, and its action is more rapid and of longer duration. However, it is less toxic than cocaine and most cocaine substitutes.

Indications: For caudal, infiltration, regional and topical anesthesia. Formulated with merthiolate to provide antiseptic effects in the prophylaxis and treatment of painful superficial infections of the cornea and conjunctiva.

Contraindications: Gross deformity or disease of spine or CNS system, local infection at site of injection, skin infections anywhere in the body, extreme obesity, profound anemia, hypersensitivity to analgesics; in obstetrics: patient psychically unsuited, large fetus and/or small vagina, floating fetal head, placenta previa, and premature separation of the placenta.

Precautions: Caudal administration should not be attempted until the physician has informed himself on all phases of the procedure. Preparations for caudal administration should not be used for spinal anesthesia. Inadvertent administration into a vein may cause a shocklike reaction, with a sharp fall in blood pressure, slow pulse, unconsciousness or even death; or nervous symptoms such as pallor, sweating, apprehension, tremors, and in severe cases, convulsions may occur.

Dosage and Administration: For infiltration anesthesia in small areas, 0.5 to 1%; solution for block anesthesia, 0.5 to 2% solution. For caudal anesthesia, initially, 8 ml of 1.5% solution. If spinal anesthesia does not occur, 22 ml is injected slowly in obstetric patients, and 42 ml in surgical patients. Supplementary injections of 20 ml every 30 to 40 minutes will maintain the anesthesia. For spinal anesthesia using saddle block technique, a single injection of 1 ml of 3% solution containing 5% dextrose is sufficient to provide anesthesia for 75 minutes. For cesarean section or other low abdominal surgery, 1.5 ml of a 3% solution containing 5% dextrose may be used; the maximal dose is 100 mg. Topically for application in the eye, 2 to 4% solution; the ointment may be applied 1 to 3 times daily. Rectally, 1 to 3 suppositories daily. For dental procedures, 1 to 2% solution. Consult package literature for complete dosage information.

Availability:
METYCAINE®: **(Lilly)**
Injection, 1.5% in vials of 200 ml; 2% in vials of 30 ml.
Powder for topical and infiltrative use in bottles of 120 mg. Solutions intended for injection should be sterilized by boiling or autoclaving.
METYCAINE and MERTHIOLATE Ophthalmic Ointment, 4% with merthiolate, 1:5000 in tubes of 3.5 gm. **(Lilly)**
METYCAINE and ZINC OXIDE COMPOUND Suppositories (OTC), 125 mg with belladonna extract, 12.5 mg; zinc oxide, 250 mg and bismuth subcarbonate, 125 mg in cartons of 12. **(Lilly)**

PIPOBROMAN

Chemical Name: 1,4-Bis(3-bromopropionyl)piperazine.

Description: Pipobroman is a dicarboxylic acid amide of piperazine with antineoplastic activity. Unlike the basic nitrogen mustards, pipobroman is a neutral amide. It occurs as a white, crystalline powder slightly soluble in water and sparingly soluble in alcohol.

Although its precise mechanism of action is unknown, it has been classified as a polyfunctional alkylating agent. Following oral administration, pipobroman is readily absorbed from the gastrointestinal tract; however, its metabolic fate and route of excretion are not known.

Indications: Primarily in the treatment of polycythemia vera. It has also been found useful in the treatment of chronic granulocytic leukemia.

Contraindications: Bone marrow depression resulting from x-ray or cytotoxic chemotherapy.

Warnings: The drug is not recommended for use in children under 15 years of age. Bone-marrow depression may not occur for 4 weeks, or more, after treatment is initiated. If the leukocyte count falls to 3000 or less, or if the platelet count falls to 150,000 or less, the drug should be discontinued temporarily. Therapy may be reinstated cautiously when these blood counts have risen. A dose-dependent anemia, which usually responds to blood transfusions and reduction in dosage, frequently develops. However, a rapid drop in hemoglobin, increased bilirubin levels, and reticulocytosis suggest a hemolytic process in which case the drug should be discontinued. Because of the potential danger of fetal death or teratogenesis associated with the use of cytotoxic agents, pipobroman should be used in women of child-bearing potential and particularly during the first trimester of pregnancy only when, in the judgment of the physician, the potential benefits outweigh the possible hazards.

Precautions: Therapy should be initiated in the hospital where the patient can be closely observed. Bone marrow determinations should be undertaken prior to therapy and again at the time of maximal hematologic response. Complete blood counts once or twice weekly, and leukocyte counts every other day, should be performed until the desired response is obtained or until significant toxic effects intervene. Ancillary laboratory studies, including liver and kidney function tests, should be carried out prior to therapy and periodically thereafter.

Adverse Reactions: Nausea, vomiting, abdominal cramping, diarrhea and skin rash. The drug should be withdrawn if these symptoms persist.

Dosage and Administration: *Orally* in divided daily doses. *Polycythemia vera:* initially, 1 mg/kg/day for at least 30 days; some patients may then be found to require 1.5 to 3 mg/kg/day. Maintenance dosage ranges from 0.1 to 0.2 mg/kg/day, and should be initiated when the hematocrit has been reduced to 50 to 55%. *Chronic granulocytic leukemia:* initially from 1.5 to 2.5 mg/kg/day, continued until a maximal clinical or hematologic response is obtained, and the leukocyte count approaches 10,000. If relapse is rapid (doubling of leukocyte count within 70 days) continuous treatment is necessary. Maintenance dosage ranges from about 7 to 175 mg daily.

Availability:
VERCYTE® Tablets, 10 and 25 mg in bottles of 100. **(Abbott)**

PITUITARY, POSTERIOR LOBE

Synonyms: Vasopressin (pitressin; pituitrin).

Description: Vasopressin, or pitressin, represents those posterior pituitary preparations which contain the pressor and antidiuretic principles and which are virtually free of the oxytocic principle. Pituitrin represents those preparations of the posterior pituitary gland which contain not only the pressor and antidiuretic principles, but the oxytocic principle as well.

Lypressin (vasopressin), the active ingredient of the nasal spray, is pharmacologically similar to parenteral vasopressin, but differs chemically in the substitution of lysine for arginine on the polypeptide nucleus. It is relatively free of oxytocic activity and possesses little pressor activity.

Vasopressin effectively lowers urine volume by increasing reabsorption of water by the renal tubule. In higher concentrations, the hormone is capable of stimulating contraction of the smooth muscle of the gastrointestinal tract and all the components of the vascular system, especially the capillaries, small arteriols and venules, with less effect on the smooth musculature of the large veins. The direct effect on the contractile elements is neither antagonized by adrenergic blocking agents nor prevented by vascular denervation.

Indications: Antidiuretic in the treatment of polyuria of diabetes insipidus. For more prolonged action, the insoluble suspension of the tannate may be used. Vasopressin is also used to raise blood pressure, increase muscular activity of the bladder and gastrointestinal tract and, in obstetrics, to stimulate uterine contractions and to control hemorrhage especially bleeding of esophageal varices. The *nasal spray* is indicated for use only in the control or prevention of the symptoms and complications of diabetes insipidus, such as polyuria, polydypsia and dehydration.

Contraindications: Abnormal sensitivity to the hormone, epilepsy, cardiorenal disease with hypertension, angina pectoris, coronary thrombosis, toxemia of pregnancy, advanced arteriosclerosis, during the first stage of labor, and contraction of the pelvis. Chronic nephritis with nitrogen retention contraindicates the use of vasopressin until reasonable nitrogen blood levels have been attained. There are no known contraindications to the nasal spray.

Warnings: It is advised to use extreme caution in patients with vascular disease, especially those of the coronary arteries, since even small doses may precipitate anginal pain. The drug may also produce water intoxication; therefore, the early signs of drowsiness, listlessness, and headache should be recognized to prevent terminal coma and convulsions. Safe use of the nasal spray during pregnancy has not been established. Before using the spray in women of childbearing potential, the anticipated benefits should be weighed against the potential hazards to mother and child.

Precautions: *Do not inject intravenously.* This agent should be used cautiously in the presence of epilepsy, migraine headache, asthma, heart failure or any condition in which a rapid addition to extracellular water may produce serious effects. Since intravenous lypressin reportedly has caused mild hypertension, the spray should be used with caution in patients with cardiovascular disease. Large intranasal doses may constrict the coronary arteries, which is why caution is advisable when treating patients with coronary artery disease. Nasal congestion, allergic rhinitis and upper respiratory tract infections may interfere with absorption of the drug by the nasal mucosa, thus minimizing the spray's efficacy. In such cases, larger doses or adjunctive therapy may be required. Patients with a known sensitivity to antidiuretic hormone should be tested for sensitivity to the nasal spray.

Adverse Reactions: Local or systemic allergic reactions may occur in hypersensitive individuals. Other complications which have been reported include tremor, sweating, vertigo, circumoral pallor, "pounding" in the head, abdominal cramps, expelling of flatus, nausea, vomiting, urticaria, bronchial constriction, anaphylaxis, and cardiac arrest. Adverse effects resulting from the use of the nasal spray have been infrequent and mild. They have included rhinorrhea, nasal congestion, irritation and pruritus of the nasal mucosa, nasal ulceration, headache, conjunctivitis, heartburn secondary to excessive usage, postnasal drip, abdominal cramps and increased bowel movements. Accidental inhalation has resulted in substernal tightness, coughing, transient dyspnea and, pronounced but transient fluid retention due to overdosage. Hypersensitivity to the nasal spray is manifested by a positive skin test.

Dosage and Administration: *Intramuscularly* or *subcutaneously.* Adults, 0.25 to 0.5 ml, repeated as indicated at intervals of 3 to 4 hours. Tannate in Oil, inject 0.3 to 1 ml *intramuscularly;* repeat as required, since the effect may be sustained for up to 96 hours. Children, proportionately less. In obstetrics, 0.2 to 1 ml (10 U.S.P. units/ml). In surgical cases, 1 to 2 ml (10 U.S.P. units/ml) or 0.5 to 1 ml of the double strength solution. *Intranasally.* One spray delivers about 2 U.S.P. posterior pituitary (pressor) units. Usual dosage is 1 or 2 sprays into each nostril 4 times daily. Dosage has ranged from 1 spray daily at bedtime to 10 sprays into each nostril every 3 to 4 hours. Patients requiring more than 2 sprays/nostril every 4 to 6 hours should reduce the interval between doses rather than increase the number of sprays each time. This is advisable to avoid postnasal wastage (see Adverse Reactions).

Availability:
DIAPID® Nasal Spray, 50 units/ml (0.185 mg/ml) in plastic squeeze bottles of 5 and 8 ml. **(Sandoz)**
PITRESSIN® Injection, 20 units/ml in ampuls of 0.5 and 1 ml. **(Parke-Davis)**
PITRESSIN (as tannate) in Oil Injection, 5 units/ml in ampuls of 1 ml. **(Parke-Davis)**
PITUITRIN® Injection (for obstetric use), 10 units/ml in ampuls of 1 ml. **(Parke-Davis)**
PITUITRIN (S) Injection (for surgical use), 20 units/ml in ampuls of 1 ml. **(Parke-Davis)**

PLASMA PROTEIN COAGULATION FACTORS, HUMAN

Description: A stable, dried, concentrated preparation containing factors II (prothrombin), VII (proconvertin), IX (PTC antihemophilic factor B), and X (Stuart-Prower factor) obtained from fresh human plasma. One factor IX unit is defined as the factor IX present in 1 ml of average normal pooled human plasma less than 1 hour old.

Indications: To control and prevent bleeding episodes due to deficiencies of these factors. It may also be used for the treatment of congenital or acquired coagulation disorders, and in certain hemorrhagic conditions of the newborn infant.

Contraindications: In patients with liver disease where there are signs of intravascular coagulation and fibrinolysis.

Warnings: Thrombin can appear spontaneously during transit or storage if this preparation is not maintained at the recommended temperature.

Precautions: It is essential to establish that the deficiency is due to one of these factors, since no benefit may be expected from this preparation when treating deficiencies due to other causes. As with other human blood derivatives, the physician must evaluate the risk that serum hepatitis may follow its use. Therefore, special consideration should be given when this preparation is to be administered to newborn infants and to patients with preexisting liver disease. Treatment should be discontinued if signs of intravascular clotting manifested by changes in blood pressure and pulse rate, respiratory distress, chest pains, and cough occur. This risk may be reduced if the patient's factor IX level is not raised to more than about 50% of normal.

Adverse Reactions: On rare occasions rapid administration can produce transient fever, chills, headache, flushing or tingling.

Dosage and Administration: *Intravenously.* Administer within 10 minutes after reconstitution. Consult package literature for specific details.

Availability:
KONYNE® in bottles of 500 units with diluent. **(Cutter)**
PROPLEX in vials of 30 ml with diluent and administration set. *Stabilized with a small amount of heparin.* **(Hyland)**

PLASMA PROTEIN FRACTION, HUMAN

Description: A buffered and stabilized solution of selected human plasma proteins (5%) consisting of approximately 88% normal human globulin, 7% alpha globulin and 5% beta globulin, as determined by electrophoresis. The concentration of these proteins is such that the solution is iso-osmotic with normal human plasma. Each liter contains approximately 110 mEq of sodium, up to 0.25 mEq of potassium and 50 mEq of chloride. Clinical experience shows that human plasma protein fraction is an adequate replacement for human plasma and is a suitable means of providing human proteins for their osmotic effect (e.g., in ascites) and nutritional value.

Indications: Emergency treatment of shock due to burns, crushing injuries, abdominal emergencies, and any other cause where there is a predominant loss of plasma fluids, rather than red blood cells. It may also be used in the emergency treatment of shock due to hemorrhage, and adjunctively in the treatment of hypoproteinemia.

Contraindications: In patients with severe anemia or cardiac failure.

Warnings: The solution should not be used if it appears turbid or if there is a sediment in the bottle. Since the product contains no preservative, it should be used promptly after opening, and any unused portion should be discarded.

Precautions: To combat the possible anemia which may result from the administration of large quantities of this product, the solution should be supplemented with or replaced by whole blood. The quick response of blood pressure which may follow rapid administration necessitates careful observation of the patient to detect bleeding areas which failed to bleed at lower blood pressure. Dehydrated patients usually require administration of additional fluids to replace the fluid withdrawn from tissues by the osmotic action of plasma protein fraction. Utmost caution should be exercised in patients with a low cardiac reserve or in those with no albumin deficiency, since a rapid increase in plasma volume may cause circulatory embarrassment or pulmonary edema. Because this product is void of coagulation factors, it should not be relied on to correct hemorrhagic states due to defects in the coagulation mechanism.

Adverse Reactions: There have been rare instances of nausea, but no causal relationship has been established.

Dosage and Administration: *Intravenously only.* Dosage is based almost entirely on the nature of the individual case and the response to therapy. *For shock:* The usual minimal dose of 250 to 500 ml, delivered at the rate of up to 17 ml/minute (1 liter/hr), has been found to be well tolerated by adults; and has also been found useful as initial therapy for shock due to dehydration and infection in infants and small children. For the treatment of acute shock states in infants, a dose of 15 ml/lb of body weight, infused at a rate of up to 5 to 10 ml/minute is recommended. *For burns:* An initial dose of 500 to 1000 ml should be followed by such quantities of solution as may be needed to prevent marked hemoconcentration, and to maintain appropriate electrolyte balance. *For hypoproteinemia:* As much as 1 to 1.5 liters of solution, which yields 50 to 75 gm of plasma proteins, may be given daily. Since blood volume in these patients may be normal, doses of more than 500 ml (0.5 liter) should be administered at a rate no faster than 500 ml in 30 to 45 minutes in order to avoid circulatory embarrassment. If less rapid administration is desired, 1000 ml may be given by continuous drip at a rate of 100 ml/hour. If sodium restriction is imperative, 25% salt poor, normal serum albumin (human) is recommended.

Availability:
PLASMANATE® Injection, 5% in bottles of 50, 250 and 500 ml with disposable administration set and airway assembly. **(Cutter)**
PLASMA-PLEX® Injection, 5% (heat-treated) in bottles of 250 and 500 ml with administration set. **(Armour)**
PROTENATE™ Injection, 5% in bottles of 250 and 500 ml with disposable administration set. **(Hyland)**

PLEXONAL Ⓒ III

Description: Each tablet contains:

Sodium diethylbarbiturate	45 mg
Sodium phenylethylbarbiturate	15 mg
Sodium isobutylallylbarbiturate	25 mg
Scopolamine hydrobromide	0.08 mg
Dihydroergotamine mesylate	0.16 mg

A balanced action is achieved through the use of 3 barbiturates with differing rates of action and dissipation, potentiated by scopolamine and dihydroergotamine.

Indications: Provides a sedative-relaxant effect for patients with anxiety, tension, nervousness, irritability, apprehension, restlessness, hyperexcitability, insomnia.

Contraindications: Severely depressed or comatose patients; hypersensitivity to any of the components.

Warnings: Barbiturates may be habit-forming.

Precautions: Should be used cautiously in the presence of hepatic disease, fever, hyperthyroidism, diabetes mellitus, or severe anemia.

Adverse Reactions: Drowsiness, skin rashes, gastrointestinal disturbances may occur.

Dosage and Administration: *Orally.* The usual adult dosage for daytime sedation, 1 tablet 2 to 4 times daily (range: 2 to 6 tablets daily); to promote sleep, 2 to 4 tablets ½ hour before retiring.

Availability:
Ⓒ III PLEXONAL® Tablets (triangular, white) in bottles of 100 and 1000. **(Sandoz)**

PNEUMOCOCCAL VACCINE, POLYVALENT

Description: A purified solution containing only the soluble polysaccharide antigens isolated from the capsules of the 14 individual types of pneumococci; it is intended for immunization against infections caused by these organisms. The product is formulated so that each 0.5 ml contains 50 mcg of each polysaccharide type dissolved in isotonic saline solution containing a suitable preservative. The vaccine affords effective protection against the 14 most prevalent capsular types accounting for at least 80% of all pneumococcal disease isolates in the United States. Onset of protection generally occurs about the third week after vaccination. Studies in humans have demonstrated the immunogenicity (antibody-stimulating capability) of each of the 14 capsular types when tested as polyvalent vaccines, and at least 90% of all adults showed a fourfold or greater increase in type-specific antibody for each vaccine capsular type. Adults of all ages and children 2 years of age and older have responded immunologically to the vaccine. The vaccine will not immunize against capsular types of pneumococci other than those contained in the vaccine, nor can it be expected to prevent pneumonia caused by organisms other than pneumococci. Furthermore, the expected serum antibody response may not be obtained if the vaccine is used in individuals receiving immunosuppressive therapy.

Indications: For immunization against pneumococcal lobar pneumonia and bacteremia, caused by those types of pneumococci included in the vaccine, in patients 2 years of age and older in whom there is an increased risk of morbidity and mortality from pneumococcal pneumonia. These include individuals with chronic debilitating diseases (heart disease, bronchopulmonary disease, renal failure); patients with diabetes mellitus, or other metabolic disorders; those residing in various institutions, or convalescing from severe illness, and individuals 50 years of age and older (especially those over 65). Preliminary data suggest that the vaccine is effective in preventing severe pneumonic disease and bacteremia in patients with sickle cell anemia and in individuals who have had a splenectomy or who have impaired splenic function. Additionally, it is expected to be found effective in preventing pneumococcal meningitis of bacteremic origin. However, it may not be effective in preventing infection resulting from basilar skull fracture or from external communication with cerebrospinal fluid. The effectiveness of the vaccine in preventing pneumococcal otitis media in infants awaits further studies.

Contraindications: Children under 2 years of age, pregnant women, and patients hypersensitive to any component of the vaccine. **Important note:** Epinephrine (1:1000) should be immediately available for use should an acute anaphylactic reaction occur.

Precautions: The vaccine should be administered subcutaneously or intramuscularly *never intravenously.* The presence of any febrile respiratory illness or other active infection is justification for delaying use of the vaccine except when, in the judgment of the physician, withholding the agent may entail an even greater risk.

Adverse Reactions: Local reactions frequently occurring are erythema and soreness at the injection site; less frequently is induration. An occasional patient may develop a low grade fever.

Dosage and Administration: *Intramuscularly or subcutaneously only.* **Not for intravenous administration.** A single 0.5-ml dose should be injected SC or IM (preferably in the deltoid muscle or midlateral thigh) with appropriate precautions to avoid intravascular administration. Available data suggest that revaccination before 3 years may result in more frequent and severe local reactions at the injection site, especially in individuals who have retained high levels of antibodies.

Availability:
PNEUMOVAX® Solution in vials of 2.5 ml (5 doses). **(Merck Sharp & Dohme)**

POISON IVY, OAK AND SUMAC ALLERGENIC EXTRACTS

Description: The active toxic principle extracted from the fresh leaves of Rhus toxicodendron, Toxicodendron radicans (poison ivy), Rhus diversiloba, Toxicodendron diversiloba (poison oak) or Rhus venenta, Toxicodendron vernix (poison sumac) in vegetable oil or in alcohol (for seasonal or preseasonal injection). Alcoholic extracts also are available for preseasonal oral treatment.

Indications. Prophylaxis and treatment of Rhus dermatitis.

Contraindications: The use of the extract should be delayed in the presence of any febrile respiratory illness or other active infection, except when in the opinion of the physician, withholding the agent entails even greater risk.

Warnings: The use of poison ivy extract for treatment of individuals with acute Rhus dermatitis is not recommended. There is some evidence that injection of immunizing agents during an epidemic of poliomyelitis may result, on rare occasions, in localization of paralysis in the inoculated arm or leg in those patients who subsequently develop paralytic poliomyelitis. Therefore, if poliomyelitis is present in the community, elective immunization should be deferred.

Precautions: Kidney damage may follow extensive dermatitis and, in the case of acute Rhus dermatitis, may be aggravated by the use of Rhus antigen. Patients with a history of sensitivity to the Rhus plant should have the dosage reduced by one-half. If signs of sensitivity are apparent, discontinue treatment until all symptoms disappear, then cautiously administer one-fourth the dosage which caused the reaction and increase gradually until reaching the point prior to the symptom-producing level. Continue with this dosage indefinitely or until immunity is definitely established. Before initiating therapy, the physician should weigh the inherent risks against the severity of the patient's allergy to, and the danger of, contracting poison oak or ivy dermatitis.

Adverse Reactions: Reactions in the mouth, skin and around the anus may occur. Traces of extract on the skin following injection may produce contact dermatitis. These should be washed with several latherings of strong soap or scrubbed thoroughly with alcohol. The development of fever, urticaria and exanthematous eruption, malaise, and constitutional reactions warrants immediate discontinuation of therapy. Local reactions may occur such as abscess, erythema, sensation of local heat, swelling and pain at the injection site, pruritus, and edema.

Dosage and Administration: Preseasonal treatment should be instituted about 4 to 6 weeks before expected exposure, *Intramuscularly*, 0.5 to 1 ml weekly for about 3 to 5 weeks.

Availability:
POISON IVY EXTRACT [Rhus Toxicodendron (poison ivy-poison oak) antigen] in sterile almond oil in vials of 1 ml. **(Parke-Davis)**
RHUS TOX ANTIGEN™ Injection (poison ivy extract) 40 mg/ml in an aqueous-alcoholic solution in vials of 1 ml in packages of 4. **(Lemmon)**

POLIOVIRUS VACCINE, LIVE, ORAL, TRIVALENT

Description: The trivalent vaccine combines in a single dose a mixture of monovalent poliovirus vaccines, Sabin strains Types 1, 2 and 3, which have been propagated on monkey kidney tissue in a medium of lactalbumin hydrolysate, antibiotics and calf serum. Potency is expressed in terms of 50% tissue culture infective doses ($TCID_{50}$). The approximate concentration of poliovirus for each strain in a single dose is: Type 1, 800,000 $TCID_{50}$; Type 2, 100,000 $TCID_{50}$; Type 3, 500,000 $TCID_{50}$. Phenol red has been added as a pH indicator and the finished product has a variable red to yellow hue. Color changes may occur on thawing or storage but have no significance providing the vaccine remains crystal clear. However, the possibility of bacterial contamination should be considered whenever a thawed and entered vial shows color changes from red or pink to yellow during subsequent storage. Under such conditions, the residual vaccine should not be used.

Indications: Active immunization against poliomyelitis caused by Types 1, 2 and 3 polioviruses. Infants 6 to 12 weeks of age, all children and adolescents through the level of high school are the usual candidates for routine prophylaxis. Nonimmunized adults who may be unduly exposed to the virus (e.g., employees of hospitals, medical laboratories, clinics, and sanitation facilities), or those who live in or travel to epidemic or endemic areas should receive the vaccine according to the schedule outlined for children and adolescents.

Contraindications: In the presence of persistent vomiting or diarrhea, and in patients with acute illnesses other than minor afebrile upper respiratory tract infections. Since infection with live attenuated polioviruses may be potentiated by severe underlying diseases such as leukemia, lymphoma, dysgammaglobulinemia, or generalized malignancy, or because of lowered resistance due to therapy with immune serum globulin, steroids, alkylating drugs, antimetabolites, or radiation, it is advised that vaccination be postponed. Simultaneous administration of live virus vaccines should be avoided, and whenever possible, should be given at least

1 month apart. However, tonsillectomy, tooth extraction, or penicillin hypersensitivity do not constitute a contraindication to the use of this vaccine. Also, the administration of Diphtheria and Tetanus Toxoids and Pertussis Vaccine and small pox vaccination are no longer considered to be contraindications. **Note:** Not to be administered parenterally.

Precautions: The vaccine's efficacy depends on the multiplication of the virus within the gastrointestinal tract; other enteroviruses including Coxsackie, ECHO (enteric cytopathogenic human orphan), and wild or other attenuated polioviruses may interfere with this multiplication. It is preferable that vaccination be carried out at a time when interference from enteroviruses is at a minimum (November through May). It has been established that attenuated poliovirus vaccine may revert to a slightly more toxic strain following multiplication in the vaccinated individual or following transmission of the organism to nonvaccinated contacts. However, it is generally agreed that there is no danger of significant reversion to virulence after human passage. May be given during pregnancy when immunization is required. Administration to the newborn (under 6 weeks) is not generally performed because of the varying persistence of maternal antibodies.

Adverse Reactions: Paralytic disease, although rare, has been reported.

Dosage and Administration: *Orally only.* The recommended dose is either 2 drops (multiple-dose vial) or the entire contents of a 0.5 ml (single-dose vial), depending on which form the physician prefers. Each dose may be administered directly from the dropper or mixed with distilled water, milk, simple syrup or **unchlorinated** tap water. Alternately, it may be absorbed on bread, cake, or cube sugar. Two doses at intervals of 8 weeks are recommended. For infants, the vaccine may be integrated with the first and third DPT (diphtheria-pertussis-tetanus) immunizations, with a third dose given at the age of 1 year to complete the primary immunization series. Two doses at intervals of 8 weeks also are indicated for those whose past immunization history against "polio" is doubtful, consisting of Salk vaccine only, or of only 1 or 2 monovalent, oral, poliovirus vaccines. Infants immunized initially with the 3 monovalent vaccines beginning at less than 6 months of age should be given a single dose of trivalent vaccine at about 1 year of age. Another dose (booster) of trivalent vaccine should be given when the child enters school and to those of unusual risk, such as those who live in epidemic areas, travel abroad, and those entering military service.

Availability:
DIPLOVAX® (Sabin strain, Types 1, 2 and 3) in pipettes of 1 dose, in vials of 10 doses and in single-dose plastic disposable droppers of 0.5 ml. **(Pfizer)**
ORIMUNE®(Sabin strain, Types 1, 2 and 3) in vials of 10 doses and in single-dose, disposable pipettes (Dispette®). **(Lederle)**

POLYMYXIN B SULFATE

Description: Polymyxin B sulfate is a basic polypeptide antibiotic derived from various strains of the spore-forming soil bacterium, *Bacillus polymyxa.* It occurs as a white to buff-color powder freely soluble in water and slightly soluble in alcohol. The antibiotic has a potency of not less than 6000 units/mg of activity, calculated on the dried basis. Dosages expressed in terms of weight refer to the pure U.S.P. reference standard which contains 10,000 units/mg; it does not refer to the actual weight of the antibiotic.

Polymyxin B sulfate increases the permeability of bacterial cell-wall membrane. In concentrations of 0.5 to 20 units/ml, polymyxin is bactericidal in vitro against most gram-negative organisms including *E. coli, Ps. aeruginosa, A. aerogenes, K. pneumoniae, H. influenzae,* and species of *Shigella; Pr. vulgaris* usually is more resistant. Bacteria initially susceptible rarely acquire resistance to the antibiotic. (All gram-positive bacteria, fungi, and gram-negative cocci, *N. gonorrhoeae,* and *N. meningitidis* are resistant to polymyxin.) If the Kirby-Bauer method of disc susceptibility testing is used, a 300 unit polymyxin B disc should give a zone of over 11 mm when tested against a polymyxin B-susceptible bacterial strain.

Polymyxin B sulfate is not absorbed from the normal alimentary tract. Since the drug loses 50% of its activity in the presence of serum, active blood levels are low. Repeated injections may give a cumulative effect. Levels tend to be higher in infants and children. The drug is excreted slowly by the kidneys; tissue diffusion is poor and the drug does not pass the blood brain barrier into the cerebrospinal fluid. In therapeutic dosage, polymyxin B sulfate causes some nephrotoxicity with tubule damage to a slight degree.

Indications: Treatment of septicemia, meningitis, urinary tract and other systemic infections and local infections due to susceptible organisms. Deep-seated or walled-off infections cannot be expected to respond to topical treatment and may require systemic therapy. Meningeal infection should be treated only by the intrathecal route.

Contraindications: Hypersensitivity to polymyxin B sulfate or to any of the components formulated with it.

Warnings: When polymyxin B sulfate is given intramuscularly and/or intrathecally, it should be administered only to hospitalized patients, so as to provide constant supervision by a physician. Renal function should be carefully determined and patients with renal damage and nitrogen retention should be given a reduced dosage. Patients with nephrotoxicity due to polymyxin B sulfate usually show albuminuria, cellular casts, and azotemia; a diminishing urine output and a rising BUN are indications for discontinuing therapy with this drug. Neurotoxic reactions may be manifested by irritability, weakness, drowsiness, ataxia, perioral paresthesia, numbness of the extremities, and blurring of vision. These are usually associated with high serum levels found in patients with impaired renal function and/or nephrotoxicity. The concurrent use of other nephrotoxic and neurotoxic drugs, particularly kanamycin, streptomycin, polymyxin E (colistin), neomycin, gentamicin, and viomycin should be avoided. The neurotoxicity of polymyxin B sulfate can result in respiratory paralysis from neuromuscular blockade, especially when the drug is given soon after anesthesia and/or muscle relaxants. The safety of this drug in women during pregnancy has not been established.

Precautions: The nephrotoxic potential of this drug should be taken into account, and baseline renal function should be done prior to therapy, with frequent monitoring of renal function and blood levels of the drug during parenteral therapy. Curariform muscle relaxants and other neurotoxic drugs such as ether, tubocurarine, succinylcholine, gallamine, decamethonium and sodium citrate should not be used concurrently with polymyxin B sulfate. If signs of respiratory paralysis appear, respiration should be assisted, and the drug withdrawn. Overgrowth of nonsusceptible organisms, including fungi, may occur and should be treated with appropriate measures.

Adverse Reactions: *Nephrotoxic reactions:* albuminuria, cylindruria, azotemia, and rising blood levels without any increase in dosage. *Neurotoxic reactions:* facial flushing, dizziness progressing to ataxia, drowsiness, peripheral paresthesias (circumoral and stocking-glove), apnea due to concurrent use of curariform muscle relaxants, other neurotoxic drugs, or inadvertent overdosage, signs of meningeal irritation with intrathecal administration, e.g., fever, headache, stiff neck and increased cell count and protein in cerebrospinal fluid. *Other reactions* occasionally reported are drug fever, urticarial rash, pain (severe) at intramuscular injection sites, thrombophlebitis at intravenous injection sites, and itching, burning or inflammation at topical application sites.

Dosage and Administration: *Intramuscularly*, for systemic, meningeal and urinary tract infections. The drug should be administered only to hospitalized patients so that there is constant supervision by the physician. The usual dosage range is 1.5 to 2.5 mg/kg of body weight daily; should not exceed 2.5 mg/kg daily or in any case, 200 mg/day. The drug has been administered at 4-, 6-, 8-, or 12-hour intervals. *Intravenous drip*, for systemic infections. The daily dosage should be approximately 2.5 mg/kg of body weight in patients with relatively normal renal function, and 1.5 mg/kg or less in patients with preexisting kidney impairment. The total daily dose should not exceed 200 mg. The total calculated daily dose may be given as a single intravenous infusion or may be divided into 2 daily infusions and administered at intervals of 8 to 12 hours. *Intrathecally*, for meningeal infections. The usual dosage for children under 2 years of age is 2 mg every day or 2.5 mg every other day. When giving 2 mg every day, the dosage may be continued for 3 or 4 days, and then 2.5 mg may be given every other day. For children over 2 years of age and for adults, the dosage is 5 mg every day for 3 or 4 days and then 5 mg every other day. Susceptible infections usually respond within 2 to 3 days, but it is recommended that therapy be continued for at least 3 days after the spinal fluid is sterile; in some cases it may be necessary to continue treatment for several weeks. *Inhalation*, for pulmonary infections. Usually 1 or 2 ml of solutions of 1 to 10 mg/ml 4 to 6 times daily. *Topically*, for local infections. Concentrations of 0.1 to 0.25% (1 to 2.5 mg/ml) applied as a wet dressing, spray, by irrigation or, in the case of the eye, ear or nose, in the form of drops 2 to 4 times daily or as directed by the physician. Treatment may continue from a few days to several weeks as required to control the infection.

Availability:

Polymyxin B Sulfate

AEROSPORIN®: **(Burroughs Wellcome)**
Otic Solution (sterile), 1 mg/ml (10,000 units/ml) in bottles of 10 ml.
Sterile Powder in 20-ml vials containing 500,000 units (50 mg).
POLYMYXIN B SULFATE Sterile Powder in vials of 500,000 units (50 mg). **(Pfizer)**

Combinations

LIDOSPORIN® Otic Solution, 1 mg/ml (10,000 units/ml) with lidocaine hydrochloride, 50 mg in bottles of 10 ml with dropper. **(Burroughs Wellcome)**
MYCITRACIN®: **(Upjohn)**
Ophthalmic Ointment in tubes of 3.5 gm with applicator tip. Each gm contains polymyxin B sulfate, 0.5 mg; bacitracin, 500 units and neomycin sulfate, 5 mg (equiv. to 3.5 mg base).
Topical Ointment (OTC) in tubes of 15 and 30 gm and in unit-dose (foil packs) of 0.001 gm. Each gm contains polymyxin B sulfate, 0.5 mg; bacitracin, 500 units and neomycin sulfate, 5 mg (equiv. to 3.5 mg of base).
NEOSPORIN®: **(Burroughs Wellcome)**
Aerosol in spray cans of 90 gm containing polymyxin B sulfate, 10 mg; zinc bacitracin, 8000 units and neomycin sulfate, 100 mg.
G.U. Irrigant (sterile) 20 mg/ml with neomycin sulfate equivalent to 40 mg of base in ampuls of 1 ml and in multi-dose vials of 20 ml.
Ophthalmic Ointment, 0.5 mg/gm with zinc bacitracin, 400 units and neomycin sulfate, 5 mg in tubes of 3.5 gm with tip.
Ophthalmic Solution, 0.5 mg/ml with neomycin sulfate, 2.5 mg and gramicidin, 0.025 mg in plastic bottles of 10 ml.
Topical Ointment (OTC) in tubes of 15 and 30 gm and in unit-dose foil packets of 0.033 gm. Each gm contains polymyxin B sulfate, 0.5 mg, neomycin sulfate, 5 mg and zinc bacitracin, 400 units.
Topical Powder, 0.5 mg/gm with zinc bacitracin, 400 units and neomycin sulfate, 5 mg in shaker-top vials of 10 gm.
NEOSPORIN®-G Cream, 1 mg/gm with neomycin sulfate, 5 mg and gramicidin, 0.25 mg in tubes of 15 gm.
OTOBIONE® Otic Suspension in amber bottles of 5 ml with sterile dropper. Each ml contains polymyxin B sulfate, 1 mg (10,000 units); neomycin sulfate, 5 mg (equiv. to 3.5 mg of base) and hydrocortisone, 10 mg. **(Schering)**
POLYCIN® Topical Ointment (OTC) in tubes of 15 gm. Each gm contains polymyxin B sulfate, 0.8 mg (8000 units) and zinc bacitracin, 400 units. **(Dow)**
POLYSPECTRIN®: **(Allergan)**
S.O.P.® Ophthalmic Ointment (sterile) in tubes of 3.5 gm. Each gm contains polymyxin B sulfate, 0.5 mg; zinc bacitracin, 400 units and neomycin sulfate, 5 mg (equiv. to 3.5 mg neomycin base).
Ophthalmic Solution, in dropper bottles of 10 ml. Each ml contains polymyxin B sulfate, 0.5 mg; neomycin sulfate, 5 mg (equiv. to 3.5 mg neomycin base) in a Liquifilm vehicle containing polyvinyl alcohol, 1.4 mg.
POLYSPORIN®: **(Burroughs Wellcome)**
Ophthalmic Ointment (sterile), 1 mg/gm with zinc bacitracin, 500 units in tubes of 3.5 gm with tip.
Topical Ointment (OTC), 1 mg/gm with zinc bacitracin, 500 units in tubes of 15 and 30 gm with tip and in unit-dose foil packets of 0.033 gm.
PYOCIDIN OTIC® Solution, 1 mg/ml with hydrocortisone, 5 mg in dropper bottles of 10 ml. **(Cooper)**
STATROL®: **(Alcon)**
Ophthalmic Ointment in tubes of 3.5 gm. Each gm contains polymyxin B sulfate, 6000 units and neomycin sulfate equiv. to 3.5 mg neomycin base.

Ophthalmic Solution in Drop-Tainer® bottles of 5 ml. Each ml contains polymycin B sulfate, 16,250 units; neomycin sulfate equiv. to 3.5 mg neomycin base and phenylephrine hydrochloride, 0.12%.

POLYSTYRENE SULFONATE SODIUM

Description: Polystyrene sulfonate sodium is a sulfonic cation exchange resin charged with sodium and occurs as a fine, light-brown to brown powder that is insoluble in water. In vitro studies indicate that the compound has an exchange capacity of about 3.1 mEq of potassium/gm (in vivo about 1 mEq/gm). The sodium content is about 100 mg/gm.

As the resin passes along the intestine or is retained in the colon after administration by enema, the sodium ions are partially released and are replaced by potassium ions. For the most part, this action occurs in the large intestine, which excretes potassium ions to a greater degree than does the small intestine. Concomitant use of cation-containing laxatives and antacids may decrease the effectiveness of this resin.

Indications: Symptomatic treatment of hyperkalemia due to acute renal failure.

Warnings: Seriously low potassium levels may occur if the effective dosage range is exceeded; thus it is imperative to determine the daily serum potassium levels. However, it should be kept in mind that severe intracellular depletion may occur in the presence of near normal serum levels. Particular caution is advisable in patients with actual or impending cardiac failure; in such instances the total fluid intake should be restricted. The resin should be administered with caution to patients with acute or chronic renal failure to avert heart failure, edema, and severe hypertension. Patients receiving repeated doses should be monitored for acid/base electrolyte and mineral status. Particular care should also be exercised in patients receiving digitalis preparations since their action may be exaggerated in the presence of hypokalemia. Electrocardiograms are of value in the diagnosis of hyper- and hypokalemia, hypocalcemia, and digitalis intoxication.

Precautions: Caution is advised when this preparation is administered to patients who cannot tolerate even a small increase in sodium loads (i.e., severe congestive heart failure, severe hypertension, or marked edema). In such instances compensatory restriction of sodium intake from other sources may be indicated. Furthermore, the clinician should be aware that the simultaneous oral administration of the resin with nonabsorbable cation-donating antacids and laxatives may result in systemic alkalosis and may reduce the resin's potassium exchange capability. One patient with chronic hypocalcemia of renal failure developed a grand mal seizure when given the resin with magnesium hydroxide as laxative. If constipation occurs, patients should be treated with a mild laxative or sorbitol (from 10 to 20 ml of 70% syrup every 2 hours or as needed to produce 1 or 2 watery stools daily), a measure which also reduces any tendency to fecal impaction.

Adverse Reactions: Anorexia, nausea, vomiting, diarrhea, and fecal impaction may occur as well as hypokalemia, hypocalcemia, and significant sodium retention. Large oral doses in elderly patients may cause fecal impaction, an effect which may be prevented by the use of the resin in enemas. Also reported was intestinal obstruction caused by concretions of aluminum hydroxide when used in combination with polystyrene sulfonate sodium.

Dosage and Administration: *Orally.* The usual dose is 15 gm 1 to 4 times daily. Infants and small children, dosage is calculated on the exchange rate of 1 mEq of potassium/gm of resin. *Rectally.* Adults, 30 to 50 gm every 6 hours, administered as a warm emulsion (at body temperature) in 100 ml of aqueous vehicle such as sorbitol. The emulsion should be agitated gently during administration. The preparation should be retained for as long as possible and should be followed by use of a cleansing enema. The resin may also be introduced into the stomach through a plastic tube and, if desired, mixed with a diet appropriate for a patient in renal failure.

Availability:

KAYEXALATE® in jars of 453.6 gm. **(Breon)**

POLYTHIAZIDE: see The Thiazide Diuretics

POTASSIUM CHLORIDE
POTASSIUM GLUCONATE

Description: Potassium is one of the principal cations of intracellular fluid and is essential for the maintenance of isotonicity and electrodynamic characteristics of the cell. It is also essential to a number of physiologic processes including the transmission of nerve impulses, contraction of cardiac, smooth and skeletal muscles, gastric secretion, and normal renal function.

Indications: Treatment of potassium and chloride deficiency which may occur in conjunction with long-term diuretic therapy, digitalis intoxication, inadequate dietary intake, loss of potassium due to vomiting and diarrhea, diabetic acidosis, hypochloremic alkalosis, corticosteroid therapy, familial periodic paralysis, as well as other causes. May also be used to treat cardiac arrhythmias due to digitalis intoxication.

Contraindications: Severe renal impairment with oliguria, anuria, or azotemia; untreated Addison's disease; adynamia episodica hereditaria; acute dehydration; heat cramps; and hyperkalemia from any cause. Potassium intensifies the symptoms of myotonia congenita. Also, potassium salts are contraindicated in patients receiving potassium-sparing agents such as aldosterone antagonists and triamterene.

Warnings: Parenteral solutions must be diluted before intravenous administration. High plasma levels of potassium ion may cause death through cardiac depression, arrhythmias, or arrest, and may complicate such conditions as chronic renal failure, acute dehydration, extensive tissue breakdown as in severe burns, and adrenal insufficiency. The drug should also be used with caution in the presence of cardiac disease and systemic acidosis, and periodic ECG and serum potassium levels should be made. Patients with chronic renal disease, or any other condition which impairs potassium excretion, requires careful monitoring of the serum potassium concentration and appropriate dosage adjustment. There have been several reports concerning nonspecific small-bowel lesions, consisting of stenosis with or without ulceration, associated with *enteric-coated* potassium tablets. These lesions have caused obstruction, hemorrhage and perforation. Surgery has often been required, and deaths have occurred. Available information tends to implicate enteric-coated potassium salts, although lesions of this type also occur spontaneously. Therefore, coated potassium tablets should be given only when indicated and should be discontinued immediately if abdominal pain, distention, nausea, vomiting, or gastrointestinal bleeding occurs; they should be used only when adequate dietary supplementation is not practical.

Precautions: Potassium must be administered cautiously, since the degree of deficiency or the ideal daily dosage often is not accurately known. Excessive dosage may result in potassium intoxication. Potassium salts should not be given intravenously unless serial electrocardiograms are taken or serial serum determinations [potassium] are made. Patients should be well hydrated and kidney function should be adequate before potassium salts are given.

Adverse Reactions: Vomiting, diarrhea, nausea, and abdominal discomfort have been reported. The signs and symptoms of potassium intoxication include paresthesia of the extremities, flaccid paralysis, listlessness, mental confusion, weakness and heaviness of the legs, fall in blood pressure, cardiac arrhythmias, heart block, hyperkalemia, and electrocardiographic abnormalities (disappearance of the P wave, depression of the S-T segment, tall and peaked T waves, spreading and slurring of the QRS complex with the development of a biphasic curve, and cardiac arrest). Late manifestations include muscle paralysis and cardiovascular collapse from cardiac arrest.

Dosage and Administration: *Intravenous* dosage usually is 1 liter of an 0.3% solution infused over a period of 4 hours at a rate of 8 to 12 ml/min. As little as 1 gm may be given. *Orally*, 1 gm up to 6 times daily; usually 1 gm 3 times daily. The packets should be dissolved in ½ glass of water or fruit juice. **Note:** A 15% solution of potassium chloride furnishes 40 mEq potassium and chloride ions. Potassium gluconate, 1.17 gm, supplies 5 mEq of potassium ion. See individual products for complete dosage recommendations.

Availability:

Potassium Chloride

KAOCHLOR® 10% Liquid, 1.5 gm/15 ml (20 mEq each of K and Cl) in bottles of 1 pint and 1 gallon, in Stat-Paks® (unit-dose) of 15 ml and in single-unit packages of 120 ml. **(Warren-Teed)**

KAOCHLOR S-F 10% Liquid (sugar free), 1.5 gm/15 ml (20 mEq each of K and Cl) in bottles of 120 ml, 1 pint and 1 gallon and in Stat-Paks (unit-dose) of 15 ml. **(Warren-Teed)**

KAON-CL-20% Liquid (sugar free), 3 gm/15 ml (40 mEq) in bottles of 120 ml, 1 pint and 1 gallon. **(Warren-Teed)**

KAON-CL TABS® Tablets, (controlled-release, sugar coated), 500 mg (6.67 mEq) in bottles of 250 and 1000. **(Warren-Teed)**

KAY-CIEL®: **(Cooper)**

Elixir, 1.5 gm/15 ml (20 mEq each of K and Cl) in bottles of 1 pint and 1 gallon.

Powder, 1.5 gm/Solodose packet (20 mEq) in cartons of 30.

K-LOR™ Powder, 1.125 gm/3-gm packet (15 mEq of K and Cl) in cartons of 100; 1.5 gm/4-gm packet (20 mEq of K and Cl) in cartons of 30 and 100. **(Abbott)**

KLORVESS® Liquid 10% (cherry flavored), 1.5 gm/15 ml (20 mEq) in bottles of 1 pint and 1 gallon. **(Dorsey)**

PAN-KLORIDE Elixir, 1.5 gm/15 ml in bottles of 1 pint and 1 gallon. **(Panray)**

PFIKLOR®: **(Pfizer)**

Liquid 10% (sugar free), 1.5 gm/15 ml (20 mEq) in bottles of 1 pint and 1 gallon.

Powder for Oral Solution, 1.5 gm/packet (20 mEq) in cartons of 30 packets.

POTASSIUM CHLORIDE:

Enseals® (enteric-coated tablets), 300 mg and 1 gm in bottles of 100 and 1000. **(Lilly)**

Injection, 10 mEq in ampuls of 5 ml; 20 mEq in ampuls of 10 ml; 30 and 40 mEq in ampuls of 20 ml. **(Abbott)**

Injection, 40 mEq in ampuls of 20 ml. **(Lilly)**

Injection, 20 mEq in ampuls of 10 ml; 40 mEq in ampuls of 20 ml. **(Various Mfrs.)**

Tablets, 300 mg and 1 gm in bottles of 100 and 1000. **(Various Mfrs.)**

Liquid, 10% and *Concentrate,* 20% in bottles of 120 ml, 1 pint and 1 gallon. **(Lederle)**

Liquid in unit-dose patient cups of 15 mEq/11.25 ml (10%); 20 mEq/15 ml (10%); 30 mEq/22.5 ml (10%); 40 mEq/30 ml (10%); 20 mEq/30 ml (5%). **(Parke-Davis)**

Liquid (sugar free), in unit-dose patient cups of 15 mEq/11.25 ml (10%); 20 mEq/15 ml (10%); 30 mEq/22.5 ml (10%); 40 mEq/30 ml (10%); 20 mEq/30 ml (5%). The 10% solution in bottles of 180 ml, 1 pint and 1 gallon; the 5% solution in bottles of 1 pint and 1 gallon. **(Philips Roxane)**

Powder (sugar free), 20 mEq/4-gm packet in cartons of 30 and 100 packets; 20 mEq/1.5-gm packet in cartons of 30. **(Philips Roxane)**

POTASSIUM TRIPLEX Liquid, 15 mEq/5 ml as furnished by 10% each of potassium acetate, potassium bicarbonate and potassium citrate in bottles of 1 pint and 1 gallon. **(Lilly)**

SLOW-K® Tablets (sugar coated) 600 mg (8 mEq) in bottles of 100 and 1000, in Accu-Paks® of 100 and in Consumer Packs of 100. **(Ciba)**

Combinations

KEFF Effervescent Tablets (sugar-free) 20 mEq each of K and Cl ion provided by potassium chloride, potassium carbonate, potassium bicarbonate and betaine hydrochloride in bottles of 60 and 240. **(Lemmon)**

KOLYUM® Liquid or Powder (sugar free). Each 15 ml of solution and each 5-gm packet contains 20 mEq of potassium ion and 3.34 mEq of chloride ion derived from 3.897 gm of potassium gluconate and 0.249 gm of potassium chloride. Liquid in bottles of 1 pint and 1 gallon; powder in packets of 5 gm. **(Pennwalt)**

KAOCHLOR-EFF™ Effervescent Tablets (sugar free). Contains 20 mEq each of K and Cl ion provided by 0.596 gm of potassium chloride; 0.216 gm of potassium citrate; 1 gm of potassium bicarbonate; 1.843 of betaine hydrochloride with 20 mg of saccharin in dispensing cartons of 60 tablets. **(Warren-Teed)**

KLORVESS®: **(Dorsey)**

Effervescent Tablets (sugar free). Contains 20 mEq each of K and Cl ions provided by 1.125 gm of potassium chloride; 0.5 gm of potassium bicarbonate and 0.913 gm of L-lysine monohydrochloride in individually foil-wrapped units of 2 tablets in cartons of 30 units.

PFIKLOR®-F Effervescent Tablets (sugar free). Contains 20 mEq of K and Cl ion provided by

1.125 gm of potassium chloride; 0.5 gm of potassium bicarbonate and 0.913 gm of L-lysine monohydrochloride in bottles of 60. **(Pfizer)**

Potassium Gluconate:

Elixir, 4.68 gm/15 ml in bottles of 1 pint and 1 gallon. **(Lederle)**

Elixir, 4.68 gm/15 ml (20 mEq) in unit-dose containers of 15 ml. **(Parke-Davis)**

Elixir, (sugar and cyclamate free), 4.68 gm/15 ml (20 mEq) in unit-dose containers of 15 ml and in bottles of 1 pint and 1 gallon. **(Philips Roxane)**

KAON®: **(Warren-Teed)**

Elixir (sugar free), 4.68 gm/15 ml (20 mEq) in bottles of 120 ml, 1 pint and 1 gallon and in Stat-Paks® of 15 ml.

S.C.T. Tablets, 1.17 gm (5 mEq) in bottles of 100 and 500 and in Stat-Paks® (unit-dose) of 100.

POTASSIUM IODIDE

Description: Potassium iodide occurs as colorless or white crystals, white granules, or powder very soluble in water and soluble in alcohol.

Indications: To facilitate cough and bronchial drainage in chronic bronchitis, bronchiectasis, pulmonary emphysema, asthma, and certain allergic manifestations of the respiratory tract characterized by difficult-to-raise sputum; for the prophylaxis of goiter and in the management of certain phases of hyperthyroidism.

Contraindications: Hypersensitivity or idiosyncrasy to iodides and in hyperkalemic states. Potassium iodide should not be administered in the presence of acute bronchitis.

Warnings: Coated potassium-containing formulations should be administered only when adequate dietary supplementation is not practicable, since these preparations have been known to cause small bowel lesions (consisting of stenosis with or without ulceration). These small bowel lesions have caused obstruction, hemorrhage, and perforation. Surgery has frequently been required, and deaths have occurred. If abdominal pain, distension, nausea, vomiting or gastrointestinal bleeding occur, therapy should be discontinued.

Precautions: Should be administered with caution during pregnancy since iodides have been associated with abnormal thyroid function and/or goiter in the newborn. Iodides should be given with utmost caution, if at all, in the presence of tuberculosis.

Adverse Reactions: Thyroid adenoma, goiter, and myxedema are possible side effects. Hypersensitivity to iodides may be manifested by angioneurotic edema, cutaneous and mucosal hemorrhages, and symptoms resembling serum sickness, such as fever, arthralgia, lymph node enlargement, and eosinophilia. Iodism or chronic iodine poisoning may occur during prolonged treatment. The symptoms of iodism include a metallic taste, soreness of the mouth, increased salivation, coryza, sneezing, and swelling of the eyelids. There may be a severe headache, productive cough, pulmonary edema, and swelling and tenderness of the salivary glands. Acneform skin lesions are seen in the seborrheic areas. Severe and sometimes fatal skin eruptions may develop. Gastric disturbance and diarrhea are common. If iodism appears, the drug should be withdrawn and the patient given appropriate supportive therapy.

Dosage and Administration: *Orally,* 300 or 600 mg 3 or 4 times daily, usually given after meals and at bedtime with milk or food. Dosage should be adjusted according to patient's response.

Availability:

POTASSIUM IODIDE Enteric Coated Tablets, 300 mg in bottles of 100 and 1000. **(Lilly)**

POTASSIUM IODIDE Liquid, 500 mg/15 ml in bottles of 1 pint and in unit-dose patient cups of 15 ml. **(Philips Roxane)**

POTASSIUM PARA-AMINOBENZOATE

Description: Potassium para-aminobenzoate is the salt of para-aminobenzoic acid. *p*-Aminobenzoic acid is a white or slightly yellow, odorless crystal or crystalline powder soluble in water and in alcohol. It crystallizes as a colorless substance that melts at 186°. It is found widely distributed in plant and animal tissue, both in the free and bound form.

p-Aminobenzoic acid appears to be an essential constituent of cellular metabolism, though its function is unknown. It is present as a component part of folic acid. It also counteracts the bacteriostatic effect of sulfanilamide and other sulfa drugs, due, presumably, to its structural similarity.

It has been suggested that the antifibrotic action of potassium *p*-aminobenzoate is due to the mediation of increased oxygen uptake at the tissue level. It has been postulated that fibrosis may occur from either too much serotonin or too little monoamine oxidase activity. MAO requires an adequate supply of oxygen to function properly, and by increasing the oxygen supply at the tissue level potassium *p*-aminobenzoate may enhance MAO activity and prevent, or bring about regression of, fibrosis.

Indications: May be of use in the treatment of Peyronie's disease, scleroderma, dermatomyositis, morphea and linear scleroderma, and pemphigus. The addition of pyridoxine hydrochloride (B-6) replenishes this vitamin which is usually depleted in serious and chronic scleroderma.

Contraindications: Not to be administered to patients taking sulfonamides, or to those hypersensitive to the components.

Precautions: If anorexia or nausea occur, therapy should be interrupted until the patient is eating normally again. This procedure permits prompt subsidence of symptoms, and also avoids the possible development of hypoglycemia. Should be given with caution to patients with renal disease.

Adverse Reactions: Anorexia, nausea, fever and rash have occurred infrequently; however, these reactions subside upon discontinuation of the drug. When desensitization is accomplished, treatment may be resumed.

Dosage and Administration: *Orally.* Usual adult dose is 4 tablets or capsules 6 times daily, or 6 tablets or capsules 4 times daily, usually with meals and at bedtime with a snack. It is advisable to dissolve the tablets in an adequate amount of liquid to prevent gastrointestinal upset. **Note:** To attain maximum response, adequate dosage should be given for a sufficient length of time.

Availability:
POTABA®: **(Glenwood)**
(contains 22.3% potassium)
Capsules, 0.5 gm in bottles of 250 and 1000.
Envules, 2 gm in cartons of 50.
Powder, pure, in containers of 100 gm and 1 and 5 lb.
Tablets, 0.5 gm in bottles of 100 and 1000.
POTABA + 6: **(Glenwood)**
(contains 22.3% potassium)
Capsules, 0.5 gm w/pyridoxine hydrochloride, 1 mg in bottles of 240 and 1000.
Tablets, 0.5 gm w/pyridoxine hydrochloride, 1 mg in bottles of 120 and 1000.

POVIDONE-IODINE

Description: Povidone-iodine, a topical antiseptic, is a virtually nonstinging, film-forming, water-soluble iodine complex that is nonstaining to skin and natural fabrics. It retains the nonselective broad-range antimicrobial activity of iodine, yet virtually without the undesirable features inherent in other iodine preparations. It kills bacteria, fungi, viruses, protozoa, and yeasts and has a more prolonged germicidal action than ordinary iodine solutions.

Indications: Management of infectious nonspecific vaginitis, monilial vaginitis, and *Trichomonas vaginalis* vaginitis.

Contraindications: Hypersensitivity to iodine.

Precautions: If irritation, redness or swelling develops, the drug should be discontinued.

Dosage and Administration: *Intravaginally.* Insert 1 applicatorful each night, followed by a douche the next morning. This regimen should be followed through the entire menstrual cycle including the days of the menses.

Availability:
BETADINE® Vaginal Gel in tubes of 18 and 90 gm with applicator. Each 5 gm (1 applicatorful) is equivalent to 50 mg of available iodine. **(Purdue Frederick)**

PRALIDOXIME CHLORIDE

Chemical Name: 2-Formyl-1-methylpyridinium chloride oxime (pyridine-2-aldoxime methochloride).

Description: Pralidoxime chloride is a cholinesterase reactivator that is used primarily in the treatment of poisoning caused by powerful anticholinesterases. It is an effective antidote in many cases of systemic poisoning by the organophosphate pesticides or related compounds. The specific activity of the drug resides in the 2-formyl-1-methylpyridinium ion and is independent of the particular salt employed. The compound occurs as a white, nonhygroscopic, crystalline powder that is soluble in water to the extent of 1 gm in less than 1 ml.

The drug acts directly by breaking the relatively irreversible binding of the phosphoryl group to cholinesterase. This chemical action regenerates the depressed enzyme activity and thus restores acetylcholinesterase. It also slows the "aging" of phosphorylated cholinesterase to a nonreactivable form. Therefore, prompt treatment is very essential, not only to overcome the effects of intoxication but also to assure that the drug reaches the phosphorylated enzyme before it becomes nonreactive. The destruction of accumulated acetylcholine can then proceed and neuromuscular junctions will again function normally.

The drug is employed to reverse respiratory muscular paralysis. Because the drug is less effective in relieving respiratory center depression, atropine, in sufficient dosage, is always required concomitantly to block the effect of accumulated acetylcholine at this site. Pralidoxime relieves muscarinic signs and symptoms, salivation, bronchospasm, etc., but this action is relatively unimportant since atropine is adequate for this purpose. It is also of value in overcoming the toxic effects on the neuromuscular junction of the carbamate anticholinesterases, neostigmine, pyridostigmine, and ambenonium, used in the treatment of myasthenia gravis. However, it is not nearly as effective as an antidote to these drugs as it is to the organophosphates.

The drug is distributed throughout the extracellular fluid; it is not bound to plasma proteins. It is rapidly excreted in the urine partly unchanged, and partly as a metabolite produced by the liver. Consequently, it is relatively short-acting and repeated doses may be necessary, especially where there is any evidence of continuing absorption of the poison.

Indications: As an antidote in the treatment of poisoning due to those pesticides and chemicals of the organophosphate class which possess anticholinesterase activity, and in the control of overdosage by anticholinesterase drugs used in the treatment of myasthenia gravis.

Contraindications: There are no known contraindications to the use of pralidoxime in patients with known organic phosphate poisoning.

Warnings: Treatment should be undertaken only under the close supervision of a physician and in the presence of readily available supportive measures. The drug is not effective in the treatment of poisoning due to phosphorus, inorganic phosphates, or organophosphates not having anticholinesterase activity. Until further information is available, no recommendation is made as to the use of pralidoxime in intoxication by pesticides of the carbamate class.

Precautions: Although the drug is well tolerated in most cases, it must be considered that the severe condition of the organophosphate-poisoned patient will generally mask minor signs and symptoms as have been noted in normal individuals. Intravenous administration should be carried out slowly and, preferably, by infusion since a too rapid rate of injection may precipitate tachycardia, laryngospasm, and muscle rigidity. Dosage should be reduced in patients with impaired renal function. Extreme caution is advised in the treatment of organophosphate overdosage in patients with myasthenia gravis since a myasthenic crisis may be precipitated. Barbiturates should be given with utmost care if the patient is having convulsions. Patients poisoned by organophosphates should not receive morphine, theophylline, aminophylline, succinylcholine, reserpine or the phenothiazine-type tranquilizers.

Adverse Reactions: Pralidoxime may cause dizziness, blurred vision, diplopia and impaired accommodation, headache, drowsiness, nausea, tachycardia, hyperventilation, and muscular weakness. However, it is very difficult to differentiate the toxic effects produced by atropine or the organophosphate compounds from those of the drug. When atropine and pralidoxime are used concomitantly, the signs of atropinization may occur earlier than might be expected when atropine is used alone. This is especially true if the total dose of atropine has been large and the administration of pralidoxime has been delayed. Excitement and manic behavior immediately following recovery of consciousness have been reported in several instances. However, similar behavior has occurred in cases of organophosphate poisoning that were not treated with pralidoxime.

Dosage and Administration: *Orally or intravenously.* Initial measures should include removal of secretions, maintenance of a patent airway, and if necessary, artificial ventilation. As soon as cyanosis has been relieved, atropine, 2 to 4 mg for adults and 0.5 to 1 mg for children should be administered *intravenously;* this dose may be repeated at 5- to 10-minute intervals for adults and 10- to 15-minute intervals for children until signs of toxicity appear. Some degree of atropinization should be maintained for at least 48 hours. If cyanosis is present, the same dose of atropine should be administered *intramuscularly.* Both pralidoxime and atropine should be given simultaneously. For adults—initially 1 to 2 gm of pralidoxime *intravenously,* preferably diluted with 100 ml of sodium chloride solution, and infused over a period of 15 to 30 minutes. If this is not practicable or if pulmonary edema is present, the dose should be given slowly by intravenous injection of a 5% solution in water over not less than 5 minutes. If the response is poor, the dose may be repeated in 1 hour. Additional doses may be given if muscle weakness persists. If intravenous administration is not feasible, *intramuscular* or *subcutaneous* injection may be employed. For children—the dose is 20 to 40 mg/kg of body weight. Treatment will be most effective if initiated within a few hours after poisoning has occurred; little will be accomplished if the drug is first administered more than 48 hours after exposure, but in severe poisoning it is, nevertheless, indicated since occasionally patients have responded after such an interval. Continued absorption of the poison may occur, and in such cases additional doses of the drug may be needed every 3 to 8 hours. In the absence of severe gastrointestinal symptoms resulting from the anticholinesterase intoxication, the drug may be administered *orally* in doses of 1 to 3 gm (2 to 6 tablets) every 5 hours. Close supervision of the patient is advised for at least 24 hours. If convulsions interfere with respiration, sodium thiopental (2.5% solution) may be given *intravenously.*

Availability:
PROTOPAM® CHLORIDE: **(Ayerst)**
Emergency Kit, vial of 20 ml containing 1 gm of powder, 20-ml vial of diluent, disposable syringe of 20 ml, needle and alcohol swab.
Injection (dry powder) in vials of 20 ml containing 1 gm of powder.
Tablets, 500 mg in bottles of 100.

PRAMET FA

Description: Each tablet provides:

Iron (as ferrous sulfate)		60 mg
Folic acid		1 mg
Vitamin A acetate	(4000 units)	1.2 mg
Ergocalciferol	(400 units)	10 μg
Ascorbic acid		100 mg
Thiamine mononitrate		3 mg
Riboflavin		2 mg
Pyridoxine hydrochloride		5 mg
Cyanocobalamin		3 μg
Niacinamide		10 mg
d-Calcium pantothenate		1 mg

Calcium (as calcium carbonate), 250 mg; copper (as cupric chloride), 0.15 mg and iodine (as calcium iodate), 0.1 mg.

Indications: Supportive nutritional supplementation during pregnancy and lactation. Elemental iron is provided in controlled-release form (Gradumet®), thereby minimizing the possibility of gastric irritation. Folic acid may be of value in protecting pregnant women against folate deficiency, including those with multiple fetuses, chronic hemolysis and megaloblastic anemia.

Contraindications: Copper is contraindicated in Wilson's disease (hepatolenticular degeneration).

Warnings: Folic acid alone is improper therapy in the treatment of pernicious anemia and other megaloblastic anemias where vitamin B-12 is deficient.

Precautions: Folic acid may obscure the symptoms of pernicious anemia by returning all hematologic parameters to normal while neuropathic manifestations continue unabated.

Adverse Reactions: Allergic sensitization has been reported following both oral and parenteral administration of folic acid.

Dosage and Administration: *Orally,* 1 tablet daily or as directed by physician. Because the iron is in a controlled-release form, the tablet may be taken while the stomach is empty.

Availability:
PRAMET® FA Filmtab® Tablets in bottles of 100. **(Ross)**

PRAMOXINE HYDROCHLORIDE

Chemical Name: 4-*n*-Butoxyphenyl gammamorpholinopropyl ether hydrochloride.

Description: Pramoxine is a surface anesthetic agent obtained from morpholine. It is chemically unrelated to the ester or amide type compounds, and because of its distinct chemical structure, it is apt to minimize the incidence of cross-sensitivity reaction in patients allergic to other local anesthetics. It appears to be well-tolerated when applied to the skin or to less delicate mucous membranes; however, it is irritant when used in the eyes and nose.

Indications: To relieve pain and discomfort associated with dermatoses, anogenital pruritus, hemorrhoids, anal fissure, following episiotomy, and hemorrhoidectomy, during and after endotracheal and intragastric intubation procedures (except bronchoscopy or gastroscopy), to reduce laryngeal reflexes for endotracheal intubation incident to surgical anesthesia. Also useful in relieving pain during rectal examination such as sigmoidoscopy, and to relieve the discomfort from cracked nipples, burns, including sunburn, and other minor injuries.

Contraindications: Hypersensitivity to pramoxine, for use in eyes and nose, and in bronchoscopy or gastroscopy procedures. *It should not be injected into the tissues.*

Precautions: Pramoxine is not intended for prolonged use, nor should it be applied to extensive areas of the skin.

Adverse Reactions: An occasional stinging sensation may occur. If redness, irritation, or pain persists or increases, therapy should be discontinued.

Dosage and Administration: *Topically.* Apply to the affected area every 3 to 4 hours as needed; however, severe cases may require application every 2 hours.

Availability:
TRONOTHANE® HYDROCHLORIDE: **(Abbott)**
Cream, 1% in tubes of 30 gm with rectal applicator.
Jelly, 1% in tubes of 30 gm with rectal applicator.

Combinations

ANUSOL® Ointment (OTC), 0.1% with benzyl benzoate, 1.2%; Peru balsam, 1.8% and zinc oxide, 11% in tubes of 30 gm with rectal applicator. **(Warner-Chilcott)**

PRAZEPAM Ⓒ

Chemical Name: 7-Chloro-1-(cyclopropylmethyl)-1,3-dihydro-5-phenyl-2H-1,4-benzodiazepin-2-one.

Description: Prazepam, a benzodiazepine derivative, is a psychotherapeutic agent structurally and pharmacologically related to diazepam and oxazepam. In common with other antianxiety agents, it shares a similar CNS-depressant action. Results of controlled clinical studies in normal individuals showed that peak blood levels occurred 6 hours after the administration of a single oral dose with significant amounts still present after 48 hours. Steady-state plasma concentrations are achieved in approximately 1 week, and the half-life of prazepam at this point is about 3 days. The primary metabolites are 3-hydroxyprazepam and oxazepam.

Indications: Symptomatic relief of anxiety conditions associated with various psychoneurotic disorders, and as an adjunct in disease states in which anxiety is manifested. It is not recommended for use in psychotic states or in those psychiatric disorders in which anxiety is not a prominent feature.

Contraindications: Hypersensitivity to prazepam and in acute narrow-angle glaucoma.

Warnings: Since drowsiness and dizziness are common reactions, patients should be advised to avoid undertaking activities that require alertness, judgment and physical coordination. Patients should also be advised against the simultaneous use of alcohol and other CNS-depressant drugs (phenothiazines, narcotics, barbiturates, MAO inhibitors and other depressants). Withdrawal symptoms (similar to those noted with barbiturates and alcohol) have occurred following abrupt discontinuance of prazepam (convulsions, tremor, abdominal and muscle cramps, vomiting and sweating). Addiction-prone individuals should be under careful supervision because of their predisposition to habituation and dependence.

Precautions: The usual precautions are indicated for severely depressed patients or those in whom there is some evidence of impending depression; particularly the recognition that suicidal tendencies may be present and protective measures may be necessary. Routine precaution should be observed in treating patients with impaired renal or hepatic function. Periodic blood counts and liver function tests are advisable during long-term therapy. In elderly and debilitated patients, dosage should be limited to the smallest effective amount to preclude the development of ataxia or oversedation. Safe use in pregnant and lactating women or in patients under 18 years of age has not been determined.

Adverse Reactions: Fatigue, dizziness, weakness, drowsiness, lightheadedness, and ataxia have been reported most frequently. Other reactions noted occasionally include headache, confusion, tremor, vivid dreams, slurred speech, palpitation, stimulation, dry mouth, diaphoresis, various gastrointestinal responses, pruritus, skin rashes (transient), swelling of feet, joint pains, various genitourinary symptoms, blurred vision, and syncope. These reactions appear to be dose-related and probably could be modified or avoided by strict adherence to the lowest possible dose with maximal effectiveness.

Dosage and Administration: *Orally* in divided doses. The usual daily dose is 30 mg, then gradually adjusted to 20 to 60 mg daily according to the response of the patient. For elderly or debilitated patients, the recommended initial dose is 10 to 15 mg daily. The drug may also be given as a single dose at bedtime, starting with 20 mg nightly and adjusted as necessary. The optimal dosage will usually range from 20 to 40 mg. Prolonged treatment (over 4 months) demands reevaluation of the clinical status of the patient.

Availability:
Ⓒ VERSTRAN® Tablets, 10 mg (light blue) in bottles of 100. **(Warner-Chilcott)**

PRAZOSIN HYDROCHLORIDE

Chemical Name: 1-(4-Amino-6, 7-dimethoxy-2-quinazolinyl)-4-(2-furanylcarbonyl)piperazine hydrochloride.

Description: Prazosin is a quinazoline derivative with antihypertensive properties. It occurs as a white, crystalline powder that is slightly soluble in water an in isotonic saline solution. Its molecular weight is 419.87.

Although its precise mechanism of action is unknown, the drug has been found to act predominantly as a smooth muscle relaxant. Reduction in blood pressure is believed to be due to a direct relaxation of peripheral arterioles, and is associated with a pronounced decrease in peripheral vascular resistance. Pharmacologic studies suggest that the therapeutic effect of prazosin may be due to the fact that it increases intracellular levels of cyclic AMP [cyclic 3′, 5′ -adenosine monophosphate] and cyclic GMP [cyclic guanosine monophosphate]. This appears to be accomplished by the apparent inhibiting action of the drug on the enzyme PDE [phosphodiesterase] which has been shown to be of prime importance in the degradation of both cyclic AMP and cyclic GMP. Also, cyclic AMP has been found to mediate smooth muscle relaxation and cyclic GMP to induce acetylcholine decreases in cardiac contraction (both rate and force), although showing little activity in arteriolar smooth muscle. Consequently, the inhibiting effect of the drug on PDE would therefore be expected to result in arteriolar vasodilation with subsequent decreases in blood pressure, while the expected reflex tachycardia due to increased levels of cyclic AMP in the heart would be prevented by the opposing effect of increased levels of cyclic GMP.

Blood pressure is lowered in both the supine and standing position, an effect that is more pronounced on the diastolic blood pressure. Pharmacologic studies revealed that prazosin does not significantly change cardiac output or heart rate. This was supported by the fact that patients with coronary artery disease who were given the drug experienced no significant problems. In addition, renal blood flow, glomerular filtration rate and kidney function remain essentially unchanged, even in patients with impaired renal function. To date, there has been no evidence of interference with sympathetic nervous system function, no apparent alpha adrenergic receptor blocking activity, no increase in plasma renin activity, and no measurable effect on the chronotropic responses to either sympathetic or vagal stimulation.

Following oral administration, plasma concentration reaches a peak at about 3 hours with a plasma half-life of 2 to 3 hours. Approximately, 97% of the drug is bound to serum protein. It appears to be metabolized primarily by demethylation and conjugation, and excreted mainly in the bile and feces. Long-term studies with rats and dogs receiving 25 mg/kg/day (60 times the maximal clinical dose) showed testicular changes, necrosis and atrophy. These effects were not evident when 10 mg/kg/day was given to the same species of animals. Thus far, testicular involvement has not been demonstrated during clinical trials with prazosin.

The incidence of orthostatic hypotension in clinical trials was 3.4%. In a small number of patients, the drug has caused syncope with sudden loss of consciousness, usually occurring within 30 to 90 minutes of the initial dose. This is believed to be due to an excessive postural hypotensive effect. The incidence was approximately 1% in patients given an initial dose of 2 mg or more. Clinical trials suggest that these episodes can be minimized by limiting the initial dose to 1 mg 3 times daily.

Although clinical experience is limited, prazosin has been administered without any observable unfavorable interactions with such drugs as cardiac glycosides (digitalis and digoxin); hypoglycemics (insulin, chlorpropamide, phenformin, tolazamide and tolbutamide); tranquilizers and sedatives (chlordiazepoxide, diazepam and phenobarbital); antigout medications (allopurinol, colchicine and probenecid); antiarrhythmics (procainamide, quinidine and propranolol); and analgesics, antipyretics and antiinflammatories (propoxyphene, aspirin, indomethacin and phenylbutazone).

Indications: Treatment of hypertension. May be used as the initial agent or combined with a diuretic and/or antihypertensive drugs.

Contraindications: Hypersensitivity to prazosin.

Warnings: Syncope with sudden loss of consciousness may occur, and may be due to an excessive postural hypotension or to severe tachycardia. Syncope may also occur when the dosage is rapidly increased or when another antihypertensive agent is added to the regimen, especially if the patient is taking large doses of prazosin. Patients on concomitant therapy with a beta-adrenergic blocking agent such as propranolol may also experience severe hypotension. If syncope occurs, the patient should be placed in the recumbent position and the necessary measures should be instituted. This adverse effect is self-limiting and in most cases does not recur after the initial period of therapy or during subsequent dosage adjustment. Patients should always be started on the 1-mg dose; the 2- and 5-mg doses are not intended for initial therapy. Since dizziness and lightheadedness may occur and may be followed by fainting, patients should be advised on the proper measures to take, and should be cautioned to avoid situations where injury could result. To date, there have been no clinical trials with the use of this drug in pediatric patients.

Adverse Reactions: Side effects most commonly noted in patients were dizziness in 10.3%, headache in 7.8%, drowsiness in 7.6%, lack of energy in 6.9%, weakness in 6.5%, palpitations in 5.3%, and nausea in 4.9%. In most instances they seem to disappear with continued treatment or have been tolerated with no adjustment in the dosage. Other reactions that may occur include vomiting, diarrhea, constipation, abdominal discomfort and/or pain; edema, dyspnea, syncope, and tachycardia; nervousness, vertigo, depression, and paresthesia; rash and pruritus; urinary frequency, and impotence. Other reactions that may develop include blurred vision, reddened sclera, epistaxis, tinnitus, dry mouth, nasal congestion, and diaphoresis. There have been single reports of pigmentary mottling and serous retinopathy, and a few reports of cataract development or disappearance. In these instances, the exact causal relationship has not been established because baseline observations were frequently inadequate. In slit-lamp and funduscopic studies, no drug-related abnormal ophthalmological findings have been reported.

Dosage and Administration: *Orally.* The initial adult dosage is 1 mg 3 times daily. The maintenance dosage may be slowly increased to a total daily dose of 20 mg given in divided doses. Higher doses usually do not increase effectiveness, however a few patients may benefit from further increases up to a daily dose of 40 mg given in divided doses. After the initial titration some patients can be maintained adequately on a twice daily dosage regimen. The addition of a diuretic or other antihypertensive agent to the dosage regimen requires that prazosin be reduced to 1 or 2 mg 3 times daily and then retitration carried out.

Availability:
MINIPRESS® Capsules, 1, 2 and 5 mg in bottles of 250 and in unit-dose packages of 100.

(Pfizer)

PREDNISOLONE: see The Adrenal Corticosteroids

PREDNISONE: see The Adrenal Corticosteroids

PREFRIN-A

Description: A decongestant-antihistaminic solution consisting of pyrilamine maleate, 0.1%; phenylephrine hydrochloride, 0.12%; antipyrine, 0.1% with benzalkonium chloride, boric acid, disodium edetate and sodium bisulfite.

Indications: Symptomatic relief of eyes affected with allergy, inflammation, and irritation of a mild to moderate degree, particularly when the allergic insult results from air pollutants or airborne pollens.

Contraindications: Because of phenylephrine, the solution should not be used in the presence of narrow-angle glaucoma. Also infections, foreign bodies or severe irritation of the eye contraindicates its use.

Warnings: Extreme caution is required when used in patients predisposed to narrow-angle glaucoma or with a history of glaucoma in order to avoid producing an acute attack. Since topical antihistamines are potential sensitizing agents, their use can cause a local reaction.

Precautions: Should sensitivity or other adverse reactions occur, the medication should be discontinued and the physician consulted.

Dosage and Administration: *Topically.* Instill 1 or 2 drops into the conjunctival sac every 3 or 4 hours or as needed.

Availability:
PREFRIN™-A Ophthalmic Solution in dropper bottles of 15 ml. **(Allergan)**

PRILOCAINE HYDROCHLORIDE

Chemical Name: 2-(Propylamino)-*o*-propionotoluidide hydrochloride.

Description: Prilocaine is a local anesthetic of the amide type and is similar structurally to lidocaine and mepivacaine. It occurs as a colorless or white, crystalline powder freely soluble in water and soluble in alcohol.

Its effectiveness as a local anesthetic is said to compare with that of lidocaine. It acts by stabilizing the neuronal membranes thus preventing the initiation and transmission of nerve impulses. The onset of action is about 2 minutes longer for prilocaine than for lidocaine, whereas the duration of action is, at least, 30 to 60 minutes longer for prilocaine in nerve blocks. The drug is metabolized in both the liver and kidneys and is excreted in the urine; it is not metabolized by plasma esterases. One of its metabolites *o*-toluidine has been found to produce methemoglobin in both in vitro and in vivo studies.

Indications: In infiltration anesthesia, therapeutic nerve blocks such as intercostal and paravertebral blocks, regional anesthesia such as brachial plexus and sciatic-femoral blocks, and blockade of major nerve trunks by way of the peridural and caudal routes. Since solutions of prilocaine, with the exception of the Forte solution, do not contain epinephrine, they may be used in patients in whom vasopressors are contraindicated.

Contraindications: In patients with known hypersensitivity to local anesthetics of the amide type, in those with congenital or idiopathic methemoglobinemia, or with severe shock or heart block, and in the presence of inflammation and/or sepsis at the injection site.

Warnings: Resuscitative equipment and medication should be readily available in the event of toxic reactions or complications. The Forte solution which contains a vasoconstrictor should be used with considerable caution in patients receiving MAO inhibitors, tricyclic antidepressants, phenothiazines, etc., since severe and sustained hypotension or hypertension may occur. Careful consideration should be given to the possible adverse effects upon fetal development before administering this drug to women of childbearing potential, and particularly during the first trimester of pregnancy. However, prilocaine has been used effectively at term for obstetrical analgesia. Adverse effects on the fetus, course of labor or delivery have rarely been observed.

Precautions: The safety and effectiveness of prilocaine depend upon proper dosage, correct technique, adequate precautions, and readiness for emergencies. The lowest dosage that results in effective anesthesia should be employed to avoid high plasma levels and serious adverse reactions. Repeated doses may cause significant increases in blood levels of the drug and its metabolites which may lead to methemoglobinemia. Patients with liver disease, or debilitated, elderly, or acutely ill patients and children should be given reduced doses commensurate with their age and physical status. Epidural or caudal anesthesia should be used with extreme caution in patients with existing neurological disease, spinal deformities, septicemia, severe hypertension, and in pediatric patients. Also, the drug should be administered with care in individuals with known drug sensitivities. Prilocaine may react with certain metals and cause the release of their respective ions which, if injected, may cause severe local irritation; therefore, adequate precaution should be taken to avoid this type of interaction. The Forte solution should be used with caution in the presence of diseases which may adversely affect the patient's cardiovascular system; also, severe cardiac arrhythmias may develop when employed during or following the administration of chloroform, halothane, cyclopropane, trichloroethylene or other related agents. Special care should be taken to avoid intravascular injection, and the rate of administration should be slow in an attempt to avoid systemic effects.

Adverse Reactions: Side effects usually result from high plasma levels due to excessive dosage, rapid absorption or inadvertent intravascular injection, or may result from a hypersensitivity, idiosyncrasy or diminished tolerance to the drug. Such reactions are systemic in nature and involve the CNS and/or the cardiovascular system. CNS reactions are both excitatory and depressant, and may be characterized by nervousness, dizziness, blurred vision and tremors, followed by drowsiness, convulsions, unconsciousness and possibly respiratory arrest. The excitatory reactions may be very brief or may not occur at all, in which case the first manifestations of toxicity may be drowsiness, merging into unconsciousness and respiratory arrest. Cardiovascular reactions are depressant, and may be manifested by hypotension, myocardial depression, bradycardia and possibly cardiac arrest. Allergic reactions are usually characterized by cutaneous lesions, urticaria, edema or anaphylactoid reactions. Detection of sensitivity by skin testing is of doubtful value. Methemoglobin formation has occurred when the maximum recommended dose of 600 mg was administered; however, in all patients, the blood levels were found to be less than 15% of the total hemoglobin content. Cyanosis has also been reported at this dosage level. A dose-response relationship appears to exist between the amount of prilocaine administered as a single injection and the incidence and degree of methemoglobin formation. Methemoglobinemia is rapidly and effectively reversed with methylene blue.

Dosage and Administration: *Parenterally.* Only the lowest concentration and volume that will produce the desired results should be used. The total dose, however, in normal healthy adults should not exceed 600 mg for any procedure. *For nerve block*, 20 to 30 ml of the 1 or 2% solution and 15 to 20 ml of the 3% solution will usually produce adequate operative anesthesia. *For therapeutic nerve block* (e.g., intercostal or paravertebral), 3 to 5 ml of the 1 or 2% solution is usually adequate. *For infiltration anesthesia*, for most surgical procedures, 20 to 30 ml of the 1 or 2% solution usually will provide adequate operative anesthesia. *For regional anesthesia* (e.g., brachial plexus or sciatic-femoral blocks), 20 to 30 ml of the 2% solution or 15 to 20 ml of the 3% solution. *For peridural anesthesia*, 20 to 30 ml of the 2% solution or 15 to 20 ml of the 3% solution. *For caudal anesthesia*, 20 to 30 ml of the 1% solution will usually provide adequate obstetrical anesthesia for most vaginal deliveries. *For surgical procedures requiring more extensive anesthesia*, 20 to 30 ml of the 2% solution or 15 to 20 ml of the 3% solution are recommended. *For dental procedures,* 0.5 to 5 ml (usually 1 to 2 ml) of the 4% (plain) solution or 0.5 to 3.6 ml of the (Forte) solution are recommended. Children under 10 years of age usually require no more than 0.9 ml. The onset and duration of anesthesia and the degree of muscular relaxation are proportional to the volume and concentration of the local anesthetic employed. **Important Note:** Injections should always be made *slowly* and with frequent aspirations so that the possibility of intravascular injection may be reduced. In addition, a test dose of 2 to 5 ml should be administered at least 5 minutes prior to injecting the total volume required for epidural or caudal anesthesia. It is important that a single-dose container be employed for epidural anesthesia.

Availability:
CITANEST® Solution, 1 and 2% in ampuls and vials of 30 ml; 3% in ampuls of 20 ml; 4% (plain) in dental cartridges of 1.8 ml. **(Astra)**

w/Epinephrine
CITANEST® Forte Solution, 4% with epinephrine, 1:200,000 in dental cartridges of 1.8 ml. **(Astra)**

PRIMAQUINE PHOSPHATE

Chemical Name: 8-(4-Amino-1-methylbutylamino)-6-methoxyquinoline phosphate.

Description: Primaquine phosphate is a synthetic 8-aminoquinoline derivative possessing potent antimalarial activity. It occurs as an orange-red, crystalline powder with a bitter taste that is moderately soluble in water. It acts by eliminating tissue (exo-erythrocytic) infections, thereby preventing the development of the blood (erythrocytic) forms of the parasite which are responsible for relapses in *P. vivax* malaria. It is also active against gametocytes of *P. falciparum.* Following oral administration, primaquine is readily absorbed and rapidly metabolized, and only a small proportion is excreted as the parent drug. The concentration of the drug in the plasma reaches a peak in about 6 hours, but falls rapidly and is barely detectable after 24 hours.

Indications: To prevent relapses and to effect a radical cure of malaria caused by *Plasmodium vivax.*

Contraindications: Because quinacrine hydrochloride appears to potentiate the toxicity of antimalarial compounds which are structurally related to primaquine, the use of quinacrine in patients receiving primaquine is contraindicated. Similarly, primaquine should not be administered to patients who have received quinacrine recently, as toxicity is increased. The drug is also contraindicated in acutely ill patients suffering from systemic disease manifested by tendency to granulocytopenia, such as rheumatoid arthritis and lupus erythematosus, and in those patients receiving concurrently other potentially hemolytic drugs or depressants of myeloid elements of the bone marrow.

Warnings: Before prescribing this drug, the physician should be well-informed of the data that appears in the manufacturer's literature. The drug should be discontinued promptly if signs suggestive of hemolytic anemia occur characterized by darkening of urine, marked fall of hemoglobin or erythrocyte count. Primaquine or related drugs may precipitate moderate or severe hemolytic anemia in certain ethnic groups (particularly in Sardinians and dark-skinned individuals and in those with a family or personal history of favism) who are deficient in the enzyme glucose-6-phosphate dehydrogenase. Its use in pregnant patients is not recommended since its effect on the fetus has not been established.

Precautions: Because anemia, methemoglobinemia, and leukopenia have been noted following administration of large doses of primaquine, the adult dosage of 1 tablet daily for 14 days should not be exceeded. It is also advisable to perform periodic blood examinations (particularly blood cell counts and hemoglobin determinations) during treatment. The patient should be closely observed for any signs of intolerance to the drug.

Adverse Reactions: Primaquine may cause nausea, vomiting, epigastric distress, and abdominal cramps. Hematologic reactions include leukopenia and hemolytic anemia in patients deficient in glucose-6-phosphate dehydrogenase, and methemoglobinemia in those deficient in nicotinamide adenine dinucleotide methemoglobin reductase. Overdosage is manifested by abdominal cramps, vomiting, burning epigastric distress, CNS and cardiovascular disturbances, cyanosis, methemoglobinemia, moderate leukocytosis, or leukopenia, and anemia. The most striking symptoms are granulocytopenia and acute hemolytic anemia in sensitive patients. Acute hemolysis occurs, but patients recover completely if the drug is withdrawn.

Dosage and Administration: *Orally*, 1 tablet daily for 14 days. Patients suffering from an attack of vivax malaria or having parasitized red blood cells should receive a course of chloroquine phosphate which quickly destroys the erythrocytic parasites and terminates the paroxysm. Concurrently primaquine should be administered to eradicate the exo-erythrocytic parasites.

Availability:
PRIMAQUINE PHOSPHATE Tablets, 26.3 mg (equal to 15 mg base) in bottles of 100.

(Winthrop)

PRIMIDONE

Chemical Name: 5-Ethyl-dihydro-5-phenyl-4,6(1H,5H)-pyrimidinedione.

Description: Primidone is a pyrimidine derivative structurally resembling phenobarbital but having different chemical and pharmacologic properties; it differs from phenobarbital only in that 2 hydrogen atoms replace the oxygen on the carbon atom of the urea moiety. It is a colorless, crystalline substance that is very slightly soluble in water and in most organic solvents.

Although the precise mode and site of action is not clear, the drug apparently acts on the motor cortex to raise seizure threshold or alter seizure pattern. Following oral administration, peak plasma levels are reached in approximately 1 hour, and maximal therapeutic effects are noted within 6 to 8 hours. About 60 to 80% of the drug is excreted in the urine within 24 hours as unchanged drug and its metabolite phenylethylmalondiamide.

Indications: To control grand mal, psychomotor, and focal epileptic seizures. May be used alone or in combination with other anticonvulsants.

Contraindications: Patients with porphyria, or who are sensitive to phenobarbital.

Warnings: The physician should keep in mind that abrupt withdrawal of anticonvulsant medication may precipitate status epilepticus. Clinical findings strongly suggest that anticonvulsant drugs are associated with an increased incidence of congenital malformation among the offspring of women who received the drug during pregnancy. Therefore, the use of these drugs in pregnant women or in women of childbearing potential requires that the anticipated benefits be weighed against the possible hazards to the patients as well as to the fetus. However, these drugs should not be discontinued in those patients predisposed to major seizures because of the strong possibility of precipitating status epilepticus with its attendant hypoxia and risk to both the mother and fetus. Nonetheless, consideration should be given to discontinuing these agents prior to and during pregnancy when the nature, frequency and severity of the seizures do not constitute a serious threat to the patient.

Precautions: Dosage exceeding 2 gm daily is not recommended. Since therapy generally extends over prolonged periods, a complete blood count and a sequential multiple analysis-12 (SMA-12) test should be performed every 6 months. Clinical evidence shows that primidone appears in the milk of nursing mothers in substantial quantities; therefore, the presence of undue somnolence and drowsiness in nursing infants is an indication that nursing should be discontinued. Neonatal hemorrhage, with a coagulation defect resembling vitamin K deficiency, has been noted in newborn infants whose mothers were taking primidone. Pregnant women under anticonvulsant therapy should receive prophylactic vitamin K therapy for 1 month prior to, and during, delivery.

Adverse Reactions: The most frequently occurring are ataxia and vertigo. These tend to disappear with continued therapy, or with reduction of initial dosage. Occasionally noted were nausea, anorexia, vomiting, fatigue, hyperirritability, emotional disturbances, impotence, diplopia, nystagmus, drowsiness, and morbilliform skin eruptions. On rare occasions, persistent or severe side effects may necessitate withdrawal of the drug. Megaloblastic anemia may occur as a rare idiosyncrasy to primidone. The anemia responds to 15 mg of folic acid daily without necessity of discontinuing medication.

Dosage and Administration: *Orally.* Adults and children over 8 years of age, initially, 250 mg daily; increase by increments of 250 mg at weekly intervals, to tolerance or therapeutic effectiveness, up to daily dosages not exceeding 2 gm. The average adult dosage is 0.75 to 1.5 gm daily. Children under 8 years of age, ½ the adult dosage. In patients already receiving other anticonvulsants, primidone should be gradually increased as dosage of the other drug is maintained or gradually decreased.

Availability:
MYSOLINE®: **(Ayerst)**
Suspension, 250 mg/5 ml in bottles of 240 ml.
Tablets, 50 mg in bottles of 100 and 500; 250 mg in bottles of 100 and 1000 and in unit-dose packages of 100.

PROBENECID

Chemical Name: 4-[(Dipropylamino)sulfonyl] benzoic acid.

Description: Probenecid, a sulfonamide derivative of benzoic acid, occurs as a fine, white or nearly white, crystalline powder practically insoluble in water and soluble in alcohol. Molecular weight is 285.36.

Probenecid is a uricosuric and renal tubular blocking agent. Reports indicate that it inhibits the tubular reabsorption of urate, thus increasing the urinary excretion of uric acid and decreasing serum uric acid levels. Effective uricosuria reduces the miscible urate pool, retards urate deposition, and promotes resorption of urate deposits.

Probenecid also inhibits the tubular secretion of penicillin and usually increases plasma levels of ampicillin, methicillin, oxacillin, cloxacillin or nafcillin by any route the antibiotic is given. In addition, the drug decreases the urinary excretion of aminosalicylic acid, aminohippuric acid, phenolsulfonphthalein, pantothenic acid, 17-ketosteroids, sodium iodomethamate, and related iodinated organic acids, sulfonamides, and sulfonylureas. It decreases both hepatic and renal excretion of sulfobromophthalein (BSP). The tubular reabsorption of phosphorus is inhibited in hypoparathyroid but not in euparathyroid individuals. It appears to produce an insignificant increase in free sulfa plasma concentrations, but a significant increase in total sulfa plasma levels. It also produces a notable increase in indomethacin or methotrexate plasma levels.

Probenecid does not influence plasma concentrations of salicylates, nor the excretion of streptomycin, chloramphenicol, chlortetracycline, oxytetracycline or neomycin.

Indications: Treatment of hyperuricemia associated with gout and gouty arthritis; as an adjuvant to therapy with penicillin. The addition of colchicine provides a specific prophylactic, suppressive effect that helps to reduce the incidence of acute attacks.

Contraindications: Hypersensitivity to probenecid or colchicine; patients with blood dyscrasias in the presence of an acute gouty attack, or uric acid kidney stones; and children under 2 years of age.

Warnings: An exacerbation of gout following therapy with probenecid may occur; in such instances colchicine or other appropriate therapy is advisable. Since salicylates antagonize the uricosuric activity of probenecid, they should not be used concomitantly with this drug during therapy. Acetaminophen is preferred when a mild analgesic agent is necessary. The appearance of a hypersensitivity reaction warrants cessation of therapy.

Precautions: When coadministered with sulfonamides, probenecid increases the amount of conjugated sulfonamide in the plasma; therefore, plasma concentrations should be determined regularly, especially if concomitant therapy is prolonged. The presence of a reducing substance in the urine of patients receiving probenecid may result in a false-positive *Benedict's* test for glycosuria. The hazard of producing hematuria, renal colic and costovertebral pain or formation of urate stones in patients with gout exists, particularly during the initial stage of therapy. These may be prevented by alkalization of the urine and a liberal fluid intake. Use with caution in patients with a history of peptic ulcer. Coadministration with penicillin is not recommended in patients with known renal impairment.

Adverse Reactions: Headache, anorexia, nausea, vomiting, increased urinary frequency; hypersensitivity reactions (including anaphylactoid, dermatitis, pruritus and fever), sore gums, flushing, dizziness, anemia, and hemolytic anemia (usually associated with a deficiency of glucose-6-phosphate dehydrogenase in red blood cells) have been reported. Nephrotic syndrome, hepatic necrosis, and aplastic anemia occur rarely. For other adverse reactions, see monograph on Colchicine.

Dosage and Administration: *Orally*, recommended adult dosage is ½ tablet (probenecid) twice daily for 1 week, followed by 1 tablet twice daily thereafter. Probenecid and colchicine, 1 tablet daily for 1 week, followed by 1 tablet twice daily thereafter. Therapy with probenecid should not be initiated until an acute gouty attack has subsided. However, if an acute attack is precipitated during therapy, the drug may be continued without changing the dosage, and full therapeutic dosage of colchicine or other appropriate therapy should be given to control the acute attack.

Availability:

BENEMID® Tablets, 0.5 gm in bottles of 100 and 1000 and in single-unit packages of 100. **(Merck Sharp & Dohme)**

PROBENECID Tablets, 0.5 gm in bottles of 100 and 1000. **(Lederle)**

ColBENEMID® Tablets, 0.5 gm with colchicine, 0.5 mg in bottles of 100. **(Merck Sharp & Dohme)**

PROBUCOL

Chemical Name: 4,4′-(Isopropylidenedithio)bis(2,6-di-t-butylphenol).

Description: Probucol is a lipophilic agent indicated primarily for the reduction of elevated serum cholesterol. Possessing a unique chemical structure that is different from that of other available cholesterol-lowering agents, it has been found useful in treating patients with primary hypercholesterolemia. The drug's mechanism of action is not known, but it has been demonstrated that there is no apparent increase in the cyclic precursors of cholesterol, namely desmosterol and 7-dehydrocholesterol. On this basis, it has been concluded that probucol probably does not interfere with the later stages of cholesterol biosynthesis.

To achieve higher and less variable blood levels of the drug. It is recommended that probucol be taken with food. During continuous administration of the recommended dosage, blood levels gradually increase in the first 3 to 4 months, and thereafter remain fairly constant. When a 12-month treatment program was discontinued in 8 patients, the average blood levels fell 60% in approximately 6 weeks and 80% in about 6 months. Results of animal studies showed that probucol sensitizes the canine myocardium to epinephrine resulting in ventricular fibrillation. This phenomenon appears to be unique to the dog since this effect was not apparent in four other species (mice, rat, monkey and pig).

At the present time it has not been established whether or not the drug-induced lowering of serum cholesterol or lipid levels has any effect, determental, beneficial or none at all, on the morbidity or mortality due to atherosclerosis or coronary heart disease.

Indications: Conditions in which the reduction in primary hypercholesterolemia is desirable. Also indicated for patients with abnormally high levels of both cholesterol and triglycerides, but not for those with primary hypertriglyceridemia alone. Should be used as an adjunct to appropriate dietary regulation and other essential measures.

Contraindications: Known hypersensitivity to probucol.

Precautions: Attempts should first be made to control serum cholesterol with appropriate dietary measures, weight reduction and the treatment of any underlying disorder which might cause the condition. Because the drug may necessarily be given for prolonged periods, adequate baseline studies should be performed to determine whether or not the patient has significantly elevated serum lipid levels. Serum cholesterol and triglyceride levels should be determined frequently during the first few months of therapy and periodically thereafter, so that by the sixth month it can be decided whether the reduction warrants further treatment; persistent hypertriglyceridemia indicates cessation of therapy. Because neither oral hypoglycemic nor oral anticoagulant agents alter the effect of probucol on serum cholesterol, the dosage of these agents is generally not modified when given concomitantly. Use of the drug in pregnant women is not recommended, and if the patient wishes to become pregnant, it is advised that the drug be withdrawn and birth control procedures be used for at least six months before conception is attempted. Additionally, it is advised that nursing mothers refrain from nursing their infants while taking this drug. Safe and effective use in children have not been established.

Adverse Reactions: During clinical trials about 2% of the patients had to discontinue treatment because of gastrointestinal reactions. Diarrhea occurs in about 10% of the patients. Other gastrointestinal reactions in descending order of frequency are flatulence, abdominal pain, nausea and vomiting. These reactions are usually transient and seldom require the drug to be withdrawn. Less frequently observed were hyperhidrosis, fetid sweat, and angioneurotic edema. An idiosyncratic reaction characterized by dizziness, palpitations, syncope, nausea, vomiting and chest pain has been reported. Headache, dizziness, paresthesias and eosinophilia were observed in about 2% of the patients; consistently low hemoglobin and/or hematocrit values were observed in about 1% of the patients. Rarely noted were rash, pruritus, impotence, insomnia, conjunctivitis, tearing, blurred vision, tinnitus, diminished sense of taste and smell, enlargement of a multinodular goiter, anorexia, heartburn, indigestion, gastrointestinal bleeding, ecchymosis and petechiae, decreased hemoglobin, thrombocytopenia, nocturia, peripheral neuritis, elevations of serum transaminases (glutamic-oxaloacetic and glutamic-pyruvic), bilirubin, alkaline phosphatase, creatine phosphokinase, uric acid, BUN and blood glucose. Although the basis for the relationship between probucol and these abnormalities is not firm, the possibility that some of these are drug-related cannot be excluded.

Dosage and Administration: *Orally.* The recommended adult dosage is 250 mg twice daily taken with the morning and evening meals.

Availability:
LORELCO® Tablets, 250 mg in bottles of 120 and in unit-dose packages of 112. **(Dow)**

PROCAINAMIDE HYDROCHLORIDE

Chemical Name: *p*-Amino-*N*-(2-diethylaminoethyl)benzamide hydrochloride.

Description: Procainamide hydrochloride is an amide analogue of procaine hydrochloride which differs structurally only in the replacement of the ester group with an amide group. It occurs as a white to tan, hygroscopic, crystalline powder very soluble in water and soluble in alcohol. Solutions of procainamide are colorless or may turn slightly yellow on standing.

Procainamide depresses the excitability of cardiac muscle to electrical stimulation, and slows conduction in the atrium, the bundle of His, and the ventricle. The refractory period of the atrium is considerably more prolonged than that of the ventricle. Contractility of the heart is usually not affected nor is cardiac output decreased to any extent unless myocardial damage exists. In the absence of any arrhythmia, the heart rate may occasionally be accelerated by conventional doses, suggesting that the drug possesses anticholinergic properties. Larger doses can induce atrioventricular block and ventricular extrasystoles which may proceed to ventricular fibrillation. These effects on the myocardium are reflected in the electrocardiogram; a widening of the QRS complex occurs most consistently; less regularly, the P-R and Q-T intervals are prolonged, and the QRS and T waves show some decrease in voltage.

The action of procainamide begins almost immediately after intramuscular or intravenous administration. Plasma levels after intramuscular injection are at their peak in 15 to 60 minutes. Following oral administration, plasma levels of the drug are comparable to those obtained parenterally and are maximal within 1 hour; therapeutic levels are usually attained in 1/2 that time.

Procainamide is less readily hydrolyzed than procaine, and plasma levels decline slowly—about 10 to 20%/hour. The drug is excreted primarily in the urine, approximately 10% as free and conjugated *p*-aminobenzoic acid and about 60% in the unchanged form. The fate of the remainder is unknown.

Indications: Treatment of ventricular extrasystoles and ventricular tachycardia. May be useful in the treatment of atrial arrhythmias such as ectopic contractions, tachycardia, flutter and fibrillation, particularly if the arrhythmia is of recent development, and during anesthesia to correct cardiac arrhythmias; prophylactically for cardiac arrhythmias which may occur during surgical anesthesia in patients with known heart conditions or those undergoing thoracic surgery.

Contraindications: Myasthenia gravis, complete atrioventricular heart block, in second and third degree atrioventricular block unless an electrical pacemaker is operative, and hypersensitivity to procainamide.

Warnings: Prolonged administration often results in the development of a positive antinuclear antibody test with or without symptoms of a lupus erythematosis-like syndrome. If the test is positive, the benefit-to-risk ratio related to continued treatment with this drug should be assessed, and may necessitate consideration of alternative antiarrhythmic therapy.

Precautions: The drug should be used with extreme caution in patients with coronary occlusion, disturbances in impulse conduction, considerable cardiac enlargement, hypotension, frank or impending congestive failure, and in the treatment of digitalis intoxication in order to avoid ventricular fibrillation or further depression of cardiac function. Procainamide should be used with utmost care in patients who have undergone electrical reversion to sinus rhythm. When used in the treatment of atrial arrhythmias, it may produce an increased ventricular rate due to a vagolytic effect. Procainamide therapy should be preceded by digitalization in the treatment of atrial arrhythmias; digitalization may reduce but does not abolish the possibility of increased ventricular rate. Cardiotonic glycosides when used in the treatment of atrial fibrillation, particularly when complicated by congestive failure, may result in forceful atrial contractions which may cause dislodgement of mural thrombi, resulting in embolization. It should be used cautiously in patients with liver or kidney disease as accumulation of the drug may occur which may produce ventricular tachycardia and severe hypotension. It is recommended that tests for lupus erythematosus should be performed regularly, and if symptoms appear, the drug should be discontinued. However, if the LE syndrome develops in a patient with recurrent life-threatening arrhythmias not controllable by other antiarrhythmic agents, steroid suppressive therapy may be used simultaneously with procainamide. Also blood count studies should be undertaken during therapy as agranulocytosis has occurred with the repeated use of this drug and deaths have been reported. Electrocardiographic monitoring of cardiac function is advised during therapy with this drug.

Adverse Reactions: Severe lowering of blood pressure and hypotension, serious disturbances in cardiac rhythm such as ventricular asystole or fibrillation has been noted. Large oral doses of procainamide may produce anorexia, nausea, vomiting, urticaria, pruritus. A lupus erythematosus syndrome, fever, chills, abdominal pain, acute hepatomegaly, rise in SGOT levels, bitter taste, diarrhea, weakness, mental depression, giddiness, psychosis with hallucinations, angioneurotic edema, maculopapular rash, and agranulocytosis have also been reported. Patients should be instructed to report any soreness of the mouth, throat or gums, unexplained fever or any symptoms of an upper respiratory tract infection. Should any of these occur, the drug is withdrawn and appropriate treatment instituted immediately.

Dosage and Administration: *Orally. For ventricular tachycardia*—1 gm initially followed thereafter by a total daily dose of 50 mg/kg of body weight given at 3-hour intervals. *For premature ventricular contractions*—the suggested dosage is 50 mg/kg of body weight daily given in divided doses at 3-hour intervals. *For atrial fibrillation and paroxysmal atrial tachycardia*—1.25 gm initially followed in 1 hour by 0.75 gm if there have been no electrocardiographic changes. A dose of 0.5 to 1 gm may then be given every 2 hours until arrhythmia is interrupted or the limit of tolerance is reached. The suggested maintenance dosage is 0.5 to 1 gm every 4 to 6 hours. *Intramuscularly*, 0.5 to 1 gm every 6 hours; usual daily dosage range is 500 mg to 2 gm. *Intravenously*, 25 to 50 mg/minute up to a total dose of 1 gm; usual dosage range is 50 to 250 mg; *For cardiac arrhythmias associated with anesthesia and surgery* —0.1 to 0.5 gm preferably administered *intramuscularly*. For more detailed dosage information, see package literature.

Availability:
PROCAINAMIDE HYDROCHLORIDE Capsules, 250 and 375 mg in bottles of 100; 500 mg in bottles of 100 and 1000. **(Lederle)**
PROCAMIDE Capsules, 250 mg in bottles of 100 and 1000. **(Amfre-Grant)**
PRONESTYL®: **(Squibb)**
Capsules, 250 and 500 mg in bottles of 100 and 1000; 375 mg in bottles of 100.
Injection, 100 mg/ml in vials of 10 ml; 500 mg/ml in vials of 2 ml.
Tablets (Filmlok®), 250 and 500 mg in bottles of 100 and 1000; 372 mg in bottles of 100.

PROCAINE HYDROCHLORIDE

Chemical Name: 2-(Diethylamino)ethyl *p*-aminobenzoate hydrochloride.

Description: Procaine hydrochloride is an effective local anesthetic when administered parenterally. It does not irritate tissues and is one of the least toxic of the injectable local anesthetics. It occurs as colorless crystals or as a white, crystalline powder readily soluble in cold water, but less soluble in alcohol. It is incompatible with caustic alkalies and their carbonates. Epinephrine prolongs its duration of action.

Procaine stabilizes the neuronal membrane and prevents the initiation and transmission of nerve impulses, thereby effecting local anesthesia. Procaine lacks surface anesthetic activity. The onset of action is rapid, approximately 2 to 5 minutes, and the duration of action is relatively short, usually 1 hour. Because it is hydrolyzed in the body to para-aminobenzoic acid, a compound that inhibits the action of sulfonamides, it should therefore not be used in any condition in which therapy with a sulfonamide is being employed.

Indications: For the production of local anesthesia by infiltration injection, nerve block, or other epidural blocks.

Contraindications: Procaine is contraindicated in patients with a known hypersensitivity (allergy) to the drug or drugs of a similar chemical configuration. Contraindications to saddle block during delivery include pelvic disproportion, placenta praevia, abruptio placentae, unengaged head, and intrauterine manipulation (e.g., podalic version).

Warnings: Resuscitative equipment and drugs should be immediately available when local anesthesia is administered. Safe use of procaine during pregnancy has not been established with respect to possible adverse effects upon fetal development. Therefore, it should not be used in women of childbearing potential and particularly during early pregnancy unless in the judgment of the physician the potential benefits outweigh the unknown hazards. Solutions containing vasopressors should be used with extreme caution in patients receiving drugs known to produce blood pressure alterations (i.e., MAO inhibitors, tricyclic antidepressants, phenothiazines, etc.) as either severe and sustained hypotension or hypertension may occur. In obstetrics, if vasopressor drugs are used either to correct hypotension or added to the local anesthetic solution, the obstetrician should be aware that some oxytocic drugs may cause severe persistent hypertension and even rupture of a cerebral blood vessel may occur during the postpartum period.

Precautions: The lowest dosage that results in effective anesthesia should be used to avoid overdosage. The safety and effectiveness of procaine are dependent on proper dosage, number of dermatomes to be blocked, correct technique, adequate precautions and readiness for emergencies. Tolerance varies with the status of the patient. The debilitated, elderly, or acutely ill patient and children should be given reduced doses commensurate with their age and physical status. Procaine should be employed cautiously in patients with known drug allergies or sensitivities. Spinal anesthesia should be administered with extreme caution, if at all, in the following conditions: Disease of the cerebrospinal system, such as meningitis, spinal fluid block, cranial or spinal hemorrhage, tumors, and syphilis; suppuration at the site of puncture; shock; profound anemia, cachexia, and when death is imminent; sepsis with positive blood cultures; high blood pressure; low blood pressure; highly nervous and sensitive individuals; visceral perforation, bowel strangulation, acute peritonitis; cardiac decompensation, massive pleural effusion, and increased intraabdominal pressure (e.g., full-term pregnancy, massive ascites, large tumor). Solutions containing a vasopressor should be used with caution in the presence of diseases which may adversely affect the patient's cardiovascular system.

Adverse Reactions: These result from high plasma levels due to excessive dosage, rapid absorption or inadvertent intravascular injection. Hypersensitivity or diminished tolerance may also be the cause of reaction. Those due to overdosage (high plasma level) are systemic and involve the CNS and the cardiovascular system. Reactions involving the CNS are characterized by excitation and/or depression. Nervousness, dizziness, blurred vision or tremors may occur followed by drowsiness, convulsions, unconsciousness and possibly respiratory arrest. Excitement may be transient or absent, and the first manifestations may be drowsiness merging into unconsciousness and respiratory arrest. Reactions involving the cardiovascular system include depression of the myocardium, hypotension, bradycardia and even cardiac arrest.

Treatment of a patient with toxic manifestations consists of maintaining an airway, and supporting ventilation using oxygen and assisted or controlled respiration as required. Supportive treatment of the cardiovascular system consists of using vasopressors, preferably those that stimulate the myocardium (e.g., ephedrine, metaraminol), and intravenous fluids. Convulsions may be controlled by the intravenous administration of small increments of an ultra-short acting barbiturate (i.e., thiopental, thiamylal) or a short-acting barbiturate if these are not available (secobarbital, pentobarbital) or a short-acting muscle relaxant (succinylcholine), together with oxygen. Muscle relaxants and intravenous barbiturates should only be used by those familiar with their use. Allergic reactions are characterized by cutaneous lesions of delayed onset, urticaria, edema or other manifestations of allergy. The detection of sensitivity by skin testing is of doubtful value.

Dosage and Administration: *For infiltration and extensive field block:* 200 to 300 ml of an 0.25 or 0.5% solution may be used; 350 to 600 mg is generally regarded to be a safe single total dose. For each 100 ml of procaine solution, 0.5 to 1 ml of epinephrine solution (1:1000) is generally added for its vasoconstrictor effect. *For conduction anesthesia* (nerve block): 1 to 2% solution with 0.05 to 0.1 ml of epinephrine solution (1:1000) in each 10 ml. *For spinal anesthesia,* depending upon extent and duration of anesthesia: from 0.5 to 2 ml of 10% solution. **Note:** The usual initial dose should not exceed 1 gm.

Availability:
NOVOCAIN® Injection, 1% in ampuls of 2 and 6 ml and in vials of 30 ml; 2% in vials of 30 ml; 10% in ampuls of 2 ml. **(Breon)**
PROCAINE HYDROCHLORIDE Injection, 1 and 2% in vials of 30 and 100 ml. **(Abbott)**

PROCARBAZINE HYDROCHLORIDE

Chemical Name: *N*-Isopropyl-α-(2-methylhydrazino)-*p*-toluamide monohydrochloride.

Description: Procarbazine, a methylhydrazine, is representative of a group of substituted hydrazines that have demonstrated an antineoplastic effect against Hodgkin's disease. The mode of cytotoxic action has not yet been clearly defined; however, there is evidence that the drug may act by inhibiting the synthesis of protein, RNA (ribonucleic acid) and DNA (deoxyribonucleic acid). No cross-resistance with other chemotherapeutic agents, radiotherapy or corticosteroids has been demonstrated.

Clinical studies, in which the duration of response is at least a month, show an over-all response rate of about 50%. This includes both objective regression of disease and associated clinical benefits. These observations have been made in patients who have had prior treatment with radiotherapy and other antineoplastic agents.

In laboratory studies, procarbazine hydrochloride produced a variety of biologic effects. Among these have been immunosuppression, teratogenesis, carcinogenesis, cytotoxicity with mitotic suppression and chromatin derangement, and an antineoplastic effect against a spectrum of transplanted tumors in mice and rats. The major drug toxicities in acute and chronic animals studies were hematologic with granulocyte depression, thrombocyte depression and anemia. Reticuloendothelial system lymphocytic depletion, marrow cell depression, testicular atrophy and mucous membrane ulceration were further evidence of in vivo cytotoxicity. Distribution of the drug in body fluids showed rapid equilibration between plasma and cerebrospinal fluid after oral administration. Pharmacological studies indicated that the drug was readily absorbed from the gastrointestinal tract. The major portion of drug was excreted in the urine as N-isopropylterephthalamic acid with approximately 25 to 42% appearing during the first 24 hours after administration.

Indications: Currently recommended for the palliative management of generalized Hodgkin's disease and in those patients who have become resistant to other forms of therapy. The drug should be used as an adjunct to standard modalities of therapy.

Contraindications: Patients with known hypersensitivity to the drug, or inadequate bone marrow reserve. Due consideration of this possible state should be given to each patient with leukopenia, thrombocytopenia or anemia.

Warnings: It is recommended that this drug be given only by or under the supervision of a physician experienced in the use of potent antineoplastic agents. Adequate clinical and laboratory facilities should be available to patients for proper monitoring of treatment. To minimize CNS depression and possible synergism, barbiturates, antihistamines, narcotics, hypotensive agents or phenothiazines should be used cautiously. Ethyl alcohol may precipitate a disulfiram-like reaction, and should therefore be avoided. Because this drug inhibits monoamine oxidase to some extent, sympathomimetic drugs, tricyclic antidepressants (e.g., amitriptyline, imipramine, etc.) and foods with a high tyramine content (e.g., ripe cheese and bananas) should be avoided. A further phenomenon of toxicity common to many hydrazine derivatives is hemolysis and the appearance of Heinz-Ehrlich inclusion bodies in erythrocytes. Teratogenicity has been reported in animals. Use of this drug during pregnancy, lactation or in women of childbearing potential requires that the potential benefits of the drug be weighed against the possible hazard to mother and child.

Precautions: Undue toxicity may occur if this drug is used in patients with known impairment of renal or hepatic function, or both. It is essential therefore that renal and hepatic function be evaluated prior to and frequently during the course of treatment. Hospitalization for the initial course of treatment should be considered. Bone marrow depression often occurs 2 to 8 weeks after the start of treatment. The patient should be hospitalized to assure appropriate treatment to prevent systemic infection. If radiation or a chemotherapeutic agent known to have marrow-depressant activity has been used, an interval of one month or longer without such therapy is recommended before starting treatment with procarbazine. The length of this interval may also be determined by evidence of bone marrow recovery based on successive bone marrow studies. Prompt cessation of therapy is recommended if paresthesias, neuropathies, or confusion; leukopenia (WBC count under 4000); thrombocytopenia (platelets under 100,000); hypersensitivity reaction; stomatitis; frequent bowel movements, or watery stools, and hemorrhage or bleeding tendencies develop.

Adverse Reactions: Leukopenia, anemia, thrombopenia occur frequently. Nausea and vomiting are the most commonly reported complaints. Less frequently reported are anorexia, stomatitis, dry mouth, dysphagia, diarrhea and constipation. Pain including myalgia and arthralgia, chills and fever, sweating, weakness, fatigue, lethargy and drowsiness are often noted. Intercurrent infections, effusion, ascites, cough and other respiratory symptoms are common. Petechiae, purpura, epistaxis, hemoptysis, hematemesis, melena, dermatitis, pruritus, herpes, hyperpigmentation, flushing, alopecia and jaundice have also been noted. Paresthesias, neuropathies, headache, dizziness, depression, apprehension, nervousness, insomnia, nightmares, hallucinations, falling, unsteadiness, ataxia, footdrop, decreased reflexes, tremors, coma, confusion, and convulsions are infrequently noted. Hoarseness, tachycardia, retinal hemorrhage, nystagmus, photophobia, photosensitivity, genitourinary symptoms, hypotension, fainting, diplopia, inability to focus, papilledema, altered hearing, and slurred speech have occurred. Coincidental onset of leukemia during therapy with procarbazine has been reported in rare instances.

Dosage and Administration: *Orally. Adults:* initially, 100 to 200 mg daily, in single or divided doses, for the first week, then 300 mg daily until the white cell count falls below 4000/cm or the platelets fall below 100,000/cm or until maximal response is obtained. When hematologic toxicity is evident, the drug should be discontinued until recovery is satisfactory. Treatment may then be resumed at 50 to 100 mg daily and maintained at this level when maximal response is obtained. *Children:* Dosage must be highly individualized. The following is only a guideline: initially, 50 mg daily for the first week, then maintained at 100 mg/sq meter of body surface (to the nearest 50 mg) until leukopenia or thrombocytopenia occurs or maximal response is obtained. When hematologic toxicity is evident, the drug should be discontinued until blood cell recovery is satisfactory. Treatment may then be resumed at 50 mg daily and maintained at this level when maximal response is obtained. For general instructions pertaining to therapy, consult package literature.

Availability:
MATULANE® Capsules, 50 mg in bottles of 100. **(Roche)**

PROCHLORPERAZINE: see The Phenothiazines

PROCYCLIDINE

Chemical Name: α-Cyclohexyl-α-phenyl-l-pyrrolidinepropanol hydrochloride.

Description: Procyclidine occurs as a white, tasteless, crystalline powder soluble in water. It is a synthetic antispasmodic compound that has been found to be useful for the symptomatic treatment of parkinsonism (paralysis agitans) and extrapyramidal dysfunction. Pharmacologic tests have shown that procyclidine exhibits an atropine-like action and exerts an antispasmodic effect on smooth muscle. It is a potent mydriatic and inhibits salivation. Doses as high as 4 mg/kg of body weight did not produce sympathetic ganglion blocking activity.

Indications: Treatment of parkinsonism including the postencephalitic, arteriosclerotic and idiopathic types. For the relief of symptoms of extrapyramidal dysfunction (dystonia, dyskinesia, akathisia, and parkinsonism) such as may be induced by the use of phenothiazines or rauwolfia compounds in the drug therapy for mental disorders, and for the control of sialorrhea resulting from neuroleptic medication.

Contraindications: Procyclidine should not be used in angle-closure glaucoma although simple-type glaucomas do not appear to be adversely affected.

Warnings: Safe use in children or in pregnant or lactating women or in women of childbearing age has not been established; therefore, the use of the drug requires that the potential benefits be weighed against the possible hazards to the child, the mother or the fetus.

Precautions: Should be given with special care in patients with tachycardia or urinary retention (such as may occur with marked prostatic hypertrophy). Hypotensive patients who receive this drug should be observed closely. Occasionally, particularly in older patients, mental confusion, and disorientation may occur with the development of agitation, hallucinations and psychotic-like symptoms. Patients with mental disorders occasionally experience a precipitation of a psychotic episode when the dosage of antiparkinsonism drugs is increased to treat the extrapyramidal side effects of phenothiazine and rauwolfia derivatives.

Adverse Reactions: Dryness of mouth, mydriasis, blurring of vision, giddiness, lightheadedness and gastrointestinal disturbances such as nausea, vomiting, epigastric distress, and constipation. Occasionally, an allergic reaction such as skin rash may be encountered. Feelings of muscular weakness may also occur. Acute suppurative parotitis as a complication of dry mouth has been reported. These can usually be minimized or eliminated by careful adjustment of dosage.

Dosage and Administration: *Orally. For parkinsonism:* The usual initial dosage is 2 to 2.5 mg 3 times daily after meals. If well tolerated, this dosage may be gradually increased to 4 to 5 mg 3 times daily; some patients may require an additional 4 to 5 mg at bedtime. Lower dosage may be used if the drug is given in conjunction with other antiparkinsonian agents. *For drug-induced extrapyramidal symptoms:* The usual initial dosage is 2 to 2.5 mg 3 times daily; may be increased in daily increments of 2 to 2.5 mg until the patient experiences satisfactory relief of symptoms. In most cases optimal therapeutic benefits are usually obtained with 10 to 20 mg daily.

Availability:
KEMADRIN® Tablets, 2 mg in bottles of 100 and 1000; 5 mg in bottles of 100, 1000 and 5000.

(Burroughs Wellcome)

PROGESTERONE

Chemical Name: Pregn-4-ene-3,20-dione.

Description: Progesterone is the natural hormone secreted by the corpus luteum which is necessary for the implantation of the fertilized ovum in the endometrium of the uterus during pregnancy and for the maintenance of pregnancy. It occurs synthetically as a white or creamy white, odorless, crystalline powder practically insoluble in water, but soluble in alcohol and sparingly soluble in vegetable oils.

Progesterone causes the secretory phase of the endometrium to develop and attain up to 10 times the original thickness, with distention and activity of the glands and profound hyperemia. Its greatest effectiveness depends upon previous priming of the endometrium with estrogens.

Indications: Habitual and threatened abortion, premature labor, functional uterine bleeding, functional dysmenorrhea, premenstrual tension, primary and secondary amenorrhea and female hypogonadism.

Contraindications: Hypersensitivity or idiosyncrasy to progesterone, in patients with impaired renal function, missed or incomplete abortion, known or suspected carcinoma of the breast, and undiagnosed genital bleeding. A history or the presence of thrombophlebitis, thromboembolic disorders, cerebrovascular accident, or pulmonary embolism also contraindicates the use of progesterone.

Warnings: Progesterone therapy should be discontinued pending examination if there is a sudden partial or complete loss of vision, or if there is a sudden onset of proptosis, diplopia or migraine. If examination reveals papilledema or retinal vascular lesions, the medication should be withdrawn. Although progesterone has been detected in the milk of nursing mothers, the long-range effects on the nursing infant is not known. Masculinization of the female fetus has occurred when progestogens have been used in pregnant women.

Precautions: Pretreatment physical examination should include breast and pelvic organs, as well as a Papanicolaou smear. Patients with a history of psychic depression should be carefully observed, and the drug withdrawn if a recurring depression develops to a serious degree. Because some degree of fluid retention may occur, conditions which may be influenced by this factor such as epilepsy, migraine, asthma, cardiac or renal dysfunction require careful observation. Progesterone will not cause a cessation of bleeding from an atrophic endometrium and is not recommended in such instances. When used in the treatment of functional uterine bleeding, genital malignancy should be excluded and diagnostic studies performed prior to therapy. The pathologist should be advised of progesterone therapy when relevant specimens are submitted. A decrease in glucose tolerance has been observed in a small percentage of patients, therefore, diabetic patients should be carefully observed during treatment with progesterone.

Adverse Reactions: Edema; urticaria; pruritus vulvae; gastrointestinal disturbances manifested by nausea, vomiting, and diarrhea; ulcerative stomatitis; headache; weight gain, and local irritation. In general, the following untoward reactions have been observed in patients taking progestogen preparations, and may possibly be noted with the use of this drug. These include breakthrough bleeding, spotting, changes in menstrual flow, amenorrhea, edema, changes in weight (increase or decrease), changes in cervical erosion and cervical secretions, cholestatic jaundice, rash (allergic) with or without pruritus, melasma or chloasma, and mental depression. Progestogens may alter the results of the pregnanediol test. In addition, the following laboratory results may be altered by the concomitant use of estrogens with progestogens: hepatic function, increase in prothrombin, Factors VII, VIII, IX, X, increase in PBI, BEI and a decrease in T_3 uptake, metyrapone test. The following adverse effects may occur with estrogen-progesterone combinations: thrombophlebitis, pulmonary embolism, and cerebral thrombosis and embolism. For this reason patients on progesterone therapy should be carefully observed. The following may also occur: neuro-ocular lesions (retinal thrombosis and optic neuritis), rise in blood pressure in susceptible individuals, premenstrual-like syndrome, changes in libido, changes in appetite, cystitis-like syndrome, headache, nervousness, dizziness, fatigue, backache, hirsutism, loss of scalp hair, erythema multiforme, erythema nodosum, hemorrhagic eruption, and itching.

Dosage and Administration: *Intramuscularly. Habitual abortion:* 5 to 20 mg 3 times weekly, beginning soon after onset of pregnancy and continuing through the eighth month. *Threatened abortion:* 25 to 50 mg daily so long as there is pain and bleeding, after which 10 to 25 mg daily maintained through the eighth month. *Premature labor:* 25 to 50 mg daily until symptoms subside. *Functional uterine bleeding:* 5 to 10 mg daily or 25 mg on alternate days, starting 8 to 10 days before expected menstruation; severe cases may require 50 mg daily. *Functional dysmenorrhea, premenstrual tension:* 10 to 25 mg daily during the last 8 to 10 days before expected menstruation. *Primary and secondary amenorrhea, female hypogonadism:* 25 mg 3 times weekly during the last 2 weeks of a calculated menstrual cycle after estrogen therapy during the first 2 weeks of the calculated cycle.

Availability:
PROGESTERONE Injection in Oil, 25 and 50 mg/ml in vials of 10 ml. **(Lilly)**
LIPO-LUTIN® Injection in Oil, 50 mg/ml in Steri-Vial®s of 5 ml. **(Parke-Davis)**

PROMAZINE HYDROCHLORIDE: see The Phenothiazines

PROMETHAZINE HYDROCHLORIDE: see The Phenothiazines

PROMETHESTROL DIPROPIONATE: see The Estrogens

PROPANTHELINE BROMIDE

Chemical Name: (2-Hydroxyethyl)diisopropylmethylammonium bromide xanthene-9-carboxylate.

Description: Propantheline bromide is an anticholinergic drug which differs structurally from methantheline bromide in the presence of two isopropyl groups in place of the two ethyl radicals on the quaternary nitrogen atom of methantheline. It occurs as a white or yellowish white, bitter, crystalline substance very soluble in water and in alcohol.

Propantheline has been noted to inhibit gastrointestinal motility and to diminish gastric acid secretion. It also inhibits the action of acetylcholine at the postganglionic nerve endings of the parasympathetic nervous system. The usual clinical dose (15 mg) reaches peak plasma concentration at 6 hours with a plasma half-life of approximately 9 hours. About 70% is excreted in the urine as metabolites and a small amount (5%) as intact drug.

Indications: May be of use as adjunctive therapy in the treatment of peptic ulcer and the irritable bowel syndrome (irritable colon, spastic colon, mucous colitis, acute enterocolitis and functional gastrointestinal disorders). The parenterally administered drug is also effective in reducing duodenal motility to facilitate the diagnostic radiologic procedure, hypotonic duodenography. The mild sedation provided by phenobarbital protects the patient against the physical and emotional stresses often present in conditions causing vagotonia and parasympathotonia. Thiopropazate hydrochloride is a phenothiazine tranquilizer which acts as adjunctive therapy in reducing ulcerogenic tensions.

Contraindications: Hypersensitivity to any of the components; glaucoma, obstructive disease of the gastrointestinal tract (pyloroduodenal stenosis, achalasia, paralytic ileus, etc.), obstructive uropathy, intestinal atony of elderly or debilitated patients, toxic megacolon, complicating ulcerative colitis, hiatal hernia associated with reflux esophagitis, unstable cardiovascular adjustment in acute hemorrhage, and myasthenia gravis.

Warnings: Phenobarbital may be habit-forming. Patients with severe cardiac disease should be given this medication with caution if even a slight increase in heart rate is undesirable. Fever and possibly heat stroke may occur due to anhidrosis, particularly when the environmental temperature is high. Overdosage may result in a curare-like action; loss of control of the voluntary muscles usually occurs, the most frequent manifestation being loss of control of the respiratory muscles. Such patients should receive prompt and continuing artificial respiration until the drug effect has been exhausted. Diarrhea in an ileostomy patient may indicate obstruction; the possibility of this problem should be considered before administering this drug.

Precautions: Since elderly patients with prostatic hypertrophy may experience varying degrees of urinary hesitancy, they should be advised to micturate at the time of taking the medication. Special care should be observed in elderly patients and in all those with autonomic neuropathy, hepatic or renal disease, hyperthyroidism, coronary heart disease, congestive heart failure, cardiac tachyarrhythmias, or hypertension. Dosage should be carefully regulated, since severe complications may occur with large doses. Thiopropazate hydrochloride should be used with caution in pregnant patients with minor tensions and in those under the effects of barbiturates, narcotics or alcohol, in patients with epilepsy (may precipitate convulsions), depression (may increase depression) or hepatic disease (may cause coma).

Adverse Reactions: Dry mouth, mydriasis, blurred vision, urinary retention, nervousness, drowsiness, dizziness, insomnia, headache, loss of taste, nausea, vomiting, constipation, impotence, and allergic dermatitis. Overdosage should be avoided in patients severely ill with ulcerative colitis. For other adverse reactions, see monograph on each of the components.

Dosage and Administration: Pro-Banthīne: *Orally*, 2 half-strength or 1 full-strength tablet 30 minutes before each meal followed by 4 half-strength or 2 full-strength tablets at bedtime. For severe manifestations, 2 tablets 4 times daily. Pro-Banthīne P.A.: 1 tablet twice daily (morning and evening); or 1 tablet every 8 hours. Tablets with Dartal: 1 tablet 3 times daily, increasing to 1 or 2 additional tablets, if required. Pro-Banthīne with Phenobarbital, 1 or 2 tablets 3 or 4 times daily. *Intravenously,* the contents of the vial should be diluted in 10 ml of Sodium Chloride Injection U.S.P. *Intramuscularly*, the contents of the vial should be diluted in 1 ml of Sterile Water for Injection U.S.P. The initial adult dose is 30 mg every 6 hours, and the maintenance dosage is 15 mg every 6 hours. For hypotonic duodenography, 30 to 60 mg intramuscularly 5 to 10 minutes prior to the diagnostic procedure, or by slow intravenous administration immediately prior to the procedure. The rate of intravenous administration should not exceed 2 ml (6 mg)/minute.

Availability:
GIQUEL Tablets, 15 mg in bottles of 100. **(Lemmon)**
PRO-BANTHĪNE®: **(Searle)**
Injection in vials of 30 mg in cartons of 5, 25 and 100.
Tablets, 7.5 mg (white) in bottles of 100 and 500; 15 mg (peach) in bottles of 100, 1000 and 2500 and in packages of 100 individually blister-sealed tablets in cartons of 10.
PRO-BANTHĪNE P.A.® Tablets (prolonged action), 30 mg in bottles of 100. **(Searle)**
PRO-BANTHĪNE with DARTAL® Tablets, 15 mg with thiopropazate hydrochloride, 5 mg in bottles of 100 and 500. **(Searle)**
PRO-BANTHĪNE with PHENOBARBITAL Tablets, 15 mg (ivory color) with phenobarbital, 15 mg in bottles of 100, 1000 and 2500 and in individually blister-sealed packages of 100 in cartons of 10. **(Searle)**
PROPANTHELINE BROMIDE:
Tablets, 15 mg in bottles of 100 and 1000. **(Lederle)**
Tablets, 15 mg in bottles of 100 and 1000 and unit-dose blister packs of 100. **(Philips Roxane)**

PROPARACAINE HYDROCHLORIDE

Chemical Name: 3-Amino-4-propoxybenzoic acid 2-(diethylamino)ethyl ester.

Description: Proparacaine hydrochloride, a topical anesthetic, occurs as a light brown solid soluble in water and in alcohol. Produces rapid corneal anesthesia thus permitting the use of ophthalmic procedures such as tonometry, gonioscopy, removal of foreign bodies, and sutures, conjunctival scraping, etc. without irritating the conjunctiva or causing dilatation or other pupillary changes, and for surgical intervention. Anesthesia usually occurs within 13 to 20 seconds and lasts for 15 minutes or longer.

Indications: Topical anesthesia in ophthalmic procedures.

Contraindications: Hypersensitivity to any of the components of the preparations.

Warnings: Prolonged use may produce permanent corneal opacification with accompanying visual loss, and therefore is not recommended.

Precautions: Proparacaine should be used cautiously and sparingly in patients with known allergies, cardiac disease, hyperthyroidism or open lesions. Local and systemic sensitivity may occur and prolonged use may delay wound healing. An occasional patient may experience pupillary dilatation or cycloplegia.

Adverse Reactions: Occasional temporary stinging, burning, and conjunctival redness have been reported, as well as a rare, severe, immediate-type, hyperallergic corneal reaction, with acute, intense and diffuse epithelial keratitis, a gray, ground-glass appearance, sloughing of large areas of necrotic epithelium, corneal filaments, and occasionally iritis with descemetitis. Also reported was an allergic contact dermatitis with drying and fissuring of the fingertips.

Dosage and Administration: *Topically into the eyes.* Deep anesthesia: 1 drop every 5 to 10 minutes for 5 to 7 doses. Removal of foreign bodies: 1 or 2 drops prior to operating. Removal of sutures: 1 or 2 drops 2 to 3 minutes before procedure. Tonometry: 1 or 2 drops immediately before measurement.

Availability:
ALCAINE™ Ophthalmic Solution, 0.5% in Drop-Tainer® dispensers of 15 ml. **(Alcon)**
OPHTHAINE® Ophthalmic Solution, 0.5% in bottles of 15 ml with dropper tip. **(Squibb)**
OPHTHETIC® Ophthalmic Solution, 0.5% in bottles of 15 ml with dropper tip. **(Allergan)**

PROPIONATE SODIUM

Description: Propionate sodium, a fatty acid salt, is a topical antifungal, antibacterial, antipruritic and antiinflammatory agent. It occurs as transparent crystals or granules freely soluble in water and soluble in alcohol.

Indications: Propionate sodium in a concentration of 1% is used to control susceptible infections in such conditions as dermatophytosis, contact dermatosis, eczema, vulvovaginitis and minor burns. A combination of 10% each of sodium and calcium propionates is used for the treatment of monilial vulvovaginitis. A combination with neomycin sulfate is used for the topical treatment of otitis externa and chronic otitis media, particularly when caused by *Ps. aeruginosa*, and hemolytic *S. aureus*.

Contraindications: Hypersensitivity to any of the components. The use of vaginal applicators is contraindicated during the last trimester of pregnancy.

Precautions: Reports in current medical literature indicate an increase in the prevalence of cutaneous hypersensitivity reactions to topical neomycin. The use of neomycin sulfate may result in the overgrowth of nonsusceptible organisms, in which case, the antibiotic should be discontinued and appropriate countermeasures instituted. The remote possibility that neomycin may cause ototoxicity should be considered, especially in patients with perforation of the tympanic membrane.

Dosage and Administration: *Topically.* To make a 1% or an 0.5% solution, dissolve 1 packet (or 1 teaspoonful of the bulk powder) in ½ or 1 pint of water respectively. The 1% solution may be used as a wet dressing, soak, mouthwash or douch. The 0.5% solution may be used for a footbath or in those conditions complicated by severe inflammation. The ointment should be applied liberally several times during the day and on retiring. *Otic Solution:* Thoroughly cleanse and dry the ear canal. Instill several drops into the auditory canal 3 or 4 times daily. A gauze wick moistened with the solution may be used. *Gel:* Insert 1 applicatorful into the vaginal vault morning and evening.

Availability:

Propionate Sodium

PROPHYLLIN® (OTC): **(Rystan)**
Ointment, 5% in tubes of 30 gm.
Powder for Solution in jars of 120 gm and in packets of 2.3 gm in cartons of 12.

Combinations

OTOBIOTIC® Otic Solution, 50 mg with neomycin sulfate, 5 mg/ml in dropper bottles of 15 ml. **(Schering)**

PROPION® GEL 10% with 10% of calcium propionate in tubes of 95 gm with applicator. **(Wyeth)**

PROPOXYPHENE Ⓒ IV

Chemical Name: *d*-4-Dimethylamino-3-methyl-1,2-diphenyl-2-butanol propionate.

Description: Propoxyphene is a synthetic analgesic structurally related to the narcotic analgesics methadone and isomethadone. Only the *alpha-dextro* steroisomer of propoxyphene possesses analgesic properties; the *levo* steroisomer is used as an antitussive. *Propoxyphene hydrochloride* occurs as a bitter, white, crystalline powder freely soluble in water and soluble in alcohol. *Propoxyphene napsylate* is a synthetic odorless, white, crystalline solid with a bitter taste. It is very slightly soluble in water and soluble in methanol, alcohol, chloroform, and acetone.

Since propoxyphene napsylate is a water-insoluble salt of propoxyphene, it thus differs from propoxyphene hydrochloride in that it provides more stable liquid and tablet formulations when used either alone or combined with aspirin. The pharmacologic properties of propoxyphene napsylate are similar to those of propoxyphene hydrochloride which produces mild to moderate analgesia. However, because of the difference in their molecular weight, the amount of propoxyphene available in 100 mg of propoxyphene napsylate is equivalent to that available in only 65 mg of propoxyphene hydrochloride.

In most individuals, recommended doses of propoxyphene have not caused clinically significant alterations of respiration, blood pressure or pulse rate.

Propoxyphene is combined with aspirin and with APC for their analgesic, antipyretic and antiinflammatory attributes.

Indications: Relief of mild to moderate pain. The combination with acetaminophen may be used when pain is accompanied by fever.

Contraindications: Hypersensitivity to any of the components; concomitant administration of propoxyphene with orphenadrine-containing compounds.

Warnings: Mental and physical abilities may be impaired, especially during the first few days of therapy; therefore, patients should be warned not to engage in activities requiring alertness or skill. Propoxyphene in combination with other CNS depressants (alcohol, tranquilizers, sedative-hypnotics, and other similarly acting drugs) significantly increases the depressant effects. Toxic reactions and fatalities have occurred following overdoses of propoxyphene alone and in combination with other CNS depressant drugs. Patients should be advised of this hazard and should be cautioned not to exceed the recommended dosage. The physician should use caution in prescribing this drug to patients with histories of emotional disturbances or suicidal tendencies and in those likely to abuse CNS-active drugs. Tolerance, psychological and physical dependence have been reported; also the liability of abuse with propoxyphene is qualitatively similar to that of codeine although quantitatively less. This drug will not support morphine dependence. Salicylates (A.S.A.) should be used with caution in the presence of gastric ulcer. Prolonged and excessive use of phenacetin may aggravate or produce renal disease, and overdosage of acetaminophen may cause hepatic necrosis. Safe use during pregnancy has not been established relative to possible adverse effects on fetal development. Instances of withdrawal symptoms in the neonate have been reported following use during pregnancy. Therefore, propoxyphene should not be used in pregnant women unless, in the judgment of the physician, the potential benefits outweigh the possible hazards. Until further experience with regard to safe and effective use in children has been gained, it is not recommended for use in patients in this age group.

Precautions: When substituting propoxyphene for analgesics used previously, withdrawal symptoms may be avoided by reducing the dosage of the latter as the former is being instituted.

Adverse Reactions: *Propoxyphene:* dizziness, sedation, somnolence, paradoxical excitement and insomnia, skin rash, lightheadedness, headache, weakness, liver dysfunction, and gastrointestinal disturbances including nausea, vomiting, abdominal pain and constipation; and euphoria, dysphoria, visual disturbances, and tolerance. Chronic ingestion of large doses (800 mg) has caused toxic psychosis and convulsions. Confusion, anxiety, and tremors have been reported in a few patients receiving propoxyphene concomitantly with orphenadrine. *Aspirin:* gastric irritation, in which case the aspirin-containing preparations should be taken with food or milk or discontinued. Salicylates may also induce hypersensitivity, urate and kidney stones, chronic gastrointestinal blood loss, tinnitus, nausea and vomiting.

The manifestations of serious overdosage with propoxyphene are similar to those of narcotic overdosage and include respiratory depression (a decrease in respiratory rate and/or tidal volume, Cheyne-Stokes respiration, and cyanosis), extreme somnolence progressing to stupor or coma, pupillary constriction, and circulatory collapse. In addition, focal and generalized convulsions constitute a pronounced characteristic in most instances of acute propoxyphene poisoning, and cardiac arrhythmias and pulmonary edema which have, on occasion, resulted in apnea, cardiac arrest and fatality have been reported. Primary attention should be given to the reestablishment of adequate respiratory exchange through provision of a patent airway and institution of assisted or controlled ventilation. Naloxone, levallorphan, and nalorphine are specific antidotes against the respiratory depression produced by this drug. In addition, the patient may require careful titration with an anticonvulsant to control convulsions. Analeptic drugs (caffeine or amphetamine) are not recommended because of their tendency to precipitate convulsions. Oxygen, intravenous fluids, vasopressors, and other supportive measures should be employed where indicated. Gastric lavage may be helpful; and activated charcoal can adsorb a significant amount of ingested propoxyphene. Dialysis is of little value with respect to this drug alone.

Dosage and Administration: *Orally for adults only.* Propoxyphene is currently not recommended for children. Usually, 32 to 65 mg 3 or 4 times daily. *Darvocet-N:* usually 2 tablets every 4 hours as needed for pain. *Darvon Compound:* usually 1 or 2 capsules 3 or 4 times daily. *Darvon Compound-65* or *Darvon with A.S.A.:* usually 1 capsule 3 or 4 times daily. *Darvo-Tran:* usually 1 capsule 3 or 4 times daily, but this dosage may be doubled when pain is severe. *Darvon-N* or *Darvon-N with A.S.A.:* usually 1 tablet 3 or 4 times daily.

Availability:

Propoxyphene Hydrochloride

Ⓒ DARVON® Pulvules® (capsules), 32 and 65 mg in bottles of 100 and 500, and in Rx Paks of 100; 65 mg tablets are also available in blister packs of 1000 and in Rx Paks of 750 (25 × 30) and 1000 (20 × 50). **(Lilly)**

Ⓒ DOLENE®-65 Capsules, 65 mg in bottles of 100 and 500 and in unit-dose packages of 25, 60 and 100 in cartons of 50. **(Lederle)**

Ⓒ SK-65® Capsules, 65 mg in bottles of 100 and 500 and in single-unit packages of 100. **(Smith Kline & French)**

Ⓒ PROPOXYPHENE HYDROCHLORIDE Capsules, 65 mg in bottles of 1000 and in unit-dose packages of 100. **(Parke-Davis)**

Ⓒ PROPOXYPHENE HYDROCHLORIDE Capsules, 65 mg in bottles of 100 and 500. **(Squibb)**

Combinations

Ⓒ DARVON® COMPOUND and DARVON COMPOUND-65 Pulvules (capsules), 32 or 65 mg with aspirin, 227 mg; phenacetin, 162 mg and caffeine, 32 mg in bottles of 100 and 500, in Identi-Dose® (unit-dose) packages of 500 and in Rx Paks of 100. **(Lilly)**

Ⓒ DARVON with A.S.A.® Pulvules (capsules), 65 mg with A.S.A. (aspirin), 325 mg in bottles of 100 and 500 and in Rx Paks of 100. **(Lilly)**

Ⓒ DOLENE AP-65 Tablets, 65 mg with acetaminophen, 650 mg in bottles of 100 and 500 and in unit-dose packages of 100 (10 × 10). **(Lederle)**

Ⓒ DOLENE COMPOUND-65 Capsules, 65 mg with aspirin, 227 mg; phenacetin, 162 mg and caffeine, 32.4 mg in bottles of 100 and 500 and in unit-dose packages of 30, 60 and 100 in cartons of 50. **(Lederle)**

Ⓒ ICN 65 COMPOUND Capsules, 65 mg with aspirin, 227 mg; phenacetin, 162 mg and caffeine, 32.4 mg in bottles of 100 and 1000. **(ICN)**

Ⓒ PROPOXYPHENE COMPOUND-65 Capsules, 65 mg with aspirin, 227 mg; phenacetin, 162 mg and caffeine, 32.4 mg in bottles of 1000 and in unit-dose cartons of 100. **(Parke-Davis)**

Ⓒ PROPOXYPHENE HYDROCHLORIDE COMPOUND-65 Capsules, 65 mg with aspirin, 227 mg; phenacetin, 162 mg and caffeine, 32.4 mg in bottles of 100 and 500 and in unit-dose cartons of 100 and 500. **(Philips Roxane)**

Ⓒ PROPOXYPHENE COMPOUND-65 Capsules, 65 mg with aspirin, 227 mg; phenacetin, 162 mg and caffeine 32.4 mg in bottles of 100 and 500. **(Squibb)**

Ⓒ SK-65 COMPOUND® Capsules, 65 mg with aspirin, 227 mg; phenacetin, 162 mg and caffeine, 32.4 mg in bottles of 100 and 500. **(Smith Kline & French)**

Ⓒ UNIGESIC-A® Tablets, 65 mg with A.S.A. (aspirin), 325 mg in bottles of 100. **(Upjohn)**

Ⓒ WYGESIC® Tablets, 65 mg with acetaminophen, 650 mg in bottles of 100 and 500 and in Redipak® (unit-dose) cartons of 100 (10 x 10). **(Wyeth)**

Propoxyphene Napsylate

Ⓒ DARVOCET-N® Tablets (dark-orange), 50 mg with acetaminophen, 325 mg in bottles of 100 and 500 and in Identi-Dose® (unit-dose) packages of 100 and 500 and in Rx Paks of 750 (25 × 30) and 1000 (20 × 50); 100 mg with acetaminophen, 650 mg in bottles of 100 and 500 and in Rx Paks of 100, 700 and 1000 and in individual blister-strips of 100 and 500. **(Lilly)**

Ⓒ DARVON-N®: **(Lilly)**

Oral Suspension, 50 mg/5 ml in bottles of 1 pint and in single-dose packs of 10 ml.

Tablets, 100 mg in bottles of 100 and 500, in Rx Paks of 750 (25 × 30) and in individual blister-strips of 10 in packages of 10 strips.

Ⓒ DARVON-N with A.S.A. Tablets, 100 mg with aspirin, 325 mg in bottles of 100 and 500, in Rx Paks of 750 (25 × 30) and in individual blister-strips of 10 in packages of 10 strips. **(Lilly)**

PROPRANOLOL HYDROCHLORIDE

Chemical Name: 1-(Isopropylamino)-3-(1-naphthyloxy)-2-propanol hydrochloride.

Description: Propranolol hydrochloride is a beta-adrenergic blocking agent possessing no other autonomic nervous system activity. It is a colorless, crystalline solid soluble in water and in alcohol.

Since only beta-adrenergic receptors are apparently present in the myocardium, they respond to their endogenous stimulators, norepinephrine and epinephrine, causing increased cardiac activity (increased rate and force of contraction). While sympathetic nervous stimulation is a significant component in supporting circulatory function, it may also play an important role in the occurrence of several types of cardiac arrhythmias.

Propranolol exerts its cardiac-antiarrhythmic effects in concentrations associated with beta-adrenergic blockade and this appears to be its principal antiarrhythmic mode of action. It specifically competes with other beta-adrenergic receptor stimulating agents for available beta-receptor sites. When access to beta-receptor sites is blocked by propranolol undesirable beta-adrenergic stimulation of the myocardium is lessened proportionately, causing a reduction in heart rate (chronotropic effect) and force of contraction (inotropic effect). This is usually of sufficient magnitude to counteract cardiac hyperactivity and irritability and, thereby, helps to abolish, control, or prevent arrhythmias. At present much of the clinical value of propranolol as a beta-blocking agent rests upon the high degree of specificity it has shown. It selectively blocks the positive inotropic and chronotropic effects of adrenergic stimuli without abolishing the inotropic action of nonadrenergic drugs, such as digitalis, on the heart muscle (*i.e.*, that of supporting the strength of myocardial contractions). It is especially effective in the management of supraventricular arrhythmias. The response of ventricular arrhythmias is generally less predictable. Propranolol has been found to be of particular value in the control of digitalis-induced arrhythmias; however, it does not interfere with the cardiotonic action of digitalis or similar drugs. This drug exerts its antiarrhythmic effects by reducing the oxygen requirement of the heart at any given level of effort by blocking catecholamine-induced increases in heart rate, systolic blood pressure, and the velocity and extent of myocardial contraction. On the other hand, propranolol may increase oxygen requirements by increasing left ventricular fiber length, end diastolic pressure, and systolic ejection period.

The mechanism by which the drug achieves its antihypertensive effects is not known, but among the factors that may be involved include decreased cardiac output and inhibition of renin release by the kidney and of tonic sympathetic nerve outflow from the vasomotor centers.

Propranolol is readily and almost completely absorbed from the gastrointestinal tract, and a portion of the drug is immediately bound by the liver. Maximal pharmacologic effect occurs within 1 to 1½ hours. The metabolic half-life ranges from 2 to 3 hours.

Indications: Management of hypertension. It is generally employed in combination with other drugs, particularly a thiazide diuretic. It is not indicated for treatment of hypertensive emergencies. Propranolol is also indicated for the treatment of angina pectoris due to coronary atherosclerosis, cardiac arrhythmias (supraventricular arrythmias and ventricular tachycardias, tachyarrhythmias of digitalis intoxication and those associated with anesthesia), hypertrophic subaortic stenosis, and as an adjunctive agent in the treatment of pheochromocytoma.

Contraindications: Bronchial asthma, allergic rhinitis, sinus bradycardia, greater than first degree heart block, cardiogenic shock, right ventricular failure secondary to pulmonary hypertension, congestive heart failure (unless the failure is secondary to a tachyarrhythmia that responds to propranolol therapy), and coadministration of adrenergic-augmenting psychotropic drugs including MAO inhibitors (within 2 weeks of withdrawal period).

Warnings: Before using propranolol, the physician should be thoroughly familiar with the basic concept of alpha and beta adrenergic receptors and the pharmacology of this drug. Propranolol should be given cautiously, preferably with digitalis, to patients with frank or incipient congestive heart failure. In patients without a history of cardiac failure, continued depression of the myocardium may lead to heart failure. Therefore, at the first sign or symptom of impending cardiac failure, patients should be fully digitalized and the response observed closely. If failure continues to progress, therapy should be withdrawn. In the presence of thyrotoxicosis, propranolol may mask the clinical signs of hyperthyroidism or its complications, and give a false impression of improvement; however, the drug does not distort thyroid-function tests. Following administration in patients with Wolff-Parkinson-White syndrome, several instances have been reported in which tachycardia was replaced by a severe bradycardia that required a demand pacemaker. In one patient this resulted after an initial dose of 5 mg of propranolol. The dose should be titrated carefully when administered for arrhythmias occurring during anesthesia. The drug should be withdrawn 48 hours prior to major surgery; however, in the case of emergency surgery, its effects can be reversed by the administration of isoproterenol or levarterenol. Nevertheless, these patients may be subjected to a prolonged severe hypotension. Difficulty in restoring and maintaining the heart beat has also been reported. It should be used with caution in patients prone to nonallergic bronchospasm such as chronic bronchitis and emphysema, since it may block bronchodilation due to stimulation of beta receptors by endogenous and exogenous catecholamines. Special care should be exercised when propranolol is given to patients subject to spontaneous hypoglycemia, to diabetics (especially labile diabetics) receiving insulin or oral hypoglycemic agents, and to patients receiving catecholamine depleting drugs. Safe use of propranolol during pregnancy or in women of childbearing potential has not been established; therefore, the potential benefits of the drug must be weighed against the possible hazards to mother and fetus.

Precautions: The physician should be aware that the drug may also produce hypotension and/or marked bradycardia resulting in vertigo, syncope or orthostatic hypotension. In patients who have undergone prolonged treatment, the dosage should be gradually reduced over a period of several weeks when it is anticipated that the administration of propranolol will be discontinued to avoid inducing or precipitating a myocardial infarction. There have been a few reports of this occurring within 2 to 3 days following discontinuation of the drug in patients with angina pectoris, but an association has not been established. As with any drug given over prolonged periods, complete laboratory studies should be performed at regular intervals. Propranolol should be used with caution in patients with impaired renal or hepatic function.

Adverse Reactions: Those reported included *Cardiovascular reactions:* bradycardia; congestive heart failure; intensification of AV block; hypotension; paresthesias of hands; and arterial insufficiency (usually of the Raynaud type). *CNS reactions:* lightheadedness; mental depression manifested by insomnia, lassitude, weakness and fatigue; reversible mental depression progressing to catatonia; visual disturbances; hallucinations; an acute reversible syndrome characterized by disorientation for time and place, amnesia (short-term), emotional lability, slightly clouded sensorium, and decreased performance on neuropsychometrics. *Gastrointestinal reactions:* nausea; vomiting; epigastric distress; abdominal cramping; diarrhea, and constipation. *Allergic reactions:* pharyngitis, agranulocytosis, erythematous rash, fever combined with aching and sore throat; laryngospasm and respiratory distress. *Respiratory reaction:* bronchospasm. *Hematological reactions:* agranulocytosis nonthrombocytopenic purpura, and thrombocytopenic purpura. *Miscellaneous reaction:* reversible alopecia. Also reported were elevated blood urea levels in patients with severe heart disease, elevated serum transaminase, alkaline phosphatase, and lactic dehydrogenase.

Dosage and Administration: *Orally. Hypertension,* initially 80 mg daily in divided doses. Dosage may be increased gradually until optimal blood pressure response is achieved. The usual effective dose ranges from 160 to 480 mg daily; however, some patients may require 640 mg daily. *Angina pectoris,* initially 10 to 20 mg 3 or 4 times daily, before meals and at bedtime. Dosage should be gradually increased at intervals of 3 to 7 days until the optimal response is obtained. Although individual patients may respond at any dosage level, the average optimal dosage appears to be 160 mg/day. The value and safety of dosage exceeding 320 mg/day have not been established. If treatment is to be discontinued, the dosage should be reduced gradually over a period of several weeks. *Arrhythmias,* 10 to 30 mg 3 or 4 times daily before meals and at bedtime. *Hypertrophic subaortic stenosis,* 20 to 40 mg 3 or 4 times daily before meals and at bedtime. *Pheochromocytoma,* 60 mg daily in divided doses for 3 days prior to surgery, administered concomitantly with an alpha-adrenergic blocking agent; *for the management of inoperable tumor,* 30 mg may be given in divided doses. *Intravenously.* This mode of administration is reserved for life-threatening arrhythmias and those occurring under anesthesia. The usual *intravenous* dose is 1 to 3 mg, administered while the patient is being monitored by ECG, at a rate not to exceed 1 ml/min. Depending upon the response, a second dose may be given after 2 minutes; additional doses should not be given within 4 hours. Data on the use of this drug in the pediatric age group are too limited to permit adequate directions for use.

Availability:
INDERAL®: **(Ayerst)**
Injection, 1 mg/ml in ampuls of 1 ml in cartons of 10.
Tablets, 10, 20, 40 and 80 mg in bottles of 100 and 1000 and in unit-dose packages of 100.

PROPYLTHIOURACIL

Chemical Name: 6-Propyl-2-thiouracil.

Description: Propylthiouracil is an antithyroid drug chemically and physiologically related to other thiouracil derivatives. It inhibits conversion of iodide to iodine, iodination of tyrosine, and formation of thyroxin from diiodotyrosine. It occurs as a white, crystalline powder, slightly soluble in water, ether, and chloroform, sparingly soluble in alcohol, and soluble in ammonia and alkali hydroxides.

The drug does not inactivate thyroxine and triiodothyronine already made and stored in colloid or circulating in the blood, nor does it alter thyroid hormones given by mouth or by injection.

Indications: Medical treatment of hyperthyroidism; preoperatively before thyroidectomy or radioactive iodine therapy.

Contraindications: Hypersensitivity or idiosyncrasy to propylthiouracil.

Warnings: Because propylthiouracil readily crosses the placental membranes and can induce goiter and even cretinism in the developing fetus, it is important that a sufficient, but not excessive, dose be given. In some instances, it may be necessary to withdraw the drug 2 or 3 weeks before delivery. The concomitant administration of thyroid during propylthiouracil therapy of the pregnant hyperthyroid patient is also recommended in order that hypothyroidism in the mother and fetus may be prevented. Administration should continue through and beyond delivery. Postpartum patients receiving this drug should not nurse their babies.

Precautions: Because agranulocytosis may occur during therapy, the drug should be administered cautiously and the patient should be instructed to report any symptoms of illness such as sore throat, skin eruptions, fever, headache, or general malaise. In such cases, white blood cell and differential counts should be made to determine whether agranulocytosis has developed. Particular care should be exercised with patients who are receiving additional drugs known to cause agranulocytosis. Furthermore, since the drug has been reported to cause hypoprothrombinemia and bleeding, prothrombin time should be monitored during therapy, especially before surgical procedures. Drug fever, severe skin reactions such as exfoliative dermatitis, and arthralgia or other joint symptoms are indications for immediate withdrawal of the drug permanently. Propylthiouracil should not be administered concurrently with sulfonamides or coal-tar derivatives such as acetanilid, antipyrine, and aminopyrine.

Adverse Reactions: Minor adverse reactions include skin rash, urticaria, nausea, vomiting, epigastric distress, arthralgia, paresthesia, loss of taste, abnormal loss of hair, myalgia, headache, pruritus, drowsiness, neuritis, edema, vertigo, skin pigmentation, jaundice, sialadenopathy, and lymphadenopathy. These occur in less than 3% of the patients. Less frequently noted but of a more serious nature include inhibition of myelopoiesis (agranulocytosis, granulopenia, and thrombocytopenia), drug fever, a syndrome resembling lupus erythematosus but without lupus cells in the blood, hepatitis, periarteritis, and hypoprothrombinemia and bleeding, It should be noted that about 10% of patients with untreated hyperthyroidism have leukopenia (white blood cell count of less than 4000/cu mm), often with relative granulopenia. Serious or severe reactions should be followed by withdrawal of the drug.

Dosage and Administration: *Orally.* The daily dosage and the length of treatment cannot be predicted with any degree of accuracy. In general, slightly larger amounts are required to treat large or nodular goiters, particularly if there has been recent treatment with iodine. The total daily dosage is usually given in 3 equal doses at approximately 8-hour intervals. For adults, initially, 300 mg for mild hyperthyroidism, 400 mg for moderately severe cases, and 600 to 900 mg in severe cases. The maintenance daily dose is usually 100 to 150 mg. For children 10 years of age and over, the initial dosage is 150 to 300 mg daily; 6 to 10 years of age, 50 to 150 mg daily. The maintenance dosage for children is determined by the response of the patient.

Availability:
PROPYLTHIOURACIL:
Tablets, 50 mg in bottles of 100 and 1000. **(Lederle)**
Tablets, 50 mg in bottles of 100 and 1000. **(Lilly)**
Tablets, 50 mg in bottles of 100 and 1000 and in unit-dose packages of 100 (10 × 10). **(Parke-Davis)**

PROTAMINE SULFATE

Description: Protamines are simple proteins of low molecular weight that are rich in arginine and are strongly basic. Protamine sulfate is prepared from the sperm or mature testes of salmon and certain other species of fish. It occurs as a fine, white or in a faintly color, amorphous or crystalline powder sparingly soluble in water, forming colorless solutions.

When administered alone, protamine has an anticoagulant effect. However, when it is given in the presence of heparin (which is strongly acidic), a stable salt is formed which results in the loss of anticoagulant activity of both drugs. Each mg of protamine sulfate neutralizes approximately 90 U.S.P. units of heparin activity derived from lung tissue or about 115 U.S.P. units of heparin activity derived from intestinal mucosa.

Indications: Treatment of heparin overdosage.

Warnings: Hyperheparinemia or bleeding has been reported in experimental animals and in some patients 30 minutes to 18 hours after cardiac surgery (under cardiopulmonary bypass) in spite of complete neutralization of heparin by adequate doses of protamine sulfate at the end of the operation. Therefore, it is important to keep such patients under close postoperative observation. Additional doses of protamine sulfate should be administered if indicated by coagulation studies, such as the heparin titration test with protamine and the determination of plasma thrombin times. There is no adequate information as to whether or not this drug may affect fertility in male or female patients or have a teratogenic potential or other harmful effect on the fetus.

Precautions: Protamine sulfate should be given by slow intravenous injection (in 1 to 3 minutes) and in doses not exceeding 50 mg in any 10-minute period. The necessary facilities to treat shock should be immediately available. Patients allergic to fish may develop hypersensitivity reactions to protamine, although to date no relationship has been established between allergic reactions to protamine and fish allergy.

Adverse Reactions: Intravenous administration may cause a sudden fall in blood pressure, bradycardia, dyspnea, or transitory flushing and a feeling of warmth.

Dosage and Administration: *Intravenously,* administered *very slowly* (1 to 3 minutes); not to exceed 50 mg in any 10-minute period. The dosage of protamine sulfate should be guided by blood coagulation studies.

Availability:
PROTAMINE SULFATE Injection, 10 mg/ml in ampuls of 5 and 25 ml. **(Lilly)**
PROTAMINE SULFATE for Injection in vials of 50 mg with a 5-ml vial of sterile water for injection. **(Upjohn)**

PROTAMINE ZINC INSULIN (PZI): see The Insulins

PROTEIN (MODIFIED FIBRIN) HYDROLYSATE

Description: A sterile, pyrogen-free hydrolysate containing essential amino acids, for intravenous use, made by the partial acid hydrolysis of animal blood fibrin and consisting of a mixture of approximately 2/3 free amino acids and 1/3 small-chain peptides. Each liter represents the equivalent of 50 gm of protein. The alpha amino nitrogen is about 55% of total nitrogen content, and the total nitrogen ranges from 6.5 to 7 gm/liter. pH ranges from 5 to 6. The solution also provides 345 calories/liter.

Indications: May be of use as adjunctive therapy in partially reversing negative nitrogen balance in patients on long-term parenteral therapy, or when there is interference with ingestion, digestion, or absorption of dietary protein for prolonged periods.

Contraindications: In patients with severe liver disease or symptoms of impending hepatic coma.

Precautions: Since free ammonia is present in fibrin hydrolysates which may produce an excess of ammonia in the plasma, blood ammonia levels should be checked regularly particularly in premature and newborn infants and in patients with liver disease. The physician is advised to administer this solution in restricted amounts to patients with acidosis, impaired renal function or azotemia, and to use it with caution in those with severe congestive heart failure. Circulatory overload should be avoided, especially in patients with cardiac or pulmonary disorders. This preparation should not be used with hypertonic concentrations of dextrose in the presence of intracranial or intraspinal hemorrhage, nor in delirium tremens if the patient is already dehydrated. Only solutions which are clear should be administered intravenously. The rate of infusion should be slow initially (no more than 2 ml/min) to permit careful observation of the patient for possible reactions.

Adverse Reactions: Excessively rapid rates of injection may produce fever, chills, nausea and vomiting. Other complications which may occur include urticarial rash, vasodilatation, abdominal pain and convulsions. Injection should be discontinued promptly if hypersensitivity is exhibited by the patient. Local phlebitis and thrombosis may occur at the site of injection or along the course of the vein used for infusion. If this occurs, another vein may be used for further administration.

Dosage and Administration: *Intravenously.* The rate of infusion initially should be 2 ml/min, and then increased gradually to tolerance if the initial rate of administration is well tolerated. Caloric intake must be maintained during administration to prevent utilization of the protein hydrolysate for energy rather than for protein synthesis. The average dosage for adults is 2 to 3 liters a day; however, larger daily amounts usually are tolerated by patients with severe protein deficiency. **Note:** antibiotics or other drugs may be added to the solution provided that they are compatible with the protein fibrin hydrolysate.

Availability:
AMINOSOL® 5% in Abbo-Vac® (partially filled) bottles of 1000 ml each containing 700 ml of solution and in D5-W Injection in Abbo-Vac® (partially filled) containers of 1000 ml each containing 750 ml of solution. Each 100 ml contains 17 mEq potassium ion, less than 10 mEq sodium ion and 5 gm of dextrose with 0.06% of potassium metabisulfate as preservative.

(Abbott)

PROTOKYLOL HYDROCHLORIDE

Chemical Name: α-[(α-Methyl-3, 4-methylenedioxyphenethylamino) methyl] protocatechuyl alcohol hydrochloride.

Description: A sympathomimetic amine, protokylol is used primarily as a bronchodilator in the treatment of asthmatic conditions. It occurs as a white, crystalline solid that is soluble in water. Because it is a long-acting derivative of isoproterenol, the drug shares the same selective β-receptor-stimulating activity of the parent compound; however, it has been reported to be much more stable in the body. When taken orally, onset of action occurs within 30 to 90 minutes and the effects persist for 3 to 4 hours.

Indications: Treatment of reversible bronchospasm associated with acute and chronic bronchial asthma, pulmonary emphysema, bronchitis and bronchiectasis.

Contraindications: Because of the cardiac accelerator action of the drug, protokylol is contraindicated in patients with cardiac arrhythmias or coronary insufficiency, or in those receiving propranolol or similar beta-blocking agents.

Warnings: If this drug is considered for administration to pregnant women or to women of childbearing potential, the possibility of risk to the fetus must be weighed against the expected therapeutic benefits.

Precautions: Protokylol should be administered with caution to patients with cardiovascular disorders including coronary insufficiency. Also, special care is advised in those with diabetes, hyperthyroidism, prostatic hypertrophy, glaucoma, and known hypersensitivity to sympathomimetic agents. The drug should be immediately withdrawn if precordial distress or anginal-type pains develop. Caution is also recommended in patients receiving other sympathomimetic amines prior to the administration of this agent.

Adverse Reactions: Side effects are similar to those of isoproterenol and are referable to the cardiovascular and central nervous systems. Although elevation of blood pressure is not usually a problem, tachycardia and palpitation may occur. The undesirable effects on the CNS include tremulousness, tension, insomnia, and dizziness. Some patients may experience weakness, nausea, and difficulty in voiding.

Dosage and Administration: *Orally.* The usual adult dosage is 1 or 2 tablets 4 times daily.

Availability:
VENTAIRE® Tablets, 2 mg in bottles of 100. **(Marion)**

PROTRIPTYLINE HYDROCHLORIDE

Chemical Name: *N*-Methyl-5H-dibenzo[a,d]cycloheptene-5-propylamine hydrochloride.

Description: Protriptyline is an antidepressant structurally and pharmacologically related to amitriptyline, imipramine, desipramine and nortriptyline. It occurs as a white to yellowish-white, crystalline powder freely soluble in water, and has a molecular weight of 299.8.

Protriptyline is a dibenzocycloheptene derivative, not an MAO inhibitor, and is characterized by a more rapid onset of initial effect than other tricyclic antidepressants. The onset of effect may be indicated by increased activity and energy which may occur within 1 week. Apathy and lethargy may be ameliorated early in the course of therapy. Clinical studies show it to be lacking in sedative and tranquilizing properties.

Well absorbed following oral use, it reaches significant plasma concentrations within 2 hours, attains maximum in 8 to 12 hours, then declines gradually since the rate of excretion is slow. Protein binding is quite high accounting for 92% of the drug.

Indications: Treatment of symptoms of mental depression in patients who are under close medical supervision. Its activating properties make it particularly suitable for withdrawn and anergic patients.

Contraindications: Patients with known hypersensitivity to the drug; those with pyloric stenosis, glaucoma, or a tendency to urinary retention; during the acute recovery phase following myocardial infarction; concomitant administration with MAO inhibitors (hyperpyretic crises, severe convulsions and death have occurred), or guanethidine and similarly acting antihypertensives.

Warnings: Because of its activating and energizing properties, protriptyline may aggravate anxiety in patients with minor functional psychoneuroses. Also, it may impair mental and/or physical abilities required for the performance of hazardous tasks requiring alertness or skill. It should be used with caution in the elderly and in those patients with cardiovascular disorders that could be aggravated by drug-induced tachycardia or postural hypotension, arrhythmias, and prolongation of the conduction time. Myocardial infarction and stroke have occurred. Hyperthyroid patients or those receiving thyroid medication may develop cardiac arrhythmias when taking protriptyline. This drug is not recommended for the pediatric age group since safety and effectiveness have not been established. Unless deemed necessary, the drug should not be used in women of childbearing potential, in nursing mothers or pregnant women unless the possible benefits are weighed against the potential risks to the mother and child.

Precautions: Psychotic symptoms may be aggravated in schizophrenics with depressive symptomatology, in which case the dose of protriptyline should be reduced, or a tranquilizer used concurrently. Patients taking large doses for prolonged periods, or in combination with other drugs, should have liver function studies and blood cell counts evaluated periodically. Protriptyline may enhance the response to alcohol and the effects of barbiturates and other CNS depressants, and may reverse the antihypertensive effects of guanethidine or similarly acting drugs. Should be used with caution in the presence of liver disease, in patients with a history of seizures and in those who are overactive or agitated, or conjunctively with anticholinergics or sympathomimetics. The drug may possibly cause symptoms of the manic phase to emerge in manic-depressive patients. Thus, when response becomes apparent in these patients, dosage should be reduced promptly and cautiously. Severely depressed patients are potential suicides, at least until significant remission occurs. It is important, therefore, to observe these patients carefully during the first few weeks of therapy, particularly as the depression lifts and the ability to act returns. Hospitalization or electroconvulsive therapy may be required in addition to protriptyline. If possible, the drug should be discontinued several days prior to elective surgery. Both elevation and lowering of blood sugar levels have been reported with the use of this drug.

Adverse Reactions: Those reported were: *Cardiovascular:* hypotension, hypertension, tachycardia, palpitation, arrhythmias. *CNS and Neuromuscular:* confusional states (especially in the elderly); disorientation; delusions; hallucinations; anxiety; agitation; restlessness; insomnia; numbness, tingling, and paresthesias of the extremities; peripheral neuropathy; incoordination; ataxia; tremor; seizures. *Anticholinergic:* dry mouth and rarely associated sublingual adenitis, blurred vision, disturbance of accommodation, mydriasis, constipation, urinary retention, dilatation of the urinary tract. *Other* reactions include: skin rash, petechiae, urticaria, itching, photosensitization (avoid excessive exposure to sunlight), edema (general, or of face and tongue), nausea, vomiting, epigastric distress, anorexia, peculiar taste, stomatitis, parotid swelling, impotence, jaundice (simulating obstructive), drowsiness, dizziness, weakness, fatigue, headache, perspiration, weight gain or loss, urinary frequency. *Withdrawal Symptoms:* In an occasional patient, abrupt cessation of treatment after prolonged administration may produce nausea, headache, and malaise. These are not indicative of addiction. The following adverse reactions have been reported less frequently: myocardial infarction, heart block, stroke, panic, nightmares, alteration in EEG patterns, hypomania, exacerbation of psychosis, extrapyramidal symptoms, tinnitus, paralytic ileus, delayed micturition, drug fever, bone marrow depression, agranulocytosis, eosinophilia, purpura, thrombocytopenia, diarrhea, abdominal cramps, black tongue, testicular swelling and gynecomastia in the male, breast enlargement and galactorrhea in the female, increased or decreased libido, altered liver function, flushing, nocturia, alopecia. High doses may cause temporary confusion, disturbed concentration, or transient visual hallucinations.

Overdosage may cause drowsiness; hypothermia; tachycardia and other arrhythmic abnormalities, for example, bundle branch block; ECG evidence of impaired conduction; congestive heart failure; dilated pupils; convulsions; severe hypotension; stupor; and coma. Other symptoms may be agitation, hyperactive reflexes, muscle rigidity, vomiting, and hyperpyrexia. Treatment is symptomatic and supportive and involves gastric lavage, maintenance of an open airway, adequate fluid intake and regulation of body temperature. Physostigmine, 1 to 3 mg intravenously, has been reported to reverse these untoward effects. Because physostigmine is rapidly metabolized, the dosage should be repeated as required particularly if life-threatening signs such as cardiac arrythmias, convulsions, and deep coma recur or persist after the initial dosage of physostigmine. Standard measures should also be employed to manage circulatory shock and metabolic acidosis. Cardiac arrhythmia may be treated with neostigmine, pyridostigmine or propranolol. Should cardiac failure occur, the use of digitalis should be considered. Close monitoring of cardiac function for not less than 5 days is advisable. Convulsions may be controlled by anticonvulsant drugs. Dialysis is of no value because of the low plasma concentration of the drug.

Dosage and Administration: *Orally* for adults and children older than 12 years. Dosage must be individualized, bearing in mind the possibility of spontaneous remission in certain instances regardless of therapy, as well as the danger of relapse. The usual dosage ranges between 5 and 10 mg 3 or 4 times daily; as much as 60 mg daily may be required, depending upon the condition being treated and its severity. Patients with insomnia should take the last dose of the day no later than midafternoon. Increases in dosage, if required, should be added to the morning dose. Since the natural course of depression persists for many months, maintenance therapy should be continued for at least 3 months after satisfactory improvement is first noticed. This will reduce the chance of relapse, which may occur if the depressive cycle is not complete.

Availability:
VIVACTIL® Tablets, 5 and 10 mg in bottles of 100 and 1000 and in single-unit packages of 100.

(Merck Sharp & Dohme)

PSEUDOEPHEDRINE HYDROCHLORIDE

Chemical Name: 1-Phenyl-2-methylamine-propanol-1 hydrochloride.

Description: Pseudoephedrine hydrochloride, a sympathomimetic amine, is the physiologically active stereoisomer of ephedrine; it occurs as a white, crystalline powder that is freely soluble in water.

Following oral administration, the therapeutic effect is usually experienced within 15 to 30 minutes with complete effect occurring in 30 to 60 minutes. Decongestion of the mucous membranes of the respiratory tract is mediated through the drug's action on the sympathetic nerves.

Indications: Symptomatic relief of nasal congestion associated with the common cold, acute respiratory infections, allergic rhinitis, vasomotor rhinitis and sinusitis. May also be used as supportive therapy in the treatment of acute serous otitis media with eustachian tube congestion. It has been found useful in the relief of mucosal congestion, croup, acute and subacute sinusitis, asthma, acute tracheobronchitis and acute otitis media as adjunctive therapy with antihistamines, antibiotics, analgesics and expectorants.

Contraindications: Pseudoephedrine should not be used in the presence of high blood pressure, heart disease, diabetes or thyroid disease unless directed by the physician. Also contraindicated in patients hypersensitive to sympathomimetic drugs, in nursing mothers, and in patients on MAO inhibitor therapy.

Warnings: The prescribed dosage should not be exceeded; and should nervousness, restlessness, or sleeplessness occur, the dosage should be reduced. Sympathomimetic amines should be used judiciously and sparingly in patients with hypertension, diabetes mellitus, ischemic heart disease, increased intraocular tension, hyperthyroidism, and prostatic hypertrophy. Symptoms of overdosage manifested by hallucinations, convulsions, CNS depression, and possibly death are more likely to occur in elderly patients. The usual precautions governing its use in pregnant patients should be exercised.

Precautions: The drug should be used with great caution, if at all, in patients with cardiovascular disease, and hyperactivity to ephedrine. Sympathomimetics may reduce the antihypertensive effects of methyldopa, mecamylamine, reserpine and veratrum alkaloids, whereas MAO inhibitors and beta-adrenergic blocking agents may enhance the effects of pseudoephedrine.

Adverse Reactions: Hyperreactive individuals may experience ephedrine-like reactions such as tachycardia, palpitations, headache, dizziness or nausea. Sympathomimetic agents have been associated with certain untoward reactions including fear, anxiety, tenseness, restlessness, tremor, weakness, pallor, respiratory difficulty, dysuria, insomnia, hallucinations, convulsions, CNS depression, arrhythmias, and cardiovascular collapse with hypotension.

Dosage and Administration: *Orally.* **Tablets and syrup:** Older children and adults, 60 mg; children 4 months to 6 years of age, 30 mg; infants up to 4 months, 15 mg. Dosage indicated may be given 3 or 4 times daily. **Sustained-release capsules and tablets:** Adults and children over 12 years of age, 1 capsule or tablet twice daily, morning and night. Should not be given to children under 12 years of age.

Availability:

Pseudoephedrine Hydrochloride

NOVAFED® Liquid, 30 mg/5 ml (alcohol 7.5%) in bottles of 120 ml. **(Dow)**

NOVAFED 120 Capsules, 120 mg (sustained-release) in bottles of 100 and in unit-dose cartons of 100. **(Dow)**

PSEUDOEPHEDRINE HYDROCHLORIDE Tablets, 30 and 60 mg in bottles of 100 and 1000. **(Lederle)**

PSEUDOEPHEDRINE HYDROCHLORIDE Tablets, 60 mg in bottles of 1000. **(Lemmon)**

SUDAFED®: **(Burroughs Wellcome)**

S.A. Capsules (sustained release), 120 mg in bottles of 100.

Syrup, 30 mg/5 ml (OTC) in bottles of 120 ml and 1 pint.

Tablets, 30 mg (OTC) in bottles of 100 and 1000 and in blister packs (unit-dose) packages of 24; 60 mg in bottles of 100 and 1000.

Combinations

COTROL-D™ Tablets, 60 mg with chlorpheniramine maleate, 4 mg in bottles of 100. **(Beecham)**

NALDEGESIC Tablets (OTC), 15 mg with acetaminophen, 325 mg in bottles of 100. **(Bristol)**

NOVAFED® A: **(Dow)**

Capsules (controlled release), 120 mg with chlorpheniramine maleate, 8 mg in bottles of 100.

Liquid (OTC), 30 mg/5 ml with chlorpheniramine maleate, 2 mg/5 ml in bottles of 120 ml.

Pseudoephedrine Sulfate

AFRINOL™ Tablets (long-acting), 120 mg in bottles of 100. **(Schering)**

PYRANTEL PAMOATE

Chemical Name: *Trans*-1,4,5,6-tetrahydro-1-methyl-2-[2-(2-thienyl)vinyl]-pyrimidine hydrogen pamoate.

Description: Pyrantel pamoate is an anthelmintic drug that appears to be selective against *Enterobius vermicularis* (pinworm) and *Ascaris lumbricoides* (roundworm). Although its exact mechanism of action is unknown, it appears to exert its anthelmintic effect by interfering with the neuromuscular function of the parasite.

Following oral administration, it is partially absorbed through the intestinal mucosa. Plasma levels of the unchanged drug are low with peak levels of 0.05 to 0.13 mcg/ml attained in 1 to 3 hours. Fifty percent or more of the drug is excreted unchanged in the feces, and about 7% or less in the urine in both unchanged form and its metabolites. Results of reproductive studies in animals did not reveal any evidence of fetal toxicity.

Indications: Treatment of roundworm and pinworm infections in adults and children.

Warnings: Safe use in pregnant women or in children under 2 years of age has not been established; therefore, the relative benefit-to-risk ratio should be considered.

Precautions: Minor transient elevations of SGOT have occurred in a small percentage of patients. Therefore, this drug should be used with caution in patients with preexisting liver dysfunction.

Adverse Reactions: The most frequently encountered were gastrointestinal reactions manifested by anorexia, nausea, vomiting, gastralgia, abdominal cramps, diarrhea, and tenesmus, and liver dysfunction manifested by elevated SGOT levels. Also noted were headache, dizziness, drowsiness, insomnia, and skin rashes.

Dosage and Administration: *Orally,* in a single dose of 11 mg (base)/kg of body weight or 1 ml/10 lbs of body weight. The maximum total dose is 1 gm. May be administered without regard to ingestion of food or time of day, and purging is not necessary prior to, during, or after therapy. It may be taken with either milk or fruit juices.

Availability:

ANTIMINTH® Suspension, 50 mg/ml (as base) in bottles of 60 ml. **(Roerig)**

PYRAZINAMIDE

Chemical Name: Pyrazinoic acid amide.

Description: Pyrazinamide, a bacteriostatic agent against *Mycobacterium tuberculosis,* is a pyrazine analogue of niacinamide. It occurs as a white to practically white, odorless, crystalline powder that is stable at room temperature and is sparingly soluble in water. Because of pyrazinamide's potential toxicity (most serious is hepatic damage) and short duration of effectiveness (resistance to the drug develops rapidly) it is considered as a secondary agent in the chemotherapy of tuberculosis.

After oral administration, pyrazinamide is well absorbed from the gastrointestinal tract and, is widely distributed throughout the body. A 1-gm dose produces blood levels of approximately 45 μg/ml at 2 hours and 10 μg/ml at 15 hours. Excretion is primarily by glomerular filtration and the major metabolite in the urine is 5-hydroxyprazinoic acid.

Indications: A tuberculostatic drug which may be administered after an adequate course of treatment with primary drugs (e.g., isoniazid, streptomycin, aminosalicylic acid) in any form of active tuberculosis. Pyrazinamide should only be given with other effective antituberculous agents.

Contraindications: Severe hepatic damage.

Warnings: Pyrazinamide should be used only when close observation of the patient is possible and when laboratory facilities are available for performing frequent, reliable liver function tests and blood uric acid determinations. The drug should be discontinued *and not be resumed* if signs of hepatocellular damage or hyperuricemia accompanied by an acute gouty arthritis become evident. Because of the potential toxicity of this drug, its use in children should be avoided unless crucial to therapy.

Precautions: Pretreatment examinations should include in vitro susceptibility tests of recent cultures of *M. tuberculosis* from the patient as measured against the usual antituberculous drugs. Liver function tests (especially SGPT, SGOT determinations) should be performed prior to and every 2 to 4 weeks during therapy. Increased difficulty in the management of patients with gout or diabetes mellitus has been reported.

Adverse Reactions: The principal untoward effect is a hepatic reaction. This varies from a symptomless abnormality of hepatic cell function, detectable by laboratory tests, through a mild syndrome of fever, anorexia, malaise, liver tenderness, hepatomegaly and splenomegaly, to more serious reactions such as clinical jaundice, and rare cases of progressive fulminating acute yellow atrophy and death. Other reactions are acute gout, sideroblastic anemia, arthralgias, anorexia, nausea and vomiting, dysuria, malaise, fever, and urticaria. Aggravation of peptic ulcer has been reported. Since there has been one report that the use of pyrazinamide increased the incidence of fatal hemoptysis, the possibility of the adverse effect of pyrazinamide on the blood clotting mechanism or vascular integrity should be borne in mind.

Dosage and Administration: *Orally.* The usual adult dosage is 20 to 35 mg/kg of body weight daily in 3 or 4 divided doses; maximal dosage is 3 gm daily; *not to be exceeded.* The drug should be administered with at least one other effective antituberculous agent.

Availability:
PYRAZINAMIDE Tablets, 0.5 gm in bottles of 500. **(Lederle)**

PYRIDOSTIGMINE BROMIDE

Chemical Name: 3-Hydroxy-1-methylpyridinium bromide dimethylcarbamate.

Description: Pyridostigmine is an analog of neostigmine and, like neostigmine, interferes with cholinesterase in its destruction of acetylcholine, thereby permitting freer transmission of nerve impulses across the myoneural junction. However, it differs from neostigmine and other members of the physostigmine group in that its action is characterized by a smoother therapeutic action and causes less gastrointestinal stimulation and other muscarinic side effects. Pyridostigmine bromide occurs as a white or nearly white, crystalline powder freely soluble in water, in alcohol and in chloroform, but is practically insoluble in ether.

Indications: Treatment of myasthenia gravis, and as a reversal agent or antagonist to nondepolarizing muscle relaxants.

Contraindications: Mechanical intestinal or urinary obstruction; the drug should be used cautiously in patients with bronchial asthma. Care should be observed in the use of atropine for counteracting side effects. Also contraindicated in patients with known hypersensitivity to anticholinesterase agents.

Warnings: Particular caution is stressed in patients with bronchial asthma or cardiac dysrhythmias. Transient bradycardia may occur and may be relieved by atropine sulfate. Care should be observed in the use of atropine for counteracting side effects; it should be administered as sparingly as possible since it may mask signs of cholinergic overdosage. When large doses of pyridostigmine are administered, the prior or simultaneous injection of atropine sulfate is advised. Increasing muscle weakness is an important sign of cholinergic overdosage as well as of impending myasthenic crisis. Respiratory distress may develop and may lead to respiratory arrest. Therefore, the differential diagnosis requires close observation of the patient with special attention to the time relationship between medication and development of weakness. Furthermore, whereas the presence of myasthenic crisis suggests the need for more intensive anticholinesterase therapy, the diagnosis of cholinergic crisis calls for prompt withdrawal of all drugs of this type. The immediate use of atropine in cholinergic crisis is also recommended. When pyridostigmine is used as an antagonist to nondepolarizing muscle relaxants, adequate recovery of voluntary respiration and neuromuscular transmission must be obtained prior to discontinuation of respiratory assistance and there should be continuous patient observation. Satisfactory recovery may be defined by a combination of clinical judgment, respiratory measurements and observation of the effects of peripheral nerve stimulation. If there is any doubt concerning adequate recovery from the effects of the nondepolarizing muscle relaxant, artificial ventilation should be continued until all doubt is removed. Safe use of this drug during pregnancy and lactation has not been established; therefore, its use in pregnant patients or those who may become pregnant is dictated by the desired therapeutic benefits as against the potential hazards to the mother and child.

Precautions: Increasing muscular weakness may be a sign of impending myasthenic crisis or of cholinergic crisis due to overdosage. It is extremely important that a distinction be made between these two crises, since increases in dosage of pyridostigmine or other similar drugs in the presence of cholinergic crisis or of a refractory state could have grave consequences. **Note:** Because of the hygroscopic nature of the Timespan tablets, mottling may occur; however, this occurrence does not affect their efficacy.

Adverse Reactions: Effects are most commonly related to overdosage and generally are of two varieties: muscarinic and nicotinic. Among these are nausea, vomiting, diarrhea, abdominal cramps, increased peristalsis, increased salivary and bronchial secretions, miosis, diaphoresis, muscle cramps, fasciculation and weakness. The use of any bromide can result in skin rash, which usually disappears when medication is discontinued.

Dosage and Administration: *Orally.* The size of the dosage and the frequency of administration must be adjusted to meet the needs of each individual patient. The average dosage is 600 mg daily, but as little as 360 mg daily in milder cases or as much as 1.5 gm daily in severe cases may be required. If the extended-release tablet is used, 1 to 3 tablets once or twice daily usually controls symptoms; the interval between doses, however, should be at least 6 hours. For optimal control, it may be necessary to use the more rapidly acting regular tablets (or syrup) in conjunction with the extended-release tablets. *Parenterally. For myasthenia gravis,* the usual adult dosage is 1/30 the oral dose administered either *intramuscularly* or *intravenously* (very slowly), and for neonates, the usual dosage requirements range from 0.05 to 0.15 mg/kg of body weight administered *intramuscularly. For reversal of nondepolarizing muscle relaxants,* usually 10 or 20 mg is administered *intravenously* (very slowly). It is recommended that atropine sulfate in a dose of 0.6 to 1.2 mg also be given *intravenously* immediately prior to the administration of pyridostigmine bromide. Although full recovery may occur within 15 minutes in most patients, others may require 1/2 hour or more. Satisfactory reversal can be evident by adequate voluntary respiration, respiratory measurements and the use of a peripheral nerve stimulator device. It is recommended that the patient be well-ventilated and a patent airway maintained until complete recovery of normal respiration is assured. Once satisfactory reversal has been attained, recurarization has not been reported. Failure of pyridostigmine bromide to provide prompt (within 1/2 hour) reversal may occur in the presence of extreme debilitation, carcinomatosis, or with concomitant use of certain broad spectrum antibiotics or anesthetic agents, notably ether. Under these circumstances ventilation must be supported by artificial means until the patient has resumed respiratory control.

Availability:
MESTINON®: **(Roche)**
Injection, 5 mg/ml in ampuls of 2 ml in cartons of 10.

Syrup, 60 mg/5 ml (alcohol, 5%) in bottles of 1 pint.
Tablets, 60 mg in bottles of 100 and 500.
Timespan® Tablets (extended-release), 180 mg in bottles of 100.
REGONOL® Injection, 5 mg/ml in ampuls of 2 ml. **(Organon)**

PYRIDOXINE HYDROCHLORIDE

Synonym: Vitamin B-6.

Chemical Name: Pyridoxol hydrochloride.

Description: Pyridoxine is a water-soluble, thermostable, photolabile, synthetic vitamin, a member of the vitamin B complex group. The exact role of pyridoxine in human nutrition is not known. In the body, pyridoxine apparently is converted to pyridoxal, a constituent of the enzyme system which plays a role in the metabolism of amino acids. The aqueous solution is acid in reaction, with a pH between 2 and 3.8.

Pyridoxine affects the metabolism of amino acids, fats, and carbohydrates. The requirement increases with the amount of protein in the diet. The coenzyme form of pyridoxine, pyridoxal phosphate (or codecarboxylase), is responsible for many enzymatic transformations in the metabolism of amino acids. The half-life of pyridoxine ranges from 15 to 20 days. It is degraded in the liver to 4-pyridoxic acid which is excreted by the kidney.

Pyridoxine is widely distributed in foods, especially in liver, vegetables, whole-grain cereals and meat.

Indications: Prophylaxis and treatment of pyridoxine deficiencies. This vitamin is said to be of value in patients taking oral contraceptives, in the treatment of irradiation sickness and in the treatment of nausea and vomiting of pregnancy; and in the prevention of the peripheral neuritis which may accompany isoniazid therapy. The toxic effects of high doses of cycloserine on the CNS have been prevented or controlled by pyridoxine alone or in combination with anticonvulsants, tranquilizers or sedatives.

Contraindications: Other than extremely rare instances of hypersensitivity, there are no known contraindications.

Adverse Reactions: Temporary burning or stinging and pain may be experienced at the site of infection. Although no untoward effects have been noted in clinical studies from daily doses of 130 mg to more than 1 gm given for periods of 6 to 21 days, long-term use may result in paresthesia, somnolence, and low folic acid levels.

Dosage and Administration: *Intramuscularly* or, slowly, by the *intravenous* route. The optimal dosage for treatment of pyridoxine deficiency has not been established; 10 to 150 mg daily or on alternate days may be considered an average dosage range.

Availability:
HEXA-BETALIN® Injection, 100 mg/ml in ampuls of 10 ml. **(Lilly)**
HEXAVIBEX® Injection, 100 mg/ml in vials of 5 ml. **(Parke-Davis)**
PYRIDOXINE HYDROCHLORIDE Injection, 100 mg/ml in vials of 10 ml. **(Abbott)**

PYRIMETHAMINE

Chemical Name: 2,4-Diamino-5-(p-chlorophenyl)-6-ethylpyrimidine.

Description: Pyrimethamine is a folic acid antagonist with antimalarial and antitoxoplasmic activity. It is related chemically to a metabolite of chloroguanide, but possesses greater potency and a much longer half-life. It occurs as a white, odorless, tasteless, crystalline powder practically insoluble in water.

Pyrimethamine appears to possess blood schizonticidal and some tissue schizonticidal activity against the malarial parasites. However, its blood schizonticidal activity may be slower than that of 4-aminoquinoline compounds. Pyrimethamine does not destroy gametocytes, but arrests sporogony in the mosquito.

The action of pyrimethamine against *Toxoplasma gondii* appears to be greatly enhanced when used in conjunction with sulfonamides. Laboratory studies demonstrated that a combination of the 2 drugs effectively prevented the development of severe uveitis in most rabbits following the inoculation of the anterior chamber of the eye with toxoplasma. Pyrimethamine, in large doses, has produced teratogenic effects in laboratory animals.

Indications: Chemoprophylaxis of malaria due to susceptible strains of plasmodia, and the treatment of toxoplasmosis. Combined with chloroquine, amodiaquine, quinacrine or quinine for the treatment of acute attacks of malaria.

Warnings: Pyrimethamine is a potent and long-acting drug. The dosage required for the treatment of toxoplasmosis is 10 to 20 times the recommended antimalarial dosage and approaches the toxic level. If signs of folic or folinic acid deficiency develop the dosage should be reduced or the drug withdrawn depending upon the response of the patient. Folinic acid (leucovorin) helps to prevent or correct the hematologic toxic effects. Patients should be cautioned to keep the drug out of reach of children since accidental ingestion has led to fatalities. The large doses required to treat toxoplasmosis should be used in pregnant patients only after a definitive diagnosis of acute toxoplasmosis has been made, and the possibility of teratogenic effects should be carefully weighed against the possible risks of damage to the fetus from the infection. Concurrent administration of folinic acid is recommended when this drug is used for treatment of toxoplasmosis during pregnancy.

Precautions: The recommended dosage for malaria suppression should not be exceeded. Patients receiving high dosages should have semi-weekly blood counts, including platelet counts, performed. In patients with convulsive disorders, a small initial dose (for toxoplasmosis) is recommended to avoid the potential nervous-system toxicity of pyrimethamine.

Adverse Reactions: Large doses may cause anorexia and vomiting. Vomiting may be minimized by taking the drug with meals, but generally disappears promptly with a reduction in dosage. Also, large doses appear to induce megaloblastic anemia, leukopenia, thrombocytopenia, pancytopenia, and atrophic glossitis. Acute intoxication may follow the ingestion of an excessive amount of pyrimethamine which may involve CNS stimulation including convulsions. In such events, parenteral barbiturates followed by folinic acid may be instituted.

Dosage and Administration: *Orally. For suppressive prophylaxis of malaria:* 25 mg for adults and children over 10 years of age; 12.5 mg for children 4 to 10 years, and 6.25 mg for children under 4 years; doses are given on a *once weekly* regimen. *Treatment of acute attack of malaria:* 25 to 50 mg daily for 2 days for adults and children over 10 years; 25 mg daily for 2 days for children 4 to 10 years. *Treatment of toxoplasmosis:* usual starting dosage for adults is 50 to 75 mg daily, together with 1 to 4 gm of trisulfapyrimidines for 1 to 3 weeks; then reduced to approximately ½ that previously given for each drug and continued for an additional 4 or 5 weeks. For children, usually 1 mg/kg of body weight daily divided into 2 equal doses together with the usual pediatric sulfonamide dosage administered for 2 to 4 days; then reduced to ½ for each drug and continued for 1 month.

Availability:
DARAPRIM® Tablets (scored), 25 mg in bottles of 100 and 1000. **(Burroughs Wellcome)**

PYRVINIUM PAMOATE

Chemical Name: Bis[6-(dimethylamino)-2-[2-(2,5-dimethyl-1-phenylpyrrol-3-yl)vinyl]-1-methylquinolinium]4,4'-methylenebis(3-hydroxy-2-naphthoate).

Description: Pyrvinium pamoate is an anthelmintic dye, and occurs as a red, crystalline powder which is stable to heat, light, and air, and is practically insoluble in water.

Pyrvinium appears to exert its anthelmintic effect by preventing the parasite from using exogenous carbohydrates, thereby causing its death. The drug is not appreciably absorbed from the gastrointestinal tract.

Indications: Treatment of enterobiasis.

Warnings: Since no laboratory or clinical studies have been performed, the use of this drug during pregnancy requires that the potential benefits be weighed against the possible hazards to the mother and fetus.

Precautions: To forestall undue concern and help avoid accidental staining, patients and parents should be informed of the staining properties of this preparation. Tablets should be swallowed whole to avoid staining the teeth. This product will color the stool a bright red, but this is not harmful to the patient. If emesis occurs, the vomitus will probably be colored red and will stain most materials.

Adverse Reactions: Nausea, vomiting, abdominal cramping, diarrhea, and hypersensitivity reactions (photosensitization and other allergic reactions) have been reported. Gastrointestinal reactions occur more often in older children and adults who have received large doses.

Dosage and Administration: *Orally* in a single dose equivalent to 5 mg (base)/kg of body weight. If necessary, the dose may be repeated in 2 or 3 weeks.

Availability:
POVAN®: **(Parke-Davis)**
Filmseals, 50 mg (equiv. to base) in bottles of 50.
Suspension, 10 mg/ml (equiv. to base) in bottles of 60 ml.

QUADRINAL

Description: Each tablet contains ephedrine hydrochloride, 24 mg; phenobarbital, 24 mg; theophylline calcium salicylate, 130 mg (provides 65 mg of anhydrous theophylline) and potassium iodide, 320 mg. Each 5 ml (teaspoonful) of the suspension is equivalent to ½ tablet.

Two bronchodilators, ephedrine and theophylline, supplement each other for sustained action. Phenobarbital serves as a mild sedative to help counteract CNS stimulation which may be caused by ephedrine. Wheezing and coughing are relieved by improved bronchodilation while expectorant action of potassium iodide helps to remove a source of irritation in the bronchial tree. Dyspnea is thus relieved or prevented and acute episodes of bronchospasm are often eliminated with consequent lessening of apprehension and distress.

Indications: Symptomatic treatment of chronic respiratory diseases in which tenacious mucus and bronchospasm are the dominant symptoms, as in bronchial asthma, chronic bronchitis and pulmonary emphysema.

Warnings: Phenobarbital may be habit-forming. When taken during pregnancy, iodine-induced goiter with hypothyroidism may appear in the newborn infant.

Precautions: Caution is recommended in patients sensitive to iodides; in those receiving potassium sparing diuretics or potassium supplements, in cardiovascular disease; in hyperthyroidism; in diabetes; in peptic ulcer and during pregnancy. In some patients, prolonged use of iodides can lead to hypothyroidism. Since salicylates block the uricosuric action of probenecid and sulfinpyrazone, special care should be exercised in patients with gout.

Adverse Reactions: Gastrointestinal irritation is rarely encountered when taken with or after meals.

Dosage and Administration: *Orally.* Adults and children over 12 years of age, 1 tablet or 2 teaspoonful of suspension 3 or 4 times daily, repeated at bedtime if necessary. Children 6 to 12 years of age, ½ tablet or 1 teaspoonful 3 times daily. Children under 6 years of age, adjust dosage according to body weight.

Availability:
QUADRINAL™: **(Knoll)**
Suspension in bottles of 1 pint.
Tablets in bottles of 100 and 1000.

QUINACRINE HYDROCHLORIDE

Chemical Name: 6-Chloro-9-[[4-(diethylamino)-1-methylbutyl]amino]-2-methoxyacridine dihydrochloride dihydrate.

Description: Quinacrine hydrochloride, an acridine derivative, occurs as a bright yellow, odorless, bitter, crystalline powder sparingly soluble in water and soluble in alcohol. It is readily absorbed from the intestinal tract, is widely distributed in the tissues from which it is very slowly liberated.

The drug exerts both suppressive and therapeutic action in malaria. It destroys erythrocytic asexual forms (trophozoites) of vivax, falciparum, and quartan malaria, and sexual forms (gametocytes) of vivax and quartan malaria; however, it is ineffective against falciparum gametocytes and against sporozoites of all forms of malaria. In addition, it eradicates certain intestinal cestodes, for example, beef tapeworm *(Taenia saginata)*, pork tapeworm *(Taenia solium)*, dwarf tapeworm *(Hymenolepis nana)*, and probably fish tapeworm *(Diphyllobothrium latum)*, and eliminates *Giardia lamblia* from the intestinal tract.

Indications: For the treatment and suppression of malaria as well as for the treatment of patients with giardiasis and cestodiasis.

Contraindications: Coadministration with primaquine, and during pregnancy when used in the treatment of intestinal cestodiasis or giardiasis.

Warnings: Patients should be strongly cautioned to keep this drug out of the reach of children. Quinacrine occasionally causes a transitory psychosis and therefore should be used with special caution in patients over 60 years of age or in those with a history of psychosis. It should be used with extreme caution, if at all, in patients with psoriasis or porphyria, since pronounced exacerbation is frequently produced. The use of quinacrine in the suppression or treatment of malaria during pregnancy should be avoided except when, in the judgment of the physician, the benefits outweigh the possible hazards.

Precautions: In recent years it has been found that certain strains of *Plasmodium falciparum* have become resistant to synthetic antimalarial compounds including quinacrine as shown by the fact that normally adequate doses have failed to prevent or cure clinical malaria or parasitemia; therefore, treatment with quinine or other specific forms of therapy is advised for patients infected with a resistant strain of parasites. Quinacrine should be used with caution in conjunction with known hepatotoxic drugs and in alcoholics or patients with hepatic disease. Periodic blood-cell counts should be made if patients are given extended suppressive therapy for malaria. Patients on prolonged therapy should be instructed to promptly report any visual disturbances and to receive periodic complete ophthalmologic examinations. Cautious use of the drug is essential in patients having G-6-PD (glucose-6-phosphate dehydrogenase) deficiency.

Adverse Reactions: The drug temporarily imparts a yellow color to the urine and skin (but does not cause jaundice). Following administration in doses adequate for the treatment of an acute malarial attack, mild and transient headache, dizziness, and gastrointestinal complaints (diarrhea, anorexia, nausea, abdominal cramps and, on rare occasions, vomiting) may occur. Other infrequent but reversible side effects include pleomorphic skin eruptions, neuropsychiatric disturbances (nervousness, vertigo, irritability, emotional change, nightmares, and transient psychosis). Aplastic anemia, hepatitis, and lichen planus like eruptions have been described, especially after long periods of malarial suppressive therapy with quinacrine. Exfoliative dermatitis can develop as a primary reaction to the drug or as a secondary response to other types of quinacrine-induced symptoms. Contact dermatitis can also occur. Epileptiform convulsions have been reported following the administration of massive doses. Corneal changes, such as transient edema or deposits of an opaque substance in the corneal epithelium, with symptoms of visual halos, focusing difficulties, and blurred vision, were rarely noted on slit-lamp examination in patients on long-term quinacrine-suppressive therapy for malaria. These reactions were reversible on cessation of therapy. Retinopathy has been reported in a small number of patients on prolonged therapy with this drug who had also received 4-aminoquinoline drugs, such as chloroquine.

Dosage and Administration: *Orally. Treatment of Malaria—Adults and children over 8 years,* 200 mg with 1 gm of sodium bicarbonate every 6 hours for 5 doses, then 100 mg 3 times daily for 6 days (total dosage 2.8 gm in 7 days). *Children from 4 to 8 years,* 200 mg 3 times the first day, then 100 mg 2 times daily for 6 days. *Children from 1 to 4 years,* 100 mg 3 times the first day, then 100 mg once daily for 6 days. Medication should be taken after meals, with a full glass of water, tea, or fruit juice. *Suppression of Malaria—Adults,* 100 mg once daily. *Children,* 50 mg daily. Medication should be maintained for 1 to 3 months. *Giardiasis—Adults,* 100 mg 3 times daily for 5 to 7 days. Children, 7 mg/kg/day in 3 divided doses (maximum 300 mg/day) after meals for 5 days. *Tapeworm (Beef, Pork, and Fish)*—(1) Preliminary bland, semisolid, nonfat diet, or milk diet on the day before medication, with fasting following the evening meal. A saline purge or purge and cleansing enema before treatment if desired. (2) *Adults,* 4 doses of 200 mg 10 minutes apart (total dose, 800 mg). Sodium bicarbonate 600 mg with each dose in order to reduce the tendency to nausea and vomiting. *Children from 5 to 10 years,* a total dose of 400 mg. *Children from 11 to 14 years,* a total dose of 600 mg, divided into 3 or 4 doses administered 10 minutes apart. Sodium bicarbonate 300 mg with each dose if desired. (3) Saline purge 1 to 2 hours later. The expelled worm is stained yellow, facilitating identification of scolex. *Dwarf Tapeworm*—(1) *Adults,* the night before medication 1 tablespoonful of sodium sulfate dissolved in water. *Children,* 1/2 adult dose. (2) *Adults,* on first day, 900 mg of the antimalarial compound, on an empty stomach, in 3 portions 20 minutes apart, with sodium sulfate purge 1 1/2 hours later. On the following 3 days, 100 mg 3 times daily. *Children from 4 to 8 years,* initial dose of 200 mg, followed by 100 mg after breakfast for 3 days. *Children from 8 to 10 years,* initial dose of 300 mg, followed by 100 mg twice daily for 3 days. *Children from 11 to 14 years,* initial dose of 400 mg, followed by 100 mg 3 times daily for 3 days.

Availability:
ATABRINE® Tablets, 100 mg in bottles of 100. **(Winthrop)**

QUINAMM

Description: Each tablet contains quinine sulfate, 260 mg and aminophylline, 195 mg. Quinine acts on skeletal muscle by two mechanisms: it prolongs the refractory period due to direct action on the muscle fiber and it decreases the excitability of the motor end-plate by a curare-like action. Although the mechanism of action of aminophylline has not been fully established, it has been postulated to be due to an increase in blood flow, a depolarization of the muscle membrane, or an increase in the muscle's metabolic rate.

Indications: Prophylaxis and treatment of nocturnal recumbency leg muscle cramps, including those associated with arthritis, diabetes, varicose veins, thrombophlebitis, arteriosclerosis, and static foot deformaties.

Contraindications: Quinine is contraindicated in women of childbearing potential, during pregnancy, in patients with known quinine sensitivity, and in those with a deficiency of the enzyme glucose-6-phosphate dehydrogenase.

Precautions: Quinine may produce thrombocytopenic purpura in highly sensitive patients; however, recovery usually follows withdrawal of the medication.

Adverse Reactions: Aminophylline may produce intestinal cramps in some instances, and quinine may produce symptoms of cinchonism, such as tinnitus, dizziness, and gastrointestinal disturbances. The drug should be withdrawn if ringing in the ears, deafness, skin rash, or visual disturbances occur.

Dosage and Administration: *Orally,* 1 tablet upon retiring. Where necessary, dosage may be increased to 1 tablet following the evening meal and 1 tablet upon retiring.

Availability:
QUINAMM™ Tablets in bottles of 100 and 500. **(Merrell-National)**

QUINETHAZONE

Chemical Name: 7-Chloro-2-ethyl-1,2,3,4-tetrahydro-4-oxo-6-sulfamyl-quinazoline.

Description: Quinethazone is a nonmercurial diuretic of the sulfonamide group, and occurs as a yellowish-white, crystalline powder practically insoluble in water and soluble in alcohol. It differs structurally from the thiazide diuretics by the nature of the cyclic ring. Its action is pharmacologically identical to the thiazide group.

Following administration, quinethazone produces urinary excretion of sodium and chloride in approximately equivalent amounts (saluresis), while potassium is excreted to a lesser degree. The saluretic effect of the drug is rapid and relatively prolonged, beginning within 2 hours, reaching a peak in 6 hours, and lasting for 18 to 24 hours. The renal excretion of sodium and chloride appears to result from inhibition of the tubular mechanism of electrolyte reabsorption. The renal effect seems to be virtually independent of alterations in acid-base balance.

In common with other drugs of this class, quinethazone inhibits the proximal reabsorption of sodium and chloride; the excretion of potassium results from increased potassium secretion by the distal tubule where potassium is exchanged for sodium. It probably exerts its antihypertensive effect either by diuresis and sodium loss or by action on vascular function to reduce peripheral resistance or both.

Indications: Treatment of all types of edema involving retention of salt, such as edema associated with congestive heart failure, nephrotic syndrome, hepatic cirrhosis, toxemia of pregnancy, premenstrual tension syndrome, menopausal syndrome, obesity, and steroid administration; it may be helpful in some cases of lymphedema, idiopathic edema, and edema due to venous obstruction. Also indicated in the treatment of hypertension with or without edema, either alone or in combination with other antihypertensive agents. Reserpine is employed as an adjunct in the treatment of hypertension and should be used only when the need for combined therapy has been established.

Contraindications: Hypersensitivity to any of the components; progressive renal disease including azotemia and anuria. The routine use of diuretics in an otherwise healthy pregnant patient with or without mild edema is contraindicated and possibly hazardous. Reserpine is contraindicated in patients with a history of mental depression or psychosis, and in those with a history of peptic or duodenal ulcer; also in those with severe hepatic disorders.

Warnings: Since enteric-coated potassium salts may cause small-bowel lesions, they should be given only when adequate dietary supplementation is not practical and should be discontinued immediately if abdominal pain, distention, nausea, vomiting or gastrointestinal bleeding occurs. Drug-induced hepatitis has been reported; therefore, quinethazone should be discontinued promptly when patients show signs of hypersensitivity such as fever, rash or pruritus. Administration to pregnant women or to women of childbearing potential requires that the potential benefits of the drug be weighed against the possible hazards to the mother and fetus. Reserpine has been reported to cause CNS depression in the newborn infant when given to the mother just prior to delivery. Thiazide diuretics have been noted to cause neonatal thrombocytopenia when administered during pregnancy, and the possibility of encountering this reaction with the use of quinethazone should be considered.

Precautions: Quinethazone should be used with caution in patients with impaired liver function or progressive liver disease, since minor alterations in fluid and electrolyte balance may precipitate hepatic coma. Caution is especially indicated during prolonged or intensive therapy and when salt intake is restricted or when steroids or ACTH is used concomitantly. The possibility of potassium depletion and its toxic sequelae must be kept in mind, particularly in patients with cirrhosis or in those receiving digitalis. In individuals with impaired renal function, azotemia and/or excessive drug accumulation may develop. When quinethazone is added to a regimen that includes ganglionic blocking agents or other antihypertensive agents, the dosage of these agents should be reduced to avoid a sudden drop in blood pressure. Increases in serum uric acid may occur, but precipitation of gout has been rare. A decreased glucose tolerance as evidenced by hyperglycemia and glycosuria has occurred which may aggravate or provoke diabetes mellitus. Quinethazone may decrease arterial responsiveness to norepinephrine; therefore, the drug should be withdrawn 48 hours before elective surgery. If emergency surgery is indicated, preanesthetic and anesthetic agents should be given in reduced dosage. Quinethazone may also increase the responsiveness to tubocurarine. The antihypertensive effects of the drug may be enhanced in the postsympathectomy patient. It should be borne in mind that hypersensitivity reactions are more likely to occur in patients with a history of allergy or bronchial asthma. The possibility of exacerbation or activation of systemic lupus erythematosus should be considered. For precautions regarding reserpine, see monograph on Reserpine.

Adverse Reactions: Anorexia, gastric irritation, nausea, vomiting, cramping, diarrhea, constipation, jaundice (intrahepatic cholestatic jaundice), pancreatitis, hyperglycemia, glycosuria, CNS, hematologic, dermatologic and hypersensitivity reactions, orthostatic hypotension (may be potentiated by alcohol, barbiturates or narcotics), muscle spasm, weakness, restlessness have been reported. For other adverse reactions, see monograph on Reserpine.

Dosage and Administration: *Orally,* 1 or 2 tablets once daily or 1 tablet twice daily; if necessary 3 or 4 tablets daily. With reserpine: initially 3 to 4 tablets daily for not more than 2 weeks. For maintenance, 1 or 2 tablets once daily.

Availability:
HYDROMOX® Tablets, 50 mg in bottles of 100 and 500. **(Lederle)**
HYDROMOX R Tablets, 50 mg with reserpine, 0.125 mg in bottles of 100 and 500. **(Lederle)**

QUINIDINE

Description: Quinidine is an alkaloid obtained from various species of Cinchona and their hybrids, or prepared from quinine. It is available as the gluconate, polygalacturonate and sulfate salts. These salts have a bitter taste; their solutions slowly acquire a brownish tint on exposure to light, and may undergo spontaneous crystallization. Quinidine polygalacturonate is a polymer of quinidine and polygalacturonic acid, and occurs as a creamy-white or tannish-white, amorphous powder very slightly soluble in water and insoluble in alcohol. It disintegrates slowly in the gastrointestinal tract and is absorbed as free quinidine.

The action of quinidine in preventing aberrant cardiac rhythms of atrial and ventricular origin resides in its ability to (1) depress excitability of cardiac muscle, (2) slow the rate of spontaneous rhythm, (3) decrease vagal tone, and (4) prolong conduction and effective refractory period. Although the precise mechanism by which quinidine acts is not fully understood, its effects on cardiac rhythm appear to be similar to those of procainamide. Also, its effects are enhanced by potassium and reduced by low plasma levels of the ion.

Following oral administration, it is readily absorbed from the gastrointestinal tract reaching maximal effect in 1 to 3 hours and maintaining therapeutic activity for 6 to 8 or more hours. The usual effective blood levels for quinidine range from 3 to 6 mg/liter of plasma; those above 8 mg/liter are sure to produce toxic reactions. Approximately 60 to 80% of the drug is bound to plasma proteins; up to 60% is excreted in the urine within 24 hours.

Indications: Restoration of normal rhythm in premature atrial and ventricular contractions, paroxysmal tachycardia of atrial or atrioventricular junctional origin, atrial flutter, paroxysmal atrial fibrillation, established atrial fibrillation when therapy is appropriate, and paroxysmal ventricular tachycardia when not associated with complete heart block. May also be used as maintenance therapy after electrical conversion of atrial fibrillation and/or flutter. Parenteral quinidine is indicated (1) when the patient with ectopic tachycardia cannot take medication by mouth because of vomiting or unconsciousness and (2) when, in the presence of very rapid heart action (especially ventricular tachycardia), it is imperative that the therapeutic effect of quinidine be obtained as quickly as possible. In the absence of an emergency, quinidine should be given orally.

Contraindications: Hypersensitivity or idiosyncrasy to quinidine or to other derivatives of cinchona, in the presence of intraventricular conduction defects, atrioventricular block, aberrant impulses and abnormal rhythms due to escape mechanisms.

Warnings: In the treatment of atrial flutter, reversion to sinus rhythm may be preceded by a progressive reduction in the degree of A-V block to a 1:1 ratio and resulting in extremely rapid ventricular rate. Quinidine has been reported to increase the hypoprothrombinemic effect of the oral anticoagulants and has been implicated in the production of frank hemorrhage on chronic oral anticoagulation. It has also been implicated as potentiating both depolarizing and nondepolarizing neuromuscular blocking agents. Acetazolamide, bicarbonate and other agents which alkalinize the urine may enhance renal tubular reabsorption of quinidine and thus could lead to increased quinidine serum levels. Concurrent administration of phenobarbital or phenytoin may significantly reduce the serum half-life of quinidine; therefore, when adding or reducing these agents, quinidine dosage adjustments may be necessary. The use of quinidine during pregnancy should be reserved only for those cases where the benefits outweigh the possible hazards to the mother and fetus.

Precautions: Parenteral quinidine should be given with extreme caution in the presence of atrioventricular block or in the absence of atrial activity. Quinidine is more hazardous in patients with extensive myocardial damage than it is in patients with a normal heart but who may experience cardiac arrhythmias. The use of quinidine in digitalis-induced arrhythmia is extremely dangerous because the cardiac glycoside may already have caused serious impairment of the intracardiac conduction system; patients must be observed closely. Frequent or continuous electrocardiograms are desirable, especially during intravenous injection, in order to detect any change in rate or rhythm. Administration of the drug must be discontinued when any one of the following occurs: (1) side effects of more than trivial nature, (2) restoration of sinus rhythm, (3) prolongation of the QRS complex in excess of 25% beyond that observed prior to the injection, (4) disappearance of the P waves, and (5) decrease in heart rate to 120 beats/minute. The presence of heart block, congestive failure, or digitalis intoxication makes the use of quinidine hazardous. The danger that a thrombus may be dislodged from the atrium, when longstanding atrial fibrillation is converted to regular rhythm, is a possibility.

Adverse Reactions: Patients should be carefully observed for signs of toxicity or idiosyncrasy manifested by nausea, vomiting, diarrhea, and increased urge to defecate or urinate, abdominal cramps, dizziness, cold sweat, respiratory distress including temporary cessation of respiration; cinchonism with disturbances of hearing and vision (not usually sufficient reason for terminating quinidine therapy); cutaneous flushing with intense pruritus; acute hemolytic anemia; hypothrombinemia; thrombocytopenic purpura; agranulocytosis; localized edema; headache; fever; apprehension; excitement; confusion; delirium, syncope; angioedema; acute asthmatic episode; vascular collapse; coma and death. Cases of quinidine-induced hypoprothrombinemic hemorrhage in patients on prolonged anticoagulant drug therapy have been reported. Too rapid injection may cause a fall in blood pressure. Large doses may have a deleterious effect on the heart and result in heart block or standstill in diastole.

Dosage and Administration: *Orally: For premature atrial and ventricular contractions,* the recommended adult dosage is 200 to 300 mg 3 or 4 times daily. *For paroxysmal supraventricular tachycardia,* 400 to 600 mg every 2 or 3 hours. *For conversion of atrial fibrillation,* generally 200 mg every 2 or 3 hours for 5 to 8 doses followed by a daily increase in the individual dose until sinus rhythm is restored or toxic effects appear. The total daily dose should not exceed 3 to 4 gm in any regimen. It is recommended that prior to quinidine administration, the ventricular rate and congestive failure, if present, should be brought under control by digitalis therapy. For maintenance, 200 to 300 mg 3 or 4 times daily. Extended-release tablets may be given every 8 or 12 hours. Gastrointestinal symptoms can be minimized by giving the drug with food. *Intramuscularly:* Initially, 600 mg followed by 400 mg every 2 hours if necessary. The amount of each dose must be gauged by the effect of the preceding dose. *Intravenously:* 330 to 750 mg depending upon the extent of the arrhythmia, administered at a rate of 1 ml/min.

Availability:

Quinidine Gluconate

QUINAGLUTE® Dura Tabs® (extended release tablets), 324 mg in bottles of 100 and 250 and in unit-dose packages of 100. **(Cooper)**

QUINIDINE GLUCONATE Injection, 80 mg/ml in ampuls of 10 ml. **(Lilly)**

Quinidine Polygalacturonate

CARDIOQUIN® Tablets, 275 mg equivalent to 200 mg of quinidine sulfate in bottles of 50 and 500. **(Purdue Frederick)**

Quinidine Sulfate

CIN-QUIN™: **(Rowell)**

Capsules, 200 mg in bottles of 100 and 1000; 300 mg in bottles of 100 and 500 and in unit-dose packages of 100.

Tablets, 100, 200 and 300 mg in bottles of 100 and 1000 and in unit-dose packages of 100.

QUINIDEX® Extentabs® (extended-release tablets), 300 mg in bottles of 100 and 250. **(Robins)**

QUINIDINE SULFATE Tablets, 200 mg in bottles of 1000. **(Beecham)**
QUINIDINE SULFATE Tablets, 200 mg in bottles of 100 and 1000 and in unit-dose packages of 90 and 120. **(ICN)**
QUINIDINE SULFATE Tablets, 200 mg in bottles of 100 and 1000 and in unit-dose packages of 5000 (50 × 100). **(Lederle)**
QUINIDINE SULFATE: **(Lilly)**
Pulvules® (Capsules), 200 mg in bottles of 100.
Tablets, 200 mg in bottles of 100 and 1000 and in individual blister-strips in cartons of 100.
QUINIDINE SULFATE Tablets, 200 mg in bottles of 100 and 1000. **(McKesson)**
QUINIDINE SULFATE Tablets, 200 mg in bottles of 100 and 1000 and in unit-dose packages of 100. **(Parke-Davis)**
QUINIDINE SULFATE Tablets, 200 mg in bottles of 1000 and in unit-dose cartons of 100; 300 mg in bottles of 100 and 1000 and in unit-dose packages of 100. **(Philips Roxane)**
QUINORA® Tablets, 200 and 300 mg in bottles of 100 and 1000. **(Key Pharm.)**
SK-QUINIDINE SULFATE™ Tablets, 200 mg in bottles of 100 and 500. **(Smith Kline & French)**

RABIES VACCINE

Description: Rabies vaccine is a sterile suspension of killed, fixed virus of rabies. The virus is obtained from the tissues of duck embryos, that have been infected with fixed rabies virus. Although beta-propiolactone has been added as a virucidal agent, it does not remain in the final product since it is hydrolyzed to nontoxic substances. The vaccine contains a suitable preservative. It has been reported to contain little or none of the paralytic factor said to be present in vaccines obtained from brain tissue, thereby significantly reducing the possibility of neurologic adverse effects.

Because of the protracted incubation period of rabies in individuals (2 weeks to several months), there usually is sufficient time for the development of immunity if the vaccine is administered promptly. It has been demonstrated that this vaccine produces antibodies in patients within 10 to 15 days after initiating a course of treatment.

Indications: Prevention of clinical symptoms of rabies in individuals bitten by animals known, or for valid reasons suspected, to be rabid, and for prophylactic immunization in high-risk individuals likely to be exposed to rabid animals.

Precautions: The vaccine should be used cautiously in patients known to be allergic to chicken or duck eggs or protein. Adrenocorticotropin and adrenal corticosteroids should not be given to patients who have been exposed to infectious agents (e.g., rabies) for which no satisfactory antimicrobial therapy is available. May be used during pregnancy if the patient is suspected of or of having contacted rabies, although safe use has not been established.

Adverse Reactions: Local reactions to vaccines of duck origin are less frequent and somewhat less severe than those seen with vaccines of brain origin. Tenderness at the injection site is common. Varying degrees of local erythema and induration have been observed; these reactions tend to appear from the 6th to the 10th day of treatment but may occur after each inoculation. Subsequent injections are likely to cause flareups at the sites of previous inoculations. Regional lymphadenopathy may occur as may sensitivity or anaphylactic reactions in patients sensitive to protein of foreign origin. Urticaria, respiratory distress (including dyspnea and bronchospasm), and gastrointestinal disorders (abdominal cramps, nausea, vomiting, and diarrhea) have been reported. Epinephrine may be helpful in controlling these complications. Patients with a history of allergy should be tested for hypersensitivity before the vaccine is administered. The development of fever, malaise and drowsiness suggests close surveillance of the patient. Minor neurological reactions, such as headache, photophobia, paresthesias, listlessness, malaise, and increased fatigability, have been reported. Rarely noted were transverse myelitis, cranial or peripheral palsy, and encephalitis; however, in the event these occur, the vaccine should be discontinued.

Dosage and Administration: *Subcutaneously,* in the outer aspect of the upper arm. *For preexposure immunoprophylaxis,* inject 1 ml every week for 3 weeks followed by a booster dose of 1 ml in 5 to 6 months after the third injection. Another method is to inject 1 ml every month for 2 months followed by a booster dose of 1 ml in 7 months. *For postexposure immuni-*

zation, usually 1 dose daily for 14 days. More intense treatment is indicated for bites associated with a relatively short incubation period (head and neck), e.g., 2 doses daily for 7 consecutive days followed by 1 dose daily for 7 consecutive days making a total of 21 doses. It is recommended that 3 supplemental doses of the vaccine should be given on the 10th, 20th and 90th day after completion of the 14-day course.

Availability:
RABIES VACCINE (duck ombryo origin), Dried Killed Virus, in single-dose vials with diluent in cartons of 7. **(Lilly)**

RAUWOLFIA SERPENTINA

Description: Rauwolfia serpentina is obtained from the dried root of a family of tropical and semitropical plants related to oleander and periwinkle. A number of related alkaloids have been isolated from rauwolfia such as reserpine, rescinnamine, deserpidine, and a synthetic analog syrosingopine that is prepared from reserpine by hydrolysis and reesterification.

Rauwolfia serpentina probably produces its antihypertensive effects through depletion of tissue stores of epinephrine and norepinephrine from peripheral sites. It lowers blood pressure and slows the pulse rate. These effects are delayed but sustained, and sudden drops and peaks in pressure are avoided. By contrast, its sedative and tranquilizing properties are thought to be related to depletion of 5-hydroxytryptamine from the cerebral areas. It alleviates such common hypertensive symptoms as anxiety, headaches, and palpitations. It does not appear to be habit-forming and tolerance has not been reported.

Indications: Treatment of mild essential hypertension, and as adjunctive therapy with other antihypertensive agents in the more severe forms of hypertension. Also for the relief of symptoms in agitated psychotic states such as schizophrenia, primarily in those individuals unable to tolerate phenothiazine derivative or those who also require antihypertensive medication. Combinations with thiazide diuretics and potassium chloride are indicated in patients who are not adequately benefited by rauwolfia alone; in hypertensive patients who show signs of congestive heart failure and edema, and in patients in whom an immediate lowering of blood pressure is essential.

Contraindications: Hypersensitivity to rauwolfia serpentina or its analogues, especially in cases where a past history of bronchial asthma or allergy is present; in patients who are mentally depressed, particularly those with suicidal tendencies; active peptic ulcer or ulcerative colitis, and in patients undergoing electroconvulsive therapy.

Warnings: Extreme caution should be exercised in treating patients with a history of mental depression. The drug should be withdrawn at the first sign of despondency, early morning insomnia, loss of appetite, impotence, or self depreciation. Drug-induced depression may persist for several months following withdrawal of the medication and may be severe enough to result in suicide. When prescribed for pregnant patients, the potential benefits of the drug should be weighed against the possible adverse effects on the fetus. The hazards of using rauwolfia preparations include increased respiratory secretions, nasal congestion, cyanosis and anorexia in infants born to mothers treated with this drug. Rauwolfia preparations cross the placental barrier and appear in cord blood and breast milk.

Precautions: Because rauwolfia preparations increase gastrointestinal motility and secretion, this drug should be used cautiously in patients with a history of peptic ulcer, ulcerative colitis, or gallstones where biliary colic may be precipitated. Patients receiving high dosages should be observed carefully at regular intervals to detect possible reactivation of peptic ulcer. Caution should also be exercised when treating hypertensive patients with renal insufficiency since they adjust poorly to lowered blood pressure levels. Special care is deemed essential when rauwolfia serpentina is used together with digitalis or quinidine, since cardiac arrhythmias have occurred with rauwolfia derivatives. Preoperative withdrawal of rauwolfia alkaloids does not insure that circulatory instability will not occur. It is important that the anesthesiologist be aware of the patient's drug intake and consider this in the overall management, since hypotension has occurred in patients receiving rauwolfia preparations. Anticholinergic and/or adrenergic drugs such as metaraminol or norepinephrine have been employed to treat adverse vagocirculatory effects.

Adverse Reactions: The following reactions are usually reversible and tend to disappear when the drug is discontinued. *Gastrointestinal:* hypersecretion, nausea, vomiting, anorexia, and diarrhea. *CNS:* drowsiness, depression, nervousness, paradoxical anxiety, nightmares, rare parkinsonian syndrome, CNS sensitization manifested by dull sensorium, deafness, glaucoma, uveitis, and optic atrophy. *Cardiovascular:* angina-like symptoms, arrhythmias, particularly when used concurrently with digitalis or quinidine, and bradycardia. *Other:* nasal congestion, pruritus, rash, dryness of mouth, dizziness, headache, dyspnea, purpura, impotence or decreased libido, dysuria, muscular aches, conjunctival injection, weight gain, and extrapyramidal tract symptoms. Rarely noted was water retention with edema in patients with hypertensive vascular disease; this condition generally clears with cessation of therapy, or with the administration of a diuretic agent.

For further information, see monographs on the individual components.

Dosage and Administration: *Orally. For hypertension.* The initial adult dose is two to four 100 mg tablets daily in single or divided doses; this dosage may be adjusted within the range of 50 to 300 mg in single or divided doses daily for maintenance. *For emotional disorders,* 200 mg daily; for maintenance, 50 to 300 mg daily given in single or divided doses. In adjusting the dosage, it is important to take into account the fact that results of therapy tend to appear slowly. Dosage for pediatric, adolescent and elderly patients should be proportionately less. Coadministration with ganglionic blocking agents, guanethidine, veratrum, hydralazine, methyldopa, chlorthalidone, or thiazides necessitates careful titration of dosage with each agent.

Availability:

Rauwolfia Serpentina

RAUDIXIN® Tablets, 50 and 100 mg in bottles of 100 and 1000. **(Squibb)**

RAUWOLFIA SERPENTINA Tablets, 50 and 100 mg in bottles of 1000 and in single-unit packages of 100. **(Lederle)**

w/Thiazides and Potassium Chloride

RAUTRAX® Tablets, 50 mg with flumethiazide, 400 mg and potassium chloride, 400 mg in bottles of 100. **(Squibb)**

RAUTRAX®-N Tablets, 50 mg with bendroflumethiazide, 4 mg and potassium chloride, 400 mg in bottles of 100 and 1000. **(Squibb)**

RAUTRAX-N Modified Tablets, 50 mg with bendroflumethiazide, 2 mg and potassium chloride, 400 mg in bottles of 100. **(Squibb)**

RAUZIDE® Tablets, 50 mg with bendroflumethiazide, 4 mg in bottles of 100 and 1000. **(Squibb)**

RECTAL MEDICONE-HC

Description: An anesthetic, antiinflammatory, antipruritic and antibacterial preparation. Each suppository contains:

Hydrocortisone acetate	10 mg
Benzocaine	130 mg
Oxyquinoline sulfate	16 mg
Zinc oxide	200 mg
Menthol	9 mg
Balsam Peru	65 mg

in a cocoa butter and vegetable and petroleum oil base.

Indications: Symptomatic therapy in hemorrhoids, acute and chronic proctitis, postoperative edema, cryptitis, pruritus ani and inflamed postoperative scar tissue. Provides temporary relief of pain, burning and itching.

Contraindications: Tuberculosis of the rectum.

Precautions: A thorough proctologic diagnosis should be made when considering the use of hydrocortisone. Caution is suggested if the patient is on other corticosteroid therapy or if infection is present or if rash or irritation develops.

Dosage and Administration: *Rectally.* Initially, 1 suppository twice daily for 3 to 6 days. For maintenance, a suitable preparation without hydrocortisone is recommended.

Availability:
RECTAL MEDICONE®-HC Suppositories (foil-wrapped) in cartons of 12. **(Medicone)**

REGULAR INSULIN: see The Insulins

RESCINNAMINE

Chemical Name: 3,4,5-Trimethoxycinnamic acid ester of methyl reserpate.

Description: Rescinnamine is a pure, crystalline alkaloid derived from the roots of a species of Rauwolfia of the dogbane family. It occurs as white, needle-shaped crystals that are insoluble in water but moderately soluble in various organic solvents.

The pharmacologic actions of rescinnamine are virtually identical to those of the parent compound *Rauwolfia serpentina.* It is readily absorbed from the gastrointestinal tract. Rescinnamine is characterized by a slow onset of action and a sustained effect. Both its cardiovascular and CNS effects may persist following withdrawal of the drug.

Indications: Treatment of mild essential hypertension. The drug is also probably effective as an adjunct to other antihypertensive agents in the more severe forms of hypertension.

For further information on the actions, uses and precautions, see the monograph on Rauwolfia Serpentina.

Dosage and Administration: *Orally.* Dosage is regulated depending upon the patient's response. To provide hypotensive or tranquilizing effects, or both, the recommended initial dosage is 0.5 mg 2 times daily. If necessary, the dosage may be increased gradually. Cautious increase of dosage up to 2 mg daily at increments of 0.25 mg daily, may be attempted. Maintenance dosage may vary from 0.25 to 0.5 mg daily. Higher doses should be used cautiously because the incidence of serious mental depression and other side effects may be increased considerably. Coadministration of rescinnamine with ganglionic blocking agents, guanethidine, veratrum, hydralazine, methyldopa, chlorthalidone, or thiazides necessitates careful titration of dosage of each agent.

Availability:
MODERIL® Tablets, 0.25 mg (yellow) and 0.5 mg (salmon) in bottles of 100. **(Pfizer)**

RESERPINE

Description: Reserpine is a pure alkaloid derived from the root of species of *Rauwolfia* or produced synthetically. It occurs as a white, pale buff or yellowish, odorless, crystalline powder insoluble in water, freely soluble in acetic acid, and very slightly soluble in alcohol. Aqueous solutions in polyethylene glycol darken on exposure to light.

In addition to sharing the clinical uses of oral rauwolfia derivatives, reserpine may be given parenterally for the treatment of hypertensive crises or encephalopathy. Following intravenous administration, reserpine begins to exert its effect within 1 hour, persisting for 6 to 8 hours. The onset is slower following intramuscular injection, but the effects persist longer (about 10 to 12 hours). Both its cardiovascular and CNS effects usually continue following withdrawal of the drug.

Indications: Treatment of mild essential hypertension. It is useful as adjunctive therapy with other antihypertensive agents in the more severe forms of hypertension. In addition, it is indicated for the relief of symptoms in agitated psychotic states such as schizophrenia, primarily in those individuals who are unable to tolerate phenothiazine derivatives or those who also require antihypertensive medication. Parenteral administration of reserpine is indicated in the treatment of hypertensive emergencies, such as acute hypertensive encephalopathy, in which it is desired to reduce the blood pressure promptly. Also, to initiate treatment in psychiatric patients who are unable to accept oral medication or to control symptoms of extreme agitation.

Contraindications: Hypersensitivity to reserpine; in patients who are mentally depressed, especially those with suicidal tendencies, active peptic ulcer or ulcerative colitis, and in patients receiving electroconvulsive therapy. Parenteral reserpine should not be used if the patient is under treatment for hypertension.

Warnings: Extreme caution should be exercised in treating patients with a history of mental depression. The drug should be withdrawn at the first sign of despondency, early-morning insomnia, loss of appetite, impotence, or self-deprecation. Drug-induced depression may persist for several months after the drug has been discontinued and may be severe enough to result in suicide. Electroconvulsive therapy should not be given concurrently with reserpine since severe and even fatal reactions have been reported. Since the safety for its use during pregnancy has not been established, reserpine may be used in pregnant patients only when its use is deemed essential to the welfare of the patient. Increased respiratory tract secretions, nasal congestion, cyanosis, and anorexia may occur in infants born to mothers treated with reserpine since this drug is known to cross the placental membrane and to appear in cord blood and breast milk.

Precautions: Reserpine may increase gastrointestinal motility and secretion, and it may precipitate biliary colic in patients with gallstones. The drug should, therefore, be used cautiously in patients with a history of peptic ulcer, ulcerative colitis or other gastrointestinal disorders. Due to the effect of catecholamine depletion, special care should be exercised when treating patients with a history of bronchial asthma; such patients are more likely to be hypersensitive, and their conditions may become aggravated. Hypertensive patients with renal insufficiency require special care, since they may adjust poorly to lowered blood pressure levels. Caution is deemed essential when reserpine is used together with digitalis or quinidine, since cardiac arrhythmias have occurred with rauwolfia derivatives. Concurrent use of rauwolfia derivatives and guanethidine may cause bradycardia, mental depression, and postural hypotension. Administration of reserpine during therapy with tricyclic antidepressant drugs has been shown to produce a stimulating effect in some depressed patients. Preoperative withdrawal of reserpine does not assure that circulatory instability will not occur. It is important that the anesthesiologist be aware of the patient's drug intake and consider this in the overall management, since hypotension has occurred in patients receiving rauwolfia preparations. Anticholinergic and/or adrenergic drugs such as metaraminol or norepinephrine have been employed to treat adverse vagocirculatory effects.

Adverse Reactions: When they occur, reactions usually are reversible and disappear when the drug is withdrawn. *Gastrointestinal:* sialorrhea, increased motility and secretion, nausea, vomiting, anorexia, aggravation of peptic ulcer or ulcerative colitis, diarrhea. *Cardiovascular:* angina-like syndrome, ectopic arrhythmias, particularly when used concurrently with digitalis, and bradycardia. *CNS:* mental depression, drowsiness, nervousness, paradoxical anxiety, nightmares which may be an early sign of mental depression, atypical parkinsonian syndrome and other extrapyramidal symptoms, CNS sensitization manifested by dull sensorium, Parkinson's syndrome (rare), deafness, glaucoma, uveitis and optic atrophy. *Dermatologic-Hypersensitivity:* pruritus, skin rash, dry mouth, dizziness, headache, syncope, purpura due to thrombocytopenia, asthma in susceptible individuals. *Miscellaneous:* nasal congestion, weight gain, impotence or decreased libido, increased susceptibility to the common cold, dysuria, conjunctival injection, dyspnea and muscular aches, rarely, water retention with edema. Impairment of consciousness may occur with acute overdosage and may range from drowsiness to coma. Flushing of the skin, conjunctival injection, and pupillary constriction are to be expected. Hypotension, hypothermia and central respiratory depression may also occur. Overdosage requires symptomatic and supportive treatment which may include gastric lavage.

Dosage and Administration: It is best to take the drug after meals in order to minimize the possible discomfort due to increased gastric secretion. The parenteral form should be reserved for patients who cannot take the drug by mouth or those in whom prompt results are imperative. *Orally. For hypertension,* the initial dose is 0.5 mg daily for 1 or 2 weeks; for maintenance, 0.1 to 0.25 mg daily. *Intramuscularly.* An initial dose of 0.5 to 1 mg is followed by doses of 2 and 4 mg at intervals of 3 hours until the blood pressure falls to the desired level. If the 4 mg dose is ineffective, other antihypertensive agents should be used. *For psychiatric disorders,* the initial *oral* dose is 0.5 mg with a range of 0.1 to 1 mg adjusted according to the patient's response. The usual *intramuscular* dose for psychiatric emergencies is from 2.5 to 5 mg, following a small initial dose to test patient responsiveness. Concomitant administration of reserpine with ganglionic blocking agents, guanethidine, veratrum, hydralazine, methyldopa, chlorthalidone, or thiazides necessitates careful titration of dosage with each agent.

Availability:

Reserpine

LEMISERP® Tablets, 0.25 mg (purple) in bottles of 1000. **(Lemmon)**
RAU-SED® Tablets, 0.25 mg in bottles of 1000 and 5000. **(Squibb)**
RESERPINE Tablets, 0.1 and 0.2 mg in bottles of 100 and 1000. **(ICN)**
RESERPINE Tablets, 0.1 and 0.25 mg in bottles of 1000 and in unit-dose packages of 100. **(Lederle)**
RESERPINE Tablets, 0.1 and 0.25 mg in bottles of 1000. **(McKesson)**
RESERPOID® Tablets, 0.25 mg in bottles of 100 and 1000. **(Upjohn)**
SANDRIL®: **(Lilly)**
Injection, 2.5 mg/ml in vials of 10 ml.
Tablets, 0.1 mg in bottles of 100; 0.25 mg in bottles of 100 and 1000.
SERPASIL®: **(Ciba)**
Elixir, 0.2 mg/4 ml in bottles of 1 pint.
Injection, 2.5 mg/ml in ampuls of 2 ml and in multiple-dose vials of 10 ml.
Tablets, 0.1 mg in bottles of 100, 500 and 1000; 0.25 mg in bottles of 100, 500, 1000 and 5000; 1 mg in bottles of 100.
SK-RESERPINE™ Tablets, 0.25 mg in bottles of 1000. **(Smith Kline & French)**
VIO-SERPINE™ Tablets, 0.1 and 0.2 mg in bottles of 100 and 1000. **(Rowell)**

RETICULOGEN

Description: Each ml contains vitamin B-12 activity (derived from liver) equiv. to cyanocobalamin, 20 mcg; thiamine hydrochloride, 5 mg. Reticulogen Fortified has the same formula except that an additional 20 mcg of cyanocobalamin (vitamin B-12 crystalline) are added.

Indications: Treatment of pernicious anemia and related macrocytic anemias; also to prevent the neurological manifestations of pernicious anemia.

Contraindications: Hypersensitivity to any of the components.

Precautions: Patients showing extensive neurological involvement or other degenerative changes usually require more than the average dose. Epinephrine should be readily available to offset an unexpected or unusual response.

Adverse Reactions: Pain and tenderness at the site of injection, fever, weakness, increased pulse rate and perspiration, drop in systolic pressure, pruritus, urticaria, and hypersensitivity reactions which may result in anaphylaxis.

Dosage and Administration: *Intramuscularly,* 0.5 ml daily for 3 successive days. For maintenance, 0.5 ml every 7 to 10 days is usually sufficient to maintain an adequate red-blood cell response.

Availability:
RETICULOGEN®/RETICULOGEN FORTIFIED Injection in ampuls of 5 ml. **(Lilly)**

Rh_0(D) IMMUNE GLOBULIN (HUMAN)

Description: A sterile solution of anti Rh_0(D) gamma globulin concentrated by cold alcohol fractionation from the venous (non-placental) blood of carefully selected donors who are nonreactive for hepatitis B surface antigen, and titrated against a DBS (Division of Biologic Standards) Reference Rh_0(D) human immune globulin. It contains approximately 16.5% gamma globulin dissolved in 0.2 to 0.3 M glycine and preserved with 1:10,000 thimerosal. The pH is adjusted with sodium carbonate.

Since Rh_0(D) hemolytic disease of the newborn is the result of the active immunization of an

Rho(D) negative mother following a previous delivery of an Rho(D) positive child, the solution acts by suppressing the stimulation of active immunity by fetal Rho(D) positive erythrocytes that may enter the mother's circulation at the time of delivery.

Indications: For the prevention of Rho(D) hemolytic disease of the newborn. Administration is recommended within 72 hours after the birth of an Rho(D) or D^u positive baby to an Rho(D) or D^u negative mother, or after a miscarriage of an Rh-positive fetus. In order for this agent to be effective, the newborn should be Rho(D) or D^u positive and should present a negative direct Coombs' test, and the mother must not have been immunized by the Rho(D) or D^u positive factor from a previous pregnancy, or by miscarriage of an Rh-positive fetus (if the blood type of the fetus is not known and cannot be determined, it should be assumed that it is Rho(D) positive), or by accidental transfusion with Rho(D) positive blood to an Rho(D) negative patient.

Contraindications: Should not be administered to an Rho(D) or D^u positive individual, to an Rho(D) or D^u negative individual who has received Rho(D) positive blood, or to anyone who has been actively immunized to the Rho(D) blood factor. **This agent should never be administered to the infant.**

Precautions: This preparation should *never* be administered intravenously, and should be given *only to the postpartum mother.* Also, it should not be administered without first performing a crossmatch test. (See package literature.)

Adverse Reactions: Noted were soreness at the injection site, and low grade fever. Repeated injections rarely caused sensitization. Serum hepatitis has not been reported.

Dosage and Administration: *Intramuscularly* **only.** Inject the entire content of the vial into the postpartum mother or in women undergoing an abortion or miscarrage up to 12 weeks gestation.

Availability:
GAMULIN® Rh Solution in vials containing a single dose and packaged with a disposable 2-ml syringe and a dropper vial of a 1:1000 dilution for the crossmatch test. **(Parke-Davis)**
HypRho®-D Solution in vials containing a single dose and packaged with a dropper-filled vial of a 1:1000 dilution for the crossmatch test. **(Cutter)**
MICRhoGAM™ Solution in vials containing a single dose and packaged with a vial of a 1:1000 solution for the cross-match test. **(Ortho)**
RhoGAM® Solution in vials containing a single dose and packaged with a dropper vial of a 1:1000 dilution for the crossmatch test. **(Ortho)**

RIFAMPIN

Chemical Name: 3-(4-Methyl-1-piperazinyliminomethyl) rifamycin SV.

Description: Rifampin is a semisynthetic derivative of rifamycin B, an antibiotic obtained from the fermentation of *Streptomyces mediterranei.* Laboratory studies, in vitro as well as in vivo, have shown the drug to be active against the tubercle bacilli. It is also active against a wide range of gram-negative and gram-positive organisms, and appears to inhibit some viruses when administered in large doses.

In susceptible cells rifampin appears to repress DNA-dependent RNA polymerase activity. It exerts its therapeutic effect primarily by interacting with bacterial RNA polymerase without suppressing the mammalian enzyme. Cross resistance has been observed to occur only with other rifamycins.

Peak blood levels are attained between 2 and 4 hours following the oral administration of a 600-mg dose. The average peak value is 7 mcg/ml; however, the peak level may vary from 4 to 32 mcg/ml. Distribution occurs throughout the body and the drug is present in effective concentrations in many organs and body fluids, including the cerebrospinal fluid.

In normal individuals the biological half-life of rifampin in the blood is approximately 3 hours; however, it may be decreased in patients receiving isoniazid concomitantly who are slow inactivators of the drug. Large quantities of the antibiotic are excreted in the bile; urinary concentrations are low.

Oral doses of 150 to 250 mg/kg/day given to pregnant rodents produced an increase in congenital malformations, primarily spina bifida and cleft palate, in the offspring of these animals. The possible teratogenic effect on the fetus of pregnant patients should be carefully considered.

Indications: Treatment of pulmonary tuberculosis, rifampin must always be used in conjunction with one or more antituberculous agents—frequently used regimens are rifampin with isoniazid or ethambutol or both. In asymptomatic carriers of *Neisseria meningitidis,* rifampin is used to eliminate meningococci from the nasopharynx; it is *not* indicated for the treatment of meningococcal infection. **Note:** To avoid indiscriminate use of the drug, diagnostic laboratory procedures, including serotyping and susceptibility testing, should be performed in order to establish the carrier state and the correct treatment. To preserve the usefulness of rifampin in the treatment of asymptomatic meningococcal carriers, it is recommended that the drug be reserved for situations in which the risk of meningococcal meningitis is high. Since small numbers of resistant cells, even when present within large populations of susceptible cells, can rapidly become the predominating type, culture and susceptibility tests should be performed in the event of persistent positive cultures.

Contraindications: A history of hypersensitivity reaction to any of the rifamycins.

Warnings: Rifampin is a potentially hepatotoxic drug. Fatalities associated with jaundice have occurred in patients with liver disease and in those receiving rifampin concomitantly with other hepatotoxic agents. In the presence of liver disease, the benefits of the drug must be weighed carefully against the risk of further liver damage, and periodic evaluation of liver function is mandatory. The effect of combinations of rifampin with other antituberculous drugs on the human fetus is not known; therefore, the possible teratogenic potential in women of childbearing age should be carefully weighed against the anticipated benefits of therapy. Since this drug has been reported to cross the placenta and appear in cord blood, neonates of rifampin-treated mothers should be carefully observed for any evidence of adverse effects.

Precautions: Rifampin is not recommended for intermittent therapy; therefore, patients should be firmly advised not to interrupt the daily dosage regimen since renal hypersensitivity has been reported when therapy was resumed in such patients. The drug has been observed to increase the requirements for anticoagulant drugs of the coumarin type. This effect was not manifested until the fifth day following the initiation of treatment. The decrease in prothrombin time usually persists for 5 to 7 days; therefore, it is recommended that patients who are receiving anticoagulants should have daily evaluation of prothrombin time until the required dose of the anticoagulant has been established. Patients should be informed that rifampin and its metabolites may impart a red-orange color to the urine, feces, saliva, sputum, sweat, and tears. The effectiveness of oral contraceptives may be altered when rifampin is used together with at least one other antituberculous drug, thus an alternative contraceptive measure may need to be considered. Also reported was that combinations of rifampin and other antituberculous agents may affect the blood concentration of methadone, oral hypoglycemics, digitalis derivatives and corticosteroids; therefore, dosage adjustment of the interacting drugs is recommended.

Adverse Reactions: Intermittent exposure to rifampin generally produces more frequent aderse reactions. A "flu-like syndrome" is most often reported in patients taking the drug on an intermittent schedule. Gastrointestinal disturbances such as heartburn, epigastric distress, anorexia, nausea, vomiting, flatulence, cramps, and diarrhea have been noted. Headache, drowsiness, fatigue, menstrual disturbances, ataxia, dizziness, inability to concentrate, mental confusion, visual disturbances, muscular weakness, fever, pains in the extremities and generalized numbness have also been noted. Pruritus, urticaria, skin rashes, eosinophilia, sore mouth, and sore tongue have occasionally been encountered. Thrombocytopenia, transient leukopenia, hemolytic anemia, and decreased hemoglobin have been observed. Thrombocytopenia has occurred when rifampin and ethambutol were given concomitantly on an intermittent dose schedule twice weekly and in high doses. Elevation of BUN and serum uric acid have occurred and, rarely observed were hemolysis, hemoglobinuria, hematuria, renal insufficiency or acute renal failure. These complications are generally considered to be hypersensitivity reactions. Transient abnormalities in liver function tests (elevations of serum bilirubin, BSP, alkaline phosphatase, and serum transaminases) have been observed.

Nausea, vomiting, and increasing lethargy are signs and symptoms of overdosage. Actual unconsciousness may occur with severe hepatic involvement. These usually occur within a short time following ingestion. Liver enlargement, possibly with tenderness, can develop within a few hours after considerable overdosage and jaundice may develop rapidly. Also, direct and total bilirubin levels may increase rapidly and hepatic enzyme levels may be affected. A direct effect upon the hematopoietic system, electrolyte levels, or acid-base balance is unlikely. Other physical findings remain essentially normal. Treatment by gastric lavage followed by the use of absorbants, antiemetic and diuretic agents help to promote the excretion of the drug.

Dosage and Administration: *Orally.* Adults, 600 mg in a single daily dose. Children, 10 to 20 mg/kg of body weight; not to exceed 600 mg/day. Dosage for children under 5 years of age has not been determined. It is recommended that rifampin be administered once daily, either 1 hour before or 2 hours after a meal. In the treatment of *pulmonary tuberculosis,* the drug must be used in conjunction with at least one other antituberculous agent, and therapy should be continued until bacterial conversion and maximal improvement have occurred. Rifampin susceptibility powders are available for both direct and indirect methods of determining the susceptibility of strains of mycobacteria. The MIC's of susceptible clinical isolates when determined in 7H10 or other nonegg-containing media have ranged from 0.1 to 2 mcg/ml. In the treatment of *meningococcal carriers,* it is recommended that the drug be given once daily for 4 consecutive days. Susceptibility discs containing 5 mcg of rifampin are available for susceptibility testing of *N. meningitidis.*

Availability:
RIFADIN® Capsules, 300 mg in bottles of 30, 60 and 100, in unit-dose strip packages of 100 (50 x 2) and in convenience packages (1-week treatment folder) containing 14 capsules of rifampin, 300 mg and 7 tablets of isoniazid, 300 mg in cartons of 2 and 5 folders. **(Dow)**
RIFAMATE™ Capsules, 300 mg with isoniazid, 150 mg in bottles of 60. **(Dow)**
RIMACTANE® Capsules, 300 mg (opaque scarlet and caramel) in bottles of 30, 60 and 100. **(Ciba)**
RIMACTANE/INH in Dual Packs each containing 2 Rimactane 300 mg capsules and 1 INH (isoniazid) 300 mg tablet in cartons of 30 Dual Packs. **(Ciba)**
RIMACTAZID® Capsules, 300 mg with isoniazid, 150 mg in bottles of 60. **(Ciba)**

RO-BILE

Description: Each yellow tablet contains pepsin, 260 mg in the outer layer surrounding an enteric-coated core of enzyme concentrate (a specially-prepared pancreatin 4X NF, with added standardized lipase), 75 mg; ox bile extract, 100 mg; dehydrocholic acid, 30 mg, and belladonna extract, 8 mg.

Indications: Indigestion due to a deficiency of digestive enzymes and bile; relieves discomfort from overeating and over-ingestion of fats.

Contraindications: Biliary obstruction and hepatitis.

Precautions: If dryness of the mouth occurs, dosage should be decreased. Therapy with this formulation should be terminated if rapid pulse, dizziness or blurred vision develops. Use with caution in glaucoma.

Dosage and Administration: *Orally,* 1 or 2 tablets with meals, or after meals, as directed by the physician.

Availability:
RO-BILE™ Tablets in bottles of 100 and 1000. **(Rowell)**

ROBITUSSIN-DAC Ⓒ

Description: Contains in each 5 ml (teaspoonful):

Guaifenesin .... 100 mg

Pseudoephedrine hydrochloride .... 30 mg
Codeine phosphate .... 10 mg
with 1.4% alcohol in a palatable, aromatic vehicle.

Indications: A combination of an expectorant with a decongestant-antitussive agent recommended for the temporary relief of cough complicated by nasal and respiratory tract congestion as may occur with the common cold or with inhaled irritants.

Contraindications: Hypersensitivity to any of the ingredients, marked hypertension, hyperthyroidism, and concomitant use with MAO inhibitors or antihypertensive medication.

Warnings: Codeine phosphate may be habit-forming. Administer with caution to children under 2 years of age or to those taking other drugs; to patients with persistent or chronic cough such as occurs with smoking, asthma, emphysema or when cough is accompanied by excessive secretions; to patients with high blood pressure, heart disease, diabetes, chronic pulmonary disease or with shortness of breath; and in the presence of prostatic hypertrophy or glaucoma. Patients should be informed that the drug may cause or aggravate constipation. **Important Note:** Guaifenesin has been shown to produce a color interference with certain clinical laboratory determinations of 5-hydroxyindoleacetic acid (5-HIAA) and vanillylmandelic acid (VMA).

Adverse Reactions: Agitation, nervousness, dizziness, insomnia, palpitation or nausea may occur. In such instances, reduction in frequency and/or quantity of the dose is recommended.

Dosage and Administration: *Orally* every 4 hours. Adults, 1 or 2 teaspoonsful, not to exceed 12 teaspoonsful in a 24-hour period. Children 6 to 12 years of age, 1 teaspoonful, not to exceed 6 teaspoonsful in a 24-hour period; 2 to 6 years of age, ½ teaspoonful, not to exceed 3 teaspoonsful in a 24-hour period; children under 2 years of age, as directed by the physician.

Availability:
Ⓒ ROBITUSSIN®-DAC Syrup in bottles of 1 pint. **(Robins)**

RUBELLA AND MUMPS VIRUS VACCINE, LIVE

Description: The vaccine is prepared from Meyer and Parkman's attenuated strain of rubella virus, HPV-77, adapted to and propagated in duck embryo cell culture; and from the Jeryl Lynn (B level) mumps strain grown in cell cultures of chick embryos free of avian leukosis, according to the general procedures used to prepare Enders' measles virus vaccine, live, attenuated. The two viruses are mixed before being lyophilized. Each dose of reconstituted vaccine contains not less than 1000 $TCID_{50}$ of rubella virus vaccine, live and 5000 $TCID_{50}$ of mumps virus vaccine, live, expressed in terms of the assigned titer of the NIH reference rubella and mumps viruses.

Indications: Simultaneous immunization of susceptible children, ages 15 months to puberty, against rubella and mumps. However, it may be given as early as 12 months if that offers greater convenience in scheduling. Children under 1 year of age may retain maternal neutralizing antibodies (rubella and mumps) which may interfere with the immune response and, therefore, should *not* receive the vaccine.

Contraindications: Pregnant women or women who might become pregnant within 3 months following vaccination; hypersensitivity to chicken or duck, chicken or duck eggs or feathers, or to neomycin (each dose contains 25 mcg of neomycin); febrile respiratory illness or other active febrile infection; patients receiving therapy with ACTH, corticosteroids, irradiation, alkylating agents or antimetabolites; those with blood dyscrasias, leukemia, lymphomas of any type, or other malignancies affecting the bone-marrow or lymphatic system, and primary immunodeficiency states, including cellular immuno deficiencies, hypogammaglobulinemia, and dysgammaglobulinemia.

Precautions: Reports indicate that attenuated, live virus mumps vaccine may temporarily depress sensitivity to tuberculin skin tests for a period of 4 weeks or longer. Such testing, if contemplated, should precede administration of mumps vaccine to circumvent the possibility of a false-negative response. The vaccine should not be given less than 1 month before or after immunization with other *live* virus vaccines. Vaccination should be deferred for at least 3 months following blood transfusions or administration of more than 0.02 ml of immune serum globulin (human)/lb of body weight, or human plasma. There have been no reports of transmission of live attenuated mumps viruses from the individual vaccinated to susceptible contacts. Epinephrine should be available for immediate use in the event of an anaphylactoid reaction.

Adverse Reactions: These may include fever and rash; mild local reactions such as erythema, induration, tenderness, and regional lymphadenopathy; parotitis; thrombocytopenia and purpura; allergic reactions such as urticaria; arthritis, arthralgia and polyneuritis and, rarely, encephalitis and other nervous system reactions.

Dosage and Administration: *Subcutaneously only; never intramuscularly or intravenously.* After suitable cleansing of the injection site, the total volume of reconstituted vaccine should be injected into the outer aspect of the upper arm. For method of reconstitution and storage, see Rubella Virus Vaccine, Live.

Availability:
BIAVAX® (lyophilized) in single-dose vials with disposable syringe containing diluent.

(Merck Sharp & Dohme)

RUBELLA VIRUS VACCINE, LIVE

Description: This is a live-virus vaccine prepared from Meyer and Parkman's attenuated strain of rubella virus (HPV-77) adapted to and propagated in cell cultures of duck embryo origin.

The vaccine has induced hemagglutination-inhibiting antibody in an average of over 96% of susceptible children. Antibody levels, following immunization, have persisted for at least 5½ years without substantial decline. The pattern of antibody response closely resembles that observed for natural rubella, although the antibody level is lower than that following the natural infection. If this pattern continues, it will provide a basis for expectation that immunity following the vaccine will be permanent. However, continued surveillance will be required to demonstrate this point.

Indications: Immunization against rubella (German measles). It is indicated in children between 15 months of age and puberty. Should not be administered to infants less than 15 months of age. Also indicated for postpubertal males and females, and those following exposure to natural rubella. Women should be tested for susceptibility by means of the hemagglutination inhibition (HI) test.

Contraindications: Pregnancy; sensitivity to chicken or ducks or their eggs or feathers, or to neomycin (each dose contains 25 mcg of neomycin); any febrile respiratory illness or other active febrile infection, unless contracting rubella involves a greater risk (vaccination should be postponed until the patient has recovered); patients with malignancies, particularly those affecting the bone marrow or lymphatic systems, or those receiving therapy with corticosteroids, irradiation, alkylating agents or antimetabolites, because of their alteration of normal defense mechanisms; and primary immunodeficiency states, including cellular immune deficiencies, hypogammaglobulinemia, and dysgammaglobulinemia.

Precautions: Epinephrine should be readily available for immediate use in case of an anaphylactoid reaction. There is the theoretical possibility that excretion of the live attenuated rubella virus from the throats of vaccinated individuals, a common occurrence, may endanger a pregnant woman who comes in contact with such individuals. When the vaccine is given to women of childbearing age, pregnancy must be ruled out, and every precaution taken to prevent conception for at least 3 months. Other than children already exposed to natural rubella, administration of the vaccine after exposure may not prevent the illness. The vaccine should be given at least 1 month before or after, but not concurrently with, other elective immunizations, with the exception of trivalent poliovirus vaccine, live, oral, which may be administered simultaneously; vaccination should be deferred for at least 3 months following blood transfusions or administration of over 0.02 ml/lb of body weight of human immune serum globulin or human plasma. There is some evidence that the injection of immunizing agents during an epidemic of poliomyelitis may result, on rare occasions, in localized paralysis in the inoculated arm or leg of those who subsequently develop paralytic polio. This vaccine is not known to have been given under these conditions, nor have there been any reports of paralysis involving this vaccine. Since the vaccine may temporarily depress skin sensitivity to the tuberculin test, this test should be performed either before or simultaneous with the vaccine.

Adverse Reactions: Mild fever unrelated to the vaccine; local reactions such as erythema, induration, tenderness and regional lymphadenopathy, thrombocytopenia, purpura, urticaria, transient arthralgia and arthritis are noted more frequently in the adult female than in the prepubertal female or in the adult male. Also noted was transient polyneuropathy manifested by intermittent pain, muscle spasm, paresthesia and, very rarely, encephalitis.

Dosage and Administration: *Subcutaneously only; never intramuscularly or intravenously.* The total volume of reconstituted vaccine should be injected into the outer aspect of the upper arm, after suitably cleansing the injection site. Only the diluent supplied should be used to reconstitute the vaccine. To reconstitute, inject all of the diluent in the syringe into the vial of lyophilized vaccine, and agitate to ensure thorough mixing. Each dose of reconstituted vaccine contains not less than 1000 $TCID_{50}$ (tissue culture infectious doses) of rubella virus vaccine expressed in terms of the assigned titer of the NIH reference rubella vaccine. If not used immediately, the reconstituted vaccine should be refrigerated, or discarded if not used within 8 hours.

Availability:
MERUVAX® (lyophilized) in single-dose vials with disposable syringe containing diluent.

(Merck Sharp & Dohme)

RYNA-CX Ⓒ

Description: Each 5 ml (teaspoonful) of syrup contains:

Codeine phosphate	10 mg
Pseudoephedrine hydrochloride	30 mg
Guaifenesin	100 mg

Formulated in a clear color, cherry-vanilla-mint flavored demulcent base containing no sugar, dyes or alcohol. Provides antitussive, decongestant and expectorant actions.

Indications: Temporary relief of the concurrent symptoms of dry, nonreproductive cough and nasal congestion.

Contraindications: Hypersensitivity to any of the components.

Warnings: Codeine phosphate may be habit-forming, and may cause or aggravate constipation. This preparation should not be used, except under the advice and supervision of a physician, in children under 2 years of age or those taking other medication; in individuals with persistent or chronic cough such as occurs with smoking, asthma, emphysema, or when attended with excessive secretions; in patients with chronic pulmonary disease, shortness of breath, high blood pressure, heart disease, diabetes, or thyroid disease, as well as those taking drugs containing MAO inhibitors.

Precautions: If the cough persists for more than 1 week, tends to recur, or is accompanied by high fever, rash, or persistent headache, the drug should be discontinued and the physician consulted.

Adverse Reactions: Dosages exceeding the recommended schedule may cause nervousness, dizziness, or sleeplessness.

Dosage and Administration: *Orally* every 4 hours; not to exceed 6 doses in a 24-hour period. Adults, 2 teaspoonsful; children 6 to 12 years of age, 1 teaspoonful; 2 to 5 years of age, ½ teaspoonful.

Availability:
Ⓒ RYNA-CX™ Syrup Rx or OTC (State laws vary) in bottles of 120 ml and 1 pint.

(Mallinckrodt)

RYNATAN

Description: Each tablet and each 5 ml of pediatric suspension contain:

	Tablet	*Pediatric Suspension*
Phenylephrine tannate	25 mg	5 mg
Pyrilamine tannate	25 mg	12.5 mg
Chlorpheniramine tannate	8 mg	2 mg

Indications: Combines antihistaminic and decongestant actions to provide symptomatic relief of coryza and nasal congestion associated with the common cold, other upper respiratory infections and allergic rhinitis.

Contraindications: Hypersensitivity to sympathomimetic drugs.

Precautions: Should be used with caution in patients with hypertension, hyperthyroidism, diabetes mellitus or coronary artery disease. Patients should be cautioned that in the event of drowsiness, they should not drive an automobile or engage in hazardous occupations requiring alertness or skill.

Adverse Reactions: Drowsiness and dryness of mouth.

Dosage and Administration: *Orally,* every 12 hours. Adults, 1 or 2 tablets. Children over 6 years of age, 1 to 2 teaspoonsful; children 2 to 6, 1/2 to 1 teaspoonful; and children less than 2 years, 1/3 teaspoonful.

Availability:
RYNATAN®: **(Mallinckrodt)**
Pediatric Suspension in bottles of 1 pint.
Tabules (tablets) in bottles of 100 and 500.

RYNATUSS

Description: Each tablet and each 5 ml of pediatric suspension contain:

	Tablet	*Pediatric Suspension*
Carbetapentane tannate	60 mg	30 mg
Chlorpheniramine tannate	5 mg	4 mg
Ephedrine tannate	10 mg	5 mg
Phenylephrine tannate	10 mg	5 mg

Indications: Relief of cough due to the common cold, asthma, and in acute and chronic bronchitis.

Contraindications: Hypersensitivity to sympathomimetic drugs.

Precautions: Use with caution in patients with hypertension, hyperthyroidism, diabetes mellitus or coronary artery disease. Patients should be warned that in the event of drowsiness, they should not engage in activities requiring alertness or skill.

Adverse Reactions: Drowsiness and dryness of mouth may occur occasionally.

Dosage and Administration: *Orally* every 12 hours. Adults, 1 or 2 tablets. Children over 6 years of age, 1 or 2 teaspoonsful; children 2 to 6 years, 1/2 to 1 teaspoonful; children under 2 years, 1/3 teaspoonful.

Availability:
RYNATUSS®: **(Mallinckrodt)**
Pediatric Suspension in bottles of 240 ml. And 1 pint.
Tabules (tablets) in bottles of 100 and 500.

SALICYLATE MAGNESIUM

Description: An analgesic-antiinflammatory agent, magnesium salicylate is utilized for the symptomatic relief of arthritis and related disorders. Its therapeutic value is due to a depressant action on the CNS and to a reduction of prostaglandins by inhibiting their synthesis. These chemical mediators have been found to reproduce some of the essential features associated with an acute inflammatory response. The drug contains neither sodium nor free salicylic acid; and has a pH of 7.1.

Indications: Symptomatic relief of mild to moderately advanced rheumatoid arthritis, osteoarthritis, and related diseases.

Contraindications: Patients with advanced renal insufficiency.

Precautions: Since salicylates may exacerbate gastric hemorrhage, the drug should be given with caution to patients with acute (corrosive) gastritis or peptic ulcer. It should be used with extreme caution, if at all, in those taking coumarin or indandione anticoagulants, or heparin. The risk of gastrointestinal bleeding is increased when salicylates are given concurrently with steroids, the butazones, or alcohol. Salicylates in low dosages can depress uric acid clearance by decreasing the uricosuric effects of probenecid and sulfinpyrazone. Until further clinical experience is gained, this drug is not recommended for use in children under 12 years of age.

Adverse Reactions: Complications rarely occur with recommended doses. Those that may occur include epigastric discomfort, nausea, anorexia, and occult blood loss. Large doses and/or prolonged therapy may result in salicylate intoxication manifested by tinnitus, headache, dizziness, confusion, fever, sweating, thirst, drowsiness, dimness of vision, impaired hearing, hyperventilation, increased pulse rate, and diarrhea.

Dosage and Administration: *Orally,* The recommended dose is 1 or 2 tablets 3 or 4 times daily. Patients with rheumatic fever may require as many as 16 tablets daily.

Availability:
CAUSALIN Tablets, 600 mg in bottles of 100 and 500. **(Amfre-Grant)**
MAGAN® Tablets, 650 mg in bottles of 100 and 500. **(Warren-Teed)**
MOBIDIN™ Tablets, 600 mg in bottles of 100 and 500. **(Ascher)**

SALSALATE

Description: An ester of salicylic acid, salsalate is an analgesic-antiinflammatory agent. The drug is slowly hydrolyzed in the small intestine to 2 molecules of free salicylic acid, and has been reported to exhibit a much longer biological half-life than that of other salicylates.

Indications: Relief of the signs and symptoms of rheumatoid arthritis, osteoarthritis and other rheumatic conditions.

Contraindications: Patients hypersensitive to salicylates.

Precautions: The usual precautions associated with salicylates should be followed in treating patients with peptic ulcers, bleeding tendencies, or those on anticoagulant therapy. Since the drug has not been evaluated in pediatric patients, no dosage recommendation can therefore be made for children under 12 years of age.

Adverse Reactions: The incidence of side effects appears to be lower with salsalate than with other salicylates. Gastrointestinal reactions manifested by nausea, dyspepsia, and heartburn are usually mild. Clinical studies suggest that the risk of significant gastric irritation, erosion and hemorrhage generally evident with acetylsalicylic acid does not exist with this drug. Salsalate has not been associated with reactions causing asthmatic attack in susceptible patients. Large doses and/or prolonged therapy may produce symptoms of salicylate intoxications manifested by tinnitus, vertigo, headache, confusion, drowsiness, sweating, hyperventilation, vomiting or diarrhea. Treatment is aimed at increasing elimination of the drug and specific therapy for any of the toxic manifestations.

Dosage and Administration: *Orally.* The usual dosage is 2 tablets 3 times daily. It is recommended that the last dose be taken at bedtime. If necessary, the frequency of dosage can be adjusted upwards or downwards depending on the response.

Availability:
DISALCID Tablets, 500 mg in bottles of 100. **(Riker)**

SANTYL

Description: Santyl contains the enzyme collagenase which is derived from the fermentation of *Clostridium histolyticum.* It catalyzes the destruction of both native and denatured collagen. Since collagen accounts for 75% of the dry weight of skin tissue, the ability of this enzyme to digest collagen in the physiological pH range and temperature makes it effective in the removal of detritus, thus contributing toward the formation of granulation tissue and the subsequent epithelization of skin ulcers and severely burned areas of the body. Each gm of ointment contains 250 units of collagenase. Its potency is based on the digestion of undenatured collagen (from bovine Achilles tendon) at pH 7.2 and 37°C for 24 hours. The number of peptides cleaved are measured by reaction with ninhydrin. Peptides released by a trypsin digestion control are subtracted. One net collagenase unit will solubilize ninhydrin reaction material equivalent to 4 micromoles of leucine.

Indications: Debridement of skin ulcers and severely burned areas of the body. In other types of necrotic skin lesions reports on the use of collagenase have been limited to clinical observations without controls.

Contraindications: Patients who have shown local or systemic hypersensitivity to this enzyme.

Precautions: Since the enzyme's optimal pH is 7 to 8, lower pH conditions have a definite adverse effect on the enzymatic activity of collagenase. This activity is also affected by detergents, hexachlorophene and heavy metal ions such as mercury and silver which are used in some antiseptics. When it is suspected that such materials have been employed, the site should be carefully cleansed by repeated washings with normal saline solution before this ointment is applied. Soaks containing metal ions or acidic solutions (low pH) such as Burow's solution should be avoided. However, hydrogen peroxide or Dakin's solution does not interfere with collagenase's activity.

Debilitated patients should be closely monitored for systemic bacterial infections because of the possibility that debriding enzymes may increase the risk of bacteremia. It is important that the drug be confined to the area of the lesion in order to avoid the risk of irritation or maceration of normal skin. A slight erythema has been noted occasionally in the surrounding tissue particularly when the enzyme was not confined to the lesion. This response can be readily controlled by protecting the healthy skin with a material such as Lassar's paste. Since the enzyme is a protein, sensitization may develop with prolonged use.

Adverse Reactions: None have been noted when used as directed.

Dosage and Administration: *Topically.* Apply directly to the lesion once daily (once every other day for outpatients) and cover with a gauze or linen dressing. At each redressing, the lesion should be irrigated with isotonic saline solution or hydrogen peroxide in order to remove any film and digested material. Should infection be present, as evidenced by positive cultures, pus, inflammation or odor, Neosporin® (neomycin-bacitracin-polymyxin) should be applied to the lesion in powder form or solution prior to the use of this ointment. If the infection does not respond, therapy with Santyl should be discontinued until remission of the infection. Treatment should be terminated when sufficient debridement of necrotic tissue has been achieved.

Availability:
SANTYL® Ointment, 250 units/gm in jars of 25 and 50 gm. **(Knoll)**

SCOPOLAMINE HYDROBROMIDE

Description: Scopolamine hydrobromide is the salt of a *levo*rotatory alkaloid obtained from *Atropa belladonna*. Scopolamine, or hyoscine, resembles atropine in its peripheral action, but it differs greatly in its central effects. Scopolamine is a primary central depressant with marked sedative and tranquilizing properties and, like atropine, it is a potent mydriatic and cycloplegic. It occurs as colorless or white crystals or as a white, granular powder freely soluble in water and soluble in alcohol.

Indications: An anticholinergic-CNS depressant; as a preanesthetic medication prior to surgery or obstetrics, alone or combined with a strong analgesic (morphine); the treatment of postencephalitic parkinsonism and paralysis agitans; in spastic states; and, topically, as a substitute for atropine in ophthalmology.

Contraindications: Glaucoma and prostatic hypertrophy.

Precautions: Should be used cautiously in patients with cardiac disease and in those over 40 years of age.

Adverse Reactions: Effects are similar to those of atropine, i.e., dry mouth, blurred vision, flushing, tachycardia, mydriasis, or urinary retention. Acute doses, in addition, may cause tachycardia, scarlatiniform rash, delirium, fever, stupor, coma, respiratory failure, and death. Occasionally, it acts as an excitant causing delirium, especially in painful conditions if analgesics are not also given.

Dosage and Administration: *Intramuscularly,* 0.4 mg ½ to 1 hour before surgery or during labor. *Subcutaneously,* 0.5 to 1 mg as a sedative and, alone or combined with morphine, for preanesthetic medication; dosage may be increased cautiously in parkinsonism and in spastic states. Children, 0.006 mg/kg of body weight ½ to 1 hour preoperatively. *Topically* as an ophthalmic solution, for local instillation into the conjunctival sac; usually 1 or 2 drops. Dosage should be adjusted according to specific requirements.

Availability:
ISOPTO® HYOSCINE Ophthalmic Solution, 0.25% in Drop-Tainer® bottles of 5 and 15 ml. **(Alcon)**
SCOPOLAMINE HYDROBROMIDE Injection, 0.43 mg /0.5 ml in ampuls of 0.5 ml; 0.54 mg/ml in multiple-dose vials of 20 ml. **(Burroughs Wellcome)**
SCOPOLAMINE HYDROBROMIDE Hypodermic Tablets, 0.4 and 0.6 mg in bottles of 100. **(Lilly)**

SECOBARBITAL Ⓒ

Chemical Name: Sodium 5-allyl-5-(1-methylbutyl) barbiturate.

Description: Secobarbital is a short-acting barbiturate and occurs as a slightly bitter, white, amorphous powder slightly soluble in water and very soluble in alcohol. The sodium salt occurs as a bitter, white, hygroscopic powder very soluble in water and soluble in alcohol.

The major action of the barbiturates is depression of the CNS. The cerebral cortex and the reticular activating system are the most sensitive to barbiturate effects; the cerebellar, vestibular and spinal systems are less sensitive; and the vital medullary systems concerned with respiration and circulation are least sensitive. The barbiturates produce sleep which closely resembles physiologic sleep, subjectively and on the EEG.

Barbiturates are respiratory depressants by virtue of their direct effect on the medullary respiratory center. They diminish and, in high doses, may abolish the sensitivity of the respiratory center to its normal stimulus, carbon dioxide. Ordinary hypnotic doses of barbiturates have no significant effect on the cardiovascular system. The barbiturates tend to decrease the tonus of the gastrointestinal musculature. They have no direct injurious effect on the normal kidney. Severe oliguria or anuria may occur in acute barbiturate poisoning, largely as a result of the marked hypotension. Clinical studies have shown that hypnotic doses tend to reduce slightly the metabolic rate; body temperature is reduced slightly owing to lessened activity and to depression of the central temperature regulatory mechanisms.

The metabolism of secobarbital takes place in large measure in the liver. Secobarbital is classified as short acting on the basis of the duration of its hypnotic action. It readily passes the placental barrier.

Indications: Insomnia, sedation in obstetrics, neuropsychiatry and dental procedures, or whenever a rapid-acting sedative or hypnotic effect is desirable. Combined with phenyltoloxamine, a long-acting tranquilizer with muscle-relaxing properties, to attain prompt and sustained sleep, especially when insomnia is due to tension and anxiety or is associated with psychiatric problems, allergic conditions, dermatosis, or musculoskeletal disorders.

Contraindications: In patients with a history of sensitivity to barbiturates, severe hepatic disease, a history of porphyria or severe respiratory or cardiac disease, during parturition, fetal immaturity, uncontrolled pain, and drug-dependence.

Warnings: May be habit-forming. Because of possible harmful effect on the fetus, special caution and judgment are essential when the drug is given to pregnant patients. In such instances, fetal heart rate should be carefully monitored, and should slowing or irregularities develop, oxygen should be administered by appropriate means. Since barbiturates stimulate the activity of hepatic microsomal enzymes responsible for drug metabolism, they may decrease the blood concentration and clinical effectiveness of various drugs when given concurrently. Also, they may lower the blood level of coumarin anticoagulants and thus shorten prothrombin time.

Precautions: Should be used with caution in patients with liver dysfunction. Intramuscular injection should be made deeply into a large muscle; the volume should not exceed 5 ml at any one site. Intravenous administration should not exceed a rate of 50 mg/second; rapid administration may cause respiratory depression, apnea, laryngospasm, or vasodilatation with a fall in blood pressure. Special care is needed when secobarbital is given concomitantly with other CNS depressants. When administered during an office procedure, the patient should not be discharged unaccompanied and should not attempt to drive a car for the remainder of the day. Intraarterial injection must be avoided since its consequences may vary from transient pain to gangrene. Untoward reactions can occur in the presence of fever, hyperthyroidism, diabetes mellitus and severe anemia. Secobarbital should be given with extreme caution to patients in shock, or with uremia or upper respiratory infection.

Adverse Reactions: Idiosyncrasy (in the form of excitement), hangover or pain may be experienced. Hypersensitivity reactions occur in some patients, especially in those with asthma, urticaria, or angioneurotic edema. Respiratory depression is the most common side effect of the intravenous use of sodium secobarbital. Overdosage or too rapid intravenous administration may induce spasm of the larynx, pharynx or both, or vasodilatation and fall in blood pressure. Cutaneous eruptions may occur in those who are allergic to barbiturates. Nausea, vomiting, vertigo, headache, postoperative atelectasis and circulatory disturbances are uncommon and are usually due to overdosage or extraneous factors. With continuous use of excessive amounts, more marked sequelae such as delirium, stupor and ataxia may occur. The drug should be discontinued if side effects occur.

Dosage and Administration: *Orally.* Insomnia: 100 mg at bedtime. Preoperatively: Adults, 200 to 300 mg; children, 50 to 100 mg 1 or 2 hours before surgery. *Rectally.* Children up to 6 months of age, 16 to 50 mg; 6 to 36 months of age, 50 to 60 mg; older children, 50 to 100 mg. Average dose is 1.8 to 2.3 mg/lb of body weight. *Intramuscularly* or *intravenously,* the usual dose is 100 to 200 mg or up to a total of 500 mg. Secobarbital-phenyltoloxamine combination: Adults and children over 12 years of age, 1 or 2 tablets at bedtime. Consult package literature for details.

Availability:

Secobarbital

Ⓒ SECONAL® Elixir, 22 mg/5 ml in bottles of 1 pint. **(Lilly)**

Secobarbital Sodium

Ⓒ SECOBARBITAL SODIUM: **(Wyeth)**

Capsules, 100 mg in Redipak® (unit-dose) cartons of 25.

Injection, 50 mg/ml in 1- and 2-ml disposable syringes with needle (Tubex®) in Tamp-R-Tel® (tamper-resistant) packages of 10.
Ⓒ III SECONAL® SODIUM: **(Lilly)**
Enseals, 100 mg in bottles of 100.
Injection, 50 mg/ml in 20-ml ampuls and 2-ml (Hyporets®) disposable syringe with needle.
Pulvules (capsules), 30 mg in bottles of 100; 50 and 100 mg in bottles of 100 and 500 and in blister-strip packages of 100.
Suppositories (rectal), 30, 60, 120 and 200 mg in cartons of 12.

Combinations

Ⓒ III HYPTRAN® Tablets, 60 mg with phenyltoloxamine, 25 mg (in the outer layer) and phenyltoloxamine, 75 mg (in the inner core) in bottles of 100. **(Wallace)**
Ⓒ III TUINAL® Capsules (Pulvules®), 50 mg in bottles of 100; 100 and 200 mg in bottles of 100 and 1000 and in unit-dose packages of 100 (10 x 10). Each capsule contains equal parts of secobarbital sodium and amobarbital sodium. **(Lilly)**

SELENIUM SULFIDE

Description: Selenium sulfide is a mixture of crystalline selenium monosulfide and a suspension of solid selenium and amorphous sulfur. It occurs as a bright orange powder that is insoluble in water and in organic solvents. Its mode of action in seborrheic dermatitis is not sufficiently known, but may be due to its antimitotic activity.

Indications: Treatment of common dandruff, and mild to moderately-severe seborrheic dermatitis of the scalp; for the control of chronic seborrheic conditions of the scalp.

Contraindications: Acute inflammation of the scalp; hypersensitivity to selenium.

Warnings: Safe use on infants has not been established.

Precautions: Conjunctivitis may follow accidental entry of selenium sulfide into the eye. If any skin reaction occurs, the medication should be discontinued. Yellow or orange discoloration of gray or white hair may occur following treatment, but may be avoided by thorough, careful rinsing of the hair. It should also be thoroughly rinsed (5 minutes under cool, running water) from the hair before dyeing, tinting or waving, and should not be applied for 4 days following any of these procedures. The preparation should not be used until all traces of any product containing metallic compounds (e.g., mercuric ointment) have been removed from the scalp. Patients should be instructed to keep this product out of the reach of children since it is readily absorbed following oral ingestion and may produce toxic results.

Adverse Reactions: The occurrence of untoward reactions with selenium sulfide is rare. Application of the lotion to an acutely inflamed scalp may result in cutaneous absorption with the production of systemic toxic effects; therefore, the product should not be used when acute inflammation is present. Increased oiliness of the hair or falling of hair may accompany treatment of the scalp.

Dosage and Administration: *Topically.* Massage about 1 or 2 teaspoonsful of the suspension into the wet scalp, *avoid contact with the eyes;* after 2 or 3 minutes, rinse scalp thoroughly and repeat procedure. Hands should be carefully washed after treatment. Two applications each week for 2 weeks will afford control. Treatment may be continued on a weekly basis, but it should be applied more frequently than that required to maintain control. Apply a sufficient amount of the lotion to cover the affected areas and lather; after 5 minutes rinse thoroughly. Use once or twice weekly.

Availability:
EXSEL® Lotion, 2.5% in plastic bottles of 120 ml. **(Herbert)**
SELSUN® Suspension, 2.5% in plastic bottles of 120 ml. **(Abbott)**
SELSUN BLUE Cream, 1% (OTC) in tubes of 105 and 165 gm. **(Abbott)**
SELSUN BLUE Lotion, 1% (OTC) in bottles of 120, 240 and 360 ml. **(Abbott)**

SIDONNA

Description: Each tablet contains simethicone, 25 mg; butabarbital sodium, 16 mg; hyoscyamine sulfate, 0.1037 mg; atropine sulfate, 0.0194 mg and scopolamine hydrobromide, 0.0065 mg.

Formulated to provide spasmolysis, mild sedation, and to combat gas pains, flatulence and distention associated with functional disorders of the gastrointestinal tract, such as the irritable bowel syndrome, spastic colon, pylorospasm, gastroenteritis, gastritis, nausea, nervous indigestion, and gastric and duodenal ulcers.

Indications: Relief of spasm, abdominal pain and gaseous distention.

Contraindications: Hypersensitivity to any of the components, glaucoma, prostatic hypertrophy, or pyloric obstruction.

Warnings: Butabarbital sodium may be habit-forming.

Precautions: The occurrence of urinary retention requires that the dose be reduced or the drug withdrawn.

Adverse Reactions: Dryness of mouth, blurred vision, dysuria, skin rash, constipation, or drowsiness may occur. If drowsiness occurs, patients should be cautioned not to engage in activities requiring alertness or skill.

Dosage and Administration: *Orally,* 1 or 2 tablets preferably before meals and at bedtime.

Availability:
SIDONNA® Tablets in bottles of 100. **(Reed & Carnrick)**

SINCALIDE

Description: Sincalide is sterile, lyophilized, white powder of the synthetic C-terminal octapeptide of cholecystokinin. Each vial provides 5 mcg of sincalide and 45 mg of sodium chloride. pH is adjusted to 5.5 to 6.5 with sodium hydroxide or hydrochloric acid. When reconstituted with 5 ml of Sterile Water for Injection U.S.P., each ml contains 1 mcg of sincalide and 9 mg of sodium chloride.

Following intravenous administration, the drug causes a prompt and diagnostically satisfactory gallbladder contraction that becomes optimal within 5 to 15 minutes, as compared with that due to a fatty meal which causes a progressive contraction that becomes maximal after about 40 minutes. The resultant evacuation of bile is similar to that which occurs in response to endogenous cholecystokinin. Generally, a 40% reduction in radiographic area of the gallbladder is considered satisfactory contraction.

In common with cholecystokinin, sincalide, when given concurrently with secretin, stimulates pancreatic secretion for analysis of its composition and examination of cytology, thus permitting assessment of specific pancreatic function. The parameters usually determined are: the volume of the secretion; the bicarbonate concentration, and the amylase content (which parallels the content of trypsin and total protein).

Indications: A diagnostic agent that provides an increased volume of bile, and in conjunction with secretin, an increased volume of pancreatic secretion for analysis and cytological examination, and for postevacuation cholecystography in cases in which the physician deems this procedure essential but wishes to avoid use of a fatty meal.

Contraindications: In patients sensitive to the drug.

Warnings: Although animal studies did not reveal any teratogenic or antifertility effects, clinical data have not been sufficient to determine safe use in pregnant women; therefore, its use should be restricted to those cases in which the benefits outweigh the possible risks to the fetus. Additionally, safe use in children has not been established.

Precautions: Drug-induced gallbladder contraction in patients with small stones could lead to the mobilization of the stones from the gallbladder to the cystic duct or the common bile duct. However, this risk is considered to be minimal since sincalide, when given as directed, does not ordinarily cause complete contraction of the gallbladder.

Adverse Reactions: Frequently occurring are gastrointestinal symptoms such as abdominal discomfort or pain, and the urge to defecate. These adverse effects are usually manifestations of the physiologic action of the drug, which includes delayed gastric emptying and increased intestinal motility, and are not to be construed as necessarily indicating an abnormality of the biliary tract unless there is other clinical or radiologic evidence of disease. Nausea, dizziness, and flushing occur occasionally.

Dosage and Administration: *Intravenously. For prompt contraction of the gallbladder,* a dose of 0.02 mcg/kg of body weight (1.4 mcg/70 kg) is injected over an interval of 30 to 60 seconds; if a satisfactory response does not occur in 15 minutes, a second dose of 0.04 mcg/kg may be given. *For visualization of the gallbladder (cholecystography),* roentgenograms are usually taken at intervals of 5 minutes after the injection. *For visualization of the cystic duct,* it may be necessary to take roentgenograms at intervals of 1 minute during the first 5 minutes after the injection. *For the secretin-sincalide test of pancreatic function,* initially, secretin in a dose of 0.25 units/kg of body weight is infused intravenously over a period of 60 minutes. Thirty minutes after the initiation of the secretin infusion, a seperate intravenous infusion of sincalide at a total dose of 0.02 mcg/kg is administered over an interval of 30 minutes. For example, the total dose for a 70 kg patient is 1.4 mcg of sincalide; therefore, dilute 1.4 ml of reconstituted solution to 30 ml with Sodium Chloride Injection U.S.P. and administer at the rate of 1 ml/minute.

Availability:
KINEVAC® Powder for Injection in vials of 5 mcg. **(Squibb)**

SINUBID

Description: Each tablet contains:

Acetaminophen	300 mg
Acetophenetidin (phenacetin)	300 mg
Phenylpropanolamine hydrochloride	100 mg
Phenyltoloxamine citrate	66 mg

Indications: Prolonged relief of symptoms associated with sinus or other frontal headache; allergic and vasomotor manifestations of upper respiratory tract disorders such as sinusitis, allergic rhinitis (hay fever, rose fever, etc.), vasomotor rhinitis, coryza; and for the relief of accompanying fever.

Contraindications: Patients whose sensitivity to small doses of sympathomimetics is manifested by insomnia, dizziness, lightheadedness, weakness, tremulousness, or cardiac arrhythmias or patients hypersensitive to any of the components.

Warnings: Patients should be cautioned that, in the event of drowsiness, they should not drive an automobile or engage in hazardous occupations requiring alertness. Neither should they ingest alcoholic beverages, MAO inhibitors, nor barbiturates while taking this preparation.

Precautions: Since safe use during pregnancy or lactation or in women of childbearing potential has not been established, potential benefits should be weighed against the possible risks to mother and child. Should be used cautiously in patients with hyperthyroidism, hypertensive-cardiovascular disease, diabetes mellitus, and liver disease. Phenacetin-containing preparations should be used with caution in patients with chronic renal disease.

Adverse Reactions: Those generally noted are due to their individual or combinations of components: *Acetaminophen*—urticaria, epigastric distress, dizziness, and palpitation. *Phenacetin*—cyanosis with methemoglobinemia, hemolytic anemia, dyspnea, headache, vascular collapse, and kidney damage from prolonged use. *Phenylpropanolamine hydrochloride* — anxiety, restlessness, tension, insomnia, tremor, weakness, headache, vertigo, sweating, arrhythmia, nausea, and vomiting. *Phenyltoloxamine citrate*—urticaria, drowsiness, disturbed coordination, inability to concentrate, dizziness, insomnia, tremors, nervousness, palpitation, convulsions, muscular weakness, gastric distress, diarrhea, intestinal cramps, blurred vision, hypotension, urinary retention, dryness of mouth, throat and nose.

Dosage and Administration: *Orally,* twice daily (every 12 hours). Adults, 1 tablet; children 6 to 12 years of age, 1/2 tablet. Tablets should not be chewed.

Availability:
SINUBID® Tablets in bottles of 100. **(Warner-Chilcott)**

SINUTAB with CODEINE Ⓒ III

Description: Each tablet contains:

Acetaminophen	150 mg
Acetophenetidin (phenacetin)	150 mg
Phenylpropanolamine hydrochloride	25 mg
Phenyltoloxamine citrate	22 mg
Codeine phosphate	15 mg

Indications: Relief of nasal congestion in severe sinus or other frontal headache; allergic and vasomotor manifestations of upper respiratory disorders such as sinusitis, allergic rhinitis, vasomotor rhinitis, coryza; facial pain and "pressure" of acute and chronic sinusitis; and for the relief of accompanying fever.

Contraindications: Patients whose sensitivity to small doses of sympathomimetic amines produces sleeplessness, dizziness, lightheadedness, weakness, tremulousness, or cardiac arrhythmias, or patients hypersensitive to any of the components.

Warnings: Codeine may be habit-forming. Patients should be instructed not to drive or operate machinery if drowsiness occurs. Neither should they ingest alcoholic beverages, MAO inhibitors, nor barbiturates while taking this medication.

Precautions: Use with caution in patients with hyperthyroidism, hypertensive-cardiovascular disease, diabetes mellitus or liver disease. Precautions regarding the chronic administration of phenacetin-containing compounds and their use in patients with chronic renal disease should be observed. Since there is no adequate experience in pregnant patients who have received this drug, safe use during gestation has not been established.

Adverse Reactions: Since the components of this product are the same as those in Sinubid with the exception of codeine, see the above monograph for possible adverse effects. In addition, codeine may also induce nausea, vomiting, constipation, sedation, and dizziness.

Dosage and Administration: *Orally.* Adults, initially 2 tablets followed, if needed, by 1 or 2 tablets every 4 hours.

Availability:
Ⓒ III SINUTAB® with CODEINE Tablets in bottles of 24. **(Warner-Chilcott)**

SITOSTEROLS

Description: Sitosterols is a mixture of plant sterols consisting of β-sitosterol (stigmast-5-en-3β-ol) and certain saturated sterols. It contains not less than 95% of total sterols and not less than 85% of unsaturated sterols calculated on the dried basis as β-sitosterol. The exact mechanism of action of sitosterols has not been confirmed but it appears to compete with cholesterol for absorption sites in the intestine. It is poorly absorbed and is excreted in the feces as unchanged drug. The effect of the drug on elevated serum cholesterol has been found to be moderate and variable. There is insufficient evidence to indicate whether or not drug-induced reduction of serum cholesterol or other lipid levels has a detrimental, a beneficial, or no effect on the morbidity or mortality of atherosclerosis or coronary heart disease. Proper assessment of the magnitude and variability of changes in serum cholesterol depends on obtaining several (usually 3 or more) base-line serum cholesterol values while the patient is on a controlled diet over a period of 1 to 3 weeks prior to treatment with this agent.

Indications: Conditions in which the reduction of hypercholesterolemia and hyperbetalipoproteinemia is desirable. Should be used as an adjunct to appropriate dietary regulation and other essential measures.

Contraindications: None known.

Warnings: Safe use during pregnancy has not been established.

Precautions: Sitosterols may interfere with the absorption of other substances and drugs besides cholesterol.

Adverse Reactions: Since sitosterols is not absorbed, the stool becomes bulky and light in color. The suspension may have a very mild laxative effect because of the methylcellulose derivative used as a dispersing agent. If the loose stools become troublesome, foods containing roughage should be restricted.

Dosage and Administration: *Orally,* mixed with liquids. Suggested dosage is 15 ml (1 tablespoonful) before meals of medium size, increased to 22 or 30 ml when large or high-fat meals are eaten. Some individuals may require up to 120 to 180 ml daily. Any additional food eaten between meals should be preceded by a whole or fractional dose of the suspension.

Availability:
CYTELLIN® Suspension, 3 gm/15 ml (4% alcohol) in bottles of 1 pint. **(Lilly)**

SMALLPOX VACCINE

Description: Smallpox vaccine is the living virus of vaccinia that has been grown in the skin of a vaccinated bovine calf, and prepared as a freeze-dried powder for reconstitution. The dried vaccine may contain traces of polymyxin B sulfate, dihydrostreptomycin sulfate, and neomycin sulfate. An antiseptic dye, brilliant green, is present in some preparations as a preservative.

Failure of smallpox vaccination to provide immunization is due almost always to failure to maintain storage temperature at 0°C. or below with resultant loss of potency, or to faulty technique. It must be remembered that immunity is not permanent; its duration varies from individual to individual and rarely persists for life. Absence of reaction is *not* necessarily evidence of immunity; it usually indicates an unsuccessful effort. *Vaccination should always be repeated.* In case of repeated failures in primary vaccinations, a fresh supply of vaccine should be used at a different site, away from the area of the previous attempts.

Indications: Production of active immunity to smallpox. It is especially recommended for all health services and medical personnel who are at high risk of exposure to the virus and for travelers to areas where smallpox has not as yet been eradicated.

Contraindications: Smallpox vaccination should not be used in the presence of eczema and other forms of chronic or contact dermatitis. Since the vaccine virus may on occasion cross the placental barrier, vaccination should be deferred until after pregnancy if no exposure is threatened. Vaccination is contraindicated in patients with leukemia, lymphoma, and other reticuloendothelial malignancies, in the presence of lowered immune responses such as dysgammaglobulinemia, and in those receiving steroid therapy, treatment with antimetabolites or irradiation. Vaccination should not be performed in children during hot weather because of the potential of skin disease or in the presence of active infections. If vaccination is absolutely essential in these individuals because of possible exposure in an endemic area, vaccinia immune globulin should be administered concurrently. Immunization in infants under 12 months of age is unwarranted unless it is deemed necessary because of high risk of exposure.

Warnings: Smallpox vaccination should not be used in patients under treatment with immunosuppressive drugs.

Precautions: The vaccinated individual should be cautioned not to touch the lesion so as to avoid spread and secondary infection, and should also be kept away from potential contacts who have eczema or severe dermatitis for at least 10 days, until the danger of contact vaccination has passed. It is generally recommended that immunization with other live virus vaccines be deferred for at least 1 month before or after vaccination with this agent. However, when the immunization program effectiveness is hindered or a threat of high-risk exposure exists, the relevant live virus vaccines may be given concurrently without significant increase in adverse reactions or depressed antibody responses.

Adverse Reactions: Transient fever and regional axillary node enlargement are occasionally observed. Accidental autoinoculation, most commonly on eyelids, conjunctivae and/or cornea; satellite lesions, secondary heteroinoculation, and keloid formation may occur. Erythema multiforme, a hypersensitivity reaction, and other rashes including roseola vaccinia have been reported. Eczema vaccinatum, generalized vaccinia and vaccinia necrosum are rare but serious complications, as is encephalitis. Rarely reported were myocarditis, osteitis, arthritis, pneumonia, and neuritis, and recently of malignant tumors in the scar at the site of vaccination.

Dosage and Administration: The vaccine is deposited in the target cells in the basal layers of the epithelium using a bifurcated needle which has been dipped into the vaccine. For primary vaccination, 5 firm punctures are made with the needle perpendicular to the skin; for revaccination 15 punctures are made. Punctures should draw a droplet of blood within 10 to 20 seconds. No pad or shield should be applied. 'Non-takes' should be revaccinated. Vaccination is best performed before the third year. Since immunity in most cases is almost completely lost after 10 years, a second vaccination is advised between the seventh and tenth year of age.

Availability:
SMALLPOX VACCINE (DRYVAX®) with brilliant green in cartons containing 1 vial of dried smallpox vaccine (calf lymph type) with 1 container (0.15 or 0.25 ml) of diluent and 25 or 100 bifurcated needles; 1 carton is sufficient for 25 or 100 vaccinations. **(Wyeth)**

SODIUM FLUORIDE: see The Fluoride-Vitamins

SOMATOTROPIN

Description: Somatotropin is a purified growth hormone processed from human pituitary glands. It is specifically indicated for treating children afflicted with hypopituitary dwarfism. Potency is determined by bioassay in hypophysectomized rats and is designated in international units (IU). Each 10-ml vial provides 10 IU of somatotropin and 40 mg of mannitol. pH is adjusted between 6 and 8 with hydrochloric acid and/or sodium hydroxide.

The drug stimulates linear growth in children who are deficient in pituitary growth hormone. The salient action of somatotropin is anabolic in that it increases intracellular transport of amino acids in addition to increasing the retention of nitrogen, phosphorus, and potassium. It also stimulates certain somatic processes such as the intestinal absorption and urinary excretion of calcium; the serum concentration of phosphorus and alkaline phosphatase; the synthesis of chondroitin sulfate and collagen, as well as the urinary excretion of hydroxyproline. Furthermore, it increases intracellular lipolysis, the plasma concentration of free fatty acids due to its adipokinetic action, and the oxidation of fatty acids. Intracellular glucose metabolism however is inhibited, and there is decreased sensitivity to the action of insulin in response to the chronic administration of this hormone.

Since somatotropin is extracted from cadaver pituitary glands, the very limited supply of this hormone restricts its use to those children whose growth failure, as evidenced by a growth rate that is subnormal for age, is caused only by a deficiency of pituitary growth hormone. This condition must be confirmed by demonstrating failure of the serum growth hormone concentration to increase above 5 to 7 ng/ml in response to two of the following standard stimuli. These include hypoglycemia, intravenous arginine, oral levodopa, intramuscular glucagon, or suitable modifications of these procedures.

Indications: Intended for use only in dwarfed children whose growth failure is a response to a deficiency of pituitary growth hormone.

Contraindications: In patients with closed epiphyses or those with an underlying progressive intracranial lesion.

Precautions: Somatotropin should be used only by physicians experienced in the diagnosis and management of patients with pituitary growth hormone deficiency. Because of its diabetogenic actions, which include the induction of hyperglycemia and ketosis, the drug should be used with caution in patients with diabetes mellitus or with a family history of this disorder. Regular urine testing for evidence of glycosuria should be carried out in all patients. Subcutaneous administration may lead to local lipoatrophy or lipodystrophy and may enhance the development of neutralizing antibodies. Administration should be made by the intramuscular route *only* and the injection site should be rotated to prevent skin atrophy. Bone age must be monitored annually during therapy, especially in patients who are pubertal and/or receiving concomitant thyroid replacement therapy, since under these circumstances, epiphyseal maturation may progress rapidly to closure. Concurrent glucocorticoid therapy may inhibit the response to therapy and should not exceed 10 to 15 mg of hydrocortisone equiv./M^2 body surface area during administration of this hormone. Patients with growth hormone deficiency secondary to an intracranial lesion should be examined frequently for progression or recurrence of the underlying disease process.

Adverse Reactions: Antibodies to somatotropin are formed in about 30 to 40% of patients. In general, these antibodies are not neutralizing and do not interfere with the response to the drug. Approximately 5% however develop neutralizing antibodies and thus fail to respond to the drug. Therefore, testing for antisomatotropin antibodies should be carried out in any patient with well-documented growth hormone deficiency who fails to respond to therapy.

Dosage and Administration: *Intramuscularly.* Each vial should be reconstituted with Bacteriostatic Water for Injection (U.S.P.) only. The recommended initial dosage is 1 ml (2 IU) 3 times a week, with a minimum of 48 hours between injections. If at any time during continuous administration the growth rate does not exceed 2.5 cm (1 inch) in a 6-month period, the dose may be doubled for the next 6 months. This may be done with or without the presence of antibodies. If there is still no satisfactory response, therapy should be discontinued and the patient reevaluated. The criteria which determines withdrawal of the medication are when the patient has reached a satisfactory adult height, when the epiphyses have fused, or when the patient ceases to respond to the drug.

Availability:
ASELLACRIN® Dry Powder (lyophilized) in vials of 10 units in cartons of 4. **(Hoechst)**

SPECTINOMYCIN DIHYDROCHLORIDE PENTAHYDRATE

Chemical Name: Decahydro-4α,7,9-trihydroxy-2-methyl-6,8-bis(methylamino)-4*H*-pyrano [2,3-*b*] (1,4)-benzodioxin-4-one dihydrochloride pentahydrate.

Description: Spectinomycin dihydrochloride pentahydrate is an aminocyclitol antibiotic obtained from the cultures of *Streptomyces spectabilis.* It occurs as a white, crystalline substance that remains stable for 3 years in the dry state.

The antibacterial action of spectinomycin is a consequence of its combination with the 30S ribosomes of the gonococcal organism, thus inhibiting protein synthesis; however, it is not significantly bound to plasma protein. Studies in vitro have shown no cross-resistance of *N. gonorrhoeae* between spectinomycin and penicillin.

Following an intramuscular injection, peak plasma levels are detectable in 1 or 2 hours and can be demonstrated at least 8 hours after administration. A single 2-gm dose produces peak serum concentration of 100 μg/ml in 1 hour, and a single 4-gm dose produces peak serum concentration of 160 μg/ml in 2 hours. Average serum concentrations of 15 μg/ml for the 2-gm dose and 31 μg/ml for the 4-gm dose were present 8 hours after administration.

Indications: Treatment of acute gonorrheal urethritis and proctitis in the male and acute gonorrheal cervicitis and proctitis in the female when due to susceptible strains of *N. gonorrhoeae.* Spectinomycin is *not* indicated for the treatment of syphilis.

Contraindications: Hypersensitivity to spectinomycin.

Warnings: Constant observation of the patient is necessary since the drug may mask or delay symptoms of syphilis; a serologic test for syphilis should be performed at the time of diagnosis and again in 3 months. Safe use in pregnant women and in infants and children has not been established.

Precautions: The usual precautions should be observed in hypersensitive patients and in those who may develop resistance to the drug.

Adverse Reactions: Noted following a single dose were soreness at the injection site, urticaria, dizziness, nausea, chills, fever, and insomnia. Repeated doses in volunteers showed a decrease in hemoglobin, hematocrit, and creatinine clearance, elevation of alkaline phosphatase, BUN and SGPT, and reduction in urine output.

Dosage and Administration: *Intramuscularly* only. Injection should be made deep into the upper outer quadrant of the gluteal muscle. Male and female patients should receive a single dose of 2 gm; those who have shown resistance to other antibiotics should receive a dose of 4 gm which may be divided into 2 intramuscular injections.

Availability:
TROBICIN® Injection, equivalent to 400 mg/ml in vials of 2 and 4 gm with diluent. **(Upjohn)**

SPIRONOLACTONE

Chemical Name: 17-Hydroxy-7α-mercapto-3-oxo-17α-pregn-4-ene-21-carboxylic acid γ-lactone acetate.

Description: Spironolactone is a synthetic steroid in which the side chain at the 17 position is replaced by a spironolactone ring. It occurs as a white, crystalline powder insoluble in water and soluble in most organic solvents.

Spironolactone blocks the activity of aldosterone through competitive binding of receptors at the aldosterone dependent sodium-potassium exchange site, and thus inhibits reabsorption of sodium and water in the distal renal tubule. Additionally, it retards excretion of potassium and may cause hyperkalemia. The drug is used primarily in conditions in which excess aldosterone is produced such as in the nephrotic syndrome or hepatic cirrhosis with ascites. The onset of diuresis is gradual with an increasing response, usually attaining maximal effect on the third day. Upon discontinuing the drug, the effects diminish gradually usually within 2 to 3 days. Spironolactone has not been reported to elevate serum uric acid, precipitate gout or interfere with carbohydrate metabolism.

Indications: Alone, or combined with hydrochlorothiazide, the drug is indicated in the treatment of severe essential hypertension, and the edema and ascites of congestive heart failure, hepatic cirrhosis, the nephrotic syndrome and in idiopathic edema. Additionally, the drug is indicated for the prophylaxis and treatment of hypokalemia when other measures are considered inappropriate or inadequate. Spironolactone is also useful in establishing a diagnosis of primary hyperaldosteronism.

Contraindications: Acute renal insufficiency, rapidly progressing impairment of renal function, anuria and hyperkalemia, hypersensitivity to the components. For other contraindications, see monograph on Hydrochlorothiazide (The Thiazide Diuretics).

Warnings: Since spironolactone retards the excretion of potassium and may cause abnormally high serum potassium levels, it should not be used in patients receiving potassium supplements unless a glucocorticoid is also given; spironolactone should be discontinued immediately if hyperkalemia develops. The drug has been shown to be tumorigenic in chronic toxicity studies performed in rats, with its proliferative effects manifested on endocrine organs and the liver. The use of this drug in pregnant women or in women of childbearing potential requires that the anticipated benefits be weighed against the possible hazards to the mother and fetus. The routine use of diuretics in an otherwise healthy pregnant woman is inappropriate and exposes the mother and fetus to unnecessary risks. Diuretics do not prevent development of toxemia of pregnancy, and there is no satisfactory evidence that they are useful in the treatment of this condition. Therefore, the drug should be used only if the clinical situation clearly justifies the need.

Precautions: Serum electrolyte determinations should be made periodically to avoid the possible development of electrolyte imbalance, especially hyponatremia and hyperkalemia. Spironolactone may also cause mild acidosis. The drug should be administered with caution to patients with severe renal disease and to those with elevated potassium levels. BUN levels may become elevated. When coadministered with other antihypertensive drugs, particularly the ganglionic blocking agents, the dosage of these other drugs should be reduced by at least one-half. The physican should be alert to the possible onset of gynecomastia. This effect appears to be related to both dosage level and duration of therapy. The condition is normally reversible upon cessation of therapy; however, in rare instances it may persist. For other precautions, see monograph on Hydrochlorothiazide (The Thiazide Diuretics).

Adverse Reactions: Drowsiness, lethargy, headache, diarrhea and other gastrointestinal symptoms, photosensitivity, maculopapular or erythematous cutaneous eruptions, urticaria, mental confusion, drug fever, ataxia, gynecomastia, inability to achieve or maintain erection, mild androgenic effects including hirsutism, irregular menses and deepening of the voice. For other adverse reactions, see monograph on Hydrochlorothiazide (The Thiazide Diuretics).

Dosage and Administration: *Orally Aldactone:* The daily adult dosage *for essential hypertension* is 50 to 100 mg in divided doses, continued for 2 weeks or more. *For other indications,* the initial adult dosage is 100 mg in divided doses for at least 5 days when given as the sole agent for diuresis. *For the diagnosis of primary hyperaldosteronism,* the drug is administered at a daily dosage of 400 mg for 4 days with proper regulation of sodium and potassium intake. A rise of serum potassium to normal levels suggests primary hyperaldosteronism. The daily dosage for children should provide 1.5 mg/lb of body weight. *Aldactazide:* Adults, 1 or 2 tablets 4 times daily. Children, 0.75 to 1.5 mg/lb of body weight. The fixed dose combination drug is not indicated for initial therapy of edema or hypertension; however, if the fixed combination represents the dosage so determined, its use may be more convenient in patient management.

Availability:
ALDACTONE® Tablets, 25 mg (light tan) in bottles of 100, 500, 1000 and 2500 and in packages of 10 cartons each containing 100 unit-dose (individually blister-sealed) tablets. **(Searle)**
ALDACTAZIDE® Tablets, 25 mg (ivory) with hydrochlorothiazide, 25 mg in bottles of 100, 500, 1000 and 2500 and in packages of 10 cartons each containing 100 unit-dose (individually blister-sealed) tablets. **(Searle)**

STANOZOLOL

Chemical Name: 17-Methyl-2′*H*-5α-androst-2-eno [3,2-*c*]pyrazol-17β-ol.

Description: Stanozolol is a steroid hormone chemically and pharmacologically related to methyltestosterone. Structurally, stanozolol is unique in that it has a pyrazol ring at the 2, 3 position. It occurs as a white, crystalline powder insoluble in water and sparingly soluble in alcohol.

Stanozolol increases retention of nitrogen and minerals; reverses tissue-depleting processes, and promotes better utilization of dietary protein. The actions of stanozolol are similar to those of the male sex hormones with the possibility of causing serious disturbances of growth and sexual development if given to young children. Anabolic steroids suppress the gonadotropic functions of the pituitary and may exert a direct effect upon the testes. Human growth hormone is the preferred treatment of pituitary dwarfism; if this hormone is not available, anabolic agents may be used to treat this condition.

Indications: May be effective in increasing hemoglobin levels in patients with aplastic (congenital or idiopathic) anemia. As adjunctive therapy in senile and postmenopausal osteoporosis. Equal or greater consideration should be given to diet, calcium balance, physiotherapy, and good general health-promoting measures. Stanozolol has no value as primary therapy. Also useful in pituitary dwarfism, where anabolic agents may be used with care until growth hormone is more available.

Contraindications: Hypersensitivity to stanozolol; male patients with carcinoma of the prostate or breast; carcinoma of the breast in some female patients; pregnancy because of masculinization of the fetus; nephrosis or the nephrotic phase of nephritis, and in severe liver damage.

Warnings: Stanozolol will not enhance athletic ability. Although rare, hepatic tumors have been noted following prolonged use of anabolic-androgenic steroids. Generally, discontinuation of these agents has resulted in tumor regression without the need for employing appropriate therapy.

Precautions: Hypercalcemia may develop, both spontaneously and as a result of hormonal therapy, in women with disseminated breast carcinoma. If it develops during therapy, the drug should be withdrawn. Caution is required in administering stanozolol to patients with cardiac, renal, or hepatic disease; edema may occur occasionally. Concomitant administration with adrenal steroids or ACTH may add to the edema. If amenorrhea or menstrual irregularities develop during treatment with this agent the drug should be discontinued until the cause is determined. Stanozolol may increase sensitivity to anticoagulants; therefore, dosage of the anticoagulant may have to be decreased in order to maintain the prothrombin time at the desired therapeutic level. Anabolic steroids have been shown to alter glucose tolerance tests. Patients with diabetes should be carefully observed and the insulin or oral hypoglycemic dosage adjusted accordingly. Since stanozolol contains a 17-α alkyl group, liver function should be checked at regular intervals in patients receiving this drug. Stanozolol should be used with caution in patients with benign prostatic hypertrophy. Serum cholesterol levels may increase or decrease during therapy; therefore, caution is required when administering to patients with a history of myocardial infarction or coronary artery disease. Serial determinations of serum cholesterol levels should be made and therapy adjusted accordingly.

Since bone growth and maturation are accelerated, certain precautions should be taken when giving this drug to infants or children in whom full growth and epiphysial closure have not yet occurred. If the bone maturation and growth of the child are essentially normal (near the 50 percentile line) therapy should not continue for more than 3 months. However, if growth and bone maturation are well below normal, therapy may be continued for a year or more, provided bone maturation is carefully checked by roentgenographic examinations every 3 to 6 months. Since skeletal stimulation may continue for 6 months after therapy has been discontinued, it is recommended that the drug be withdrawn well before bone maturation reaches the norm for the chronologic age of the child.

Adverse Reactions: Reactions reported include nausea and vomiting; diarrhea; increased or decreased libido; acne (especially in females and prepubertal males); habituation; excitation and insomnia; chills; bleeding in patients on concomitant anticoagulant therapy; premature closure of epiphyses in children; and jaundice with, rarely, hepatic necrosis and death. Also, there have been rare reports of hepatic tumors, histologically hepatocellular carcinoma, in patients taking 17-alkyl androgenic-anabolic steroids usually for prolonged periods. In some cases discontinuation of steroids resulted in tumor regression. Phallic enlargement and increased frequency of erections have occurred in prepubertal males. Inhibition of testicular function, testicular atrophy and oligospermia, impotence, chronic priapism, gynecomastia, and epididymitis and bladder irritability have occurred in postpubertal males. In females, hirsutism, male pattern baldness, deepening of the voice, and clitoral enlargement have occurred. These changes are usually irreversible even after prompt discontinuance of therapy, and are not prevented by concomitant use of estrogens. Menstrual irregularities have also occurred.

Therapy with anabolic steroids has caused alterations in the metyrapone test; the fasting blood sugar and glucose tolerance test; and the thyroid and liver function tests [decrease in protein-bound iodine (PBI), thyroxine-binding capacity, and radioactive iodine (RAI) uptake, and increase in T_3 uptake by the red blood cells or resin]. Free thyroxine is normal and the altered tests usually persist for 2 to 3 weeks after therapy has been discontinued. Alterations in liver function tests include increased bromsulphalein (BSP), increased or decreased serum cholesterol, increased serum glutamic oxaloacetic transaminase (SGOT), increased serum bilirubin, and increased alkaline phosphatase. Also noted were retention of electrolytes including sodium, chlorides, potassium, phosphates, calcium, and water; suppression of clotting factors II, V, VII, and X; increased creatine and creatinine excretion lasting up to 2 weeks after discontinuance of therapy; and decreased 17-ketosteroid excretion.

Dosage and Administration: *Orally.* Adults: Initially, 1 tablet 3 times daily just before or with meals. Children under 6 years of age, ½ tablet twice daily. Children 6 to 12 years of age, 1 tablet 3 times daily. For young women particularly susceptible to the androgenic effects of the drug, 1 tablet twice daily, increased to 1 tablet 3 times daily, if necessary. Duration of therapy depends upon the therapeutic response and the appearance of adverse reactions. The diet should be well-balanced.

Availability:
WINSTROL® Tablets, 2 mg in bottles of 100 and 1000. **(Winthrop)**

STAPHYLOCOCCUS TOXOID

Description: Sterile solutions of bacteria-free filtrates of 3 strains of *Staphylococcus aureus* cultures, containing dermonecrotic toxins treated with formaldehyde (or by pepsin digestion) so that their toxicity is markedly decreased but specific antigenicity is retained. The preparations are standardized, their potency per ml being expressed in the number of dermonecrotic units of toxin from which the toxoid was derived. The formaldehyde treated filtrate is diluted with physiological saline solution to the standard concentration, and preserved with thimerosal 1:10,000. The digest-modified filtrate is undiluted and is preserved with phenol, 0.25% and phenylmercuric borate 1:50,000. Stimulates formation of antibodies to staphylococcus organisms.

Indications: For the prophylaxis and treatment of staphylococcal infections, including recurrent boils, carbuncles, styes, and pustular acne. It is recommended that treatment be combined with appropriate antibacterial agents.

Contraindications: Patients sensitive to protein, or who have a history of allergic or anaphylactic reaction to injections and vaccinations.

Warnings: The clinician should keep in mind that some patients may exhibit a high susceptibility to staphylococcus antigens or toxoids which may be expressed by severe local or constitutional reactions.

Precautions: The parenteral administration of any biological agent should be attended by every known precaution for the prevention and arrest of allergic and other untoward reactions. A careful history should review possible sensitivity of the patient to the type of protein to be injected. A separate heat-sterilized syringe and needle should be used for each individual patient to prevent transmission of homologous serum hepatitis and other infectious agents from one patient to another.

Dosage and Administration: *Intramuscularly* or *subcutaneously.* Sensitivity to the toxoid should be determined prior to treatment by injecting intradermally 0.1 ml of a 1:10 dilution of Dilution No. 1 or 0.1 ml of a 1:100 dilution of Dilution No. 2. The formation and extent of the presenting erythema provides a basis for subsequent treatment. The toxoid is then administered in dosages indicated for each preparation. Initially, 0.1 ml of Dilution No. 1 or 0.01 ml of Dilution No. 2 followed by successive injections in increments of 0.2 or 0.02 ml respectively at intervals of 2 to 7 days until a maximum of 1 ml is reached. When the highest dose (usually 1 ml of Dilution No. 2) is reached, it may be repeated at weekly intervals until clinical recovery is attained. The digest modified toxoid should begin with 0.1 ml of the undiluted solution or of that dilution which has been shown not to produce excessive reaction. Injection should be made twice weekly in increments of 0.1 or 0.2 ml with each injection until the patient is receiving 1 ml of the undiluted toxoid. The 1 ml dose may then be repeated as often as necessary. Intervals between injections may be increased to 1 or 2 weeks when the full dose of 1 ml is being used.

Availability:
STAPHYLOCOCCUS TOXOID Injection (formaldehyde modified), 100 units/ml (Dilution No. 1) and 1000 units/ml (Dilution No. 2) in vials of 5 ml. **(Lederle)**
STAPHYLOCOCCUS TOXOID Injection (digest modified), 10,000 units/ml in vials of 5 ml. **(Lederle)**

STREPTOKINASE

Description: A proteolytic enzyme elaborated by group C beta-hemolytic streptococci, streptokinase has been found to possess effective thromboembolytic activity. It combines with plasminogen to produce an activator complex that then converts residual plasminogen into the proteolytic enzyme plasmin which digests fibrin into a number of soluble fragments. Both plasminogen and streptokinase dissolve into the thrombus/embolus, the activator is incorporated throughout the clot, and there, within a self-contained system, the resulting plasmin lyses the fibrin clot. The drug has been used for a variety of thromboembolic disorders, but its most favorable effects have been observed in acute, extensive thrombi of the deep veins; acute, massive pulmonary emboli; and the clearing of occluded arteriovenous cannulae. Treatment should be instituted as soon as possible, preferably within several days—5 days is the limit in pulmonary emboli—after onset of symptoms, since older thrombi are more resistant, and positive results from lytic therapy decline rapidly with increasing age of the lesion. Comparative studies with heparin have demonstrated that streptokinase provides a much more rapid dissolution of recent pulmonary emboli, and that recent thrombotic occlusions of deep veins are more susceptible to complete lysis with streptokinase, but whether or not morbidity or mortality occur less frequently has not been established.

Following intravenous administration, the effect on coagulation generally persists for up to 12 hours. Studies with radioactive drug indicate 2 disappearance rates: a fast half-life of approximately 18 minutes due to the action of antibodies, and a slow half-life, operative in the absence of antibodies, of about 83 minutes. Effective blood levels and disappearance rates are dependent upon the availability of substrates and, thus, are only relative indices of the pharmacologic effects of the drug.

Indications: Streptokinase is used primarily for the lysis of objectively diagnosed acute, massive pulmonary emboli and may be used for embolization accompanied by unstable hemodynamics; for the lysis of objectively diagnosed acute, extensive deep vein thrombosis, but not for superficial thrombophlebitis; and for the clearing of totally or partially occluded arteriovenous cannulae as an alternative to surgical revision when acceptable flow cannot otherwise be achieved. Approximatley 50% of totally occluded cannulae and 80% of partially occluded cannulae can be cleared sufficiently to resume dialysis. Its value in the treatment of septic thrombophlebitis remains to be established.

Contraindications: Because thrombolytic therapy increases the risk of bleeding, streptokinase is inadvisable for use within 10 days of surgery or other invasive procedures (hepatic or renal biopsy, parturition, intraarterial procedures). This drug is contraindicated in cases involving an ulcerative wound; recent trauma; visceral carcinoma, ulcerative colitis or diverticulitis; hypertension; liver or kidney disease; thrombocytopenia, or other evidence of defective hemostasis; active tuberculosis; subacute, bacterial endocarditis; gastrointestinal bleeding (within 6 months); in patients with a predisposition to systemic infection, and in those with a history of previous severe allergic reaction to the drug or who present a significant risk of an allergic response. Also, it should not be used within 2 months following a cerebrovascular accident (embolic, thrombolic, or hemorrhagic) because patients with cerebral infarction remain at risk of bleeding into the infarcted tissue for an indefinite period.

Warnings: Activation of the fibrinolytic system with streptokinase results in a more profound alteration of the hemostatic status of the patient than does anticoagulant therapy with heparin or coumarin compounds. Although therapy is aimed at producing sufficient amounts of plasmin for dissolving intravascular fibrin deposits, other fibrin deposits, including those which provide hemostasis from cuts, needle puncture, etc. are also affected and bleeding from such sites may occur. Unnecessary handling of the patient should be avoided since there is a significant possibility of bruising or hematoma formation, especially with intramuscular injection; the high risk of developing a hematoma precludes this mode of administration. Because bleeding can occur at sites of recent invasive procedures, arterial invasive procedures must also be avoided before and during treatment with streptokinase. However, should an arterial puncture be absolutely necessary, the radial or brachial artery should be used, *not the femoral artery*, and the procedure should be done carefully by a clinician experienced in the management of thrombotic disease. Pressure should be applied for at least 15 minutes, followed by a pressure dressing, and the puncture site checked frequently for evidence of bleeding. Also, invasive venous procedures should be performed as carefully and as infrequently as possible, and if bleeding from an invasive site is not serious, treatment may be continued accompanied by close clinical observation, and the immediate application of local measures. Spontaneous bleeding from internal sites not accessible for pressure application may also occur. Since the risk of spontaneous bleeding is greater in patients with histories suggestive of prior hemostatic defects, with or without demonstrable abnormalities in platelet count, prothrombin time, partial thromboplastin time, or bleeding time, such patients should be assessed carefully before treatment, and should serious spontaneous bleeding occur, the use of the infusion should be terminated immediately and the proper treatment instituted. In addition to its fibrinolytic action, plasmin also degrades fibrinogen, Factor V, Factor VIII and other proteins. The products of plasmin degradation of fibrinogen and fibrin possess anticoagulant effects, and bleeding, should it occur, may be difficult to control. It is advised that serial thrombin time determinations be carefully monitored. Treatment of patients with atrial fibrillation or other conditions in which there is a possible risk of cerebral embolism may be hazardous because of the risk of bleeding into the infarcted area. Because of the drug's antigenic nature, allergic, and possibly anaphylactic, reactions may occur. Since there is no reliable test with which to predict allergic responses, patients should be observed carefully during the first few hours of infusion. Patients with known allergies to other antigens are more likely to react adversely to the drug. If significant changes in blood pressure (elevation or lowering of more than 25 mm Hg systolic) or asthmatic symptoms occur, which might be due to allergy, the infusion should be discontinued and symptomatic treatment employed. Other mild allergic manifestations such as rash, musculoskeletal pain, flushing, itching, nausea, and chills have been observed, but generally are not serious enough to warrant withdrawal of the medication. Concurrent use of anticoagulants with streptokinase is not recommended and may be hazardous. Before initiating therapy with streptokinase in patients being treated with heparin, the effects of heparin should be allowed to diminish with time. As a general rule, a thrombin time of less than twice the normal control value is adequate for starting the infusions safely. Similarly, heparin should not be administered following streptokinase therapy until the thrombin time has returned to less than twice the normal control value. While rethrombosis has been observed after termination of therapy, this risk may be minimized by strict adherence to the details of anticoagulation. The use of intravenous heparin followed by oral anticoagulant therapy is considered a necessary adjunct following therapy with streptokinase. Safe and effective use in pregnant patients and in children has not been established, and its use in such patients is therefore not recommended.

Precautions: In order to determine the proper loading dose for patients who have had a recent streptococcal infection or recent treatment with streptokinase (high antibody titer), determination of the patient's resistance to the drug is recommended. Patients showing a streptokinase resistance test exceeding 1,000,000 units are not considered suitable candidates for treatment since the drug is unlikely to be active in these patients. Since the infusions have been associated with altered platelet function, concurrent use of drugs that may potentiate this effect, such as aspirin, indomethacin and phenylbutazone, should be avoided.

Adverse Reactions. Severe spontaneous bleeding, including cerebral bleeding, retroperitoneal or gastrointestinal bleeding has been documented in 6 of 292 patients, and cerebral hemorrhage has accounted for several fatilities. Superficial hematoma, hematuria, and hemoptysis are less severe and have been observed to occur about twice as often with streptokinase than with heparin. In several instances, spontaneous bleeding has been traced to concomitant anticoagulant treatment. Oozing of blood from sites of percutaneous trauma is frequent, hence all invasive procedures must be avoided and intravenous punctures kept to a minimum before and during therapy. The drug must be discontinued in the event of serious bleeding. If very rapid reversal of the fibrinolytic state is required, treatment with aminocaproic acid can be instituted. A loading dose of 5 gm intravenously or orally, followed by 1 gm/hour for the next 2 to 4 hours can be considered. Plasma volume expanders are indicated to replace blood volume deficit. If blood loss has been considerable, human red blood cells or whole blood may also be indicated. Allergic reactions determined to represent possible anaphylaxis have been observed in 2.4% of the patients. These ranged in severity from minor breathing difficulty to bronchospasm, periorbital swelling or angioneurotic edema. Other milder allergic effects such as urticaria, pruritus, flushing, nausea, headache, and musculoskeletal pain have been observed in approximately 12% of patients. There was no apparent relationship to dosage. Transient elevation or lowering of systolic blood pressure of greater than 25 mm Hg has been observed in less than 2% of patients. Mild to moderate reactions may be managed with concomitant antihistamine or corticosteroid therapy or both without interrupting treatment; however, severe allergic responses require immediate discontinuation of streptokinase, with corticosteroids administered intravenously as required. Although the drug has been reported to be nonpyrogenic, approximately ⅓ of patients have shown increases in body temperature of 1.5° F or more; the incidence of fever of 104° F or greater was 3.4%. Symptomatic treatment with acetaminophen rather than with aspirin is recommended and is usually sufficient to alleviate discomfort. Phlebitis near the site of intravenous infusion has occurred in less than 2% of patients. Further dilution of the streptokinase solution is generally adequate for management.

Dosage and Administration: *Intravenously.* The recommended treatment of venous thrombosis and pulmonary embolism begins with a loading dose of 250,000 IU administered by intravenous infusion over a 30-minute period, followed by a sustaining infusion of 100,000 IU/hour using an infusion pump. Thrombin time should be determined at 4 hours, 12 hours and twice daily thereafter. The drug should be used within 24 hours following reconstitution. The physician is urged to refer to the package literature for comprehensive details.

Availability:
STREPTASE® Lyophilized White Powder in color-coded labeled vials of 6.5 ml representing 100,000 IU (yellow), 250,000 IU (green) and 750,000 IU (blue) in packages of 10. **(Hoechst)**

STREPTOKINASE-STREPTODORNASE

Description: A mixture composed of extracellular enzymes derived from the growth of a strain of *Streptococcus hemolyticus. Streptokinase* is an extracellular enzyme activator and is unique in its specificity and the rapidity with which it transforms plasminogen to plasmin. It changes plasminogen into the active enzyme plasmin which then causes fibrinolysis. Under the influence of plasmin, insoluble fibrin and soluble fibrinogen undergo a mild proteolysis to smaller soluble proteins or large polypeptides with only approximately 10% evolved as nonprotein nitrogen. Antistreptokinase antibodies may develop in patients treated with streptokinase and may persist for at least 2 years after therapy. In some instances, patients treated with the enzymes developed anaphylactoid reactions. Its potency is standardized on the basis of units. One unit is defined as the activity contained in an amount of solution which will cause lysis of a standard fibrin clot in 10 minutes.

Streptodornase is a deoxyribonuclease and acts directly upon a substrate of deoxyribonucleoprotein and deoxyribonucleic acid, which are the chief components of the nuclei and constitute 30 to 70% of the sediment of thick purulent exudates. Its action requires the presence of the magnesium ion that is universally present in tissues. The nucleoprotein is split into free purine bases and pyrimidine nucleosides, thus lowering the viscosity of purulent material. In addition to its depolymerizing action, there is a progressive liberation of acid-soluble phosphorus and nitrogen from the substrate, with no increase in uric acid. Thus, the enzyme produces a striking decrease in degenerated leukocytes and a rapid disappearance of all extracellular deoxyribonucleoprotein. It acts only on extracellular nucleoprotein or nuclei of degenerating cells; it does not attack the nuclei or nucleoprotein of living cells and there is no evidence of species specificity. Potency is standardized on the basis of units. One unit is defined as that amount of enzyme that will bring about a change in the relative viscosity of an 0.15% solution of deoxyribonucleic acid from 5 to 4 in 10 minutes at 30° C.

Indications: Topical agent to remove clotted blood or fibrinous or purulent accumulations present following trauma or inflammation. It is also used as an adjunct in the treatment of hemothorax, hematoma, empyema, and chronic suppuration involving draining sinuses, osteomyelitis, infected wounds or ulcers and other common suppurative lesions. As an adjunct to surgery in the care of chronic suppuration, the enzymes may aid in making secondary closure more effective and may be of value in preventing postoperative adhesions. However, their use in surgical debridement and drainage should be more as supplements rather than substitutes. The enzymes do not act upon fibrous tissues, mucoproteins, or collagen; thus, when an area of hemorrhage or pyogenic exudate is developing, their action is less efficacious. Intramuscular use is proposed for the treatment of edema and trauma in such conditions as thrombophlebitis, epididymitis and cellulitis, with concomitant use of a broad spectrum antibiotic agent. Oral administration is helpful as an adjunct to standard therapeutic procedures in reducing soft tissue inflammation and edema associated with traumatic injuries such as contusions, sprains, ecchymoses, and hematomas; in localized inflammation such as abscesses, phlebitis, thrombophlebitis, dermatoses, cellulitis, and diabetic and vascular ulcers; in induced trauma following dental, obstetrical, genitourinary, plastic, and general surgical procedures; and to liquefy upper respiratory tract secretions as in bronchitis and chronic bronchiectasis.

Contraindications: Intravenous administration; in patients with reduced plasminogen or fibrinogen levels.

Precautions: Because streptokinase-streptodornase does not act upon fibrous tissues, mucoproteins, or collagen, its use in conditions involving scarring, organized exudate or organized blood clots is not recommended. Allergic manifestations are rare, but proper precautions should be taken. Prolonged therapy may produce anti-streptokinase antibodies. The antibody titer apparently is not harmful, but higher dosage is necessary.

Adverse Reactions: Nausea, vomiting, diarrhea, skin rash and urticaria following oral administration have been reported but rarely required withdrawal of therapy. A pyrogenic reaction is the most common effect from topical administration that is usually minimized when closed areas are drained regularly. Pain at the site of injection or a febrile reaction has occurred after intramuscular administration.

Dosage and Administration: *Intramuscularly.* The recommended dosage is 0.5 ml (streptokinase, 5000 units and streptodornase, 1250 units) twice daily. *Orally.* The suggested dosage is 1 tablet (streptokinase, 10,000 units and streptodornase, 2500 units) 4 times daily. *Topically.* A solution of the enzymes is prepared by adding enough isotonic sodium chloride solution to the vial to provide approximately 5000 to 10,000 units of streptokinase and 1000 to 2000 units of streptodornase/ml. For closed cavity conditions such as hemothorax and empyema, initial doses of 200,000 and 50,000 units of streptokinase and streptodornase, respectively, are suggested; instillation by means of a thoracotomy tube. For use in smaller spaces such as in maxillary sinus empyema, proportionately smaller doses of 10,000 units of streptokinase and 2500 units of streptodornase are used. In order to maintain debriding activity in closed spaces, the enzyme must be aspirated and replenished regularly because of the increase in fluid volume resulting from liquefaction of the exudate. In chronic suppurations, such as draining sinuses or open wounds, and in ulcers, this preparation is administered by *instillation* or by *direct application* with gauze dressings. Repeated application is necessary to maintain enzymatic activity.

Availability:
VARIDASE®: **(Lederle)**
Intramuscular Injection in vials of 25,000 units.
Oral Tablets, 12,500 units in bottles of 24 and 100
Topical Solution in vials of 125,000 units.
With Carboxymethylcellulose (CMC) Jelly in a combination package consisting of 1 vial of Varidase (125,000 units) and 1 jar of CMC jelly (4.5%), 15 ml.

STREPTOMYCIN SULFATE

Description: Streptomycin is a water-soluble aminoglycoside antibiotic derived from *Streptomyces griseus.* Since it is not absorbed from the gastrointestinal tract when given orally, streptomycin should be administered parenterally for systemic action.

In recommended doses, streptomycin is active against susceptible strains of many gram-negative and gram-positive organisms, including the tubercle bacillus. When used alone, bacterial resistance has been shown to develop rapidly. Therefore, in the treatment of tuberculosis, it should be used in combination with other antituberculous drugs. In therapeutic doses, streptomycin is bactericidal; the mode of action is the interference with normal protein synthesis and production of "faulty proteins."

Following intramuscular injection of 1 gm of the drug, a peak serum level of 25 to 50 mcg/ml is reached within 1 hour, diminishing slowly to about 50% after 5 to 6 hours. Appreciable concentrations are found in all organ tissues except the brain. Significant amounts have been found in pleural fluid and tuberculous cavities. Streptomycin passes through the placenta with serum levels in the cord blood similar to maternal levels. Small amounts are excreted in milk, saliva, and sweat. It is excreted rapidly in the urine by glomerular filtration. In patients with normal kidney function, between 29 and 89% of a single 0.6-gm dose is excreted within 24 hours. Any reduction of glomerular activity results in decreased excretion of the drug and concurrent rise in serum and tissue levels. If the Kirby-Bauer method of disc sensitivity is used, a 10-mcg streptomycin disc should give a zone of over 15 mm when tested against streptomycin-sensitive bacterial strain.

Indications: Treatment of all types of tuberculosis. Used alone or in combination with other drugs or antibiotics, streptomycin may be useful in the treatment of urinary tract infections, tularemia, plague, bacterial endocarditis, enterococcal endocarditis, brucellosis, pneumonia, gonorrhea, granuloma inguinale, and other infections caused by susceptible organisms.

Contraindications: Patients with a history of ototoxic reactions or other hypersensitivity reactions to streptomycin.

Warnings: The risk of severe neurotoxic reactions is sharply increased in patients with impaired kidney function or prerenal azotemia. These include disturbances of the auditory nerve, optic nerve, peripheral neuritis, arachnoiditis, and encephalopathy. Renal function should be carefully determined and patients with renal damage and nitrogen retention should be given reduced dosage. The peak serum concentration in individuals with kidney damage should not exceed 20 to 25 mcg/ml.

The concurrent systemic use of other neurotoxic and/or nephrotoxic drugs, particularly kanamycin, polymyxin B, polymyxin E (colistin), neomycin, and viomycin, should be avoided. The neurotoxicity of streptomycin can result in respiratory paralysis from neuromuscular blockade, especially when the drug is given soon after anesthesia and the use of muscle relaxants.

The administration of streptomycin in parenteral form should be reserved for patients where adequate laboratory facilities are available and constant supervision of the patient is possible. This antibiotic may frequently affect the vestibular branch of the auditory nerve causing severe nausea, vomiting, and vertigo. The incidence is directly proportional to duration and amount of the drug administered. Advanced age and renal impairment predispose to ototoxicity. Symptoms subside and recovery is usually complete following discontinuance of the drug. Loss of hearing has been reported following long-term therapy; however, ototoxic effect on the auditory branch of the eighth nerve is infrequent and usually is preceded by vestibular symptoms. Hearing loss, when extensive, is usually permanent. Since streptomycin readily crosses the placental barrier, cautious use of the drug is important to prevent ototoxicity in the fetus.

Solutions should *never* be injected intravenously or intrathecally. Special care should be taken to avoid contact with or inhalation of this antibiotic.

Precautions: Baseline and periodic caloric stimulation tests and audiometric tests are advisable with extended streptomycin therapy. Tinnitus, roaring noises, or a sense of fullness in the ears indicates need for audiometric examination or termination of therapy or both. Care should be taken by individuals handling or preparing streptomycin for injection to avoid skin-sensitivity reactions. As with other antibiotics, use of this drug may result in overgrowth of nonsusceptible organisms, including fungi. If superinfection occurs, appropriate therapy should be instituted. When treating patients with gonorrhea, granuloma inguinale or chancroid, if a concomitant syphilitic condition is suspected, the clinician should initiate such laboratory procedures as a dark field examination prior to treatment, and thereafter, a monthly serologic test should be performed for at least 4 successive months.

Adverse Reactions: Commonly noted were ototoxicity manifested by nausea, vomiting, and vertigo; paresthesia of the face; rash; fever; urticaria, angioneurotic edema; and eosinophilia. Those less frequently noted were deafness, exfoliative dermatitis, anaphylaxis, azotemia, leukopenia, thrombocytopenia, pancytopenia, hemolytic anemia, muscular weakness, and amblyopia.

Dosage and Administration: *Intramuscularly* only. *For active pulmonary tuberculosis,* 1 gm daily during the early months of initial therapy. This dosage can be reduced to 1 gm 2 or 3 times weekly after the disease is controlled. Streptomycin should be administered concurrently with isoniazid and/or other antituberculous agents. For elderly patients or those with auditory or renal function impairment, lower daily doses (0.5 gm) are recommended. *For unusually severe pulmonary, meningeal, miliary or genitourinary tuberculosis,* 1 to 2 gm daily of streptomycin together with full doses of isoniazid and/or PAS should be initiated and maintained until a remission has been established; streptomycin dosage may then be intermittent (twice weekly). *For nontuberculous infections,* 1 gm daily in divided doses; therapy with streptomycin alone is rarely indicated beyond 7 to 10 days. Brucellosis should be treated over a period of 3 weeks with 2 gm of streptomycin daily for the first week and 1 gm daily for the remaining 2 weeks in conjunction with 2 gm of tetracycline hydrochloride daily. The individual dose of streptomycin for children may be calculated as 10 mg/lb of body weight to a maximum of 20 mg/lb of body weight daily in equally divided doses at 6- to 8-hour intervals. Particular care should be taken to avoid excessive dosage in children.

Availability:
STREPTOMYCIN SULFATE Injection, 0.5 gm/ml in ampuls of 2 and 10 ml. **(Lilly)**
STREPTOMYCIN SULFATE Powder for Injection in ampuls of 1 and 5 gm. **(Lilly)**
STREPTOMYCIN SULFATE Injection, 1 gm/2.5 ml in vials of 2.5 and 12.5 ml; 1 gm/2 ml in Isoject® (disposable prefilled syringes and needle unit) of 2 ml. **(Pfizer)**
STREPTOMYCIN SULFATE Powder for Injection in vials of 1 and 5 gm. **(Pfizer)**

STUART PRENATAL with FOLIC ACID

Description: Each tablet contains:

Vitamin A acetate	(6000 U.S.P. units)	1.8 mg
Vitamin D (ergocalciferol)	(400 U.S.P. units)	10 μg
Ascorbic acid		100 mg
Thiamine mononitrate		3 mg
Riboflavin		3 mg
Pyridoxine hydrochloride		10 mg
Cyanocobalamin (vitamin B-12)		5 μg
Niacinamide		20 mg
Pantothenic acid (from 5.44 mg calcium pantothenate)		5 mg
Folic acid		0.3 mg
Iron (from 197 mg ferrous fumarate)		65 mg
Calcium (from 1.2 gm calcium sulfate)		350 mg

Indications: Vitamin-mineral supplement for use during pregnancy and lactation. Folic acid is added to aid in the prevention of megaloblastic anemia.

Precautions: Folic acid may partially correct the hematological damage due to vitamin B-12 deficiency of pernicious anemia while the associated neurological damage progresses.

Dosage and Administration: *Orally.* One tablet daily after a meal, or as directed by the physician.

Availability:
STUART PRENATAL® with FOLIC ACID Tablets in bottles of 100. **(Stuart)**

SUCCINYLCHOLINE CHLORIDE

Chemical Name: bis(2-Dimethylaminoethyl)succinate bis(methochloride).

Description: Succinylcholine chloride is a synthetic quaternary ammonium compound which produces rapid and complete relaxation of skeletal muscle for brief periods. It produces muscular relaxation by inducing depolarization of motor end-plates at the myoneural junction. The drug has no demonstrable effect on consciousness, the pain threshold or on cerebration, and no direct effect on the myocardium, smooth muscles or the uterus. Since the drug is highly ionized and has a low lipid solubility, it does not readily cross the placenta and may, therefore, be employed in obstretrical anesthesia. It occurs as a white, odorless, slightly bitter powder that is very soluble in water. The drug is unstable in alkaline solutions, but is relatively stable in acid solutions depending upon the concentration of the solution and the storage temperature. To preserve its potency, it should be stored under refrigeration. Each ml of aqueous solution contains the equivalent of 20, 25, 50 or 100 mg of anhydrous salt.

Succinylcholine produces skeletal muscle paralysis by blocking neural transmission at the myoneural junction. It competes with acetylcholine for the cholinergic receptors of the motor end plate. The neuromuscular block so achieved produces a flaccid paralysis of skeletal muscles. Succinylcholine is dissipated through the enzymatic action of pseudocholinesterase at such a rate that the effect of a single paralyzing dose of the drug generally disappears within 8 to 10 minutes. When a single effective dose of the drug is given intravenously, muscular relaxation occurs within 1 minute, persists for about 2 minutes and returns to normal within 8 to 10 minutes. If a paralyzing dose is given intramuscularly, the onset of action may be delayed for 2 to 3 minutes. When given by intravenous drip, a predetermined degree of muscular relaxation can be closely approximated by adjusting the rate of flow of the infusion.

Succinylcholine differs from tubocurarine in that it is not generally antagonized by anticholinesterases. On the contrary, such drugs as physostigmine, neostigmine and procaine usually prolong the action of succinylcholine. The drug is rapidly hydrolyzed by pseudocholinesterase to succinylmonocholine (a weak nondepolarizing type of muscle relaxant), and then more slowly to the normal metabolites succinic acid and choline. However, about 10% of the drug is excreted unchanged in the urine. Compounds such as magnesium sulfate, quinine and quinidine have been reported to potentiate the neuromuscular blockade produced by succinylcholine; diazepam to reduce the duration of the blockade. Succinylcholine's action may be additionally altered by acetylcholine, anticholinesterases, dehydration, hypothermia, electrolyte imbalance, antibiotics other than the penicillin group, some carcinomas, procaine-type local anesthetics or the administration of other nondepolarizing or depolarizing muscle relaxants.

Indications: Adjunct to anesthesia to induce skeletal muscle relaxation. May also be employed to reduce the intensity of muscle contractions of pharmacologically or electrically induced convulsions.

Contraindications: In patients with known hypersensitivity to the drug.

Warnings: Succinylcholine should be administered *only* by anesthesiologists or those qualified to manage patients during apnea, and *only* when apparatus for assisted or controlled respiration with oxygen is available. Because the drug is readily hydrolyzed in alkaline solutions, it is incompatible with barbiturates; therefore, separate injections are mandatory. Safe use during pregnancy has not been established, and should not be used in women of childbearing potential and particularly during the first trimester of pregnancy unless in the judgment of the physician the potential benefits outweigh the unknown hazards.

Precautions: Low levels, or abnormal variants of plasma pseudocholinesterase may be associated with prolonged respiratory depression or apnea following the use of succinylcholine. Low levels of the enzyme may occur in patients with severe liver disease or cirrhosis, severe anemia, malnutrition, severe dehydration, changes in body temperature, exposure to neurotoxic insecticides, those receiving antimalarial drugs, or those with a recessive hereditary trait. Succinylcholine should be administered with extreme care to such patients and dosage should be minimal. If low plasma pseudocholinesterase activity is suspected, a small test dose of from 5 to 10 mg of succinylcholine may be administered, or relaxation may be produced by the cautious administration of an 0.1% solution of the drug by intravenous drip. Drugs which either inhibit plasma cholinesterase, such as neostigmine, or compete with succinylcholine for the enzyme, as does intravenous procaine, should not be given concurrently with succinylcholine.

The clinician is urged to use special care in patients with cardiovascular, hepatic, pulmonary, metabolic, or renal disorders, those with severe burns, those recovering from severe trauma, those suffering from electrolyte imbalance, those who have been digitalized recently or who may have digitalis toxicity as serious cardiac arrhythmias or cardiac arrest may result. Utmost caution should be observed also in patients with preexisting hyperkalemia or who are paraplegic, have suffered spinal neuraxis injury, or have degenerative or dystrophic neuromuscular disease, as such patients tend to become severely hyperkalemic when succinylcholine is given. When the drug is given over a prolonged period of time, the characteristic depolarization block of the myoneural junction may change to a nondepolarizing block which results in prolonged respiratory depression or apnea. Succinylcholine should be used with caution during ocular surgery and in patients with glaucoma. The drug should be employed with caution in patients with fractures or muscle spasm as the muscle fasciculations may cause additional trauma. Muscle fasciculations and hyperkalemia may be reduced by administering a small dose of a nondepolarizing relaxant. If other relaxants are to be used during the same procedure, the possibility of a synergistic or antagonistic effect should be considered. The sudden development of severe, malignant hyperthermia has been reported to occur in patients receiving potent anesthetics such as halothane, methoxyfluothane, cyclopropane, and diethyl ether as well as succinylcholine. Although the etiology is unknown, the syndrome appears to have a genetic basis and to occur in male and female patients of all ages. Because of the seriousness of this adverse effect and the need for early effective treatment, it is strongly advised that the patient's temperature be continuously monitored throughout such procedures.

Adverse Reactions: These consist primarily of an extension of the pharmacologic actions of the drug. Profound and prolonged muscle relaxation may occur, resulting in respiratory depression to the point of apnea. Also, it has been reported to cause both decreases and increases in heart rate and blood pressure. Initially, a transient bradycardia accompanied by hypotension, arrhythmias and even a sinus arrest may occur due to an increase in vagal tone. This is noted particularly in children and is more apparent with repetitive administration. These effects are enhanced by cyclopropane and halothane and are inhibited by thiopental and atropine. Transient increase in intraocular pressure, hypertension, tachyphylaxis (following repeated administration), cardiac arrest, respiratory depression, apnea, hyperthermia, muscle fasciculation, postoperative muscle pain, myoglobinemia and myoglobinuria, especially in children, and excessive salivation were also noted.

Dosage and Administration: *Intravenously* or *intramuscularly.* Dosage is essentially individualized, and the drug should be administered only after unconsciousness has been induced. Initially, a test dose of 10 mg may be used to determine the patient's response and recovery time. *For short surgical procedures*, the usual adult dose is 40 mg given *intravenously* as a single injection; the optimum dose will vary from 20 to 80 mg. *For prolonged surgical procedures,* sustained relaxation may be obtained with continuous *intravenous drip* infusion at the rate of 2.5 mg/minute for adult patients. A solution of 0.1 or 0.2% in either 5% dextrose or sodium chloride injection is employed. *Intermittent intravenous* injection may also be used to provide muscular relaxation for long procedures. Initially, 20 to 80 mg followed at appropriate intervals by further injections of 3 to 5 mg so that the desired degree of relaxation required will be maintained. The intravenous dose for infants and children is 1 to 2 mg/kg of body weight. Succinylcholine may be given *intramuscularly* to infants, older children or adults when a suitable vein is inaccessible. A dose of up to 2.5 mg/kg is given, but no more than a total dose of 150 mg should be administered.

Availability:

ANECTINE®: **(Burroughs Wellcome)**
Injection, 20 mg/ml in multi-dose vials of 10 ml.
Powder for Injection in Flo-Pack® vials of 0.5 and 1 gm.

QUELICIN® Injection, 20 mg/ml in Fliptop vials of 10 ml; 50 mg/ml in ampuls of 10 ml; 100 mg/ml in ampuls of 10 ml, in half-filled Fliptop vials of 20 ml and in half-filled Pintop vials of 10 and 20 ml. **(Abbott)**

SUCCINYLCHOLINE CHLORIDE Injection, 20 mg/ml in multiple-dose vials of 10 ml. **(Organon)**

SUCOSTRIN® Injection, 20 mg/ml in vials of 10 ml; 50 mg/ml in ampuls of 10 ml; 100 mg/ml in vials of 10 ml. **(Squibb)**

SULADYNE: see The Sulfonamides

SULFACETAMIDE SODIUM: see The Sulfonamides

SULFACHLORPYRIDAZINE: see The Sulfonamides

SULFACYTINE: see The Sulfonamides

SULFADIAZINE: see The Sulfonamides

SULFAMETER: see The Sulfonamides

SULFAMETHIZOLE: see The Sulfonamides

SULFAMETHOXAZOLE: see The Sulfonamides

SULFAMETHOXYPYRIDAZINE: see The Sulfonamides

SULFASALAZINE: see The Sulfonamides

SULFINPYRAZONE

Chemical Name: 1,2-Diphenyl-4-(2′-phenylsulfinylethyl)-3,5-pyrazolidinedione.

Description: Sulfinpyrazone is a sulfoxide analog of phenylbutazone and is a potent uricosuric agent, but lacks the clinically impressive antiinflammatory and analgesic properties of the parent compound. It occurs as a white, bitter, odorless, crystalline powder slightly soluble in water and in alcohol. Its molecular weight is 404.4.

Clinical observations suggest that sulfinpyrazone produces its uricosuric effect by preventing tubular reabsorption of uric acid, without affecting the rate of glomerular filtration.

Following oral administration, the drug is rapidly and completely absorbed from the gastrointestinal tract. Its uricosuric effect may persist for as long as 10 hours. Approximately 98 to 99% is bound to plasma proteins. About ½ of the orally administered dose appears in the urine in 24 hours; 90% of the drug is eliminated in unchanged form, and the remainder as N_1-p-hydroxyphenyl metabolite which is also an active uricosuric substance. Studies with animals have not produced conclusive evidence of teratogenic potential.

Indications: Management of chronic gout; it is not intended for the relief of an acute attack. By reducing the serum urate level, the drug materially reduces or abolishes the number and severity of acute attacks in both chronic tophaceous and acute intermittent gout. **Note:** In the initial stages of therapy, because of the drug's ability to mobilize urates, acute attacks of gouty arthritis may be precipitated.

Contraindications: Active peptic ulcer; coadministration with salicylates.

Warnings: Sulfinpyrazone should be used cautiously in pregnant patients and the anticipated therapeutic benefits of the drug should be weighed against the possible hazards to the fetus.

Precautions: It should be used with caution in patients with known sensitivity to phenylbutazone and other pyrazoles. It may be administered with care to patients with a history of healed peptic ulcer. Constant medical supervision and periodic blood counts are recommended. Special care is required when administered concurrently with sulfonamides, the sulfonylurea hypoglycemic agents and insulin. The hazard of precipitating renal calculi and causing renal colic exists, particularly during the initial stages of therapy; therefore, an adequate fluid intake and alkalinization of the urine are recommended. In patients with significant renal impairment, renal function should be evaluated periodically. Sulfinpyrazone may accentuate the action of coumarin-type anticoagulants and further depress prothrombin activity when these medications are employed simultaneously.

Adverse Reactions: Most frequently observed are upper gastrointestinal disturbances (should be administered with food, milk or antacids), aggravation or reactivation of peptic ulcer. Less than 3% of the patients experienced skin rash which in most instances did not require discontinuation of therapy. Blood dyscrasias manifested by anemia, leukopenia, agranulocytosis and thrombocytopenia have been noted. Overdosage is characterized by nausea, vomiting, diarrhea, epigastric pain, ataxia, labored respiration, convulsions, and coma. Other possible reactions that may occur include anemia, jaundice, and ulceration. Since there is no specific antidote, treatment involves inducing emesis or instituting gastric lavage, intravenous glucose infusions and analeptics.

Dosage and Administration: *Orally.* Initially, 200 to 400 mg daily in 2 divided doses, with meals or milk, gradually increasing to full maintenance level in 1 week. Maintenance, 400 mg daily (200 to 800 mg may be given if necessary) in 2 divided doses. Treatment should be continued without interruption even in the event of acute exacerbations which can be concomitantly treated with phenylbutazone or colchicine.

Availability:
ANTURANE®: **(Ciba)**
Capsules, 200 mg in bottles of 100.
Tablets, 100 mg in bottles of 100.

SULFISOXAZOLE: see The Sulfonamides

SULFOBROMOPHTHALEIN

Chemical Name: Disodium phenoltetrabromophthalein-3′,3″-disulfonate.

Description: Sulfobromophthalein occurs as a white, crystalline, hygroscopic powder soluble in water and insoluble in alcohol. Following intravenous injection, the dye is bound to plasma proteins and transported to the liver where about 80% is biotransformed into conjugated compounds which are then excreted in the bile. The rate of clearance from the blood provides a useful test of hepatic excretory function.

Indications: To test the functional capacity of the liver, particularly to detect hepatic disease with little or no associated jaundice.

Contraindications: Hypersensitivity to sulfobromophthalein or a history of allergy, urticaria, atrophy or asthma; injection into an artery or muscle.

Precautions: Since anaphylactoid reactions have occurred, the dye should be administered only by highly qualified persons and should be injected slowly over a period of 5 minutes. Extravasation should be avoided and when observed, administration of the dye should be terminated. Vigorous resuscitation should be attempted in the event of an anaphylactoid reaction and epinephrine and antihistaminics should be readily available. Patients with a history of allergy or extreme drug sensitivities should be given an intradermal test (0.1 ml of a 1:100 dilution) before BSP determination is made. Concentrations stronger than 1:100 dilution should not be used intradermally as such concentrations may confuse the sensitivity test. It should be used with extreme caution, if at all, in patients in whom repeated sulfobromophthalein tests have been done. Because the dyes used in gallbladder tests interfere with the excretion and clearance of sulfobromophthalein, the BSP determination should either precede gallbladder tests or be delayed for at least 1 week. Morphine, pethidine, amidone, and amine oxidase inhibitors may give slightly elevated readings, and anabolic steroids, certain estrogens, androgens and oral contraceptive agents interfere with BSP readings. **Note:** The solution approaches the limit of solubility of the dye. Ampuls should be stored in a warm place to prevent crystallization; should crystals form they may readily be redissolved by immersing the ampul in warm (not hot) water. Because this product is an indicator dye, very small difference in pH affects the tint of the solution; slight variations of tint in different lots are not, however, of any practical significance.

Adverse Reactions: Nausea and thrombophlebitis.

Dosage and Administration: *Intravenously* only. Inject 5 mg/kg of body weight slowly into an arm vein. At the end of 45 to 60 minutes, 5 ml of blood is withdrawn from a vein in the opposite arm and the amount of dye retained in the blood is estimated by comparisons with standards. For alternate methods, see package literature.

Availability:
BROMSULPHALEIN® (BSP®) Solution, 50 mg/ml in ampuls of 3, 7.5 and 10 ml.

(Hynson, Westcott & Dunning)

THE SULFONAMIDES, ANTIBACTERIAL

All of the antibacterial sulfonamides are closely related chemical compounds. They exist in the blood as free, conjugated (acetylated and possibly other forms) and protein-bound forms. The "free" form is considered to be the therapeutically active form. It has been shown that approximately 70% is protein bound in the blood, and of the unbound portion 80 to 90% is in the nonacetylated form. Excretion of sulfonamides is chiefly by the kidneys with glomerular filtration as the primary mechanism.

The systemic sulfonamides are bacteriostatic agents. The spectrum of activity is similar for all. Sulfonamides competitively inhibit bacterial synthesis of folic acid from para-aminobenzoic acid. Resistant strains are capable of utilizing folic acid precursors or preformed folic acid.

They vary in effectiveness against various bacterial organisms in the rate of absorption and excretion, solubility, rate and degree of hepatic acetylation, degree of plasma binding, and in toxicity. Those sulfonamides with a free amino group on the benzene ring, such as sulfadiazine, exert their bacteriostatic effect by acting as a competitive antimetabolite. Some bacteria, by altering their metabolic pathways, can develop a high degree of resistance to these drugs during therapy, and cross resistance to all sulfonamides must then be expected. Hepatic acetylation of the free amino group is the usual means of detoxication, although for some compounds glucuronide conjugation is more important. Either type of detoxication inactivates the drug, and may increase or decrease its solubility in the urine.

Indications: The short-acting systemic sulfonamides appear to be indicated in the following conditions: acute, recurrent and chronic urinary tract infections (primarily pyelonephritis, pyelitis, cystitis) due to susceptible organisms (such as *E. coli, Klebsiella-Aerobacter, Staphylococcus aureus, Proteus mirabilis* and, less frequently, *Proteus vulgaris*), meningococcal meningitis where the organisms are susceptible, *Haemophilus influenzae* meningitis (as an adjunct to parenteral streptomycin), meningococcal meningitis group A strains, toxoplasmosis (as an adjunct to pyrimethamine therapy), acute otitis media due to *H. influenzae* as adjunct to penicillin, chancroid, trachoma, inclusion conjunctivitis, corneal ulcer and other superficial ocular infections, nocardiosis, as adjunctive therapy in malaria due to chloroquine-resistant strains of *Plasmodium falciparum* and, as an alternative to the preferred penicillin, in the prophylaxis of rheumatic fever (sulfadiazine only).

Use of the less hazardous short-acting sulfonamides is preferred over the long-acting systemic group.

According to the U.S. Food and Drug Administration, the systemic sulfonamides are probably not indicated in common respiratory, skin, soft tissue, gastrointestinal and chronic obstructive urinary tract infections because of potential adverse side effects and lack of evidence of effectiveness. Except for sulfadiazine in rheumatic fever, the sulfonamides are not indicated for prophylactic use.

Those preparations which are not absorbed from the gastrointestinal tract may be utilized either in an attempt to sterilize the gut preoperatively or to treat specific infections of the intestinal tract, or for the management of specific diseases such as ulcerative colitis (sulfasalazine).

In vitro sulfonamide sensitivity tests are not always reliable. The test must be carefully coordinated with bacteriologic and clinical response. When patients are taking sulfonamides, follow-up cultures should have aminobenzoic acid added to the culture media. **Important Note:** The increasing frequency of resistant organisms is a limitation of the usefulness of antibacterial agents including the sulfonamides, especially in the treatment of chronic and recurrent urinary tract infections.

Contraindications: Hypersensitivity to sulfonamides including antibacterials, oral hypoglycemics, and thiazide diuretics. In infants less than 2 months of age, except in the treatment of congenital toxoplasmosis as adjunctive therapy with pyrimethamine. In patients with intestinal or urinary obstruction, or in those with porphyria, since these drugs may precipitate an acute attack. Pregnancy at term and during the nursing period, because sulfonamides pass the placenta and are excreted in the milk and may result in kernicterus in the infant by displacing protein-bound bilirubin. Because of their tendency to produce crystalluria, the sulfonamides may be contraindicated in patients with only one kidney or when adequate urinary volume cannot be maintained.

Warnings: Safe use of sulfonamides during pregnancy has not been established, and their use should be limited only to those cases in which a definite need has been confirmed. Laboratory studies have indicated a significant increase in the incidence of cleft palate and other bony abnormalities in the offspring of mice and rats. Sulfonamides are not recommended for the treatment of group A beta-hemolytic streptococcal infections because they will not eradicate the organisms and, therefore, will not prevent the subsequent development of such conditions as rheumatic fever and glomerulonephritis. Deaths from hypersensitivity reactions, agranulocytosis, aplastic anemia, and other blood dyscrasias, irreversible neuromuscular and CNS changes, and fibrosing alveolitis have been reported. Fatalities have also occurred due to the development of the Stevens-Johnson syndrome following the use of sulfonamides; therefore, the patient must be closely observed and should a rash develop during therapy, the drug should be discontinued immediately. The presence of clinical signs such as sore throat, fever, pallor, purpura or jaundice may be early indications of serious blood disorders; therefore, complete blood counts should be performed frequently in patients receiving sulfonamides. To prevent crystalluria and stone formation, it is essential that sufficient fluid intake be maintained. Also, urinalysis with careful microscopic examination should be obtained frequently in patients receiving these agents.

Precautions: As with all drugs that are largely excreted in the urine, the absorbable sulfonamides must be given with caution in the presence of impaired renal or hepatic function. The urinary volume must be adequate (about 1.5 liters/day) before therapy is even begun, and if the urine is highly acidic, sodium bicarbonate should be given concomitantly. Since some sulfonamides may form an insoluble precipitate with formaldehyde in the urine, it is probable that no methenamine compound should be given during sulfonamide therapy. Sulfonamides may also cause kernicterus in newborn or jaundiced infants; presumably, therefore, these drugs should never be given to premature or full-term infants less than 1 or 2 weeks of age. Sulfonamides that produce prolonged blood levels in pregnant women near term are not advisable, since these drugs may persist in the infant after birth. That detoxication of these drugs is decreased in patients with severe hepatic dysfunction should be kept in mind. Individuals with congenital deficiency of erythrocytic glucose-6 phosphate dehydrogenase (G-6-PD), which most frequently occurs in Negroes and people of Mediterranean racial descent, may develop hemolytic anemia if treated with sulfonamides; this reaction is frequently dose-related. Because of the possible occurrence of blood dyscrasias, blood cell studies should be made during prolonged therapy with any sulfonamide. Caution is essential when giving these agents to patients with a history of sensitization to any sulfonamide, especially to those patients with severe allergy or bronchial asthma.

Adverse Reactions: Allergic reactions, such as skin rashes, pruritus and fever, are the most common untoward effects; nausea, vomiting, diarrhea, anorexia, pancreatitis, stomatitis, headache, lassitude, dizziness, tinnitus, insomnia, peripheral neuritis, convulsions, ataxia, hallucinations, mental depression, abdominal pain, epidermal necrolysis, urticaria, anaphylactoid reactions, periorbital edema, conjunctival and scleral injection, arthralgia, allergic myocarditis, and photosensitization may also occur. Less common reactions include hepatotoxicity and jaundice, serious blood dyscrasias (granulocytopenia, agranulocytosis, aplastic or hemolytic anemia, leukemia, methemoglobinemia, thrombocytopenia, hypoprothrombinemia), cyanosis, purpura, central and peripheral neurotoxicity (psychoses, neuritis), toxic nephrosis with oliguria or anuria, periarteritis nodosa, lupus erythematosus, serum-sickness syndrome, and severe exfoliative dermatitis. Gross or microscopic hematuria, with or without crystalluria, is especially likely to occur in patients with oliguria or acidic urine. The long-acting sulfonamides may occasionally cause the severe skin eruption of Stevens-Johnson syndrome (erythema multiforme exudativum); this reaction appears to occur most commonly in children. Rarely noted were development of goiter, diuresis or hypoglycemia. Because some fatalities have been reported, patients receiving the long-acting sulfonamides should be observed closely; if a skin rash develops, therapy should be discontinued immediately.

Dual or triple sulfonamides (e.g., trisulfapyrimidines) may lower the incidence of renal complications. They are given in the usual dosage; however, a lesser amount of each component sulfonamide is present in the combination. It has been said that combinations of sulfonamides possess some inherent hazards as well as advantages. For example, the incidence of fever, rash and conjunctivitis is greater when sulfonamides are used in combination than it is when a single agent is employed. Also, it has been suggested that the antibacterial activity of various mixtures is unpredictable.

Dosage and Administration: *Orally, parenterally* and *topically*. Effective blood concentrations have been estimated at various levels between 1 and 12 mg/100 ml. Dosage must be adequate to prevent the utilization of available *p*-aminobenzoic acid in the body. Low dosage results only in bacteriostasis and may lead to an increase in resistant pathogenic bacteria; high dosages are bactericidal to susceptible organisms.

The preceding was a general discussion of the sulfonamides as a group. The monographs that follow deal specifically with each of the following:

Phthalysulfathiazole
Suladyne
Sulfacetamide Sodium
Sulfachlorpyridazine
Sulfacytine
Sulfadiazine
Sulfameter
Sulfamethizole
Sulfamethoxazole
Sulfamethoxypyridazine
Sulfasalazine
Sulfisoxazole
Sultrin

PHTHALYLSULFATHIAZOLE

Chemical Name: 4′-(2-Thiazolylsulfamyl)phthalanilic acid.

Description: Phthalylsulfathiazole is a dicarboxylic derivative of sulfathiazole and occurs as a white or faintly yellowish-white, crystalline powder that is practically insoluble in water, but soluble in solutions of alkali hydroxides and carbonates, and in hydrochloric acid. It is a bacteriostatic agent with activity limited essentially to the intestinal tract.

Phthalylsulfathiazole is not absorbed from the gastrointestinal tract to any appreciable degree, so that a high concentration is maintained in the bowel and systemic reactions are rare. It is hydrolyzed by bacteria in the large intestine to sulfathiazole which is poorly absorbed in the colon, thus reaching concentrations of 1 gm% in the feces with minimal risk of toxicity. Following administration of full doses of the drug, blood concentrations rarely exceed

1.5 mg%. Since little of the drug is absorbed from the gastrointestinal tract, the major portion of a therapeutic dose is excreted in the feces; only about 5% is excreted in the urine.

Indications: Preoperative preparation and postoperative management of patients requiring surgery of the intestinal tract. In nonspecific ulcerative colitis, particularly the acute form, phthalylsulfathiazole together with the usual supportive and dietary measures may help to relieve abdominal cramps, decrease blood and pus in the feces, and decrease diarrhea by producing a formed stool.

The drug shares with other antibacterial sulfonamides the potential hazards associated with its use.

Adverse Reactions: Headache, malaise, anorexia, nausea, vomiting, diarrhea, hepatitis, pancreatitis, blood dyscrasias, neuropathy, drug fever, skin rash, injection of the conjunctiva and sclera, petechiae, purpura, hematuria and crystalluria.

Dosage and Administration: *Orally. For pre- and postoperative treatment:* Initially, 125 mg/kg of body weight, then 125 mg/kg daily in 3, 4, or 6 divided doses. The daily dosage should not exceed 8 gm. *For ulcerative colitis:* The usual dosage is 50 to 100 mg/kg of body weight daily in 3 to 6 divided doses. The initial course of 2 to 4 weeks should be followed by a rest period of 5 to 10 days. The usual supportive and dietary measures should be employed.

Availability:
SULFATHALIDINE® Tablets, 0.5 gm in bottles of 100. **(Merck Sharp & Dohme)**

SULADYNE

Description: Each tablet contains sulfamethizole, 125 mg; sulfadiazine, 125 mg and phenazopyridine hydrochloride, 75 mg.

Indications: Treatment of acute urinary tract infections (cystitis, urethritis, pyelitis, pyelonephritis and prostatitis) when caused by organisms susceptible to sulfonamides; and for the symptomatic relief of associated pain, burning, frequency and urgency.

Contraindications: Hepatic or renal failure, glomerulonephritis, pyelonephritis of pregnancy with gastrointestinal disturbances, pregnant women approaching or at term; hypersensitivity to sulfonamides.

Precautions: The high solubility of this drug in both acid and alkaline body fluids minimizes the hazards of crystalluria or renal tubule obstruction. However, the usual precautions exercised with sulfonamide therapy such as maintaining an adequate liquid intake should be observed. Patients should be forewarned that this product imparts an orange-red color to the urine.

Adverse Reactions: Occasionally, anorexia, nausea, vomiting, urticaria, pruritus, rash, malaise or hematuria may occur. In such instances, the drug should be discontinued immediately.

Dosage and Administration: *Orally.* Adults, 2 tablets 4 times daily.

Availability:
SULADYNE® Tablets in bottles of 100. **(Stuart)**

SULFACETAMIDE SODIUM

Chemical Name: Sodium *N*-sulfanilylacetamide.

Description: Sulfacetamide, a highly soluble sulfonamide, occurs as a white, odorless, bitter, crystalline powder freely soluble in water and sparingly soluble in alcohol. The drug is bacteriostatic against a wide spectrum of sensitive ocular pathogens and against gram-positive pyogenic cocci.

Indications: Treatment of conjunctivitis, corneal ulcer, and other superficial ocular infections due to susceptible microorganisms, and as adjunctive treatment in systemic sulfonamide therapy of trachoma. Also for topical application in scaling dermatoses, seborrheic dermatitis, seborrhea sicca, and bacterial infections of the skin.

Precautions: Solutions of sulfacetamide sodium are incompatible with silver preparations. The ointments may retard corneal healing. Nonsusceptible organisms, including fungi, may proliferate. Sulfonamides are inactivated by the para-aminobenzoic acid present in purulent exudates. When using the lotion, particular care is required if areas of denuded or abraded skin are involved. The 30% solution has been reported to cause local irritation manifested by a transient stinging or burning sensation.

For further information, see general statement.

Dosage and Administration: *Topically. For conjunctivitis or corneal ulcer:* Instill 1 drop of the 30% solution into the lower conjunctival sac every 2 hours for severe infections, and the same amount 3 or 4 times daily for chronic infections. For prophylaxis, 1 drop 4 to 6 times daily. *For trachoma:* Instill 2 drops of the 30% solution every 2 hours, concomitant systemic sulfonamide therapy is indicated, or 1 or 2 drops of the 10% solution into the lower conjunctival sac every 2 or 3 hours during the day and less often at night. A small amount of the ointment may be applied 4 times daily and at bedtime; may be used conjunctively with either solution. *For seborrheic dermatitis:* Apply lotion to the scalp at bedtime and allow to remain overnight; repeat for 8 to 10 nights. Thereafter, repeat 1 or 2 times weekly or every other week. *For primary and secondary skin bacterial infections:* Apply lotion 2 to 4 times daily.

Availability:
BLEPH®-10/-30 Ophthalmic Solution, 10% in bottles of 5 and 15 ml; 30% in dropper bottles of 15 ml. Both products are formulated with polyvinyl alcohol (Liquifilm®), 1.4%. **(Allergan)**
CETAMIDE™ Sterile Ophthalmic Ointment, 10% in tubes of 3.5 gm. **(Alcon)**
ISOPTO® CETAMIDE Ophthalmic Solution, 15% in Drop-Tainer® bottles of 5 and 15 ml. **(Alcon)**
SEBIZON® Lotion, 10% in plastic-squeeze tubes of 90 gm. **(Schering)**
SULAMYD® SODIUM: **(Schering)**
Ophthalmic Ointment, 10% in tubes of 3.75 gm. **Note:** Is nonsterile; contains less than 5 microorganisms/gm.
Ophthalmic Solution, 10% in dropper bottles of 5 and 15 ml; 30% in dropper bottles of 15 ml.
SULF-10™ Ophthalmic Solution, 10% in dropper bottles of 15 ml and in Dropperettes® applicators of 1 ml. **(Smith, Miller & Patch)**

Combinations

VASOCIDIN® Ophthalmic Solution, 10% with prednisolone sodium phosphate, 0.25% and phenylephrine hydrochloride, 0.125% in dropper bottles of 5, 10 and 15 ml. **(Smith, Miller & Patch)**
VASOSULF® Ophthalmic Solution, 15% with phenylephrine hydrochloride, 0.125% in dropper bottles of 5 and 15 ml. **(Smith, Miller & Patch)**

SULFACHLORPYRIDAZINE

Chemical Name: N^1-(6-Chloro-3-pyridazinyl)sulfanilamide.

Description: Sulfachlorpyridazine is an antibacterial sulfonamide closely related chemically to, but differing structurally from, sulfamethoxypyridazine in that a chlorine atom has replaced a methoxy group at position 6 on the pyridazine ring. At pH 5.5 to 7.4, it is slightly less soluble than sulfisoxazole, but more soluble than sulfamethoxypyridazine or sulfadiazine. It occurs as a pale yellow, crystalline powder that is sparingly soluble in water and soluble in alcohol.

It is readily absorbed following oral administration, attaining peak blood levels of about 21.7 mg/100 ml, of which 18 mg/100 ml is in the free form, at 3 hours following a 4-gm dose. After 24 hours, the blood level usually averages 5.8 mg/100 ml, of which 4 mg/100 ml is in the free form. The free form is considered to be the therapeutically active form. Maximal urine concentration occurs within 3 to 6 hours after ingestion. Approximately 60% of the dose is eliminated in the urine within 12 hours, and of this only 24% is in the conjugated form. The conjugated form is cleared at a rate of about 2½ times faster than that of the free form.

Indications: Treatment of acute recurrent or chronic urinary tract infections, primarily cystitis pyelitis and pyelonephritis when due to susceptible organisms. See general statement for other uses.

The usual precautions applicable to sulfonamides should be observed. See general statement.

Dosage and Administration: *Orally.* Treatment should be continued for 5 to 7 days or until urinary cultures are sterile. *Adults:* 2 to 4 gm initially, then 2 to 4 gm daily in 3 to 6 divided doses. *Children and infants over 2 months of age,* 75 mg/kg of body weight initially, then 150 mg/kg daily, up to a maximum of 6 gm, in 4 to 6 divided doses.

Availability:
NEFROSUL® Tablets, 0.5 gm in bottles of 100. **(Riker)**
SONILYN® Tablets, 0.5 gm in bottles of 100 and 500. **(Mallinckrodt)**

SULFACYTINE

Chemical Name: 1-Ethyl-*N*-sulfanilylcytosine.

Description: Sulfacytine is a soluble, short-acting, antibacterial sulfonamide that is similar in action to sulfadiazine and sulfisoxazole. However, studies with infections in mice have found it to be 2 to 3 times as active as sulfisoxazole. It occurs as a white, crystalline solid that is very slightly soluble in water and freely soluble in boiling alcohol. The bacteriostatic activity of sulfacytine is limited essentially to the genitourinary tract.

When given orally in single doses of 0.5, 1, 2 and 4 gm, the drug is rapidly and adequately absorbed from the gastrointestinal tract, and reaches peak blood levels within 2 to 3 hours, with a half-life of 4 hours. Clinical studies showed that an oral dosage of 250 mg 4 times daily for 7 days will produce a mean total sulfonamide plasma level of 16.8 mcg/ml, and a mean free plasma level of 16.5 mcg/ml for 2 to 7 days. Of the total amount of sulfacytine found in the urine, as determined by chromatographic analysis, about 79% is in the free form, whereas 10% is acetylated and approximately 11% is present as *N*-glucuronides. The drug is bound to plasma proteins to the extent of 86%, but it is readily released as the concentration of unbound sulfonamide falls. Kidney excretion is rapid with approximately 88% of a single 500-mg dose appearing in the urine at the end of 24 hours and 95% at the end of 5 days. Following the recommended dosage schedule, the urinary concentration of free sulfacytine was found to be over 10 times the highest minimal inhibitory concentration (MIC) for sensitive strains of Escherichia coli, Enterobacter and Proteus organisms.

Indications: Treatment of acute urinary infections such as pyelonephritis, pyelitis, and cystitis due to susceptible strains of the following microorganisms: *Escherichia coli, Klebsiella-Enterobacter, Staphylococcus aureus, Proteus mirabilis,* and *Proteus vulgaris.* It should not be used if obstructive uropathy or foreign bodies are present.

The drug shares with other antibacterial sulfonamides the potential contraindications, warnings, precautions and adverse reactions. See general statement.

Dosage and Administration: *Orally.* The usual adult dose is 500 mg as an initial loading dose, then 250 mg 4 times daily for 10 days. Due to lack of clinical experience with sulfacytine in the pediatric age group, it is not recommended for use in children under 14 years of age.

Availability:
RENOQUID® Tablets, 250 mg in bottles of 100, in unit-dose packages of 100 (10 × 10) and in Therapy Packs of 41 tablets (10 days dosage regimen). **(Parke-Davis)**

SULFADIAZINE

Chemical Name: 2-Sulfanilamidopyrimidine.

Description: Sulfadiazine occurs as a white or slightly yellow powder insoluble in water and sparingly soluble in alcohol. The sodium salt of sulfadiazine is freely soluble in water and slightly soluble in alcohol.

In controlled studies in adult volunteers given a single oral dose of 2 gm, peak serum levels of 6.04 mg/100 ml, of which 4.65 mg/100 ml is in the free form, were attained in 4 hours and approximately 50% was recovered in the urine within the 24-hour period following administration. It readily diffuses into cerebrospinal fluid and is the sulfonamide of choice in treating meningococcal meningitis. Protein binding ranges from 38 to 48%.

Indications: Sulfadiazine alone or in combination with other sulfonamides is used in the treatment of infections caused by susceptible gram-negative and gram-positive organisms as well as being effective against yeasts. Included are bacillary dysentery, meningococcemia, acute infections of the urinary tract, shigellosis and some *Salmonella* infections. In conjunction with antibiotics, it is used in meningitis caused by meningococci, pneumococci, *H. influenzae* and other organisms. Otitis media, tonsillitis, pneumonia, and skin and soft-tissue infections frequently are caused by sulfonamide-sensitive organisms. For prophylaxis against recurrences of rheumatic fever as an alternative to penicillin, and as adjunctive therapy with pyrimethamine for the treatment of toxoplasmosis. Silver sulfadiazine is employed for topical use as adjunctive therapy for the prevention and treatment of wound sepsis in patients with second and third degree burns. See general statement for other uses.

Precautions: The silver sulfadiazine may inactivate topically applied proteolytic enzymes when used in conjunction with this agent. The usual precautions applicable to sulfonamides should be observed. See the general statement for adverse reactions usually associated with sulfonamides.

Dosage and Administration: *Orally. Adults,* the usual initial dose is 2 to 4 gm, then 2 to 4 gm daily divided into 3 to 6 doses. *Children and infants,* the usual initial dose is 75 mg/kg of body weight, then 150 mg/kg daily divided into 4 to 6 doses. The maximum daily dose is 6 gm. For rheumatic fever prophylaxis, patients weighing under 30 kg (66 lbs) should receive 0.5 gm/day and those weighing 30 kg or more should receive 1 gm/day. *Parenterally.* The usual initial dose is 50 mg/kg of body weight, followed by 100 mg/kg daily divided into 3 doses if given subcutaneously or into 4 doses if given by slow intravenous infusion. Systemic sulfonamides are contraindicated in infants under 2 months of age, except in the treatment of congenital toxoplasmosis as adjunctive therapy with pyrimethamine. *Topically.* The cream should be applied 1 or 2 times daily to a thickness of approximately 1/16 of an inch.

Availability:
Sulfadiazine
SULFADIAZINE:
Tablets (Dulcet®), 300 mg in bottles of 100. **(Abbott)**
Tablets, 0.5 gm in bottles of 100 and 1000. **(Lederle)**
Tablets, 0.5 gm in bottles of 100. **(Lilly)**
w/Sulfamerazine
SULFONAMIDES DUPLEX Suspension, 250 mg/5 ml each of sulfadiazine and sulfamerazine in bottles of 1 pint. **(Lilly)**
Trisulfapyrimidines
By official definition, a mixture of equal parts of sulfadiazine, sulfamerazine and sulfamethazine. Expressed in terms of total sulfonamide content.
NEOTRIZINE®: **(Lilly)**
Suspension, 0.5 gm/5 ml in bottles of 1 pint.
Tablets, 0.5 gm in bottles of 100 and 1000.
SULFOSE®: **(Wyeth)**
Suspension, 0.5 gm/5 ml in bottles of 1 pint.
Tablets, 0.5 gm in bottles of 100.
TERFONYL®: **(Squibb)**
Oral Suspension, 0.5 gm/5 ml in bottles of 1 pint.
Tablets, 0.5 gm in bottles of 100.
TRIPLE SULFAS: **(Lederle)**
Oral Suspension, 0.5 gm/5 ml in bottles of 1 pint.
Tablets, 0.5 gm in bottles of 1000.

TRISEM: **(Beecham)**
Oral Suspension, 0.5 gm/5 ml in bottles of 1 pint.
Tablets, 0.5 gm in bottles of 100.

Silver Sulfadiazine

SILVADENE® Cream (micronized), 10 mg/gm in jars of 50 and 400 gm. **(Marion)**

SULFAMETER

Chemical Name: 2-Sulfanilamido-5-methoxypyrimidine.

Description: Sulfameter is a long-acting antibacterial sulfonamide similar in action to sulfadimethoxine and sulfamethoxypyridazine. It occurs as a white, crystalline powder that is insoluble in water and slightly soluble in alcohol.

Following oral administration, the drug is readily absorbed from the gastrointestinal tract. Measurable amounts are detected in the plasma in about 2 hours and peak levels are attained within 4 to 8 hours. Ingestion of a 1-gm dose produced maximal plasma levels averaging approximately 6 to 10 mg/100 ml, which then gradually decreased to about 4 to 7 mg/100 ml after 24 hours. Sulfameter is distributed to most body tissues; however, it is poorly diffused into the cerebrospinal fluid. The drug is actively metabolized by both the liver and kidneys. It is excreted in the urine in the free form and as metabolites; there appears to be a high degree of tubular reabsorption of the free form. Measurable amounts of the drug can be found in the body 96 hours following an oral dose; approximately 90% of the drug in the plasma is nonacetylated.

Indications: Treatment of acute and chronic urinary tract infections. It is more effective when the causative organism is *Escherichia coli, Klebsiella-aerobacter, Paracolon* species, *Streptococcus* species, and *Proteus* species. It is not effective in viral or richettsial infections, and is not recommended for generalized bacterial infections including meningitis.

Warnings: Fatalities have occurred due to the development of Stevens-Johnson syndrome following the use of sulfameter; therefore, the patient must be closely observed and should a rash develop during therapy, the drug should be discontinued immediately. Because of the hazard of severe hypoglycemic reactions, this sulfonamide should be administered with caution to patients receiving oral hypoglycemic agents of the sulfonylurea type.

Dosage and Administration: *Orally.* The following dosage schedule is recommended to rapidly obtain and maintain a peak serum level of approximately 10 $\pm$ 3 mg%. (medication given preferably after breakfast). Patients over 100 lbs or 12 years of age—loading dose (first day only, single dose) of 1.5 gm (3 tablets) and daily maintenance (single dose at 24-hour intervals) of 500 mg (1 tablet). **Note:** Pending additional clinical experience, the drug should be directed primarily toward those urinary tract infections requiring short-term or intermittent therapy. In any event continuous administration should not, at the present time, exceed 180 days. Since there has been limited experience in younger age groups, the drug is not recommended for children under 12 years of age.

Availability:
SULLA® Tablets (pale green, scored), 500 mg in bottles of 100 and 500. **(Robins)**

SULFAMETHIZOLE

Chemical Name: N[1]-(5-Methyl-1,3,4-thiadiazol-2-yl)sulfanilamide.

Description: Sulfamethizole occurs as a light-buff or white, crystalline powder that is sparingly soluble in alcohol; solubility in water depends on pH. This sulfonamide has been found to be highly soluble in body fluids and urine, is noncumulative and is rapidly excreted. About 90% of the drug in the urine is in the active form, which is highly soluble in acid urine. Since crystalluria with this agent is rare, alkalinization of the urine is generally considered unnecessary.

Indications: Treatment of acute or recurrent, chronic urinary tract infections caused by organisms sensitive to sulfonamides. Formulated with phenazopyridine hydrochloride, a urinary tract analgesic, for the relief of pain, burning, frequency, and urgency that generally accompanies such infections.

Sulfamethizole shares the actions, uses and adverse reactions of other sulfonamides. The usual precautions associated with sulfonamides should be observed. See general statement.

Dosage and Administration: The usual adult *oral* dosage is 0.5 to 1 gm 3 or 4 times daily. The dosage for infants (over 2 months) and children is based on 30 to 45 mg/kg of body weight daily in 4 divided doses. The usual dosage for sulfamethizole combined with phenazopyridine hydrochloride is 2 tablets for adults and 1 tablet for children (9 to 12 years of age) 4 times daily.

Availability:
Sulfamethizole
THIOSULFIL®: **(Ayerst)**
Oral Suspension, 250 mg/5 ml in bottles of 1 pint.
Tablets, 250 mg in bottles of 100 and 1000.
Tablets Forte, 500 mg in bottles of 100 and 1000 and in unit-dose packages of 100.
Combinations
THIOSULFIL®-A: **(Ayerst)**
Tablets, 250 mg with 50 mg of phenazopyridine hydrochloride in bottles of 100 and 1000.
Tablets Forte, 500 mg with 50 mg of phenazopyridine hydrochloride in bottles of 100 and 1000.
THIOSULFIL® DUO-PAK® in units consisting of Bottle No. 1 (24 yellow tablets of Thiosulfil-A Forte) and Bottle No. 2 (32 white tablets of Thiosulfil Forte).

SULFAMETHOXAZOLE

Chemical Name: N[1]-(5-Methyl-3-isoxazolyl)sulfanilamide.

Description: Sulfamethoxazole is an intermediate-acting sulfonamide closely related chemically to sulfisoxazole. It occurs as an almost white, odorless, tasteless compound.

Sulfamethoxazole has been reported to be effective both in vitro and in vivo against commonly encountered gram-positive and gram-negative organisms. It is rapidly absorbed and has an intermediate rate of excretion, permitting a convenient twice-a-day dosage schedule for the treatment of susceptible infections. Since it is highly soluble at the critical pH range of 5.5 to 7.4, the risk of crystalluria is minimal. It has been shown that approximately 70% of sulfamethoxazole is bound to protein in the blood, and that 80 to 90% of the unbound portion is in the nonacetylated form.

Indications: Treatment of acute, recurrent or chronic urinary tract infections (primarily pyelonephritis, pyelitis, and cystitis) due to susceptible organisms. Formulated with phenazopyridine for the relief of associated dysuria, burning and frequency.

The usual precautions associated with sulfonamides should be observed. See general statement for other indications, precautions and adverse reactions.

Dosage and Administration: *Orally.* Adults, 2 gm initially then 1 gm every 12 hours. Children and infants over 2 months of age, 50 to 60 mg/kg of body weight, then 25 to 30 mg/kg every 12 hours. Maximum dose should not exceed 75 mg/kg/daily. In severe infections, maintenance doses may be given 3 times daily. With phenazopyridine hydrochloride, 4 tablets initially, followed by 2 tablets twice daily (morning and evening).

Availability:
GANTANOL®: **(Roche)**
DS Tablets, 1 gm in bottles of 100 and in Tel-E-Dose® (single unit-dose) cartons of 100.
Suspension, 500 mg/5 ml in bottles of 1 pint.

Tablets, 500 mg in bottles of 100 and 500, in Tel-E-Dose® (single-unit dose) cartons of 100 and in Prescription Paks of 50 and 500.
AZO GANTANOL® Tablets, 500 mg with 100 mg of phenazopyridine hydrochloride in bottles of 100 and 500. **(Roche)**

SULFAMETHOXYPYRIDAZINE

Chemical Name: N'-(6-Methoxy-3-pyridazinyl)sulfanilamide.

Description: Sulfamethoxypyridazine is an antibacterial sulfonamide that is slowly excreted in the urine and hence is long-acting. It occurs as a white or yellowish-white, crystalline powder that is very slightly soluble in water and sparingly soluble in alcohol.

When given orally, sulfamethoxypyridazine is readily absorbed from the gastrointestinal tract. Approximately 40 to 70% of the total administered dose is excreted in the urine in the acetylated form and about 30 to 60% in the free form. Following administration of a single oral dose, peak blood levels are achieved in 1 to 2 hours, and this level is maintained for about 10 hours. Thereafter, blood levels fall slowly and at the end of 24 to 48 hours, blood levels are approximately one-half the maximum level. Since about 85% of the drug is bound to plasma protein, only a small percentage is available for glomerular filtration. In addition, the free form of the drug is readily reabsorbed by the renal tubules.

Indications: Treatment of urinary tract infections, upper respiratory tract infections, bacillary dysenteries, surgical and soft tissue infections due to sulfonamide-sensitive organisms.

Warnings: Fatalities have occurred due to the development of the Stevens-Johnson syndrome (erythema multiforme exudativum) following the use of sulfamethoxypyridazine. Patients should be closely observed during treatment, and if a rash develops, the drug should be discontinued immediately.

Adverse Reactions: Erythema multiforme exudativum, urticaria, exfoliative dermatitis, toxic hepatitis, isolated myocarditis, lupus erythematosus, aplastic anemia, leukopenia, pancytopenia, thrombocytopenic purpura, and hemolytic anemia, including that associated with a deficiency of erythrocytic glucose-6-phosphate dehydrogenase. Also noted were headache and drug fever. Relief of headache may be obtained by reducing the dosage or by discontinuation of the drug. The appearance of a rash indicates the need for immediate withdrawal of the drug. Other complications included nausea, vomiting, mental depression, agranulocytosis, serum-sickness syndrome, photosensitivity, abdominal pain, peripheral neuritis, arthralgia, albuminuria, and crystalluria.

For further information on the indications, precautions and adverse reactions, see general statement.

Dosage and Administration: *Orally,* once every 24 hours immediately after a meal. Therapy should continue for 5 to 7 days or until the patient is asymptomatic for 48 to 72 hours. Adequate fluid intake must be maintained during and for at least 24 to 48 hours after treatment. The average adult dose for mild to moderate infections is 1 gm the 1st day, followed by 0.5 gm every day thereafter. The recommended 1st day dosage for infants and children is 30 mg/kg of body weight. The dosage for each day thereafter is ½ the initial dose, or 15 mg/kg of body weight. The dosage varies from the adult dosage since children generally require proportionately larger doses of antibacterials than adults. Higher dosages are not recommended. *Prophylaxis of streptococcal infection:* A single weekly dose of 2 to 3 gm depending on the weight of the patient. Therapeutic blood levels are generally maintained for 5 days or more on this regimen.

Availability:
MIDICEL® Tablets, 0.5 gm in bottles of 100 and 1000. **(Parke-Davis)**

SULFASALAZINE

Chemical Name: 5-[[p-(2-Pyridylsulfamoyl)phenyl]azo]salicylic acid.

Description: Sulfasalazine is produced synthetically by diazotization of sulfapyridine and coupling of the diazonium salt with salicylic acid. Reductive splitting of the azo linkage yields sulfapyridine and 5-aminosalicylic acid. It occurs as a brownish-yellow, odorless powder slightly soluble in alcohol and practically insoluble in water.

The precise mode of action of sulfasalazine has not been established. Rapid absorption of the sulfapyridine moiety accounts for recovery in the urine of up to 85% of ingested drug during continued administration. Doses of 4 gm daily result in steady-state serum levels averaging 12 mcg/ml of sulfasalazine and its conjugates and 50 mcg/ml of sulfapyridine and its conjugates. Only small amounts of 5-aminosalicylic acid are recovered from the urine, indicating that this metabolite is excreted largely unabsorbed in the feces.

Indications: Adjunctive treatment of ulcerative colitis, presumably because of its particular affinity for connective tissue. It is especially useful when prolonged therapy is indicated.

The drug shares with other antibacterial sulfonamides the potential toxicities. See general statement.

Dosage and Administration: *Orally.* The usual dosage for adults, initially, is 4 to 8 gm in divided doses daily or as indicated up to 12 gm daily, in 4 to 8 equally divided doses. In severe colitis, it is often advisable to start therapy (in adults) with 8 gm daily and to adjust the dosage upward to 12 gm daily, depending upon individual response. Children, 75 to 150 mg/kg of body weight daily in 3 to 6 equally divided doses. Adults can be maintained on 0.5 gm 4 times daily, and children on 40 mg/kg/day divided into 4 doses. Response to therapy and adjustment of dosage should be governed by the findings of proctoscopic and sigmoidoscopic examinations. If diarrhea recurs, dosage should be increased to previous effective levels. The enteric-coated tablet may be preferred to the regular tablet in those patients demonstrating gastric intolerance. Patients should be forewarned that sulfasalazine produces an orange-yellow color when the urine is alkaline; a similar discoloration of the skin has also been reported. The drug may be discontinued altogether when remission from active disease has been achieved.

Availability:

AZULFIDINE®: **(Pharmacia)**

Entabs (enteric-coated tablets), 500 mg in bottles of 100 and 500.

Tablets, 500 mg in bottles of 100 and 500 and in unit-dose packages of 100 and 1000.

S.A.S.-500® Tablets, 500 mg (scored) in bottles of 100 and 1000 and in unit-dose packages of 100. **(Rowell)**

SULCOLON® Tablets (brown, scored), 500 mg in bottles of 500. **(Lederle)**

SULFISOXAZOLE

Chemical Name: N^1-(3,4-Dimethyl-5-isoxazolyl)sulfanilamide.

Description: Sulfisoxazole occurs as a white to slightly yellowish, odorless, slightly bitter, crystalline powder very slightly soluble in water and freely soluble in boiling alcohol. N^1-acetylsulfisoxazole is the tasteless form of sulfisoxazole, and is believed to be metabolized to sulfisoxazole in the gastrointestinal tract by means of enzymatic splitting which is presumed to be responsible for the delayed absorption and attainment of blood levels. With continued administration of N^1-acetylsulfisoxazole, blood levels approximate those of sulfisoxazole.

Sulfisoxazole is highly soluble in neutral and in slightly acidic body fluids, thus reducing the likelihood of renal blockage or crystalluria. Supplemental alkali therapy, therefore, is not necessary. Its distribution in body tissue differs from that of other sulfonamides in that it apparently is confined to extracellular body fluids. Thus, the same amount of drug will yield a concentration in plasma of about twice that of sulfadiazine or sulfamerazine.

Indications: Treatment of acute and chronic urinary tract infections caused by susceptible gram-positive and gram-negative organisms. It is said to be particularly effective against *B. proteus.* The drug is used also in systemic infections caused by gram-positive streptococci, staphylococci, and by gram-negative meningococci, *H. influenzae.* Formulated with phenazopyridine hydrochloride when urinary tract infections are associated with pain and discomfort. The diolamine salt of sulfisoxazole is used in the treatment of superficial infections of the eye, caused by susceptible gram-negative and gram-positive organisms and as an adjunct in systemic sulfonamide therapy in trachoma.

For further information regarding the antimicrobial activity, uses, precautions and adverse reactions, see general statement. The usual precautions associated with sulfonamides should be observed.

Dosage and Administration: *Orally, parenterally* and *topically.* For adults, the initial *oral* dosage is 2 to 4 gm, followed by 1 to 2 gm every 4 hours until the temperature has been normal or until urinary cultures have been sterile for at least 2 days. For children, the initial oral dosage is 75 mg/kg of body weight, followed by 150 mg/kg of body weight daily in divided doses every 4 to 6 hours. An emulsion of acetylsulfisoxazole yields higher and more prolonged blood levels than an equal amount of an aqueous suspension; 75 mg/kg twice daily provides therapeutic blood levels for a period of 24 hours. The drug is not intended for use in children under 2 months of age. *With phenazopyridine hydrochloride,* the recommended adult dosage is 4 to 6 tablets initially followed by 2 tablets 4 times daily for up to 3 days. If pain persists, causes other than infection should be sought. After relief of pain has been obtained, continued treatment of the infection with sulfisoxazole alone may be considered. The diolamine salt, 400 mg, is administered by slow *subcutaneous, intramuscular* or *intravenous* injection every 8 to 12 hours if oral therapy is not feasible. Not more than 5 ml should be injected *intramuscularly* into any one site. When administered *subcutaneously,* the drug should be diluted to a concentration of 5% or less. *Topically,* in the form of ophthalmic ointment or solution, or vaginal cream, from 1 to 4 times daily.

Availability:

Sulfisoxazole

GANTRISIN®: **(Roche)**

Tablets, 0.5 gm in bottles of 100, 500 and 1000, in drums of 5000 and in Tel-E-Dose® (unit-dose) packages of 100 and in Prescription Paks of 100 and 1000.

Vaginal Cream, 10% in tubes of 90 gm with applicator.

KORO-SULF Vaginal Cream, 10% in tubes of 85 gm with applicator. **(Holland-Rantos)**

SK-SOXAZOLE™ Tablets, 0.5 gm in bottles of 100. **(Smith Kline & French)**

SOSOL® Tablets, 0.5 gm in bottles of 100, 1000 and 5000. **(McKesson)**

SULFALAR® Tablets, 500 mg in bottles of 1000 and in unit-dose packages of 100 (10 × 10). **(Parke-Davis)**

SULFISOXAZOLE Tablets, 500 mg in bottles of 1000 and in unit-dose packages of 100. **(Lederle)**

w/Phenazopyridine Hydrochloride

AZO GANTRISIN® Tablets, 0.5 gm with 50 mg of phenazopyridine hydrochloride in bottles of 100 and 500. **(Roche)**

Acetyl Sulfisoxazole

GANTRISIN®: **(Roche)**

Pediatric Suspension, 0.5 gm/5 ml in bottles of 120 ml and 1 pint.

Syrup, 0.5 gm/5 ml in bottles of 1 pint.

LIPO GANTRISIN® Emulsion, 1 gm/5 ml in bottles of 1 pint.

Sulfisoxazole Diolamine

GANTRISIN®: **(Roche)**

Injectable, 400 mg/ml in ampuls of 5 and 10 ml.

Ophthalmic Ointment, 4% in tubes of 3.75 gm.

Ophthalmic Solution, 4% in dropper bottles of 15 ml.

SULTRIN

Description: Cream and each vaginal tablet contain:

	Cream	*Tablet*
Sulfathiazole	3.42%	172.5 mg
Sulfacetamide	2.86%	143.75 mg
Sulfabenzamide	3.7%	184 mg
Urea	0.64%	13 mg

Indications: Treatment of vaginitis due to *Haemophilus vaginalis.* May also be used as a deodorant for saprophytic infection following radiation therapy.

Contraindications: Kidney disease and hypersensitivity to any of the components.

Dosage and Administration: *Intravaginally.* Insert 1 tablet twice daily for 10 days; or 1 applicatorful twice daily for 4 to 6 days. Dosage may then be reduced by ½ to ¼.

Availability:
SULTRIN®: **(Ortho)**
Cream in tubes of 78 gm with measured-dose applicator.
Vaginal tablets in packages of 20 with vaginal applicator.

SULFOXONE SODIUM

Chemical Name: Disodium [sulfonylbis(*p*-phenylenimino)]dimethanesulfinate.

Description: Sulfoxone sodium, a disubstituted derivative of dapsone, occurs as a white to pale yellow powder with a characteristic odor and is very soluble in water and slightly soluble in alcohol.

Following oral administration, sodium sulfoxone undergoes hydrolysis and is absorbed chiefly in the form of the parent compound. It is distributed throughout the body fluids, but only a small amount enters the cerebrospinal fluid. Approximately 48% of an orally administered dose is excreted in the urine and about 44% in the feces. Available evidence indicates that the beneficial effects of the drug most likely result from increasing host resistance to the organism.

Indications: Treatment of all forms of leprosy; also indicated in dermatitis herpetiformis.

Contraindications: In patients hypersensitive to sulfones and in those with advanced renal amyloidosis, which is sometimes seen in patients with leprosy.

Warnings: Severe anemia should be treated prior to initiation of therapy. At the very first sign of a hypersensitivity reaction (including a lepra reaction), or if severe anemia develops, the drug should be discontinued and appropriate treatment initiated. Safe use during pregnancy has not been established.

Precautions: Normocytic anemia and methemoglobinemia may occur during the initial stages of treatment but do not indicate withdrawal of the drug unless these conditions become acute. Periodic blood studies should be performed and therapy should be discontinued or the dosage greatly reduced only if the red and/or white cell count falls below the critical level, or remains persistently low after 6 weeks of therapy. Treatment should be suspended if a lepra reaction (e.g., erythema nodosum, erythema multiforme, erythema necrotans) appears. Signs of jaundice or liver damage may appear after prolonged therapy with high dosages, in which case therapy should be withdrawn.

Adverse Reactions: Dose-related hemolysis and hemolytic anemia, in patients with or without glucose-6-phosphate-dehydrogenase deficiency, are the most common toxic effects noted. The occurrence of leukopenia, granulocytopenia, agranulocytosis, allergic dermatitis (sometimes exfoliative with concomitant liver damage), jaundice, hematuria, motor neuropathy, and psychosis (rare) may necessitate immediate withdrawal of the drug, as well as macrocytic anemia if it does not respond to vitamin B therapy. There have been reports of erythema multiforme and toxic epidermal necrolysis occurring with the use of sulfone preparations. Since toxic epidermal necrolysis is a potentially fatal reaction, treatment may have to be terminated immediately and appropriate measures instituted. Cyanosis as a consequence of methemoglobinemia is common, but does not require withdrawal of the medication unless very severe. Headache, giddiness and tachycardia may be avoided if the dosage is gradually increased. A lepra reaction may be precipitated by infection, excessive antilepra medication or appear without apparent cause. Anorexia, nausea and vomiting are uncommon if the dosage is increased gradually.

Dosage and Administration: *Orally. For the treatment of leprosy,* the recommended adult dosage for the 1st and 2nd week is 330 mg 2 times a week (alternate 165 mg 4 times a week); if no symptoms of intolerance develop, then for the 3rd and 4th week, 330 mg 4 times a week (alternate 165 mg daily); in the absence of any serious side effects, the 5th and succeeding weeks 330 mg daily for 6 days, 1 day rest period and continue. Children, 4 years of age or older, ½ the adult dosage. *For the treatment of dermatitis herpetiformis,* the recommended adult dosage is 330 mg daily for the 1st week, increased to 660 mg daily if necessary; maintenance dose is 330 mg daily.

Availability:
DIASONE® SODIUM Enterab® (enteric-coated tablets), 165 mg in bottles of 100. **(Abbott)**

SULINDAC

Chemical Name: (Z)-5-Fluoro-2-methyl-1-[[*p*-(methylsulfinyl)phenyl]methylene]-1*H*-indene-3-acetic acid.

Description: Sulindac is a synthetic, nonsteroidal, antiinflammatory, antiarthritic compound with analgesic and antipyretic activity. An indene derivative, it is chemically unrelated to salicylates, pyrazoline or propionic acid. Classified as a weak organic acid, it occurs as a yellow, crystalline substance with a molecular weight of 356.42, is insoluble in water below pH 4.5, but soluble as the sodium salt, or in buffers of pH 6 or higher. Following absorption, sulindac undergoes 2 major biotransformations resulting in a reversible reduction to the biologically active sulfide metabolite and an irreversible oxidation to the biologically inactive sulfone metabolite. The analgesic and antiinflammatory actions are thought to be the result of inhibition of the production of prostaglandin in various tissues by the sulfide metabolite. Standard daily doses of sulindac have demonstrated similar antiinflammatory activity when compared to daily doses of 2.4 to 4.8 gm of aspirin in the treatment of rheumatoid arthritis and osteoarthritis; to 75 to 150 mg of indomethacin and to 400 to 600 mg of phenylbutazone in the treatment of ankylosing spondylitis; to 600 mg of phenylbutazone in the treatment of acute gouty arthritis, and to 400 to 600 mg of oxyphenbutazone in the treatment of acute painful shoulder. When compared to aspirin, the proposed advantages of sulindac are a lower incidence of adverse effects including tinnitus and gastrointestinal intolerance, less effect on platelet function and bleeding time, and a longer plasma half-life.

Among the criteria used to measure the clinical effects of sulindac were a reduction in the number of inflamed joints; relief of pain, swelling and tenderness; delay in the onset of fatigue; decrease in morning stiffness; increase in joint motion and in functional capacity as indicated by a progressive increase in grip strength. Although the drug did not alter the course of the fundamental disorder, its ability to provide effective symptomatic relief was confirmed by the parameters evaluated.

Approximately 90% of the drug is absorbed following oral administration. The biologically active sulfide metabolite reaches peak plasma concentration within 2 hours in the fasting subject and within 3 to 4 hours when the drug is taken with meals. The mean half-life of unchanged drug is 7.8 hours while the mean half-life of the sulfide metabolite is 16.4 hours; the latter being responsible for prolonged antiarthritic action, thereby sustaining beneficial relief on a twice-a-day dosage schedule. The rationale for sustained plasma levels is probably due to extensive enterohepatic circulation of sulindac and its 2 metabolites in addition to reversible metabolism of the active sulfide metabolite.

Approximately 50% of the administered dose is excreted in the urine with the sulfone metabolite accounting for the major portion and the sulfide metabolite for less than 1%. About 25% is found in the feces primarily as the sulfone and sulfide metabolites. The bioavailability of sulindac, as assessed by urinary excretion, was not changed by concomitant administration of antacids containing magnesium and aluminum hydroxides. In healthy subjects, the average fecal blood loss, measured over a 2-week period during administration of 400 mg daily of sulindac, was similar to that for placebo, and was statistically less than that resulting from 4.8 gm of aspirin.

Although the drug and its sulfide metabolite are highly bound to protein, studies have shown no clinically significant interaction with oral anticoagulants or oral hypoglycemic agents. However, until wider clinical experience is obtained, sulindac should be used with caution in patients receiving such medications. The plasma levels of the active sulfide metabolite were significantly reduced when aspirin was given concomitantly with sulindac, but were only slightly reduced, while the plasma levels of the free drug and the sulfone metabolite were increased when coadministered with probenecid. Additionally, sulindac was shown to produce a modest reduction in the uricosuric action of probenecid. Neither propoxyphene hydrochloride nor acetaminophen had any effect on the plasma levels of sulindac or its sulfide metabolite. The administration of aspirin with sulindac is not recommended until further clinical studies demonstrate either favorable or unfavorable combined effects.

In experiments with pregnant animals, it has been observed that drugs which inhibit prostaglandin synthetase also cause prolonged gestation, and may cause dystocia and delayed parturition. Additional studies in animals exposed to high doses (2.5 to 5 times the maximal daily clinical dose) of sulindac revealed visceral and skeletal malformations, a decrease in average fetal weight, and an increase in the number of dead offspring.

Indications: For acute and long-term use in the relief of the signs and symptoms of osteoarthritis, rheumatoid arthritis, ankylosing spondylitis, acute painful shoulder (acute subacrominal bursitis and supraspinatus tendinitis) and acute gouty arthritis. It is not recommended for rheumatoid arthritis in patients with functional class IV disease, i.e., those who are incapacitated, largely or wholly bedridden or confined to a wheel chair with little or no ability to care for themselves.

Contraindications: Unusual sensitivity to sulindac, and in patients in whom acute asthmatic attacks, urticaria or rhinitis is precipitated by aspirin or by other nonsteroidal antiinflammaory agents.

Warnings: Since peptic ulceration and gastrointestinal bleeding have been reported, it is therefore advisable to use sulindac cautiously in patients with gastrointestinal bleeding, an active peptic ulcer, or a history of such conditions. Careful monitoring of the patient's progress with special regard to possible adverse reactions is also recommended.

Precautions: Decreased platelet aggregation and prolonged bleeding time; abnormalities in liver function tests, primarily manifested by increased levels of alkaline phosphatase; eye changes, and peripheral edema may accompany the use of sulindac; therefore, adequate precautions and careful monitoring of the patient, particularly those who may be adversely affected, are essential. If a significant abnormality in liver function persists, the drug should be withdrawn. Patients with compromised cardiac function, hypertension or other conditions predisposing to fluid retention, and those with significantly impaired renal function require special care and adequate adjustment of the dosage. In chronic studies in mice, rats and monkeys exposed to high dosages, there were occasional occurrences of mild renal toxicity as evidenced by papillary edema or mild interstitial nephritis in some animals. Papillary necrosis occurred infrequently in mice and rats. However, there has been no evidence to date of renal toxicity in clinical studies. Sulindac may allow a reduction in dosage or the elimination of chronic corticosteroid therapy in some patients with rheumatic arthritis, but in order to avoid an exacerbation of the disease or the signs and symptoms of adrenal insufficiency, it is generally necessary to reduce the corticosteroids gradually over a period of several months. Abrupt withdrawal is usually not recommended even when patients have had a serious complication as a result of prolonged corticosteroid therapy. The use of sulindac in pregnant patients is not recommended, nor should nursing be undertaken while a patient is taking the drug. Pediatric indications and dosage have not been established, but studies in juvenile rheumatoid arthritis are in progress.

Adverse Reactions: The most frequently occurring include gastrointestinal pain, dyspepsia, nausea with or without vomiting; diarrhea, pruritus; dizziness, headache, nervousness; tinnitus; edema. Those less frequently occurring include gastritis or gastroenteritis, peptic ulcer, rarely, gastrointestinal bleeding; stomatitis, sore or dry mucous membranes; vertigo; hypersensitivity. Hypertension; paresthesias, neuritis; transient visual disturbances, decreased hearing; epistaxis; depression have also been noted but a causal relationship to the drug has not been confirmed. In the event of overdosage, the stomach should be emptied by inducing vomiting or by gastric lavage, and the patient carefully observed and given symptomatic and supportive management.

Dosage and Administration: *Orally* twice daily with meals. For osteoarthritis, rheumatoid arthritis, and ankylosing spondylitis, the recommended initial dose is 300 mg daily divided into 2 equal doses. The dose may then be increased or decreased depending upon the patient's response. For acute painful shoulder or acute gouty arthritis, the recommended dose is 400 mg daily divided into 2 equal doses. Therapy for 7 to 14 days is usually adequate for painful shoulder, and for 7 days for gouty arthritis. Daily doses above 400 mg is not recommended until further clinical experience assures safe use.

Availability:
CLINORIL® Tablets, 150 and 200 mg in bottles of 100. **(Merck Sharp & Dohme)**

SULISOBENZONE

Chemical Name: 5-Benzoyl-4-hydroxy-2-methoxybenzenesulfonic acid.

Description: Contains sulizobenzone, 10% in a heavy lotion base that is odorless, colorless, nongreasy, nonoccluding, nonstaining and bitter to taste.

A benzophenone sunscreen agent, sulisobenzone provides solar protection in the wave lengths significantly higher than 3100 Angstrom units.

Indications: To prevent sunburn, freckling and aging of the skin caused by overexposure to sunlight.

Contraindications: Hypersensitivity to sulisobenzone.

Precautions: Accidental contact with the eyes may cause slight burning due to pH. If skin irritation or sensitivity develops, discontinue use.

Dosage and Administration: *Topically.* Should be applied evenly to exposed skin, rubbed in well and allowed to dry. To maintain maximum protection, reapply after swimming or after excessive perspiring.

Availability:
UVAL® Lotion (OTC) in squeeze bottles of 75 and 165 gm. **(Dorsey)**

SULTRIN: see The Sulfonamides

SUTILAINS

Description: Sutilains are proteolytic enzymes derived from a strain of *Bacillus subtilis.* One gm of ointment provides 82,000 casein units of proteolytic activity. A casein unit is the amount of enzyme required to produce the same optical density at 275 mμ as that of a solution of 1.5 mcg tyrosine/ml after the enzyme has been incubated with 35 mg of casein at 37° C for 1 minute. The debriding properties of proteolytic enzymes promote normal granulation, accelerate epithelization, reduce putrefactive odors, and minimize the incidence of scarring.

Sutilains dissolve and facilitate the removal of proteinaceous material, such as clotted blood, purulent exudate and necrotic tissue, resulting from burns, trauma or inflammation. They act most effectively within a pH range of 6 to 6.8, and improvement is usually noted within 24 hours of treatment. The enzymes are virtually inactive on viable tissue.

Following topical application, the optimal activity period occurs within the first 6 hours, and putrefaction often will be eliminated within 72 hours. If there is no demonstrable debriding action within 24 to 48 hours, further application is unlikely to have any effect.

Indications: Recommended as an adjunctive therapeutic agent in the management of wound debridement in second and third degree burns, decubitus ulcers, incisional, traumatic, and pyogenic wounds, and in ulcers secondary to peripheral vascular disease.

Contraindications: Its use is contraindicated for wounds communicating with major body cavities, for those containing exposed major nerves or nervous tissue, for fungating neoplastic ulcers; and in women of childbearing potential (its effect on the fetus remains to be established).

Warnings: Contact with the eyes should be avoided; however, should this occur, the eyes should be copiously rinsed with water (preferably sterile water).

Precautions: Since moisture draws the enzyme into intimate contact with necrotic tissue, a moist environment is therefore essential to the optimal activity of this agent. It has been observed that enzymatic activity may be impaired by various agents. In vitro studies suggest that several detergents and antiseptics (i.e., benzalkonium chloride, hexachlorophene, iodine, and nitrofurazone) render the substrate unresponsive to the action of the enzyme. Compounds containing metallic ions (i.e., thimerosal) appear to interfere directly with enzymatic activity, whereas neomycin, sulfamylon, streptomycin, and penicillin do not affect this activity. Therefore, wounds must be well-cleansed of antiseptics or heavy-metal antibacterial agents which may denature the enzymes or alter substrate characteristics. It is recommended that concurrent use of an appropriate systemic antibiotic should be instituted in the presence of a threatening invasive infection. Although there have been no reports of systemic allergic reactions in clinical experience with this drug, studies have shown that there may be an antibody response to absorbed enzyme material.

Adverse Reactions: Those reported consist of mild, transient pain, (controlled with mild analgesics), paresthesias, bleeding and transient dermatitis. Occasionally, untoward reactions, severe enough to warrant discontinuation of therapy, have occurred. If bleeding or dermatitis appear, therapy should be withdrawn. No systemic toxicity has been observed as a result of the topical application of this drug.

Dosage and Administration: *Topically.* Strict adherence to the following is required for effective results of treatment: (1) thoroughly cleanse and irrigate the wound area with sodium chloride or water solutions; (2) thoroughly moisten wound area through tubbing, showering, or wet soaks with either sodium chloride or water solutions; (3) apply ointment in a thin layer extending to 1/4 to 1/2 inch beyond the area to be treated, thus assuring intimate contact with necrotic tissue and complete wound coverage; (4) apply loose wet dressings; and (5) repeat the entire procedure 3 or 4 times daily for optimal results.

Availability:
TRAVASE® Ointment, 82,000 casein units/gm in tubes of 14.2 gm. **(Flint)**

SYNALGOS

Description: Each capsule contains:

Promethazine hydrochloride	6.25 mg
Aspirin	194.4 mg
Phenacetin	162 mg
Caffeine	30 mg

Each Synalgos-DC capsule contains, in addition, dihydrocodeine bitartrate, 16 mg.

Indications: May be of use in the control of mild to moderate or severe pain, and for those conditions in which a mild sedative effect is desired.

Contraindications: Hypersensitivity or intolerance to any of the ingredients. Prolonged use of phenacetin is contraindicated in patients with renal disease.

Warnings: Dihydrocodeine bitartrate may be habit-forming. Salicylates should be used with special care in patients with peptic ulcer or blood coagulation disorders. Promethazine should be administered with caution to patients with cardiovascular or liver disease. Dihydrocodeine can produce drug dependence of the codeine type and therefore has the potential for drug abuse. Psychic dependence, physical dependence and tolerance may develop upon repeated administration of this compound; therefore, it should be prescribed and administered with the same degree of caution appropriate to the use of other oral narcotic-containing medications. The sedative effects of dihydrocodeine and promethazine may represent a hazard in ambulatory patients whose activities require alertness and motor coordination. Patients receiving other centrally acting depressants (i.e., other narcotic analgesics, general anesthetics, hypnotics, alcohol, etc.) may experience an additive CNS depression. When such combined therapy is contemplated, the dose of one or both agents should be reduced. Since no adequate data are available on its teratogenic potential, it should be given to pregnant patients only when the therapeutic benefits outweigh the possible hazard to the fetus. Use in children is not recommended until safe and effective results have been established.

Precautions: Salicylates may enhance the effects of anticoagulants, and may also inhibit the effects of uricosuric agents. Prolonged and excessive use of either product may result in anemia, methemoglobinemia, hypersensitivity and renal disease. Hydrocodeine should be given with caution to elderly or debilitated patients, and to those with hypothyroidism, Addison's disease, prostatic hypertrophy, or urethral strictures. Phenacetin in excessive amounts may impair renal function.

Adverse Reactions: The most frequently observed reactions include drowsiness, lightheadedness, dizziness, sedation, nausea, vomiting, constipation, pruritus, skin reactions and, rarely, hypotension.

Dosage and Administration: *Orally.* The usual adult dosage is 2 capsules every 4 hours as needed for pain. Dosage should be adjusted according to the severity of the pain and the response of the patient.

Availability:

SYNALGOS® Capsules in bottles of 100 and 500. **(Ives)**

Ⓒ III SYNALGOS-DC Capsules in bottles of 100 and 500. **(Ives)**

TABRON

Description: Each tablet contains:

Thiamine mononitrate	6 mg
Riboflavin	6 mg
Pyridoxine hydrochloride	5 mg
Vitamin B-12 (crystalline cyanocobalamin)	25 μg
Folic acid	1 mg
Niacinamide	30 mg
Ascorbic acid	500 mg
Calcium pantothenate	10 mg
Vitamin E (*dl*-alpha tocopheryl acetate)	30 IU
Ferrous fumarate (represents 100 mg elemental iron)	304.2 mg
Dioctyl sodium sulfosuccinate	50 mg

Indications: Prevention and treatment of iron and folate deficiency anemias.

Precautions: Folic acid may obscure the presence of pernicious anemia in that the peripheral blood picture may revert to normal while the neurological manifestations progress.

Dosage and Administration: *Orally.* Usual dose is 1 tablet daily or as directed by the physician.

Availability:
TABRON® Tablets (Filmseal®) in bottles of 100 and in unit-dose packages of 100.

(Parke-Davis)

TALBUTAL Ⓒ

Chemical Name: 5-Allyl-5-*sec*-butylbarbituric acid.

Description: Talbutal is a short- to intermediate-acting barbiturate and occurs as a white, crystalline powder very slightly soluble in water and soluble in alcohol.

Indications: Hypnotic for the treatment of insomnia.

Contraindications: Hypersensitivity or idiosyncrasy to barbiturates, porphyria, marked impairment of kidney or liver function, and respiratory disease when dyspnea or obstruction is evident, and in the presence of uncontrolled pain.

Warnings: May be habit-forming. Prolonged use may produce psychic and physical dependence in susceptible patients.

Precautions: Cautious use is essential in patients with liver disease. If confusion develops in elderly patients, the dosage should be decreased or the drug discontinued. Barbiturates may increase the metabolism of some drugs, including anticoagulants.

Adverse Reactions: Slight hangover, drowsiness, headache, rash, emesis, paradoxical excitation, and hypersensitivity reactions. Manifestations of overdosage include CNS depression, respiratory depression, depression of superficial and deep reflexes, constriction of the pupils, decreased urine formation, lowered body temperature and coma. General management should consist of symptomatic and supportive therapy, including gastric lavage, administration of intravenous fluids, and maintainance of blood pressure, body temperature, and adequate respiratory exchange. Dialysis will increase the rate of removal of barbiturates from the body fluids.

Dosage and Administration: *Orally.* The full hypnotic dose for adults is 120 mg 15 to 30 minutes before retiring. Normal sleep occurs in 15 to 30 minutes and lasts 6 to 8 hours.

Availability:
Ⓒ LOTUSATE® Caplets® (Tablets), 120 mg in bottles of 100. **(Winthrop)**

TAMOXIFEN CITRATE

Chemical Name: (Z)-2-[4-(1,2-Diphenyl-1-butenyl)phenoxy]-N,N-dimethylethanamine-2-hydroxy-1,2,3-propanetricarboxylate (1:1).

Description: A synthetic, nonsteroidal compound with antiestrogen effects intended for the palliative treatment of advanced breast cancer in postmenopausal women. It occurs as a crystalline substance that is very soluble in water. Molecular weight was found to be 563.62.

The antiestrogenic action of tamoxifen appears to be related to its ability to compete with estrogen for binding sites, thereby depriving the normal target tissues of estradiol. By inhibiting estrogen from binding within those breast cancer cells that contain estrogen receptors, the drug inhibits not only estrogen receptor protein formation but also cell division. Therefore, patients with tumors that are estrogen-receptor-positive appear more likely to have a favorable response to therapy. Studies with rats demonstrated that tamoxifen inhibits the induction of mammary carcinoma caused by dimethylbenzanthracene (DMBA) and influences the regression of established DMBA-induced tumors. It was also demonstrated that the drug can cause teratogenic, mutagenic, and carcinogenic effects, and that it affects the reproductive function in rats at dose levels in excess of those recommended for clinical use.

Following oral administration of radiolabeled drug in doses of approximately 0.3 mg/kg of body weight, peak plasma values of 0.06 to 0.14 mcg/ml were attained within 4 to 7 hours with only 20 to 30% present as unchanged drug. The initial biologic half-life of tamoxifen and its metabolites tends to range from 7 to 14 hours with secondary peaks occurring 4 or more days later. While only small amounts of the drug can be recovered from the urine, the major portion is slowly excreted in the feces chiefly as conjugates, with unchanged drug and hydroxylated metabolites accounting for 30% of the total dose. The prolongation of blood levels and fecal excretion is believed to be due to enterohepatic circulation.

Indications: Palliative treatment of advanced breast cancer in postmenopausal women. Available evidence indicates that patients who have had a recent negative estrogen receptor assay are unlikely to respond to the drug.

Contraindications: None known.

Warnings: Safe use during pregnancy has not been established.

Precautions: Tamoxifen should be used cautiously in patients with existing leukopenia or thrombocytopenia. Occasionally, these abnormalities have occurred during treatment, but whether or not they were drug-related has not been confirmed. Transient decreases in platelet counts, usually to 50,000 to 100,000/cu mm, infrequently lower, have been reported. No hemorrhagic tendency has been noted and the platelet counts returned to normal levels even though treatment with the drug continued. Periodic blood cell and platelet counts are nevertheless advised.

Adverse Reactions: Those most frequently occurring are the familiar menopausal symptoms such as hot flushes, nausea, and vomiting, and may occur in up to 25% of the patients; less frequently occurring are vaginal bleeding or discharge, menstrual irregularities, and skin rash. Rarely, are these severe enough to warrant a reduction of dosage or withdrawal of the drug. Increased bone and tumor pain, and local flare-up of the disease, which are sometimes associated with good tumor response, have occurred. Patients with soft tissue disease may experience sudden increases in the size of preexisting lesion, which at times may be accompanied by marked erythema within and surrounding the lesions and/or may develop new lesions. If bone pain or disease flare-up occurs, they usually do so shortly after initiating therapy and generally subside rapidly. Other adverse reactions that may occur are hypercalcemia, peripheral edema, distaste for food, pruritus vulvae, depression, dizziness, lightheadedness, and headache. If adverse reactions are severe, it is sometimes possible to control them by reducing the dosage without losing control of the disease. Overdosage in patients has not been reported. Animals given maximum doses responded with respiratory distress and convulsions. Since there is no known specific treatment for overdosage, treatment is therefore symptomatic.

Dosage and Administration: *Orally.* The recommended dosage is 1 or 2 tablets twice daily in the morning and evening.

Availability:
NOLVADEX® Tablets, 10 mg in containers of 60. **(Stuart)**

TERBUTALINE SULFATE

Chemical Name: α-[(Tert-butylamino)methyl]-3,5-dihydroxybenzyl alcohol sulfate.

Description: Terbutaline is a synthetic sympathomimetic amine used primarily for its bronchodilating effects. It occurs as a colorless, crystalline solid that is soluble in water. The drug has been shown by in vitro and in vivo studies in animals to exert a preferential effect on β_2 adrenergic receptors such as those located in the bronchial smooth muscle. However, this particular action did not appear to occur during controlled clinical studies in patients who were given the drug subcutaneously. In chronic obstructive pulmonary disease, it relieves bronchospasm manifested by a clinically significant increase in pulmonary function.

Following oral administration, measurable therapeutic effects are usually noticeable within ½ hour, significant effects within 1 to 2 hours and maximal effects within 2 to 3 hours. The drug also produces a significant decrease in airway and pulmonary resistance which persists for 4 hours or more. Following a subcutaneous dose of 0.25 mg, a measurable change in flow rate is usually observed within 5 minutes, and a clinically significant increase in FEV_1 occurs in about 15 minutes following the injection. The maximal effect usually occurs within 30 to 60 minutes and therapeutic activity has been observed to persist for up to 4 hours in some patients. The usual cardiovascular effects commonly associated with sympathomimetic amines were also observed with terbutaline.

Indications: Treatment of bronchial asthma and for reversible bronchospasm which may occur in association with bronchitis and emphysema.

Contraindications: In patients known to be hypersensitive to sympathomimetic amines.

Warnings: Although animal reproduction studies have not revealed any adverse effects upon fetal development, the safe use of this drug in pregnant or lactating women or in women of childbearing potential has not been established. Until further clinical experience is gained, terbutaline is not recommended for use in children under 12 years of age.

Precautions: The physician is advised to use caution when giving this drug to patients with diabetes, hypertension, hyperthyroidism, or cardiac disorders, especially those associated with arrhythmias. The concomitant use of this drug with other sympathomimetic agents is not recommended, since their combined effect on the cardiovascular system may be harmful to the patient.

Adverse Reactions: Those commonly observed were increases in heart rate, nervousness, tremor, palpitations, and dizziness. These were more frequently noted when the doses were injected in amounts in excess of 0.25 mg. Other reported reactions include headache, drowsiness, nausea and vomiting, and anxiety. These reactions are transient in nature and usually do not require treatment.

Dosage and Administration: *Orally.* Adults: The recommended dosage is 5 mg 3 times daily at 6-hour intervals. If side effects are particularly disturbing, the dose may be decreased to 2.5 mg 3 times daily. The total daily dose should not exceed 15 mg. Children 12 to 15 years of age: The recommended dosage is 2.5 mg 3 times daily. The total daily dose should not exceed 7.5 mg. Currently, the drug is not recommended for use in children under 12 years of age. *Subcutaneously.* The usual dose is 0.25 mg injected into the lateral deltoid area. If significant clinical improvement does not occur within 15 to 30 minutes, a second dose of 0.25 mg may be administered. A total dose of 0.5 mg should not be exceeded within a 4-hour period. If the patient fails to respond to a second dose of 0.25 mg within 15 to 30 minutes, other therapeutic measures should be considered.

Availability:
BRETHINE™: **(Geigy)**
Injection, 1 mg/ml in ampuls of 2 ml each containing 1 ml of solution in packages of 10.
Tablets, 2.5 and 5 mg (equiv. to 2.05 and 4.1 mg of base, respectively) in bottles of 100 and 1000 and in unit-dose packages of 100.
BRICANYL®: **(Astra)**
Solution (isotonic), 1 mg (equiv. to 0.82 mg of base) in ampuls of 2 ml each containing 1 ml of solution in packages of 10.
Tablets, 2.5 and 5 mg (equiv. to 2.05 and 4.1 mg in base, respectively) in bottles of 100 and 1000 and in unit-dose packages of 100. The 5 mg tablets are also available in bottles of 500.

TESTOLACTONE

Chemical Name: D-Homo-17α-oxaandrosta-1,4-diene-3,17-dione (1-dehydrotestolactone).

Description: Testolactone is a chemotherapeutic agent whose chemical configuration is similar to that of certain androgenic hormones but, paradoxically, is devoid of androgenic activity in the doses commonly employed. It occurs as a white, odorless, crystalline solid soluble in alcohol and slightly soluble in water.

The precise mechanism by which testolactone exerts its antineoplastic effects clinically is unknown at present. The drug was found to be effective in approximately 15% of the patients with advanced or disseminated mammary cancer evaluated according to the following criteria: 1) those with a measurable decrease in size of all demonstrable tumor masses; 2) those in whom more than 50% of nonosseous lesions decreased in size although all bone lesions remained static, and 3) those in whom more than 50% of total lesions improved while the remainder were static.

Indications: Adjunctive therapy in the palliative treatment of advanced or disseminated mammary cancer in postmenopausal women when hormonal therapy is indicated. **Note:** It may also be used in women who were diagnosed as having had disseminated mammary carcinoma when premenopausal and in whom ovarian function has been subsequently terminated.

Contraindications: Treatment of breast cancer in male patients.

Warnings: Since safe use of testolactone has not been established with respect to adverse effects upon fetal development, and since this preparation is intended for use only in postmenopausal women, the drug should not be used during pregnancy.

Precautions: Plasma calcium levels should be determined routinely in any patient being treated for mammary cancer, particularly during periods of active remission of bony metastases. If hypercalcemia occurs, appropriate measures should be instituted.

Adverse Reactions: Intramuscular injection may result in slight pain at the injection site, local inflammation and/or irritation. Reported reactions include maculopapular erythema, increased blood pressure, paresthesias, aches and edema of extremities, glossitis, anorexia, nausea, vomiting, and rarely, alopecia with or without disturbances in nail growth.

Dosage and Administration: *Deep intramuscular injection,* preferably into the upper outer quadrant of the gluteal muscle. The usual precautions relevant to intramuscular injections should be observed. The recommended dosage is 100 mg 3 times weekly for at least 3 months, unless there is active progression of the disease. Alternate injection sites should be used for each injection. The recommended *oral* dosage is 250 mg 4 times daily. Oral doses up to 2 gm daily have been used although no dose-response relationship has been established.

Availability:
TESLAC®: **(Squibb)**
Aqueous Suspension, 100 mg/ml in multiple-dose vials of 5 ml.
Oral Tablets, 50 and 250 mg in bottles of 100.

TESTOSTERONE

Chemical Name: 17β-Hydroxy-4-androsten-3-one. **Methyltestosterone:** 17β-Hydroxy-17-methylandrost-4-en-3-one.

Description: Testosterone, a steroid compound, is the principal hormone of the testes. It occurs as a stable, white or slightly yellow, crystalline substance that is insoluble in water but freely soluble in alcohol, ether, vegetable oils, and other organic solvents. It is prepared either synthetically or isolated from bull testes. In humans, testosterone is the male sex hormone which is secreted by the interstitial cells under the influence of the anterior pituitary, and is responsible for the development and maintenance of accessory male organs and characteristics.

Testosterone is primarily used for its protein anabolic effect and its catabolic inhibiting effect on tissue. Nitrogen balance is improved but only when there is sufficient intake of calories and protein. Whether this positive nitrogen balance is of primary benefit in the utilization of protein-building dietary substances has not been established. Enhancement of protein anabolism is manifested by the conservation of sodium, nitrogen, phosphorus, potassium, sulfur, and water in the proportions of physiologic protein tissues, and of calcium with additional phosphorus in the proportion of physiologic bone tissue.

The actions of the anabolic steroids are therefore similar to those of male sex hormones with the possibility of causing serious disturbances of growth and sexual development if given to young children. They suppress the gonadotropic functions of the pituitary and may exert a direct effect upon the testes.

The cypionate, enanthate and propionate esters of testosterone produce a longer-lasting effect than does that of the free compound. Testosterone propionate is more effective for parenteral use because its absorption is delayed by its combination with propionic acid; its effect lasts for 1 to 2 days. Buccal administration permits the testosterone to be absorbed directly into the systemic venous return so that the active hormone is carried directly to the tissues. Testosterone cypionate is qualitatively similar to testosterone and its esters in physiologic activity. In hypogonadal males, the effect of a single injection of 200 to 400 mg of the cypionate in oil was observed to be maintained for 2 to 4 weeks, which is 2 to 4 times longer than the effect produced by a comparable dose of the propionate ester. Testosterone is readily absorbed from the gastrointestinal tract, but is metabolized by the liver before reaching the systemic circulation.

Indications: *In the male:* Replacement therapy in eunuchoidism and eunuchism; male climacteric symptoms; impotence, postpubertal cryptorchidism with evidence of hypogonadism, and other conditions due to loss, atrophy, or hypofunction of the testes. *In the female:* As androgen therapy in dysmenorrhea and premenstrual tension, functional uterine bleeding, menopause, endometriosis, frigidity, postpartum breast pain, and inoperable breast carcinoma and metastases in women who are more than 1 year but less than 5 years postmenopausal.

Contraindications: Severe liver damage; in male patients with suspected or proved carcinoma of the prostate or of the male breast; in patients with nephroses or the nephrotic phase of nephritis; a history of hypersensitivity or idiosyncrasy to testosterone; cardiac, hepatic or renal decompensation; hypercalcemia; prepubertal males; in patients easily stimulated; during pregnancy, or in lactating women who are breast feeding their infants.

Warnings: Female patients should be observed carefully for symptoms or signs of virilization such as hoarseness or deepening of the voice, oily skin, acne, hirsutism, enlarged clitoris, stimulation of libido, and menstrual irregularities. Some of these manifestations may be irreversible even after the drug has been discontinued. Testosterone should not be given to elderly asthenic males who may react adversely to overstimulation by androgens. Cholestatic hepatitis with jaundice and altered liver function tests such as increased BSP retention and increased SGOT levels have been reported during treatment with methyltestosterone. These changes appear to be dose-related. If variations occur in liver function tests, the drug should be withdrawn. Anabolic steroids may increase sensitivity to anticoagulant drugs, may alter glucose tolerance tests, and may cause edema when used concomitantly with adrenal corticosteroids or ACTH.

Precautions: Testosterone, through its metabolic effects, stimulates the nervous, mental, and physical activities of the patient. Therefore, it should be used with caution in the presence of cardiovascular and renal diseases, especially in the elderly male. Care should be taken in the treatment of adolescent or preadolescent males so that premature epiphyseal closure or precocious sexual development may be avoided. Prolonged administration or excessive dosage may cause inhibition of testicular function. As a result, oligospermia may develop, and there may be a decrease in ejaculatory volume. If priapism or other signs of excessive sexual stimulation develop, discontinue treatment with testosterone. Anaphylactoid reactions, although rare, may also occur, and treatment should be readily available. Hypersensitivity reactions, including rash and dermatitis, have been reported. PBI may be decreased in patients taking androgens. Hepatocellular carcinoma and peliosis hepatis (a rare condition of unknown etiology consisting of blood-filled cysts in the liver) have been observed in patients with congenital and acquired aplastic anemia treated with androgens for prolonged periods. In some cases withdrawal of the drug has been associated with regression of the hepatic lesions.

Adverse Reactions: Occasionally, patients complain of local irritation, redness, and pain at the site of injection of testosterone propionate, even though it is given by the intramuscular route. The administration of testosterone may result in renal reabsorption of electrolytes. Sodium retention may cause edema, especially in individuals with cardiovascular or renal disease. Hypercalcemia may occur in patients with metastatic bone lesions from a breast malignancy; this usually indicates progression of the disease. Patients with osteolytic neoplastic lesions who are bedfast or only semiambulatory may develop nephrocalcinosis when given androgens. There is a possibility of gynecomastia during the initial phase of testosterone therapy, but it usually recedes with continued administration. Other reactions that may occur include inhibition of testicular function, testicular atrophy and oligospermia, impotence, chronic priapism, epididymitis, and bladder irritability. In addition, the following reactions are known to occur with anabolic steroids: increased or decreased libido, flushing of the skin, acne, habituation, excitation and sleeplessness, chills, leukopenia, and bleeding in patients on concomitant anticoagulant therapy. Alterations may occur in the following clinical laboratory tests: metyrapone test, fasting blood sugar and glucose tolerance tests, thyroid function tests (decrease in protein bound iodine, thyroxine-binding capacity, and radioactive iodine uptake, and an increase in T^3 uptake by the red blood cells or resin: free thyroxine levels remain normal and the altered tests usually persist for 2 to 3 weeks after discontinuation of anabolic therapy), blood coagulation tests (increase in clotting factors II, V, VII, X), and miscellaneous laboratory tests (decreased creatinine and creatine excretion lasting up to 2 weeks after withdrawal of the drug and increased 17-ketosteroid excretion).

Dosage and Administration: *Intramuscularly* only. *For androgen deficiency,* 10 to 25 mg 2 or 3 times a week. *For postpartum breast engorgement,* 25 to 50 mg for 3 to 4 days, beginning at the time of delivery. *For palliation of mammary cancer,* the usual dosage is 100 mg 3 times a week for as long as improvement is maintained. *Subcutaneous implantation. For male hypogonadism,* the average total daily dose is 2 to 6 pellets implanted every 3 to 6 months. Pellets are inserted into the medial aspect of the thighs by means of a pellet injector. When optimal clinical improvement has been obtained, dosage may be decreased in accordance with the requirements of the patient. *Orally,* for maintenance therapy, 10 to 40 mg, up to 80 mg daily or every other day.

Availability:

Testosterone

NEO-HOMBREOL® F Aqueous Suspension, 25 and 50 mg/ml in vials of 10 ml. **(Organon)**
ORETON® Pellets for Subcutaneous Implantation in vials of 75 mg. **(Schering)**
TESTOSTERONE Aqueous Suspension, 25 and 50 mg/ml in ampuls of 10 ml. **(Lilly)**

Testosterone Cypionate

DEPO®-TESTOSTERONE CYPIONATE Injection, 50 mg/ml in vials of 10 ml; 100 and 200 mg/ml in vials of 1 and 10 ml. **(Upjohn)**

Testosterone Enanthate

DELADUMONE® Injection in oil, 90 mg with 4 mg/ml of estradiol valerate in vials of 5 ml and in 1-ml disposable syringe. **(Squibb)**
DELADUMONE® OB Injection, 180 mg with 8 mg/ml of estradiol valerate in vials of 2 ml and in 2-ml disposable syringe. **(Squibb)**
DELATESTRYL® Injection in oil, 200 mg/ml in vials of 5 ml and in 1-ml disposable syringe (Unimatic®). **(Squibb)**

Testosterone Propionate

NEO-HOMBREOL® Injection in Oil, 50 mg/ml in vials of 10 ml. **(Organon)**
TESTOSTERONE PROPIONATE Injection in Oil, 50 mg/ml in ampuls of 10 ml. **(Lilly)**

Methyltestosterone

METANDREN®: **(Ciba)**
Linguets® Sublingual Tablets, 5 and 10 mg in bottles of 100.
Oral Tablets, 10 and 25 mg in bottles of 100.
ORETON® METHYL: **(Schering)**
Buccal Tablets, 10 mg in bottles of 100.
Oral Tablets, 10 and 25 mg in bottles of 100.
TESTRED® Capsules, 10 mg in bottles of 100, 500 and 1000. **(ICN)**

TETANUS IMMUNE GLOBULIN (HUMAN)

Description: Tetanus immune globulin is a sterile solution of globulins derived from the blood plasma of adult human donors who have been hyperimmunized with tetanus toxoid, and whose plasma has been found to be nonreactive when tested for hepatitis B surface antigen. It contains not less than 15 gm and not more than 18 gm of protein/100 ml, of which not less than 90% is globulin. It contains a suitable preservative and may contain glycine as a stabilizing agent. It provides protective levels of circulating antitoxin for a longer period at considerably lower dosage levels than that found following administration of equine or bovine antitoxin. It has a half-life of 4 weeks and shows significant serum levels for up to 14 weeks.

Indications: To provide passive immunity to tetanus in patients with a tetanus-prone injury who are not known to be immune to tetanus. It has also been used for the treatment of active tetanus infection.

Contraindications: Intravenous administration.

Precautions: It is important to use a separate heat-sterilized syringe and needle for each patient to prevent transmission of homologous serum hepatitis and other infectious agents from one individual to another. Passive immunization with this agent should not be considered a substitute for active immunization with tetanus toxoid before injury, nor as a substitute for adequate medical and surgical care of contaminated or potentially contaminated wounds. It is therefore recommended that active immunization with tetanus toxoid be completed in all patients either immediately or shortly thereafter because passive immunization is only a temporary and partial substitute for active immunization. Since anaphylactic reactions may occur, the necessary precautions should be maintained. **Note:** Skin tests for sensitivity are not recommended because the inflammatory reactions that may occur are almost always false-positive reactions.

Adverse Reactions: Local tenderness and stiffness, erythema, low-grade fever and, rarely, sensitivity.

Dosage and Administration: *Intramuscularly* only. The usual prophylactic dose is 250 units; children may be given 4 units/kg of body weight. May be repeated in 1 month for additional protection. Doses of 400 to 500 units have been recommended for patients who are grossly overweight and in those with extremely tetanus-prone wounds or when longer than 1 day has elapsed between the time of injury and treatment. For the treatment of tetanus, it is recommended that 500 units be given daily until 3000 to 6000 units have been given, but optimal dosage schedules have not been established.

Availability:
AR-TET® in vials and in disposable syringes of 250 units. **(Armour)**
HU-TET in vials and prefilled disposable syringes of 250 units. **(Hyland)**
HYPER-TET® in vials and in prefilled disposable syringes of 250 units. **(Cutter)**
IMMU-TETANUS® in vials and in prefilled disposable syringes of 250 units. **(Parke-Davis)**
TETANUS IMMUNE GLOBULIN, 250 units in 2-ml disposable syringe and needle (Tubex®). **(Wyeth)**
T-I-GAMMAGEE® in disposable syringes of 250 units. **(Merck Sharp & Dohme)**

TETANUS TOXOID

Description: Tetanus toxoid is a sterile solution of the formaldehyde-treated products of growth of the tetanus bacillus, *Clostridium tetani.* It contains not more than 0.02% of residual free formaldehyde, and contains a suitable preservative.

Adsorbed tetanus toxoid is a sterile suspension of tetanus toxoid precipitated or adsorbed by the addition of alum, aluminum hydroxide, or aluminum phosphate to a formaldehyde-treated solution of the products of growth of the tetanus bacillus, *Clostridium tetani.*

Provides highly effective immunization and ensures protection against tetanus for 10 years or more.

Indications: Active immunization against tetanus.

Contraindications: Treatment of actual tetanus infections, and the immediate prophylaxis of nonimmunized individuals.

Precautions: Suitable medication should be available in case of anaphylaxis. Local and systemic reactions may occur more frequently and may be more severe following numerous previous injections of tetanus toxoid. Immunization should be deferred in the presence of any acute respiratory disease or other active infections, in patients receiving immunosuppressive agents or irradition treatment, and in those with immunologic deficiency disease. As with all intramuscular injections, aspiration is necessary to help avoid inadvertant instillation into a blood vessel.

Adverse Reactions: These may be local or systemic and are usually low in incidence and relatively mild. Local redness and/or edema, pain, tenderness and a nodule at the site of injection which may be accompanied by regional adenopathy have been reported. Systemic effects of chills, fever and malaise can also occur, as well as anaphylaxis or anaphylactoid reactions. It is advisable that epinephrine be readily available at all times. The possible occurrence of postvaccinal neurologic disorders should be considered.

Dosage and Administration: For active immunization, 2 doses of the suspension are given *intramuscularly* 4 to 6 weeks apart, or 3 doses of the solution are given *subcutaneously* or *intramuscularly* at intervals of 3 to 4 weeks. A booster dose may be given 1 year later and every 10 years thereafter. In case of possible infection with tetanus, a single dose of the solution rather than the suspension is recommended. However, this is justified only if it can be definitely established that the patient has been actively immunized against tetanus and that at least 1 month has elapsed since immunization has been completed.

Availability:

Tetanus Toxoid Purified, Fluid

Purogenated® in vials of 7.5 ml and in (Lederject®) 0.5-ml disposable syringes with needle. **(Lederle)**

Vials of 1.5 and 7.5 ml and in 0.5-ml Hyporet® (disposable syringes) with needle. **(Lilly)**

Vials of 0.5 and 7.5 ml and in M-N-L Ject (prefilled syringes) of 0.5 ml. **(Merrell-National)**

Vials of 7.5 ml and in 0.5-ml disposable syringes with needle (Tubex®). **(Wyeth)**

Tetanus Toxoid, Aluminum Phosphate Adsorbed

Purogenated® in vials of 5 ml and in 0.5-ml Lederject® (disposable syringes with needle.) **(Lederle)**

Vials of 1 and 5 ml and in 0.5 ml Hyporet® (disposable syringes with needle). **(Lilly)**

Vials of 5 ml. **(Merck Sharp & Dohme)**

Vials of 0.5 and 5 ml and in M-N-L Ject (prefilled syringes) of 0.5 ml. **(Merrell-National)**

Vials of 5 ml and in 0.5-ml Steri-Dose® (disposable syringe with needle). **(Parke-Davis)**

Vials of 5 ml and in 0.5-ml disposable syringes with needle (Tubex®). **(Wyeth)**

TETRACAINE HYDROCHLORIDE

Chemical Name: 2-(Dimethylamino)ethyl-*p*-(butylamino)benzoate hydrochloride.

Description: Tetracaine is a local anesthetic and occurs as a white, odorless, crystalline powder, readily soluble in water, physiologic salt solution, and dextrose solution. Aqueous solutions are stable and can be sterilized by brief boiling.

Tetracaine is a long-acting local anesthetic, more effective than cocaine topically for mucous membranes and the eyes (in which it is nonmydriatic, noncycloplegic, and does not raise intraocular pressure). Following subarachnoid or caudal injection or infiltration, tetracaine provides anesthesia of 2 to 3 hours or more in duration, thus reducing the number of injections when continuous or intermittent techniques are used.

Indications: Topical anesthesia of the eye, nose, mouth, and throat, and for prolonged spinal anesthesia and continuous caudal analgesia.

Contraindications: *For spinal anesthesia* includes diseases of the cerebrospinal system, such as meningitis, spinal fluid block, cranial or spinal hemorrhage, tumors, and syphilis; suppuration at the site of puncture; in the presence of shock, profound anemia, cachexia, and when death is imminent; sepsis with positive blood cultures; high or low blood pressure; in highly nervous and sensitive individuals; in visceral perforation, bowel strangulation, acute peritonitis; cardiac decompensation, massive pleural effusion, and increased abdominal pressure. Contraindications to *saddle block during delivery* include pelvic disproportion, placenta praevia, abruptio placentae, unengaged head, and intrauterine manipulation (e.g., podalic version). *Continuous caudal anesthesia* is contraindicated in the presence of placenta praevia, inertia uteri, uncontrollable hysteria, and disproportion between child and pelvis, also in extremely obese individuals in whom the sacral hiatus cannot be palpated, and in women with a history of instability.

Warnings: When there is a possibility of systemic involvement, resuscitative equipment and drugs should be immediately available. The patient's blood pressure should be carefully monitored during the procedure. Vomiting, restlessness, pallor, and a weak pulse with shallow respiration usually accompany a marked decrease in blood pressure; if these occur a parenteral pressor agent should be administered. Safe use has not been established with respect to adverse fetal affects. Therefore, it should not be used in women of childbearing potential, and particularly during the first trimester of pregnancy, unless the potential benefits outweigh the unknown hazards. The eye ointment is incompatible with sulfonamides, mercury or silver salts. For anesthetizing the larynx, trachea, or esophagus, the total absorbed dose should not exceed 20 mg except in special techniques that have been carefully worked out.

Precautions: To combat the vasodepressor effects of tetracaine hydrochloride, especially when used for spinal anesthesia, a long-acting vasoconstrictor may be injected intramuscularly or intravenously, and the necessary equipment should be readily available for emergency use. Hypotension should be corrected promptly, especially if it develops during spinal anesthesia for normal vaginal delivery, since hypoxic fetal bradycardia may occur. If a vasoconstrictor is given to correct the hypotension, the addition of an oxytocic drug of the ergot type may result in severe, persistent hypertension with possible rupture of a cerebral blood vessel during the postpartum period. Topical anesthetics should be applied sparingly on open lesions. Careful use is advised in patients with known allergies, in those with cardiac or hepatic disease, hyperthyroidism, or other endocrine disorders, and in patients who are emaciated. Prolonged applications of topical anesthetics to the eye is not recommended because it may cause corneal inflammation or damage.

Adverse Reactions: CNS stimulation followed by depression, vasomotor paralysis, respiratory paralysis, meningitis, palsies, paralysis of extraocular muscles and, rarely, of other cranial nerves, headache, nausea and vomiting, and systemic side effects. Other reactions that may occur are skin rashes or urticaria. Topical applications to the eye may cause transient smarting when concentrations higher than 0.5% are used. On rare occasions lacrimation, photophobia, and chemosis in sensitive patients have been noted. Administration of a barbiturate preoperatively tends to prevent or to reduce the severity of reactions. In allergic individuals a skin test should be employed as an additional safeguard; although the test is not always accurate, it will detect hypersensitivity in some patients.

Dosage and Administration: *Intraspinal.* The suggested dosage for *saddle block anesthesia* is 1 to 2 ml of the 0.2% solution; for *low spinal anesthesia,* 1 to 2 ml of the 0.3% solution; for *median spinal anesthesia,* 3 to 4 ml of the 0.3% solution, and for *high spinal anesthesia,* 5 ml of the 0.3% solution. *Topically.* For application to eye, 0.5% solution; to nose, throat and mouth, 2% solution. For specific dosages in specific indications, see package literature.

Availability:
TETRACAINE HYDROCHLORIDE:
Ophthalmic Solution, 0.5% in Steri-Units® of 2 ml and in Drop-Tainer® (dropper-bottles) of 15 ml. **(Alcon)**
Ophthalmic Solution, 0.5% in sterile pack Dropperettes® applicators of 1 ml. **(Smith, Miller & Patch)**
PONTOCAINE®: **(Breon)**
Compound Ointment, 0.5% in tubes of 30 gm with pile pipe.
Cream, 1% in tubes of 30 gm with pile pipe.
Dry Powder for Injection (for spinal use) in Niphanoid® ampuls of 20 mg.
Ophthalmic Ointment, 0.5% in tubes of 3.75 gm.
Solution for Injection (for spinal use), 0.2% with 6% dextrose in ampuls of 2 ml; 0.3% with 6% dextrose in ampuls of 5 ml; 1% in ampuls of 2 ml.
Topical Solution, 0.5% in Mono-Drop® bottles of 15 ml and in bottles of 60 ml; 2% in bottles of 30 and 120 ml.

TETRACYCLINE HYDROCHLORIDE

Chemical Name: 4-Dimethylamino-1,4,4α,5,5α,6,11,12α-octahydro-3,6,10,12,12α-pentahydroxy-6-methyl-1,11-dioxo-2-naphthacenecarboxamide hydrochloride.

Description: Tetracycline hydrochloride is prepared by the catalytic hydrogenation (removal of chlorine) of chlortetracycline or by fermentation. It is freely soluble in water and more stable in aqueous solution than the hydrochlorides of chlortetracycline or oxytetracycline. Citrates, phosphates, glucosamine and other agents have been added to tetracycline preparations in an effort to increase their absorption from the gastrointestinal tract. Such buffering, or the use of tetracycline phosphate complex, may produce somewhat higher blood levels but well-controlled studies have not confirmed these claims and any increased absorption is probably clinically insignificant. Tetracycline generally is bacteriostatic rather than bactericidal in action and has a broad antimicrobial spectrum. They are readily absorbed and are bound to plasma proteins in varying degrees.

The mechanism of action remains obscure; however, on the basis of present observations, tetracycline may interfere with bacterial protein synthesis or with cellular oxidative metabolism. Resistance develops in a slow, step-wise fashion. Organisms made resistant to one tetracycline are usually cross resistant to others. Those found to be resistant include streptococci, staphylococci, pneumococci, gonococci, and other gram-negative organisms. Therefore, culture studies and sensitivity testing are advised before initiating therapy, and to determine the susceptibility of the infecting organism. Readily absorbed from the gastrointestinal tract, peak serum levels are attained in about 2 to 4 hours and are maintained for 6 hours or more following single oral doses. Intravenously, maximum serum concentrations are attained in about 5 minutes and detectable levels remain as long as 12 hours. Intramuscularly, peak plasma levels are reached in 1 hour and detectable amounts remain for 12 hours or longer. Intramuscular preparations, although generally compounded with solubilizing agents and local anesthetics, are not quite satisfactory because full doses require frequent, painful injections. After absorption, tetracycline is concentrated in the liver and excreted in the bile; it is partially excreted in the urine, and fairly large amounts can be recovered from the stool.

Indications: Recommended primarily for the treatment of gram-negative bacillary infections, rickettsial diseases, gram-positive infections resistant to penicillin, and susceptible bacterial infections in patients who are hypersensitive to other antibiotics. It is effective against staphylococci, pneumococci, *alpha*- and *beta*-hemolytic streptococci, nonhemolytic streptococci, gram-negative rods, rickettsiae, spirochetes, and some large viruses. However, tetracycline should not be used for streptococcal disease unless the organism has been demonstrated to be sensitive. It is not considered the drug of choice in the treatment of any type of staphylococcal infections. For upper respiratory infections due to Group A beta-hemolytic streptococci, penicillin is the drug of choice, including prophylaxis of rheumatic fever. Tetracycline is also effective in the treatment of urinary tract and other infections caused by *E. coli, A. aerogenes,* and tetracycline-susceptible staphylococci. It has limited value in the treatment of *Salmonella* infections, and little or no activity against most strains of *Proteus vulgaris* and *Pseudomonas aeruginosa.* Besides its value in the treatment of gram-negative and gram-positive organisms, tetracycline has also been found useful as an alternative drug, in those cases in which penicillin is contraindicated in the treatment of *N. gonorrhoeae, T. pallidum* and *pertenue* (syphilis and yaws), *Listeria monocytogenes,* Clostridia, *B. anthracis,* Fusobacterium (Vincent's infection), and Actinomyces; as adjunctive therapy in acute intestinal amebiasis, and in severe acne. It is indicated in the treatment of trachoma, although the infectious agent is not always eliminated, as determined by immunofluorescence. Inclusion conjunctivitis may be treated with oral tetracycline or with a combination of oral and topical agents. The topical solution is recommended for the treatment of acne vulgaris.

Contraindications: Coadministration with other potentially hepatotoxic drugs; hypersensitivity or idiosyncrasy to tetracycline; daily dosages exceeding 2 gm.

Warnings: The use of tetracycline during tooth development (last half of pregnancy, infancy, and childhood to the age of 8 years) may cause permanent discoloration of the teeth (yellow-gray-brown). This adverse reaction is more common during long-term use of the drugs but has been observed following repeated short-term courses. Enamel hypoplasia has also been reported. Tetracycline drugs, therefore, should not be used in this age group unless other drugs are not likely to be effective or are contraindicated. If renal impairment exists, even usual oral or parenteral doses may lead to excessive systemic accumulation of the drug and possible liver toxicity. Intravenous tetracycline therapy has been associated with deaths through liver failure, particularly in pregnant patients. This occurs most commonly with doses of 2 gm daily but it has been reported to occur with doses as low as 1 gm daily. Under such conditions, lower than usual doses are indicated, and, if therapy is prolonged, serum level determinations of the drug may be advisable. Photosensitivity manifested by an exaggerated sunburn reaction has been observed in some individuals taking tetracyclines. Patients who may be exposed to direct sunlight or ultraviolet light should be advised that this reaction can occur with tetracycline and treatment should be discontinued at the first evidence of skin erythema. The antianabolic action of the tetracyclines may cause an increase in BUN. While this is not a problem in those with normal renal function, in patients with significantly impaired function, higher serum levels of tetracycline may lead to azotemia, hyperphosphatemia, and acidosis. Therefore, 1/2 or 1/4 of the usual dose should be given to patients with renal disease or azotemia, and the blood level should be monitored at frequent intervals. Results of animal studies indicate that tetracyclines cross the placenta, are found in fetal tissues and can have toxic effects on the developing fetus (often related to retardation of skeletal development). Evidence of embryotoxicity has also been noted in animals treated early in pregnancy. Tetracycline forms a stable calcium complex in any bone-forming tissue. A decrease in the fibula growth rate has been observed in premature infants given oral tetracycline in doses of 25 mg/kg every 6 hours. However, this reaction was shown to be reversible when the drug was discontinued. It should be noted that tetracycline has been found to be present in the milk of lactating women.

Precautions: Since bacteriostatic agents may interfere with the bactericidal action of penicillin, it is advisable not to administer tetracycline in conjunction with penicillin. When given for prolonged periods, tetracycline has been found to produce a brown-black microscopic discoloration of the thyroid gland; however, no abnormality in thyroid function was noted. In venereal diseases when coexistent syphilis is suspected, darkfield examination should be performed before initiating treatment and serologic tests repeated monthly for a minimum of 4 months. Because tetracycline has been shown to depress plasma prothrombin activity, patients who are taking anticoagulant drugs may require a downward adjustment of the anticoagulant dosage. As with other antibiotics, the use of tetracycline occasionally may result in overgrowth of nonsusceptible organisms, including fungi. Constant observation of the patient is essential. If new infections appear during therapy, the drug should be discontinued and appropriate measures should be taken. In long-term therapy, periodic laboratory evaluation of organ systems, including hematopoietic, renal and hepatic studies should be performed. All infections due to Group A beta hemolytic streptococci require a minimum of 10 days of treatment.

Adverse Reactions: Some local pain has been experienced following intramuscular injection. Deep injection in the gluteal region is recommended, but proper precautions should be taken to avoid the sciatic nerve and intravascular administration. Thrombophlebitis, a possibility with all intravenous therapy, should be guarded against by strict attention to preparation of the solution and the technique of inserting and fixing the position of the needle; too rapid administration should be avoided. If large doses are necessary, the serum concentration of tetracycline should be monitored and the dose lowered if the concentration exceeds 16 mcg/ml of serum. Gastrointestinal involvement is manifested by anorexia, nausea, vomiting, diarrhea, glossitis, dysphagia, enterocolitis, and inflammatory lesions (with monilial overgrowth) in the anogenital region. These reactions have been caused by both the oral and parenteral administration of tetracyclines. Reactions involving the skin include maculopapular and erythematous rashes, exfoliative dermatitis (rare), and photosensitivity. Renal toxicity usually causes a rise in BUN and is apparently dose-related. Hypersensitivity reactions may include urticaria, angioneurotic edema, anaphylaxis, anaphylactoid purpura, pericarditis, and exacerbation of systemic lupus erythematosus. Tetracyclines have been reported to cause increased intracranial pressure and tense bulging of the fontanels in young infants, even when given the usual therapeutic doses. Discontinuation of therapy produces prompt return of the pressure to normal. Hemolytic anemia, thrombocytopenia, neutropenia, and eosinophilia have also been reported in patients sensitive to these agents.

Dosage and Administration: *Orally.* Adults, 250 mg every 6 hours around the clock, or 2 *bid*Caps twice daily, in patients with an acute illness of more than average severity, or if there is no clinical response within 24 hours, it is advisable to increase the number of daily doses to 6 or 8. Children, 25 mg/kg of body weight daily in 4 equally divided doses. Children weighing more than 40 kg should receive the adult dose. Iron, aluminum, calcium, and magnesium interfere significantly with absorption; therefore, oral doses should be given on an empty stomach and milk, food, or such agents as alumina gel, magnesia gel or dicalcium phosphate should be withheld for at least 1 hour after administration. *Intramuscularly.* Recommended dosage is 100 mg every 8 to 12 hours; in severe infections, dosages up to 250 mg every 12 hours may be given. Children, 15 to 25 mg/kg of body weight in 2 or 3 divided doses. Children weighing more than 40 kg should receive the adult dose. *Intravenously.* Adults, 250 to 500 mg may be given every 6 to 12 hours. Children, 10 to 20 mg/kg of body weight daily in 2 divided doses. **Note:** Whatever the route of administration, therapy should be continued for 24 to 48 hours after symptoms and fever have subsided. *Topically.* In treating superficial infections of the eye, ear, nose, throat and skin due to susceptible organisms, applications may be made locally from 1 to 3 times daily according to the needs and response of the patient.

Availability:

ACHROMYCIN®: **(Lederle)**
Intramuscular (powder) in vials of 100 and 250 mg buffered with ascorbic acid.
Intravenous in vials of 250 and 500 mg buffered with ascorbic acid.
Ointment, 3% (30 mg/gm) in tubes of 15 and 30 gm.
Ophthalmic Suspension, 1% in plastic dropper bottles of 4 ml.
Ophthalmic Ointment, 1% in tubes of 3.75 gm.

ACHROMYCIN® V: **(Lederle)**
Capsules, 100 mg in bottles of 100; 250 and 500 mg in bottles of 100 and 1000 and in unit-dose packages of 100.
Syrup, 125 mg/5 ml in bottles of 60 ml and 1 pint.

BRISTACYCLINE® Capsules, 250 mg in bottles of 100 and 1000; 500 mg in bottles of 100. **(Bristol)**

CYCLOPAR® Capsules, 250 mg in bottles of 100 and 1000 and in unit-dose (individual blisters) packages of 100; 500 mg in bottles of 100 and in unit-dose packages of 100. **(Parke-Davis)**

KESSO-TETRA®: **(McKesson)**
Capsules, 250 mg in bottles of 100, 1000 and 5000 and in unit-dose packages of 100; 500 mg in bottles of 100.
Syrup, 125 mg/5 ml in bottles of 60 ml and 1 pint.

PANMYCIN®: **(Upjohn)**
Capsules, 250 mg in bottles of 100 and 1000.
Syrup, 125 mg/5 ml in bottles of 60 ml and 1 pint.
Tablets, 250 mg in bottles of 1000; 500 mg in bottles of 100.

ROBITET®: **(Robins)**
Capsules, 250 mg in bottles of 100 and 1000; 500 mg in bottles of 100 and 500.
Syrup, 125 mg/5 ml in bottles of 1 pint.

SK-TETRACYCLINE™: **(Smith Kline & French)**
Capsules, 250 mg in bottles of 100 and 1000; 500 mg in bottles of 100.
Syrup, 125 mg/5 ml in bottles of 1 pint.

SUMYCIN®: **(Squibb)**
Capsules, 250 mg in bottles of 100 and 1000 and in Unimatic®s (unit-dose) of 100; 500 mg in bottles of 100 and 500 and in Unimatic®s of 100.
Syrup, 125 mg/5 ml in bottles of 60 ml and 1 pint.
Tablets, 250 and 500 mg in bottles of 100 and 1000.

TETRACYCLINE Capsules, 250 mg in bottles of 1000; 500 mg in bottles of 50 and 250. **(Philips Roxane)**

TETRACYCLINE Capsules, 250 mg in bottles of 100 and 1000; 500 mg in bottles of 100. **(Wyeth)**

TETRACYN®: **(Pfipharmecs)**
Capsules, 250 mg in bottles of 100 and 1000 and in unit-dose packages of 100; 500 mg in bottles of 100 and in unit-dose packages of 100.
Syrup, 125 mg/5 ml in bottles of 60 ml and 1 pint.

TETRACYN®: **(Pfizer)**
Intramuscular in vials of 100 and 250 mg.
Intravenous in vials of 250 and 500 mg.

TETREX® Capsules, 250 mg in bottles of 100; 500 mg (*bid*Caps®) in bottles of 50 and 100. **(Bristol)**

TOPICYCLINE® Topical Solution, 2.2 mg/ml in bottles of 70 ml. **(Proctor & Gamble)**

w/Amphotericin B

MYSTECLIN® F: **(Squibb)**

Capsules, 125 mg with 25 mg of amphotericin B in bottles of 100; 250 mg with 50 mg of amphotericin B in bottles of 16 and 100.

Syrup, 125 mg with 25 mg/5 ml of amphotericin B in bottles of 60 and 240 ml.

w/Nystatin

ACHROSTATIN® V Capsules, 250 mg with 250,000 units of nystatin in bottles of 16 and 100. **(Lederle)**

COMYCIN® Capsules, 250 mg with 250,000 units of nystatin in bottles of 100. **(Upjohn)**

TETRASTATIN® Capsules, 250 mg with 250,000 units of nystatin in bottles of 100. **(Pfipharmecs)**

TETRAHYDROZOLINE HYDROCHLORIDE

Chemical Name: 2-(1,2,3,4-Tetrahydro-1-naphthyl)-2-imidazoline hydrochloride.

Description: Tetrahydrozoline hydrochloride is a sympathomimetic amine structurally and pharmacologically related to naphazoline. It occurs as a white, odorless powder freely soluble in water and in alcohol. Possesses vasoconstrictor and decongestant actions when applied to the nasal mucosa, resulting in constriction of the smaller arterioles of the nasal passages thus reducing congestion or swelling.

Indications: Temporary relief of nasal and nasopharyngeal congestion.

Contraindications: In patients receiving monoamine oxidase inhibitors (MAOI); hypersensitivity to the drug; infants under 2 years of age; the 0.1% solution is contraindicated in children under 6 years of age.

Warnings: Safe use during pregnancy has not been established. Excessive application, or high concentrations of the drug may produce severe drowsiness and profuse sweating.

Precautions: The recommended dosage schedule should not be exceeded. Hypotension and shock may occur with improper use of the drug in children. Also, rebound congestion may occur with prolonged use. Use cautiously in patients with cardiovascular disease (e.g., coronary artery disease, hypertension), and metabolic-endocrine disease (e.g., hyperthyroidism, diabetes).

Adverse Reactions: Frequently reported were burning, stinging, sneezing, dryness, headache, drowsiness, weakness, tremors, lightheadedness, insomnia, and palpitations. Excessive overdosage may result in a shock-like syndrome with hypotension and bradycardia.

Dosage and Administration: *Intranasally.* Adults and children 6 years of age and over, 2 to 4 drops of the 0.1% solution. Children 2 to 6 years of age, 2 to 3 drops of the 0.05% solution. Should never be administered more often than every 3 hours.

Availability:

TYZINE®: **(Key Pharm.)**

Nasal Solution, 0.1% in plastic spray bottles of 15 ml, in bottles of 1 pint and in dropper bottles of 30 ml.

Pediatric Nasal Drops, 0.05% in squeeze bottles of 15 ml.

THEOBROMINE MAGNESIUM OLEATE

Chemical Name: Magnesium 3, 7-dimethylxanthine oleate.

Description: Theobromine magnesium oleate, a compound containing the magnesium double salt of theobromine and oleic acid, has been reported to promote diuresis by increasing renal blood flow, to produce coronary and peripheral arterial vasodilatation, and to stimulate the myocardium, thereby increasing cardiac output and improving the general circulation. It also relieves the pain and discomfort of angina pectoris and coronary disease and other symptoms of general arteriosclerosis. The addition of magnesium nicotinate stimulates the peripheral circulation and increases the serum magnesium level.

Indications: Treatment of arteriosclerosis and its manifestations including myocardial insufficiency, thromboangiitis obliterans, and xanthomatosis, and as an adjunct to the usual therapeutic measures in diabetic endarteritis.

Contraindications: Serious kidney disease and obstructive lesions of the genitourinary tract.

Adverse Reactions: Gastric upset may occur, although rarely encountered. The component magnesium nicotinate may produce flushing (a sensation of warmth) and pruritus, but these reactions are transient and apparently harmless.

Dosage and Administration: *Orally.* The usual dosage is 1 or 2 tablets 3 times daily. An alternative dosage regimen is 2 tablets 3 times daily for 6 to 8 weeks, then 1 tablet 3 times daily.

Availability:
ATHEMOL® Tablets, 200 mg in bottles of 100 and 500. **(Meyer)**
ATHEMOL-N Tablets, 200 mg with magnesium nicotinate, 100 mg (equiv. to 75 mg of nicotinic acid) in bottles of 100 and 500. **(Meyer)**

THEOKIN

Description: Each 15 ml (1 tablespoonful) and each tablet contain theophylline calcium salicylate 448.5 mg (equiv. to 225 mg of anhydrous theophylline) and potassium iodide, 450 mg. The elixir also contains 9.5% alcohol.

Indications: Symptomatic treatment of bronchial asthma, chronic bronchitis and chronic obstructive pulmonary emphysema when reversible bronchospasm and thickened mucus secretions are evident.

Contraindications: Hypersensitivity or idiosyncrasy to iodides; concurrent use with other preparations containing theophylline.

Warnings: Caution is recommended during pregnancy, and when administering to children.

Precautions: Should be used with care in patients sensitive to iodides, salicylates, in the presence of hyperthyroidism, in pregnant patients (iodide-induced goiter with hypothyroidism may occur in the newborn). Prolonged use of iodides can lead to hypothyroidism. Coadministration with other xanthine preparations should be avoided. Should be used sparingly and with caution in patients with hypertension, cardiac arrhythmias, acute cardiac infarction, congestive heart failure, hepatic dysfunction, and peptic ulcer. Since salicylates block the action of probenecid and sulfinpyrazone, particular care should be exercised in patients with gout. Recent reports suggest that troleandomycin reduces the clearance of theophylline by 50% resulting in a doubling of theophylline blood levels. The effect of concomitant administration of other macrolide antibiotics, such as erythromycin, is not known.

Adverse Reactions: Gastric irritation, nausea, vomiting, diarrhea, palpitations, restlessness, insomnia, headache, and CNS stimulation. Taking the drug with or after meals, as well as adjusting the dosage and monitoring blood levels may help to alleviate or avoid such symptoms. If vomiting occurs, the drug should be withdrawn.

Dosage and Administration: *Orally,* 1 tablet or 1 tablespoonful of elixir 2 to 3 times daily, increased by 1/2 in severe attacks. Children 6 to 12 years of age, 1/2 tablet/45 lb of body weight or 1 teaspoonful/30 lb of body weight; children under 6 years of age, 1/2 teaspoonful/15 lb of body weight once or twice daily. Administer preferably on an empty stomach, and at intervals of not less than 6 hours.

Availability:
THEOKIN®: **(Knoll)**
Elixir in bottles of 1 pint.
Tablets in bottles of 100.

THEOPHYLLINE

Chemical Name: 1,3-Dimethylxanthine.

Description: Theophylline, an alkaloid of the xanthine group, is isomeric with theobromine. It occurs as a bitter, white, odorless, crystalline powder slightly soluble in water and sparingly soluble in alcohol. Theophylline relaxes smooth muscle constriction of the smaller bronchi, promotes dilatation of the small pulmonary arteries, increases cardiac output and is a mild diuretic.

Indications: Symptomatic relief of acute bronchial asthma, and for reversible bronchospasm associated with chronic bronchitis and emphysema; paroxysmal cardiac dyspnea; and edema of congestive heart failure. It provides rapid relief of acute asthmatic attacks. When combined with sympathomimetic agents, the effect is more pronounced than when either drug is used alone. The addition of potassium iodide or iodinated glycerol provides a liquefying action when tenacious mucus obstruction is a severe symptom. Formulated with a barbiturate to allay and control the undesirable CNS stimulating effects of the xanthine group and to reduce the anxiety and tension which frequently accompany diseases of the cardiovascular system.

Contraindications: Peptic ulcer, gout, and hypersensitivity to theophylline or to any component formulated with it. As with other xanthine medications, it should not be administered to patients with coronary artery disease or angina pectoris where, in the physician's judgment, myocardial stimulation might prove harmful.

Warnings: Barbiturates may be habit-forming.

Precautions: Coadministration with other xanthine preparations should be avoided. Theophylline should be used with caution in pregnant patients. In some patients prolonged use of iodides may lead to hypothyroidism. Should be used with caution in the presence of severe cardiac disease, acute myocardial injury, congestive heart failure, severe hypertension, hyperthyroidism, and peptic ulcer. Toxic synergism with ephedrine and other sympathomimetic bronchodilator drugs may occur.

Adverse Reactions: Because of the pharmacologic similarities among the xanthine group of drugs, the following adverse reactions should be anticipated when theophylline is administered. These include *gastrointestinal effects* manifested by nausea, vomiting and epigastric pain, generally preceded by headache, hematemesis, and diarrhea; *CNS effects* by irritability, restlessness, insomnia, reflex hyperexcitability, muscle twitching, clonic and tonic generalized convulsions, and agitation; *cardiovascular effects* by palpitation, tachycardia, extrasystoles, flushing, marked hypotension, and circulatory failure; *respiratory effects* by tachypnea, and respiratory arrest; *renal effects* by albuminuria, and hematuria; *miscellaneous effects* by fever and dehydration. Overdosage in children is manifested by agitation, headache, hyperreflexia, fasciculations, and clonic and tonic convulsions; in adults by nervousness, insomnia, nausea, vomiting, tachycardia, and extrasystoles. Treatment involves inducing emesis, initiating supportive treatment for hypotension, seizure, arrhythmias, and dehydration; sedatives to control CNS stimulation; lactate or bicarbonate to restore the acid-base balance, and oxygen and antibiotics as additional supportive measures.

For additional contraindications, warnings, precautions and adverse reactions, see the specific monograph on the individual components.

Dosage and Administration: *Orally* every 6 to 8 hours. Adults, 1 or 2 capsules, tablets or teaspoonsful of elixir. Children 8 to 12 years of age, 1 capsule or teaspoonful; children under 8 years of age, 3 to 5 mg/kg of body weight. The sustained-release capsule is administered every 8 to 12 hours. With potassium iodide: Adults, 30 ml 3 times daily; children, 0.2 ml/lb of body weight 3 times daily. Adults, 1 or 2 tablets 4 times daily. Dosage should not exceed 2 tablets in any 4-hour period. Children 6 to 12 years of age, ½ tablet 4 times daily; children under 6 years of age, dosage should be adjusted proportionately.

Availability:
ACCURBRON™ Liquid, 50 mg/5 ml in bottles of 1 pint with graduated measuring spoon. *Contains 7.5% alcohol.* **(Dow)**

BRONKODYL®: **(Breon)**
Capsules (micro-pulverized), 100 and 200 mg in bottles of 100.
Elixir, 80 mg/15 ml in bottles of 1 pint. *Contains 20% alcohol.*
ELIXICON™ Suspension, 100 mg/5 ml in bottles of 240 ml. *(Alcohol and dye free).* **(Cooper)**
ELIXOPHYLLIN®: **(Cooper)**
Capsules, 100 and 200 mg (anhydrous) in a suspension of polyethylene glycol 400; the 100 mg capsules in bottles of 100; the 200 mg capsules in bottles of 100 and 500 and in unit-dose cartons of 100.
Elixir, 80 mg/15 ml (20% alcohol) in pints, quarts and gallons.
SR Capsules (sustained release), 125 and 250 mg in bottles of 100 and 500.
Pediatric Suspension, 100 mg/5 ml in bottles of 240 ml. *(Alcohol and dye free).*
SOMOPHYLLIN® Capsules, 100, 200 and 250 mg in bottles of 100. **(Fisons)**
THEOBID® Capsules (Duracap®), 260 mg in bottles of 60 and 500. **(Meyer)**
THEO-DUR™ Tablets (sustained action), 100, 200 and 300 mg in bottles of 100 and 1000. **(Key Pharm.)**
THEOLAIR™: **(Riker)**
Liquid, 80 mg/15 ml in bottles of 1 pint and 1 gallon.
Tablets, 125 and 250 mg (anhydrous) in unit-dose (sealed aluminum foil pouches) in cartons of 100 and 250.
THEOPHYL™: **(Knoll)**
Chewable Tablets, 100 mg in bottles of 100.
Elixir, 225 mg/30 ml (anhydrous) in bottles of 1 pint. *Contains 5% alcohol.*
SR Capsules (sustained release), 125 and 250 mg in bottles of 100.
Tablets, 225 mg (anhydrous) in bottles of 100.
THEOPHYLLINE Elixir, 80 mg/15 ml in Abbo-Pac®s (unit-dose) of 15 and 30 ml. **(Abbott)**
THEOPHYLLINE Elixir, 80 mg/15 ml in unit-dose (Aluminum Cups) of 15 and 30 ml. **(Parke-Davis)**
THEOPHYLLINE Elixir, 80 mg/15 ml in unit-doses (Patient Cups) of 15 and 30 ml and in bottles of 1 pint and 1 gallon. **(Philips Roxane)**

Combinations

BRONCHOBID® Capsules (Duracap®), 260 mg with pseudoephedrine hydrochloride, 50 mg in bottles of 60 and 500. **(Meyer)**
DUOVENT® Tablets, 130 mg with ephedrine hydrochloride, 24 mg; guaifenesin, 100 mg and phenobarbital, 8 mg in bottles of 100. **(Riker)**
ELIXOPHYLLIN® KI Liquid, 80 mg/15 ml with potassium iodide, 130 mg in bottles of 240 ml and 1 gallon. **(Cooper)**
MARAX®: **(Roerig)**
Syrup, 32 mg/5 ml with ephedrine sulfate, 6.25 mg and hydroxyzine hydrochloride, 2.5 mg in pints and gallons.
Tablets in bottles of 100 and 500. Each tablet is equivalent to 20 ml of syrup.
MARAX-DF Syrup, 32.5 mg/5 ml with ephedrine sulfate, 6.25 mg; hydroxyzine hydrochloride, 2.5 mg and alcohol, 5% v/v in bottles of 1 pint and 1 gallon. **(Roerig)**
QUIBRON®: **(Mead Johnson)**
Capsules, 150 mg with guaifenesin, 90 mg in bottles of 100 and 1000 and in unit-dose packages of 100.
300 Capsules, 300 mg with guaifenesin, 180 mg in bottles of 100.
Elixir, 50 mg/5 ml with guaifenesin, 30 mg in pints and gallons.
QUIBRON PLUS: **(Mead Johnson)**
Capsules, 150 mg with guaifenesin, 100 mg; ephedrine hydrochloride, 25 mg and butabarbital, 20 mg in bottles of 100.
Elixir, 150 mg/15 ml with guaifenesin, 100 mg; ephedrine hydrochloride, 25 mg; butabarbital, 20 mg and alcohol, 15% in bottles of 1 pint.
TEDRAL®: **(Warner-Chilcott)**
Elixir in a dark red, cherry-flavored vehicle. Each 5 ml contains theophylline, 32.5 mg, ephedrine hydrochloride, 6 mg; phenobarbital, 2 mg and alcohol, 15% in bottles of 1 pint.
Expectorant Tablets, 130 mg with ephedrine hydrochloride, 24 mg; guaifenesin, 100 mg and phenobarbital, 8 mg in bottles of 100.
Tablets, 130 mg with ephedrine hydrochloride, 24 mg and phenobarbital, 8 mg in bottles of 100 and 1000 and in unit-dose packages of 100.

SA Tablets (sustained-action), 180 mg with ephedrine hydrochloride, 48 mg and phenobarbital, 25 mg in bottles of 100 and 1000 and in unit-dose packages of 100.
Suspension, 65 mg/5 ml with ephedrine hydrochloride, 12 mg and phenobarbital, 4 mg in bottles of 240 ml and 1 pint.
25 Tablets, 130 mg with ephedrine hydrochloride, 24 mg and butabarbital, 25 mg in bottles of 100. Other dosage forms do not require a prescription.
THEO-NAR Tablets (timed release), 100 and 200 mg with noscapine, 15 and 30 mg, respectively in bottles of 100 and 500. **(Key Pharm.)**
THEO-ORGANIDIN® Elixir, 120 mg/15 ml with iodinated glycerol, 30 mg (equiv. to 15 mg of organically bound iodine) and alcohol, 15% in bottles of 1 pint and 1 gallon. **(Wallace)**

THIABENDAZOLE

Chemical Name: 2-(4-Thiazolyl)benzimidazole.

Description: Thiabendazole is an anthelmintic that occurs as a white crystalline substance that is insoluble in water but soluble in dilute acid or alkali solutions.

Although the exact mechanism of anthelmintic activity has not been determined, it has been postulated that thiabendazole probably interferes with the metabolic pathways essential for a variety of helminths.

Following oral administration, the drug is rapidly absorbed and peak plasma levels are attained within 1 to 2 hours. It is metabolized almost completely to the 5-hydroxy form which appears in the urine as glucuronide or sulfate conjugates. Within 48 hours, approximately 5% of the administered dose is recovered from the feces and approximately 90% from the urine.

Indications: Treatment of enterobiasis, strongyloidiasis, ascariasis, uncinariasis, trichuriasis, and cutaneous larva migrans (creeping eruption). Therapeutic effect in trichuriasis is limited. May also be used for alleviating symptoms of trichinosis during the invasive phase of the disease.

Contraindications: A history of hypersensitivity to thiabendazole.

Warnings: The drug should be discontinued immediately and not be resumed if a hypersensitivity reaction occurs. Erythema multiforme, and in severe cases Stevens-Johnson syndrome that resulted in fatalities have been reported. Patients should be cautioned that in the event of drowsiness or dizziness they should not engage in hazardous occupations requiring alertness or coordination. Safe use in pregnant and lactating patients has not been confirmed.

Precautions: Patients who are anemic, dehydrated or malnourished should be given supportive therapy prior to treatment with this drug. Careful monitoring of patients with renal or hepatic dysfunction is indicated.

Adverse Reactions: The most frequently encountered side reactions are anorexia, nausea, vomiting and dizziness. Less frequently, diarrhea, epigastric distress, pruritus, weariness, drowsiness, giddiness, and headache have occurred. Those rarely occurring are tinnitus, hyperirritability, numbness, abnormal sensation in eyes, blurring of vision, xanthopsia; hypotension, collapse; enuresis; transient rise in cephalin flocculation and SGOT levels; perianal rash, cholestasis and parenchymal liver damage; hyperglycemia; transient leukopenia; malodor of the urine, crystalluria, hematuria; appearance of live Ascaris in the mouth and nose. Hypersensitivity reactions include fever, facial flush, chills, conjunctival injection, angioedema, anaphylaxis, skin rashes, erythema multiforme (including Stevens-Johnson syndrome), and lymphadenopathy.

Dosage and Administration: *Orally*, preferably after meals. The usual dosage schedule for all conditions is 2 doses daily for 2 successive days; the recommended maximum daily dose is 3 gm. The size of the dose is determined by the patient's weight. Patients weighing less than 150 lbs, the dose is 10 mg/lb of body weight or 25 mg/kg of body weight. Patients weighing 150 lbs and over, the dose is 1.5 gm.

Availability:
MINTEZOL®: **(Merck Sharp & Dohme)**

Chewable Tablets, 500 mg in cartons of individually foil-wrapped tablets in a strip of 36 tablets.
Oral Suspension, 500 mg/5 ml in bottles of 120 ml.

THIAMINE HYDROCHLORIDE

Synonym: Vitamin B-1.

Chemical Name: 3-(4-Amino-2-methylpyrimidyl-5-methyl)-4-methyl-5(β-hydroxyethyl)thiazolium chloride hydrochloride.

Description: The readily water-soluble hydrochloride of pure, synthetic vitamin B-1; it occurs as white crystals or crystalline powder that is very soluble in water.

Thiamine is the prosthetic group of the enzyme, carboxylase. This enzyme promotes the decarboxylation of alpha keto acids such as pyruvic acid. It therefore serves an important function in the intermediary metabolism of carbohydrate. In thiamine deficiency, the oxidation of alpha keto acids is impaired, and an increase in the level of pyruvic acid of the blood is one of the diagnostic signs of the deficiency state. It has also been definitely established that the requirement for thiamine is related to metabolic rate and is greatest when carbohydrate is a source of energy.

Indications: Prophylaxis and treatment of vitamin B-1 deficiency and treatment of beriberi.

Contraindications: Patients who have shown a history of sensitivity to thiamine hydrochloride.

Warnings: Parenteral administration of solutions containing this vitamin may cause severe allergic reactions or anaphylaxis, some of which have been fatal. Therefore, sensitivity tests should be performed before administering a therapeutic dose. Intravenous injections should be administered slowly.

Precautions: Simple vitamin B-1 deficiency rarely occurs. Multiple vitamin deficiencies should be suspected in any case of dietary inadequacy.

Adverse Reactions: Feeling of warmth, pruritus, urticaria, weakness, sweating, nausea, restlessness, tightness of the throat, angioneurotic edema, cyanosis, pulmonary edema, hemorrhage into the gastrointestinal tract, collapse, and death have been reported.

Dosage and Administration: *Intramuscularly* or *intravenously.* The daily average dose is 30 to 60 mg divided into 3 equal doses.

Availability:
BETALIN®S Injection, 100 mg/ml in ampuls of 1 ml and in vials of 10 and 30 ml. **(Lilly)**
THIAMINE HYDROCHLORIDE:
Injection, 100 mg/ml in Steri-vials of 10 and 20 ml. **(Parke-Davis)**
Injection, 100 mg/ml in Tubex® (disposable syringes and needle unit) of 1 ml fill in 2 ml. **(Wyeth)**

THIAMYLAL SODIUM Ⓒ III

Chemical Name: Sodium 5-allyl-5-(1-methylbutyl)-2-thiobarbiturate.

Description: Thiamylal sodium is an ultrashort-acting barbiturate primarily used for intravenous anesthesia alone in procedures of relatively short duration, as a supplement to other anesthetic agents, or as a means for inducing a hypnotic state. It occurs as a pale yellow, hygroscopic powder having a disagreeable odor. It is readily soluble in water or other parenteral solutions customarily used for this type of preparation. It has been found to be less cumulative and to have an anesthetic potency of about 1.5 times that of thiopental sodium. Following administration, anesthesia usually occurs within 20 to 60 seconds while recovery occurs within 10 to 30 minutes after the last injection, depending upon the amount administered.

Indications: When a rapid, ultra-short acting anesthetic is required.

Contraindications: Hypersensitivity to barbiturates, latent or manifest porphyria, and when general anesthesia is contraindicated.

Warnings: Standard equipment for endotracheal intubation, oxygen therapy, artifical respiration and drugs should be present. To be administered only by those qualified in the use of intravenous anesthetics. Repeated or continuous infusion may cause cumulative effects resulting in prolonged somnolence, respiratory and circulatory depression. Since safe use of thiamylal sodium has not been established with respect to adverse effects upon fetal development, this anesthetic should not be used in women of childbearing potential and particularly during the first trimester of pregnancy unless, in the judgment of the physician, the expected benefits outweigh the potential hazards.

Precautions: Caution should be exercised in debilitated patients, or in those with impaired function of respiratory, circulatory, renal, hepatic, and endocrine systems. Extreme caution is required in patients with status asthmaticus. Extravascular injection may cause pain, swelling, ulceration and necrosis. Intraarterial injection is dangerous and may produce gangrene of an extremity.

Adverse Reactions: Reported were circulatory depression, thrombophlebitis, pain at injection site, respiratory depression including apnea, laryngospasm, bronchospasm, salivation, hiccups, emergence delirium, headache, injury to nerves adjacent to injection site, skin rashes, urticaria, nausea, and emesis.

Dosage and Administration: *Intravenously*. For induction, 3 to 6 ml of a 2.5% solution is administered at the rate of 1 ml every 5 seconds; maintenance 0.5 to 1 ml as required. When used in conjunction with other anesthetic agents, an 0.3% solution is administered by *continuous intravenous drip*. For complete details on procedure, see package literature.

Availability:
Ⓒ III SURITAL® in ampuls of 5 gm and in Steri-Vials® of 1, 5 and 10 gm. **(Parke-Davis)**

THE THIAZIDE DIURETICS

Description: The benzothiadiazine, or thiazide, diuretics include those compounds derived from the heterocyclic sulfonamide, 1,2,4-benzothiadiazine-7-sulfonamide 1,1-dioxide and consequently have the same basic molecular structure. The difference structurally of the individual derivatives occurs at position 3-4 and at positions 6, 3 and 2 of the parent molecule. Chlorothiazide is the prototype of the thiazide diuretics. In general, the thiazides occur as white, crystalline solids that are very slightly soluble in water.

The differences that have been demonstrated among the various agents in this group of similarly-acting oral diuretics involve only dosages and duration of action; in other respects they are almost identical. These drugs share a common mechanism of action in that they increase the urinary excretion of water, sodium, chloride and, to a lesser degree, potassium and bicarbonate ions. The thiazides also have antihypertensive properties and may be used for this purpose either alone in the presence of mild hypertension, or with other antihypertensive drugs in patients with severe hypertension or in those who are not controlled by the diuretic alone. The mechanism by which the benzothiadiazines produce a reduction of elevated blood pressure has not been clearly defined, but it may be related to depletion of extracellular volume, depletion of sodium, or to a direct effect on vascular smooth muscle. Their advantage is due to the fact that they lower both standing and supine blood pressures, the antihypertensive effect is maintained during prolonged administration, and they enhance the effect of other antihypertensive drugs, thereby permitting a reduction in dose, thus reducing the incidence and severity of unpleasant reactions. They are rapidly absorbed from the gastrointestinal tract, and the diuresis they produce lasts from 12 to 72 hours, varying with the compound used.

It has been postulated that the thiazides act by inhibiting the reabsorption of electrolytes in the proximal renal tubule, thus promoting their urinary excretion. Carbonic anhydrase inhibitory activity is relatively weak and generally does not contribute significantly to diuretic effectiveness. However, inhibition of carbonic anhydrase may be largely responsible for the extent to which these compounds increase potassium and bicarbonate loss. The diuretic effect of the thiazides is apparent within 2 hours and reaches its maximum in 4 to 6 hours following oral administration; they are excreted by the kidneys.

Indications: All the thiazide diuretics produce diuresis that results in weight loss and symptomatic improvement in patients with edema associated with various disorders. Thus they are useful as adjuncts in the management of congestive heart failure. They may be given to initiate diuresis and maintain the edema-free state in all types and degrees of severity of cardiac decompensation. However, patients with the most severe forms of the disease may not respond to their action, particularly when the glomerular filtration rate is reduced. These agents are satisfactory as replacement for other oral diuretics and can often be used in place of those organic mercurials that must be administered parenterally. The thiazide diuretics are also useful in many patients who either fail to respond or become refractory to other diuretics. Although thiazide therapy is not intended to serve as a replacement for a low-sodium diet, administration of these agents makes it possible to liberalize the salt intake in selected patients with congestive heart failure. The thiazides have also been used in patients with edema associated with nephrosis and certain types of nephritis; liver disease, particularly portal cirrhosis; obesity; the premenstrual syndrome, and edema induced by the administration of corticotropin, adrenal corticosteroids, and some estrogens. However, the results in these conditions have been less successful. Edema during pregnancy generally responds well to thiazides except when due to renal disease. Hypertension associated with pregnancy also responds well, but toxemia (eclampsia) may require more potent diuretics. Nonetheless, the routine use of these compounds are not recommended in pregnant women with mild edema who are otherwise healthy.

The thiazides can be used alone or in combination with other drugs such as reserpine and deserpidine for the treatment of mild to moderate hypertension. They can also be used with more potent hypotensive agents including hydralazine, guanethidine, pargyline, and the ganglionic blocking agents for the treatment of more severe hypertension. However, because of a potentiating effect, the dosage of these other agents should be reduced considerably; this decreases or even eliminates some of their more troublesome reactions, including those resulting from parasympathetic ganglionic blockade.

Contraindications: All diuretics, including the thiazide diuretics, are contraindicated in anuria. If increasing azotemia and oliguria occur during treatment of severe progressive renal disease, therapy with diuretics should be discontinued. They are also contraindicated in patients known to be sensitive to these or other sulfonamide-derived compounds. The routine use of diuretics in otherwise healthy pregnant women with or without edema is contraindicated and possibly hazardous.

Warnings: Minor alterations of fluid and electrolyte balance may precipitate hepatic coma. Periodic determinations of serum electrolytes to detect possible electrolyte imbalance should be performed at appropriate intervals. These are especially indicated for patients with severe derangement of metabolic processes, e.g., surgery, vomiting or parenteral fluid therapy. Electrolyte imbalance may also be caused by such diseases as cirrhosis, or it may result from drug therapy, such as therapy with corticosteroids. Patients with cirrhosis who are continually receiving thiazide medication should be observed carefully for the development of hepatic precoma or coma. Indications of impending hepatic failure are tremor, confusion, drowsiness, and hepatic fetor. Also impaired renal function may precipitate azotemia or may lead to the development of cumulative effects of the drug. Sensitivity reactions may occur in patients with a history of allergy or bronchial asthma. The possibility of exacerbation or activation of systemic lupus erythematosus has been reported. Thiazides may be additive or may potentiate the action of other antihypertensive drugs, such as the ganglionic or peripheral adrenergic blocking agents.

Available information tends to implicate enteric-coated potassium salts with or without thiazides in the etiology of nonspecific small bowel lesions consisting of ulceration with or without stenosis, causing obstruction, hemorrhage and perforation, and frequently requiring surgery. Deaths due to these complications have been reported. Enteric-coated potassium salts should be used only when adequate dietary supplementation is not practical and should be discontinued immediately if abdominal pain, distention, nausea, vomiting or gastrointestinal bleeding occur.

Thiazides require cautious use when administered to pregnant women or nursing mothers since they cross the placental barrier and appear in cord blood and in breast milk. The use of thiazides may result in fetal or neonatal jaundice, bone marrow depression, thrombocytopenia, and possibly other adverse reactions which have occurred in the adult. Altered carbohydrate metabolism has been noted in newborn infants of mothers manifesting a decreased glucose intolerance. Intravenous use in infants and children has been limited and is generally not recommended.

Precautions: Patients in whom the excretion of potassium is likely to be excessive (elderly debilitated patients, those with hepatic cirrhosis, and those who are receiving digitalis, adrenal corticosteroids, or corticotropin) should receive supplementary potassium as a salt or preferably foods high in potassium content (e.g., orange juice). However, enteric-coated potassium tablets should be used only when dietary supplementation is not practical, and with the accepted warnings. Hypokalemia may also result in increased sensitivity to the action of digitalis; (digitalis therapy may exaggerate the metabolic effects of hypokalemia especially with reference to myocardial activity); thus, changes in the dosage requirements of both drugs must be anticipated. Patients with myocardial ischemia resulting from coronary artery disease may also have a predisposition to serious cardiac arrhythmias if hypokalemia occurs. Less frequently, thiazides may produce a hypochloremic alkalosis with hypokalemia in patients who have an additional loss of chloride and potassium due to vomiting, diarrhea, other gastrointestinal drainage, sweating, paracentesis, or potassium-depleting disorders of the kidney. A chloride salt should be given to compensate for the chloride deficit; however, ammonium chloride should not be given to patients with hepatic insufficiency. Occasionally, sodium depletion occurs in patients with dietary restriction of sodium, and produces drowsiness, weakness, and mental confusion.

Occasionally, a dilutional hyponatremia can occur as a complication of thiazide therapy in patients with severe congestive heart failure and marked edema. When this occurs as the result of dietary restriction of sodium, it may be necessary to treat it by restricting the intake of water. The thiazides should be given cautiously or, in some instances, may even be contraindicated in patients with severe renal or hepatic impairment in whom depletion of potassium may already exist. Nitrogen retention may indicate the onset of renal impairment, and dosage should be adjusted or the drug discontinued if this occurs. These patients should be observed for signs of impending hepatic coma or uremia, which is presaged by fetor hepaticus, flapping tremor, confusion, and drowsiness. Since the thiazides decrease the renal excretion of uric acids, they may aggravate gout or interfere with its treatment with uricosuric agents. When these diuretics are given with other potent hypotensive agents (e.g., guanethidine, mecamylamine, hydralazine), the doses of the latter should be reduced by at least 50% to prevent excessive hypotensive effects, especially in the upright position.

In elderly patients with advanced arteriosclerosis, the use of these drugs may precipitate coronary or cerebral thrombosis due to severe orthostatic hypotension, especially if the patient is receiving a ganglionic blocking agent or has undergone a sympathectomy in the past. Since these patients may have a marked hypotensive response, the usual doses should be reduced by ½. The thiazides should not be used indiscriminately in patients with edema and toxemia of pregnancy because of the lack of information concerning their possible adverse effects on the fetus and neonate. These hazards include their potential for causing both electrolyte disturbances and other reactions such as neonatal thrombocytopenia. Clinical reports have indicated that the thiazides may decrease arterial responsiveness to pressor amines (e.g., levarterenol) and augment the paralyzing action of tubocurarine in surgical patients. It is suggested that administration of these drugs be discontinued 1 week prior to elective surgery. Thiazides may decrease serum PBI levels without signs of thyroid disturbance. They have been reported on occasion to elevate serum calcium to hypercalcemic levels; this condition returned to normal upon discontinuation of the drug. Nevertheless, thiazides should be discontinued before carrying out tests for parathyroid function. Also, the response to tubocurarine may be aggravated.

Adverse Reactions: Molecular modification has not affected the occurrence of the untoward effects most frequently associated with chlorothiazide. Because of their effect on renal function, all of these agents may produce electrolyte imbalances. Therefore, all patients receiving thiazide therapy should be observed for clinical signs of fluid and electrolyte imbalance (hyponatremia, hypochloremic alkalosis, and hypokalemia). Serum and electrolyte determinations are particularly important when the patient is vomiting excessively or receiving parenteral fluids. Medications such as digitalis may also influence serum electrolytes. Warning signs irrespective of the cause are usually manifested by dryness of mouth, thirst, weakness, lethargy, drowsiness, restlessness, muscle pains or cramps, muscular fatigue, hypotension, oliguria, and tachycardia may occur. Other reactions that may be noted include anorexia, gastric irritation, nausea, vomiting, cramping, diarrhea, constipation, and jaundice (intrahepatic cholestatic jaundice); fever, dizziness, vertigo, paresthesias, headache, and xanthopsia; purpura, rash, and urticaria, exfoliative dermatitis, and glomerulonephritis. Orthostatic hypotension may occur and may be aggravated by alcohol, barbiturates, or narcotics. If these persist, they may be controlled by reducing the dose. Photosensitivity reactions and pancreatitis have occurred rarely. Because of the tendency of these drugs to cause elevated uric acid levels in the serum, asymptomatic hyperuricemia has been observed commonly, but acute gouty arthritis has occurred infrequently except in patients already subject to attacks. Thiazides and related diuretics may produce a necrotizing vasculitis of the skin and kidney in elderly patients. The results following the administration of small test doses to a single patient seem to support these observations. Blood dyscrasias (leukopenia, aplastic anemia, thrombocytopenia with purpura, and agranulocytosis) have been reported infrequently with the older agents and not, as yet, with every one of these drugs. However, because of the similarities in molecular structure of the drugs, the physician should be aware that these adverse effects may occur. Development of hyperglycemia in patients with latent diabetes and aggravation of preexisting diabetes have been noted occasionally with all of these agents. The hyperglycemic action of these drugs should not preclude their use in diabetic patients, but blood sugar levels should be determined regularly during their prolonged administration. Increased doses of hypoglycemic agents may be needed to control the elevated blood sugar concentrations. Hypotensive episodes under anesthesia have been observed in some patients receiving thiazides. Ulceration of the small intestine has been reported in patients taking a thiazide with potassium chloride in enteric-coated form. Potassium chloride should be given with a thiazide only when there is a specific indication for its use and when dietary measures are inadequate. If supplementation is in fact necessary, the use of liquid preparations of potassium chloride is suggested.

The preceding discussed the chemical, pharmacologic and clinical similarities of the thiazide diuretics as a group. In the discussions that follow, each individual monograph deals specifically with each of the following:

Bendroflumethiazide
Benzthiazide
Chlorothiazide
Cyclothiazide
Hydrochlorothiazide
Hydroflumethiazide
Methyclothiazide
Polythiazide
Trichlormethiazide

BENDROFLUMETHIAZIDE

Chemical Name: 3,4-Dihydro-3-(phenylmethyl)-6-(trifluoromethyl)-2H-1,2,4-benzothiadiazine-7-sulfonamide 1, 1-dioxide.

Description: Bendroflumethiazide is a thiazide diuretic that differs structurally from hydroflumethiazide in that a benzyl group has been substituted for hydrogen at position 3 on the hydroflumethiazide molecule. The pharmacologic actions of bendroflumethiazide are essentially the same as those of the prototype, chlorothiazide. When the maximal effective dose is exceeded, no further increases in water and electrolyte loss occur. Serum electrolyte concentrations are not altered appreciably. The drug is readily absorbed from the gastrointestinal tract and is excreted chiefly by tubular secretion.

Indications: Bendroflumethiazide shares the actions and uses of other drugs in this group. Diuresis occurs within 2 hours and lasts for 18 to 24 hours.

For the action, clinical uses, precautions and adverse reactions, see general statement.

Dosage and Administration: *Orally.* To induce diuresis in the treatment of edema, the usual initial dosage is 5 mg once daily, preferably given in the morning. This dose may be increased to 20 mg administered as a single dose or in 2 divided doses. For maintenance therapy after diuresis has been established, the dose is 2.5 to 5 mg daily depending upon the patient's response. In the treatment of hypertension, the usual initial dosage is 5 to 20 mg daily for 1 week and the maintenance dosage is 2.5 to 15 mg daily depending upon the patient's response. Compound with potassium, 1 to 4 tablets daily.

Availability:
NATURETIN® Tablets, 2.5 and 10 mg in bottles of 100; 5 mg in bottles of 100 and 1000. **(Squibb)**
NATURETIN with K Tablets, 2.5 mg with 500 mg of potassium chloride in bottles of 100; 5 mg with 500 mg of potassium chloride in bottles of 100 and 1000. **(Squibb)**

BENZTHIAZIDE

Chemical Name: 6-Chloro-3-[[(phenylmethyl)thio]methyl]-2H-1,2,4-benzothiadiazine-7-sulfonamide 1, 1-dioxide.

Description: Benzthiazide is a thiazide diuretic that differs structurally from chlorothiazide in that a benzylthiomethyl group is attached at position 3. It occurs as a white, bitter, crystalline compound with a characteristic odor, practically insoluble in water but readily soluble in alkaline solutions. Rapidly absorbed from the gastrointestinal tract, the drug induces diuresis within 2 hours, reaches a peak effect in 4 to 6 hours, and the action persists for about 12 to 18 hours. Serum electrolyte levels usually are not affected by therapeutic doses used for brief periods.

Indications: In addition to its use as a diuretic, benzthiazide also may be of use in the control of hypertension and toxemia of pregnancy, and for the relief of angina when due to congestive heart failure and/or hypertension.

For the action, clinical uses, precautions and adverse reactions, see general statement.

Dosage and Administration: *Orally.* In the treatment of edematous states, the initial daily adult dosage may vary from 50 to 200 mg. Maintenance dosage usually is in the range of 50 to 150 mg daily. The maximal single effective dose is about 100 mg; when daily dosage exceeds this amount, divided doses are preferred. In the treatment of hypertension, the usual adult initial dosage is 50 mg once or twice daily. Dosage may be decreased, or increased to as much as 200 mg daily, for maintenance. Therapy should never be initiated with the fixed-ratio combination, and should be employed only when the amounts therein meet the requirement of the individual patient.

Availability:
AQUASTAT Tablets, 50 mg in bottles of 100. **(Lemmon)**
EXNA® Tablets, 50 mg in bottles of 100 and 500. **(Robins)**
EXNA-R Tablets, 50 mg with 0.125 mg of reserpine in bottles of 100 and 500. **(Robins)**

CHLOROTHIAZIDE

Chemical Name: 6-Chloro-2H-1,2,4-benzothiadiazine-7-sulfonamide 1,1-dioxide.

Description: Chlorothiazide is the prototype of all the thiazide diuretics. It occurs as a white, crystalline compound with low solubility in water, but is readily soluble in dilute sodium hydroxide solution. Rapidly and uniformly absorbed from the gastrointestinal tract, the diuretic effects produced by the drug are apparent within 2 hours, reach a peak in 4 hours and persist for about 6 to 12 hours. Intravenous administration of the drug as the sodium salt produces a response within 15 minutes, reaches a peak effect in 30 minutes, and persists for about 2 hours. Chlorothiazide is eliminated rapidly by the kidney. Its rate of elimination is decreased somewhat by the coadministration of probenecid without, however, an accompanying reduction of diuresis.

Indications: In addition to its use as a diuretic, chlorothiazide also may be used alone for the treatment of mild to moderate hypertension or combined with more potent hypotensive agents for the treatment of the more severe types.

For the actions, clinical uses, precautions and adverse reactions, see general statement.

Dosage and Administration: *Diuresis:* The usual *intravenous* or *oral* dosage for adults is 0.5 to 1 gm once or twice daily. A total daily dosage of 1 gm or more usually is given in 2 divided doses. The usual oral dosage for children is 22 mg/kg daily in 2 divided doses. In infants under 6 months of age it may be necessary to increase this dosage to 33 mg/kg of body weight daily in 2 divided doses to achieve the desired effect. *Hypertension:* The initial oral dosage ranges from 0.5 to 1 gm daily as a single or divided dose, then increased or decreased according to the response of the patient. Careful observation for changes in blood pressure must be made when the product containing reserpine is used with other antihypertensive drugs. The dosage of these other agents must be reduced at least 50% to prevent an excessive drop in blood pressure. A continuing drop in blood pressure warrants further reduction in dosage or discontinuation of the other antihypertensive agent.

Availability:
CHLOROTHIAZIDE Tablets, 250 and 500 mg in bottles of 100 and 1000. **(Lederle)**
DIURIL®: **(Merck Sharp & Dohme)**
Oral Suspension, 250 mg/5 ml in bottles of 237 ml.
Powder for Injection (Diuril Sodium), 0.5 gm in vials of 20 ml.
Tablets, 250 mg in bottles of 100 and 1000 and in single-unit dispenser packages of 100; 500 mg in bottles of 100, 1000 and 5000 and in single-unit dispenser packages of 100.
DIUPRES® Tablets, 250 mg or 500 mg with 0.125 mg of reserpine in bottles of 100 and 1000. **(Merck Sharp & Dohme)**
SK-CHLOROTHIAZIDE™ Tablets, 250 and 500 mg in bottles of 100 and 1000. **(Smith Kline & French)**

CYCLOTHIAZIDE

Chemical Name: 3-Bicyclo[2,2,1]hept-5-en-2-yl-6-chloro-3,4-dihydro-2H-1,2,4-benzothiadiazine-7-sulfonamide 1, 1-dioxide.

Description: Cyclothiazide is a thiazide diuretic with antihypertensive action. It differs chemically from the other thiazides in that it has a complex ring structure at the 3 position on the benzothiadiazine nucleus. It occurs as a white to nearly white powder that is practically insoluble in water and sparingly soluble in alcohol. A notable advantage is its once-a-day dosage schedule and a prolonged duration of action (approximately 18 to 24 hours).

Indications: In addition to its usefulness in the treatment of edema associated with various forms of renal dysfunction, such as the nephrotic syndrome, acute glomerulonephritis, and chronic renal failure, it is also of value as adjunctive therapy in edema due to congestive heart failure, hepatic cirrhosis, and corticosteroid and estrogen therapy.

For contraindications, warnings, precautions and adverse reactions, see general statement.

Dosage and Administration: *Orally. For diuretic effect,* the usual adult dosage is ½ to 1 tablet (1 or 2 mg) once daily, preferably early in the morning in order to obtain daytime diuresis without disturbing the patient's rest at night. *For maintenance therapy,* ½ to 1 tablet given on alternate days or 2 to 3 times a week may be sufficient. *For antihypertensive effect,* the usual dosage is 1 tablet (2 mg) once daily; in some cases it may be necessary to give 1 tablet 2 or 3 times daily.

Availability:
ANHYDRON® Tablets, 2 mg (pink) in bottles of 100 and 1000. **(Lilly)**

HYDROCHLOROTHIAZIDE

Chemical Name: 6-Chloro-3,4-dihydro-2H-1,2,4-benzothiadiazine-7-sulfonamide 1,1-dioxide.

Description: Hydrochlorothiazide is the 3,4-dihydro derivative of chlorothiazide. It produces both diuretic and antihypertensive effects. Well absorbed after oral ingestion, the diuretic effect of hydrochlorothiazide occurs within 2 hours, reaches a peak effect in about 4 hours, and some residual effect may persist for 12 hours or longer. The drug is eliminated by the kidney largely in unchanged form.

Indications: In addition to treatment of edema associated with congestive heart failure, premenstrual tension, toxema of pregnancy (including eclampsia), or that due to liver cirrhosis, renal dysfunction, such as the nephrotic syndrome, acute glomerulonephritis, chronic nephritis, and corticosteroid and estrogen therapy, it is also useful in the management of mild to moderate hypertension or combined with more potent hypotensive agents for the treatment of severe hypertension.

For the action, clinical uses, precautions and adverse reactions, see general statement.

Dosage and Administration: *Orally.* The initial adult dosage to induce *diuresis* is 25 to 200 mg daily; the average maintenance dosage is 25 to 100 mg. For children, the recommended dosage is about 2 mg/kg daily, given in 2 divided doses. Infants under 6 months of age may require up to 3 mg/kg daily, in 2 divided doses. *Hypertension:* The usual dosage is 25 to 50 mg once or twice daily, but some patients may require as much as 200 mg daily in divided doses. Careful observation for changes in blood pressure must be made when the product containing reserpine is used with other antihypertensive drugs. The dosage of these other agents must be reduced at least 50% to prevent an excessive drop in blood pressure. A continuing drop in blood pressure warrants further reduction in dosage or discontinuation of the other antihypertensive agent.

Availability:

Hydrochlorothiazide

ESIDRIX® Tablets, 25 and 50 mg in bottles of 100, 1000 and 5000, in Accu-Pak®s (unit-dose) dispensers of 100 and in Consumer Packs of 30, 60 and 100; 100 mg in bottles of 100. **(Ciba)**
HydroDIURIL® Tablets, 25 and 50 mg in bottles of 100 and 1000 and in single-unit packages of 100; 100 mg in bottles of 100. **(Merck Sharp & Dohme)**
HYDROCHLOROTHIAZIDE Tablets, 25 and 50 mg in bottles of 100 and 1000. **(Lederle)**
HYDROCHLOROTHIAZIDE Tablets, 25 and 50 mg in bottles of 1000 and 5000 and in ready-to-dispense prepack cartons of 100 and in unit-dose cartons of 100 (10 x 10). **(Philips Roxane)**
LEXOR™ Tablets, 50 mg (green) in bottles of 100 and 1000. **(Lemmon)**
ORETIC® Tablets, 25 and 50 mg in bottles of 100 and 1000 and in Abbo-Pac®s (unit-dose) packages of 100. **(Abbott)**
THIURETIC® Tablets, 25 mg in bottles of 100 and in unit-dose packages of 100; 50 mg in bottles of 100 and 1000 and in unit-dose packages of 100. **(Parke-Davis)**

Combinations

Ⓒ III BUTISERPAZIDE® Tablets (Prestabs®), 25 mg (green) or 50 mg (orange) with 30 mg of butabarbital (**Warning:** may be habit-forming) and 0.1 mg of reserpine in bottles of 100 and 500. **(McNeil)**
HYDROCHLOROTHIAZIDE with RESERPINE Tablets, 25 or 50 mg with reserpine, 0.125 mg in bottles of 100 and 1000 and in unit-dose cartons of 100 (10 x 10). **(Philips Roxane)**
HYDROPRES® Tablets, 25 or 50 mg with 0.125 mg of reserpine in bottles of 100 and 1000. **(Merck Sharp & Dohme)**
SERPASIL®-ESIDRIX® Tablets, 25 or 50 mg with 0.1 mg of reserpine in bottles of 100 and 1000. **(Ciba)**

HYDROFLUMETHIAZIDE

Chemical Name: 3,4-Dihydro-6-(trifluoromethyl)-2H-1,2,4-benzothiadiazine-7-sulfonamide 1, 1-dioxide.

Description: Hydroflumethiazide is the 3,4-dihydro derivative of flumethiazide. It occurs as a white or cream-color crystalline powder that is very slightly soluble in water and soluble in alcohol. Diuresis begins within 2 hours after oral ingestion, reaches a peak in 6 to 12 hours, and lasts for 18 to 24 hours.

For the action, clinical uses, precautions and adverse reactions, see general statement.

Warnings: The fixed combination drug is not to be used for initial therapy, since hypertension requires therapy titrated to the individual patient. However, if the fixed combination represents the dosage so determined, its use may be more convenient in patient management.

Dosage and Administration: *Orally.* The usual *diuretic* dosage is 50 mg daily but, depending upon the individual response, this may be reduced to a minimum of 25 mg or increased to 200 mg in divided doses. A total daily dose of 100 mg or more is preferably given in 2 divided doses. *Hypertension:* The initial dosage is 50 mg twice daily; maintenance dosage is determined by the patient's blood pressure, but usually ranges from 50 to 100 mg daily. Dosage should not exceed 200 mg/day. *With reserpine,* 2 tablets daily.

Availability:
DIUCARDIN® Tablets, 50 mg in bottles of 100 and 1000. **(Ayerst)**
SALURON® Tablets, 50 mg in bottles of 100. **(Bristol)**
SALUTENSIN® Tablets, 50 mg with 0.125 mg of reserpine in bottles of 100 and 1000. **(Bristol)**
SALUTENSIN-DEMI™ Tablets, 25 mg with 0.125 mg of reserpine in bottles of 100 and 1000. **(Bristol)**

METHYCLOTHIAZIDE

Chemical Name: 6-Chloro-3-(chloromethyl)-3,4-dihydro-2-methyl-2H-1,2,4-benzothiadiazine -7-sulfonamide1,1-dioxide.

Description: Methyclothiazide is a synthetic saluretic-antihypertensive agent. It belongs to the benzothiadiazine (thiazide) family and is a potent analog of hydrochlorothiazide. Significant natriuresis and diuresis occurs within 2 hours after administration of a single dose, reaches a peak in approximately 6 hours and persists for about 24 hours. It is excreted unchanged by the kidneys. The excretion of sodium chloride is greatly enhanced; potassium excretion is low; urinary excretion of bicarbonate is increased slightly, usually causing no significant change in urinary pH. The mechanism by which methyclothiazide produces a reduction of elevated blood pressure has not been established; however, sodium depletion is thought to be of primary importance.

Warnings: Methyclothiazide combined with either reserpine or deserpidine is not indicated for initial treatment of hypertension since this condition requires that therapy be titrated to the individual patient. However, if the fixed combination represents the dosage so determined, its use may be more convenient in patient management.

For actions, clinical uses, contraindications, other warnings, precautions and adverse reactions, see general statement.

Dosage and Administration: *Orally.* The usual adult dosage ranges from 2.5 to 10 mg once daily. To maintain an edema-free state or as an adjunct in the management of hypertension, 2.5 to 5 mg once daily is often adequate. The maximal effective single dose is 10 mg; larger single doses do not accomplish greater diuresis, and are not recommended. Combined with deserpidine or reserpine—the usual adult dosage is 1 to 4 tablets daily depending on the clinical response. Dosage should be determined by individual titration with careful adjustment of both components to the needs of the individual. Since at least 10 to 14 days may elapse before the full effects of the drugs become manifest, the dosage of the fixed combination should not be adjusted more frequently. There is no contraindication in combining the administration of methyclothiazide with other antihypertensive agents; however, their addition to the regimen should be gradual. Ganglionic blocking agents should be given at only 1/2 the usual dose since their effect is potentiated by these compounds.

Availability:
AQUATENSEN® Tablets, 5 mg (pink) in bottles of 100 and 500. **(Mallinckrodt)**
ENDURON® Tablets, 2.5 mg in bottles of 100 and 1000; 5 mg in bottles of 100, 1000 and 5000 and in Abbo-Pac® (unit-dose) packages of 100 (10 × 10). **(Abbott)**

Combinations
DIUTENSEN®-R Tablets (round, scored, mottled), 2.5 mg with reserpine, 0.1 mg in bottles of 100 and 500. **(Mallinckrodt)**
ENDURONYL®/FORTE Tablets, 5 mg with either 0.25 or 0.5 mg of deserpidine in bottles of 100 and 1000 and in Abbo-Pac® (unit-dose) packages of 100 (10 × 10). **(Abbott)**

POLYTHIAZIDE

Chemical Name: 6-Chloro-3,4-dihydro-2-methyl-3-[[(2,2,2-trifluoroethyl)thio]methyl]-2H-1,-2,4-benzothiadiazine-7-sulfonamide 1,1-dioxide.

Description: Polythiazide is the longest-acting of the thiazide diuretics. It differs structurally from trichlormethiazide in that the dichloromethyl group has been replaced by a trifluoroethylthiomethyl chain at position 3 on the benzothiadiazine nucleus.

Oral administration produces natriuresis within 2 hours, reaches a peak in 6 hours and lasts for 24 to 48 hours. Studies with animals showed that polythiazide is almost equally potent when administered orally or intravenously, thus indicating virtually complete absorption from the gastrointestinal tract. Diuresis is obtained with a dose as low as 6 mcg/kg of body weight.

For actions, clinical uses, contraindications, warnings, precautions and adverse reactions, see general statement.

Dosage and Administration: *Orally. Diuresis:* The usual initial dose ranges from 1 to 4 mg daily; in some cases, it may be necessary to give up to 8 mg daily. The usual maintenance dose ranges from 0.5 to 4 mg daily. Doses in excess of 12 mg daily are not recommended. *Hypertension:* The usual initial dose ranges from 2 to 4 mg daily. The combination drug may be used when the amounts therein conform to those of the individual components established during titration. Maintenance dosage may then range from 1/2 to 2 tablets daily.

Availability:
RENESE® Tablets, 1, 2 and 4 mg in bottles of 100 and 1000. **(Pfizer)**
RENESE-R Tablets, 2 mg with 0.25 mg of reserpine in bottles of 100 and 1000. **(Pfizer)**

TRICHLORMETHIAZIDE

Chemical Name: 6-Chloro-3-(dichloromethyl)-3,4-dihydro-2H-1,2,4-benzothiadiazine-7-sulfonamide 1,1-dioxide.

Description: Trichlormethiazide is a thiazide diuretic which differs structurally from hydrochlorothiazide in that the hydrogen at position 3 on the latter's molecule has been replaced by a dichloromethyl group.

Following the oral ingestion of a single therapeutic dose, its duration of action may be prolonged for 24 hours or longer. In other essential respects, trichlormethiazide is similar to other thiazide diuretics. The fixed combination of trichlormethiazide and reserpine is not indicated for initial therapy of hypertension. If the fixed combination represents the dosage so determined, its use may be more convenient in patient management.

For action, clinical uses, precautions and adverse reactions, see general statement.

Dosage and Administration: *Orally.* The usual adult *diuretic* dosage is 1 to 4 mg once a day after breakfast, but some patients may require as much as 8 mg daily. The usual maintenance dosage is 2 mg daily. The usual adult *antihypertensive* dosage is 2 to 4 mg daily. Total dosage in excess of 8 mg daily should be divided into equal parts.

Availability:

Trichlormethiazide

METAHYDRIN® Tablets, 2 and 4 mg in bottles of 100 and 1000. **(Merrell-National)**

NAQUA® Tablets, 2 and 4 mg in bottles of 100 and 1000. **(Schering)**

w/Reserpine

METATENSIN® Tablets, 2 and 4 mg with 0.1 mg of reserpine in bottles of 100 and 1000. **(Merrell-National)**

NAQUIVAL® Tablets, 4 mg with 0.1 mg of reserpine in bottles of 100 and 500. **(Schering)**

THIETHYLPERAZINE MALEATE: see The Phenothiazines

THIOGUANINE

Chemical Name: 2-Aminopurine-6-mercaptopurine.

Description: Thioguanine is an antimetabolite which blocks purine metabolism. It is chemically related to mercaptopurine and differs only in the presence of an amino group at the 2 position on the purine nucleus. It occurs as a yellow, crystalline powder insoluble in water.

The mode of action of thioguanine appears to cause depletion of human bone marrow producing neutropenia, reticulopenia, anemia, thrombocytopenia, and prolongation of clotting time. The protracted but reversible aplasia of bone marrow closely resembles the effects of ionizing radiation. Clinical evidence indicates that thioguanine is extensively converted to 2-amino-6-methylmercaptopurine which is much less toxic and less effective than the parent compound, but unlike mercaptopurine and azathioprine, its metabolic process is not inhibited by the xanthine oxidase inhibitor, allopurinol.

Cross-resistance exists between thioguanine and mercaptopurine and generally it is not to be expected that patients who no longer respond to mercaptopurine will respond to thioguanine, or vice versa.

Indications: Treatment of acute leukemia. It has also been used in the treatment of chronic granulocytic (myelocytic, myeloid, myelogenous) leukemia. It may be useful during periods of thrombocytopenia induced by busulfan or other therapy. Thioguanine is not indicated for the treatment of chronic lymphocytic leukemia or solid tumors.

Contraindications: Hepatitis with jaundice.

Warnings: The drug should be used with caution in patients who have preexisting liver dysfunction. Whenever possible, thioguanine should be deferred until after the first trimester of pregnancy.

Precautions: Occasionally, a patient taking thioguanine has developed jaundice. Since it is possible that toxic hepatitis may be related to thioguanine, it is suggested that the drug be withheld if jaundice does appear. Since this compound may have a delayed and prolonged action, it is important to withdraw the drug temporarily at the first sign of an abnormally large fall in the white cell count or of abnormal bone-marrow depression. Although the effect usually occurs slowly over a period of 2 to 4 weeks, occasionally there may be a rapid fall in leukocyte count within 1 or 2 weeks. This may occur in some adults with acute leukemia and high total leukocyte counts as well as in certain adults with chronic granulocytic leukemia. For this reason, it is important to observe such patients closely, and blood counts should be done at least once a week. The drug should be used with caution, and in smaller doses, in patients with impaired renal function and preexisting liver dysfunction. Because there is no known antagonist to thioguanine, prompt withdrawal of the drug is essential to avoid irreversible depression of bone marrow.

Adverse Reactions: Nausea, vomiting, anorexia and stomatitis may occur.

Dosage and Administration: *Orally.* The usual initial dose is 2 mg/kg of body weight/day. If after 4 weeks on this dosage there is no clinical improvement and no leukocyte depression, the dosage may be increased cautiously to 3 mg/kg/day. The total daily dose, usually calculated to the closest multiple of 20 mg, may be given at one time. Maintenance dosage, usually 2 mg/kg/day, is advisable to provide a sustained remission and to avoid early relapse. Treatment may be continued in the usual dosage when allopurinol is used conjointly to inhibit uric acid formation.

Availability:
THIOGUANINE Tabloid® (Tablets), 40 mg in bottles of 25. **(Burroughs Wellcome)**

THIOPENTAL SODIUM Ⓒ III

Chemical Name: Sodium 5-ethyl-5-(1-methylbutyl)-2-thiobarbiturate.

Description: Thiopental sodium, an ultrashort-acting anesthetic, occurs as a yellowish-white hygroscopic powder with a sulfurous odor and is very soluble in water and soluble in alcohol.

Thiopental induces hypnosis and anesthesia, but not analgesia. Hypnosis occurs within 30 to 40 seconds following intravenous administration, and within 8 to 10 minutes following rectal instillation. Recovery after a small dose is rapid, with some somnolence and retrograde amnesia remaining. Repeated intravenous administration causes prolonged anesthesia due to the fact that fatty tissues act as a reservoir in that they accumulate thiopental in concentrations 6 to 12 times greater than does plasma. The drug is then released slowly to cause prolonged anesthesia.

Indications: Thiopental may be used: (1) as the sole anesthetic agent for brief surgical procedures, (2) for the induction of anesthesia prior to the administration of other anesthetic agents, (3) to supplement regional anesthesia or low potency agents such as nitrous oxide, (4) for the control of convulsive states, and (5) for narcoanalysis and narcosynthesis in psychiatric disorders. The rectal suspension is indicated whenever it is desirable to produce preanesthetic sedation or basal narcosis by the rectal route. It is particularly recommended for preanesthetic sedation in children. In selected minor procedures (in which profound muscular relaxation or a high degree of analgesia is not required) it has been used as the sole agent. Such procedures include cystoscopy, cardiac catheterization, lumbar puncture, dressing of burns, and minor surgical procedures.

Contraindications: Complete absence of suitable veins (applies only to intravenous administration), allergy or hypersensitivity to barbiturates, status asthmaticus, and latent or manifest porphyria. Rectal administration also is contraindicated in patients who are to undergo rectal surgery, or in the presence of inflammatory, ulcerative, bleeding or neoplastic lesions of the lower bowel. Thiopental is relatively contraindicated in severe cardiovascular disease; hypotension or shock; conditions in which the hypnotic effect may be prolonged or potentiated such as excessive premedication, Addison's disease, hepatic or renal dysfunction, myxedema, increased blood urea, and severe anemia; increased intracranial pressure; asthma; and myasthenia gravis.

Warnings: May be habit-forming. Repeated or continuous infusion may cause cumulative effects resulting in prolonged somnolence and respiratory and circulatory depression. Safe use during pregnancy with respect to adverse effects upon fetal development has not been established.

Precautions: Since thiopental is a potent respiratory depressant, special care is required in patients with any degree of respiratory embarrassment or obstruction. Since respiratory depression may result from either an unusual responsiveness to thiopental or an overdosage, the drug should not be administered without the ready availability of resuscitative equipment including that necessary for endotracheal intubation. In this regard, thiopental should be considered to have the same potential as an inhalation anesthetic, and patency of the airway must be maintained at all times. The drug may also cause laryngeal spasm and bronchospasm. Utmost care is essential in patients with preexisting hypotension, renal or hepatic disease, advanced cardiac disease, increased intracranial pressure, asthma, myasthenia gravis, and insufficiency of the pituitary, thyroid, adrenal and pancreatic glands. Extravasation or intraarterial injection should be avoided.

Adverse Reactions: Intravenous administration may produce respiratory depression, myocardial depression, cardiac arrhythmias, prolonged somnolence and recovery, sneezing, coughing, bronchospasm, laryngospasm, and shivering. Hypersensitivity reactions have been reported. Rectal administration may cause urticarial skin rash, rectal irritation, diarrhea, cramping, and rectal bleeding. If evacuation of the inserted dose should occur, the effects of any retained portion should be assessed before a repeat dose is administered.

Dosage and Administration: *Intravenously* only. A test dose may be helpful in determining individual tolerance which varies widely. Administer 25 to 75 mg and wait at least 60 seconds to observe the effects on the patient. Observe patient for signs indicating changes in the eyes, pulse rate, blood pressure, muscle tone, and respiration and adjust rate of administration according to the reaction of the patient. For induction of anesthesia, adults, 2 to 3 ml (25 to 75 mg) of a 2.5% solution is injected intermittently every 20 to 40 seconds. Once anesthesia is established, additional injections of 25 to 50 mg can be given whenever required. *For control of convulsive states,* adults, 3 to 5 ml (75 to 125 mg) of a 2.5% solution. *For narcoanalysis and narcosynthesis in psychiatric disorders,* adults, 4 ml/minute (100 mg/minute) of a 2.5% solution. The injection may be preceded by the administration of an anticholinergic agent and a test dose of thiopental sodium. Alternately, the drug may be given by rapid intravenous drip of 50 ml/minute of an 0.2% concentration in a 5% dextrose solution. Children, a 2 or 2.5% solution is injected intermittently at intervals of 30 seconds. Dosage is determined according to the weight of the child. *Rectally.* For preanesthetic sedation, the average dose is 1 gm/34 kg of body weight; for deeper sedation up to 1 gm/22.5 kg may be administered. Consult package literature for details.

Availability:
Ⓒ III PENTOTHAL® Sodium: **(Abbott)**
Powder for Injection in Fliptop vials of 0.5 and 1 gm; in 250 and 500 ml containers of 5 and 10 gm respectively, with diluent, and in partially filled, plastic-squeeze containers of 100 and 200 ml each containing 2.5 and 5 gm respectively.
Rectal Suspension, 400 mg/gm in Abbo-Sert® (disposable syringes) of 2.4 gm with graduated plunger and stop device.

THIORIDAZINE HYDROCHLORIDE: see The Phenothiazines

THIOTEPA

Chemical Name: N,N',N'' Triethylenethiophosphoramide.

Description: Thiotepa is a cytotoxic agent of the polyfunctional alkylating type (more than one reactive ethylenimine group) related chemically and pharmacologically to nitrogen mustard. Its radiomimetic action is believed to occur through the release of ethylenimine radicals which have deleterious effects on actively dividing cells. On the basis of tissue concentration studies, it is reported that thiotepa seems to have no differential affinity for neoplasms. Most of the drug appears to be excreted unchanged in the urine.

Indications: Palliative treatment of a variety of neoplastic diseases such as adenocarcinoma of the breast and ovary, malignant lymphomas, bronchogenic carcinoma, and for controlling intracavitary effusions secondary to diffuse or localized neoplastic disease of various serosal cavities.

Contraindications: Therapy is contraindicated in cases of existing hepatic, renal, or bone-marrow damage. However, if the need outweighs the risk in such patients, the drug may be used in low dosage, and accompanied by hepatic, renal, and hemopoietic function tests. It is also contraindicated in patients with a known hypersensitivity (allergy) to the drug.

Warnings: If used in pregnant patients, it must be considered that this drug is actively teratogenic. Also, it is highly toxic to the hematopoietic system. A rapidly falling white blood cell or platelet count indicates the necessity for discontinuing or reducing the dosage. Weekly blood and platelet counts are recommended during therapy and for at least 3 weeks after the drug has been withdrawn.

Precautions: The serious complication of excessive therapy or sensitivity to the drug's effects is bone-marrow depression manifested by leukopenia, thrombocytopenia, anemia, bleeding, and fever. Unless checked promptly, this may lead to death. It is important that administration of the drug should not follow x-ray therapy, nitrogen mustard administration, or therapy with other radiomimetic drugs, until the full effects of such treatments have been observed. The leukocyte count appears to be the best index of such effects and, accordingly, thiotepa should not be administered until the leukocyte count begins to recover from the bone-marrow depression induced by previous therapy.

In the presence of infection, the drug should be used with caution and antimicrobial therapy considered. Prophylactic antibiotics may be used if the blood count falls below 3000. Coadministration with other bone-marrow depressive drugs should be avoided. It should be kept in mind that some degree of systemic absorption occurs after local administration. There is no known antidote for overdosage with thiotepa.

Adverse Reactions: Local pain, nausea, vomiting, tightness of throat, dizziness, headache, amenorrhea, and anorexia are possible side effects. Symptoms sometimes encountered (such as febrile reaction and weeping from a subcutaneous lesion) may be due to breakdown of tumor tissue. Intestinal perforation through cytolysis within a lesion may occur. Allergic reactions are rare, but hives and skin rash have been noted occasionally. There is some evidence pointing to interference with spermatogenesis and ovarian function. Lesions in a heavily irradiated area may show a slow or lessened response, with accompanying enhanced toxic reaction, due to the radiomimetic effect of thiotepa. Other reported adverse reactions include hyperuricemia with uric acid nephropathy; anaphylactoid reactions; thrombocytopenia resulting in hemorrhage; leukopenia predisposing to infections.

Dosage and Administration: The drug may be given by the following routes: *intravenous, intratumor, intrapleural, intraperitoneal, intrapericardial, intraserosal, intracerebral, transrectal, transvaginal* and into the *surgical site* or by a combination of these after reconstitution, as directed. Adults and children over 12 years of age: initially, 60 mg except in cases of marked debility or asthenia, chronic cardiovascular or renal disease or surgical shock, in which case only 45 mg should be administered. For subsequent therapy, if given at weekly intervals, the dosage should be adjusted to a pretreatment white blood count, and may range from 5 to 60 mg. Children under 12 years of age may be given ½ the adult dosage. For intravenous administration, ½ the initial and maintenance dosage should be employed at 1- to 4-week intervals except in cases of advanced bronchogenic carcinoma in which case patients should be treated every 5th day until improvement has been achieved.

Availability:
THIOTEPA Parenteral (dry powder) in vials of 15 mg. **(Lederle)**

THIOTHIXENE

Chemical Name: N, N-Dimethyl-9-[3-(4-methyl-1-piperazinyl)propylidene]thioxanthene-2-sulfonamide.

Description: Thiothixene is a psychotherapeutic agent related structurally and pharmacologically to chlorprothixene. Structurally, thiothixene differs from chlorprothixene in the replacement of a chlorine atom with a dimethylsulfamyl group at the 2 position on the thioxanthene nucleus and in the replacement of a dimethyl group with a methylpiperazinyl group on the propylidene side chain. It differs from the phenothiazine group by the replacement of nitrogen in the central ring with a carbon-linked side chain fixed in space in a rigid structural conformation. The nucleus is activated by the addition of a dimethylsulfonamide group. The drug's action by which it produces its clinical effects has not been established. Thiothixene occurs as a white, crystalline powder insoluble in water.

Indications: Management of the manifestations of psychotic disorders. It is not recommended for the management of behavioral problems in mentally retarded patients.

Contraindications: Hypersensitivity to thiothixene, circulatory collapse, comatose state, CNS depression due to any cause, blood dyscrasias, and in children under 12 years of age until safe use and proper dosage has been established.

Warnings: Thiothixene should be used in women of childbearing potential only when, in the judgment of the physician, it is necessary for the welfare of the patient. It should be used with extreme caution in patients with a history of convulsive disorders or those in a state of alcohol withdrawal, since the drug is capable of lowering the convulsive threshold. Caution as well as careful adjustment of dosage is indicated when used in conjunction with other CNS depressants other than anticonvulsant drugs. Until their response to the drug has been determined, patients should be advised to refrain from engaging in any activity requiring alertness and physical coordination.

Precautions: The possibility that there may be a cross-sensitivity between thiothixene and the phenothiazines should be considered. As with most antipsychotic agents thiothixene may potentiate the effects of alcohol and other CNS depressants, atropine, and phosphorus and may reverse the effect of epinephrine, when these drugs are given simultaneously with thiothixene. Careful observation should be made for pigmentary retinopathy, and lenticular pigmentation (fine lenticular pigmentation has been noted in a small number of patients treated with thiothixene for prolonged periods), blood dyscrasias (agranulocytosis, pancytopenia, thrombocytopenic purpura), and liver damage (jaundice, biliary stasis), since these have been reported with related drugs. Cardiac arrhythmia or the aggravation of preexisting cardiac abnormality has been noted in some patients. Although it exhibits weak anticholinergic properties, thiothixene should be used judiciously in patients who are known or suspected to have glaucoma, who might be exposed to extreme heat or who are receiving atropine or related drugs. Because of a possible antiemetic effect, the drug may mask signs of overdosage of toxic substances and may obscure various disorders such as intestinal obstruction and brain tumor. Patients should be advised to avoid undue exposure to sunlight, since a photosensitive reaction may occur. As with all intramuscular preparations, the drug should be injected deeply into a large muscle, preferably the upper outer quadrant of the buttock (i.e., gluteus maximus) or the mid-lateral thigh. The deltoid area should be used only if it is well developed, and then only with considerable care to avoid radial nerve injury. Intramuscular injection should *not* be made into the lower or mid-section of the upper arm. Aspiration is necessary to help avoid inadvertent injection into a blood vessel.

Adverse Reactions: Since thiothixene has certain chemical and pharmacological similarities to the potent phenothiazine-psychotherapeutic agents, all of the known adverse effects and toxicity of that class of drugs should be borne in mind. For adverse reactions, see the general statement on the Phenothiazines.

Dosage and Administration: *Orally.* For mild conditions, an initial dosage of 2 mg 3 times daily may be given. If indicated, a subsequent increase to 15 mg daily is often effective. For severe conditions, initially, 5 mg twice daily. The usual optimal dose is 20 to 30 mg daily; may be increased to 60 mg daily but doses in excess of 60 mg/day rarely increase the beneficial response. *Intramuscularly.* The usual dosage is 4 mg 2 to 4 times daily. In general, small doses should be used initially and then gradually increased to the patient's optimal effective level. Most patients are controlled on a total daily dosage of from 16 to 20 mg daily. The maximal recommended dosage is 30 mg/day. The oral form should supplant the injectable form as soon as possible, and an adjustment of dosage may be necessary. **Note:** Not to be administered to children under 12 years of age.

Availability:
NAVANE®: **(Roerig)**
Capsules, 1, 2, 5 and 10 mg in bottles of 100 and 1000; 20 mg in bottles of 100 and 500.
Concentrate, 5 mg/ml (as hydrochloride) in bottles of 30 and 120 ml with calibrated dropper.
Solution, 2 mg/ml in vials of 2 ml.

THROMBIN

Description: Thrombin is a sterile plasma protein substance prepared from prothrombin of bovine origin through interaction with added thromboplastin in the presence of calcium. It is capable, without the addition of other substances, of causing the clotting of whole blood, plasma or a solution of fibrinogen. It may contain a suitable antibacterial agent. Potency is expressed in terms of NIH (National Institute of Health) units. Approximately 2 units are required to clot 1 ml of oxalated human plasma in 15 seconds. Thrombin occurs as a white or grayish, amorphous substance dried from the frozen state.

Indications: To control capillary bleeding or oozing in surgery, dental extraction, epistaxis; also in fibrin fixation of skin grafts and "fibrin suture" of tissue surfaces and wound edges. Also may be used orally to control hemorrhage of the upper gastrointestinal tract.

Contraindications: Parenteral administration; known hypersensitivity to substances of bovine origin.

Warnings: Extreme care should be exercised to prevent the substance from entering or infiltrating large blood vessels, since extensive intravascular clotting and death may result. Since antigenic reactions have occurred in animals, an allergic phenomenon is a potential possibility in patients being treated with this agent.

Precautions: Solutions of thrombin should be used within a few hours after preparation. If several hours are to elapse between time of preparation and time of use, the solution should be refrigerated or preferably frozen and not used after 48 hours. Dilute acid, alkalies, heat and salts of heavy metals are detrimental to thrombin activity. Prior to oral use for gastrointestinal bleeding, stomach acids should be neutralized.

Adverse Reactions: An allergic type reaction following the use of thrombin for treatment of epistaxis has been noted. Febrile reactions have also been observed following the use of this preparation in certain surgical procedures but whether or not they were due to the drug has not been established.

Dosage and Administration: *Topically.* The intended use determines the strength of solution to be used. For hemostasis, a solution of 1000 units/ml should be sprayed on the bleeding surface immediately following removal of excess blood (by sponging). For fibrin fixation of tissue surfaces, the solution is mixed with blood plasma to form a fibrin "glue." More concentrated solutions may be required if cut surfaces are anticipated in more vascular tissues such as the liver or spleen. *Orally.* After the patient has taken about 60 ml of milk or cream, and after a lapse of about 5 minutes, the patient then takes 10,000 to 20,000 units in another 60 ml of milk or cream. This is repeated 3 times a day for 4 or 5 days or until bleeding has been controlled.

Availability:
THROMBIN Topical (bovine origin) in vials of 1000 and 10,000 units and in a package containing a vial of 5000 units of thrombin and a 5-ml vial of diluent. **(Parke-Davis)**

THYROGLOBULIN

Description: Thyroglobulin is obtained from the purified extract of fresh frozen hog thyroid gland. It is a polypeptide with a high molecular weight. Levothyroxine and sodium liothyronine are present in thyroglobulin in a ratio of approximately 2.5 to 1, respectively, combined in peptide linkages. Potency of thyroglobulin is standardized to meet U.S.P. requirements for iodine content and by animal bioassay. Thyroglobulin occurs as a tan powder insoluble in water and in alcohol.

The actions of the thyroid hormone(s) involve the maturation and proper function of such organ systems as the endocrine, nervous, skeletal, reproductive, and gastrointestinal. The calorigenic and other actions of thyroid hormone(s) are instrumental in maintaining the normal functional capacity of tissues in organ systems throughout the body.

Indications: Replacement therapy for all forms of hypothyroidism including that resulting from surgical ablation and radiation. It may also be used for thyroid-suppression therapy in selected cases of nontoxic goiter and as adjunctive treatment of secondary (pituitary) myxedema.

Contraindications: Uncorrected adrenal insufficiency.

Warnings: Extreme care should be exercised in patients with hypertension or cardiovascular disorders. When severe myxedema, heart disease or treated adrenal insufficiency exists, the initial dose should be small and then gradually increased in small increments. Thyroglobulin should not be used in the presence of cardiovascular disease unless thyroid replacement therapy is clearly indicated. Morphologic hypogonadism and nephroses should be ruled out before the drug is administered. In patients in whom hypothyroidism and adrenal insufficiency exist concomitantly, the adrenal insufficiency must be treated before attempting thyroid replacement therapy. Patients with myxedema may be especially sensitive to thyroid.

Precautions: If chest pains or signs of aggravation of cardiovascular disease such as tachycardia develop, the dosage should be reduced. As with all thyroid preparations, this preparation will alter results of thyroid function tests.

Adverse Reactions: Overdosage or too rapid increase in dosage may result in signs and symptoms of hyperthyroidism, such as menstrual irregularities, nervousness, cardiac arrhythmias, and angina pectoris. Headache, instability, nervousness, sweating, tachycardia, unusual bowel motility, angina pectoria or congestive heart failure (induced or aggravated) and shock are manifestations of overdosage. Massive overdosage may result in symptoms resembling thyroid storm. Chronic excessive dosage will produce signs and symptoms of hyperthyroidism. Supportive measures should be utilized in the event of shock, and treatment of unrecognized adrenal insufficiency should be considered.

Dosage and Administration: *Orally.* Dosage should be started in small amounts, and increased gradually with increments at intervals of 1 to 2 weeks. The usual maintenance dose is 32 to 200 mg daily.

Availability:
PROLOID® Tablets, 16 mg (1/4 gr), 32 mg (1/2 gr), 65 mg (1 gr, scored), 100 mg (1 1/2 gr), 200 mg (3 gr) and 325 mg (5 gr, scored) in bottles of 100 and 1000; 130 mg (2 gr, scored) in bottles of 100. **(Warner-Chilcott)**

THYROID

Description: Thyroid is prepared by a special process from the fresh desiccated thyroid glands of domesticated animals. Thus the active thyroid hormones *l*-thyroxine (T_4) and *l*-triiodothyronine (T_3) are available in their natural state and ratio for full therapeutic availability. It is standardized to contain no less than 0.17% and no more than 0.23% iodine.

The principal effect of thyroid hormones is to accelerate cellular metabolic rate processes, thus increasing the metabolic rate of body tissues. The effect develops slowly but is prolonged. Following oral administration, the increase in metabolic rate usually begins within 48 hours and reaches a maximum in approximately 8 to 10 days although the full effects of continued administration may not be evident for several weeks.

Thyroid hormones are also concerned with the growth and differentiation of tissues. In deficiency states in the young there is retardation of growth and failure of maturation of the skeletal and other body systems, especially in failure of ossification in the epiphyses and in the growth and development of the brain. Thyroid increases the basal metabolic rate, and also increases the protein-bound iodine in the blood; however, the blood cholesterol level is lowered. Euthyroid individuals often tolerate large doses of thyroid without an increase in metabolism.

Indications: Replacement therapy in hypothyroidism (cretinism, myxedema), and after surgery following complete thyroidectomy, and as an adjunct to the use of thyroid-inhibiting agents when decreased release of thyrotropic hormones is desired.

Contraindications: In thyrotoxicosis, angina pectoris, myocardial infarction, hypertension unless complicated by hypothyroidism, and uncorrected adrenal insufficiency.

Warnings: Thyroid should be used with the greatest caution in patients who have cardiovascular disease, including hypertension. The development of chest pains or other aggravation of cardiovascular disease, such as tachycardia, requires a reduction of dosage. Morphologic hypogonadism and nephroses should be ruled out before the drug is administered. Injection of epinephrine in patients with coronary artery disease may precipitate an episode of coronary insufficiency; this may be enhanced in patients receiving thyroid preparations. Patients with coronary artery disease should be carefully observed during surgery since the possibility of precipitating cardiac arrhythmias may be greater in those treated with this hormone. Thyroid replacement may potentiate the anticoagulant effects of such agents as warfarin or bishydroxycoumarin; therefore, the anticoagulant dosage should be reduced by 1/3 upon initiating thyroid therapy. Subsequent anticoagulant-dosage adjustment should be made on the basis of frequent prothrombin determinations. When adrenal insufficiency and hypothyroidism coexist, the adrenal insufficiency should be corrected before administering thyroid hormones.

Precautions: Patients with myxedema are particularly sensitive to thyroid preparations so that treatment should begin with small doses and increments should be gradual. In patients with diabetes mellitus, the addition of thyroid may cause an increase in the required dosage of insulin or oral hypoglycemic agents. Conversely, decreasing the dose of thyroid may cause a hypoglycemic reaction if the dosage of insulin or oral hypoglycemic agents is not adjusted. As with all thyroid preparations, this drug will alter the results of thyroid function tests.

Adverse Reactions: Palpitation, tachycardia, cardiac arrhythmias, weight loss, elevated blood pressure, angina pectoris, tremors, headache, diarrhea, nervousness, insomnia, fever, sweating, intolerance to heat, and changes in appetite are usually indicative of overdosage. In such instances temporary discontinuance of medication is advisable; therapy may be reinstituted at a lower dosage level after symptoms subside.

Dosage and Administration: *Orally.* The dosage should be titrated to the individual's needs. The response of the patient is determined by clinical judgment in conjunction with laboratory findings. Generally, thyroid therapy is instituted at low dosage levels and increased in small increments at intervals until the desired effect is obtained. It is usually given as a single dose, preferably before breakfast. *Adult myxedema,* the usual dosage regimen is 15 mg/day for 2 weeks, increased to 30 mg/day for 2 or more weeks, and then 60 mg/day. It is advised that the patient be carefully assessed after 1 month of treatment with the 60 mg dose and again after an additional month's treatment. If necessary, the dose may then be increased to 120 mg/day for 2 months and the examination repeated. If the values of the laboratory test used are low or if the clinical reponse is inadequate, the dose may be increased to 180 mg/day. Further increases, when necessary, may be made in increments of 30 or 60 mg/day. The usual maintenance dose is from 60 to 180 mg/day, but it may vary in individual patients. *Adult hypothyroidism without myxedema,* the usual initial dosage regimen is 60 mg/day, increasing by 60 mg every 30 days until the maintenance dose is determined. *Cretinism or severe hypothyroidism in children,* the dosage regimen is the same as for adults with myxedema; however, each dosage increment should be made at intervals of 2 weeks. The final maintenance dose may be greater in the growing child than in the adult. The sleeping pulse and the basal morning temperature are useful guides to treatment.

Availability:
THYRAR® Tablets (bovine origin), 32, 60 and 130 mg in bottles of 100. **(Armour)**
THYROCRINE® Tablets, 130, 150, 195 and 325 mg in bottles of 1000. **(Lemmon)**
THYROID:
Enseals, 30, 120 and 200 mg in bottles of 100; 60 mg in bottles of 100 and 1000. **(Lilly)**
Tablets, 15, 30 and 120 mg in bottles of 100 and 1000; 60 mg in bottles of 100, 1000 and 5000. **(Lilly)**
Tablets, 15 and 180 mg in bottles of 100 and 1000; 240 and 300 mg in bottles of 100; 30, 60 and 120 mg in bottles of 100 and in Armadose® (unit-dose) packages of 100; 30, 60, 100 and 200 mg in handy packages of 100. **(Armour)**
Tablets, 30, 60 and 120 mg in bottles of 100 and 1000. **(ICN)**
Tablets, 30, 60, 120 and 200 mg in bottles of 1000. **(Lederle)**
Tablets, 16, 32, 65 and 130 mg in bottles of 1000. **(McKesson)**
Tablets, 15, 30, 60 and 125 mg in bottles of 100 and 1000. The 60 mg tablets are also available in unit-dose packages of 100. **(Marion)**

Tablets (Strong), 32, 65, and 130 mg in bottles of 100 and 1000; 200 mg in bottles of 100. **(Marion)**
Tablets, 60 mg in bottles of 1000 and in unit-dose blister packs of 100. **(Philips Roxane)**
Tablets, 65 mg in bottles of 1000. **(Upjohn)**

THYROTROPIN

Description: Thyrotropin is a thyroid stimulating hormone prepared in a highly purified form from bovine anterior pituitary glands. The potency of thyrotropin is designated in terms of international thyrotropin units, and is free from significant amounts of adrenocorticotropic, gonadotropic, somatotropic and posterior pituitary hormones. It is soluble throughout a wide pH range and is stable at room temperatures when kept in the dry state. It dissolves readily in physiologic saline solution but will retain its potency for 2 weeks only if refrigerated.

Thyrotropin appears to act by increasing the iodine uptake in the thyroid gland, the formation of thyroid hormone, secretion or release of thyroid hormone and by causing a hyperplasia of thyroid cells.

Indications: To determine subclinical (borderline to obscure) hypothyroidism or low thyroid reserve; to differentiate between primary and secondary hypothyroidism; to evaluate the need for thyroid medication in patients who are receiving thyroid therapy, and to aid in detection of remnants and metastases of thyroid carcinoma. It is also used for the management of certain types of thyroid carcinoma and consequent metastases, and is used in conjunction with I^{131} to enhance the uptake of the radioactive substance by the thyroid.

Contraindications: Coronary thrombosis, adrenal insufficiency, hypersensitivity to thyrotropin.

Precautions: Should be used with caution in the presence of angina pectoris, cardiac failure and hypopituitarism.

Adverse Reactions: An occasional mild reaction at the injection site has been reported. Nausea, vomiting, urticaria, transitory hypotension, tachycardia, atrial fibrillation, irregular menses, fever, headache, and swelling of the thyroid gland have been reported. Administration of an antihistamine ½ hour before injection of thyrotropin will tend to prevent any serious reaction. A few instances of anaphylactoid reactions have also been reported. Angina pectoris or congestive heart failure may be induced or aggravated with large doses. Shock may also develop. Chronic excessive dosage will usually produce signs and symptoms of hyperthyroidism.

Dosage and Administration: *Intramuscularly* or *subcutaneously. For diagnosis,* 10 units for 1 to 3 days. *For treatment,* 10 units daily for 3 to 8 days prior to a therapeutic dose of radioactive iodine.

Availability:
THYTROPAR® Lyophilized in vials of 10 units with a vial of sodium chloride diluent. **(Armour)**

TICARCILLIN: see The Penicillins

TIMOLOL MALEATE

Chemical Name: S-(-)-1-(tert-Butylamino)-3-[(4-morpholino-1,2,5-thiadiazol-3-yl)oxy]-2-propanol maleate.

Description: Timolol is a beta-adrenergic blocking agent with clinical value in the treatment of glaucoma. When applied topically in the eye, it reduces elevated as well as normal intraocular pressure, whether or not glaucoma is present. Its action compares favorably with that of epinephrine and pilocarpine, but timolol appears to be better tolerated, causing fewer and less severe side effects. Moreover, the drug has no effect on pupil size or visual acuity, nor does it have any significant intrinsic sympathomimetic, direct myocardial depressant, or local anesthetic activity.

The precise mechanism of the ocular hypotensive action is not clearly understood, but clinical tonographic and fluorophotometric studies suggest that it may be related to reduced aqueous formation and to a slight increase in aqueous outflow. In controlled clinical studies in patients with untreated intraocular pressures of 22 mmHg or greater, timolol solution, 0.25 or 0.5% administered twice a day produced a greater reduction in intraocular pressure than did a pilocarpine solution, 1, 2, 3 or 4% administered 4 times a day or an epinephrine solution, 0.5, 1 or 2% administered twice a day. Following a single application, onset of therapeutic action occurs within 1/2 hour, reaches a peak in 1 to 2 hours, and continues for up to 24 hours. No evidence of diminished responsiveness has been reported, and repeated observations over a period of 1 year indicate that the intraocular pressure lowering effect is well maintained.

Since timolol is compatible with other antiglaucoma agents, it can be used successfully with such compounds as pilocarpine, epinephrine, and acetazolamide, thus intensifying the ocular hypotensive action, which may then benefit some patients who responded inadequately to previous polyantiglaucoma drug therapy.

Long-term studies did not reveal any adverse ocular effects in rabbits and dogs given topical application of the drug. However, rats and mice receiving oral administration of the drug showed some evidence of mammary fibroadenomas in rats and hepatomas in mice.

Indications: For reduction of elevated intraocular pressure. It is not currently indicated for use in narrow-angle glaucoma or angle-closure glaucoma until sufficient clinical data have been obtained to assure safe and effective use in these conditions.

Contraindications: Hypersensitivity to timolol.

Precautions: Should be used with special care in patients with known contraindications to the systemic use of beta-adrenergic receptor blocking agents. These include bronchial asthma, sinus bradycardia and greater than first degree heart block, cardiogenic shock, right ventricular failure secondary to pulmonary hypertension, congestive heart failure, in addition to concomitant use with adrenergic-augmenting psychotropic drugs. It is recommended that the pulse rate be checked regularly in patients with a history of severe cardiac disease. It is well to bear in mind that concomitant use with orally administered beta-adrenergic blocking agents may have an additive effect either on intraocular pressure or on the known systemic effects of beta blockade activity, and that tolerance to drug therapy may develop with the simultaneous use of other antiglaucoma agents. Its use in pregnant patients requires that the anticipated benefits be weighed against the potential hazards. Until clinical response and proper dosage have been determined, it is not recommended for use in children.

Adverse Reactions: Occasionally observed were signs and symptoms of mild ocular irritation as well as a slight reduction of the resting heart rate (mean reduction of 2.9 beats/minute with a standard deviation of 10.2); rarely observed were hypersensitivity reactions.

Dosage and Administration: *Topically.* The usual initial dose is 1 drop of the 0.25% solution in each eye twice daily. If reduction in intraocular pressure is not adequate, the dosage may be changed to 1 drop of the 0.5% solution in each eye twice daily. If the pressure is maintained at satisfactory levels, the dosage schedule may then be changed to 1 drop in each eye once daily. Because of diurnal variations in intraocular pressure, satisfactory response to the once daily regimen is best determined by measuring the pressure at various times throughout the day. Dosages above 1 drop of 0.5% solution twice daily generally have not been shown to produce further reduction in intraocular pressure. It the patient's response is still not satisfactory, concomitant therapy with pilocarpine and other miotics, and/or epinephrine or systemically administered carbonic anhydrase inhibitors, such as acetazolamide, can be instituted. To transfer patients from current therapy to timolol, on the initial day continue with the medication already being used and add 1 drop of 0.25% timolol solution in each eye twice daily; then on the second day, discontinue the previously administered medication altogether and continue the timolol regimen. If a higher dosage of timolol is required, substitute 1 drop of 0.5% solution in each eye twice daily.

Availability:

TIMOPTIC™ Ophthalmic Solution, 0.25 and 0.5% in Ocumeter® (plastic dispensers with controlled tip) of 5 ml. **(Merck Sharp & Dohme)**

TINVER

Description: The formulation provides sodium thiosulfate, 25%; salicylic acid, 1% and isopropyl alcohol N.F., 10% in an aqueous vehicle containing propylene glycol U.S.P., disodium edetate, colloidal alumina and purified water.

Indications: Treatment of tinea versicolor (Malassezia furfur) infection.

Precautions: Discontinue use upon the appearance of any symptoms suggesting sensitivity or irritation. Avoid contact with the eyes.

Dosage and Administration: *Topically.* The affected areas should be thoroughly washed, rinsed and dried before applying the medication. A thin film of lotion should then be applied to cover the affected areas and other susceptible areas twice daily. Although diagnostic evidence of the disease may disappear in a few days, it is advisable to continue treatment for a much longer period. Clothing should be boiled to prevent reinfection.

Availability:
TINVER® Lotion in plastic bottles of 180 ml. **(Barnes-Hind)**

TOBRAMYCIN SULFATE

Description: Tobramycin is a water soluble, aminoglycoside antibiotic derived from *Streptomyces tenebrarius.* Solutions of the drug are clear, colorless and stable and require no refrigeration.

In vitro tests demonstrate that the drug is bactericidal and that it acts by interfering with protein synthesis in bacterial cells. It exhibits a broad range of activity against gram-positive and gram-negative organisms. Sensitive bacteria include *Pseudomonas aeruginosa,* Proteus species (indole-positive and indole-negative), including *Pr. mirabilis, Pr. morganii, Pr. rettgeri.* and *Pr. vulgaris, Escherichia coli,* Klebsiella-Enterobacter-Serratia group, Citrobacter and Providencia species, Staphylococci including *Staphylococcus aureus* (coagulase-positive and coagulase-negative), and some strains of group D streptococci. The combination of penicillin G and tobramycin results in a synergistic bactericidal effect against certain strains of *Streptococcus faecalis,* but not against closely related organisms such as *Str. faecium.*

Following an intramuscular injection of 1 mg/kg of body weight, the drug yields a peak serum level of about 4 mcg/ml within 30 to 90 minutes, and measurable levels for as long as 8 hours; also, the urine concentration reaches peak values of 75 to 100 mcg/ml. After several days of treatment, the amount of the antibiotic excreted in the urine approaches the daily dose administered. Similar serum concentrations of the drug may also be obtained by intravenous infusion of 1-hour duration.

Ultrafiltration studies demonstrate that practically no serum protein binding occurs. Repeated injections (every 8 hours) do not lead to accumulation of the antibiotic in the blood in patients with normal renal function except neonates. However, in those with reduced renal function and in neonates accumulation tends to be higher and can be measured for longer periods of time. Tobramycin is eliminated almost exclusively by glomerular filtration. Renal clearance is similar to that of endogenous creatinine. In patients with normal renal function, up to 84% of the dose is recoverable from the urine in 8 hours and up to 93% in 24 hours. The serum half-life in normal individuals is 2 hours.

Tobramycin diffuses into tissues and body fluids, and appears in low concentration in the cerebrospinal fluid following parenteral administration. It also has been found in the sputum, peritoneal fluid, and abcess fluids and it crosses the placental membranes. Concentrations in bile and feces ordinarily have been low, which suggests minimal biliary excretion.

If the Bauer-Kirby-Sherria-Truck method of disc susceptibility testing is used, a disc containing 10 mcg of tobramycin should give a zone of at least 14 mm when tested against susceptible organisms and a zone of 13 mm or less against resistant organisms.

Indications: The use of this antibiotic should be restricted to the treatment of serious infections caused by susceptible bacteria. Septicemia; CNS infections, including meningitis; neonatal sepsis; lower respiratory tract infections; gastrointestinal infections, including peritonitis; and skin, bone, and soft-tissue infections, including burns usually respond to treatment with tobramycin. It has also been found effective in the treatment of serious, complicated, recurrent urinary tract infections due to susceptible organisms; nevertheless, it is not indicated in uncomplicated initial episodes of urinary tract infections unless the causative organisms do not respond to treatment with other less toxic antimicrobial agents. It may also be considered for use in serious staphylococcal infections in cases in which penicillin or other less toxic drugs are contraindicated and when bacterial susceptibility testing and clinical judgment indicate its use.

Contraindications: A history of hypersensitivity to tobramycin.

Warnings: Patients should be under close clinical observation because nephrotoxicity and ototoxicity (vestibular and auditory) can occur, primarily in those with preexisting renal damage. Serum concentrations should be monitored when feasible and prolonged concentrations above 12 mcg/ml are not advised. Patients initially showing normal renal function may develop signs of malfunction characterized by clindruria, oliguria, proteinuria, or evidence of nitrogen retention manifested by increasing levels of BUN, NPN, or creatinine. Evidence of impairment in renal, vestibular or auditory function requires adjustment of dosage or withdrawal of the drug. In the event of overdose or toxic reactions, peritoneal dialysis or hemodialysis will aid in the removal of the drug from the blood. Concurrent and sequential use of other neurotoxic and/or nephrotoxic antibiotics, particularly streptomycin, neomycin, kanamycin, gentamicin, cephaloridine, paromomycin, viomycin, polymyxin B, and polymyxin E (colistin), should be avoided. It should not be given concurrently with potent diuretics since certain diuretics by themselves may cause ototoxicity. In addition, diuretics when given intravenously may effect a rise in the serum and tissue levels of tobramycin and thus potentiate neurotoxicity. Premature and neonatal infants require special care due to their renal immaturity and the resulting prolongation of the serum half-life of the drug. Safe use during pregnancy has not been established.

Precautions: Neuromuscular blockade and respiratory paralysis have been reported in cats receiving very high doses of tobramycin (40 mg/kg). The possibility that prolonged or secondary apnea may occur should be considered if the drug is administered to anesthetized patients who are also receiving neuromuscular blocking agents, such as succinylcholine or tubocurarine. Cross-allergenicity among the aminoglycoside antibiotics has been demonstrated. As with other antibiotics, use of this drug may result in overgrowth of nonsusceptible organisms. If superinfection occurs, appropriate therapy should be instituted.

Adverse Reactions: Those commonly noted are nephrotoxic reactions which are manifested by increased levels of BUN, NPN, and serum creatinine, and by oliguria, cylindruria, and increased proteinuria, and ototoxic reactions, which involve both the vestibular and auditory branches of the eight nerve, and usually produce such symptoms as dizziness, vertigo, tinnitus, roaring in the ears, and hearing loss. These usually develop in patients with poor kidney function, or those who receive higher than the recommended dosage regimen. Other reported reactions possibly related to tobramycin include increased serum transaminase (SGOT, SGPT) and increased serum bilirubin; anemia, granulocytopenia, and thrombocytopenia; fever, rash, itching, urticaria, nausea, vomiting, headache, and lethargy.

Dosage and Administration: *Intramuscularly or intravenously.* The patient's pretreatment body weight should be obtained for calculation of correct dosage. The recommended dosage for adults, children, and older infants with normal renal function is 3 mg/kg/day administered in 3 equal doses every 8 hours; if the infection is life-threatening up to 5 mg/kg/day may be given. To prevent increased toxicity due to excessive blood levels, dosage should not exceed 5 mg/kg/day unless serum levels are monitored. For neonates 1 week of age or less, dosages up to 4 mg/kg/day may be given in 2 equal doses every 12 hours. The usual duration of treatment is 7 to 10 days; however, if treatment is to extend beyond 10 days, it is advised that renal, auditory, and vestibular functions be checked. In patients with renal impairment, an initial dose of 1 mg/kg of body weight is administered and subsequent dosages are then adjusted either with reduced dosage given at 8-hour intervals or with normal doses given at extended intervals. For intravenous administration, the usual volume for adult doses is 50 to 100 ml and for children proportionately less. The solution should be infused for a period of 20 to 60 minutes. Tobramycin should not be physically premixed with other drugs but should be administered separately according to the recommended dose and route.

Availability:
NEBCIN® injection in ampuls of 20 and 80 mg and in Hyporets® (disposable syringes) of 60 and 80 mg. **(Lilly)**

TOLAZAMIDE

Chemical Name: 1-(Hexahydro-1H-azepin-1-yl)-3-(p-tolylsulfonyl)urea.

Description: Tolazamide is an orally active hypoglycemic agent useful in the management of selected cases of diabetes mellitus. It is a sulfonylurea compound related structurally and pharmacologically to tolbutamide, chlorpropamide, and acetohexamide. It occurs as a white or creamy-white powder slightly soluble in water and in alcohol. Its molecular weight is 311.40.

The primary mechanism by which tolazamide lowers blood sugar levels appears to be by stimulating the beta cells of the pancreatic islets to secrete endogenous insulin; it is not effective in the absence of functioning beta cells.

Tolazamide is well absorbed with peak blood levels occurring in 4 to 8 hours. Approximately 85% of the drug is excreted in the urine. Its biological half-life was found to be 7 hours.

Indications: Primarily for the stable or maturity-onset type of mild or moderately severe diabetes mellitus. Approximately 35% of diabetic patients assumed to be primary or secondary failures with other sulfonylurea agents reportedly have responded satisfactorily to this agent. Some patients who have developed significant adverse effects or intolerance to other similar drugs may subsequently be successfully maintained on tolazamide.

Contraindications: Diabetic patients with infection, severe trauma or who are about to receive surgical intervention, those with ketosis, acidosis or coma or those with a history of ketoacidosis or coma. It should not be used to treat diabetes of the juvenile or labile (brittle) type. Neither should it be used in diabetic patients who are pregnant, or those with hepatic, renal or endocrine disease, nor in the presence of uremia. Serious consideration should be given to the possible hazards if used in women of childbearing potential.

Precautions: Patients must be fully informed as to the nature of their disease, what they must do to prevent and detect complications, and how to control the condition. When indicated, thiazide diuretics should be used cautiously because they have been known to aggravate the diabetic state. Patients must be under continuous medical supervision, particularly during the first 6 weeks of therapy. Close observation and careful adjustment of dosages is essential in debilitated and malnourished patients. Severe hypoglycemia, though uncommon, may occur and may mimic acute neurological disorders such as cerebral thrombosis. Patients with hepatic or renal disease, those who are malnourished, or who are debilitated, geriatric patients, alcoholics and patients with adrenal and pituitary insufficiency are particularly susceptible to hypoglycemia and should be treated cautiously. Also, drugs such as insulin, sulfonamides, oxyphenbutazone, phenylbutazone, salicylates, probenecid, and MAO inhibitors may prolong and enhance the action of tolazamide and thereby increase the risk of hypoglycemia developing.

Adverse Reactions: The incidence of adverse effects has been extremely low. Those reported include dosage-related hypoglycemia, nausea, vomiting, flatulence, skin rash, pruritus, urticaria, morbilliform or maculopapular eruptions, weakness, fatigue, dizziness, and rarely, vertigo, malaise, headache, photosensitivity, altered liver function tests, (bilirubin, cholesterol, SGOT, SGPT, etc.), cholestatic jaundice, aplastic anemia, hemolytic anemia, thrombocytopenia, agranulocytosis, pancytopenia, and leukopenia. Disulfiram-like reactions following ingestion of alcohol are possible and should be kept in mind.

Dosage and Administration: *Orally.* In the newly diagnosed diabetic patient: no initial loading or priming dose is necessary. The following is a suggested initial dosage schedule for the mild to moderately severe, adult-onset type: (1) if the fasting blood sugar value is less than 200 mg%, start with 100 mg daily as a single dose with breakfast, (2) if the fasting blood sugar value is greater than 200 mg%, start with 250 mg/day as a single dose. Dosage then is either increased or decreased accordingly at weekly intervals by amounts of 100 or 250 mg daily. If more than 500 mg daily is required, the dosage should be divided and given twice daily. It is doubtful that doses in excess of 1 gm daily will improve control of the disease. In underweight, undernourished or geriatric patients, dosage increments should be on the order of 50 or 125 mg daily at weekly intervals to help avoid hypoglycemic reactions. Consult package literature for other dosage considerations.

Availability:
TOLINASE® Tablets, 100 mg in bottles of 100; 250 mg in bottles of 100, 200 and 1000 and in unit-dose (blister strip) packages of 100; 500 mg in bottles of 50; 250 and 500 mg in unit-dose bottles of 30. **(Upjohn)**

TOLAZOLINE HYDROCHLORIDE

Chemical Name: 2-Benzyl-2-imidazoline hydrochloride.

Description: Tolazoline is an alpha-adrenergic blocking agent related structurally to both histamine and epinephrine. The drug acts both centrally and locally to dilate peripheral blood vessels and to increase the flow of blood. It also blocks impulses at sympathetic nerve terminals, and interferes with the vasoconstrictor action of epinephrine and levarterenol. It occurs as a white or creamy white, crystalline powder whose solution is slightly acid to litmus; it is freely soluble in water and in alcohol, but insoluble in ethyl acetate. The drug is well absorbed following oral and parenteral administration and is largely excreted unchanged by the renal tubules.

Indications: May be of use in spastic peripheral vascular disorders which may be associated with acrocyanosis, acroparesthesia, arteriosclerosis obliterans, Buerger's disease, causalgia, diabetic arteriosclerosis, gangrene, endarteritis, frostbite (sequelae), postthrombotic conditions (thrombophlebitis), Raynaud's disease, and scleroderma.

Contraindications: Following a cerebrovascular accident and in patients with known or suspected coronary artery disease; hypersensitivity to tolazoline.

Warnings: Because tolazoline stimulates gastric activity and increases the flow of hydrochloric acid, the drug should be used cautiously in patients with gastritis or peptic ulcer or in those with suspected peptic ulcer. Patients with known or suspected mitral stenosis should receive special attention, since the drug may either increase or decrease pulmonary arterial pressure and total pulmonary resistance, particularly following parenteral administration.

Adverse Reactions: *Oral or parenteral:* Although side reactions are generally mild and may decrease progressively during continued therapy, cardiac arrhythmias, anginal pain, and marked hypertension have been reported. Exacerbation of peptic ulcer has also occurred. Other complications include nausea, vomiting, diarrhea, epigastric discomfort, tachycardia, flushing, slight rise or fall in blood pressure, and increased pilomotor activity with tingling or chilliness. Intraarterial administration, in addition, may also produce a feeling of warmth or a "burning" sensation in the injected extremity, transient weakness, postural vertigo, palpitations, formication, and apprehension. Rarely, a paradoxical response (further decrease in an already impaired blood supply) may occur in a seriously damaged limb with incipient or established gangrene. This usually disappears with continued treatment and may usually be prevented by prior administration of histamine. Overdosage is usually manifested by increased pilomotor activity, peripheral vasodilatation, skin flushing, and in rare instances, severe hypotension which may progress to shock levels.

Dosage and Administration: *Orally.* Dosage should be individualized carefully. Usually, 25 mg 4 to 6 times daily is sufficient; if necessary, dosage may be increased gradually up to 50 mg 6 times daily. Or 80 mg in the form of a long-acting tablet may be given every 12 hours to achieve the same results. *Subcutaneously, intramuscularly or intravenously,* 10 to 50 mg 4 times daily. Keeping the patient warm will frequently enhance the effects of the drug. *Intra-arterial* administration should be reserved for selected patients. Since a special technique and aseptic precautions are required, this route of administration should be used only by those experienced in the procedure and, preferably, in a hospital or clinic. Initially, a test dose of 25 mg is injected slowly to determine patient's reponse. Subsequently, the average single dose may be 50 to 75 mg/injection. To achieve an initial maximal response, 1 or 2 injections daily are usually required. For maintenance, 2 or 3 injections weekly may be sufficient to sustain improved circulation, but more may be needed. Oral tolazoline may also be given to help maintain vasodilatation between intraarterial injections.

Availability:
PRISCOLINE®: **(Ciba)**
Lontabs® (long-acting tablets), 80 mg in bottles of 100.
Parenteral, 25 mg/ml in multiple-dose vials of 10 ml.
Tablets, 25 mg in bottles of 100 and 1000.

TOLBUTAMIDE

Chemical Name: 1-Butyl-3-(*p*-tolylsulfonyl)urea.

Description: Tolbutamide is an orally effective hypoglycemic agent useful in the management of selected cases of diabetes mellitus. It is a sulfonylurea compound related structurally and pharmacologically to chlorpropamide, acetohexamide and tolazamide. It is related chemically to the antibacterial sulfonamides, but possesses no antibacterial activity itself. It differs structurally in that it has a methyl group instead of an amino group in the para position of the benzine ring. It occurs as a slightly bitter, odorless, white or practically white, crystalline powder insoluble in water and soluble in alcohol. Molecular weight is 270.34.

The primary mechanism by which tolbutamide lowers blood sugar levels appears to be by stimulating the synthesis and release of insulin from the beta cells of the pancreatic islets; it is ineffective in the absence of functioning beta cells. The blood sugar lowering effect is independent of the pituitary, adrenocortical, and neural mechanisms that exert a regulatory effect on carbohydrate metabolism. Additionally, it neither inhibits the hyperglycemic response induced by epinephrine or glucagon nor exerts an effect on the renal threshold for glucose excretion. Following oral administration of a 3-gm dose, maximal response occurs within 5 to 8 hours, following which the blood sugar rises gradually until at 24 hours it reaches pretreatment levels. The *p*-methyl group is oxidized to form a carboxyl group, converting tolbutamide into a totally inactive metabolite, which can be recovered in the urine within 24 hours in amounts accountable for up to 75% of the administered dose.

Indications: The principal clinical indication is diabetes mellitus of the stable type without acute complications such as acidosis or ketosis. This form of diabetes has been variously described as relatively mild adult, maturity-onset, or nonketotic type. In certain patients with labile diabetes, its use as a supplement to insulin therapy may effect stabilization of the diabetic condition and reduce insulin requirement.

Contraindications: Tolbutamide alone is not effective in juvenile or growth-onset diabetes nor in diabetes of the unstable, brittle type. Treatment of such cases, therefore, requires insulin, although tolbutamide may be used adjunctively when indicated. Tolbutamide should not be used in diabetes complicated by acidosis, ketosis or coma; and in patients with severe renal insufficiency. In the presence of acute complications such as fever, severe trauma or infections, diabetics may require appropriate doses of insulin to ensure continued control.

Precautions: Tolbutamide presently is not recommended for use in pregnant diabetics. Patients must be fully informed as to the nature of their disease, what they must do to prevent and detect complications, and how to control the condition. When indicated, thiazide diuretics should be used cautiously because they have been known to aggravate the diabetic state. Concomitant use of insulin, sulfonamides, oxyphenbutazone, salicylates, probenecid, monoamine oxidase inhibitors, phenylbutazone, bishydroxycoumarin, and phenyramidol may prolong or enhance the action of tolbutamide and thereby increase the risk of hypoglycemia, and *beta* blocking agents may decrease the patient's response to the drug. Severe hypoglycemia, though uncommon, may occur and may mimic acute neurological disorders such as cerebral thrombosis. Patients with hepatic and/or renal disease, those who are malnourished, or who are debilitated, geriatric patients, alcoholics and patients with adrenal and pituitary insufficiency are particularly prone to hypoglycemia and should be treated cautiously. Photosensitivity reactions and disulfiram-like reactions following ingestion of alcohol have been reported in patients taking this drug. Care must be exercised in the presence of severe trauma, infections or surgical procedures. In these circumstances, it may be necessary, temporarily, to use insulin, or to use insulin in addition to tolbutamide.

Adverse Reactions: Paradoxically severe hypoglycemia, reduction of radioactive iodine uptake after long-term use, gastrointestinal disturbances, headache, allergic skin manifestations, liver dysfunction, jaundice, leukopenia, agranulocytosis, thrombocytopenia, hemolytic anemia, aplastic anemia, pancytopenia, hepatic porphyria, and porphyria cutanea tarda.

Dosage and Administration: As with insulin, dosage must be individualized. The average initial *oral* dosage is 1 to 2 gm daily, increased or decreased according to patient response. The ideal dosage is the smallest amount necessary to maintain optimal control. This will vary considerably among patients, and may be as little as 250 mg or as much as 3 gm. The total daily dose may be taken either in the morning or in divided doses throughout the day. Consult package literature for other dosage considerations.

Availability:
ORINASE®: **(Upjohn)**
Diagnostic, Sterile (for intravenous diagnostic use) in vials of 1 gm with a 20-ml ampul of sterile water for injection.
Tablets, 250 mg in bottles of 100; 500 mg in bottles of 30, 50, 100, 200, 500 and 1000 and in unit-dose (blister-strip) packages of 100.

TOLMETIN SODIUM

Chemical Name: 1-Methyl-5-(p-toluoyl)-pyrrole-2-acetate dihydrate sodium.

Description: A synthetic, nonsteroidal antiinflammatory drug with analgesic and antipyretic properties. Tolmetin is related to the indoles but lacks their serotonin-like nucleus and is therefore classed as a pyrrole; its unique molecule makes it chemically distinct from other antiinflammatory compounds currently used in the treatment of rheumatoid arthritis. The precise mode of action is not known; however, clinical studies have revealed that the therapeutic effect is *not* mediated through pituitary-adrenal stimulation, but may be due to a reduction in prostaglandin synthesis. In studies with rats, the drug was noted to prevent the development of experimentally induced polyarthritis and to decrease established inflammation. Its antirheumatic activity was reported to be comparable to aspirin and to indomethacin, but the incidence of tinnitus and gastrointestinal intolerance and toxicity appeared less than in aspirin-treated patients, and the CNS reactions (headache, dizziness, lightheadedness) also appeared less than in indomethacin-treated patients. Whether or nor there is less peptic ulceration with tolmetin than with the other two drugs is not known.

In clinical trials, the drug was observed to decrease the duration of morning stiffness and to increase functional capacity as indicated by a progressive increase in grip strength. Among the additional criteria used to measure the effects of tolmetin were a reduction in the number of inflamed joints; relief of pain, swelling and tenderness; a delay in the onset of fatigue; and an increase in joint motion. Although the drug did not alter the course of the underlying disease, its ability to provide effective symptomatic relief was confirmed by the parameters evaluated.

Under fasting conditions, tolmetin is rapidly and almost completely absorbed, achieving peak plasma levels of 40 mcg/ml within 30 to 60 minutes of oral administration of a 400-mg dose; biological half-life is approximately 1 hour. Essentially, all of the administered dose is recovered in the urine within 24 hours either as an inactive oxidative metabolite or as conjugates of tolmetin. Therapeutic response usually occurs within a few days to a week.

In contrast to most nonsteroidal antiinflammatory agents, tolmetin does not potentiate coumarin-type drugs, thus suggesting safe use in patients on anticoagulant therapy, nor does it alter the clinical effects of sulfonylureas or insulin. Studies lasting from 4 to 6 days demonstrated that the degree of fecal blood loss was less with this drug than with aspirin. Also, it does not interfere with the clinical assessment of the tuberculin skin or the immediate-type hypersensitivity skin test, nor does it appear to interfere with the immune mechanism as measured by skin-testing.

Indications: For relief of the signs and symptoms of rheumatoid arthritis. It is indicated in the treatment of acute flareups and in the long-term management of the disease. May be used as the sole therapeutic agent or in combination with gold or corticosteroids. It is not recommended for patients who are severely incapacitated, bedridden or confined to a wheelchair until safe and effective use has been established.

Contraindications: Patients with known hypersensitivity to the drug. Tolmetin should not be given to patients in whom aspirin and other nonsteroidal antiinflammatory drugs induce the symptoms of asthma, rhinitis, or urticaria.

Warnings: Patients with a history of upper gastrointestinal tract disorders should be under close supervision since peptic ulceration and gastrointestinal bleeding, sometimes severe, have been reported. In these instances attempts should be made to treat the arthritis with nonulcerogenic drugs such as gold salts.

Precautions: Although clinical evidence to date has not demonstrated drug-induced eye changes or renal toxicity, the possibility should be kept in mind. Therapy should therefore be guided by periodic eye examinations and frequent assessment of kidney function. The drug has been found to prolong bleeding time, and to cause sodium and water retention with peripheral edema in about 2% of patients; therefore, those with compromised cardiac function require utmost care. In individuals receiving combined tolmetin-steroid therapy, any reduction in steroid dosage should be gradual to avoid the possible complications of sudden steroid withdrawal.

The urinary metabolites of this drug tend to show positive results for proteinuria when employing tests which rely on acid precipitation (e.g. sulfosalicylic acid) as their endpoint; however, this phenomenon does not occur when dye-impregnated reagent strips such as Albustix®, Uristix®, or other such agent is used. Adult diabetic patients receiving a sulfonylurea agent or insulin in addition to tolmetin experienced no observable change in the clinical effects of either drug. Reproduction studies in rats and rabbits at doses up to 1.7 times the maximal clinical dose did not yield evidence of impaired fertility or teratogenesis. However, as with other nonsteroidal antiinflammatory agents known to inhibit prostaglandin synthesis, an increased incidence of dystocia and delayed parturition occurs in rats, but these effects were absent when the drug was discontinued 24 hours prior to expected delivery. Until clinical data is available to ascertain its safe use during pregnancy, the drug should not be given to pregnant patients unless the clinical situation justifies the risk, and then only with extreme caution. For the present, it is recommended that lactating mothers refrain from nursing their infants while on this medication.

Adverse Reactions: All of the following adverse reactions are presented in their decreasing order of frequency and their occurrence in an approximate number of patients: Epigastric or abdominal pain or discomfort (1 in 6); nausea (1 in 25); vomiting (1 in 30); indigestion and heartburn (1 in 50); constipation (1 in 60); dyspepsia (1 in 100). In clinical studies in 1359 patients treated for up to two years, peptic ulcer occurred in 27 patients (an incidence of about 1 in 50); eleven of the 27 patients (41%) had either a prior history of peptic ulcer and/or were receiving concomitant antiinflammatory drugs, including corticosteroids, known to produce peptic ulceration. Significant gastrointestinal bleeding without evidence of peptic ulceration has been reported (1 in 250). In clinical trials with tolmetin, about 10% of the patients discontinued treatment because of adverse reactions, mostly gastrointestinal in nature. Other adverse reactions are headache (1 in 15); dizziness and lightheadedness (1 in 25); tension, nervousness, and drowsiness (1 in 50); rash, including maculopapular eruptions or urticaria (1 in 30); pruritus (1 in 50); however, no vesicular or desquamative rashes were observed; tinnitus (1 in 10); mild edema (1 in 50). Small and transient decreases in hemoglobin and hematocrit (not associated with gastrointestinal bleeding) and a few cases of granulocytopenia have been observed.

Dosage and Administration: *Orally.* To achieve optimal therapeutic effect the dose should be adjusted according to the patient's response. The recommended initial dose is 400 mg (2 tablets) 3 times daily, preferably in the morning, during the day and at bedtime. Control is usually achieved at doses of 600 to 1800 mg daily in 3 or 4 divided doses; up to, but no more than 2000 mg (2 gm) daily may be given. Until further experience with regard to safe and effective use has been gained, this drug is not recommended for use in children.

Availability:
TOLECTIN® Tablets, 200 mg in bottles of 100 and 500. **(McNeil)**

TOLNAFTATE

Chemical Name: *m,N*-Dimethylthiocarbanilic acid *O*-2-naphthylester.

Description: Tolnaftate is a synthetic antifungal agent, and occurs as a white, crystalline powder slightly soluble in water and soluble in alcohol. The cream and solution afford effective topical treatment for athlete's foot, jock itch, and ringworm, and will begin to relieve the accompanying itching, burning and soreness within 24 hours.

Indications: Topical treatment of tinea pedis, tinea cruris, tinea corporis, and tinea manuum due to infection by *T. rubrum, T. mentagrophytes, T. tonsurans, M. canis, M. audouini, E. floccosum,* and for tinea versicolor due to infection by *Malassezia furfur.* It may also be useful in the control of recent, mild fungus infection of the scalp (tinea capitis). When tolnaftate is used to treat onychomycosis and chronic infections of the scalp, or chronic refractory fungus infections of the palms and soles, concomitant use of a systemic antifungal agent is required.

Warnings: Avoid contact with the eyes. If irritation or hypersensitivity develops, or if the patient's skin condition becomes worse, treatment should be discontinued.

Precautions: If the patient shows no improvement after 4 weeks of treatment, the diagnosis should be reevaluated; and if the patient's condition becomes more severe the drug should be withdrawn. In mixed infections where bacteria or nonsusceptible fungi such as *Candida albicans* are present, supplementary topical or systemic antibacterial therapy is indicated.

Adverse Reactions: A few instances of local irritation and sensitization have been noted, but whether or not these were drug-related has not been confirmed.

Dosage and Administration: *Topically,* 1 to 3 drops of the solution, or a small amount of the cream or powder are rubbed into the lesion twice daily for 2 to 3 weeks, although treatment for 4 to 6 weeks may be required occasionally.

Availability:
TINACTIN®: **(Schering)**
Cream, (OTC), 1% in tubes of 15 gm with dispensing tip.
Powder, (OTC), 1% in containers of 45 gm.
Solution, (OTC), 1% in squeeze bottles of 10 ml.
Spray Powder (OTC), in aerosol containers of 120 gm.

TRANYLCYPROMINE

Chemical Name: 2-Phenylcyclopropylamine.

Description: Tranylcypromine is a nonhydrazine monoamine oxidase inhibitor related structurally to amphetamine differing only in that its side chain is cyclic. Onset of action is more rapid than that of the hydrazine group of MAO inhibitors. It occurs as a white, crystalline powder soluble in water and insoluble in alcohol.

Tranylcypromine increases the concentration of epinephrine, norepinephrine, and serotonin in storage sites throughout the nervous system, and in theory, this increased concentration of the drug in the brainstem is the basis for its antidepressant activity. When tranylcypromine is withdrawn, monoamine oxidase activity is recovered within 3 to 5 days, although the drug is excreted in 24 hours.

Indications: Relief of symptoms of severe reactive or endogenous depression in patients for whom electroconvulsive therapy is not indicated and who have been found not to respond satisfactorily to other antidepressant therapy.

Contraindications: Patients over 60 years of age or those with a confirmed or suspected cerebrovascular defect or patients with cardiovascular disease, hypertension or a history of headache; pheochromocytoma; liver dysfunction; in combination with other MAO inhibitors, dibenzazepine derivatives, sympathomimetics including amphetamines, and drugs such as cold, hay fever or reducing preparations that contain vasoconstrictors; narcotics; alcohol; hypotensive agents; cheese or other foods that contain a high tyramine content. Additionally, excessive use of caffeine in any form should be avoided.

Warnings: Tranylcypromine is a potent drug with the capability of producing serious side effects. It should be reserved for patients who are either hospitalized or under close supervision and who have not responded satisfactorily to other antidepressants. Use of the drug during pregnancy, lactation, or in women of childbearing potential requires that the anticipated benefits be weighed against the possible hazards to the mother or child.

Precautions: Caution should be exercised if patients are given tranylcypromine and antiparkinsonian drugs concomitantly, since severe reactions have been reported. Intracranial bleeding (sometimes fatal) associated with paradoxical hypertension, severe occipital headache that may radiate frontally, palpitation, stiffness or soreness of the neck, nausea, vomiting, sweating, fever, cold clammy skin, photophobia, tachycardia, bradycardia, constricting chest pains, and dilated pupils may occur. It is recommended that the drug be discontinued when any of these signs or symptoms appear. Since tranylcypromine can also cause postural hypotension, it should not be used concomitantly with other antihypertensive agents. The usual precautions should be observed in patients with impaired renal function because of the possibility of cumulative effects. It should be used cautiously in patients with epilepsy or diabetes. Because hypertensive crises have sometimes occurred during tranylcypromine therapy after ingestion of foods containing a high tyramine content, patients should be instructed not to take such foods as cheese (particularly the strong and aged varieties), sour cream, chianti or sherry wine, beer, yeast extracts, pickled herring, chicken livers, canned figs, raisins, chocolate, soy sauce, or the pods of broad beans. In general, the patient should avoid protein foods in which aging or protein breakdown is used to increase flavor. Special care is advised in patients who are hyperthyroid because of their increased sensitivity to pressor amines.

Adverse Reactions: Overstimulation which may include increased anxiety, agitation and manic symptoms, restlessness, insomnia, weakness, drowsiness, dizziness, dry mouth, nausea, diarrhea, abdominal pain, constipation, tachycardia, anorexia, edema, palpitation, blurred vision, chills, impotence, headaches, hepatitis, skin rash, tinnitus, muscle spasm, tremors, paresthesia, and urinary retention.

Dosage and Administration: *Orally.* The recommended initial dosage is 20 mg daily, 10 mg in the morning and 10 mg in the afternoon for 2 weeks. If no response is noted, the dosage may be increased to 30 mg daily, 20 mg in the morning and 10 mg in the afternoon for 1 week. If no improvement occurs continued administration is unlikely to be beneficial. When a satisfactory response is obtained, dosage may be reduced to a maintenance level. Dosage increases should be made in increments of 10 mg daily at intervals of 1 to 3 weeks. It is important that the lowest effective dose be used.

Availability:
PARNATE® Tablets, 10 mg in bottles of 100 and 1000. **(Smith Kline & French)**

TRETINOIN

Chemical Name: *All trans* retinoic acid; vitamin A acid.

Description: Tretinoin is a topical acne medication. The commercial product contains 0.05% tretinoin incorporated in a base of polyethylene glycol 400, butylated hydroxytoluene and 55% alcohol.

Following application to the affected area, therapeutic results should be apparent after 2 to 3 weeks of therapy; however, optimal results may not be noted until after 6 weeks. During the early weeks of treatment, an *apparent* exacerbation of inflammatory lesions may occur. This usually is due to the action of tretinoin on deep, previously unseen comedones and papules.

Indications: Treatment of acne vulgaris, primarily grades I through III in which comedones, papules and pustules predominate. **Note:** It is not effective in most cases of severe pustular and deep cystic nodular varieties of acne (acne conglobata).

Contraindications: Hypersensitivity to any of the components.

Warnings: Tretinoin should not be permitted to come in contact with the eyes, mouth, angles of the nose or mucous membranes. Topical use may induce severe local erythema and peeling at the site of application. If undue irritation occurs, patients should be instructed to use the medication less frequently, discontinue use temporarily, or withdraw the medication completely. Since the drug has been reported to cause severe irritation on eczematous skin, tretinoin should be used with utmost caution in patients with this condition.

Precautions: Concomitant topical medication should be used with care because of possible interaction with tretinoin. Particular caution is required when using preparations containing peeling agents, such as sulfur, resorcinol, benzoyl peroxide, salicylic acid, or those containing a strong drying effect such as medicated or abrasive soaps, cleansers, cosmetics, or products with a high concentration of alcohol with this agent. Before treatment is initiated, it is advisable to "rest" the patient's skin until the effects of peeling agents subside. Exposure to sunlight, including sunlamps, should be minimized and patients with sunburn should be advised not to use tretinoin until fully recovered because of heightened susceptibility to sunlight. Patients whose occupation exposes them to a considerable amount of sun should be particularly careful. Excessive application will not produce faster or better results and may cause marked redness, peeling or discomfort.

Adverse Reactions: The skin of sensitive individuals may become excessively red, edematous, blistered or crusted. If these effects occur, treatment should be either discontinued until the integrity of the skin is restored or adjusted to a level the patient can tolerate. Temporary hyper- or hypopigmentation has been reported with repeated application. To date, all adverse reactions have been reversible upon discontinuance of therapy.

Dosage and Administration: *Topically.* Apply once daily before retiring, using enough of the medication to cover the effected area lightly. Care should be taken not to extend into areas in which treatment is not intended. Cosmetics may be used, but before applying the medication, the area to be treated should be cleansed thoroughly.

Availability:
ABEREL® Saturated Swabs, 0.05% in cartons of 30. **(McNeil)**
RETIN-A: **(Johnson & Johnson)**
Cream, 0.05 and 0.1% in tubes of 20 gm; 0.05% also available in tubes of 45 gm.
Gel, 0.01% in tubes of 15 gm; 0.025% in tubes of 15 and 45 gm.
Liquid, 0.05% in bottles of 28 ml.
Saturated Swabs, 0.05% in cartons of 30.

TRIAMCINOLONE: see The Adrenal Corticosteroids

TRIAMINIC

Description: An orally effective sympathomimetic amine has been combined with 2 antihistamines in the following dosage forms:

	Tablets	*Juvelets*	*Oral Infant Drops/ml*
Phenylpropanolamine hydrochloride	50 mg	25 mg	20 mg
Pheniramine maleate	25 mg	12.5 mg	10 mg
Pyrilamine maleate	25 mg	12.5 mg	10 mg

Indications: Symptomatic treatment of colds, nasal allergies, sinusitis, rhinitis and postnasal drip. These preparations decongest and normalize respiratory passages, reduce irritating secretions, combat allergic symptoms and improve drainage of sinuses.

Precautions: Should be used cautiously in patients with hypertension, cardiovascular disease, diabetes or hyperthyroidism. Patients should be cautioned that in the event of drowsiness, they should not operate a motor vehicle or engage in any hazardous occupation requiring alertness or skill.

Adverse Reactions: Drowsiness, blurred vision, cardiac palpitations, flushing, dizziness, nervousness or gastrointestinal disturbances. These may occur occasionally.

Dosage and Administration: *Orally. Tablets:* adults, 1 tablet swallowed intact 3 times daily. *Juvelets:* children 6 to 12 years of age, 1 tablet swallowed intact 3 times daily; adults, 2 tablets on the same dosage schedule. *Oral Infant Drops:* 1 drop/2 lb of body weight given 4 times daily.

Availability:
TRIAMINIC®: **(Dorsey)**
Juvelets (timed-release tablets) in bottles of 50.
Oral Infant Drops in dropper bottles of 15 ml.
Tablets (timed-release) in bottles of 100 and 250.

TRIAMINIC EXPECTORANT DH (C-III)

Description: Each teaspoonful (5 ml) contains:

Hydrocodone bitartrate	1.67 mg
Phenylpropanolamine hydrochloride	12.5 mg
Pheniramine maleate	6.25 mg
Pyrilamine maleate	6.25 mg
Guaifenesin	100 mg

with 5% alcohol in a mint-flavored vehicle.

Indications: Relief of cough and nasal congestion associated with the common cold, nasal allergies, sinusitis and postnasal drip. May also be used for the relief of severe, prolonged or refractory cough associated with other respiratory infections.

Warnings: Hydrocodone is a narcotic and may be habit-forming.

Precautions: Should be used cautiously in patients with hypertension, cardiovascular disease, diabetes or hyperthyroidism. Patients should be cautioned that in the event of drowsiness, they should not operate a motor vehicle or engage in any hazardous occupation requiring alertness or skill.

Adverse Reactions: Occasional drowsiness, blurred vision, palpitations, flushing, dizziness, nervousness or gastrointestinal disturbances.

Dosage and Administration: *Orally,* every 4 hours. Adults, 2 teaspoonsful; children 6 to 12 years of age, 1 teaspoonful; children 1 to 6 years, ½ teaspoonful.

Availability:
(C-III) TRIAMINIC® EXPECTORANT DH in bottles of 1 pint. **(Dorsey)**

TRIAMTERENE

Chemical Name: 2,4,7-Triamino-6-phenylpteridine.

Description: Triamterene is not a thiazide diuretic, nor an altered thiazide molecule or steroid. It is a pteridine derivative and is an orally effective diuretic. It occurs as a yellow, crystalline powder very slightly soluble in water and in alcohol.

Its mode of action is unique in that it interferes with the exchange of sodium for potassium and hydrogen ions, an action which is independent of aldosterone. Thus, triamterene promotes the excretion of sodium and chloride and, by reducing the transportation of potassium from the cell to the lumen of the distal segment of the renal tubules, it minimizes the risk of hypokalemia frequently observed with other diuretics. However, triamterene occasionally does in fact cause an increase in serum potassium which, in some instances, can result in hyperkalemia. Because it does not cause excessive excretion of titratable acid and ammonia, the incidence of alkalosis is not very likely.

Following oral ingestion, onset of action occurs in about 2 to 4 hours. Most patients usually respond to triamterene during the 1st day of treatment; however, maximum therapeutic effect may not be seen for several days. Duration of diuresis depends on several factors, especially renal function, but the diuretic action generally tapers off about 7 to 9 hours after taking the drug.

Indications: Treatment of edema associated with congestive heart failure, cirrhosis and the nephrotic syndrome. It is also indicated in steroid-induced edema, idiopathic edema and edema due to secondary hyperaldosteronism. It is especially useful when patients become resistant or only partially responsive to other diuretics and in cases where sodium-retaining steroids are present. Since hydrochlorothiazide further promotes excretion of sodium and water by acting primarily at the proximal tubule and Henle's loop, the combination of triamterene and hydrochlorothiazide is employed for the treatment of mild to moderate hypertension. This fixed combination drug is not indicated for initial therapy of edema or hypertension, since these conditions require that treatment be titrated to the individual patient. However, if the fixed combination represents the dosage so determined, then its use may be more convenient to patient management. The routine use of diuretics in otherwise healthy pregnant women is inappropriate and exposes the mother and fetus to unnecessary hazards. Since they do not prevent the development of toxemia of pregnancy and there is no satisfactory evidence that they are useful in the treatment of actual toxemia; therefore, they should be used only if the clinical situation clearly justifies the need.

Contraindications: Hypersensitivity to either component, anuria or progressive renal disease or dysfunction with the possible exception of nephrosis; severe hepatic disease; hypersensitivity to the drug; patients with preexisting elevated serum potassium levels as is seen occasionally in the presence of impaired renal function, oliguria and increasing azotemia or in patients who develop hyperkalemia while on the drug.

Warnings: Patients should be observed regularly for signs of blood dyscrasias, liver damage or other idiosyncratic reactions. Serum potassium and BUN values should be determined periodically to assess kidney function, especially in patients with suspected or confirmed renal insufficiency and in the elderly. The drug should be used during pregnancy or in women of childbearing potential only when, in the judgment of the physician, its use is deemed essential to the welfare of the patient. Since it may appear in the milk of lactating women, infants should not be nursed during drug treatment. When triamterene is added to other diuretic therapy, or when a patient is transferred to triamterene from another diuretic, all potassium supplementation should be discontinued.

Precautions: Although unlikely when urinary output is adequate, the possibility that large doses of triamterene used for prolonged periods may cause hyperkalemia should be considered, and the drug should be discontinued if this occurs. However, if withdrawal is abrupt, a rebound kaliuresis could occur; withdrawal in these patients should, therefore, be gradual. Also, if triamterene is used concomitantly with spironolactone, the physician should frequently determine serum potassium levels, since both of these agents can cause potassium retention and, in some instances, hyperkalemia. Electrolyte imbalance may be aggravated or caused independently by any diuretic agent, including this agent. Mild, reversible nitrogen retention is a possibility. Periodic blood studies are suggested, particularly in patients with cirrhosis and splenomegaly. Although triamterene is not considered an antihypertensive agent, the physician should be aware, nonetheless, that blood pressure may be lowered and that concomitant administration of antihypertensive drugs may result in an additive effect. Since triamterene and quinidine have a similar fluorescence spectra, this drug will therefore interfere with the fluorescent measurement of quinidine.

Adverse Reactions: Diarrhea or constipation, nausea, vomiting, other gastrointestinal disturbances, muscle cramps, weakness, dizziness, headache, dry mouth, anaphylaxis, photosensitivity, purpura, rash, urticaria, and elevated uric acid levels in patients predisposed to gouty arthritis. Thiazides have been known to cause necrotizing vasculitis, paresthesias, icterus, pancreatitis, and xanthopsia, and occasionally, allergic pneumonitis. In rare instances, newborn infants, whose mothers had received thiazides during pregnancy, have developed thrombocytopenia and pancreatitis.

Dosage and Administration: *Orally. For edema,* the usual initial dosage for adults is 100 mg twice daily after meals. Maintenance, 100 mg daily or every other day. Total daily dosage should not exceed 300 mg daily. *For hypertension,* the usual initial dosage is 1 capsule of

Dyazide twice daily after meals. Total dose should not exceed 4 capsules daily. Adequate information for use in children is not available.

Availability:
DYRENIUM® Capsules, 50 mg in bottles of 100 and in single-unit packages of 100; 100 mg in bottles of 100 and 1000 and in single-unit packages of 100. **(Smith Kline & French)**
DYAZIDE® Capsules, 50 mg with 25 mg of hydrochlorothiazide in bottles of 100 and 1000 and in single-unit packages of 100 **(Smith Kline & French)**

TRICHLORMETHIAZIDE: see The Thiazide Diuretics

TRICLOFOS SODIUM

Chemical Name: 2,2,2-Trichloroethanol dihydrogen phosphate.

Description: Triclofos, a hypnotic agent, is the phosphate ester of trichlorethanol. Triclofos sodium is the sodium salt of trichlorethyl phosphate.

It is rapidly dephosphorylated, primarily in the intestine, yielding high blood levels of trichlorethanol which is the same pharmacologically active metabolite obtained from chloral hydrate.

Peak serum levels are reached in about 1 hour and the half-life is approximately 11 hours. A dose of 1.5 gm is equivalent to 1 gm of chloral hydrate. Triclofos produces minimal effects on the various stages of normal sleep, including REM sleep. However, the precise clinical significance of changes in REM sleep has not been determined.

In animal studies triclofos appears to increase the content of slow-wave, high-voltage spontaneous cortical EEG activity concomitant with normal sleep. The arousal threshold on electrical stimulation of the midbrain reticular formation appears to be increased; whether this effect is responsible for the hypnotic action of this drug has not been established.

Indications: Treatment of insomnia characterized by difficulty in falling asleep, frequent nocturnal awakenings, or early morning awakening. May also be used to induce sleep in patients undergoing electroencephalography.

Contraindications: In patients with marked renal or hepatic impairment, in those known to be sensitive or allergic to chloral hydrate or triclofos, in women at labor and in the neonate.

Warnings: Triclofos may be habit-forming; therefore, caution should be exercised when administering this drug to patients known to be addiction prone. Repeated use of the drug is advisable only under careful medical supervision. Response to concomitantly administered oral anticoagulants may be modified by triclofos. Careful monitoring of prothrombin time with adjustment of anticoagulant dosage is advised throughout therapy and following withdrawal of this drug. Safe use in pregnant women or in nursing mothers has not been established. The drug is not currently recommended for use in children under 12 years of age except for single-dose administration for sleep induction in electroencephalography.

Precautions: Patients should be cautioned that triclofos may increase the CNS depressant effects of such drugs as alcohol, barbiturates and tranquilizers. In the event of drowsiness, patients should be warned not to engage in activities requiring alertness or skill. The drug should be used with caution in patients with cardiac arrhythmias or with severe cardiac disease. Periodic blood counts should be performed when prolonged use is necessary. Data on the effectiveness of therapy with triclofos for periods exceeding 6 weeks have not been obtained.

Adverse Reactions: Headache, hangover, drowsiness, gastrointestinal upset, "gas," flatulence, nausea and vomiting, staggering gait, ataxia, "bad taste," ketonuria, relative eosinophilia, urticaria, lightheadedness, vertigo, nightmares, malaise, and reduction in total white blood cell count have been noted. Excitement and delirium, since they have been observed with chloral hydrate, are possible occurrences.

Dosage and Administration: *Orally.* The usual hypnotic dosage is 2 tablets or 1 tablespoonful of liquid taken 15 to 30 minutes before retiring. The usual dose for sleep induction in electroencephalography in children under 12 years of age is 0.1 ml/lb of body weight.

Availability:
TRICLOS®: **(Merrell-National)**
Liquid, 1.5 gm/15 ml in bottles of 240 ml.
Tablets, 0.75 gm in bottles of 100 and 500.

TRIDIHEXETHYL CHLORIDE

Chemical Name: (3-Cyclohexyl-3-hydroxy-3-phenylpropyl) triethylammonium chloride.

Description: Tridihexethyl chloride is a synthetic quaternary ammonium anticholinergic compound closely related structurally and pharmacologically to oxyphenonium, hexocyclium, and tricyclamol. It occurs as a bitter, white crystalline powder freely soluble in water and in alcohol.

Relieves pain and spasm by reducing the frequency and force of smooth muscle contractions in the gastrointestinal tract.

Indications: Adjunctive treatment of peptic ulcer, gastric hyperacidity and hypermotility, and parenterally in acute pancreatitis. May also be useful in gastrointestinal spastic conditions, such as spastic and irritable colon, mucous colitis, acute enterocolitis, and functional gastrointestinal disorders; in neurogenic bowel disturbances, including the splenic flexure syndrome, which are not associated with organic change. Phenobarbital is added to provide sedative action, or meprobamate is added as an adjunctive measure when anxiety and emotional distress are present which may adversely affect the underlying conditions.

Contraindications: Allergic or idiosyncratic reaction to tridihexethyl or to any of the components. Glaucoma; obstructive uropathy (bladder neck obstruction due to prostatic hypertrophy); achalasia, paralytic ileus, pyloroduodenal stenosis; intestinal atony of the elderly or debilited patient; unstable cardiovascular status in acute hemorrhage; severe ulcerative colitis; toxic megacolon complicating ulcerative colitis; and myasthenia gravis. Phenobarbital and meprobamate are contraindicated in acute intermittent porphyria.

Warnings: Use of the drug during pregnancy, lactation, or in women of childbearing potential, requires that the potential benefit be weighed against its possible hazards to the mother and child. Also, an inhibiting effect on lactation may occur. Heat prostration manifested by fever and heat stroke due to decreased sweating may occur in high environmental temperatures. Diarrhea may be an early symptom of incomplete intestinal obstruction, especially in patients with ileostomy or colostomy. In this instance treatment with this drug would be inappropriate and possibly harmful. Phenobarbital may be habit-forming.

Precautions: The drug should be discontinued if severe reactions or idiosyncrasy occurs. Tridihexethyl chloride should be administered with caution, if at all, to the elderly, the depressed, and to patients with cardiac arrhythmias (especially tachycardia since the drug may increase heart rate), decompensation and coronary artery disease. Caution is also essential in patients with hypertension, autonomic neuropathy, early evidence of ileus as in peritonitis, ulcerative colitis (large doses may suppress intestinal motility to the point of producing a paralytic ileus, thus the use of this drug may precipitate or aggravate the serious complication of toxic megacolon), hiatal hernia associated with reflux esophagitis, and nonobstructing prostatic hypertrophy. It should be noted that the use of anticholinergic drugs in the treatment of gastric ulcer may produce a delay in gastric emptying time and may complicate such therapy (antral stasis). Overdosage may precipitate a curare-like action. Preparations containing phenobarbital should be used with caution in patients with hyperthyroidism, high fever, diabetes mellitus, marked anemia, and severe hepatic and renal disease. Psychic dependence may develop from prolonged use. Since phenobarbital may decrease the action of anticoagulant drugs, the dose of these drugs may have to be increased in order to maintain their optimal effect. Patients should be cautioned that in the event of drowsiness or dizziness, they should not operate a motor vehicle or engage in any hazardous occupation requiring alertness or skill.

Adverse Reactions: Complications produced by anticholinergic drugs include xerostomia; urinary hesitancy and retention; blurred vision and tachycardia; palpitations; mydriasis; dilation of the pupil; cycloplegia; increased ocular tension; loss of taste; headaches; nervousness; drowsiness; weakness; dizziness; insomnia; nausea; vomiting; decreased sweating; impotence; suppression of lactation; constipation; bloated feeling; severe allergic reaction or drug idiosyncrasies including anaphylaxis; urticaria and other dermal manifestations; some degree of mental confusion and/or excitement especially in elderly patients. Acute toxic reactions are manifested by dry mouth, difficulty in swallowing, marked thirst; blurred vision, photophobia; flushed, hot, dry skin; rash; hyperthermia; tachycardia with weak pulse, elevated blood pressure; urinary urgency with difficulty in micturition; abdominal distention; restlessness, confusion, delirium and other signs suggestive of an acute organic psychosis. Gastric lavage, supportive and symptomatic therapy are indicated. For complete data on any of the components, see their individual monographs.

Dosage and Administration: Pathilon: *Orally.* Tablets, the average adult dosage is 25 to 50 mg, with or without 15 or 45 mg phenobarbital, 3 or 4 times daily. The usual bedtime dose is 50 mg. Dosage may range from 10 mg 3 times daily to 75 mg 4 times daily. The suggested initial dosage is 25 mg 3 times daily before meals and 50 mg at bedtime. Sequels, 75 mg every 6 or 12 hours. *Intravenously, intramuscularly or subcutaneously,* 10 to 20 mg every 6 hours. Pathibamate: *Orally,* 1 tablet 3 times daily with meals and 2 tablets at bedtime. Not recommended for use in children under 12 years of age.

Availability:
PATHILON®: **(Lederle)**
Parenteral Solution, 10 mg/ml in ampuls of 1 ml.
Sequels® (sustained-release capsules), 75 mg in bottles of 30.
Sequels, 75 mg with phenobarbital, 45 mg in bottles of 30.
Tablets, 25 mg in bottles of 100 and 1000.
Tablets, 25 mg with phenobarbital, 15 mg in bottles of 100 and 1000.
PATHIBAMATE®-200 Tablets, 25 mg with meprobamate, 200 mg in bottles of 100 and 1000. **(Lederle)**
PATHIBAMATE-400 Tablets, 25 mg with meprobamate, 400 mg in bottles of 100, 1000 and 5000. **(Lederle)**

TRIFLUOPERAZINE: see The Phenothiazines

TRIFLUPROMAZINE HYDROCHLORIDE: see The Phenothiazines

TRIHEMIC 600

Description: Each tablet contains:

Ascorbic acid (vitamin C)	600 mg
Vitamin B-12 (cobalamin concentrate, N.F.)	25 μg
Intrinsic factor concentrate	75 mg
Folic acid	1 mg
Vitamin E (*d*-alpha tocopheryl acid succinate)	30 IU
Elemental iron (as ferrous fumarate, 350 mg)	115 mg
Dioctyl sodium sulfosuccinate U.S.P.	50 mg

Provides a combination of ingredients essential to normal erythropoiesis in addition to a stool softener to counteract the constipating effects of iron.

Indications: Treatment of most megaloblastic, macrocytic and iron-deficiency anemias, in the anemias of pregnancy and in those due to the malabsorption syndromes. A useful adjuvant in patients in whom erythropoiesis is suppressed due to severe infections, malignancies or to the toxic effects of certain chemotherapeutic agents. The addition of vitamin E—as an aid in decreasing the fragility of the red blood cells, and vitamin C—as an aid in the effective absorption of iron.

Precautions: Not all patients with pernicious anemia show satisfactory therapeutic responses to oral vitamin B-12 with intrinsic factor preparations. Some patients with an initial good response appear to become refractory to intrinsic factor following varying periods of oral therapy. Periodic examinations and laboratory studies of pernicious anemia patients are essential and recommended. This preparation should be discontinued if signs of sensitivity occur. Folic acid may obscure the presence of pernicious anemia, in that the hematological remission may occur while the neurological manifestations remain progressive.

Adverse Reactions: Gastrointestinal reactions manifested by nausea, vomiting, diarrhea or abdominal pain may occur. Also, skin rashes of various types have been noted. Alterations in dosage and usage may be necessary. Allergic sensitization has been reported following both oral and parenteral use of folic acid.

Dosage and Administration: *Orally*, 1 tablet daily, or as directed by the physician.

Availability:
TRIHEMIC® 600 Tablets in bottles of 30 and 500. **(Lederle)**

TRIHEXYPHENIDYL HYDROCHLORIDE

Chemical Name: 3-(1-piperidyl)-1-phenyl-cyclohexyl-1-propanol hydrochloride.

Description: Trihexyphenidyl hydrochloride, a synthetic antispasmodic drug, is a tertiary amine anticholinergic compound incompatible with oxidizing agents. It occurs as a white or slightly off-white, crystalline powder with a bitter taste that is followed by local tingling and numbness in the mouth, and is slightly soluble in water and soluble in alcohol. Following oral administration, trihexyphenidyl exerts a direct inhibitory effect upon the parasympathetic nervous system. It also appears to have a relaxing effect on smooth musculature, exerted both directly upon the muscle tissue itself and indirectly through an inhibitory effect upon the parasympathetic nervous system. Its therapeutic properties are similar to those of atropine, although undesirable side effects are ordinarily less frequent and less severe than those of atropine.

Indications: Treatment of all forms of parkinsonism (postencephalitic, arteriosclerotic, and idiopathic) as well as the control of extrapyramidal disorders due to drugs that act on the CNS, such as the phenothiazines, thioxanthenes and butyrophenones.

Contraindications: Hypersensitivity to the drug.

Warnings: The benefits of therapy must be carefully weighed when evaluating patients with glaucoma, urinary retention, cardiac arrhythmias, or any other condition that would be adversely affected by anticholinergic action. Since trihexyphenidyl may impair mental and/or physical abilities, patients should be cautioned not to engage in activities requiring alertness or skill. Safe use during pregnancy has not been established, and the drug should not be administered unless the expected benefits outweigh the potential risks.

Precautions: Patients with a history of drug idiosyncrasies or arteriosclerosis may exhibit mental confusion, agitation or nausea and vomiting. While hypertension, cardiac, kidney, or liver disorders are not contraindications, patients with these conditions should be observed carefully. Incipient glaucoma may be precipitated; therefore, it is advised that all patients undergo periodic gonioscopic evaluations. It should be used with caution in patients with obstructive disease of the gastrointestinal or genitourinary tracts, and in elderly male patients with possible prostatic hypertrophy. Older patients, particularly those over the age of 60 years, frequently develop increased sensitivity to the actions of this drug, and hence, require strict dosage regulation.

Adverse Reactions: Isolated instances of suppurative parotitis secondary to excessive dryness of mouth, skin rashes, dilatation of the colon, paralytic ileus, and psychiatric manifestations such as disorientation, confusion, excitement, delirium, delusions and hallucinations, plus one doubtful case of paranoia have been reported. Minor side effects such as dryness of the mouth, blurring of vision, lightheadedness, dizziness, memory loss, mild nausea or nervousness, will be experienced in some patients. These patients should be allowed to develop a tolerance through small initial doses with gradual increase until an effective level is reached. If a severe reaction should occur, the drug should be discontinued for a few days and then resumed at a lower dosage. Constipation, drowsiness, urinary hesitancy or retention, tachycardia, dilation of the pupil, increased intraocular tension, weakness, vomiting and headache are potential side effects and must be considered. The occurrence of angle-closure glaucoma due to prolonged use has been reported.

Dosage and Administration: *Orally. For parkinsonism:* Initially, 1 mg the first day, then increased by 2-mg increments at intervals of 3 to 5 days until a total of 6 to 10 mg are given daily in divided doses. Some patients may require 12 to 15 mg daily. Concomitant use with levodopa requires careful dosage adjustment of both drugs. *For control of extrapyramidal conditions:* The total daily dosage usually ranges between 5 and 15 mg, although some patients may respond satisfactorily to as little as 1 mg daily.

Availability:
ARTANE®: **(Lederle)**
Elixir, 2 mg/5 ml in bottles of 1 pint.
Sequels (sustained-release capsules), 5 mg in bottles of 30 and 500.
Tablets, 2 and 5 mg in bottles of 100 and 1000 and in unit-dose packages of 100 (10 × 10).
TREMIN® Tablets, 2 and 5 mg in bottles of 100. **(Schering)**

TRIMEPRAZINE TARTRATE: see The Phenothiazines

TRIMETHADIONE: see Paramethadione

TRIMETHAPHAN CAMSYLATE

Chemical Name: (+)-1,3-Dibenzyldecahydro-2-oxoimidazo[4,5-c]thieno[1,2-a]thiolium 2-oxo-10 bornanesulfonate.

Description: Trimethaphan, a nonquaternary ammonium ganglionic blocking agent, is a thiophanium derivative and occurs as a white, crystalline powder freely soluble in water and in alcohol. Its molecular weight is 596.80.

The drug produces ganglionic blockade by occupying receptor sites on the ganglion cells and by stabilizing the postsynaptic membranes against the action of acetylcholine liberated from the presynaptic nerve endings. These effects are achieved without: altering membrane potentials of ganglionic cells; modifying conduction of impulses in the pre- and postganglionic neurons; or preventing the release of acetylcholine by preganglionic neurons. By producing a direct peripheal vasodilator effect, it causes pooling of blood in the dependent periphery and the splanchnic system. Vasodilatation results in lowered blood pressure. The drug also liberates histamine. Some animal studies have indicated that excessive dosage administration may result in respiratory failure.

Indications: Production of controlled hypotension where indicated, e.g., during a surgical procedure, or in pulmonary edema resulting from pulmonary hypertension associated with systemic hypertension, or to control dangerous systemic hypertension.

Contraindications: Those conditions where hypotension may subject the patient to undue risk, e.g., uncorrected anemia, hypovolemia, incipient and frank shock, asphyxia, or uncorrected respiratory insufficiency. Inadequate availability of fluids and inability to replace blood for technical reasons also may constitute contraindications.

Warnings: Trimethaphan is a potent hypotensive drug and should always be diluted before use. Adequate clinical and laboratory facilities should be available to patients for proper monitoring of treatment. Sufficient oxygenation must be assured throughout the treatment period, especially in regard to coronary and cerebral circulation. The drug should be used with extreme caution in patients with arteriosclerosis, cardiac disease, hepatic or renal disease, degenerative disease of the CNS, Addison's disease, diabetes and in patients treated with steroids. The induction of hypotension in a gravid patient may have serious consequences on the fetus.

Precautions: Should be used cautiously in patients receiving antihypertensive drugs, when used concurrently with anesthetic agents (especially spinal anesthetics), in the elderly or debilitated patient, or in children. Because of its histamine-liberating potential, the drug should be used with caution in allergic individuals. Diuretic agents may enhance the responses evoked by ganglionic blocking drugs. Also, concomitant use with other drugs can significantly modify the dose of trimethaphan necessary to achieve the desired hypotensive response. **Note:** Pupillary dilatation does not necessarily indicate anoxia or depth of anesthesia, since trimethaphan appears to have a specific effect on the pupil. Although a causal relationship has not been confirmed, respiratory arrest has occurred; therefore, it is advised that the patient's respiratory status be monitored closely, particularly if large doses are to be used.

Adverse Reactions: Undesirable low blood pressure.

Dosage and Administration: *By intravenous infusion.* The contents of 1 ampul are diluted to 500 ml using *only* 5% dextrose injection (1 mg/ml) and the infusion is started at an average rate of 60 drops (3 to 4 mg)/minute. The rate of administration is then adjusted to maintain the desired level of hypotension, and should be accompanied by frequent blood pressure determinations to maintain proper control. When used during a surgical procedure, administration of the drug should be stopped prior to wound closure in order to permit blood pressure to return to normal levels. A systolic pressure of 100 mm usually will be attained within 10 minutes after discontinuing the drug. Vasopressor agents may be used to correct undesirable low pressures during surgery or to effect a more rapid return to normotensive levels. Phenylephrine hydrochloride or mephentermine sulfate should be tried initially and norepinephrine should be reserved for refractory cases.

Availability:
ARFONAD® Injection, 50 mg/ml in ampuls of 10 ml. **(Roche)**

TRIMETHOBENZAMIDE HYDROCHLORIDE

Chemical Name: *N*-[*p*-[2-(Dimethylamino)-ethoxy]benzyl]-3,4,5-trimethoxybenzamide hydrochloride.

Description: Trimethobenzamide is an antiemetic agent structurally similar to the dimethylaminoethyl antihistamines (e.g., diphenhydramine) and similar in action to the antiemetic phenothiazines. It occurs as a white, odorless, crystalline powder freely soluble in water. Its molecular weight is 424.93.

The drug appears to exert its action directly on the chemoreceptor trigger zone of the medulla oblongata through which emetic impulses are conveyed to the vomiting center; however, direct impulses to the vomiting center are not similarly inhibited. It has little or no value in the prophylaxis and treatment of motion sickness.

Animal studies reveal that pretreatment with trimethobenzamide afforded protection against the erratic response to apomorphine but produced little or no protection against emesis induced by intragastric copper sulfate.

Indications: For the control of nausea and vomiting.

Contraindications: Parenterally in children, rectally in premature or newborn infants, and in patients known to be hypersensitive to trimethobenzamide. *Since the suppositories contain benzocaine, they should not be used in patients known to be sensitive to this or similar local anesthetics.*

Warnings: In the event of drowsiness, patients should be cautioned not to operate a motor vehicle or engage in any hazardous occupation requiring alertness or skill. The development of Reye's syndrome characterized by an abrupt onset (shortly following a nonspecific febrile illness) of persistent, severe vomiting, lethargy, irrational behavior, progressive encephalopathy leading to coma, convulsion and death has been associated with the use of this drug. However, its contribution, if any, to the cause and course of the disease has not been established. Before using the drug during pregnancy or lactation, the potential benefits should be weighed against the possible hazards to the mother and child.

Precautions: Should be used cautiously in patients who have recently received other centrally acting drugs (phenothiazines, barbiturates, belladonna derivatives), particularly when these patients have an acute febrile illness, encephalitis, gastroenteritis, electrolyte imbalance or are dehydrated. Severe vomiting should not be treated with antiemetic drugs alone; where possible, the cause of vomiting should be established. Primary emphasis should be focused on restoring body fluids and electrolyte balance, relieving fever and relieving the causative disease process. Overhydration should be avoided since it may result in cerebral edema. The antiemetic effect of this drug may render diagnosis more difficult in such conditions as an acute abdomen, and may obscure the signs of toxicity due to overdosage with other drugs.

Adverse Reactions: Generally noted were hypersensitivity reactions, parkinsonian symptoms, hypotension, blood dyscrasias, blurred vision, coma, convulsions, extrapyramidal symptoms, depressed mood, diarrhea, disorientation, dizziness, drowsiness, headache, jaundice, muscular cramps, opisthotonos, and allergic-type skin reactions which necessitate prompt withdrawal of medication at the first sign of sensitization.

Dosage and Administration: *Orally,* adults, usually 250 mg 3 or 4 times daily. During pregnancy, 250 mg upon arising and again at bedtime; up to 1 gm if needed. Children 30 to 90 lb of body weight, 100 or 200 mg 3 or 4 times daily. *Rectally,* adults, usually 1 suppository 3 or 4 times daily. Children under 30 lb, 1 suppository 3 or 4 times daily; 30 to 90 lb, 1 or 2 suppositories 3 or 4 times daily. Not recommended for use in premature or newborn infants. *Intramuscularly* only, adults, usually 200 mg 3 or 4 times daily. Not recommended for use in children. To avoid the usual reactions to intramuscular administration, injection should be made deep into the upper outer quadrant of the gluteal region.

Availability:
TIGAN®: **(Beecham)**
Capsules, 100 mg in bottles of 100; 250 mg in bottles of 100 and 500.
Injection, 100 mg/ml in ampuls of 2 ml, in multiple-dose vials of 20 ml and in Thera-Ject™ (disposable syringes) of 2 ml.
Rectal Suppositories, 100 mg (pediatric) in cartons of 10; 200 mg in cartons of 10 and 50.

TRIMETHOPRIM with SULFAMETHOXAZOLE

Chemical Name: 2, 4-Diamino-5 (3, 4, 5-trimethoxybenzl) pyrimidine.

Description: Trimethoprim, chemically related to pyrimethamine, is an inhibitor of the enzyme dihydrofolate reductase. It occurs as a white to light yellow, odorless, bitter, crystalline solid with a molecular weight of 290.3. It is a weak base and forms stable salts in a variety of acids, most of which have low water solubility. A 1% aqueous suspension has a pH of 7.5 to 9. It is used in conjunction with sulfonamides in the therapy of chronic urinary tract infections.

When trimethoprim is employed with sulfamethoxazole, the combination interferes with the cellular metabolism of folic acid in the bacterial cell due to the blocking of 2 consecutive steps in the biosynthesis of nucleotides that are essential to many bacteria. *Sulfamethoxazole* inhibits bacterial synthesis of dihydrofolic acid by competing with *para*-aminobenzoic acid and *trimethoprim* binds to and reversibly inhibits the required enzyme, dihydrofolate reductase, thus blocking the production of tetrahydrofolic acid from dihydrofolic acid. In this manner, the combination of these 2 drugs results in a synergism which renders them effective in the treatment of urinary tract infections. In vitro studies have shown that bacterial resistance also develops more slowly when these drugs are used conjunctively than when either one is used alone.

Trimethoprim with sulfamethoxazole has also been found useful in the treatment of *Pneumocystis carinii* pneumonitis in patients who are receiving immunosuppressive cancer chemotherapy. *Pneumocystis carinii* pneumonitis is a serious pulmonary infection usually seen in newborn or debilitated infants and adults with altered immunologic response commonly associated with a malignancy. The incidence of this highly fatal disease has been found to be increased in patients who are immunodeficient, particularly children with acute lymphoblastic leukemia. To date, this drug has been tried only in patients 9 months to 16 years of age, and the recovery rate was reported to be approximately 80%.

Additionally, this combination produces clinically effective results in the treatment of enteritis caused by susceptible strains of *Shigella flexneri* and *Shigella sonnei*.

Following oral administration, the drug is rapidly absorbed from the gastrointestinal tract. Detectable levels of the 2 components appear in the blood in 5 minutes, significant levels within 1 hour and peak levels within 1 to 4 hours. Approximately 40 to 50% of trimethoprim is excreted unchanged in the urine within 24 hours and 80% within 48 hours. About 60% of sulfamethoxazole is also excreted in the urine within 48 hours in both the free and acetylated forms. Excretion is chiefly by the kidney through both glomerular filtration and tubular secretion. Urine concentrations of both drugs are considerably higher than are the concentrations in the blood. Neither component affects the urinary excretion pattern of the other. The half-lives, 10 and 16 hours respectively, are relatively the same regardless of whether these compounds are administered individually or together.

Sulfamethoxazole is present in the blood as free, conjugated and protein-bound forms and trimethoprim as free, protein-bound and metabolized forms. The free forms are considered to be the therapeutically active forms. It has been demonstrated that 44% of trimethoprim and 70% of sulfamethoxazole exists in the protein-bound form. Blood levels of free sulfamethoxazole and trimethoprim are proportionately dose-dependent. On repeated administration, the steady-state ratio of trimethoprim to sulfamethoxazole levels is about 1:20. The presence of 10 mg% sulfamethoxazole in plasma decreases the protein-binding of trimethoprim to an insignificant degree. However, trimethoprim does not influence the protein-binding of sulfamethoxazole.

In reproduction studies in rats, doses of 533 mg/kg of sulfamethoxazole or 200 mg/kg trimethoprim produced teratological effects manifested mainly as cleft palates. The highest dose which did not cause cleft palates in rats was 512 mg/kg sulfamethoxazole or 192 mg/kg trimethoprim when administered separately. In 2 studies with rats, no teratological effects were observed when 512 mg/kg of sulfamethoxazole was used in combination with 128 mg/kg of trimethoprim. However, in one study, cleft palates were observed in 1 litter out of 9 when 355 mg/kg of sulfamethoxazole was used in combination with 88 mg/kg of trimethoprim. When trimethoprim was administered by intubation to rabbits from days 8 to 16 of pregnancy at dosages up to 500 mg/kg, higher incidences of dead and resorbed fetuses were noted, particularly at the 500 mg/kg dose. However, there were no significant drug-related teratological effects.

The drug passes the blood-brain barrier, although the concentration of both drugs is lower than their plasma levels. However, the level is in the range of therapeutic effectiveness.

Indications: Treatment of chronic urinary tract infections manifested by persistent bacteriuria (symptomatic or asymptomatic), frequent recurring infections (relapse or reinfection), or infections associated with urinary tract complications such as obstruction. Primarily for use in pyelonephritis, pyelitis and cystitis due to susceptible organisms (i.e., *E. coli, Klebsiella-Enterobacter, Proteus mirabilis, Proteus vulgaris,* and *Proteus morganii.* **Note: The increasing frequency of resistant organisms limits the usefulness of these agents, especially in the treatment of chronic and recurrent urinary tract infections.** It is also indicated for the treatment of *Pneumocystis carinii* pneumonitis in patients who are receiving immunosuppressive cancer chemotherapy and for acute otitis media in children due to susceptible strains of *Haemophilus influenzae* or *Streptococcus pneumoniae.* The drug is not indicated for prophylactic or prolonged administration in otitis media at any age. It is also recommended for use in the treatment of enteritis caused by susceptible strains of *Shigella flexneri* and *Shigella sonnei.*

Contraindications: Hypersensitivity to either component; in pregnant women and lactating mothers and in infants under 2 months of age.

Warnings: Fatalities associated with the administration of sulfonamides have been reported due to hypersensitivity reactions; agranulocytosis, aplastic anemia, and other blood dyscrasias. Occasionally, trimethoprim has been noted to interfere with hematopoiesis; in elderly patients, who are concurrently receiving diuretics (primarily thiazides), an increased incidence of thrombopenia with purpura has been observed. The development of sore throat, fever, pallor, purpura or jaundice may be early symptoms of serious blood disorders; therefore, complete blood counts should be done frequently in patients receiving this drug. If a significant reduction in the count of any formed blood element is noted, therapy should be discontinued.

Precautions: Cautious use is required in patients with impaired renal or hepatic function, in those with possible folate deficiency, and in those with severe allergy or bronchial asthma. Hemolysis, a reaction which is frequently dose-related, may occur in patients who are deficient in the enzyme glucose-6-phosphate dehydrogenase. The patient should be cautioned to take adequate fluids in order to prevent crystalluria and stone formation. Urinalysis with careful microscopic examination and renal function tests should be performed during therapy, particularly for those patients with impaired renal function.

Adverse Reactions: The following are the major reactions usually noted with the use of sulfonamides or trimethoprim, although they may not be noted when used concomitantly. *Blood dyscrasias:* Agranulocytosis, aplastic anemia, megaloblastic anemia, thrombopenia, leukopenia, hemolytic anemia, purpura, hypoprothrombinemia and methemoglobinemia. *Allergic reactions:* Erythema multiforme, Stevens-Johnson syndrome, generalized skin eruptions, epidermal necrolysis, urticaria, serum sickness, pruritus, exfoliative dermatitis, anaphylactoid reactions, periorbital edema, conjunctival and scleral injection, photosensitization, arthralgia and allergic myocarditis. *Gastrointestinal reactions:* Glossitis, stomatitis, nausea, emesis, abdominal pains, hepatitis, diarrhea and pancreatitis. *CNS reactions:* Headache, peripheral neuritis, mental depression, convulsions, ataxia, hallucinations, tinnitus, vertigo, insomnia, apathy, fatigue, muscle weakness and nervousness. *Miscellaneous reactions:* Drug fever, chills, and toxic nephrosis with oliguria and anuria. Also periarteritis nodosa and L.E. phenomenon have occurred. Although rare, the development of goiter, diuresis, and hypoglycemia have occurred in patients receiving sulfonamides. Cross-sensitivity may exist with these agents.

Dosage and Administration: *Orally.* For urinary tract infections and shigellosis: The usual adult dosage is 2 tablets or 4 teaspoonsful (20 ml) or 1 DS tablet every 12 hours for 10 to 14 days for urinary tract infections and 5 days for shigellosis. The recommended dosage regimen for patients with renal impairment: if the creatinine clearance is above 30 ml/min, the usual standard regimen; if 15 to 30 ml/min, 2 tablets or 4 teaspoonsful (20 ml) or 1 DS tablet every 24 hours; if below 15 ml/min, the drug should not be administered. For *Pneumocystis carinii* pneumonitis: The daily recommended dosage is 20 mg/kg trimethoprim and 100 mg/kg sulfamethoxazole given in equally divided doses every 6 hours for 14 days. Children weighing 36.2 kg (80 lbs) should be given 1 double strength tablet every 6 hours for 14 days. *For otitis media* and *shigellosis:* The dose for children under 12 years of age is calculated according to body weight and is usually 8 mg/kg trimethoprim and 40 mg/kg sulfamethoxazole daily given in 2 divided doses for 10 days for otitis media and 5 days for shigellosis.

Availability:
BACTRIM™: **(Roche)**
Oral Suspension, 40 mg with 200 mg of sulfamethoxazole/5 ml in bottles of 1 pint.
Tablets, 80 mg with 400 mg of sulfamethoxazole in bottles of 100 and 500, in Tel-E-Dose® (unit-dose packages) of 100 and in Prescription Paks (unit-dose packages) of 40 in units of 1 and in trays of 10.
DS Tablets (double-strength), 160 mg with 800 mg of sulfamethoxazole in bottles of 100, in Tel-E-Dose packages of 100 and in Prescription Paks (unit-dose) packages of 100.
SEPTRA®: **(Burroughs Wellcome)**
Oral Suspension, 40 mg with 200 mg of sulfamethoxazole/5 ml in bottles of 450 ml.
Tablets, 80 mg with 400 mg of sulfamethoxazole in bottles of 40, 100, 500 and 1000 and in unit-dose packages of 100 (10 x 10).
DS Tablets (double-strength), 160 mg with 800 mg of sulfamethoxazole in bottles of 60, in unit-dose packages of 100 and in Compliance Pak®s of 20.

TRINSICON

Description: Each Pulvule contains:

Special liver-stomach concentrate (containing intrinsic factor) .... 240 mg

Cobalamin concentrate, N.F.	7.5 μg
(The total vitamin B-12 activity is 15 μg)	
Iron, elemental (as ferrous fumarate)	110 mg
Ascorbic acid (vitamin C)	75 mg
Folic acid	0.5 mg

Trinsicon M differs from Trinsicon only in that it contains no folic acid.

Indications: For anemias treatable with oral hematinics, including pernicious anemia and other megaloblastic anemias and iron-deficiency anemia.

Contraindications: Hemochromatosis and hemosiderosis are contraindications to iron therapy.

Precautions: The use of folic acid without adequate vitamin B-12 therapy in patients with pernicious anemia may result in hematologic remission but neurologic progression. Not all patients with pernicious anemia show satisfactory therapeutic responses to oral vitamin B-12—intrinsic factor preparations. In addition, some patients with an initial good response appear to become refractory to intrinsic factor after varying periods of oral therapy. If resistance develops, parenteral therapy, or oral therapy with massive doses of vitamin B-12 may be necessary for adequate treatment of the patient. Periodic examinations and laboratory studies of pernicious anemia patients are essential and recommended.

Adverse Reactions: In rare instances iron in therapeutic doses may produce gastrointestinal reactions, such as diarrhea or constipation. Reducing the dose and administering it with meals will minimize these effects in iron sensitive patients. Folic acid may cause skin rash suggesting an allergic response. Symptoms of overdosage include pallor and cyanosis, vomiting, hematemesis, diarrhea, melena, shock, drowsiness, and coma. Treatment involves exchange transfusion and chelating agents. For general management, gastric and rectal lavage with sodium bicarbonate solution or milk, administration of intravenous fluids and electrolytes, and the use of oxygen.

Dosage and Administration: *Orally,* 1 pulvule twice daily.

Availability:
TRINSICON® Pulvules® in bottles of 500, in Rx Paks (prescription packages) of 60 and in individual blister packs of 100 (10 × 10). **(Dista)**
TRINSICON® M Pulvules® in Rx Paks of 60. **(Dista)**

TRIOXSALEN

Chemical Name: 6-Hydroxy-β,2,7-trimethyl-5-benzofuranacrylic acid, o-lactone.

Description: Trioxsalen is a synthetic melanizing agent related structurally and pharmacologically to methoxsalen. It occurs as a white to cream-color, crystalline powder very slightly soluble in water and slightly soluble in alcohol.

It is said to increase the production of melanin in the skin when exposed to ultraviolet light. Melanin is formed by the oxidation of tyrosine to DOPA (dihydroxyphenylalanine), with tyrosinase as catalyst. However, this enzymatic reaction must be activated by radiant energy in the form of ultraviolet light, preferably between 2900 and 3800 angstroms (black light). The precise mode of action in the process of melanogenesis is not known; however, it has been suggested that the drug may have a direct effect on the melanocytes themselves, or that an antiinflammatory reaction is the primary response to the drug and that the process of melanogenesis is secondary. Although it possesses greater activity, its median lethal dose is 6 times that of methoxsalen.

Indications: To facilitate repigmentation of idiopathic vitiligo, to increase tolerance to direct sunlight, and to enhance pigmentation.

Contraindications: Those diseases associated with photosensitivity such as porphyria, acute lupus erythematosus, hydroa, polymorphic light eruptions, leukoderma of infectious origin and in albinism. Safe use in children under 12 years of age has not yet been established.

Warnings: Because it is a potent drug, strict adherence to dosage and length of exposure to the sun must be followed in order to prevent serious burning and blistering of the skin. When used to increase tolerance to sunlight or to accelerate tanning, the total dosage should not exceed 28 tablets. These should be taken in single doses of 2 tablets daily on a continuous or intermittent schedule.

Precautions: Photosensitizing preparations, internal or external, should not be used concomitantly with this drug. If overdosage of trioxsalen or overexposure to sunlight occurs, vomiting should be induced and the patients should remain in a darkened room for 8 hours or until cutaneous reactions subside. The treatment of severe reactions resulting from overdosage or overexposure should follow accepted procedures for treatment of severe burns. The physician should warn the patient that the consumption of furocoumarin-containing foods such as limes, figs, parsley, parsnips, mustard, carrots and celery might be dangerous and may contribute to the development of severe reactions.

Adverse Reactions: Occasional gastric discomfort, nausea, nervousness, insomnia or depressed mood. These reactions can be minimized by taking the medication either with milk or after a meal.

Dosage and Administration: *Orally.* Adults and children over 12 years of age, 10 mg taken 2 hours before exposure. Those who cannot tolerate a 10-mg dose will achieve the same therapeutic results with 5 mg, but more slowly. Sunglasses should be worn during exposures and the lips protected with a light-screening lipstick. Suggested exposure guide is available in package literature.

Availability:
TRISORALEN® Tablets, 5 mg in bottles of 28 and 100. **(Elder)**

TRIPELENNAMINE

Chemical Name: 2-[Benzyl(2-dimethylaminoethyl)amino]pyridine.

Description: Tripelennamine is a synthetic, antihistaminic compound of the ethylenediamine type and is classified pharmacologically as a histamine-antagonizing agent. It is available as the citrate and hydrochloride, both of which occur as white, crystalline powders freely soluble in water and in alcohol. Because of the difference in their molecular weights, 30 mg of the citrate is equivalent to 20 mg of the hydrochloride.

Tripelennamine antagonizes most, but not all, of the pharmacological effects of histamine. Antihistaminic effects are noted within 15 to 30 minutes following oral administration and generally last up to 4 to 8 hours depending upon the preparation ingested.

Indications: Symptomatic relief of a variety of allergic disorders responsive to antihistamines, as in perennial and seasonal allergic rhinitis; vasomotor rhinitis; allergic conjunctivitis due to inhalant allergens and foods; mild, uncomplicated allergic skin manifestations of urticaria and angioedema; amelioration of allergic reactions to blood or plasma; dermographism; anaphylactic reactions as adjunctive therapy to epinephrine and other standard measures after the acute manifestations have been controlled. With codeine, it is useful in controlling the cough reflex.

Contraindications: Hypersensitivity to tripelennamine; in premature infants, neonates, or in nursing mothers; patients with narrow-angle glaucoma, stenosing peptic ulcer, symptomatic prostatic hypertrophy, bladder neck obstruction, pyloroduodenal obstruction, lower respiratory tract complications (including asthma), and in those receiving MAO inhibitors.

Warnings: Patients should be cautioned that in the event of drowsiness, they should not operate a motor vehicle or engage in any hazardous occupation requiring alertness or skill, and that the CNS effects of this drug may be additive with those of other CNS depressants such as hypnotics, sedatives, tranquilizers, and antianxiety agents. Histamine antagonizing agents occasionally may produce signs and symptoms of excitation, particularly in children, and are more likely to cause dizziness, sedation, and hypotension in geriatric patients. Safe use of the drug during pregnancy or lactation has not been established; therefore, the expected benefits must be weighed against the potential hazards.

Precautions: Since tripelennamine possesses atropine-like, anticholinergic activity, it should be used with utmost care in patients with increased intraocular pressure, hyperthyroidism, cardiovascular disease, hypertension, or with a history of bronchial asthma. Hallucinations, convulsions and/or death may occur in infants and children receiving excessive doses.

Adverse Reactions: The most frequent side effects observed were sedation and drowsiness; dryness of mouth, nose, and throat; thickening of bronchial secretion; dizziness; disturbed coordination, and epigastric distress. Other reactions which may occur include fatigue; chills; confusion; restlessness; excitation; hysteria; nervousness; irritability, insomnia; euphoria; anorexia; nausea; vomiting; diarrhea; constipation; hypotension; tightness in the chest; wheezing; blurred vision; diplopia; vertigo; tinnitus; convulsion; headache; palpitations; tachycardia; extrasystoles; nasal stuffiness; urinary frequency; difficult urination; urinary retention; hemolytic anemia; leukopenia; thrombocytopenia; agranulocytosis; allergic or hypersensitivity reactions, including drug rash, urticaria, anaphylactic shock, and photosensitivity. Excessive perspiration, tremor, paresthesias, acute labyrinthitis, neuritis, and early menses have been reported to occur with other antihistaminics and may possibly occur with tripelennamine. Overdosage may precipitate acute signs of depression or stimulation or both characterized by hallucinations, ataxia, incoordination, athetosis, and convulsions followed by postictal depression; also dry mouth, fixed dilated pupils, flushing of the face, and fever are common and resemble the syndrome of atropine poisoning. Death may occur following deep coma and cardiovascular collapse. Since there is no specific therapy to counteract acute overdosage, general symptomatic and supportive measures should be instituted promptly and maintained for as long as required.

Dosage and Administration: *Orally.* Usual dosage for adults is 25 to 50 mg every 4 to 6 hours, but doses may range from 25 to 600 mg daily. For infants and children, 5 mg/kg/day up to a maximum, but not exceeding, 300 mg daily divided into 4 to 6 doses. Longtabs: For adults, 2 tablets in the morning and 2 tablets in the evening are generally adequate for daily protection. For children, 1 tablet in the morning and 1 tablet in the evening, although some children may require 1 tablet every 8 hours. *Tablets with ephedrine:* Adults, 1 or 2 tablets every 4 hours; older children, 1 tablet 4 times daily. *Expectorant with codeine or ephedrine:* Adults, 1 or 2 teaspoonsful; children, 1/2 to 1 teaspoonful every 3 or 4 hours.

Availability:

Tripelennamine Citrate

PYRIBENZAMINE®: **(Ciba)**

Elixir, 30 mg/4 ml in bottles of 1 pint.

Ⓒ *Expectorant with Codeine,* 30 mg/4 ml with codeine phosphate, 8 mg; ephedrine sulfate, 10 mg and ammonium chloride, 80 mg in bottles of 1 pint.

Expectorant with Ephedrine, 30 mg/4 ml with ephedrine sulfate, 10 mg and ammonium chloride, 80 mg in bottles of 1 pint.

Tripelennamine Hydrochloride

PBZ-SR™ Tablets (sustained-release), 100 mg in bottles of 100. **(Ciba)**

PYRIBENZAMINE®: **(Ciba)**

Lontabs® (long-acting tablets), 50 mg in bottles of 100.

Tablets, 25 mg in bottles of 100; 50 mg in bottles of 100 and 1000.

Tablets with Ephedrine, 25 mg with ephedrine sulfate, 12 mg in bottles of 100.

TRIPROLIDINE HYDROCHLORIDE

Chemical Name: trans-2-[3-(1-Pyrrolidinyl)-1-*p*-tolylpropenyl]pyridine hydrochloride.

Description: Triprolidine is an antihistamine related structurally to the diarylpropylamine group including pheniramine, pyrrobutamine, chlorpheniramine and brompheniramine. It occurs as a bitter, white, crystalline powder freely soluble in water and in alcohol.

The drug resembles chlorpheniramine pharmacologically. In addition to its antihistaminic properties, it exhibits local anesthetic and slight anticholinergic activity. Following oral ingestion, its onset of action is relatively rapid; effects are discernible within 30 minutes, reach their peak in about 3 to 4 hours, and persist for about 12 hours.

Indications: May be of use in the symptomatic treatment of seasonal and perennial allergic rhinitis and vasomotor rhinitis, allergic conjunctivitis, mild uncomplicated allergic skin manifestations of urticaria and angioedema, and for the amelioration and prevention of allergic reactions to blood or plasma in patients with a known history of such reactions. Combined with a decongestant and a stimulating expectorant, it is useful for the prophylaxis and treatment of symptoms associated with the common cold including cough, acute bronchitis, allergic asthma, bronchiolitis, croup, emphysema or tracheobronchitis.

Contraindications: Hypersensitivity to any of the components.

Warnings: Safe use in pregnant women has not been established.

Precautions: Although pseudoephedrine is virtually free of pressor effects in normotensive individuals, caution is advisable in patients with hypertension. Despite its low incidence of drowsiness, patients taking triprolidine should be cautioned to postpone engaging in hazardous activities requiring alertness or skill.

Adverse Reactions: Only certain patients, sensitive to one or another of the components, may experience mild stimulation or sedation or drowsiness.

Dosage and Administration: *Orally,* 2 or 3 times daily. *Actidil:* adults, 2.5 mg; children over 2 years of age, 1.25 mg; infants, 0.6 mg. *Actifed:* adults and older children, 1 tablet or 2 teaspoonsful; children 4 months through 6 years of age, 1/2 tablet or 1 teaspoonful; infants up to 4 months, 1/2 teaspoonful. These doses may be given 3 or 4 times daily. *Actifed-C:* adults and children over 12 years of age, 2 teaspoonsful; children 7 to 12 years, 1 teaspoonful; children 2 to 6 years, 1/2 teaspoonful. These doses may be given 4 times daily, or 1/2 the recommended dose may be given every 3 hours. The *Expectorant* should not be given to children under 2 years of age.

Availability:

Triprolidine Hydrochloride

ACTIDIL®: **(Burroughs Wellcome)**
Syrup, 1.25 mg/5 ml in bottles of 1 pint.
Tablets, 2.5 mg in bottles of 100.

Combinations:

ACTIFED®: **(Burroughs Wellcome)**
Syrup, 1.25 mg/5 ml with pseudoephedrine, 30 mg in bottles of 120 ml and 1 pint.
Tablets, 2.5 mg with pseudoephedrine hydrochloride, 60 mg in bottles of 20, 30, 100 and 1000 and in unit-dose packages of 100.

Ⓒ ACTIFED-C® Expectorant in bottles of 1 pint. Each 5 ml (teaspoonful) contains triprolidine hydrochloride, 2 mg; codeine phosphate, 10 mg (**Warning:** May be habit-forming); pseudoephedrine hydrochloride, 30 mg and guaifenesin, 100 mg. **(Burroughs Wellcome)**

ELDEFED Tablets, 2.5 mg with pseudoephedrine hydrochloride, 60 mg in bottles of 1000. **(Elder)**

TROLEANDOMYCIN

Description: Troleandomycin is a synthetically derived acetylated ester of oleandomycin, an antibiotic elaborated by a species of *Streptomyces antibioticus.* It is related chemically and in antibacterial activity to the erythromycins, since these compounds contain a large lactone ring in their molecular structure. It occurs as a white, crystalline compound that is insoluble in water, but readily soluble and stable in the presence of gastric juice. It has a molecular weight of 814.

Troleandomycin has been shown to be active in vitro against the following gram-positive organisms: *Staphylococcus pyogenes* and *Diplococcus pneumoniae.* If the Kirby-Bauer method of disc sensitivity is used, a 15 mcg oleandomycin disc should give a zone of over 18 mm when tested against a troleandomycin-sensitive bacterial strain.

Indications: Treatment of acute, severe infections caused by susceptible strains of pneumococcal pneumonia and group alpha- and beta-hemolytic streptococcal infections of the upper respiratory tract. Troleandomycin has also been found to be effective in the eradication of streptococci from the nasopharynx. However, its effectiveness in the subsequent prevention of rheumatic fever has not been established.

Contraindications: In patients with known hypersensitivity to the drug.

Warnings: Safe use during pregnancy has not been established. The use of this antibiotic should be limited to those infections in which sensitivity testing proves them resistant to other less toxic antibiotics. Liver function should be evaluated periodically during the course of therapy. When administered for 2 weeks or more, or in repeated courses, disturbances of liver function were manifested by jaundice accompanied by right upper quadrant pain, fever, nausea, vomiting, eosinophilia, and leukocytosis. These symptoms have been reversible when the drug was discontinued. Concurrent use of ergotamine-containing preparations may induce ischemic reactions and should therefore be avoided. Simultaneous use with theophylline may result in elevated serum concentrations of theophylline; therefore, asthmatic patients should be observed for signs of toxicity, and therapy should be appropriately modified if such signs develop.

Precautions: Since troleandomycin is principally excreted by the liver, caution should be exercised in administering this antibiotic to patients with impaired hepatic function.

Adverse Reactions: The most frequent side effects are gastrointestinal manifested by abdominal cramping and discomfort. Less frequently noted were nausea, vomiting, and diarrhea. During prolonged or repeated therapy, there is the possibility of overgrowth of nonsusceptible bacteria or fungi. Mild allergic reactions such as urticaria and other skin rashes have been reported. Also, an anaphylactoid reaction in a hypersensitive individual may occur.

Dosage and Administration: *Orally.* Adult dosage ranges from 250 to 500 mg 4 times daily. When used in streptococcal infections, therapy should be continued for 10 days to prevent the development of rheumatic fever or glomerulonephritis. The usual pediatric dosage ranges from 125 to 250 mg (3 to 5 mg/lb or 6.6 to 11 mg/kg of body weight) every 6 hours.

Availability:
TAO®: **(Roerig)**
Capsules, 250 mg in bottles of 100.
Oral Suspension, 125 mg/5 ml in bottles of 60 ml and 1 pint.

TROMETHAMINE

Chemical Name: 2-Amino-2-(hydroxymethyl)-1,3-propanediol.

Description: Tromethamine, an organic amine proton receptor, occurs as a white, crystalline solid that is very soluble in water.

When administered intravenously, the drug becomes a component of the body's buffering system. It acts as a proton acceptor and prevents or corrects acidosis by actively binding hydrogen ions (H^+). It binds not only cations of fixed or metabolic acids, but also hydrogen ions of carbonic acid, thus increasing bicarbonic anion (HCO_3^-). It also acts as an osmotic diuretic, increasing urine flow, urinary pH, and excretion of fixed acids, carbon dioxide and electrolytes. Potassium and sodium chloride have been added to the lyophilized tromethamine to correct the loss of these electrolytes by diuresis. A significant fraction of tromethamine (30% at pH 7.4) is not ionized and therefore is capable of reaching equilibrium in total body fluids. This portion may penetrate cells and may neutralize acidic ions of the intracellular fluid.

Tromethamine is rapidly eliminated by the kidneys with 75% or more appearing in the urine after 8 hours. Urinary excretion usually continues over a period of 3 days.

Indications: Prevention and correction of systemic acidosis such as the metabolic acidosis associated with cardiac bypass surgery, correction of acidity of ACD blood in cardiac bypass surgery, and the metabolic acidosis associated with cardiac arrest.

Contraindications: In anuria and uremia.

Warnings: Individually adjusted dosage is necessary to avoid increasing the blood pH above normal limits; and to prevent alkalosis and potential hypoglycemia. Care must be exercised to prevent perivascular infiltration which can cause tissue irritation. Venospasm and intravenous thrombosis may occur during infusion. Use with caution in patients with reduced urinary output or with renal disease because of potential hyperkalemia. Except in dire situations, the solution should not be given for more than one day. Blood pH, pCO_2, bicarbonate, glucose, and electrolyte determination should be performed before, during and following administration of the solution. Its effect upon fetal development has not been established clinically or in animals.

Precautions: Although not noted clinically, the drug has been reported to increase coagulation time in studies with dogs. Hypoglycemia may occur when administered to premature or full-term infants.

Adverse Reactions: Generally, complications have been infrequent and of minor consequence. Transient hypoglycemia may occur. Respiratory depression may result from excessive dosage in patients who have chronic hypoventilation or in those who have been treated with drugs which depress respiration. In patients with associated respiratory acidosis, tromethamine should be administered with mechanical ventilation.

Dosage and Administration: *Intravenously.* The average dose is the least amount required to increase the blood pH to normal limits (7.35 to 7.45). To correct systemic acidosis during cardiac surgery, the average single dose is 9 ml/kg (324 mg) with an average total dose of 500 ml. Larger single doses (up to 1000 ml) may be required in unusually severe cases. When given to correct the acidity of ACD priming blood, from 15 to 77 ml should be added for each 500 ml of blood—although 60 ml added to 500 ml of ADC blood usually is adequate. In cardiac arrest, the solution should be administered simultaneously with other standard resuscitative measures, including manual systole. Doses ranging from approximately 3.5 to 6 ml/kg of body weight have been employed for injection into a peripheral vein. Additional amounts may be required to control systemic acidosis persisting after cardiac arrest is reversed. It has been suggested that repeated determinations of pH and other clinical observations should be used as a guide to the need for repeat doses.

Availability:
THAM Solution, 0.3 M in single-dose (Abbo-Vac®) containers of 500 ml each containing 18 gm (150 mEq) of tromethamine and 3 gm (50 mEq) of acetic acid. **(Abbott)**
THAM-E™ Lyophilized Powder (anhydrous) in Non-Vac® single-dose containers of 150 ml each containing 36 gm of tromethamine, 1.75 gm of sodium chloride and 0.37 gm of potassium chloride. **(Abbott)**

TROPICAMIDE

Chemical Name: *N*-Ethyl-2-phenyl-*N*-(4-pyridylmethyl)hydracrylamide.

Description: Tropicamide is a parasympatholytic drug derived from tropic acid. It occurs as a white, crystalline powder slightly soluble in water and soluble in acid solution. Maximal mydriasis and cycloplegia is reached in about 20 to 25 minutes, persisting for about 20 minutes, followed by a rapid return to normal.

Indications: As a mydriatic and cycloplegic in diagnostic procedures. The 1% solution can be used in cases where cycloplegia is desired; for mydriasis alone, the 0.5% solution is adequate.

Contraindications: Hypersensitivity or idiosyncrasy to the drug, and in patients with known or suspected glaucoma.

Precautions: Tropicamide has virtually no tendency to increase intraocular pressure, but as with any mydriatic, it should be used cautiously in patients in whom the pressure is not known, or in those in whom the pressure is high or the anterior chamber is shallow.

Adverse Reactions: Tropicamide has rarely caused systemic reactions.

Dosage and Administration: *Topically. For mydriasis,* instill 1 or 2 drops of the 0.5% solution; may be repeated every 30 minutes if necessary. To speed recovery from mydriasis, a miotic such as pilocarpine may be used. *For cycloplegia,* instill 1 or 2 drops of the 1% solution, repeat in 5 minutes. The examination must be performed no later than 30 minutes after the second instillation.

Availability:
MYDRIACYL® Ophthalmic Solution, 0.5 and 1% in Drop-Tainer® bottles of 15 ml. **(Alcon)**

TUBERCULIN, OLD

Description: Old Tuberculin is a sterile solution of the concentrated, soluble products of growth of the tubercle bacillus (*Mycobacterium tuberculosis*) adjusted to standard potency by addition of glycerin and isotonic sodium chloride solution. Its final glycerin content is approximately 50%. Old Tuberculin, in diluted form, suitable for injection is prepared in a buffered diluent.

A positive test consists of an area of inflammation with a definitely palpable induration or edema, the latter measuring at least 5 mm in diameter. It usually appears in 6 to 8 hours, reaches its maximum in 24 to 48 hours, and disappears in 6 to 10 days. To differentiate it from a nonspecific reaction, the tuberculin test should be read 48 to 72 hours after the injection is made. Even in the presence of tuberculosis, the skin test may not be positive in patients who are moribund, recovering from measles, or receiving adrenal corticosteroids or other immunosuppressive agents.

Indications: As a skin test in the diagnosis of past or present tuberculosis.

Adverse Reactions: Highly sensitive individuals may experience vesiculation, ulceration, or necrosis at the test site which may be accompanied by pain, pruritus, and discomfort; these can usually be relieved by applying cold packs or a topical glucocorticoid ointment or cream. Transient bleeding may be observed at the puncture site, but this has no significance on interpretation of the test.

Dosage and Administration: For the Mantoux test, 0.1 ml of the desired dilution is administered *intracutaneously* in the flexor surface of the forearm. Readings are usually made after an interval of 48 hours. A positive test consists of a papule at least 5 mm in diameter surrounded by an erythematous area. For the tine test, the 4 impregnated tines should be applied to the forearm for 1 second. Sufficient pressure should be exerted so that the 4 puncture sites and a circular depression of the skin from the plastic base are visable. Readings are usually made after an interval of 48 to 72 hours. A positive reaction consists of a palpable induration of 2 mm or more around 1 or more puncture sites, and is clinically comparable to a zone of 5 mm or more as that produced by the Mantoux test.

Availability:
TUBERCULIN, OLD, TINE TEST® (Rosenthal) with OLD TUBERCULIN in packages of 5 and jars of 25 tests; 100 tests with induration indicator cards and bin packages of 250 individual tests. **(Lederle)**
TUBERCULIN, OLD, HUMAN for Mantoux Test in vials of 1 mg (10 tests) with vial of diluent. **(Lilly)**

TUBERCULIN, PURIFIED PROTEIN DERIVATIVE (P.P.D.)

Description: An aqueous solution of the active principle of tuberculin is a highly purified protein fraction isolated from the culture filtrates of human-type strains of *Mycobacterium tuberculosis.* It is prepared by the F.B. Siebert method, stabilized with polysorbate 80, buffered with potassium and sodium phosphates and is preserved with phenol. It is equivalent in potency to standard tuberculin PPD-S of the U.S. Public Health Service and the National Center for Disease Control. Each 0.1 ml provides 5 TU and is ready for immediate use without further dilution.

The test is read 48 to 72 hours after administration of the tuberculin. Sensitivity is indicated by induration, usually accompanied by erythema. Any palpable induration measuring 10 mm or over is considered to be a positive reaction. *All positive tuberculin test results must be verified by further diagnostic tests.*

Indications: A test agent for the diagnosis of tuberculosis.

Warnings: Inadvertent subcutaneous injection of the test dose may produce a general febrile reaction and/or an acute inflammation around old tuberculous lesions without the development of a local reaction. The syringe used for tuberculin should not be used for histoplasmin, blastomycin, or other materials. A separate unit should be used for each patient in order to prevent possible transmission of homologous serum hepatitis virus and other infectious agents from one individual to another.

Precautions: Epinephrine and other supportive measures should be immediately available in the event of an anaphylactoid or acute hypersensitivity reaction. Sensitivity may decrease or disappear temporarily during or immediately following severe febrile illness; measles and other exanthemas; live virus vaccination; and the administration of corticosteroids or immunosuppressive drugs, or in the presence of severe malnutrition.

Adverse Reactions: Highly sensitive individuals may experience a strong positive reaction, including vesiculation, ulceration or necrosis with possible scarring at the test site. Cold packs or topical steroid preparations may be employed for symptomatic relief of the associated pain, pruritus and discomfort. Slight bleeding may occur at the puncture site, but this does not affect interpretation of the test.

Dosage and Administration: *Intradermally* into the flexor surface of the forearm. Inject 0.1 ml of the solution; or apply the Aplitest unit to the test area with sufficient pressure to assure that all 4 tines have penetrated the skin and hold for about 1 second. If results are positive, an induration of 10 mm or more will develop. An induration of less than 5 mm indicates a lack of hypersensitivity to the tuberculoprotein and tuberculous infection is highly unlikely. Induration only is considered in interpreting the test.

Availability:
APLISOL® Solution (diluted) in vials of 1 ml (10 tests) and 5 ml (50 tests) and in Aplitest® (multiple puncture device) of 25 tests in packages of 5 stacks of 5 units and in dispensing packages of 25 individually capped units. **(Parke-Davis)**

TUBOCURARINE

Description: *Tubocurarine chloride* is a curare alkaloid extracted from the plant *Chondodendron tomentosum.* It occurs as white or yellowish-white to grayish-white, odorless, crystals soluble in water and sparingly soluble in alcohol. The sterile isotonic solution for injection is so standardized that each ml contains an amount of crystalline alkaloid equivalent to 20 units, or 3 mg, of tubocurarine chloride.

Dimethyl tubocurarine iodide, the dimethyl ether of *d*-tubocurarine iodide, is similar in action and uses to tubocurarine chloride. It occurs as an odorless, white or pale yellow, crystalline powder slightly soluble in water and very slightly soluble in alcohol. The iodide differs from the chloride in that it produces respiratory paralysis less frequently and it has a longer duration of action. Clinically, the ratio of potency of the iodide to the chloride is about 3:1

Tubocurarine is a nondepolarizing skeletal muscle relaxant. It competes with acetylcholine at the cholinergic receptors of the skeletal muscle endplate and prevents acetylcholine-induced changes in permeability of the myoneural membrane and development of the electric potential, thereby inhibiting neuromuscular transmission and causing flaccid paralysis of all skeletal muscles. Its action commences within seconds following intravenous injection, reaches a peak within 2 to 3 minutes and usually lasts for 25 to 90 minutes. Substantial amounts of injected tubocurarine may be retained in various organs of the body long after the neuromuscular block appears to have dissipated. The drug is slowly and only partly metabolized, most of it being eliminated unchanged in the urine.

Tubocurarine has no known effect on consciousness, the pain threshold or cerebration; or any direct action on the myocardium. Hypotension may ensue due to a histamine release, or ganglionic blockade, or to the effects of concomitant positive pressure respiration. Tubocurarine has no direct effect on the uterus or other smooth muscle structures. It readily crosses the placental barrier and neonates are especially sensitive to the drug.

Indications: The chloride and iodide share the same actions and uses. They are indicated whenever it is desirable to provide skeletal muscle relaxation as in surgery. They are valuable adjuncts to anesthesia and are useful in softening the convulsions induced in electroconvulsive therapy. The chloride, in addition, is used to treat spastic states in children. Because it aggravates the symptoms of myasthenia gravis, tubocurarine is also used as a diagnostic measure in this disease. It may also be employed to facilitate the management of patients undergoing mechanical ventilation.

Contraindications: In patients who are hypersensitive to tubocurarine, and in those in whom a histamine release is a definite hazard.

Warnings: Tubocurarine is a potent drug, and serious consequences may result if it is used other than under constant medical supervision. Dosage must be carefully adjusted and administered by clinicians who are familiar with its actions and the possible complications that might occur following its use. Prolonged apnea with its attendant hazards due to hypoxia may result from overdosage. Therefore, the drug should not be administered unless facilities for intubation, artificial respiration, oxygen therapy, and antidotes are instantaneously available. The clinician must be prepared to assist or control respiration. Cautious use is advised in patients with myasthenia gravis. The administration of quinidine during the postoperative recovery period to patients who have received this drug may result in recurarization which can progress to respiratory paralysis. It should not be administered to women of childbearing potential and particularly during early pregnancy, unless in the judgment of the physician, the therapeutic benefits outweigh the potential hazards to the fetus.

Precautions: This drug should be used with caution in patients with impaired cardiovascular, renal, hepatic, or pulmonary function; large doses may cause hypotension. The drug accumulates in body tissues and may be present in some quantity for several hours after the effects are not clinically apparent. This should be kept in mind should a patient require successive doses or a second anesthesia after having previously received this drug. The action of tubocurarine may be altered by electrolyte imbalance (hypokalemia potentiates the paralysis), abnormal states (acidosis), neuromuscular disease, renal disease, aminoglycoside antibiotics, thiobarbiturates, narcotic analgesics, droperidol, or prior administration of succinylcholine, and by certain anesthetic agents such as ether, enflurane, methoxyflurane, halothane, and, to a lesser extent, cyclopropane (the effects of ethylene and nitrous oxide are negligible). The possibility that diazepam also may potentiate the intensity and duration of neuromuscular block produced by tubocurarine has been reported. Since the drug readily crosses the placental barrier, utmost caution is required in obstetric usage.

Adverse Reactions: These consist primarily in the extension of the drug's pharmacologic actions. Overdosage may cause temporary respiratory paralysis. Idiosyncrasy, interference with physical signs of anesthesia, circulatory depression, ganglionic blockade, and the release of histamine are complications that can result from the use of tubocurarine.

Dosage and Administration: Iodide: *intravenously* over a period of 15 to 30 seconds. The type of anesthetic used will influence the size of the initial dose; dosage may range from 1.5 to 7 mg. Relaxation following the initial dose may be expected to be effective for periods of 25 to 90 minutes, with a mean average of about 1 hour. Supplemental injections of 0.5 to 1 mg may be made as required and indicated by the depth of relaxation. In electroconvulsive therapy the doses required range from 1.75 to 5.5 mg. **Chloride:** *intramuscularly* or *intravenously*, injected over a period of 60 to 90 seconds. The package literature should be consulted for specific details.

Availability:

Tubocurarine Chloride

Injection, 3 mg/ml in multiple-dose vials of 10 and 20 ml; 15 mg/ml in ampuls of 1 ml. **(Abbott)**
Injection, 3 mg/ml in multiple-dose ampuls of 10 ml. **(Lilly)**
Injection, 3 mg/ml in multiple-dose vials of 10 and 20 ml. **(Squibb)**

Dimethyl Tubocurarine Iodide

METUBINE® IODIDE Injection, 2 mg/ml in multiple-dose ampuls of 20 ml. **(Lilly)**

TUSSAMINIC

Description: Each tablet contains:

Phenylpropanolamine hydrochloride	50 mg
Pheniramine maleate	25 mg
Pyrilamine maleate	25 mg
Dextromethorphan hydrobromide	30 mg
Terpin hydrate	300 mg

Indications: Relief of cough and nasal congestion due to the common cold, nasal allergies, sinusitis, and postnasal drip.

Precautions: Since drowsiness may occur, patients should be cautioned not to engage in activities requiring alertness or mechanical coordination such as driving a motor vehicle. Routine caution is advised in the presence of hypertension, hyperthyroidism, cardiovascular disorders, or diabetes.

Adverse Reactions: Occasionally observed were drowsiness, blurred vision, cardiac palpitations, flushing, dizziness, nervousness, and gastrointestinal upsets.

Dosage and Administration: *Orally.* The usual adult dosage is 1 tablet 3 times daily (morning, midafternoon and at bedtime). *Tablets should be swallowed whole.*

Availability:
TUSSAMINIC® Tablets (timed-release, green) in bottles of 50. **(Dorsey)**

TUSSI-ORGANIDIN Ⓒ

Description: Each 5 ml of expectorant contains codeine phosphate, 10 mg; chlorpheniramine maleate, 2 mg and iodinated glycerol, 30 mg (equiv. to 15 mg organically-bound iodine) and alcohol, 15% in a sugar-free vehicle. The **DM expectorant** contains the same amounts of ingredients except that dextromorphan hydrobromide is substituted for the codeine phosphate. Combines sedative, antihistaminic and mucolytic action to provide antitussive effects. It acts by suppressing irritating, nonproductive cough and promoting easy expectoration. Tenacious mucus is mobilized by increased drainage of respiratory exudates.

Indications: Symptomatic treatment of coughs due to bronchitis, bronchial asthma, tracheobronchitis, emphysema and the common cold. Also relieves coughs due to laryngitis, pharyngitis, pertussis and croup.

Contraindications: Patients with marked sensitivity to iodides or to any of the components or related compounds.

Warnings: Codeine phosphate may be habit-forming. The drug should be withdrawn if a rash or other evidence of hypersensitivity appears. Since the antihistaminic component may produce various degrees of drowsiness, patients should be cautioned not to engage in potentially hazardous activities requiring alertness or skill, such as operating a motor vehicle, until their response to the drug has been determined. The CNS effects of antihistamines and alcohol or other CNS depressants (hypnotic, sedatives, tranquilizers) may be enhanced.

Precautions: Antihistamines may cause excitation, particularly in children and the elderly. Chronic use of inorganic iodides may cause dermatitis and other reversible manifestations of iodism, particularly in patients sensitive to iodine. Also, preparations containing iodine have been found to interfere with laboratory determinations of PBI.

Adverse Reactions: Gastrointestinal irritation, rash, drowsiness, sedation, dry mouth, nausea, restlessness, drying of mucous membranes, dizziness, headache, heartburn, dysuria, polyuria, visual disturbances, excitation (particularly in children), vomiting, constipation, and miosis. Extremely high doses of dextromorphan may precipitate respiratory depression.

Dosage and Administration: *Orally,* Adults, 1 to 2 teaspoonsful and children, ½ to 1 teaspoonful every 4 hours.

Availability:
Ⓒ TUSSI-ORGANIDIN® Expectorant in bottles of 1 pint and 1 gallon. **(Wallace)**
TUSSI-ORGANIDIN-DM Expectorant in bottles of 1 pint. **(Wallace)**

TUSS-ORNADE

Description: Each Spansule and each 5 ml (teaspoonful) of liquid contains:

	Spansule	*Liquid*
Caramiphen edisylate	20 mg	5 mg
Chlorpheniramine maleate	8 mg	2 mg
Phenylpropanolamine hydrochloride	50 mg	15 mg
Isopropamide iodide*	2.5 mg	0.75 mg

*Released from Spansule immediately upon ingestion.

Indications: Relief of coughing, upper respiratory tract congestion and hypersecretion associated with the common cold, sinusitis, vasomotor and allergic rhinitis.

Contraindications: Hypersensitivity to any of the components, concurrent therapy with MAO inhibitors, severe hypertension, bronchial asthma, coronary artery disease, stenosing peptic ulcer, pyloroduodenal or urinary bladder neck obstruction. The Spansule should not be given to children under 12 years of age.

Warnings: Patients should be cautioned that in the event of drowsiness, they should not operate a motor vehicle or engage in any hazardous occupation requiring alertness or physical coordination. Patients should also be cautioned about the additive effects of alcohol and other CNS-depressant drugs. Safe use during pregnancy has not been established; therefore, the drug should be used during pregnancy, in nursing mothers or in women of childbearing potential only when its potential benefits have been weighed against the possible hazards to mother and child. As with all anticholinergic agents, an inhibitory effect on lactation may occur.

Precautions: Use cautiously in the presence of cardiovascular disorders, hyperthyroidism, glaucoma, and prostatic hypertrophy. The iodine in isopropamide iodide may alter PBI determination, and will suppress radioactive iodine uptake. Therefore, thyroid function tests unaffected by exogenous iodides should be employed.

Adverse Reactions: Drowsiness; excessive dryness of nose, mouth, or throat; nervousness; insomnia; epigastric distress; nausea; vomiting; diarrhea; rash; dizziness; weakness; tightness of chest; anginal pain; abdominal pain; irritability; palpitation; headache; incoordination; tremor; difficulty in urination; dysuria; thrombocytopenia; leukopenia; convulsions; hypertension; hypotension; anorexia, constipation, and visual disturbances have been reported. Isopropamide iodide may cause signs of iodide toxicity such as acne and parotitis. Symptoms of overdosage may include dryness of mouth, dysphagia, thirst, blurred vision, mydriasis, photophobia, fever, rapid pulse and/or respiration, disorientation, dizziness, nausea, fainting, tachycardia, and either CNS excitation or depression. Treatment is symptomatic and supportive and consists of gastric lavage, oxygen, and CNS stimulants or depressants.

Dosage and Administration: *Orally.* Spansules: Adults and children over 12 years of age, 1 capsule every 12 hours. Liquid: Adults and children over 12 years of age, 1 to 2 teaspoonsful; children over 25 lbs, 1 teaspoonful; children 15 to 25 lbs, ½ teaspoonful; dosage may be repeated every 3 to 4 hours. Not recommended for children under 15 lbs or less than 6 months of age.

Availability:
TUSS-ORNADE®: **(Smith Kline & French)**
Liquid in bottles of 1 pint. *Contains 7.5% alcohol.*
Spansules® (sustained-release capsule) in bottles of 50 and 500.

TYBAMATE

Chemical Name: Carbamate of 2-(hydroxymethyl)-2-methylpentyl ester of butylcarbamic acid.

Description: Tybamate is a CNS depressant related structurally and pharmacologically to meprobamate, mebutamate and carisoprodol. It occurs as a white, crystalline powder very slightly soluble in water and soluble in alcohol.

Tybamate is a tranquilizing agent which acts subcortically to stabilize emotional circuits through an effect on the hippocampal and limbic structures of the brain.

Indications: For the symptomatic improvement in a variety of psychoneurotic disorders, especially in the treatment of the anxiety and tension components of psychoneuroses. Anxiety states manifested somatically have responded to the drug. Tybamate has been useful in controlling agitation in the elderly and in alleviating some of the adverse emotional problems accompanying senility. The drug has also been of benefit in the treatment of depressive symptoms associated with anxiety and other symptoms of psychoneuroses. However, it is not indicated for primary treatment of depressive states. It is not an antipsychotic agent, although it has been used as adjunctive therapy in some psychotic patients.

Contraindications: Acute intermittent porphyria as well as allergic or idiosyncratic reactions to the drug or to related compounds.

Warnings: Patients should be cautioned that this drug may impair the mental and/or physical abilities required for the performance of potentially hazardous tasks such as driving a motor vehicle or operating machinery. Simultaneous administration to psychotic patients of tybamate with phenothiazines and other CNS-depressant agents has in a few instances been associated with the occurrence of grand mal or petit mal seizures. Although not reported to have occurred with the administration of tybamate alone; nonetheless, the drug should be used cautiously in individuals who are receiving other CNS depressants or who have a history of convulsive seizures. Also, it should be borne in mind that the concomitant administration of this drug with alcohol or with other psychotropic agents, particularly phenothiazines or MAO inhibitors, which are known to potentiate the action of other drugs, may result in additive effects. Safe use in pregnant or lactating women and in children under 6 years of age has not been established.

Precautions: The lowest effective dose should be administered, particularly to elderly and/or debilitated patients, in order to preclude oversedation. It should also be kept in mind that discontinuing the drug after prolonged use may result in withdrawal symptoms; abrupt withdrawal should therefore be avoided. As with other psychotherapeutic agents, tybamate should be used cautiously in addiction-prone individuals. The possibility of suicide attempts should be considered and the least amount of the drug should be dispensed at any one time. Since the drug is metabolized in the liver and excreted by the kidney it is therefore essential that caution be exercised in patients with compromised liver or kidney function to avoid its excess accumulation in the system.

Adverse Reactions: Reports have included drowsiness, fatigue, dizziness, vertigo, ataxia, depressive reaction, confusion, panic reaction, insomnia, euphoria, hyperactivity, paresthesias, headache, and grand mal or petit mal seizures; urticaria, pruritus, skin rash; flushing, tachycardia, hypotension, and syncope, nausea, anorexia, dry mouth, and glossitis. Overdosage may be characterized by stupor, coma, shock, respiratory depression; and death may result from acute toxic doses.

Dosage and Administration: *Orally.* Adults: 250 or 500 mg 3 or 4 times daily or 350 mg 3 times daily and 700 mg at bedtime. Children 6 to 12 years of age, 20 to 35 mg/kg of body weight in 3 or 4 equally divided doses is suggested. Not recommended for children under 6 years of age. A daily dosage in excess of 3 gm is not recommended.

Availability:
TYBATRAN® Capsules, 250 and 350 mg in bottles of 100 and 500. **(Robins)**

TYLOXAPOL

Chemical Name: Oxyethylated tertiary octylphenol formaldehyde polymer.

Description: Tyloxapol is a nonionic surfactant with detergent properties. The drug facilitates expectoration by lowering the surface tension and reducing the viscosity of thick, tenacious sputum. It occurs as a pure, viscous, amber-color liquid which is slowly but freely soluble in water. Solutions of tyloxapol are compatible with penicillin and with streptomycin but are incompatible with the tetracyclines.

Indications: Treatment of patients with diseases and disorders of the lung accompanied or complicated by the presence of excessive or thickened bronchopulmonary secretions, in chronic pulmonary disease or in any condition in which the normal mechanism for the elimination of secretions is diminished or absent. Also aids in the removal of troublesome secretions which may be associated with general anesthesia, thoracic surgical procedures, tracheotomy, inhalation of noxious gases or dust and aspiration of foreign material or gastric contents. Its value in the treatment of hyaline membrane disease in infants has not been determined. Concurrent use with antituberculous agents in patients with tuberculosis should be considered in order to avoid spread of the disease.

Precautions: As with all aerosols, the possibility of bronchial asthma occurring in certain asthmatic patients should be considered. The product does not contain an antiseptic preservative; therefore, if the entire contents of the bottle has not been administered, the unused portion should be kept no longer than 2 or 3 days.

Adverse Reactions: Prolonged use may irritate the respiratory tract.

Dosage and Administration: *Inhalation:* Should be administered full strength by an aerosol nebulizer delivering a fine mist. The nebulizer is attached to an oxygen supply tank or suitable air compressor. The rate of gas flow to the nebulizer will depend on the type used; most nebulizers deliver from 2 to 12 liters/minute. The vapor may be inhaled directly from the nebulizer, by means of a face mask, or it may be delivered into an open top tent, croup tent, incubator or special tent. For full details on administration, see package literature.

Availability:
ALEVAIRE® Solution, 0.125%, with sodium bicarbonate, 2% and glycerin, 5% in bottles of 60 and 500 ml. **(Breon)**

TYMPAGESIC

Description: Contains phenylephrine hydrochloride, 0.25%, antipyrine, 5%, benzocaine, 5% in propylene glycol.

Indications: To relieve pain and reduce swelling in acute nonsuppurative otitis media as well as otitis externa.

Contraindications: Hypersensitivity to any of the components.

Adverse Reactions: Rarely noted was dermatitis.

Dosage and Administration: *Topically.* With the affected ear turned upward, fill ear canal and plug with cotton. If necessary, repeat every 4 hours.

Availability:
TYMPAGESIC® Liquid in dropper bottles of 13 ml. **(Warren-Teed)**

TYPHOID VACCINE

Description: Typhoid vaccine is a sterile suspension, in buffered, isotonic sodium chloride solution or other suitable diluent, of killed typhoid bacilli *Salmonella typhosa* (Ty 2 strain), a strain selected for high antigenic efficiency. It contains not more than 1000 million typhoid organisms in each ml. It contains, in each ml, not more than 35 mcg of total nitrogen. It may contain a suitable preservative. The potency of the vaccine is standardized to a level of 8 protective units/ml.

Indications: Prevention of typhoid fever by active immunization.

Contraindications: In the presence of acute respiratory or other active infection, and coadministration of adrenocorticotropin or adrenal corticosteroids.

Precautions: Corticosteroids should not be administered following exposure to infectious agents (mumps, rabies, tetanus) for which no satisfactory antimicrobial therapy is available. Because of a possible anaphylactic reaction, epinephrine (1:1000) and other emergency drugs and facilities should be readily available.

Adverse Reactions: Erythema, induration and tenderness at the injection site accompanied by pain. Systemic reactions may include fever, malaise, headache, and nausea. Postvaccinal neurological disorders have been reported.

Dosage and Administration: *Subcutaneously.* Primary immunization: Adults and children over 10 years of age, 0.5 ml followed in 4 or more weeks by another 0.5 ml injection. Booster injections of 0.5 ml should be administered at least every 3 years. Children 6 months to 10 years of age, 0.25 ml followed in 4 or more weeks by another injection of 0.25 ml. Booster injections of 0.25 ml should be administered at least every 3 years.

Availability:
TYPHOID VACCINE in multiple-dose vials of 5, 10 and 20 ml. **(Wyeth)**

TYPHUS VACCINE

Description: Typhus Vaccine is a sterile suspension of the killed organisms of a strain or strains of epidemic typhus rickettsiae (*Rickettsia prowazekii*) selected for antigenic efficiency. Typhus Vaccine consists of refined material derived from an aqueous suspension of the infected yolk sac membrane, and the rickettsiae are killed by means of a suitable chemical agent. It contains a suitable preservative.

Indications: An active immunizing agent for and the prophylaxis against, but not for the treatment of, louse-borne (epidemic) typhus. It does not protect against murine typhus or scrub typhus. It is indicated for persons entering endemic zones, and for special-risk groups (scientific investigators, medical personnel and laboratory personnel working with *Rickettsia prowazekii*).

Contraindications: Extreme hypersensitivity to egg protein, acute infection, tuberculosis, debilitating diseases, other latent or active infections, and coadministration of adrenocorticotropin or adrenal corticosteroids.

Warnings: The parenteral administration of any biological product should be associated with every known precaution for the prevention and treatment of allergic and other untoward reactions.

Precautions: When administered to patients who are moderately hypersensitive to egg protein, the initial dose should be small enough to avoid reaction. If no reaction occurs, the dose may be doubled at intervals of 20 minutes until a reaction occurs or until the full dose has been given.

Adverse Reactions: Postvaccinal neurological disorders have been reported.

Dosage and Administration: *Subcutaneously.* The recommended dosage for adults and children 10 years of age and over is 1 ml followed in 4 or more weeks by another 1 ml injection. Booster injections of 0.5 to 1 ml should be administered every 6 to 12 months. Children less than 10 years of age should receive 0.5 ml. Each dose should be given in a site not previously used for a vaccine or toxoid.

Availability:
TYPHUS VACCINE (epidemic type) in vials of 1 ml. **(Lederle)**
TYPHUS VACCINE (prophylaxis type) in vials of 2 ml. **(Lilly)**

TYROPANOATE SODIUM

Chemical Name: 2-(3-Butyramido-2,4,6-triiodobenzyl)-butanoate sodium.

Description: Tyropanoate sodium is a cholecystographic agent. It occurs as an off-white, hygroscopic, odorless solid possessing a molecular weight of 663.1. It contains 57.4% iodine, and is soluble in water to 14.7%.

Following oral administration, tyropanoate sodium is absorbed from the duodenum into the blood stream. The liver converts it primarily into radiopaque glucuronic acid conjugates, which are concentrated by the functioning gallbladder. These conjugates provide visualization of the gallbladder and may, upon contraction of the gallbladder, provide visualization of the extrahepatic ducts.

Indications: For radiographic delineation of the gallbladder.

Contraindications: Advanced hepatorenal disease, severe impairment of renal function, or severe gastrointestinal disorders that prevent absorption of the medium.

Warnings: Although no teratogenic effects attributable to this agent have been observed in animals, safe use of tyropanoate sodium during pregnancy has not been established. Before cholecystography with this compound is performed in women of childbearing potential, the benefits should be weighed against the possible risks to the mother and child. Use in children under 12 years of age is not recommended since clinical trials have not been performed in this age group. Elevation of protein-bound iodine for several months and false-positive urine albumin tests for several days may occur following ingestion of cholecystographic media.

Precautions: A history of iodine sensitivity implies greater than usual risk to the patient; therefore, caution should be exercised when administering this drug to patients with known iodine sensitivity and also to those with symptoms of coronary artery disease. Severe, advanced liver disease may interfere with metabolism of the radiopaque medium, and thus, a greater amount of unchanged tyropanoate sodium may be diverted to the kidney. Renal function in patients with severe, advanced liver disease should be assessed before cholecystography, and renal output and hepatic function should be observed for a few days after the procedure. Patients with these conditions should *not* be dehydrated prior to administration and should be advised to drink liberal amounts of fluids after taking the capsules. The uricosuric effect of the medium should be considered when given to patients with impaired renal function. Also, the recommended dose should not be exceeded in such patients since possible renal irritation could result in reflex vascular spasm with partial or complete renal shutdown.

Adverse Reactions: The most common reactions noted have been mild and transient *gastrointestinal disturbances* including nausea, abdominal cramps, diarrhea, vomiting, weakness and abdominal discomfort. *Allergic reactions* included rash, pruritus, and unspecified allergic responses. A variety of reactions, which have occurred infrequently, include dysuria, dyspnea, difficulty in swallowing, headache, perspiration, dizziness, fatigue, lightheadedness, pain or cramps in limbs and, rarely, laryngotracheal edema. Rare instances of disturbances in hepatic, renal, or cardiovascular function have been noted.

Dosage and Administration: *Orally.* For routine cholecystography, a single dose of 3 gm (4 capsules) is recommended for adults. Optimal visualization generally occurs in 10 to 12 hours, although satisfactory results may occur as early as 4 to 6 hours. If adequate visualization is not obtained initially, a repeat examination with a 3-gm dose may be performed on the following day. *Increasing* the amount of the repeat dose is not recommended. The meal immediately before ingestion of the capsules should be fat free. However, to reduce the incidence of a false-negative nonvisualization in patients who have been on fat-free diets, a diet containing some fat should be eaten for 1 or 2 days prior to the cholecystographic visualization. Preparatory dehydration of the patient is unnecessary and undesirable, particularly in elderly patients. For additional information, see package literature.

Availability:

BILOPAQUE® SODIUM Capsules, 750 mg in bottles of 500 with 150 dispensing envelopes and in envelopes of 4 capsules in cartons of 5 and 25 envelopes. **(Winthrop)**

URACIL MUSTARD

Chemical Name: 5-[Bis(2-chloroethyl)amino]uracil.

Description: Uracil mustard is a polyfunctional alkylating agent. It occurs as a cream-white, odorless, crystalline powder slightly soluble in water and very slightly soluble in alcohol. Uracil mustard is a member of the nitrogen mustards, synthesized in an attempt to improve the antitumor effects of nitrogen mustard without increasing toxicity.

The drug is well absorbed from the gastrointestinal tract. Its cytotoxic effect is believed to be due to its action on deoxyribonucleic acid.

Indications: Uracil mustard is used primarily for the palliative treatment of neoplasms of the reticuloendothelial and hematopoietic tissues. The drug has been shown to produce objective improvement in some patients with chronic lymphocytic leukemia, and with lymphomas including Hodgkin's disease, lymphosarcoma, lymphoblastoma, giant follicular lymphoma, and reticulum cell sarcoma. Uracil has also produced remissions or regressions in some cases of chronic granulocytic leukemia, mycosis fungoides, and polycythemia vera. Subjective improvement and, rarely, objective improvement in patients with multiple myeloma have occurred with uracil mustard therapy. Although the drug is only helpful occasionally in the palliative treatment of solid tumors, objective remission of ovarian carcinoma and some other solid tumors has been reported. Uracil mustard is not effective in acute leukemia. In some patients, the drug appears to act slowly and response may not be noted for 2 to 3 months after therapy has been initiated.

Contraindications: Pronounced leukopenia, thrombocytopenia, aplastic anemia, and when the bone-marrow has been infiltrated with malignant cells.

Warnings: Drugs of the nitrogen mustard group have been shown to produce fetal abnormalities in experimental animals when given during pregnancy. Therefore, this drug should not be given to pregnant patients unless in the opinion of the physician the potential benefits outweigh the possible hazards.

Precautions: Uracil mustard is a very toxic drug with a low therapeutic index. Hematopoietic toxicity of the drug is cumulative; as the total accumulated dose approaches 1 mg/kg of body weight, irreversible damage to the bone marrow may occur. Complete blood counts should be done once or twice weekly during and at least 1 month following therapy, since maximal bone marrow depression may not occur until 2 to 4 weeks after the drug has been withdrawn. If formed elements show a sharp drop, the drug should be withdrawn. If uracil mustard therapy follows treatment by irradiation or another antineoplastic drug, 2 or 3 weeks should elapse between the maximal bone-marrow depressant effect of previous therapy and the initial doses of this agent.

Adverse Reactions: Nausea, vomiting or diarrhea, and suppression of bone marrow activity usually occur and may be severe enough to warrant discontinuation of the medication. Other reactions, some of which may or may not be associated with the drug, include nervousness, irritability or depression, various skin reactions such as pruritus, dermatitis, and some loss of hair; however, frank alopecia has not been reported to date.

Dosage and Administration: *Orally.* Dosage must be tailored according to the degree of depression of bone marrow function produced by the drug. The gradual dosage schedule consists of 1 or 2 mg daily until clinical improvement is noted or until hematopoietic toxicity occurs. If remission is obtained, 1 mg daily should be given for 3 out of each 4 weeks. Alternatively, 3 to 5 mg daily is given initially for the first 7 days, followed by 1 mg daily. Indications for interrupting or continuing therapy, and the dosage for maintenance in remission, are the same as with the more gradual dosage schedule. It is well to bear in mind the fact that continuous therapy may appear to maintain a patient who is actually in remission.

Availability:
URACIL MUSTARD Capsules, 1 mg in bottles of 50. **(Upjohn)**

UREA

Chemical Name: Carbonyldiamide.

Description: An osmotic diuretic that induces its effect as a result of the limited capacity of the renal tubule to concentrate urine. The commercial product is a synthetic, lyophilized, sterile powder form of urea to be reconstituted with dextrose or invert sugar solution for intravenous administration.

Urea rapidly increases blood tonicity due to a greater urea concentration gradient in the blood than in the extravascular fluid. This results in transudation of fluid from the tissues, including the brain and cerebrospinal fluid, into the blood. The increasing concentration of urea in the glomerular filtrate prevents reabsorption of a proportional amount of water in the proximal tubule, thereby increasing the rate and volume of urine flow.

Indications: For the reduction of intracranial pressure (in the control of cerebral edema) and of intraocular pressure.

Contraindications: Severely impaired renal function, active intracranial bleeding, marked dehydration, and frank liver failure.

Warnings: Urea should not be infused into the veins of the lower extremities because superficial and deep thrombosis may occur especially in elderly patients. Electrolyte depletion resulting in hyponatremia or hypokalemia may occur. Early signs such as muscle weakness may indicate the need for supplementation of any depleted essential ions. Extravasation of urea can cause local reactions ranging from mild irritation to tissue necrosis. Should be administered with considerable caution in the presence of liver impairment to prevent elevated blood ammonia levels. Routine caution is essential when administrating this drug to pregnant or lactating women or to women of childbearing potential.

Precautions: An indwelling urethral catheter should be employed in comatose patients receiving this drug to insure satisfactory emptying of the bladder. To avoid hemolysis, the rate of infusion should not exceed 4 ml/minute and the drug should never be mixed with blood in the transfusion set. The reduced brain edema induced by urea may result in a reactivation of intracranial bleeding. Cautious use is essential in the presence of kidney disease; however, mild elevation of BUN does not preclude its use or continued use, but frequent laboratory studies should be made to determine if kidney function is adequate. If diuresis does not occur within 6 to 12 hours, the drug should be withdrawn pending further evaluation of renal function. Should excessive loss of blood occur within a short period of time, adequate replacement may be given simultaneously with the infusion of urea. Concomitant hypothermia may increase the risk of venous thrombosis and hemoglobinuria.

Adverse Reactions: Headache, nausea and vomiting, occasionally syncope, disorientation, and transient agitated confusional states have been reported. Infrequently noted were phlebitis and thrombosis at the injection site.

Dosage and Administration: *Slow intravenous infusion* of a 30% solution. The injection is prepared by adding an appropriate volume of 5 or 10% dextrose injection or 10% invert sugar in water. To prepare 135 ml of a 30% solution of sterile urea, the contents of one 40-gm vial are mixed with 105 ml of the diluent. Each milliliter of 30% solution provides 300 mg of urea. Solution should be freshly prepared in each case and any unused portion should be discarded. To reduce intracranial or intraocular pressure, adults, 1 to 1.5 gm (3.3 to 5 ml)/kg of body weight. Children, 0.5 to 1.5 gm/kg of body weight. Children under 2 years of age, as little as 0.1 gm/kg may be adequate.

Availability:
UREAPHIL® Dry Powder, 40 gm with citric acid buffer, 1 mg in Non-Vac® (single-dose) containers of 150 ml. **(Abbott)**

UROBIOTIC

Description: A combination of oxytetracycline hydrochloride equivalent to 250 mg of the antibiotic, oxytetracycline, with 250 mg of the antibacterial sulfonamide, sulfamethizole and 50 mg of the urinary antiseptic and analgesic, phenazopyridine hydrochloride.

Indications: Treatment of a number of genitourinary infections including pyelonephritis, pyelitis, ureteritis, cystitis, prostatitis and urethritis. Both antibacterial components are active against the most common urinary pathogens including *E. coli, Ps. aeruginosa, A. aerogenes, S. faecalis, S. hemolyticus* and *M. pyogenes.* The drug is particularly useful in infections in which the organism is more sensitive to the combination than to either component alone. It is also of value in mixed infections, and in those instances where the causative organism is unknown pending laboratory isolation.

Contraindications: Hypersensitivity to any of the ingredients. Because of the sulfonamide component, the drug should not be used during pregnancy at term, in premature infants, or in neonates during the first week of life.

For warnings, precautions and adverse reactions, see the monographs on each of the constituents.

Dosage and Administration: *Orally.* Adults, a dosage of 1 capsule 4 times daily is suggested, depending upon the severity and response of the infection; refractory cases may require 2 capsules 4 times daily. Therapy should be continued for at least 7 days or until bacterial cultures are sterile in acute infections. To aid absorption of the drug, it should be given at least 1 hour before or 2 hours after meals. Aluminum hydroxide gel given with antibiotics decreases their absorption and is therefore contraindicated.

Availability:
UROBIOTIC®-250 Capsules in bottles of 50 and in unit-dose packages of 100. **(Roerig)**

UROKINASE

Description: Urokinase, a blood-clot-dissolving agent, is a naturally occurring human enzyme (protein) produced by the kidneys and isolated from the urine or from kidney cells grown in tissue culture. The drug is a potent activator of the fibrinolytic system, and in contrast to the anticoagulant heparin, which prevents clots from forming, it dissolves clots already formed by converting plasminogen to the proteolytic enzyme plasmin. Plasmin is an active fibrinolytic (thrombolytic) substance that degrades fibrin as well as fibrinogen and other plasma proteins into soluble matter thus achieving dissolution of the clot. Therapy with urokinase is directed towards the production of sufficient amounts of plasmin for the lysis of intravascular deposits of fibrin. Since plasminogen is present in the thrombus/embolus, activation by the drug occurs within the occlusive lesion as well as on its surface. The major clinical application has been in the treatment of acute pulmonary embolism and the accompanying adverse hemodynamic effects. Resolution of the embolus has been shown to be more rapid in those receiving urinary urokinase than in those receiving heparin as the sole agent. The white, lyophilized powder is dissolved in 5.2 ml of Sterile Water for Injection, U.S.P., forming a clear, practically colorless solution containing in each ml 50,000 IU of urokinase, 0.5% mannitol and 0.9% sodium chloride. The pH is adjusted with sodium hydroxide and/or hydrochloric acid prior to lyophilization. It is recommended for use only by physicians experienced in the management of thrombotic disease and in hospitals where clinical and laboratory monitoring can be performed.

Treatment should be instituted as soon as possible, preferably within 12 hours, but no later than 5 days, after onset of the embolic episode. Intravenous infusion is promptly followed by increased fibrinolytic activity and its effect may persist for up to 12 hours after discontinuation. It is excreted in the urine either as unchanged drug or as metabolites. Angiographic and hemodynamic measurements have demonstrated a more rapid improvement during the first 24 hours of therapy than with heparin therapy. Whether or not treatment with urokinase decreases the morbidity or mortality when compared to heparin has not been established.

Indications: For the lysis of acute, massive pulmonary emboli, defined as obstruction or significant filling defects involving 2 or more lobar pulmonary arteries or an equivalent amount of emboli in other vessels, and for the lysis of pulmonary emboli accompanied by unstable hemodynamics i.e., failure to maintain blood pressure without supportive measures. The diagnosis should be confirmed by objective means, preferably pulmonary arteriography. Because thrombolytic therapy increases the risk of bleeding, urokinase is not indicated in patients presenting with conditions in which hemorrhage might constitute a significant hazard or be particularly difficult to control.

Since the contraindications, warnings, precautions and adverse reactions are generally those associated with Streptokinase, see the monograph on Streptokinase.

Dosage and Administration: *Intravenously.* Only Sterile Water for Injection, U.S.P. is the medium used for reconstitution. The recommended treatment for pulmonary embolism begins with a priming dose of 2000 IU/lb of body weight (4400 IU/Kg) administered by intravenous infusion over a period of 10 minutes, followed by continuous infusion of 2000 IU/lb/hour (4400 IU/Kg/hour) over a period of 12 hours. The total volume of fluid administered should not exceed 200 ml. Urokinase should be administered by means of a constant infusion pump that is capable of delivering a total volume of 195 ml. At the end of urokinase therapy, treatment with heparin by continuous intravenous infusion is recommended. However, heparin treatment should not begin until the thrombin time has decreased to *less than twice* the normal control value. The physician is advised to refer to the package literature for additional details on dosage recommendations and other pertinent information.

Availability:
ABBOKINASE® Lyophilized White Powder in vials of 250,000 IU. **(Abbott)**

VAGILIA

Description: The cream contains sulfisoxazole, 10%; aminacrine hydrochloride, 0.2% and allantoin, 2% in a water-miscible base. Each suppository contains sulfisoxazole, 600 mg; aminacrine hydrochloride, 12 mg and allantoin, 120 mg. The formulation combines the complementary bacteriostatic effect of sulfisoxazole with the antibacterial and antifungal actions of aminacrine hydrochloride. Sulfisoxazole is believed to act by blocking certain metabolic processes essential for the growth of microorganisms and aminacrine by interfering or competing with hydrogen ions in microbial enzyme systems. The addition of allantoin aids in debridement of necrotic tissue and the proliferation of healthy vaginal epithelium. The drug provides effective activity against gram-positive and gram-negative bacteria, trichomonads, moniliasis (C. albicans) and other susceptible microorganisms usually associated with vaginal infections.

Indications: Treatment of vaginitis and cervicitis.

Contraindications: Known or suspected sensitivity to sulfa drugs.

Precautions: Although some absorption of the sulfisoxazole may occur, systemic reactions are rarely seen. The development of local reactions such as increased discomfort or a burning sensation require the usual sulfonamide precautions.

Adverse Reactions: Patients should be observed for manifestations of skin rash or other evidence of systemic toxicity; if these occur, it is advised to discontinue the medication.

Dosage and Administration: *Intravaginally.* One applicatorful or 1 suppository should be inserted high into the vaginal vault once or twice daily. Improvement will often be apparent within a few days but treatment should be continued until the pathogens have been eliminated or a clinical cure or remission is achieved. Adequate control or eradication of monilia and trichomonads usually requires prolonged treatment. Exacerbation may occur during the menstrual period; for such infections it is, therefore, advisable to continue the applications for at least 1 month or through 1 complete menstrual cycle. Vaginal applicators should not be used after the seventh month of pregnancy.

Availability:
VAGILIA®: **(Lemmon)**
Vaginal Cream in tubes of 90 gm with applicator.
Vaginal Suppositories in cartons of 16 with applicator.

VAGISEC PLUS

Description: Each 3-gm suppository contains polyoxyethylene nonyl phenol, 5.25 mg; sodium edetate, 0.66 mg; sodium dioctyl sulfosuccinate, 0.07 mg and 9-aminoacridine hydrochloride, 6 mg in a polyethylene glycol base containing glycerin and citric acid.

Indications: Treatment of vaginitis caused by *Trichomonas vaginalis,* or vaginal infections complicated by mixed bacterial organisms.

Contraindications: Because they are spermicidal, the suppositories should not be used on days when the patient is trying to conceive.

Precautions: No patient should be considered cured until vaginal smears or cultures, taken at monthly intervals for 3 months following treatment, show absence of trichomonads and a return to a normal vaginal flora. Recurrence of vaginitis often indicates extravaginal foci of infection in cervical, vestibular and urethral glands, etc., or reinfection by the sexual partner. It is recommended that the patient refrain from intercourse, or the husband wear a prophylactic. Douching is not recommended for pregnant patients.

Adverse Reactions: Rare instances of vaginal irritation.

Dosage and Administration: *Intravaginally,* 2 suppositories daily. For complete information on office and home procedures for treatment, consult package literature.

Availability:
VAGISEC® PLUS Suppositories in cartons of 28 foil wrapped with inserter **(Schmid)**

VAGITROL

Description: The buffered cream contains sulfanilamide, 15%; aminacrine hydrochloride, 0.2% and allantoin, 2% with lactose in a water-miscible base. Each suppository contains sulfanilamide, 1.05 gm, aminacrine hydrochloride, 0.014 gm and allantoin, 0.14 gm.

The combination of an antibacterial (sulfanilamide) with an antimicrobial (aminacrine) agent provides effective activity against *Haemophilus vaginalis, Candida albicans, Trichomonas vaginalis* and other susceptible microorganisms. Allantoin is included to assist in the removal of necrotic debris and to stimulate the growth of healthy tissue.

Indications: Treatment of vaginitis, trichomoniasis and vulvovaginal candidiasis due to *Haemophilus vaginalis* or other susceptible organism.

Contraindications: Hypersensitivity to sulfonamides or to any of the components, and in the presence of kidney disease.

Warnings: Safe use during pregnancy has not been established. Because of the sulfonamide content, its usefulness is limited due to the increasing frequency of resistant organisms. Deaths associated with the administration of sulfonamides have been reported from hypersensitivity reactions, agranulocytosis, aplastic anemia, and other blood dyscrasias. The presence of clinical signs such as sore throat, fever, pallor, purpura, or jaundice may be early indications. The medication should be discontinued at the first sign of systemic toxicity.

Precautions: Routine caution is necessary when sulfonamides are given to patients with impaired renal or hepatic function and to those with severe allergy or bronchial asthma. Adequate fluid intake must be maintained in order to prevent crystalluria and stone formation. Hemolysis may occur in patients deficient in the enzyme glucose-6-phosphate dehydrogenase; this reaction is frequently dose-related.

Adverse Reactions: *Blood dyscrasias:* Agranulocytosis, aplastic anemia, thrombocytopenia, leukopenia, hemolytic anemia, purpura, hypoprothrombinemia and methemoglobinemia. *Allergic reactions:* Erythema multiforme (Stevens-Johnson syndrome), generalized skin eruptions, epidermal necrolysis, urticaria, serum sickness, pruritus, exfoliative dermatitis, anaphylactoid reactions, periorbital edema, conjunctival and scleral injection, photosensitization, arthralgia, and allergic myocarditis. *Gastrointestinal reactions:* Nausea, emesis, abdominal pains, hepatitis, diarrhea, anorexia, pancreatitis, and stomatitis. *CNS reactions:* Headache, peripheral neuritis, mental depression, convulsions, ataxia, hallucinations, tinnitus, vertigo, and insomnia. *Miscellaneous reactions:* Drug fever, chills, and toxic nephrosis with oliguria and anuria. Periarteritis nodosa and lupus erythematosus have occurred. The sulfonamides bear certain chemical similarities to some goitrogens, diuretics (acetazolamide and the thiazides), and oral hypoglycemic agents. Although rare, the development of goiter, diuresis, and hypoglycemia have occurred in patients receiving sulfonamides. Long-term administration produced thyroid malignancies in the rat species of animals.

Dosage and Administration: *Intravaginally.* The usual adult dosage is 1 applicatorful of cream or 1 suppository once or twice daily. Treatment should be continued until the pathogens have been eliminated or a clinical cure or remission is achieved. Monilial and trichomonal infections should be treated for a minimum of 1 month or through 1 menstrual cycle. If no response is apparent within a few days, or if symptoms recur, the drug should be discontinued and another attempt should be made by appropriate laboratory methods to isolate the offending organism.

Availability:
VAGITROL®: **(Syntex)**
Vaginal Cream in tubes of 120 gm with applicator.
Vaginal Suppositories in cartons of 16 with applicator.

VALPROIC ACID/VALPROATE SODIUM

Chemical Name: 2-Propylpentanoic acid/sodium.

Description: An antiepileptic drug structurally unrelated to currently available compounds in that it lacks the nitrogen and aromatic components in its molecule that are the characteristic features of other anticonvulsant agents. Its most prominent applications have been in absence seizures in which it has been found to provide satisfactory control in patients inadequately controlled with other agents. *Valproic acid* occurs as a colorless liquid that is slightly soluble in water and very soluble in organic solvents. *Valproate sodium* occurs as a white powder that is highly hygroscopic. Since the valproate ion is the circulating active principle, the 2 compounds are therefore bioequivalent when given in equivalent amounts. The drug's precise biochemical action has not been established, but its anticonvulsant effect is thought to be associated with an increase in the level of gamma-aminobutyric acid (GABA) in the brain due to inhibition of the enzyme GABA transaminase. The effect on the neuronal membrane is not known. It has been reported to produce little or no effect on the autonomic nervous system, does not appear to markedly influence respiration or body temperature and to lack significant cardiovascular, smooth muscle or renal effects. Additionally, it is devoid of antiinflammatory, analgesic and antihistaminic activity.

Following ingestion of a single dose, the drug is rapidly and completely absorbed from the gastrointestinal tract, attaining maximum serum levels within 1 to 4 hours. Therapeutic blood levels appear to be about 50 to 100 mcg/ml in most patients receiving daily doses of 1.2 to 1.5 gm. It is rapidly distributed and approximately 90% of the drug is strongly bound to serum proteins and about 60% to serum albumin. The biological half-life of valproic acid is estimated to range from 8 to 12 hours. It is metabolized primarily in the liver and eliminated principally in the urine with only minor amounts appearing in the feces and exhaled air. Urine content consists chiefly of the glucuronide conjugate, with lesser amounts of the oxidative metabolites, and only detectable amounts of the intact parent drug.

Valproate sodium has been found to produce dose-related dysmorphogenic effects in mice, rats, and rabbits characterized by kidney defects, cleft palates, encephaloceles, ablepharia, and fusion of ribs and vertebrae. Reduced spermatogenesis and testicular atrophy observed in rats and dogs require thorough clinical investigation. Thus far, no evidence of carcinogenic or mutagenic effects have been noted.

Indications: Treatment of simple and complex absence seizures, including petit mal. The drug may be introduced alone or added to existing antiepileptic medication. May also be used in combination with other anticonvulsant agents in patients with multiple seizures which include absence seizures.

Contraindications: Known hypersensitivity to the drug.

Warnings: Liver dysfunction including hepatic failure resulting in fatalities has occurred in a few patients receiving valproic acid and concomitant anticonvulsant drugs. These incidences have occurred during the first six months of treatment with this drug. Although a causal relationship has not been established, liver function tests should be performed prior to therapy and every two months thereafter. Extreme caution should be observed when administering valproic acid to patients with preexisting liver disease. Clinical reports suggest an association between the use of anticonvulsant agents in women with epilepsy and an increased incidence of birth defects in the offspring. However, such reports cannot be regarded as adequate to verify a definite cause-and-effect relationship since genetic factors or the epileptic condition itself may be more significant than drug therapy in the development of birth defects. The reports also indicate that the great majority of pregnant women receiving anticonvulsant medication deliver normal infants. It is strongly advised that anticonvulsant therapy not be discontinued abruptly because of the potential of precipitating status epilepticus with attendant hypoxia and threat to both the mother and unborn child. When withdrawal of the medication would not constitute a serious threat to the patient, discontinuation of the drug may be considered prior to and during gestation, although even mild seizures may be hazardous to the developing embryo or fetus. These considerations should be weighed in the treatment and counseling of epileptic women of childbearing potential.

Precautions: A few instances of drug-induced faulty platelet aggregation, thrombocytopenia and elevated liver enzymes have been reported; therefore, it is deemed essential to perform tests to evaluate these parameters before initiating therapy and periodically thereafter. Additionally, periodic serum level determinations of concomitant anticonvulsant drugs are also recommended during the early course of treatment. Simultaneous administration with drugs known to affect coagulation, such as aspirin and warfarin require special care. The clinician should be aware that the drug is partially eliminated in the urine as a ketone-containing metabolite and that this event may lead to a false interpretation of the urine ketone test. Since valproic acid may produce CNS depression, particularly when combined with another CNS depressant such as alcohol, patients should be advised not to engage in hazardous occupations requiring alertness and skill until their response to the drug has been established. The drug has been found to increase the serum level of phenobarbital and of phenytoin; therefore, the dosage of these drugs should be adjusted as required by the clinical response. Absence status may be induced by the concomitant use of valproic acid and clonazepam. Because the drug is excreted in breast milk and its effect on the nursing infant is not known, it is therefore generally accepted that nursing should not be undertaken while a patient is receiving this drug. Chronic toxicity studies in juvenile and adult rats and dogs have demonstrated reduced spermatogenesis and testicular atrophy at doses proportionately in excess of the recommended clinical dose, the effect on the development of the testes and on sperm production and fertility in humans awaits further studies.

Adverse Reactions: The true incidence of adverse effects is difficult to assess, since the drug is generally used in combination with other anticonvulsant preparations. Nausea, vomiting and indigestion are the most commonly reported, are usually transient, and only rarely require withdrawal of the drug. Diarrhea, abdominal cramps and constipation have also been reported. Both anorexia and increased appetite with resultant change in weight may also occur. *CNS effects* usually consist of drowsiness, and sedation, rarely, ataxia, headache, nystagmus, diplopia, asterixis (spots before the eyes), tremor, dysarthria, dizziness, and incoordination. Rare cases of coma have been noted in patients also on phenobarbital therapy. *Dermatologic effects* are manifested by hair loss, rarely, skin rash, and petechiae; *psychiatric effects* by emotional upset, depression, psychosis, aggression, hyperactivity, and behavioral deterioration; *musculoskeletal effects* by weakness; *hematopoietic effects* by inhibition of the secondary phase of platelet aggregation, lymphocytosis, mild thrombocytopenia, and leukopenia; *hepatic effects* by increases in serum alkaline phosphatase and elevations of serum glutamic oxaloacetic transaminase (SGOT), and isolated instances of severe hepatotoxicity.

Dosage and Administration: *Orally.* The recommended initial dose is 15 mg/kg/day, increasing at 1-week intervals by 5 to 10 mg/kg/day until seizures are controlled or side effects preclude further increases. The maximum recommended dosage is 30 mg/kg/day. If the total daily dose exceeds 250 mg, it should be given in a divided regimen. The capsules should be swallowed whole (not chewed) to avoid local irritation of the mouth and throat.

Availability:
DEPAKENE®: **(Abbott)**
Capsules (as valproic acid), 250 mg in bottles of 100.
Syrup (as sodium valproate), 250 mg/5 ml in bottles of 1 pint.

VANCOMYCIN HYDROCHLORIDE

Description: Vancomycin is a glycopeptide antibiotic obtained from strains of *Streptomyces orientalis*. It is bactericidal as well as bacteriostatic, particularly against gram-positive cocci due to its inhibitory function in bacterial cell-wall synthesis. It is bactericidal, both in vitro and in vivo, against streptococci, pneumococci and staphylococci. Cross resistance has not been observed between vancomycin and other antibiotics. It occurs as a white powder that is very soluble in water and practically insoluble in alcohol.

Vancomycin is poorly absorbed from the gastrointestinal tract. A 1-gm intravenous dose produces serum levels averaging 25 mcg/ml in 2 hours; its half-life in the circulation is about 6 hours. Less than 10% of the antibiotic is bound to plasma proteins. Clinically effective concentrations of the antibiotic in the blood are usually achieved and maintained by intravenous administration, and inhibitory concentrations can be demonstrated in pleural, pericardial, ascitic, and synovial fluids and in the urine. Vancomycin does not diffuse across normal meninges into the spinal fluid, but readily does so when they are inflamed. About 80% of injected drug is excreted by the kidneys. If the Kirby-Bauer method of disc sensitivity is used, a 30-mcg disc of vancomycin should produce a zone of more than 11 mm when tested against a vancomycin-sensitive bacterial strain.

Indications: Orally for the treatment of staphylococcal enterocolitis *only*. Parenterally for the treatment of staphylococcal endocarditis, osteomyelitis, pneumonia, septicemia, and soft-tissue infections.

Contraindications: Hypersensitivity to vancomycin.

Warnings: Because of ototoxic and nephrotoxic potential, vancomycin should not be used in patients with renal insufficiency or with previous loss of hearing. Since the drug may impair auditory acuity, audiometric tests should be conducted prior to and during therapy. Dosage should be well regulated and periodic determination of the drug level in the blood should be performed, since the risk of serious toxicity which may lead to permanent deafness and fatal uremia can occur with large doses, long-term use or in the presence of abnormal renal function. A dose of less than 2 gm daily will usually provide satisfactory blood levels. Concurrent or sequential use of other neurotoxic and/or nephrotoxic antibiotics, particularly streptomycin, neomycin, kanamycin, gentamicin, cephaloridine, paromomycin, viomycin, polymyxin B sulfate, colistin, and tobramycin should be avoided. As with any potent drug, special caution and judgment are essential during pregnancy.

Precautions: Evaluation of hepatic and renal function, and hematologic studies should be conducted frequently during therapy, especially if the patient is over 60 years of age, has renal dysfunction or borderline renal disease, or if the drug is administered in doses greater than 2 gm daily or for prolonged periods. The use of antibiotics may result in the overgrowth of nonsusceptible organisms, in which case appropriate measures should be taken if new infections due to bacteria or fungi appear during therapy. Intravenous administration is preferred since the drug is highly irritating and causes tissue necrosis when given by the intramuscular route.

Adverse Reactions: Chills, fever, urticaria, macular rash, nausea, hearing loss, renal toxicity, elevated BUN levels, eosinophilia, anaphylactoid reactions, pain and thrombophlebitis at the injection site have been reported.

Dosage and Administration: *Orally* or *intravenously*. Usual adult daily dosage is 2 gm; this is generally administered in doses of 500 mg every 6 hours or 1 gm every 12 hours by continuous infusion. Higher doses of 3 to 4 gm daily should be used only in desperately ill patients who have normal renal function. The daily dosage for children is 20 mg/lb of body weight administered in divided doses. When intended for oral use, the contents of the bottle should be mixed with 115 ml of distilled or deionized water. This mixture may be kept for 1 week in the refrigerator without significant loss of potency. **Note:** Thrombophlebitis, which may be associated with repeated or prolonged intravenous administration, can be minimized by using a dilute solution and alternating the sites of injection. Extravasation outside the vein should be avoided. Rapid administration may produce a feeling of warmth and generalized tingling.

Availability:
VANCOCIN®: **(Lilly)**
For Injection (dry powder) in vials of 500 mg (10 ml).
For Oral Use (dry powder) in bottles of 10 gm (110 ml).

VIDARABINE

Synonyms: Adenine arabinoside; Ara-A.

Chemical Name: 9-β-D-Arabinofuranosyladenine.

Description: Vidarabine, an antiviral agent for ophthalmic use, is a purine nucleoside obtained from fermentation cultures of *Streptomyces antibioticus.* Its viricidal action against herpes simplex types 1 and 2, varicella-zoster and vaccinia has been determined by both in vitro and in vivo studies. Except for rhabdovirus and oncornavirus, it does not display in vitro activity against other RNA or DNA viruses, including adenovirus. The drug has been found to have no clinical value for corneal infections due to bacterial, fungal or chlamydial organisms or for nonviral trophic ulcers. Although the precise mechanism of action has not been determined, the drug appears to interfere with the early stages of viral DNA synthesis.

Vidarabine is rapidly deaminated in the gastrointestinal tract to arabinosylhypoxanthine (Ara-Hx) the principle metabolite which also possesses some antiviral activity. Because of its low solubility, systemic absorption of the drug should not be expected to occur following ocular administration and possible swallowing of lacrimal secretion. If the corneal epithelium is defective; trace amounts of both vidarabine and metabolite can be recovered from the aqueous humor, but if it is normal, only trace amounts of the metabolite (Ara-Hx) can be recovered. In contrast to topical idoxuridine, vidarabine has demonstrated less cellular toxicity in the regenerating corneal epithelium of the rabbit.

In controlled and uncontrolled clinical trials, an average of 7 and 9 days of continuous treatment were required before signs of corneal re-epithelialization appeared. In the controlled trials, 70 of 81 patients (86%) and in the uncontrolled trials 101 of 142 patients (71%) achieved complete re-epithelialization at the end of 3 weeks of therapy. Also noted was that 75% of the patients in the uncontrolled trials either had not responded or had become allergic to topical idoxuridine therapy. When administered in the recommended concentration and course of treatment, the significant toxic reactions often seen with prolonged use of idoxuridine have not been observed with vidarabine. This probably is due to low tissue penetration and rapid conversion to less active metabolites, resulting in unsustained plasma and tissue levels of the fully active drug. It is therefore useful in herpetic keratitis which does not respond to topical idoxuridine or when toxic or hypersensitivity reactions to idoxuridine occur.

Parenteral administration in rodents and rabbits showed that vidarabine has teratogenic and oncogenic capabilities. When administered intramuscularly in mice, liver and renal tumors were noted, and in rats, intestinal, testicular, and thyroid tumors developed. Hepatic megalocytosis, associated with vidarabine treatment, has also been found in both short- and long-term studies with rodents. It is not clear whether or not this represents a preneoplastic change. A high concentration (10%) of the ointment when applied to 10% of body surface during organogenesis induced fetal abnormalities in rabbits, but when applied to only 2 or 3% of body surface no apparent abnormalities occurred. Results of in vitro experiments indicate that the drug can be incorporated into mammalian DNA and can induce mutation in mammalian cells, and when added to human leukocytes, it causes the chromosomes to break and separate.

Indications: *Topically* for the treatment of acute keratoconjunctivitis and recurrent epithelial keratitis due to herpes simplex virus types 1 and 2. The drug's effectiveness against stromal keratitis and uveitis due to herpes simplex virus has not been established. The following topical antibiotics: gentamicin, erythromycin and chloramphenicol; or topical steroids: prednisolone and dexamethasone have been administered concurrently with vidarabine without an increase in adverse reactions. It should be kept in mind however that corticosteroids alone are contraindicated in the treatment of herpes simplex virus infections; therefore, the concurrent topical application of both drugs may result in corticosteroid-induced ocular side effects. These generally include glaucoma or cataract formation and progression of a bacterial or viral infection. *Intravenously* for the treatment of herpes simplex encephalitis in adults.

Contraindications: Known hypersensitivity to vidarabine.

Warnings: Cautious use is advised when administering to pregnant women or nursing mothers. Too frequent administration should be avoided.

Precautions: It is recommended that the diagnosis of keratoconjunctivitis due to herpes simplex be firmly established before prescribing this drug. Patients should be forewarned that the ointment may produce a temporary visual haze. Although not reported to date, the possibility of resistant viral strains developing has been suggested.

Adverse Reactions: These are usually local in nature and include lacrimation, foreign body sensation, conjunctival injection, burning, irritation, superficial punctate keratitis, pain, photophobia, punctal occlusion, .and sensitivity. The following have also occurred but appear to be related to the disease rather than to the drug: uveitis, stromal edema, secondary glaucoma, trophic defects, corneal vascularization, and hyphema. Acute massive overdosage by oral ingestion of the ointment has not occurred, and overdosage by ocular instillation is unlikely because any excess should be quickly expelled from the conjunctival sac.

Dosage and Administration: *Topically.* Apply approximately ½ inch of the ointment inside the lower conjunctival sac 5 times daily at 3-hour intervals. If there are no signs of improvement after 7 days, or complete re-epithelialization has not occurred by 21 days, other forms of therapy should be considered. However, some severe cases may require longer treatment. After re-epithelialization has occurred, treatment for an additional 7 days at a reduced dosage (such as twice daily) is recommended in order to prevent recurrence of the infection. *Intravenously.* A regimen of 10 doses of 5-ml vials administered by infusion. The calculated dose is 15 mg/kg/day for 10 days; infusion should be maintained for 12 to 24 hours; a bolus injection should be avoided. The drug should be diluted prior to use according to the manufacturer's recommendations.

Availability:
VIRA-A®: **(Parke-Davis)**
Ophthalmic Ointment, 3% (30 mg/gm) in tubes of 3.5 gm.
Suspension (for IV infusion), 200 mg/ml in Steri-Vial®s of 5 ml.

VI-DAYLIN/F: see The Fluoride-Vitamins

VI-DAYLIN/F ADC: see The Fluoride-Vitamins

VI-FLOR(S): see The Fluoride-Vitamins

VINBLASTINE SULFATE

Description: Vinblastine sulfate, a salt of a dimeric alkaloid extracted from the periwinkle plant. *Vinca rosea* Linn., has shown varying degrees of antineoplastic activity. Experimental studies indicate that vinblastine may interfere with the metabolic pathways of amino acids. Other studies suggest that the drug affects cell-energy production required for mitosis, and that it interferes with the synthesis of nucleic acid. It occurs as a slightly yellow or off-white, amorphous powder freely soluble in water and insoluble in alcohol. Studies have shown that glutamic acid and tryptophan reverse the antitumor effect of the drug, and that glutamic acid and aspartic acid protect mice from lethal doses of vinblastine; although aspartic acid showed relatively little effect in reversing the antitumor effect. Studies with animals show metaphase arrest and degenerative changes in germ cells.

Indications: Palliative treatment of generalized Hodgkin's disease (stages 3 and 4), lymphocytic lymphoma, histiocytic lymphoma, mycosis fungoides (advanced stages), advanced carcinoma of the testis, kaposis sarcoma, and Letterer-Siwe disease (histiocytosis X). Malignancies less frequently responsive to vinblastine are choriocarcinoma resistant to other chemotherapeutic agents and carcinoma of the breast unresponsive to appropriate endocrine surgery and hormonal therapy.

Contraindications: Leukopenia and bacterial infections.

Warnings: Although no abnormalities in the human fetus have been reported thus far, caution is necessary when oncolytic agents are administered during pregnancy. Aspermia may occur in male patients treated with this drug.

Precautions: White blood cell counts should be evaluated regularly and if leukopenia with less than 2000 white blood cells/cu mm occurs, the patient should be observed carefully for signs of infection. Because of the greater likelihood that severe leukopenia may develop in older patients, especially if they are cachectic or have skin ulcers, the use of vinblastine in these patients should be avoided. The drug may also produce a precipitous fall in the leukocyte and platelet counts in patients whose bone marrow has been infiltrated with malignant cells. If this occurs therapy should be discontinued. Recommended dosage schedules must be strictly adhered to and all precautions should be observed. Serious toxicity including convulsions, CNS damage, and death have resulted from overdosage. Care must be taken to avoid contamination of the eye. Extravasation of the drug should be avoided since this causes severe irritation and pain, and may result in phlebitis or cellulitis at the site of injection. If extravasation occurs, the injection should be discontinued at once. and another vein used to complete the dose. Cold wet compresses or ice packs may be used to help disperse the drug and relieve pain.

Adverse Reactions: Prior to the use of the drug, patients should be informed of the possibility of untoward symptoms. In general, the incidence of adverse reactions appear to be related to the size of the dosage employed. With the exception of epilation, leukopenia, and neurological effects, adverse reactions usually have not persisted for longer than 24 hours. These include nausea, vomiting, constipation, vesiculation of the mouth, ileus, diarrhea, anorexia, abdominal pain, rectal bleeding, pharyngitis, hemorrhagic enterocolitis, bleeding from peptic ulcer; numbness, paresthesias, peripheral neuritis, mental depression, loss of deep-tendon reflexes, headache, convulsions; malaise, weakness, dizziness, pain in tumor site, and vesiculation of the skin. Nausea and vomiting are usually controlled with antiemetic agents. When epilation develops, it frequently is not total; and, in some cases, hair regrows while maintenance therapy continues.

Dosage and Administration: *Intravenously, only once every 7 days.* The doses following the initial injection of 0.1 mg/kg of body weight are successively increased by increments of 0.05 mg/kg until the white blood count falls to 3000/cu mm or the size of the tumor decreases, or until a maximal dose of 0.5 mg/kg is reached. A maintenance dosage, reduced by 1 increment (0.05 mg/kg), may be given at intervals of 7 to 14 days. The requirements of individual patients vary; in most cases the desired response is achieved when a dose of 0.15 to 0.2 mg/kg of body weight is achieved. An alternative approach is to use the body surface area (bsa) of the patient to calculate the appropriate dose. The adult doses following the initial injection of 3.7 mg/M² bsa are successively increased by weekly increments of 1.85 mg/M² and the children's doses following the initial injection of 2.5 mg/M² are successively increased by weekly increments of 1.25 mg/M². These increments may be applied until a maximum dose not exceeding 18.5 mg/M² for adults and 12.5 mg/M² for children is reached. It should be emphasized that even though 7 days have elapsed, the next dose should not be administered until the white blood cell count has returned to at least 4000/cu mm. A maintenance dosage reduced by 1 increment (1.85 mg/M²) for adults and (1.25 mg/M²) for children may be given at intervals of 7 days.

Availability:
VELBAN® (dry powder) for Injection in vials of 10 mg (10 ml). **(Lilly)**

VINCRISTINE SULFATE

Description: Vincristine sulfate is the salt of an alkaloid obtained from a common flowering herb, the periwinkle plant (*Vinca rosea* Linn.). It is structurally similar to vinblastine except that a formyl group replaces the methyl group on the vinblastine molecule; however, there appears to be no cross resistance between the 2 compounds. Vincristine sulfate occurs as colorless crystals; the lyophilized dosage form is a white, crystalline powder freely soluble in water.

The mode of action of vincristine is not known. Treatment of neoplastic cells in vitro demonstrated that the drug may cause an arrest of mitotic division at the metaphase stage of the dividing cell. CNS leukemia has been reported to progress in patients undergoing therapy with vincristine. This suggests that the drug does not penetrate well into the cerebrospinal fluid.

Indications: Treatment of acute leukemia. It has also been shown to be useful in combination with other oncolytic agents in Hodgkin's disease, lymphosarcoma, reticulum-cell sarcoma, rhabdomyosarcoma, neuroblastoma, and Wilm's tumor.

Contraindications: Although preexisting leukopenia does not necessarily contraindicate the initiation of therapy, the occurrence of leukopenia, or a complicating infection, during treatment warrants careful consideration before administration of the next dose.

Warnings: Since reproduction studies in animals have not been performed, there is no adequate information as to whether or not this drug may affect fertility in male or female patients or have teratogenic or other adverse effects on the fetus.

Precautions: The monitoring of serum uric acid levels and forced fluid intake to maintain adequate hydration and urinary output should serve to prevent acute uric acid nephropathy. Particular attention should be given to dosage and to neurological complications if the drug is administered to patients with preexisting neuromuscular disease and also when other drugs with neurotoxic potential are being used. In some instances, it may be advisable to administer alkali to increase the solubility of urates in the urine. If CNS leukemia is diagnosed, additional agents and routes of administration may be required, since vincristine does not appear to cross the blood-brain barrier in adequate amounts.

Adverse Reactions: In general, adverse reactions are reversible and are related to dosage. The most common side effect is hair loss while the most troublesome are neuromuscular in origin. Leukopenia, neuritic pain, constipation and difficulty in walking occur with the administration of single weekly doses and are generally of short duration (less than 7 days). These reactions tend to lessen or disappear when the dosage is reduced, but seem to be increased when the calculated amount is given in divided doses. Other complications such as hair loss, sensory impairment, paresthesia, slapping gait, loss of deep tendon reflexes, and muscle wasting may persist for at least as long as therapy is continued. In most instances, these have disappeared by about the sixth week after discontinuance of treatment, but in some patients the neuromuscular difficulties may persist for prolonged periods. Convulsions, frequently with hypertension, have also been reported. Severe constipation, sometimes resulting in colickly abdominal pain and obstruction may be prevented by a prophylactic regimen of laxatives and hydrophilic agents. In addition to constipation, paralytic ileus may occur, particularly in young children. The syndrome of hyponatremia associated with high urinary sodium excretion and inappropriate antidiuretic hormone secretion has been observed occasionally. Other adverse effects that have been noted include abdominal cramps, ataxia, foot drop, weight loss, fever, cranial nerve manifestations, paresthesia and numbness of the digits, polyuria, dysuria, oral ulceration, headache, vomiting, and diarrhea. The drug does not appear to have any constant or significant effect upon the platelets or the red blood cells. Thrombocytopenia, if present when therapy is initiated, may actually improve before the appearance of bone marrow remission.

Dosage and Administration: *Intravenously at weekly intervals.* **Extreme care must be used in calculating and administering the dose of vincristine, since overdosage may have a very serious or fatal outcome.** The usual dosage range for children is 0.05 to 0.15 mg/kg of body weight/week. Initially, 0.05 mg is given, then increased by increments of 0.025 mg/kg up to a maximum of 0.15 mg/kg of body weight. Following remission, the dosage may then be reduced, in some instances, to a maintenance level of 0.05 to 0.75 mg/kg/week. The usual dosage range for adults is 0.01 to 0.05 mg/kg of body weight. Initially, 0.01 mg is given, then increased by increments of 0.01 mg/kg up to a maximum of 0.05 mg/kg of body weight. Following remission, the dosage may then be reduced, in some instances, to a maintenance level of 0.02 to 0.05 mg/kg/week. **Note:** Extravasation during intravenous injection may cause considerable irritation. The injection should be discontinued immediately, and any remaining portion of the dose should then be introduced into another vein.

Availability:
ONCOVIN® (dry powder) for Injection in vials of 1 and 5 mg with 10-ml ampuls of diluent. **(Lilly)**

VI-PENTA F: see The Fluoride-Vitamins

VI-SYNERAL INJECTABLE

Description: Each 2 ml provides:

Vitamin A	(5000 U.S.P. units)	1.5 mg
Ergocalciferol	(400 U.S.P. units)	12.5 μg
Ascorbic acid		25 mg
Thiamine hydrochloride		5 mg
Riboflavin		0.5 mg
Niacinamide		10 mg
Pyridoxine hydrochloride		1.5 mg
Dexpanthenol		2.5 mg
Vitamin E (*dl*-α-tocopheryl acetate)		1 IU

Indications: The various conditions known to interfere with the oral intake, absorption or utilization of fat-soluble or water-soluble vitamins, or both. The preparation is valuable for the rapid replenishment of depleted tissue levels of vitamins.

Precautions: Intravenous administration of solutions containing thiamine has been known to cause an allergic reaction. It should not be given as a direct undiluted intravenous injection as it may give rise to dizziness, faintness, etc.

Dosage and Administration: *Intramuscularly,* 2 ml on alternate days, or more often as necessary. Injections should not exceed 2 ml/dose and should not be given more frequently than once daily, nor continued beyond the time required for adequate saturation of tissue, especially of vitamins A and D. *Intravenous infusion,* 2 ml daily, added directly to intravenous dextrose, saline, or similar infusion solutions, e.g., plasma, protein hydrolysates, etc. Each 2 ml of this preparation should be added to not less than 300 ml of infusion fluid.

Availability:
VI-SYNERAL® INJECTABLE Aqueous in ampuls of 2 ml and in multiple-dose vials of 10 ml.
(Fisons)

VITAMIN A

Description: Vitamin A, one of the fat-soluble vitamins, is practically free from vitamin D and is prepared synthetically or obtained from the livers of sea-water fish rich in vitamin A content. It includes vitamin A itself as well as its precursors, *alpha, beta* and *gamma* carotene and cryptoxanthin. Absorption from an aqueous vehicle is greater than from an oily solution. Vitamin A is assayed biologically and is expressed in terms of international units. One international unit equals 1 U.S.P. unit which is equal to 0.3 mcg of vitamin A alcohol, 0.34 mcg of vitamin A acetate or 0.6 mcg of beta carotene.

Beta-carotene, retinol and retinal possess effective and reliable vitamin A activity. Retinal and retinol are in chemical equilibrium in the body and possess equivalent antixerophthalmic activity. Retinal combines with the rod pigment opsin in the retina to form rhodopsin, necessary for visual dark adaptation. Vitamin A promotes normal growth and development, and is essential for the functional and structural integrity of epithelial cells. Storage of vitamin A in normal adult liver is sufficient to satisfy bio-requirements for 2 years.

Vitamin A is readily absorbed from the normal gastrointestinal tract, and plasma levels reach a peak within 3 to 5 hours. Carotene is absorbed more slowly and usually reaches its maximum in approximately 7 to 8 hours. Normal plasma levels are about 130 units/100 ml.

Animal reproduction studies have shown fetal abnormalities in several species associated with overdosage of this vitamin. Malformations of the CNS, the eye, palate, and urogenital tracts have been reported.

Indications: Vitamin A is essential to the growth and development of children, and is given as a dietary supplement. It is used to correct the deficiency which may lead to a characteristic eye disease, xerophthalmia; a type of night blindness, nyctalopia, which responds to vitamin A therapy; certain types of hyperkeratosis of the skin due to vitamin A deficiency; and lowered resistance to infections in general.

Contraindications: Hypervitaminosis A; malabsorption syndrome; intravenous administration; sensitivity to vitamin A or to any ingredient in the preparation.

Warnings: Overdosage should be avoided. Preparations containing this vitamin should be kept out of reach of children. Safe use of amounts exceeding 6000 units daily during pregnancy has not been established, and doses in excess of the recommended dietary allowance during normal pregnancy should be avoided.

Precautions: When vitamin A in high dosage is given for a prolonged period, it is advisable that treatment be interrupted at intervals to avoid possible hypervitaminosis. It has been observed that female patients on oral contraceptives have shown a significant increase in plasma vitamin A levels. Patients who are on a prolonged daily dose of over 25,000 U.S.P. units should be under close supervision. Blood-level assays are not a direct measure of liver storage, and liver storage should be adequate before discontinuing therapy.

Adverse Reactions: Anaphylactic shock and death have been reported using the intravenous route. General manifestations of acute toxicity are fatigue, malaise, lethargy, abdominal discomfort, anorexia, and vomiting. Specific manifestations include slow growth of skeletal bones, hard, tender cortical thickening over the radius and tibia, migratory arthralgia, and premature closure of epiphysis; irritability, headache, and increased intracranial pressure as manifested by bulging fontanels, papilledema, and exophthalmos; fissures of lips, drying and cracking of skin, alopecia, scaling, massive desquamation, and increased pigmentation; hypomenorrhea, hepatosplenomegaly, jaundice, leukopenia, and vitamin A plasma level in excess of 1200 IU/100 ml. Discontinuance of the vitamin results in prompt disappearance of symptoms.

Dosage and Administration: *Orally* or *parenterally*. Therapeutic daily dosage should be at least 4500 units for infants, 9000 units for children, and 12,000 units for adults. These dosages are about 3 times the M.D.R. *Intramuscularly,* 2 ml on alternate days, or at the discretion of the physician. Dosage ordinarily should not exceed an average of 50,000 units/day. Injection should be made *slowly* deep in the upper outer quadrant of the gluteus muscle or deep in the outer aspect of the thigh, changing the site for each injection. Because of the greater absorption of aqueous A, dosage should be adjusted according to individual response.

Availability:

AQUASOL® A: **(USV)**

Capsules, 25,000 units in bottles of 100; 50,000 units in bottles of 100 and 500.

Parenteral, 50,000 units/ml in vials of 5 ml.

VI-DOM-A®: **(Dome)**

Capsules, 50,000 units in bottles of 100.

Troches, 50,000 units in bottles of 25.

VITAMIN B COMPLEX, PARENTERAL

Description: A complex of vitamin B factors including thiamine, riboflavin, pyridoxine, niacin, niacinamide, cyanocobalamin, pantothenic acid, biotin and many other substances. Products supplying the vitamin B complex may be prepared from mixtures of crystalline synthetic factors; from special strains of dried brewer's yeast, alone or fortified with added crystalline factors; or from concentrates of yeast, liver, or rice polishings, alone or fortified with added crystalline factors.

Commercially available preparations employ many of the B factors, in a variety of combinations, and in varied amounts.

Indications: Prevention and treatment of vitamin B complex deficiencies. Parenteral administration of these factors is necessary in severe vitamin depletion states in which absorption from the gastrointestinal tract is likely to be impaired; it is particularly indicated when the condition of the patient suggests that a large supply of these factors be made available for the immediate demands of metabolism. Since several of the vitamin B factors are involved with carbohydrate metabolism, parenteral vitamin B complex is useful both preoperatively and postoperatively when administered concurrently with dextrose infusions.

Contraindications: Individuals who are allergic to any of the components.

Warnings: Prior to administration, an evaluation of the hematopoietic function should be made. Also, any medication the patient may be taking must be evaluated for possible vitamin interaction.

Precautions: The patient should be advised as to proper dietary habits during treatment so that relapses will be less likely to occur when dosage is reduced or therapy is withdrawn. Increased carbohydrate intake without adequate supplementation with vitamin B complex factors may rapidly precipitate an acute deficiency.

Adverse Reactions: Some individuals may develop a sensitivity or intolerance to thiamine and/or vitamin B-12, especially after repeated intravenous administrations. Since anaphylactic shock and death have been reported, it is therefore recommended that an intradermal test dose be given prior to administration of the full therapeutic dose. Some tenderness and induration may follow intramuscular injection. Other reported reactions included generalized flushing, skin rash, and pruritus.

Dosage and Administration: *Intramuscular* injection is preferred. The amount to be administered will depend upon an appraisal of the vitamin B content of the diet that the patient can and will employ, his condition, and whether it is prophylaxis or treatment that is required. Ordinarily, 2 ml should be adequate, although 5 ml or even more may be given if indicated. Dosage depends, of course, upon the composition of the preparation being used. When used with dextrose injection or other *intravenous* infusion solutions for prophylaxis, 2 to 10 ml for each liter of 5 or 10% solution may be used.

Availability:

BEJECTAL® Injection in 2 vials of 10 ml each. One vial provides in each ml thiamine HCl, 10 mg; riboflavin, 2 mg (as 5′-phosphate sodium); pyridoxine HCl, 5 mg; niacinamide, 75 mg and *d*-sodium pantothenate, 5 mg. When mixed with the contents of the second vial (preservatives and stabilizers), the combined solution is stable for 2 months at room temperature. **(Abbott)**

BEJECTAL with VITAMIN C Injectable in 2-compartment vial of 10 ml. When mixed, each ml provides thiamine HCl, 20 mg; riboflavin, 3 mg (as 5′-phosphate sodium), pyridoxine HCl, 5 mg; cyanocobalamin, 2 mcg; niacinamide, 75 mg; *d*-sodium pantothenate, 5 mg and ascorbic acid, 100 mg. After mixing, the resultant solution is stable for 2 weeks in a refrigerator. **(Abbott)**

BEJEX® Injectable in single-dose, 2-compartment vial of 5 ml. When mixed, each ml provides thiamine HCl, 2 mg; riboflavin, 2 mg (as 5′-phosphate sodium); pyridoxine HCl, 1 mg; cyanocobalamin, 5 mcg; niacinamide, 50 mg; *d*-sodium pantothenate, 10 mg and ascorbic acid, 100 mg. After mixing, the resultant solution is stable for 1 week in a refrigerator. **(Abbott)**

BEROCCA®-C Injection in ampuls of 2 ml and in multiple dose vials of 20 ml. Each 2 ml contains thiamine HCl, 10 mg; riboflavin, 10 mg (as 5′-phosphate sodium); pyridoxine HCl, 20 mg; niacinamide, 80 mg; panthenol, 20 mg (equivalent to 23.2 mg of calcium pantothenate); *d*-biotin, 0.2 mg and ascorbic acid, 100 mg. **(Roche)**

BEROCCA-C 500 Injectable in duplex packages of 2 ampuls of 2 ml each. When mixed, each 4 ml of the resultant solution contains thiamine HCl, 10 mg; riboflavin, 10 mg (as 5′-phosphate sodium); pyridoxine HCl, 20 mg; niacinamide, 80 mg; D-panthenol, 20 mg (equivalent to 23.2 mg of calcium pantothenate); *d*-biotin, 0.2 mg and ascorbic acid, 500 mg. Four ml of this solution may then be added to 1 liter of infusion liquid. **(Roche)**

BETALIN® COMPLEX Injection in ampuls of 2 ml and in multiple-dose vials of 10 ml. Each ml provides thiamine HCl, 5 mg; riboflavin, 2 mg (as 5′-phosphate sodium); pantothenic acid, 2.5 mg (as panthenol); pyridoxine HCl, 5 mg; cyanocobalamin, 2.5 mcg and niacinamide, 75 mg. *Solution should be kept refrigerated.* **(Lilly)**

BETALIN COMPLEX F.C. Injection in ampuls of 2 ml and in multiple-dose vials of 10 ml. Each ml provides thiamine HCl, 12.5 mg; riboflavin, 3 mg (as 5′-phosphate sodium); pyridoxine HCl, 5 mg; niacinamide, 50 mg; pantothenic acid, 2.5 mg (as panthenol) and ascorbic acid, 75 mg. *Solution should be kept refrigerated.* **(Lilly)**

FOLBESYN® PARENTERAL. In single-dose ampuls of 2 ml containing thiamine HCl, 10 mg; riboflavin, 10 mg (as 5′-phosphate sodium); pyridoxine HCl, 15 mg; vitamin B-12, 15 mcg; niacinamide, 75 mg; sodium pantothenate, 10 mg and ascorbic acid, 300 mg. An ampul of diluent contains folic acid, 1 mg. *Solution should be protected from light and kept refrigerated.* **(Lederle)**

KREMPLEX-B-12-1000 Injectable in vials of 10 ml. Each ml contains thiamine HCl, 100 mg; niacinamide, 50 mg; riboflavin, 5 mg; pyridoxine HCl, 2 mg; dexpanthenol, 5 mg; vitamin B-12, 1 mg (1000 mcg); chlorobutanol, 5 mg; benzyl alcohol, 2% in an isotonic solution of sodium chloride. **(Kremers-Urban)**

LYO B-C® with B-12 for Injection (lyophilized) with and without diluent. When reconstituted with 7 ml of diluent, each vial provides thiamine HCl, 100 mg; riboflavin, 10 mg; pyridoxine HCl, 10 mg; cyanocobalamin, 25 mcg; panthenol, 50 mg (equivalent to 58 mg of calcium pantothenate); niacinamide, 250 mg and ascorbic acid, 200 mg. **(Merck Sharp & Dohme)**

LYO B-C® FORTE with B-12 for Injection (lyophilized) with and without diluent. When reconstituted with 7 ml of diluent, each vial is identical in composition to LYO B-C with B-12 for Injection, except that the amounts of niacinamide and ascorbic acid have been increased to 500 mg. **(Merck Sharp & Dohme)**

PARLITE® for Injection in single-dose vials. When reconstituted with a suitable diluent, each vial provides thiamine HCl, 10 mg; riboflavin, 10 mg (as 5′-phosphate sodium); pyridoxine HCl, 5 mg; vitamin B-12, 25 mcg; sodium pantothenate, 10 mg; niacinamide, 150 mg and ascorbic acid, 500 mg. **(Lederle)**

PLEBEX® Injection in vials of 10 and 30 ml. Each ml contains thiamine HCl, 10 mg; riboflavin, 2 mg; pyridoxine HCl, 5 mg; niacinamide, 100 mg and calcium pantothenate, 5 mg. **(Wyeth)**

SOLU-B® for Injection in Mix-O-Vials® of 2 ml with diluent. When reconstituted, each Mix-O-Vial contains thiamine HCl, 10 mg; riboflavin, 10 mg; pyridoxine HCl, 5 mg; niacinamide, 250 mg and calcium pantothenate, 50 mg. **(Upjohn)**

SOLU-B with ASCORBIC ACID for Injection with a 5-ml ampul of ascorbic acid solution, 500 mg and in Mix-O-Vials of 5 ml with transfer needle. When reconstituted, each vial is identical in composition to Solu-B, plus ascorbic acid. When mixed, each Mix-O-Vial provides thiamine HCl, 10 mg; riboflavin, 10 mg (as 5′-phosphate sodium); pyridoxine HCl, 5 mg; niacinamide, 250 mg; sodium pantothenate, 50 mg and ascorbic acid, 500 mg. **(Upjohn)**

SOLU-B FORTE® for Injection in Mix-O-Vials of 10 ml with transfer needle. When mixed, each vial provides thiamine HCl, 250 mg; riboflavin, 50 mg; pyridoxine HCl, 50 mg; niacinamide, 1.25 gm; sodium pantothenate, 500 mg and ascorbic acid, 1 gm. **(Upjohn)**

VITAMIN B COMPLEX, PARENTERAL in Steri-Vials® of 10 ml. Each ml of sterile solution contains thiamine HCl, 10 mg; riboflavin, 2 mg; pyridoxine HCl, 5 mg; niacinamide, 50 mg and *d*-panthenol, 10 mg (equivalent to 10.7 mg of pantothenic acid). **(Parke-Davis)**

VITAMIN B COMPLEX with B-12 for injection in Tubex® (needle-cartridge unit) of 1 ml. Each ml contains thiamine HCl, 10 mg; riboflavin, 5 mg; niacinamide, 100 mg; pyridoxine HCl, 5 mg; cyanocobalamin, 7.5 mcg and d-pantothenyl alcohol, 5 mg. **(Wyeth)**

VITAMIN B COMPLEX with VITAMIN C for injection in Tubex® (needle-cartridge unit) of 2 ml. Each ml contains thiamine HCl, 10 mg; riboflavin, 2.5 mg; niacinamide, 50 mg; pyridoxine HCl, 2.5 mg; d-pantothenyl alcohol, 2.5 mg and ascorbic acid, 75 mg. **(Wyeth)**

VITAMIN B-12 with INTRINSIC FACTOR

Description: Vitamin B-12 with intrinsic factor is a complex prepared from vitamin B-12 and the intrinsic factor obtained from the stomach of hogs. Intrinsic factor may be defined as one of the factors of Castle, the absence of which is responsible for the development of pernicious anemia. The normal gastric juice of man contains a mucoprotein (intrinsic factor) which is necessary for the assimilation and absorption of oral cyanocobalamin.

Statements concerning the amount of vitamin B-12 present are excluded in some instances to avoid the misconception that this represents additional hematopoietic activity in excess of the number of units indicated on the package label. The potency of vitamin B-12 with intrinsic factor is expressed in terms of the U.S.P. oral units of hematopoietic activity.

Indications: Treatment and maintenance in common anemias including hypoferric anemia, anemia associated with chronic blood loss, megaloblastic anemias of pregnancy, and those of nutritional origin. All of the other means that are recognized as suited to the treatment of these anemias should also be employed (e.g., cyanocobalamin, iron salts, folic acid). Patients resistant to this form of therapy require further study to determine the etiology, followed by additional therapeutic measures.

Contraindications: In the treatment of patients with disease associated with increased iron storage (hemochromatosis). Hypersensitivity to any of the components.

Warnings: Folic acid is improper therapy in the treatment of pernicious anemia and other megaloblastic anemias where vitamin B-12 is deficient. *Store out of reach of children.*

Precautions: Some patients with pernicious anemia may not respond to oral vitamin B-12 with intrinsic factor and there is no way known to predict which patients will respond and which patients may become refractory. Periodic examinations and laboratory studies of these patients are essential and recommended. If any symptoms of intolerance occur, the drug should be discontinued, temporarily or permanently. Folic acid may obscure pernicious anemia in that the blood status in the periphery may revert to normal while neurologic manifestations may remain progressive. Supplemental folic acid should not be relied on to correct the serious folic acid deficiency characterizing sprue or the malabsorption syndromes. In these conditions, therapeutic amounts of folic acid should be given. Iron compounds taken orally can impair the absorption of tetracycline and its derivatives. In addition, antacids when given together with iron compounds will decrease the absorption of iron.

Adverse Reactions: Rare instances of gastric irritation, nausea, constipation, and diarrhea have been noted. Allergic sensitization has been reported following both oral and parenteral administration of folic acid. Overdosage of compounds containing elemental iron are usually characterized primarily by vomiting, diarrhea, and melena. Shock, dyspnea, lethargy, and coma may ensue followed by metabolic acidoses.

Dosage and Administration: *Orally.* The average daily dosage of vitamin B-12 with intrinsic factor for the treatment of pernicious anemia and related macrocytic anemias is 0.5 oral U.S.P. unit before breakfast and before dinner. A more rapid response may be obtained in severe cases by doubling the dose for the first week or two of treatment. Capsules, 1 daily with or after meals.

Availability:

Combinations

FERGON® PLUS Caplets (tablets), ½ oral unit with ferrous gluconate, 500 mg and ascorbic acid, 75 mg in bottles of 100 and 500. **(Breon)**

PRONEMIA® Capsules, vitamin B-12 (as cobalamin concentrate), 15 mcg; intrinsic factor concentrate, 75 mg; ferrous fumarate, 350 mg (elemental iron, 115 mg); ascorbic acid, 150 mg and folic acid, 1 mg in bottles of 100 and 500. **(Lederle)**

RETICULEX® Capsules (Pulvules), vitamin B-12 (as cobalamin concentrate), 10 mcg; intrinsic factor concentrate, 222 mg; ferrous sulfate, 75 mg; ascorbic acid, 50 mg and folic acid, 0.3 mg in bottles of 100. **(Lilly)**

TOLFRINIC™ Tablets, 1 oral unit with ferrous fumarate, 600 mg (equiv. to 200 mg elemental iron) and ascorbic acid 100 mg in bottles of 100. **(Ascher)**

VITRON-C-PLUS

Description: Each tablet contains:

Ferrous fumarate (equiv. to 132 mg elemental iron)	400 mg
Ascorbic acid	250 mg

Cobalamin concentrate (B-12)	25 μg
Folic acid	1 mg

Indications: Prophylaxis and treatment of anemia including iron deficiency anemia, megaloblastic anemia due to a deficiency of folic acid as may be noted in tropical or nontropical sprue; and anemias of nutritional origin.

Contraindications: In the presence of hemochromatosis and hemosiderosis; cirrhosis of the liver; unusual sensitivity to any of the components. Folic acid is contraindicated in patients with untreated and uncomplicated pernicious anemia, and in those with anaphylactic sensitivity to folic acid.

Warnings: Folic acid may mask unsuspected early pernicious anemia by correcting or preventing the hematological manifestations, while the neurological manifestations progress. Periodic examinations and laboratory studies of pernicious anemia patients are essential. Resistance to treatment may be due to depressed hematopoiesis, alcoholism, antimetabolic drugs, a deficiency of vitamin E or an increased requirement for vitamin B-6.

Precautions: In the treatment of anemia of any type a correct diagnosis is essential to determine the underlying cause. Prolonged therapeutic use of iron salts may result in iron shortage disease.

Adverse Reactions: An occasional patient may experience gastrointestinal reactions, such as diarrhea or constipation. These reactions may be alleviated by taking the drug with meals and by reducing the dose. Sensitivity to folic acid may occur on rare occasions.

Dosage and Administration: *Orally.* Adults and children over 6 years of age, 1 tablet daily.

Availability:
VITRON-C-PLUS® Tablets (maroon) in bottles of 30, 100 and 500. **(Fisons)**

VŌSOL OTIC SOLUTION
VŌSOL HC OTIC SOLUTION

Description: A nonaqueous solution of acetic acid, 2% in a propylene glycol vehicle containing propylene glycol diacetate, 3%; benzethonium chloride, 0.02% and sodium acetate, 0.015%. Vōsol HC contains in addition hydrocortisone, 1% and citric acid, 0.2%. Solutions have antibacterial and antifungal properties; are hydrophylic, have an acid pH and a low surface tension. The addition of hydrocortisone, an adrenal corticosteroid, affords antiinflammatory and antipruritic activity.

Indications: Vōsol is indicated for the treatment of superficial infections of the external auditory canal caused by organisms susceptible to the action of acetic acid. May be used prophylactically in patients who are susceptible to recurrent swimmer's ear. Vōsol HC is indicated when the otitis is complicated by inflammation.

Contraindications: Hypersensitivity to any of the components; perforated tympanic membranes. Hydrocortisone is contraindicated in vaccinia and varicella.

Precautions: Safe use of topical steroids during pregnancy has not been fully established; therefore; they should not be used for prolonged periods in pregnant patients. The possibility of systemic effects should be considered, particulary when used for extended periods of time. The medication should be discontinued promptly if sensitization or irritation develops.

Dosage and Administration: *Topically.* Adults and children: For treatment of external otitis, 5 drops instilled into ear canal 3 or 4 times daily. If perferred, a saturated gauze wick kept moist with the drops may be used for the first 24 hours. For prophylaxis of external otitis (Vōsol only), 2 drops into ear canal morning and evening.

Availability:
VŌSOL®: **(Wallace)**
Otic Solution in plastic bottles of 15 and 30 ml with calibrated dropper.
HC Otic Solution in plastic bottles of 7.5 ml with calibrated dropper.

WARFARIN

Chemical Name: 3-(α-Acetonylbenzyl)-4-hydroxycoumarin.

Description: Warfarin is a synthetic coumarin drug that depresses the formation of prothrombin in the liver, and interferes with the production of factors VII, IX, and X, thereby minimizing intravascular clotting. The inhibition of prothrombin involves interference with the action of vitamin K, and it has been postulated that warfarin, like bishydroxycoumarin, competes with vitamin K for an enzyme essential for prothrombin synthesis.

Warfarin is readily absorbed from the gastrointestinal tract. Maximal plasma levels are attained within 2 to 8 hours, peak effect in 36 to 72 hours, with effects on prothrombin time persisting for about 4 to 5 days following a single therapeutic dose.

Since coumarin anticoagulants are extensively bound to plasma proteins (97%), the displacement of only a relatively small proportion of coumarin may greatly increase the concentration of unbound coumarin, causing an unexpected prolongation of the prothrombin time. Fatalities have been reported from interactions affecting the metabolism of coumarin anticoagulants or their binding to plasma proteins. Drugs which may stimulate metabolic degradation of warfarin include phenobarbital, as well as other barbiturates, glutethimide, meprobamate, ethchlorvynol, and griseofulvin. In addition, oral contraceptives have been reported to reduce the response to coumarin anticoagulants. Patients receiving these drugs may require larger doses of warfarin to achieve an optimal anticoagulant effect. Drugs which may displace warfarin from protein binding sites in blood plasma, thus making increased quantities of free coumarin available, include aspirin, chloral hydrate, clofibrate, phenylbutazone, oxyphenbutazone, diazoxide, and mefenamic, ethacrynic, and nalidixic acids. Drugs such as quinidine and quinine as well as salicylates in large doses depress prothrombin formation in the liver, and thus may increase the patient's sensitivity to warfarin and cause hemorrhage. Other drugs which have been reported to cause an exaggerated response and a prolonged prothrombin time include methylthiouracil, propylthiouracil, methyldopa, phenyramidol, disulfiram, dextrothyroxine, and various anabolic steroids, as well as some radioactive compounds. The coumarin anticoagulants are known to potentiate the hypoglycemic effects of tolbutamide by inhibiting its degradation in the liver.

Indications: Prophylaxis and treatment of pulmonary embolism, venous thrombosis and its extension, and the treatment of atrial fibrillation with embolization, and as an adjunct in the treatment of coronary occlusion.

Contraindications: In the presence of bleeding or a tendency to bleed (hemorrhage), blood dyscrasias, purpura, open ulcerative, traumatic, or surgical wounds, ulcerations of the gastrointestinal tract, visceral carcinoma, diverticulitis, colitis, or subacute bacterial endocarditis, threatened abortion, recent surgery on the eye, brain, or spinal cord, regional and lumbar block anesthesia, vitamin K deficiency, severe hypertension, severe hepatic or renal disease, and when there is continuous tubal drainage of the gastrointestinal and urinary tracts.

Warnings: Warfarin is a potent drug, and its effects tend to be cumulative and prolonged; at the earliest sign of bleeding the drug should be withdrawn. Prothrombin time must be evaluated as often as necessary to determine dosage requirements; evaluation of clotting and bleeding times are not effective procedures in establishing proper dosage. When sodium heparin is given with warfarin, the one-stage prothrombin time determination should be delayed for a period of from 4 to 5 hours after the last intravenous dose and from 12 to 24 hours after the last subcutaneous dose of sodium heparin. During pregnancy both the mother and fetus are subject to the risks of anticoagulant therapy; fetal hemorrhage and intrauterine death have occurred. Malformations characterized by hypoplastic nasal structures in infants born to mothers with prosthetic heart valves who have been treated with coumarin anticoagulants during the first trimester of pregnancy have been reported. However, it has not been determined if the anticoagulant was the responsible agent. The risk of withholding the drug should be weighed against the possible hazards entailed in administering it. Since the drug appears in the mother's milk, the nursing infant should be observed for evidence of unexpected bleeding.

Precautions: Warfarin should be prescribed with care, and suitable laboratory facilities should be available for accurate control of therapy. The drug should be administered with caution in patients with active tuberculosis, moderate hypertension, mild liver or kidney disease, severe diabetes, indwelling catheters, during menstruation and in the postpartum period, in patients with a past history of ulcerative disease of the gastrointestinal tract, or those in occupations which carry a hazard of significant physical injury. Patients with congestive heart failure frequently require a reduction in dosage. Careful management of the patient is essential if prothrombin activity falls below 15% of normal or if hemorrhage occurs. The drug should be withdrawn temporarily and the administration of vitamin K or transfusion of whole blood may be required depending upon the clinical situation. Usually an overly prolonged prothrombin time or minor hemorrhage will respond satisfactorily to withdrawal of therapy alone. The drug should be withdrawn prior to surgery involving the CNS or eye. Following surgery within the gastrointestinal tract, the stools should be checked frequently for traces of blood. Any change in vitamin K or dietary fat intake may alter anticoagulant response to warfarin; therefore, periodic determinations of prothrombin time is essential. Cautious use is deemed necessary in debilitated or cachectic patients as well as in those with hepatic dysfunction. The newborn infant, due to vitamin K deficiency, is particularly sensitive to the drug. Renal insufficiency, fever, alcoholism, and scurvy enhance or prolong the anticoagulant response, and exposure to x-ray may lead to a prolonged prothrombin time. Conversely, diarrhea may cause a decreased response due to reduced absorption of orally administered warfarin.

Adverse Reactions: Excessive doses may cause hematuria, bleeding from mucous membranes, hemorrhage from a wound or an ulcerative lesion, or widespread petechial and purpuric hemorrhages. Paralytic ileus and intestinal obstruction have been reported from submucosal or intramural hemorrhage. Excessive uterine bleeding has occurred, but menstrual flow is usually normal. Bleeding following oral coumarin anticoagulant therapy does not always correlate with prothrombin activity. The occurrence of significant gastrointestinal or urinary tract bleeding during warfarin therapy may indicate the presence of an underlying occult lesion. If major hemorrhagic complications occur, the drug should be discontinued immediately. Bleeding episodes of any type indicate the need for critical evaluation of the patient's condition.

In addition to hemorrhage and hemorrhagic manifestations, dermatitis, urticaria, alopecia, and priapism have rarely been reported. Other less commonly reported side effects include fever and gastrointestinal symptoms varying from nausea and vomiting to abdominal cramping and diarrhea. Hemorrhagic necrosis (bleeding into the skin and subcutaneous tissue with necrosis, vasculitis, and thrombosis) of the female breast and other areas has been reported in association with oral anticoagulant therapy.

For complete information on potential drug interactions, see monograph on Bishydroxycoumarin.

Dosage and Administration: *Orally, intravenously* or *intramuscularly.* Dosage must be individualized with frequent prothrombin times being used as a guide until maintenance dosage is established. As a general guide, approximately 40 to 60 mg is a satisfactory initial dose, with 2 to 10 mg as a maintenance dose. For elderly or debilitated patients, 20 to 30 mg. The aim of therapy is to reduce prothrombin activity to 20 or 30% of normal. However, the range of 15 to 35% of normal is almost as satisfactory and may be more practicable in some cases.

Availability:

Warfarin Potassium

ATHROMBIN®-K Tablets, 5 mg in bottles of 25, 100 and 1000; 10 mg in bottles of 100 and 1000. **(Purdue Frederick)**

Warfarin Sodium

COUMADIN® (crystalline, as isopropanol elathrate): **(Endo)**

Injection in vials of 50 mg (dry) with ampuls of 2 ml of diluent.

Tablets, 2, 2.5, 5, 7.5, 10 and 25 mg in bottles of 100 and 1000 and in blister-pack cartons of 100.

PANWARFIN® Tablets, 2, 2.5, 5, and 7.5 mg in bottles of 100 and 500; 10 and 25 mg in bottles of 100. All potencies except the 25 mg are available in Abbo-Pac® (unit-dose) packages of 100. **(Abbott)**

WYANOIDS HC

Description: Each suppository contains:

Hydrocortisone acetate	10 mg
Belladonna extract (total alkaloids, 0.19 mg)	15 mg
Ephedrine sulfate	3 mg
Zinc oxide	176 mg
Boric acid	543 mg
Bismuth oxyiodide	30 mg
Bismuth subcarbonate	146 mg

with balsam of Peru, 30 mg in cocoa butter and beeswax.

Indications: Treatment of proctitis especially that secondary to ulcerative colitis.

Contraindications: Hydrocortisone should not be used until a diagnosis has been established. It is contraindicated in the presence of such conditions as tuberculosis, fungal infections, acute herpes simplex, vaccinia and varicella. Belladonna is contraindicated in glaucoma or organic pyloric stenosis.

Precautions: Other specific measures against infections, allergy and other causal factors must not be overlooked. Since safe use has not been established during pregnancy, compounds containing hydrocortisone should not be used unnecessarily in pregnant patients. Routine caution is advised if the patient is taking other corticosteroid drugs. Also, prolonged and excessive use might produce systemic corticosteroid effects. Belladonna should be used cautiously in the presence of prostatism, urinary retention, in the elderly and in children under 6 years of age. Patients should be cautioned not to exceed the prescribed dose, to decrease the dose if dryness of the mouth occurs, and to discontinue use if rapid pulse, blurring of vision or dizziness occurs. Frequent or prolonged use of belladonna should be avoided.

Dosage and Administration: One suppository inserted *rectally* twice daily for 6 days or as required.

Availability:
WYANOIDS® HC Rectal Suppositories in packages of 12 and in Redipak® cartons of 25.

(Wyeth)

XYLOMETAZOLINE HYDROCHLORIDE

Chemical Name: 2-(4′-*tert*-Butyl-2′,6′-dimethylbenzyl)-2-imidazoline monohydrochloride.

Description: Xylometazoline hydrochloride is a sympathomimetic amine related structurally and pharmacologically to naphazoline and tetrahydrozoline. It occurs as a white, crystalline powder sparingly soluble in water and freely soluble in alcohol. Its sympathomimetic action constricts the smaller arterioles of the nasal passages, effecting a decongesting action. This vasoconstriction results from alpha-adrenergic receptor stimulation of vascular smooth muscle.

Indications: Symptomatic relief of nasal and nasopharyngeal congestion associated with the common cold, hay fever, sinusitis and allergic conditions.

Contraindications: Hypersensitivity to xylometazoline, narrow-angle glaucoma, concurrent use with MAO inhibitors or tricylic antidepressants.

Warnings: Overdosage may produce a profound CNS depression in children, possibly requiring intensive supportive treatment. Safe use of xylometazoline during pregnancy has not been established with respect to adverse effects upon fetal development; therefore, the drug should not be used in women of childbearing potential and particularly during the first trimester of pregnancy unless, in the judgment of the physician, the potential benefits outweigh the possible hazards.

Precautions: Prolonged or excessive use may cause rebound congestion. It should be given sparingly to patients with hyperthyroidism, advanced arteriosclerotic conditions, coronary artery disease, and hypertension, and to infants, children, and elderly or debilitated patients.

Adverse Reactions: Sensitivity to even small doses of adrenergic substances are manifested by insomnia, dizziness, lightheadedness, weakness, tremulousness, or cardiac arrythmias. Other reactions that may occur include burning, stinging, dryness of the nasal mucosa, sneezing, palpitations, tachycardia, cardiac arrhythmias, increase in blood pressure, headache, nervousness, blurred vision, drowsiness, and CNS depression. Overdosage may be characterized by somnolence, sedation or deep coma. With severe systemic toxicity profound CNS depression may develop accompanied by hypertension, bradycardia, and decreased cardiac output, which may be followed by rebound hypotension and cardiovascular collapse. Also CNS respiratory depression may occur. Intensive supportive care is required to sustain respiratory and cardiovascular function, especially following marked overdosage.

Dosage and Administration: *Locally.* Adults, instill 2 or 3 drops of the solution, or 1 or 2 applications of the spray into each nostril every 4 to 6 hours. Children under 12 years of age, instill 2 or 3 drops of the Pediatric Solution into each nostril every 4 to 6 hours. One drop of the 0.05% solution every 6 hours should be used in infants under 6 months of age.

Availability:
OTRIVIN®: **(Geigy)**
Nasal Solution, 0.1% in dropper bottles of 30 ml and 1 pint.
Nasal Spray, 0.1% in plastic squeeze bottles of 15 ml.
Pediatric Nasal Solution, 0.05% in dropper bottles of 30 ml.

ZINC INSULIN(S): see The Insulins

ADDENDUM

CEFOXITIN SODIUM

Chemical Name: 3-(Hydroxymethyl)-7α-methoxy-8-oxo-7-[2-(2-thienyl)acetamido]-5-thia-1-azabicyclo [4,2.0] oct-2-ene-2-carboxylate carbamate ester sodium.

Description: Cefoxitin sodium is a semisynthetic, broad-spectrum cepha antibiotic for parenteral administration in hospitalized patients afflicted with a variety of serious and life-threatening infections caused by single or multiple aerobic and anerobic bacterial species. It is derived from cephamycin C which is produced by *Streptomyces lactamdurans*. In common with the penicillins and cephalosporins of the beta-lactam family, the bactericidal action results from inhibition of cell wall synthesis. It is particularly active both in vitro and in vivo against most aerobic pathogens, gram-positive and gram-negative organisms including indole-positive Proteus, and most strains of anerobic organisms including the Peptococcus, Peptostreptococcus and Bacteroides species including the *B. fragilis* group. It is not active in vitro against most strains of *Pseudomonas aeruginosa* and enterococci (*Streptococcus faecalis*) and many strains of *Enterobacter cloacae*. Methicillin-resistant staphylococci are almost uniformly resistant to cefoxitin. A major feature of the drug is the possession of a methoxy group in the 7-alpha position of its molecular structure. This 5-atom chain physically protects it from bacterial enzymatic destruction, thereby providing the antibiotic with a high degree of stability in the presence of beta-lactamases (both penicillinases and cephalosporinases) of gram-negative organisms. Each gm of the drug contains approximately 53.8 (2.3 mEq) of sodium, and the pH of a freshly prepared solution usually ranges from 4.2 to 7.

In normal subjects, a 1-gm intramuscular dose yielded peak serum levels of 24 mcg/ml within 20 to 30 minutes, and a half-life of 64.8 minutes. The same amount given intravenously yielded peak serum levels of 110 mcg/ml within 5 minutes which declined to less than 1 mcg/ml within 4 hours, and a half-life of 41 to 59 minutes. Approximately 85% of the drug is excreted unaltered by the kidney over a 6-hour period resulting in high urinary concentrations. Following an intramuscular injection of a 1-gm dose, urinary levels greater than 3000 mcg/ml were observed. The addition of probenecid to the therapeutic regimen helps to slow tubular excretion, to produce higher serum levels and to increase the duration of measurable serum concentrations.

Cefoxitin diffuses into pleural and joint fluids and is detectable in antibacterial concentrations in the bile. Clinical experience has demonstrated that the drug can be given to patients who are receiving carbenicillin or aminoglycoside antibiotics (kanamycin, gentamicin, tobramycin or amikacin); however, cefoxitin should not be added to solutions containing the aminoglycosides. If the Bauer-Kirby-Sherris-Turck method of disc susceptibility testing is used, a disc containing 30 mcg of cefoxitin should give a zone of at least 18 mm or more for highly susceptible organisms, a zone of 15 to 17 mm for intermediate susceptible organisms (those harboring partial resistance), and a zone of 14 mm or less for resistant organisms.

Indications: The drug is recommended for the treatment of serious infections caused by susceptible strains of organisms including lower respiratory tract infections caused by *Streptococcus pneumoniae* and other streptococci (excluding the enterococci), Staphylococcus aureus (penicillinase- and nonpenicillinase-producing organisms), *Escherichia coli*, Klebsiella species, *Haemophilus influenzae*, and Bacteroides species; urinary tract infections caused by *E. coli*, Klebsiella species, *Proteus mirabilis*, indole-positive *Proteus* (*P. morganii, rettgeri,* and *vulgaris*), and Providencia species; intraabdominal infections, including peritonitis and abscess, caused by *E. coli*, Klebsiella species, Bacteroides species (including the fragilis group, and Clostridium species); and gynecologic infections, septicemia, bone and joint infections, and skin structure infections caused by various organisms. Many infections caused by aerobic and anaerobic gram-negative pathogens resistant to some cephalosporins respond to cefoxitin, as do bacterial infections resistant to the penicillins.

Contraindications: In patients hypersensitive to cephalosporins or those who have shown an unusual response to cefoxitin.

Warnings: Patients with a history of allergy, particularly to drugs, and penicillin-sensitive individuals require utmost care. It is advised that the physician, by careful inquiry, determine whether or not the patient has had a previous hypersensitivity reaction to this antibiotic, to cephalosporins, penicillins or other medications. An unusual response warrants immediate withdrawal of the drug. Epinephrine and other emergency measures should be readily available in the event of an acute reaction.

Precautions: A reduction in the recommended total daily dose should be prescribed for patients with renal insufficiency manifested by transient or persistent reduction of urinary output in order to avert the high and prolonged serum antibiotic concentrations that usually occur in such individuals. As with other antibiotics, long-term use may result in overgrowth of resistant organisms; therefore, repeated evaluation of the patient's condition is essential. If superinfection occurs, appropriate measures should be instituted. Increased nephrotoxicity has been reported following concomitant administration of cephalosporins and aminoglycoside antibiotics. A false-positive reaction for glucose in urine has been observed with Clinitest® reagent tablets. Administration to pregnant or lactating women or to women of childbearing potential requires that the anticipated benefits be weighed against the possible risks; it has been found that low levels of the drug appear in the milk of nursing mothers. It is not recommended for administration to children until safe use and proper dosage have been established.

Adverse Reactions: The most common adverse reactions have been reactions following intravenous or intramuscular injection, including thrombophlebitis, pain, induration, and tenderness. *Allergic reactions* are commonly manifested by rash, pruritus, eosinophilia, fever, and other similar effects; *gastrointestinal* by nausea, vomiting, and diarrhea; *hematologic* by transient leukopenia, neutropenia, and hemolytic anemia; *hepatic* by transient elevations in SGOT, SGPT, serum lactic dehydrogenase and alkaline phosphatase; *renal* by elevations in serum creatinine and/or blood urea nitrogen levels. A positive direct Coomb's test may develop in some individuals, especially those with azotemia.

Dosage and Administration: *Intramuscularly* or *intravenously*. For uncomplicated infections, 1 gm every 6 to 8 hours intravenously or intramuscularly; for moderately severe or severe infections, 1 gm every 4 hours or 2 gm every 6 to 8 hours, intravenously; for very severe infections, 2 gm every 4 hours or 3 gm every 6 hours intravenously. In patients with renal insufficiency, an initial loading dose of 1 to 2 gm may be given, followed by a maintenance dosage of 1 to 2 gm every 8 to 12 hours for mild impairment (creatinine clearance 50 to 30 ml/minute); 1 to 2 gm every 12 to 24 hours for moderate impairment (creatinine clearance 29 to 10 ml/minute); 0.5 to 1 gm every 12 to 24 hours for severe impairment (creatinine clearance 9 to 5 ml/minute); and 0.5 to 1 gm every 24 to 48 hours for essentially no function (creatinine clearance less than 5 ml/minute). In patients undergoing hemodialysis, a loading dose of 1 to 2 gm should be given after each hemodialysis, and the maintenance dose should be given according to the schedule recommended for renal impairment. In group A beta-hemolytic streptococcal infections, therapy should be maintained for at least 10 days to guard against the risk of rheumatic fever or glomerulonephritis. The package literature should be consulted for complete instructions on procedures for dilution and administration and other pertinent information.

Availability:
MEFOXIN® Dry Powder in vials of 1 and 2 gm. **(Merck Sharp & Dohme)**

CISPLATIN

Chemical Name: cis-Diamminedichloroplatinum.

Description: An oncolytic agent with effective chemotherapeutic usage in advanced testicular and ovarian carcinomas, cisplatin is a heavy metal compound belonging to a group of platinum coordination complexes. It occurs as a white lyophilized powder that is freely soluble in water or in saline solutions and very soluble in dimethylformamide. Molecular weight has been found to be 300.1.

The drug's biochemical properties are similar to those of the bifunctional alkylating agents. It demonstrates a selective inhibition of DNA synthesis, manifested by interstrand and intrastrand cross-linkages, with no cell-cycle specificity. Following intravenous administration, the major portion of the drug is distributed in the kidneys, liver and intestinal tract with the lowest concentration appearing in the CNS. Approximately 90% of the drug is bound to protein. Pharmacodynamic studies showed that it exhibits a biphasic half-life with an initial half-life of 25 to 49 minutes and a secondary half-life of 58 to 75 minutes. Excretion is chiefly in the urine; however, this is incomplete since only 27 to 43% of the drug is excreted within the first 5 days following administration. Data are insufficient to determine whether or not biliary or intestinal excretion takes place.

Indications: Palliative treatment of metastatic testicular or ovarian tumors. It is employed in established combination therapy with other approved chemotherapeutic agents in patients who have already received appropriate surgical and/or radiotherapeutic procedures. An established combination therapy for patients with testicular tumors consists of cisplatin, bleomycin sulfate and vinblastine sulfate, and for those with ovarian tumors it consists of cisplatin and doxorubicin hydrochloride or cisplatin alone as secondary therapy in patients refractory to standard chemotherapeutic agents, and who have not been previously treated with this drug.

Contraindications: In the presence of renal dysfunction, myelosuppression or hearing impairment.

Warnings: Nephrotoxicity, ototoxicity and anaphylactic-like reactions have been reported with cisplatin. Therefore careful monitoring of serum creatinine, BUN, creatinine clearance, and hearing status should be performed prior to initiating therapy and before each subsequent dose of the drug. The anaphylactic-like reactions are generally controlled by the intravenous administration of epinephrine, corticosteroids or antihistamines. (See Adverse Reactions.) Preclinical studies have found the drug to be mutagenic, teratogenic and embryotoxic and to cause chromosome aberrations. Therefore, utmost consideration should be given to this hazard when intended for use in pregnant patients. Additionally, a carcinogenic potential may exist since compounds with similar mechanisms of action and mutagenicity have been reported to be carcinogenic.

Precautions: Peripheral blood count, liver function, and neurologic examinations should be performed at the designated intervals.

Adverse Reactions: Dose-related and cumulative renal insufficiency is the major dose-limiting toxicity of cisplatin. Renal toxicity has been noted in 28 to 36% of patients treated with a single dose of 50 mg/M². It is usually noted during the second week of treatment and is manifested by an increased BUN and serum creatinine, hyperuricemia, and/or decreased creatinine clearance. Renal toxicity has been associated with renal tubular damage, and becomes more prolonged and severe with repeated courses; therefore, renal function must return to normal before another dose can be administered. Renal toxicity may be reduced by the simultaneous infusion of intravenous fluids and mannitol over a 6- to 8-hour period. However, renal toxicity still can occur after utilization of these procedures. Ototoxicity has been observed in up to 31% of patients treated with a single dose of 50 mg/M², and is manifested by tinnitus and/or hearing loss in the high frequency range (4000 to 8000 Hz). Decreased ability to hear normal conversational tones may occur occasionally. Ototoxic effects may be more severe in children. Hearing loss may be either unilateral or bilateral and tends to become more frequent and severe with repeated doses. It is unclear whether or not drug-induced ototoxicity is reversible. Myelosuppression occurs in 25 to 30% of patients. The nadirs in circulating platelets and leukocytes occur between day 18 to 23 (range 7.5 to 45) with most patients recovering by day 39 (range 13 to 62). Leukopenia and thrombocytopenia are more pronounced at higher doses (greater than 50 mg/M²). Anemia (decrease of greater than 2 gm hemoglobin/100 ml) occurs at approximately the same frequency and with the same timing as do leukopenia and thrombocytopenia. Marked nausea and vomiting occur in almost all patients and are occasionally so severe that the drug must be withdrawn. Nausea and vomiting usually begin within 1 to 4 hours after treatment and last up to 24 hours. Various degrees of nausea and anorexia may persist for up to 1 week. Hyperuricemia has been reported to occur at approximately the same frequency as do the increases in BUN and serum creatinine. It is more pronounced after doses greater than 50 mg/M², and peak levels of uric acid generally occur between 3 to 5 days after the administered dose. Allopurinol therapy for hyperuricemia effectively reduces uric acid levels. Neurotoxicity, usually characterized by peripheral neuropathies has occurred, and preliminary evidence suggests that they may be irreversible in some patients. Loss of taste, and seizures have also been reported. Neuropathies resulting from drug treatment may occur after prolonged therapy (4 to 7 months); however, neurologic symptoms have been noted after a single dose. Cisplatin therapy should be discontinued when the symptoms are first observed. Anaphylactic-like reactions, consisting of facial edema, wheezing, tachycardia and hypotension, have been reported in patients previously exposed to the drug, and may occur within a few minutes of drug administration. Other toxicities infrequently reported are cardiac abnormalities, anorexia, and elevated SGOT.

Dosage and Administration: *Intravenously.* The recommended combination regimen for the treatment of metastatic testicular tumors consists of: cisplatin, 20 mg/M² IV daily for 5 consecutive days (days 1 to 5) every 3rd week for 3 courses; bleomycin sulfate, 30 units IV weekly on the 2nd day of each week for 12 consecutive doses, and vinblastine sulfate, 0.15 to 0.2 mg/kg IV twice weekly on the 1st and 2nd day of every 3rd week for 4 courses (a total of 8 doses). Maintenance therapy for patients who respond to this schedule consists of: vinblastine sulfate, 0.3 mg/kg IV every 4th week for a total of 2 years. The recommended combination regimen for the treatment of metastatic ovarian tumors consists of: cisplatin, 50 mg/M² IV once on the 1st day of every 3rd week, and doxorubicin hydrochloride, 50 mg/M² once on the 1st day of every 3rd week. The drugs are administered sequentially. As a single agent, cisplatin should be administered at a dose of 100 mg/M² IV once every 4th week. Pretreatment hydration with 1 to 2 liters of fluid infused for 8 to 12 hours prior to the cisplatin dose is recommended. The drug is then diluted in 2 liters of 5% Dextrose Solution or in 1/2 or 1/3 Normal Saline Solution containing 37.5 gm of mannitol, and infused over a period of 6 to 8 hours. Adequate hydration and urinary output must be maintained during the following 24 hours.

Availability:
PLATINOL™ Dry Powder in amber vials of 10 mg. **(Bristol)**

SERACTIDE ACETATE

Description: A highly purified synthetic polypeptide containing 39 amino acids in the same sequence as those described for human corticotropin, seractide acetate performs its action by stimulating the functioning adrenal cortex to produce and secrete its entire spectrum of adrenocortical hormones. Onset of action and duration of effect are similar to those of corticotropin (H.P. Actar® Gel). Each ml contains the labeled activity of corticotropin formulated with 16% gelatin and 0.5% phenol. pH is adjusted with acetic acid and sodium hydroxide.

Indications: The drug's primary indication is for diagnostic testing of adrenocortical function. It has limited therapeutic value and should be used only as an adjunct in conditions responsive to corticosteroid therapy. Seractide acetate may be employed in the following conditions:
Endocrine disorders: Nonsuppurative thyroiditis; hypercalcemia associated with cancer.
Rheumatic disorders: As adjunctive therapy for short-term administration in the acute stage or exacerbation of psoriatic arthritis; rheumatoid arthritis, including juvenile rheumatoid arthritis (selected cases may require low-dose maintenance therapy); ankylosing spondylitis; acute and subacute bursitis; acute nonspecific tenosynovitis; acute gouty arthritis; posttraumatic arthritis; synovitis of osteoarthritis; epicondylitis.
Collagen diseases: During an exacerbation or as maintenance therapy in selected cases of systemic lupus erythematosus; systemic dermatomyositis (polymyositis); acute rheumatic carditis.
Dermatologic diseases: Pemphigus; bullous dermatitis herpetiformis; severe erythema multiforme (Stevens-Johnson syndrome); exfoliative dermatitis; severe psoriasis; severe seborrheic dermatitis; mycosis fungoides.
Allergic states: Control of severe or incapacitating allergic conditions intractable to adequate trials of conventional treatment. These include seasonal or perennial allergic rhinitis; bronchial asthma; contact dermatitis; atopic dermatitis; serum sickness.
Ophthalmic diseases: Severe acute and chronic allergic and inflammatory processes involving the eye and its adnexia such as allergic conjunctivitis; keratitis; herpes zoster ophthalmicus; iritis and iridocyclitis; diffuse posterior uveitis and choroiditis; optic neuritis; sympathetic ophthalmia; chorioretinitis; anterior segment inflammation; allergic corneal marginal ulcers.
Respiratory diseases: Symptomatic sarcoidosis; Loeffler's syndrome not manageable by other means; berylliosis; fulminating or disseminated pulmonary tuberculosis when used concurrently with antituberculous chemotherapy; aspiration pneumonitis.

Hematologic disorders: Acquired (autoimmune) hemolytic anemia; secondary thrombocytopenia in adults; erythroblastopenia (RBC anemia); congenital (erythroid) hypoplastic anemia.
Neoplastic diseases: For palliative management of leukemias and lymphomas in adults; acute leukemia in children.
Edematous state: To induce diuresis or remission of proteinuria in the nephrotic syndrome without uremia of the idiopathic type or that due to lupus erythematosus.
Gastrointestinal diseases: During the critical period of ulcerative colitis; regional enteritis.
Miscellaneous: Tuberculous meningitis with subarachnoid block or impending block when concurrently accompanied by appropriate antituberculous chemotherapy; trichinosis with neurologic or myocardial involvement.

Contraindications: Seractide acetate is contraindicated in patients with scleroderma, osteoporosis, systemic fungal infections, ocular herpes simplex, recent surgery, a history or presence of peptic ulcer, congestive heart failure, hypertension, or sensitivity to the proteins of porcine gelatin in the vehicle. Furthermore, it should not be used to treat the approved conditions if they are accompanied by primary adrenocortical insufficiency or hyperfunction. Intravenous administration is contraindicated for all of the drug's therapeutic uses.

The warnings, precautions and adverse reactions are generally the same as those accompanying the systemic use of the synthetic adrenal corticosteroids. See general statement on the Adrenal Corticosteroids.

Dosage and Administration: *Intramuscularly* or *subcutaneously* every 24 to 72 hours in doses of 40 to 80 units. Only a gradual change in dosage schedule should be attempted after the full effects of the drug have become apparent, and may be accomplished by either increasing the duration between injections or by decreasing the quantity injected or both. An important fact to bear in mind is that chronic administration of more than 40 units/day may be associated with uncontrollable adverse effects.

Availability:
ACTHAR® Gel, 40 units/ml in vials of 1 ml and in multiple-dose vials of 5 ml. **(Armour)**

INDICES

—A—

—B—

—N—

—P—

—R—

—S—

—T—

—W—

—X—

—A—

MANUF. INDEX

MANUF. INDEX

MANUF. INDEX

—M—

MALLINCKRODT PHARMACEUTICALS
3600 N. Second Street, P.O. Box 5439
St. Louis, Mo. 63147

MANUF. INDEX

PROCTER & GAMBLE
P.O. Box 85507
Cincinnati, Oh. 45201

PURDUE FREDERICK CO., THE
50 Washington Street
Norwalk, Ct. 06856

—R—

REED & CARNRICK
30 Boright Avenue
Kenilworth, N.J. 07033

RIKER LABORATORIES, INC.
Sub. 3M Co.
19901 Nordhoff Street
Northridge, Ca. 91324

ROBINS CO., A.H.
1407 Cummings Drive
Richmond, Va. 23220

—A—

—C—

—D—

—E—

—F—

—G—

—H—

—I—

—J—

—K—

—N—

—Q—

—R—

—S—

—U—